Campbell-Walsh UROLOGY

NINTH EDITION REVIEW

EDITOR-IN-CHIEF

Alan J. Wein, MD, PhD (Hon)
Professor and Chair
Division of Urology
University of Pennsylvania School of Medicine
Chief of Urology
University of Pennsylvania Medical Center
Philadelphia, Pennsylvania

EDITORS

Louis R. Kavoussi, MD
Chairman, The Arthur Smith Institute for Urology
North Shore-Long Island Jewish Health System
Manhasset, New York
Professor of Urology, New York University School of Medicine
New York, New York

Alan W. Partin, MD, PhD
David Hall McConnell Professor and Director
James Buchanan Brady Urological Institute
The Johns Hopkins Medical Institutions
Baltimore, Maryland

Andrew C. Novick, MD
Chairman, Glickman Urological Institute
Cleveland Clinic Foundation
Professor of Surgery, Cleveland Clinic Lerner College of
Medicine of Case Western Reserve University
Cleveland, Ohio

Craig A. Peters, MD
John E. Cole Professor of Urology
University of Virginia Health System
Charlottesville, Virginia

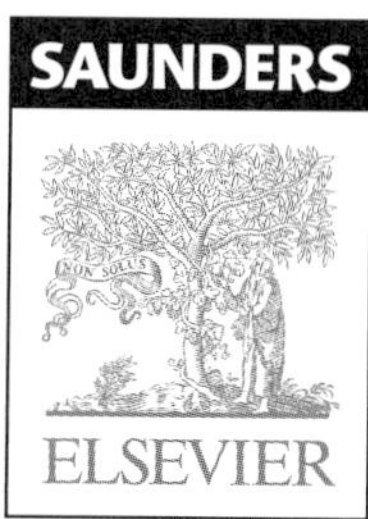

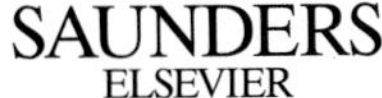

SAUNDERS
ELSEVIER

1600 John F. Kennedy Blvd.
Ste 1800
Philadelphia, PA 19103-2899

CAMPBELL-WALSH UROLOGY NINTH EDITION REVIEW

ISBN-13: 978-1-4160-3155-0
ISBN-10: 1-4160-3155-3

Notice

Neither the Publisher nor the Editors assume any responsibility for any loss or injury and/or damage to persons or property arising out of or related to any use of the material contained in this book. It is the responsibility of the treating practitioner, relying on independent expertise and knowledge of the patient, to determine the best treatment and method of application for the patient.

The Publisher

Library of Congress Cataloging-in-Publication Data

Campbell-Walsh urology ninth edition review / editor-in-chief, Alan J. Wein ; editors, Louis R. Kavoussi ... [et al.].
p. ; cm.
Companion v. to: Campbell-Walsh urology. 9th ed. / editor-in-chief, Alan J. Wein ; editors, Louis R. Kavoussi ... [et al.]. c2007.
ISBN 1-4160-3155-3
1. Urology--Examinations, questions, etc. I. Wein, Alan J. II. Campbell-Walsh urology. III. Title: Urology ninth edition review.
[DNLM: 1. Urogenital Diseases. 2. Urology--methods. WJ 100 C1905 2007]
RC871. C33 2007 Suppl.
616.6--dc22

2006029598

Acquisitions Editor: Rebecca Schmidt Gaertner
Developmental Editor: Anne Snyder
Publishing Services Manager: Tina Rebane
Project Manager: Mary Anne Folcher
Design Direction: Ellen Zanolle
Marketing Manager: Matt Latuchie

Printed in the United States of America

Last digit is the print number: 9 8 7 6 5 4 3 2 1

CONTRIBUTORS

Paul Abrams, MD, FRCS
Professor of Urology
Bristol Urological Institute
Southmead Hospital
Bristol, United Kingdom
Overactive Bladder

Mark C. Adams, MD
Professor of Urologic Surgery and Professor of Pediatrics
Vanderbilt Children's Hospital
Vanderbilt University Medical Center
Nashville, Tennessee
Urinary Tract Reconstruction in Children

Mohamad E. Allaf, MD
Assistant Professor
James Buchanan Brady Urological Institute
Johns Hopkins Medical Institutions
Baltimore, Maryland
Diagnosis and Staging of Prostate Cancer

Karl-Erik Andersson, MD, PhD
Professor
Lund University
Head Physician
Clinical Chemistry and Pharmacology
Lund University Hospital
Lund, Sweden
Pharmacologic Management of Storage and Emptying Failure

Kenneth W. Angermeier, MD
Associate Professor
Prosthetic Surgery and Genitourethral Reconstruction
Glickman Urological Institute
Cleveland Clinic Foundation
Cleveland, Ohio
Surgery of Penile and Urethral Carcinoma

Rodney A. Appell, MD
Professor
Scott Department of Urology
Baylor College of Medicine
F. Bantley Scott Chair in Urology
St. Luke's Episcopal Hospital
Houston, Texas
Injection Therapy for Urinary Incontinence

Dean G. Assimos, MD
Professor
Division of Surgical Sciences
Head
Section of Endourology and Nephrolithiasis
Department of Urology
Wake Forest University School of Medicine
Winston-Salem, North Carolina
Pathophysiology of Urinary Tract Infections

Anthony Atala, MD
William Boyce Professor and Chair
Department of Urology
Wake Forest University School of Medicine
Director
Wake Forest Institute for Regenerative Medicine
Winston-Salem, North Carolina
Tissue Engineering and Cell Therapy: Perspectives for Urology

Darius J. Bägli, MDCM, FRCSC, FAAP, FACS
Associate Professor of Surgery
Institute of Medical Science
University of Toronto
Staff Urologist and Director of Urology Research
The Hospital for Sick Children
Toronto, Ontario, Canada
Reflux and Megaureter

John M. Barry, MD
Professor of Surgery
Chairman,
Division of Urology and Renal Transplantation
Staff Surgeon, Doernbecher Children's Hospital
The Oregon Health and Science University School of Medicine
Portland, Oregon
Renal Transplantation

Georg Bartsch, MD
Professor and Chairman
Department of Urology
Medical University of Innsbruck
Innsbruck, Austria
Surgery of Testicular Tumors

Stuart B. Bauer, MD
Professor of Surgery (Urology)
Harvard Medical School
Senior Associate in Urology
Children's Hospital
Boston, Massachusetts
Anomalies of the Upper Urinary Tract
Voiding Dysfunction in Children: Non-Neurogenic and Neurogenic

Clair J. Beard, MD
Assistant Professor
Harvard Medical School
Vice-Chair
Division of Radiation Oncology
Dana-Farber Cancer Institute
Brigham and Women's Hospital
Boston, Massachusetts
Radiation Therapy for Prostate Cancer

Arie S. Belldegrun, MD, FACS
Roy and Carol Doumani Chair in Urologic Oncology
Professor of Urology
Chief, Division of Urologic Oncology
Department of Urology
David Geffen School of Medicine at University of California, Los Angeles
Los Angeles, California
Cryotherapy for Prostate Cancer

Mark F. Bellinger, MD
Professor of Urology
University of Pittsburgh Medical Center
Children's Hospital of Pittsburgh
Pittsburgh, Pennsylvania
Abnormalities of the Testes and Scrotum and Their Surgical Management

Mitchell C. Benson, MD
George F. Cahill Professor and Chairman
Department of Urology
Herbert Irving Comprehensive Cancer Center
Columbia University Medical Center
New York, New York
Cutaneous Continent Urinary Diversion

Sam B. Bhayani, MD
Assistant Professor of Surgery Department of Urology
Washington University School of Medicine
Saint Louis, Missouri
Urinary Tract Imaging: Basic Principles

Jay T. Bishoff, MD
Director, Endourology Section
Wilford Hall Medical Center
Lackland AFB, Texas
Associate Clinical Professor of Surgery
Urology/Transplantation
University of Texas Health Science Center
San Antonio, Texas
Laparoscopic Surgery of the Kidney

Jerry G. Blaivas, MD
Clinical Professor of Urology
Weill Medical College of Cornell University
Attending
New York-Presbyterian Hospital
Lenox Hill Hospital
New York, New York
Urinary Incontinence: Epidemiology, Pathophysiology, Evaluation, and Management Overview

Jon D. Blumenfeld, MD
Associate Professor of Medicine
Weil Medical College of Cornell University
Director of Hypertension
Director of The Susan R. Knafel Polycystic Kidney Disease Center
The Rogosin Institute
Associate Attending Physician
New York-Presbyterian Hospital
New York, New York
The Adrenals

Michael L. Blute, MD
Professor of Urology
Mayo Medical School
Chairman
Department of Urology
Mayo Clinic Foundation
Rochester, Minnesota
Surgery of the Adrenal Glands

Joseph G. Borer, MD
Assistant Professor of Surgery
Department of Urology
Harvard Medical School
Assistant in Urology
Children's Hospital
Boston, Massachusetts
Hypospadias

George J. Bosl, MD
Chairman
Department of Medicine
Patrick M. Byrne Chair in Clinical Oncology
Memorial Sloan-Kettering Cancer Center
New York, New York
Surgery of Testicular Tumors

Charles B. Brendler, MD
Professor and Chief
Section of Urology
Pritzger School of Medicine, University of Chicago
Chicago, Illinois
Evaluation of the Urologic Patient: History, Physical Examination, and Urinalysis

Gregory A. Broderick, MD
Professor of Urology
Mayo Medical School
Department of Urology
Mayo Clinic Foundation
Jacksonville, Florida
Evaluation and Non-Surgical Management of Erectile Dysfunction and Premature Ejaculation

James D. Brooks, MD
Assistant Professor of Urology
Associate Chief of Urologic Oncology
Department of Urology
Stanford University School of Medicine
Stanford, California
Anatomy of the Lower Urinary Tract and Male Genitalia

Ronald M. Bukowski, MD
Professor of Medicine
Cleveland Clinic Lerner College of Medicine of Case Western Reserve University
Director
Experimental Therapeutics
Cleveland Clinic Taussig Cancer Center
Cleveland, Ohio
Renal Tumors

Arthur L. Burnett, MD
Professor of Urology, Cellular and Molecular Biology
Department of Urology
Johns Hopkins University School of Medicine
Staff Urologist
Johns Hopkins Hospital
Baltimore, Maryland
Priapism

Anthony A. Caldamone, MD
Professor of Surgery and Pediatrics
Department of Urology
Brown University School of Medicine
Head of Pediatric Urology
Hasbro Children's Hospital
Providence, Rhode Island
Prune Belly Syndrome

Steven C. Campbell, MD, PhD
Professor of Surgery
Cleveland Clinic Lerner College of Medicine of Case Western Reserve University
Section of Urological Oncology
Glickman Urological Institute
Cleveland Clinic Foundation
Cleveland, Ohio
Renal Tumors
Non-Muscle-Invasive Bladder Cancer (Ta, T1, and Tis)

Douglas A. Canning, MD
Professor of Urology
University of Pennsylvania School of Medicine
Director, Pediatric Urology
Children's Hospital of Philadelphia
Philadelphia, Pennsylvania
Evaluation of the Pediatric Urology Patient

Michael Carducci, MD
Associate Professor of Oncology and Urology
Departments of Oncology and Urology
Sidney Kimmel Comprehensive Cancer Center at Johns Hopkins
Johns Hopkins University School of Medicine
Baltimore, Maryland
Treatment of Hormone-Refractory Prostate Cancer

Michael C. Carr, MD, PhD
Associate Professor of Surgery in Urology
University of Pennsylvania School of Medicine
Attending Surgeon, Pediatric Urology
Children's Hospital of Philadelphia
Philadelphia, Pennsylvania
Anomalies and Surgery of the Ureteropelvic Junction in Children

Peter R. Carroll, MD
Professor and Chair
Department of Urology
University of California, San Francisco, School of Medicine
Surgeon in Chief, Comprehensive Cancer Center
San Francisco, California
Treatment of Locally Advanced Prostate Cancer

H. Ballentine Carter, MD
James Buchanan Brady Urological Institute
Johns Hopkins Medical Institutions
Baltimore, Maryland
Basic Instrumentation and Cystoscopy
Diagnosis and Staging of Prostate Cancer

Anthony J. Casale, MD
Professor and Chairman
Department of Urology
University of Louisville School of Medicine
Chair of Urology
Kosair Children's Hospital
Louisville, Kentucky
Posterior Urethral Valves

William J. Catalona, MD
Department of Urology
Feinberg School of Medicine
Northwestern University
Feinberg School of Medicine
Director, Clinical Prostate Cancer Program
Robert H. Lurie Comprehensive Cancer Center
Northwestern Memorial Hospital
Chicago, Illinois
Definitive Therapy of Localized Prostate Cancer: Overview

David Y. Chan, MD
Director of Outpatient Urology
Assistant Professor of Urology and Pathology
James Buchanan Brady Urological Institute
Johns Hopkins Medical Institutions
Baltimore, Maryland
Basic Instrumentation and Cystoscopy

Michael B. Chancellor, MD
Professor of Urology
McGowan Institute of Regenerative Medicine
University of Pittsburgh School of Medicine
Pittsburgh, Pennsylvania
Physiology and Pharmacology of the Bladder and Urethra

C. R. Chapple, MD, FRCS (Urol), FEBU
Visiting Professor of Urology
Sheffield Hallam University
Honorary Senior Lecturer in Urology
Sheffield University
Consultant Urological Surgeon
Royal Hallamshire Hospital
Sheffield Teaching Hospitals NHS Foundation Trust
Sheffield, United Kingdom
Retropubic Suspension Surgery for Incontinence in Women

Robert L. Chevalier, MD
Benjamin Armistead Shepherd Professor and Chair
Department of Pediatrics
University of Virginia Health System
Pediatrician in Chief
University of Virginia Medical School
Charlottesville, Virginia
Renal Function in the Fetus, Neonate, and Child
Congenital Urinary Obstruction: Pathophysiology

Ben H. Chew, MD, MSc, FRCSC
Assistant Professor of Urology
University of British Columbia Faculty of Medicine
Vancouver, British Columbia, Canada
Ureteroscopy and Retrograde Ureteral Access

George K. Chow, MD
Assistant Professor
Department of Urology
Mayo Clinic Foundation
Rochester, Minnesota
Surgery of the Adrenal Glands

Ralph V. Clayman, MD
Professor of Urology
University of California, Irvine Medical Center
Chair of the Department of Urology
University of California, Irvine, School of Medicine
Orange, California
Basics of Laparoscopic Urologic Surgery

Craig V. Comiter, MD
Chief, Section of Urology
Director, Female Urology and Urodynamics
Associate Professor of Surgery/Urology
Instructor of Obstetrics and Gynecology
University of Arizona Health Sciences Center
Tucson, Arizona
Surgical Treatment of Male Sphincteric Urinary Incontinence: The Male Perineal Sling and Artificial Urinary Sphincter

Michael J. Conlin, MD
Associate Professor of Surgery
Director, Minimally Invasive Urologic Surgery
Division of Urology and Renal Transplantation
The Oregon Health and Science University School of Medicine
Portland, Oregon
Renal Transplantation

Juanita Crook, MD
Associate Professor of Radiation Oncology
University of Toronto Faculty of Medicine
Radiation Oncologist
University Health Network
Princess Margaret Hospital
Toronto, Ontario, Canada
Radiation Therapy for Prostate Cancer

Douglas M. Dahl, MD
Assistant Professor of Surgery
Department of Urology
Harvard Medical School
Assistant in Urology
Massachusetts General Hospital
Boston, Massachusetts
Use of Intestinal Segments and Urinary Diversion

Anthony V. D'Amico, MD, PhD
Professor of Radiation Oncology
Harvard Medical School
Professor and Chief of Genitourinary Radiation Oncology
Dana-Farber Cancer Institute
Brigham and Women's Hospital
Boston, Massachusetts
Radiation Therapy for Prostate Cancer

John W. Davis, MD
Assistant Professor of Urology
University of Texas M. D. Anderson Cancer Center
Houston, Texas
Tumors of the Penis

John D. Denstedt, MD
Professor of Urology
Chairman, Department of Surgery
Schulich School of Medicine and Dentistry
The University of Western Ontario
London, Ontario, Canada
Ureteroscopy and Retrograde Ureteral Access

Theodore L. DeWeese, MD, PhD
Professor of Oncology
Radiation Oncologist in Chief
Department of Radiation Oncology and Molecular Radiation Science
Johns Hopkins Medical Institutions
Baltimore, Maryland
Radiation Therapy for Prostate Cancer

David A. Diamond, MD
Associate Professor of Surgery (Urology)
Harvard Medical School
Associate in Urology
Children's Hospital
Boston, Massachusetts
Sexual Differentiation: Normal and Abnormal

Roger R. Dmochowski, MD
Professor
Vanderbilt University Medical Center
Director
Vanderbilt Continence Center
Nashville, Tennessee
Tension-Free Vaginal Tape Procedures

Steven G. Docimo, MD
Professor of Urology
Vice Chairman of Urology
University of Pittsburgh School of Medicine
Director of Urology
Division of Pediatric Urology
Children's Hospital of Pittsburgh
Pittsburgh, Pennsylvania
Pediatric Endourology and Laparoscopy

Marcus Drake, DM, MA
Consultant Urological Surgeon
Bristol Urological Institute
Southmead Hospital
Bristol, United Kingdom
Overactive Bladder

James A. Eastham, MD
Associate Member
Memorial Sloane-Kettering Cancer Center
New York, New York
Expectant Management of Prostate Cancer

Louis Eichel, MD
Clinical Associate Professor of Urology
University of Rochester School of Medicine and Dentistry
Director of Minimally Invasive Surgery
Center for Urology
Rochester, New York
Basics of Laparoscopic Urologic Surgery

Mario A. Eisenberger, MD
R. Dale Hughes Professor of Oncology and Urology
The Sidney Kimmel Comprehensive Cancer Center at Johns Hopkins
Johns Hopkins Medical Institutions
Baltimore, Maryland
Treatment of Hormone-Refractory Prostate Cancer

Alaa El-Ghoneimi, MD
Professor of Pediatric Surgery
University of Paris
Senior Surgeon
Hospital Robert Debré
Paris, France
Anomalies and Surgery of the Ureteropelvic Junction in Children

Jack S. Elder, MD
Carter Kissell Professor of Urology
Professor of Pediatrics
Vice Chairman
Department of Urology
Case Western Reserve University School of Medicine
Director of Pediatric Urology
Rainbow Babies and Children's Hospital
Cleveland, Ohio
Abnormalities of the Genitalia in Boys and Their Surgical Management

Jonathan I. Epstein, MD
Professor of Pathology, Urology, and Oncology
The Reinhard Professor of Urologic Pathology
Johns Hopkins University School of Medicine
Director of Surgical Pathology
Johns Hopkins Medical Institutions
Baltimore, Maryland
Pathology of Prostatic Neoplasia

Andrew P. Evan, PhD
Chancellor's Professor
Department of Anatomy and Cell Biology
Indiana University School of Medicine
Indianapolis, Indiana
Surgical Management of Upper Urinary Tract Calculi

Robert L. Fairchild, PhD
Professor of Pathology
Case Western Reserve University School of Medicine
Staff, Department of Immunology
Glickman Urological Foundation
Cleveland Clinic Foundation
Cleveland, Ohio
Basic Principles of Immunology

Amr Fergany, MD
Staff, Section of Urologic Oncology
Section of Laparoscopic Surgery and Robotics
Cleveland Clinic Foundation
Glickman Urological Institute
Cleveland, Ohio
Renovascular Hypertension and Ischemic Nephropathy

James H. Finke, PhD
Professor of Molecular Medicine
Joint Appointment
Department of Hematology/Oncology
Glickman Urological Institute
Cleveland Clinic Lerner College of Medicine of Case
Western Reserve University
Staff Member
Department of Immunology
Lerner Research Institute
Cleveland Clinic
Cleveland, Ohio
Basic Principles of Immunology

John M. Fitzpatrick, MCh, FRCSI, FRCS(Glas), FRCS
Professor of Surgery
Department of Surgery
University College of Dublin School of Medicine
and Medical Science
Consultant Urologist
Mater Misericordiae University Hospital
Dublin, Ireland
Minimally Invasive and Endoscopic Management of Benign Prostatic Hyperplasia

Robert C. Flanigan, MD, FACS
Albert J. Jr. and Claire R. Speh Professor and Chair
Department of Urology
Stritch School of Medicine
Loyola University
Chair of the Department of Urology
Loyola University Medical Center
Maywood, Illinois
Urothelial Tumors of the Upper Urinary Tract

Stuart M. Flechner, MD
Professor of Urology
Cleveland Clinic Lerner College of Medicine of Case
Western Reserve University
Director of Clinical Research
Section of Renal Transplantation
Glickman Urological Institute
Cleveland Clinic Foundation
Cleveland, Ohio
Basic Principles of Immunology

Tara Frenkl, MD, MPH
Assistant Professor of Urology
Director, Female Urology and Reconstructive Surgery
Robert Wood Johnson Medical School
University of Medicine and Dentistry of New Jersey
New Brunswick, New Jersey
Sexually Transmitted Diseases

Dominic Frimberger, MD
Assistant Professor of Urology
University of Oklahoma Health Sciences Center
Pediatric Urologist
Children's Hospital of Oklahoma
Oklahoma City, Oklahoma
Bladder Anomalies in Children

John P. Gearhart, MD
Professor of Pediatric Urology
Johns Hopkins University School of Medicine
Chief of Pediatric Urology
Johns Hopkins Hospital
Baltimore, Maryland
Exstrophy-Epispadias Complex

Glenn S. Gerber, MD
Associate Professor
Section of Urology, Department of Surgery
University of Chicago School of Medicine
Chicago, Illinois
Evaluation of the Urologic Patient: History, Physical Examination, and Urinalysis

Inderbir S. Gill, MD, MCh
Professor of Surgery
Head, Section of Laparoscopic and Robotic Urology
Glickman Urological Institute
Cleveland Clinic Foundation
Cleveland, Ohio
Laparoscopic Surgery of the Urinary Bladder

Kenneth I. Glassberg, MD
Professor of Urology
Department of Urology
Columbia University College of Physicians and Surgeons
Director, Division of Pediatric Urology
Morgan Stanley Children's Hospital of New York-Presbyterian
New York, New York
Renal Dysgenesis and Cystic Disease of Kidney

David A. Goldfarb, MD
Head, Section of Renal Transplantation
Glickman Urological Institute
Cleveland Clinic Foundation
Cleveland, Ohio
Etiology, Pathogenesis, and Management of Renal Failure

Irwin Goldstein, MD
Editor in Chief
The Journal of Sexual Medicine
Milton, Massachusetts
Urologic Management of Women with Sexual Health Concerns

Marc Goldstein, MD
Professor of Urology and Reproductive Medicine
Surgeon in Chief, Male Reproductive Medicine and Surgery
Executive Director, Men's Service Center
Cornell Institute for Reproductive Medicine
Weil Medical College of Cornell University
Senior Scientist, Center for Biomedical Research
The Population Council
New York, New York
Male Reproductive Physiology
Surgery of Scrotum and Seminal Vesicles

Leonard J. Gomella, MD
Bernard W. Godwin Professor of Prostate Cancer
Chairman
Department of Urology
Thomas Jefferson University School of Medicine
Director
Jefferson Prostate Diagnostic Center
Kimmel Cancer Center
Thomas Jefferson University Hospital
Philadelphia, Pennsylvania
Ultrasonography and Biopsy of the Prostate

Mark L. Gonzalgo, MD, PhD
Associate Professor of Urology and Oncology
Johns Hopkins Medical Center
Baltimore, Maryland
Management of Invasive and Metastatic Bladder Cancer

Richard W. Grady, MD
Associate Professor of Urology
University of Washington School of Medicine
Interim Chief, Pediatric Urology
Children's Hospital and Regional Medical Center
Seattle, Washington
Surgical Techniques for One-Stage Reconstruction of the Exstrophy-Epispadias Complex

Matthew B. Gretzer, MD
Assistant Professor of Clinical Surgery
Department of Surgery/Urology
University of Arizona Health Sciences Center
Tucson, Arizona
Prostate Cancer Tumor Markers

Mantu Gupta, MD
Associate Professor
Columbia University College of Physicians and Surgeons
Director of Endourology and Director of Kidney Stone Center
Columbia University Medical Center of New York
Presbyterian Hospital
New York, New York
Percutaneous Management of the Upper Urinary Tract

Ethan J. Halpern, MD
Professor of Radiology and Urology
Thomas Jefferson University School of Medicine
Co-Director
Jefferson Prostate Diagnostic Center
Philadelphia, Pennsylvania
Ultrasonography and Biopsy of the Prostate

Misop Han, MD
Assistant Professor
Department of Urology
James Buchanan Brady Urological Institute
Johns Hopkins Medical Institutions
Baltimore, Maryland
Retropubic and Suprapubic Open Prostatectomy
Definitive Therapy of Localized Prostate Cancer: An Overview

Philip M. Hanno, MD, MPH
Professor of Surgery in Urology
University of Pennsylvania School of Medicine
Safety Officer for the Clinical Practices of the
University of Pennsylvania
Philadelphia, Pennsylvania
Painful Bladder Syndrome/Interstitial Cystitis and Related Disorders

Matthew P. Hardy, PhD
Professor
Department of Urology
Weill Medical College of Cornell University
Member, Population Council
The Rockefeller University
New York, New York
Male Reproductive Physiology

David M. Hartke, MD
Resident Physician
Department of Urology
University Hospitals of Cleveland
Case Western Reserve University School of Medicine
Cleveland, Ohio
Radical Perineal Prostatectomy

Jeremy P. W. Heaton, MD, FRCSC, FACS
Professor of Urology
Assistant Professor of Pharmacology and Toxicology
Queens University
Kingston, Ontario, Canada
Androgen Deficiency in the Aging Male

Sender Herschorn, MDCM, FRCSC
Professor and Chairman
Division of Urology
Martin Barkin Chair in Urological Research
University of Toronto Faculty of Medicine
Attending Urologist
Director
Urodynamics Unit
Sunnybrook Health Sciences Center
Toronto, Ontario, Canada
Vaginal Reconstructive Surgery for Sphincteric Incontinence and Prolapse

Khai-Linh V. Ho, MD
Endourology Fellow
Mayo Clinic Foundation
Rochester, Minnesota
Lower Urinary Tract Calculi

Thomas H. S. Hsu, MD
Assistant Professor of Urology
Director, Section of Laparoscopic and Minimally Invasive Surgery
Department of Urology
Stanford University School of Medicine
Director, Laparoscopic, Robotic, and Minimally Invasive Urologic Surgery
Stanford University Medical Center
Stanford, California
Management of Upper Urinary Tract Obstruction

Mark Hurwitz, MD
Assistant Professor
Harvard Medical School
Director, Regional Program Development
Department of Radiation Oncology
Dana-Farber Brigham and Women's Cancer Center
Boston, Massachusetts
Radiation Therapy for Prostate Cancer

Douglas Husmann, MD
Professor of Urology
Vice Chairman
Department of Urology
Mayo Clinic Foundation
Rochester, Minnesota
Pediatric Genitourinary Trauma

Jonathan P. Jarow, MD
Professor of Urology
James Buchanan Brady Urological Institute
Johns Hopkins Medical Institutions
Baltimore, Maryland
Male Infertility

Thomas W. Jarrett, MD
Professor of Urology
Chairman, Department of Urology
George Washington University School of Medicine and Health Sciences
Washington, DC
Management of Urothelial Tumors of the Renal Pelvis and Ureter

Christopher W. Johnson, MD
Clinical Instructor of Urology
Weill Medical College of Cornell University
New York
Assistant Attending
North Shore-Long Island Jewish Health System
Manhasset, and St. Francis Hospital
Roslyn, New York
Tuberculosis and Parasitic and Fungal Infections of the Genitourinary System

Warren D. Johnson, Jr., MD
B. H. Kean Professor of Tropical Medicine
Chief, Division of Internal Medicine and Infectious Diseases
Weill Medical College of Cornell University
Attending Physician
New York-Presbyterian Hospital, Cornell Campus
New York, New York
Tuberculosis and Parasitic and Fungal Infections of the Genitourinary System

Deborah P. Jones, MD
Associate Professor of Pediatrics
University of Tennessee Health Science Center
Attending, Le Bonheur Children's Medical Center
Children's Foundation Research Center
Memphis, Tennessee
Renal Disease in Childhood

J. Stephen Jones, MD, FACS
Associate Professor of Surgery (Urology)
Vice Chairman, Glickman Urological Institute
Cleveland Clinic Lerner College of Medicine of Case Western Reserve University
Cleveland Clinic Foundation
Cleveland, Ohio
Non-Muscle-Invasive Bladder Cancer (Ta, T1, and Tis)

Gerald H. Jordan, MD, FACS, FAAP
Professor of Urology
Department of Urology
Eastern Virginia Medical School
Norfolk, Virginia
Peyronie's Disease
Surgery of the Penis and Urethra

Mark L. Jordan, MD
Harris L. Willits Professor and Chief
Division of Urology
University of Medicine and Dentistry of New Jersey
New Jersey Medical School
Chief of Urology
University Hospital
Newark, New Jersey
Renal Transplantation

David B. Joseph, MD
Professor of Surgery
University of Alabama at Birmingham
Chief of Pediatric Urology
Children's Hospital of Alabama
Birmingham, Alabama
Urinary Tract Reconstruction in Children

John N. Kabalin, MD
Adjunct Assistant Professor of Surgery
Section of Urologic Surgery
University of Nebraska College of Medicine
Omaha
Regional West Medical Center
Scottsbluff, Nebraska
Surgical Anatomy of the Retroperitoneum, Adrenals, Kidneys, and Ureters

Martin Kaefer, MD
Associate Professor
Indiana University School of Medicine
Riley Hospital for Children
Indianapolis, Indiana
Surgical Management of Intersexuality, Cloacal Malformation, and Other Abnormalities of the Genitalia in Girls

Irving Kaplan, MD
Assistant Professor of Radiation Oncology
Harvard Medical School
Radiation Oncologist
Department of Radiation Oncology
Beth Israel Deaconess Medical Center
Boston, Massachusetts
Radiation Therapy for Prostate Cancer

Louis R. Kavoussi, MD
Chairman, The Arthur Smith Institute for Urology
North Shore-Long Island Jewish Health System
Manhassett, New York
Professor of Urology
New York University School of Medicine
New York, New York
Laparoscopic Surgery of the Kidney

Mohit Khera, MD, MBA, MPH
Fellow, Division of Male Reproductive Medicine and Surgery
Scott Department of Urology
Baylor College of Medicine
Houston, Texas
Surgical Management of Male Infertility

Antoine Khoury, MD FRCSC, FAAP
Professor
Department of Surgery
University of Toronto Faculty of Medicine
Head
Division of Urology
Hospital for Sick Children
Toronto, Ontario, Canada
Reflux and Megaureter

Adam S. Kibel, MD
Associate Professor
Division of Urologic Surgery
Washington University School of Medicine
St. Louis, Missouri
Molecular Genetics and Cancer Biology

Roger Kirby, MD, FRCS
Professor and Director
The Prostate Centre
Visiting Professor
St. George's Hospital
Institute of Urology
London, United Kingdom
Evaluation and Nonsurgical Management of Benign Prostatic Hyperplasia

Eric A. Klein, MD
Professor of Surgery
Cleveland Clinic Lerner College of Medicine of Case Western Reserve University
Head, Section of Urologic Oncology
Glickman Urological Institute
Cleveland Clinic Foundation
Cleveland, Ohio
Epidemiology, Etiology, and Prevention of Prostate Cancer

John N. Krieger, MD
Professor
Department of Urology
University of Washington School of Medicine
Chief of Urology
VA Pugent Sound Health Care System
Attending Physician
University Hospital and Harbor View Medical Center
Seattle, Washington
Urological Implications of AIDS and HIV Infection

Bradley Kropp, MD
Professor of Urology
University of Oklahoma Health Science Center
Chief, Pediatric Urology
Children's Hospital of Oklahoma
Oklahoma City, Oklahoma
Bladder Anomalies in Children

John S. Lam, MD
Clinical Instructor in Urology
Department of Urology
David Geffen School of Medicine at
University of California-Los Angeles
Attending Urologist
University of California, Los Angeles, Medical Center
Los Angeles, California
Cryotherapy for Prostate Cancer

Herbert Lepor, MD
Professor and Martin Spatz Chair
Department of Urology
New York University School of Medicine
Chief of Urology
New York University Medical Center
New York, New York
Evaluation and Nonsurgical Management of Benign Prostatic Hyperplasia

Ronald W. Lewis, MD
Professor of Surgery (Urology) and Physiology
Witherington Chair in Urology
Chief of Urology
Medical College of Georgia
Augusta, Georgia
Vascular Surgery for Erectile Dysfunction

James E. Lingeman, MD
Volunteer Clinical Professor
Indiana University School of Medicine
Director of Research
Methodist Hospital Institute for Kidney Stone Disease
Indianapolis, Indiana
Surgical Management of Upper Urinary Tract Calculi

Richard E. Link, MD, PhD
Associate Professor of Urology
Director, Division of Endourology and Minimally Invasive Surgery
Scott Department of Urology
Baylor College of Medicine
Houston, Texas
Cutaneous Diseases of the External Genitalia

Larry I. Lipshultz, MD
Professor of Urology
Scott Department of Urology
Lester and Sue Smith Chair in Reproductive Medicine
Chief, Division of Male Reproductive Medicine and Surgery
Baylor College of Medicine
Houston, Texas
Surgical Management of Male Infertility

Mark S. Litwin, MD, MPH
Professor of Urology and Health Services
David Geffen School of Medicine, University of California, Los Angeles
University of California, Los Angeles, School of Public Health
Los Angeles, California
Outcomes Research

Yair Lotan, MD
Assistant Professor
Department of Urology
University of Texas Southwestern Medical Center
Dallas, Texas
Urinary Lithiasis: Etiology, Epidemiology, and Pathophysiology

Tom F. Lue, MD
Professor and Vice Chair
Emil Tanagho Endowed Chair
Department of Urology
University of California School of Medicine, San Francisco
San Francisco, California
Physiology of Penile Erection and Pathophysiology of Erectile Dysfunction
Evaluation and Non-Surgical Management of Erectile Dysfunction and Premature Ejaculation

Donald F. Lynch, Jr., MD
Professor and Chairman
Department of Urology
Professor of Obstetrics and Gynecology
Eastern Virginia School of Medicine
Urologic Oncologist
Sentara Hospitals
Consultant Urologist
Jones Institute for Reproductive Medicine
Norfolk, Virginia
Tumors of the Penis

Michael Marberger, MD
Professor and Chairman
Department of Urology
Medical University of Vienna
Vienna, Austria
Ablative Therapy of Renal Tumors

Brian R. Matlaga, MD, MPH
Assistant Professor
James Buchanan Brody Urological Institute
Johns Hopkins University School of Medicine
Director of Stone Disease
Johns Hopkins Bayview Medical Center
Baltimore, Maryland
Surgical Management of Upper Urinary Tract Calculi

Fray F. Marshall, MD
Professor and Chairman
Department of Urology
Emory University School of Medicine
Atlanta, Georgia
Surgery of Bladder Cancer

Ranjiv Mathews, MD
Associate Professor of Pediatric Urology
James Buchanan Brady Urological Institute
Johns Hopkins Medical Institutions
Baltimore, Maryland
Exstrophy-Epispadias Complex

Julian Mauermann, MD
Senior Resident
Department of Urology
Medical University of Vienna
Vienna, Austria
Ablative Therapy of Renal Tumors

Sarah J. McAleer, MD
Chief Resident
Department of Urology
Brigham and Women's Hospital
Boston, Massachusetts
Tuberculosis and Parasitic and Fungal Infections of the Genitourinary System

Jack W. McAninch, MD
Professor of Urological Surgery
Department of Urology
University of California, San Francisco, School of Medicine
Chief of Urology
San Francisco General Hospital
San Francisco, California
Renal and Ureteral Trauma

John D. McConnell, MD
Professor of Urology
Executive Vice President for Health Systems Affairs
Department of Urology
University of Texas Southwestern Medical Center
Dallas, Texas
Benign Prostatic Hyperplasia: Etiology, Pathophysiology, Epidemiology, and Natural History

W. Scott McDougal, MD
Professor of Urology
Harvard Medical School
Chief of Urology
Massachusetts General Hospital
Boston, Massachusetts
Use of Intestinal Segments and Urinary Diversion

Elspeth M. McDougall, MD, FRCSC,
Professor of Urology
University of California, Irvine Medical Center
Irvine, California
Basics of Laparoscopic Urologic Surgery
Percutaneous Management of the Upper Urinary Tract

Edward J. McGuire, MD
Professor
Department of Urology
University of Michigan Medical School
Ann Arbor, Michigan
Pubovaginal Sling

James M. McKiernan, MD
Assistant Professor
Department of Urology
Herbert Irving Comprehensive Cancer Center
Columbia University Medical Center
Assistant Attending Physician
New York-Presbyterian Hospital
New York, New York
Cutaneous Continent Urinary Diversion

Alan W. McMahon, MD
Associate Professor
Department of Medicine
Division of Nephrology and Transplant Immunology
University of Alberta Faculty of Medicine
Edmonton, Alberta, Canada
Renal Physiology and Pathophysiology

Maxwell V. Meng, MD
Assistant Professor
Department of Urology
University of California, San Francisco
San Francisco, California
Treatment of Locally Advanced Prostate Cancer

Edward M. Messing, MD
W. W. Scott Professor
Department of Urology
Professor of Pathology and Oncology
University of Rochester School of Medicine
Rochester, New York
Urothelial Tumors of the Bladder

Michael E. Mitchell, MD
Professor and Chief of Pediatric Urology
University of Washington School of Medicine
Children's Hospital & Regional Medical Center
Seattle, Washington
Surgical Techniques for One-Stage Reconstruction of the Exstrophy-Epispadias Complex

Drogo K. Montague, MD
Professor of Surgery
Cleveland Clinic Lerner College of Medicine of
Case Western Reserve University
Head, Section of Prosthetic Surgery and Genitourethral
Reconstruction
Glickman Urological Institute
Cleveland Clinic Foundation
Cleveland, Ohio
Prosthetic Surgery for Erectile Dysfunction

Alvaro Morales, MD, FRCSC, FACS
Professor
Queen's University
Director
Center for Advanced Urological Research
Attending Physician
Kingston General Hospital and Hotel Dieu Hospital
Kingston, Ontario, Canada
Androgen Deficiency in the Aging Male

Allen F. Morey, MD
Clinical Associate Professor of Urology
University of Texas Health Science Center
Chief
Urology Service
Brooke Army Medical Center
San Antonio, Texas
Genital and Lower Urinary Tract Trauma

John Morley, MB, BCh
Professor
St. Louis University Medical Center
Attending Physician
St. Louis VA Medical Center
St. Louis, Missouri
Androgen Deficiency in the Aging Male

Michael J. Morris, MD
Assistant Member
Memorial Sloan-Kettering Cancer Center
Instructor in Medicine
Joan and Sanford I. Weill Medical College of Cornell University
Assistant Attending Physician
Memorial Hospital for Cancer and Allied Disease
New York, New York
The Clinical State of the Rising PSA Following Definitive Local Therapy: A Practical Approach

M. Louis Moy, MD
Assistant Professor
Division of Urology
University of Pennsylvania Medical School
Philadelphia, Pennsylvania
Additional Therapies for Storage and Emptying Failure

Ricardo Munarriz, MD
Associate Professor of Urology
Boston University School of Medicine
Boston, Massachusetts
Vascular Surgery for Erectile Dysfunction

Stephen Y. Nakada, MD
Associate Professor of Surgery
Chairman of Urology
The Uehling Professor of Urology
Department of Urology
University of Wisconsin School of Medicine and Public Health
Madison, Wisconsin
Management of Upper Urinary Tract Obstruction

Joseph V. Nally, Jr., MD
Department of Nephrology and Hypertension
Cleveland Clinic Foundation
Cleveland, Ohio
Etiology, Pathogenesis, and Management of Renal Failure

Joel B. Nelson, MD
Frederic N. Schwentker Professor
Chair
Department of Urology
University of Pittsburgh School of Medicine
Chairman of Urology
University of Pittsburgh Medical Center
Co-Chair
Prostate and Urological Diseases Program
University of Pittsburgh Cancer Institute
Pittsburgh, Pennsylvania
Hormone Therapy for Prostate Cancer

Michael T. Nguyen, MD
Fellow, Pediatric Urology
The Children's Hospital of Philadelphia
Philadelphia, Pennsylvania
Evaluation of the Pediatric Urology Patient

J. Curtis Nickel, MD
Professor of Urology
Queen's University
Staff Urologist
Department of Urology
Kingston General Hospital
Kingston, Ontario, Canada
Inflammatory Conditions of the Male Genitourinary Tract: Prostatitis and Related Conditions, Orchitis, and Epididymitis

Peter T. Nieh, MD
Assistant Professor
Department of Urology
Emory University School of Medicine
Atlanta, Georgia
Surgery of Bladder Cancer

Victor W. Nitti, MD
Associate Professor and Vice Chairman
Department of Urology
New York University School of Medicine
New York, New York
Urinary Incontinence: Epidemiology, Pathophysiology, Evaluation, and Management Overview

H. Norman Noe, MD
Professor of Urology
Chief, Pediatric Urology
University of Tennessee College of Medicine
Saint Jude's Children's Research Hospital
Memphis, Tennessee
Renal Disease in Childhood

Andrew C. Novick, MD
Chairman, Glickman Urological Institute
Cleveland Clinic Foundation
Professor of Surgery
Cleveland Clinic Lerner College of Medicine of
Case Western Reserve University
Cleveland, Ohio
Renovascular Hypertension and Ischemic Nephropathy
Open Surgery of the Kidney
Renal Tumors

Seung-June Oh, MD, PhD
Associate Professor
Department of Urology
Seoul National University College of Medicine
Seoul National University Hospital
Seoul, Korea
Pubovaginal Sling

Carl A. Olsson, MD
John K. Lattimer Professor and Chairman Emeritus
Columbia University College of Physicians and Surgeons
Attending Physician
New York-Presbyterian Hospital
New York, New York
Cutaneous Continent Urinary Diversion

Michael C. Ost, MD
Fellow, Endourology and Laparoscopy
Institute of Urology
North Shore-Long Island Jewish Medical Center
New Hyde Park, New York
Percutaneous Management of the Upper Urinary Tract

Vernon M. Pais Jr., MD
Assistant Professor of Surgery
Department of Urology
University of Kentucky College of Medicine
Lexington, Kentucky
Pathophysiology of Urinary Tract Infection

John M. Park, MD
Associate Professor of Urology
University of Michigan Medical School
Chief of Pediatric Urology
University of Michigan Health Systems
Ann Arbor, Michigan
Normal Development of the Urogenital System

Alan W. Partin, MD, PhD
David Hall McConnell Professor and Director
James Buchanan Brady Urological Institute
Johns Hopkins Medical Institutions
Baltimore, Maryland
Prostate Cancer Tumor Markers
Retropubic and Suprapubic Open Prostatectomy
Diagnosis and Staging of Prostate Cancer
Anatomic Radical Retropubic Prostatectomy

Christopher K. Payne, MD
Associate Professor of Urology
Director
Female Urology and Neurology
Stanford University Medical School
Stanford, California
Conservative Management of Urinary Incontinence: Behavioral and Pelvic Floor Therapy, Urethral and Pelvic Devices

Margaret S. Pearle, MD, PhD
Professor of Urology and Internal Medicine
Department of Urology
University of Texas Southwestern Medical Center
Dallas, Texas
Urinary Lithiasis: Etiology, Epidemiology, and Pathophysiology

Craig A. Peters, MD
John E. Cole Professor of Urology
Department of Urology
University of Virginia Health System
Charlottesville, Virginia
Congenital Urinary Obstruction: Pathophysiology
Perinatal Urology
Pediatric Endourology and Laparoscopy

Andrew C. Peterson, MD, FACS
Assistant Professor of Surgery
Uniformed Services University of the Health Sciences
Bethesda, Maryland
Program Director
Urology Residency
Madigan Army Medical Center
Tacoma, Washington
Urodynamic and Videourodynamic Evaluation of Voiding Dysfunction

Curtis A. Pettaway, MD
Associate Professor of Urology
Associate Professor of Cancer Biology
University of Texas M. D. Anderson Cancer Center
Houston, Texas
Tumors of the Penis

Paul K. Pietrow, MD
Director of Minimally Invasive Urology
Hudson Valley Urology
Kingston, New York
Medical Management of Urinary Lithiasis

Louis L. Pisters, MD
Associate Professor of Urology
Department of Urology
University of Texas M. D. Anderson Cancer Center
Houston, Texas
Cryotherapy for Prostate Cancer

Elizabeth A. Platz, ScD, MPH
Associate Professor
Department of Epidemiology
Johns Hopkins Bloomberg School of Public Health
Johns Hopkins Medical Institutions
Baltimore, Maryland
Epidemiology, Etiology, and Prevention of Prostate Cancer

Jeannette Potts, MD
Senior Clinical Instructor
Department of Family Medicine
Cleveland Clinic Lerner College of Medicine
of Case Western Reserve University
Staff Physician
Glickman Urological Institute
Cleveland Clinic Foundation
Cleveland, Ohio
Sexually Transmitted Diseases

Glenn M. Preminger, MD
Professor of Urologic Surgery
Duke University Medical Center
Durham, North Carolina
Medical Management of Urinary Lithiasis

Raymond R. Rackley, MD
Professor of Surgery (Urology)
Cleveland Clinic Lerner College of Medicine
of Case Western Reserve University
Co-Head, Section of Female Urology and Voiding Dysfunction
Glickman Urological Institute
Cleveland Clinic Foundation
Cleveland, Ohio
Electrical Stimulation for Storage and Emptying Disorders

John R. Ramey, MD
Jefferson Prostate Diagnostic Center
Departments of Urology and Radiology
Kimmel Cancer Center
Thomas Jefferson University School of Medicine
Philadelphia, Pennsylvania
Ultrasonography and Biopsy of the Prostate

Neil M. Resnick, MD
Director
University of Pittsburgh Institute on Aging
Chief
Division of Gerontology and Geriatric Medicine
Professor of Medicine
University of Pittsburgh and University of Pittsburgh Medical Center
Pittsburgh, Pennsylvania
Geriatric Incontinence and Voiding Dysfunction

Martin I. Resnick, MD
Lester Persky Professor and Chair
Department of Urology
Cleveland Clinic Lerner College of Medicine
of Case Western Reserve University
Cleveland Clinic Foundation
Cleveland, Ohio
Radical Perineal Prostatectomy

Alan B. Retik, MD
Professor of Surgery (Urology)
Harvard Medical School
Chief, Department of Urology
Children's Hospital
Boston, Massachusetts
Hypospadias
Ectopic Ureter, Ureterocele, and Other Anomalies of the Ureter

Jerome P. Richie, MD
Elliott C. Cutler Professor of Urologic Surgery
Chairman, Harvard Program in Urology
Harvard Medical School
Brigham and Women's Hospital
Boston, Massachusetts
Neoplasms of the Testis

Richard Rink, MD
Professor
Indiana University School of Medicine
Riley Hospital for Children
Indianapolis, Indiana
Surgical Management of Intersexuality, Cloacal Malformation, and Other Abnormalities of the Genitalia in Girls

Michael L. Ritchey, MD
Professor of Urology
Mayo Clinic
Phoenix, Arizona
Pediatric Urologic Oncology

Ronald Rodriguez, MD, PhD
Assistant Professor of Urology, Medical Oncology, Cellular and Molecular Medicine, Viral Oncology Director, Urology Residency Program
Johns Hopkins University School of Medicine
Baltimore, Maryland
Molecular Biology, Endocrinology and Physiology of the Prostate and Seminal Vesicles

Claus G. Roehrborn, MD
Professor and Chairman
Department of Urology
University of Texas Southwestern Medical Center at Dallas
Dallas, Texas
Benign Prostatic Hyperplasia: Etiology, Pathophysiology, Epidemiology, and Natural History

Jonathan A. Roth, MD
Assistant Professor of Urology and Pediatrics
Temple University Medical School
Temple University Children's Hospital
Philadelphia, Pennsylvania
Renal Function in the Fetus, Neonate, and Child

Eric S. Rovner, MD
Associate Professor of Urology
Department of Urology
Medical University of South Carolina
Charleston, South Carolina
Urinary Tract Fistula
Bladder and Urethral Diverticula

Thomas A. Rozanski, MD
Professor
Department of Urology
University of Texas Health Science Center at San Antonio
Chief
Medical Operations
University Hospital
San Antonio, Texas
Genital and Lower Urinary Tract Trauma

Arthur I. Sagalowsky, MD
Paul C. Peters Chair in Urology in Memory of Rumsey and Louis Strickland
Professor of Urology
Department of Urology
University of Texas Southwestern Medical Center
Chief of Urologic Oncology
Zale Lipshy Hospital
Dallas, Texas
Management of Urothelial Tumors of the Renal Pelvis and Ureter

Jay I. Sandlow, MD
Associate Professor and Vice Chairman
Department of Urology
Medical College of Wisconsin
Director
Andrology and Male Infertility
Reproductive Medicine Center
Froedtert and Medical College of Wisconsin
Milwaukee, Wisconsin
Surgery of Scrotum and Seminal Vesicles

Richard A. Santucci, MD
Associate Professor and Chief of Urology
Department of Urology
Wayne State University School of Medicine
Detroit, Michigan
Renal and Ureteral Trauma

Peter T. Scardino, MD
Chair
Department of Surgery
Head
Prostate Cancer Program
Memorial Sloan-Kettering Cancer Center
New York, New York
Expectant Management of Prostate Cancer

Harriette Scarpero, MD
Assistant Professor
Vanderbilt School of Medicine
Attending Urologist
Vanderbilt University Medical Center
Nashville, Tennessee
Tension-Free Vaginal Tape Procedures

Anthony J. Schaeffer, MD
Herman I. Kretschmer Professor and Chair
Department of Urology
Northwestern University Feinberg School of Medicine
Chief of Urology
Northwestern Memorial Hospital
Chicago, Illinois
Infections of the Urinary Tract

Edward M. Schaeffer, MD, PhD
Department of Urology
James Buchanan Brady Urological Institute
Johns Hopkins Medical Institutions
Baltimore, Maryland
Infections of the Urinary Tract

Howard I. Scher, MD
Professor of Medicine
Joan and Sanford I. Weill Medical College of Cornell University
Chief
Genitourinary Oncology Service
Wayne Calloway Chair in Urologic Oncology
Memorial Sloan-Kettering Cancer Center
Attending Physician
Memorial Hospital for Cancer and Allied Diseases
New York, New York
The Clinical State of the Rising PSA Following Definitive Local Therapy: A Practical Approach

Peter N. Schlegel, MD
Professor and Chairman
Department of Urology
Professor of Reproductive Medicine
Weill Medical College of Cornell University
Staff Scientist, The Population Council
Urologist in Chief, New York-Presbyterian Hospital
Associate Physician, Rockefeller University Hospital
New York, New York
Male Reproductive Physiology

Steven M. Schlossberg, MD
Professor
Eastern Virginia Medical School
Norfolk, Virginia
Surgery of the Penis and Urethra

Richard N. Schlussel, MD
Assistant Professor
Division of Pediatric Urology
Columbia University College of Physicians and Surgeons
Morgan Stanley Children's Hospital of New York-Presbyterian
Columbia University Medical Center
New York, New York
Ectopic Ureter, Ureterocele, and Other Anomalies of the Ureter

Francis X. Schneck, MD
Associate Professor of Urology
Children's Hospital of Pittsburgh
University of Pittsburgh Medical Center
Pittsburgh, Pennsylvania
Abnormalities of the Testes and Scrotum and Their Surgical Management

Mark P. Schoenberg, MD
Professor of Urology and Oncology
Director of Urologic Oncology
James Buchanan Brady Urological Institute
Johns Hopkins Medical Institutions
Baltimore, Maryland
Management of Invasive and Metastatic Bladder Cancer

Martin J. Schreiber, Jr., MD
Chairman
Department of Nephrology and Hypertension
Cleveland Clinic Foundation
Cleveland, Ohio
Etiology, Pathogenesis, and Management of Renal Failure

Joseph W. Segura, MD
Consultant in Urology
Carl Rosen Professor of Urology
Department of Urology
Mayo Clinic Foundation
Rochester, Minnesota
Lower Urinary Tract Calculi

Jay B. Shah, MD
Chief Resident
Department of Urology
Columbia University College of Physicians and Surgeons
Columbia University Medical Center
New York, New York
Percutaneous Management of the Upper Urinary Tract

Robert C. Shamberger, MD
Robert E. Gross Professor of Surgery
Harvard Medical School
Chief of Surgery
Children's Hospital
Boston, Massachusetts
Pediatric Urologic Oncology

David S. Sharp, MD
Glickman Urological Institute
Cleveland Clinic Foundation
Cleveland, Ohio
Surgery of Penile and Urethral Carcinoma

Joel Sheinfeld, MD
Vice-Chairman
Department of Urology
Memorial Sloan-Kettering Cancer Center
New York, New York
Surgery of Testicular Tumors

Linda M. Dairiki Shortliffe, MD
Professor and Chair
Department of Urology
Stanford University School of Medicine
Chief of Pediatric Urology
Stanford Hospital and Clinics
Lucile Salter Packard Children's Hospital
Stanford, California
Infection and Inflammation of the Pediatric Genitourinary Tract

Daniel A. Shoskes, MD, FRCSC
Professor of Surgery
Cleveland Clinic Lerner College of Medicine of Case Western Reserve University
Urologist, Glickman Urological Institute
Cleveland Clinic Foundation
Cleveland, Ohio
Renal Physiology and Pathophysiology

Cary L. Siegel, MD
Associate Professor of Radiology
Division of Diagnostic Radiology
Washington University School of Medicine
St. Louis, Missouri
Urinary Tract Imaging: Basic Principles

Mark Sigman, MD
Associate Professor of Surgery (Urology)
Brown Medical School
Providence, Rhode Island
Male Infertility

Jennifer D. Y. Sihoe, BMBS(Nottm), FRCSEd(Paed), FHKAM(Surg)
Specialist in Pediatric Surgery
Division of Pediatric Surgery and Pediatric Urology
Chinese University of Hong Kong
Prince of Wales Hospital
Hong Kong
Voiding Dysfunction in Children: Non-Neurogenic and Neurogenic

Donald G. Skinner, MD
Professor and Chair
Department of Urology
Keck School of Medicine of the University of Southern California, Norris Cancer Center
Los Angeles, California
Orthotopic Urinary Diversion

Arthur D. Smith, MD
Professor
Department of Urology
Albert Einstein School of Medicine
New York, New York
Chairman Emeritus
Department of Urology
North Shore-Long Island Jewish Medical Center
New Hyde Park, New York
Percutaneous Management of the Upper Urinary Tract

Joseph A. Smith, Jr., MD
Professor
Department of Urologic Surgery
Vanderbilt University School of Medicine
Vanderbilt University Medical Center
Nashville, Tennessee
Laparoscopic and Robotic-Assisted Laparoscopic Radical Prostatectomy and Pelvic Lymphadenectomy

Jonathan Starkman, MD
Clinical Instructor
Department of Urologic Surgery
Vanderbilt University School of Medicine
Vanderbilt University Medical Center
Nashville, Tennessee
Tension-Free Vaginal Tape Procedures

David R. Staskin, MD
Director
Section of Voiding Dysfunction
Female Urology and Urodynamics
New York Hospital–Cornell
Associate Professor
Urology and Obstetrics and Gynecology
Weill Medical College of Cornell University
New York, New York
Surgical Treatment of Male Sphincteric Urinary Incontinence: The Male Perineal Sling and Artificial Urinary Sphincter

Graeme S. Steele, MD
Assistant Professor of Surgery
Harvard Medical School
Division of Urologic Surgery
Brigham and Women's Hospital
Boston, Massachusetts
Neoplasms of the Testis

John P. Stein, MD
Associate Professor in Urology
Department of Urology
Keck School of Medicine of the University of Southern California, Norris Cancer Center
Los Angeles, California
Orthotopic Urinary Diversion

John T. Stoffel, MD
Assistant Professor
Tufts University School of Medicine
Boston, Massachusetts
Senior Staff Consultant
Department of Urology
Lahey Clinic Medical Center
Burlington, Massachusetts
Pubovaginal Sling

Jack W. Strandhoy, PhD
Professor
Department of Physiology and Pharmacology
Wake Forest University School of Medicine
Winston-Salem, North Carolina
Pathophysiology of Urinary Tract Infections

Stevan B. Streem, MD *(deceased)*
Head, Section of Endourology
Cleveland Clinic Foundation
Cleveland, Ohio
Management of Upper Urinary Tract Obstruction

Li-Ming Su, MD
Associate Professor of Urology
Director of Laparoscopic and Robotic Urologic Surgery
James Buchanan Brady Urological Institute
Johns Hopkins Medical Institutions
Baltimore, Maryland
Laparoscopic and Robotic-Assisted Laparoscopic Radical Prostatectomy and Pelvic Lymphadenectomy

Anthony J. Thomas, Jr., MD
Head, Section of Male Infertility
Glickman Urological Institute
Cleveland Clinic Foundation
Faculty
Cleveland Clinic Lerner College of Medicine of Case Western Reserve University
Cleveland, Ohio
Surgical Management of Male Infertility

Ian M. Thompson, MD
Glenda and Gary Woods Distinguished Chair in Genitourinary Oncology
Henry B. and Edna Smith Dielman Memorial Chair in Urologic Science
University of Texas Health Science Center
San Antonio, Texas
Epidemiology, Etiology, and Prevention of Prostate Cancer

Sandip P. Vasavada, MD
Associate Professor of Surgery (Urology)
Cleveland Clinic Lerner College of Medicine of Case Western Reserve University
Co-Head, Section of Female Urology and Voiding Dysfunction
Glickman Urological Institute
Cleveland Clinic Foundation
Cleveland, Ohio
Electrical Stimulation for Storage and Emptying Disorders

E. Darracott Vaughan, Jr., MD
James J. Colt Professor and Chairman Emeritus of Urology
Department of Urology
Weill Medical College of Cornell University
New York-Presbyterian Hospital
New York, New York
The Adrenals

Robert W. Veltri, PhD
Associate Professor of Urology
Johns Hopkins University School of Medicine
Department of Urology
The Brady Urological Research Institute
Director
Fisher Biomarker Research Laboratory
Baltimore, Maryland
The Molecular Biology, Endocrinology, and Physiology of the Prostate and Seminal Vesicles

Patrick C. Walsh, MD
University Distinguished Service Professor of Urology
James Buchanan Brady Urological Institute
Johns Hopkins Medical Institutions
Baltimore, Maryland
Anatomic Radical Retropubic Prostatectomy

George D. Webster, MD
Professor of Urologic Surgery
Department of Urology
Duke University Medical Center
Durham, North Carolina
Urodynamic and Videourodynamic Evaluation of Voiding Dysfunction

Alan J. Wein, MD, PhD (Hon)
Professor and Chair
Division of Urology
University of Pennsylvania School of Medicine
Chief of Urology
University of Pennsylvania Medical Center
Philadelphia, Pennsylvania
Pathophysiology and Classification of Voiding Dysfunction
Pharmacologic Management of Storage and Emptying Failure
Lower Urinary Tract Dysfunction in Neurologic Injury and Disease
Additional Therapies for Storage and Emptying Failure

Robert M. Weiss, MD
Donald Guthrie Professor and Chair
Section of Urology
Yale University School of Medicine
New Haven, Connecticut
Physiology and Pharmacology of the Renal Pelvis and Ureter

Howard N. Winfield, MD, FRCS
Professor, Department of Urology
Director, Laparoscopy and Minimally Invasive Surgery
University of Iowa Hospitals and Clinics
Iowa City, Iowa
Surgery of Scrotum and Seminal Vesicles

J. Christian Winters, MD
Associate Chairman
Department of Urology
Director of Urodynamics and Female Urology
Ochsner Clinic Foundation
New Orleans, Louisiana
Injection Therapy for Urinary Incontinence

John R. Woodard, MD
Formerly: Clinical Professor of Urology
Director of Pediatric Urology
Emory University School of Medicine
Formerly: Chief of Urology
Henrietta Egleston Hospital for Children
Atlanta, Georgia
Prune Belly Syndrome

Subbarao V. Yalla, MDc
Professor of Surgery (Urology)
Harvard Medical School
Chief, Urology Division
Boston Veterans Affairs Medical Center
Boston, Massachusetts
Geriatric Incontinence and Voiding Dysfunction

C. K. Yeung, MBBS, MD, FRCSE, FRCSG, FRACS, FACS, FHKAM(Surg), DCH(Lond)
Chair and Professor of Surgery
Chinese University of Hong Kong
Director, Minimally Invasive Surgical Skills Center
Director, Children's Continence Care Center
Consultant, Pediatric Surgery and Pediatric Urology
Prince of Wales Hospital
Hong Kong
Voiding Dysfunction in Children: Non-Neurogenic and Neurogenic

Naoki Yoshimura, MD, PhD
Associate Professor of Urology and Pharmacology
University of Pittsburgh School of Medicine
Pittsburgh, Pennsylvania
Physiology and Pharmacology of the Bladder and Urethra

CONTENTS

VOLUME I

VOLUME II

VOLUME III

VOLUME IV

SECTION 17

PEDIATRIC UROLOGY 435

SECTION I

ANATOMY

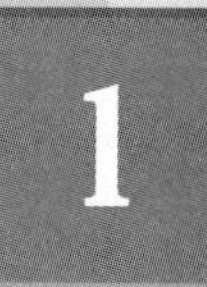

Surgical Anatomy of the Retroperitoneum, Adrenals, Kidneys, and Ureters

JOHN N. KABALIN

QUESTIONS

1. The lumbodorsal fascia originates from the:
   a. latissimus dorsi muscle.
   b. lower rib cage posteriorly.
   c. lumbar vertebrae.
   d. iliac crest.
   e. rectus sheath.
2. The lumbodorsal fascia consists of:
   a. a single layer.
   b. two distinct layers.
   c. three distinct layers.
   d. four distinct layers.
   e. five distinct layers.
3. The lumbodorsal fascia is contiguous anteriorly with the:
   a. transversalis fascia.
   b. aponeurosis of the transversus abdominis muscle.
   c. internal oblique fascia.
   d. external oblique fascia.
   e. rectus sheath.
4. The dorsal lumbotomy incision to expose the kidney:
   a. requires incision of the latissimus dorsi muscle.
   b. requires incision of the quadratus lumborum muscle.
   c. splits the lumbodorsal horizontally from posterior to anterior.
   d. splits the lumbodorsal fascia vertically without incising muscle.
   e. requires excision of the 12th rib.
5. The psoas major muscle:
   a. flexes the thigh at the hip.
   b. extends the thigh at the hip.
   c. adducts the thigh at the hip.
   d. abducts the thigh at the hip.
   e. assists in full contraction of the diaphragm.
6. Which of the following muscles is NOT a boundary of the retroperitoneum?
   a. The psoas muscle
   b. The iliacus muscle
   c. The quadratus lumborum muscle
   d. The diaphragm
   e. The rectus muscle
7. In a subcostal flank approach to the kidney, which of the following may be incised to increase upward mobility of the 12th rib?
   a. The intercostal muscles between the 11th and 12th ribs
   b. The latissimus dorsi muscle
   c. The lumbodorsal fascia
   d. The quadratus lumborum muscle
   e. The costovertebral ligament
8. The first arterial branch(es) from the abdominal aorta is(are):
   a. the paired renal arteries.
   b. the right adrenal artery.
   c. the inferior phrenic artery.
   d. the hepatic artery.
   e. the superior mesenteric artery.
9. Which of the following arteries branches from the celiac arterial trunk?
   a. The left gastric artery
   b. The right gastric artery
   c. The pancreaticoduodenal artery
   d. The superior mesenteric artery
   e. The inferior phrenic arteries

10. The renal arteries typically branch from the abdominal aorta at the level of the:
    a. 12th thoracic vertebral body.
    b. 1st lumbar vertebral body.
    c. 2nd lumbar vertebral body.
    d. 3rd lumbar vertebral body.
    e. 4th lumbar vertebral body.

11. The testicular arteries most commonly originate from the:
    a. renal arteries.
    b. adrenal arteries.
    c. abdominal aorta above the superior mesenteric artery.
    d. abdominal aorta below the renal arteries.
    e. common iliac arteries.

12. A 20-year-old man is undergoing retroperitoneal dissection for a testicular germ cell tumor. The inferior mesenteric artery is divided during reflection of the intestines to expose the retroperitoneum. This can be expected to result in:
    a. ischemia of the descending colon.
    b. ischemia of the sigmoid colon.
    c. ischemia of the rectum.
    d. ischemia of the transverse colon.
    e. none of the above.

13. Which of the following vessels drain(s) into the inferior vena cava?
    a. Renal veins
    b. Superior mesenteric vein
    c. Inferior mesenteric vein
    d. Splenic vein
    e. All of the above

14. The left gonadal vein typically drains into the:
    a. anterior aspect of the inferior vena cava.
    b. left lateral aspect of the inferior vena cava.
    c. inferior aspect of the left renal vein.
    d. left adrenal vein.
    e. inferior aspect of the common iliac vein.

15. The left renal vein crosses the abdominal aorta:
    a. anteriorly, just above the superior mesenteric artery.
    b. anteriorly, just below the superior mesenteric artery.
    c. posteriorly, at the level of the superior mesenteric artery.
    d. anteriorly, just below the inferior mesenteric artery.
    e. anteriorly, just above the inferior mesenteric artery.

16. Which of the following vessels commonly drains into the left renal vein?
    a. The left adrenal vein
    b. The second lumbar vein
    c. The left internal spermatic vein
    d. All of the above
    e. None of the above

17. On a CT scan, a male patient is found to have enlarged lymph nodes along the abdominal aorta between the left renal hilum and the inferior mesenteric artery. Sites of malignancy that would commonly drain directly to these lymph nodes would NOT include the:
    a. colon.
    b. left kidney.
    c. left testis.
    d. left renal pelvis.
    e. bladder.

18. Lymph flow in the lumbar lymphatic chains of the retroperitoneum proceeds:
    a. in a cephalad direction.
    b. in a cephalad direction and from right to left.
    c. in a cephalad direction and from left to right.
    d. caudally.
    e. caudally and from left to right.

19. The cisterna chyli is typically located at approximately the level of the first lumbar vertebral body:
    a. posterior to the inferior vena cava.
    b. posterior to the aorta.
    c. closely approximated to the posterior surface of the right adrenal gland.
    d. associated with the superior mesenteric artery.
    e. posterior to the right renal hilum.

20. The primary lymph node drainage site for the right testis is the:
    a. superficial right inguinal lymph nodes.
    b. deep right inguinal lymph nodes.
    c. right common iliac lymph nodes.
    d. lymph nodes at the right renal hilum.
    e. interaortocaval lumbar lymph nodes.

21. The lumbar sympathetic chains:
    a. run vertically in the retroperitoneum, medial to the psoas muscles.
    b. contain numerous sympathetic ganglia.
    c. are closely associated with the lumbar blood vessels.
    d. contain postganglionic sympathetic neurons supplying the lower extremities.
    e. all of the above.

22. Disruption of which sympathetic nervous plexus on the anterior abdominal aorta during retroperitoneal dissection will probably cause loss of seminal emission in a male patient?
    a. Celiac plexus
    b. Renal plexus
    c. Superior mesenteric plexus
    d. Superior hypogastric plexus
    e. All of the above

23. In the lateral abdominal wall, the iliohypogastric nerve will be found coursing in the plane:
    a. deep to the transversalis fascia.
    b. between the transversalis fascia and the transversus abdominis muscle.
    c. between the transversus abdominis and internal oblique muscles.
    d. between the internal oblique and external oblique muscles.
    e. superficial to the external oblique muscle.

24. The cremaster muscle is innervated by the:
    a. ilioinguinal nerve.
    b. iliohypogastric nerve.
    c. obturator nerve.
    d. genital branch of the genitofemoral nerve.
    e. femoral branch of the genitofemoral nerve.

25. In the retroperitoneum, where can the genitofemoral nerve be found?
    a. Posterior to the psoas muscle
    b. On the anterior surface of the psoas muscle.
    c. Lateral to the psoas muscle.
    d. Medial to the psoas muscle.
    e. The genitofemoral nerve is not typically found in the retroperitoneum.

26. The descending duodenum:
    a. lies within the retroperitoneum.
    b. receives the common bile duct.
    c. lies lateral to the head of the pancreas.
    d. lies anterior to the right renal hilum.
    e. all of the above.

27. The posterior surface of the tail of the pancreas is closely associated with the:
    a. splenic artery.
    b. splenic vein.
    c. upper pole of the left kidney.
    d. left adrenal gland.
    e. all of the above.

28. In cases of renal ectopia, the ipsilateral adrenal gland is typically:
    a. absent.
    b. found in its normal anatomic position in the upper retroperitoneum.
    c. found in association with the contralateral adrenal gland.
    d. found closely applied to the superior pole of the ectopic kidney.
    e. found closely associated with the ipsilateral renal artery.

29. In cases of unilateral renal agenesis, the ipsilateral adrenal gland is commonly:
    a. absent.
    b. found in its normal anatomic position in the upper retroperitoneum.
    c. found in association with the contralateral adrenal gland.
    d. found just inside the ipsilateral internal inguinal ring.
    e. found in an ectopic, intrathoracic location.

30. Which of the following statements is NOT true?
    a. The right renal vein is much shorter than the left renal vein.
    b. The right adrenal vein is much shorter than the left adrenal vein.
    c. The right kidney is typically located lower in the retroperitoneum than the left kidney.
    d. The right adrenal gland is typically located lower in the retroperitoneum than the left adrenal gland.
    e. Both c and d.

31. As one proceeds outward from the adrenal medulla, the three separate functional layers of the adrenal cortex are, in correct order:
    a. zona reticularis, zona fasciculata, then zona glomerulosa.
    b. zona fasciculata, zona reticularis, then zona glomerulosa.
    c. zona glomerulosa, zona fasciculata, then zona reticularis.
    d. zona glomerulosa, zona reticularis, then zona fasciculata.
    e. zona reticularis, zona glomerulosa, then zona fasciculata.

32. Which of the following statements is (are) NOT true?
    a. The adrenal medulla produces catecholamines in response to stimulation from the sympathetic nervous system.
    b. The zona glomerulosa produces aldosterone in response to angiotensin II.
    c. The zona reticularis of the adrenal cortex produces androgens in response to luteinizing hormone (LH).
    d. The zona fasciculate of the adrenal cortex produces glucocorticoids in response to adrenocorticotropic hormone (ACTH).
    e. Both b and c.

33. The adrenal arteries are branches from:
    a. the aorta.
    b. the inferior phrenic arteries.
    c. the renal arteries.
    d. the celiac arterial trunk.
    e. a, b, and c.

34. The kidney produces:
    a. renin.
    b. angiotensin.
    c. erythropoietin.
    d. both a and c.
    e. a, b, and c.

35. The normal kidney in an average-sized adult man weighs approximately:
    a. 1200 grams.
    b. 600 grams.
    c. 300 grams.
    d. 150 grams.
    e. 50 grams.

36. Persistent fetal lobation identified in the kidney of an adult patient:
    a. indicates the presence of a congenital renal disorder.
    b. indicates childhood renal injury due to infection.
    c. is observed only with long-standing obstructive uropathy.
    d. is normal.
    e. is never seen.

37. The upper pole of the kidney lies anterior to:
    a. the 12th rib.
    b. the diaphragm.
    c. the pleura.
    d. all of the above.
    e. none of the above.

38. Which of the following statements regarding the typical anatomic positioning of the kidney is TRUE?
    a. The lower pole of the kidney lies more anterior than the upper pole.
    b. The lower pole of the kidney lies more lateral than the upper pole.
    c. The medial aspect of the kidney lies more anterior than its lateral aspect.
    d. The anterior renal calyces lie lateral to the posterior renal calyces.
    e. All of the above.

39. During left radical nephrectomy performed via a transabdominal approach, excessive traction on which of the following structures might be expected to produce a significant injury to the spleen?
    a. Left adrenal gland
    b. Splenorenal ligament
    c. Splenocolic ligament
    d. Both b and c
    e. a, b, and c

40. Gerota's fascia envelops and contains the:
    a. adrenal gland.
    b. kidney.
    c. ureter.
    d. gonadal vessels.
    e. all of the above.

41. After blunt trauma to the right kidney, with a major laceration to the renal parenchyma and ongoing hemorrhage, the expanding hematoma contained within Gerota's fascia will tend to extend:
    a. across the midline into Gerota's fascia surrounding the left (contralateral) kidney.
    b. downward into the pelvis.
    c. upward into the thorax.
    d. anterolaterally, deep to the transversalis fascia.
    e. anterolaterally, between the peritoneum and transversalis fascia.

42. Proceeding from posterior to anterior, the structures encountered in the renal hilum are, in correct order, the:
    a. renal artery, renal vein, and renal pelvis.
    b. renal pelvis, renal artery, and renal vein.
    c. renal pelvis, renal vein, and renal artery.
    d. renal vein, renal artery, and renal pelvis.
    e. renal artery, renal pelvis, and renal vein.

43. The first branch segmental artery from the main renal artery is typically the:
    a. the apical anterior segmental artery.
    b. lower anterior segmental artery.
    c. posterior segmental artery.
    d. upper anterior segmental artery.
    e. middle anterior segmental artery.

44. During pyeloplasty, the posterior segmental renal artery is inadvertently divided. This will produce:
    a. no effect on the kidney.
    b. ischemic loss of a large posterior segment of the renal parenchyma.
    c. ischemic loss of a small posterior segment of the renal parenchyma.
    d. ischemic loss of a segment of upper pole renal parenchyma.
    e. ischemic loss of a segment of lower pole renal parenchyma.

45. The sequential branches of the renal artery are, in order, the:
    a. segmental, interlobar, arcuate, interlobular, and afferent arteriole.
    b. segmental, interlobular, arcuate, interlobar, and afferent arteriole.
    c. segmental, subsegmental, interlobar, interlobular, arcuate, and afferent arteriole.
    d. segmental, arcuate, interlobar, interlobular, and afferent arteriole.
    e. segmental, interlobar, interlobular, arcuate, and afferent arteriole.

46. During pyeloplasty, a large anterior segmental renal vein is inadvertently torn and subsequently ligated to control hemorrhage. This will produce:
    a. no effect on the kidney.
    b. segmental renal venous congestion and chronic pain.
    c. ischemic loss of a large anterior segment of the renal parenchyma.
    d. ischemic loss of a small anterior segment of the renal parenchyma.
    e. ischemic loss of a segment of lower pole renal parenchyma.

47. Which of the following vessels commonly drains into the right renal vein?
    a. The right adrenal vein
    b. The second lumbar vein
    c. The right gonadal vein
    d. All of the above
    e. None of the above

48. The most common renal vascular anomaly is a:
    a. supernumerary left renal artery.
    b. supernumerary right renal artery.
    c. supernumerary left renal vein coursing anterior to the aorta.
    d. supernumerary left renal vein coursing posterior to the aorta.
    e. supernumerary right renal vein.

49. After involvement of lymph nodes directly at the renal hilum, the primary lymph node drainage site for the left kidney is the:
    a. left lateral para-aortic lymph nodes.
    b. interaortocaval lymph nodes.
    c. right paracaval lymph nodes.
    d. left retrocrural lymph nodes.
    e. all of the above.

50. In a typical human kidney, there are approximately how many renal papillae and corresponding minor calyces?
    a. 3 to 5
    b. 7 to 9
    c. 11 to 12
    d. 14 to 15
    e. 17 to 18

51. A compound renal papilla and calyx:
    a. is protective against ascending infection.
    b. is least common at the upper pole of the kidney.
    c. is a rare finding.
    d. is commonly associated with formation of kidney stones.
    e. none of the above.

52. The ureteral smooth muscle consists of:
    a. a single layer of longitudinally oriented muscle bundles.
    b. a single layer of circular and obliquely oriented muscle bundles.
    c. a single layer of randomly oriented muscle bundles
    d. two layers—an inner layer of longitudinal muscle and an outer layer of circular and oblique muscle.
    e. two layers—an inner layer of circular and oblique muscle and an outer layer of longitudinal muscle.

53. The ureter receives its blood supply from the:
    a. renal artery.
    b. aorta.
    c. common iliac artery.
    d. gonadal artery.
    e. all of the above.

54. An invasive transitional cell carcinoma is diagnosed in the left proximal ureter, at the level of the third lumbar vertebral body. The primary site of potential nodal metastases from this lesion will be the:
    a. left para-aortic lymph nodes.
    b. interaortocaval lymph nodes.
    c. left common iliac lymph nodes.
    d. lymph nodes at the left renal hilum.
    e. left external iliac lymph nodes.

55. During surgical dissection, the ureter can be identified as it enters the pelvis:
    a. at the aortic bifurcation.
    b. crossing the superior border of the sacrum.
    c. crossing the common iliac artery at the branching of the internal iliac artery.
    d. crossing the uterine artery.
    e. at the internal inguinal ring.

56. A young man with right-sided abdominal pain is diagnosed with right hydroureteronephrosis by renal ultrasonography. Which of the following inflammatory processes might impinge upon the right ureter and cause obstruction?
    a. Acute appendicitis
    b. Crohn's ileitis
    c. Perforated cecal carcinoma
    d. All of the above
    e. None of the above

57. Narrowing of the ureteral luminal caliber naturally occurs at the:
    a. ureteropelvic junction.
    b. crossing of the iliac vessels.
    c. ureterovesical junction.
    d. all of the above.
    e. none of the above.

58. Sympathetic nerve input to the kidney typically travels through the:
    a. celiac plexus.
    b. superior mesenteric plexus.
    c. superior hypogastric plexus.
    d. inferior hypogastric plexus.
    e. none of the above.

59. Ureteral peristalsis requires:
    a. intact sympathetic input.
    b. intact parasympathetic input.
    c. both sympathetic and parasympathetic input.
    d. intact spinal cord.
    e. intrinsic smooth muscle pacemakers in the renal collecting system.

60. The pain caused by an obstructing ureteral stone:
    a. is primarily related to distention of the collecting system above the stone.
    b. is transmitted via nerves from the eighth thoracic through the second lumbar spinal segments.
    c. may be referred over the somatic distribution of the subcostal, iliohypogastric, or ilioinguinal nerves.
    d. may be referred over the distribution of the genitofemoral nerve.
    e. all of the above.

ANSWERS

1. **c. lumbar vertebrae.** The lumbodorsal fascia originates from the lumbar vertebrae.
2. **c. three distinct layers.** There are three distinct layers of the lumbodorsal fascia.
3. **b. aponeurosis of the transversus abdominis muscle.** All three layers of the lumbodorsal fascia join to form a single thick aponeurosis lateral to the quadratus lumborum muscle before extending further anterolaterally, where they are contiguous with the aponeurosis of the transversus abdominis muscle.
4. **d. splits the lumbodorsal fascia vertically without incising muscle.** A vertical incision that parallels the lateral borders of the sacrospinalis and quadratus lumborum can be made through this lumbodorsal fascia, posteromedial to the first transverse muscle fibers of the transversus abdominis muscle, to gain surgical access to the retroperitoneum and kidney without cutting muscle (the so-called lumbodorsal approach, or dorsal lumbotomy) (see Fig. 1-7).
5. **a. flexes the thigh at the hip.** The psoas major joins the iliacus muscle, which originates broadly over the inner aspect of the iliac wing of the pelvis, to become the iliopsoas and insert on the lesser trochanter of the femur and flex the thigh at the hip.
6. **e. The rectus muscle.** The posterior surface of the retroperitoneum is formed by the lumbar vertebral bodies in the midline, which are covered by the shiny, longitudinal fibers of the anterior spinous ligament. These are flanked bilaterally by the psoas muscles. The psoas muscles are covered by a glistening white fibrous fascia, the so-called psoas sheath, which is contiguous with the transversalis fascia. As one moves laterally, the lateral portion of the quadratus lumborum extends from behind the lateral margin of the psoas. The anterior layer of the lumbodorsal fascia covers this muscle and continues as the aponeurosis of the transversus abdominis muscle. Farther laterally, the transversus abdominis muscle proper is encountered. Superiorly, the posterior wall of the retroperitoneum is formed by the posterior insertion of the diaphragm along the lower ribs. Inferiorly, below the level of the iliac crest, the iliopsoas muscle forms the posterior confine of the retroperitoneum.
7. **e. The costovertebral ligament.** The costovertebral, or lumbodorsal, ligament is a strong fascial attachment between the inferior margin of the 12th rib and the transverse processes of the first and second lumbar vertebrae (see Fig. 1-5). It is encountered only in posterior approaches to the kidney and can be incised to produce greater mobility of the 12th rib and provide greater exposure and access to the structures of the upper retroperitoneum.
8. **c. the inferior phrenic arteries.** The first abdominal branches of the aorta are the paired inferior phrenic arteries.
9. **a. The left gastric artery.** The short celiac arterial trunk trifurcates into common hepatic, left gastric, and splenic branches.
10. **c. 2nd lumbar vertebral body.** Usually overlying the second lumbar vertebral body, but subject to considerable variation, the paired renal arteries emanate laterally from the aorta.
11. **d. abdominal aorta below the renal arteries.** The paired gonadal arteries arise from the anterolateral aorta—in atypical cases, from a single anterior trunk—at a level somewhat below the renal vessels.
12. **e. none of the above.** The inferior mesenteric artery, especially in younger individuals without atherosclerotic occlusive arterial disease, can almost always be sacrificed without complication.
13. **a. Renal veins.** Inferior mesenteric, superior mesenteric, and splenic veins join to form the portal vein and drain proximally into the liver rather than directly into the inferior vena cava.
14. **c. inferior aspect of the left renal vein.** The left gonadal vein usually enters the inferior aspect of the left renal vein.
15. **b. anteriorly, just below the superior mesenteric artery.** The left renal vein crosses the aorta anteriorly below the takeoff of the superior mesenteric artery.
16. **d. All of the above.** The left renal vein commonly receives a lumbar vein (usually the second lumbar) on its posterior aspect. In addition, the left gonadal vein typically drains into its inferior margin and the left adrenal vein into its superior margin.
17. **e. bladder.** These lumbar nodal chains are extraregional or secondary drainage sites for any metastatic process arising from the lower pelvis.
18. **b. in a cephalad direction and from right to left.** It is important that most of the lateral flow between ascending lymphatics moves from right to left ascending lumbar trunks.
19. **b. posterior to the aorta.** The structure known as the cisterna chyli truly lies within the thorax, posterior to the aorta or slightly to the right, in a retrocrural position, usually anterior to the first or second lumbar vertebral body.

20. **e. interaortocaval lumbar lymph nodes.** The right testis drains primarily to the interaortocaval region.

21. **e. all of the above.** The sympathetic trunks course vertically along the anterolateral aspect of the spinal column, in the retroperitoneum lying within the groove between the medial aspect of the ipsilateral psoas muscle and the spine, in some cases covered by the psoas. The lumbar arteries and veins, coursing posteriorly, are very closely associated with the sympathetic trunks, crossing them perpendicularly and at times proceeding directly through split portions of the sympathetic chain. The lumbar sympathetic trunks contain variable numbers of ganglia of variable size and position. Some of the preganglionic fibers of the sympathetic trunks synapse within these ganglia with postganglionic sympathetic neurons supplying the body wall and lower extremities.

22. **d. Superior hypogastric plexus.** At the lower extent of the abdominal aorta, much of the sympathetic input to the pelvic urinary organs and genital tract travels through the superior hypogastric plexus, which lies on the aorta anterior to its bifurcation and extends inferiorly on the anterior surface of the fifth lumbar vertebra. This plexus is contiguous bilaterally with inferior hypogastric plexuses, which extend into the pelvis. Disruption of the sympathetic nerve fibers that travel through these plexuses during retroperitoneal dissection can cause loss of seminal vesicle emission and/or failure of bladder neck closure, which results in retrograde ejaculation.

23. **c. between the transversus abdominis and internal oblique muscles.** The iliohypogastric nerve and the ilioinguinal nerve originate together as a common extension from the first lumbar spinal nerve before splitting. These somatic nerves cross the anterior or inner surface of the quadratus lumborum muscle before piercing the transversus abdominis muscle and continuing their course between this and the internal oblique muscle.

24. **d. genital branch of the genitofemoral nerve.** The genital branch of the genitofemoral nerve supplies the cremaster and dartos muscles.

25. **b. On the anterior surface of the psoas muscle.** The genitofemoral nerve lies directly atop and parallels the psoas muscle throughout most of its retroperitoneal course.

26. **e. all of the above.** The second (descending) part of the duodenum descends vertically, directly anterior to the right renal hilum, and thus is intimately related on its posterior aspect to the medial margin of the right kidney, right renal vessels, renal pelvis, ureteropelvic junction, and often the upper right ureter. The common bile duct also lies posterior to and drains into this part of the duodenum. Directly medial and intimately related to the descending duodenum lies the head of the pancreas.

27. **e. all of the above.** The tail of the pancreas on the left is related posteriorly to the left adrenal gland and upper portion of the left kidney. The splenic vein runs directly posterior to the pancreas, and the splenic artery runs just superior to the vein.

28. **b. found in its normal anatomic position in the upper retroperitoneum.** In cases of renal ectopia, the adrenal gland is usually found in approximately its normal anatomic position.

29. **b. found in its normal anatomic position in the upper retroperitoneum.** In cases of renal agenesis, the adrenal gland on the involved side is typically present.

30. **d. The right adrenal gland is typically located lower in the retroperitoneum than is the left adrenal gland.** The right adrenal tends to lie more superiorly in the retroperitoneum than does the left adrenal.

31. **a. zona reticularis, zona fasciculata, then zona glomerulosa.** Three cell layers can be identified in the adrenal cortex. The outermost layer is the zona glomerulosa, which produces aldosterone in response to stimulation by the renin-angiotensin system. Centripetally located are the zona fasciculata and zona reticularis, which produce glucocorticoids and sex steroids, respectively.

32. **c. The zona reticularis of the adrenal cortex produces androgens in response to luteinizing hormone (LH).** The function of production of sex steroids by the zona reticularis is regulated by pituitary release of adrenocorticotropic hormone (ACTH).

33. **e. a, b, and c.** Multiple small arteries supply each adrenal gland (see Fig. 1-21). These are branch vessels, which can be traced to three major arterial sources for each gland: (1) superior branches from the inferior phrenic artery, (2) middle branches directly from the aorta, and (3) inferior branches from the ipsilateral renal artery (see Fig. 1-10).

34. **d. both a and c.** The kidneys play a central role in fluid, electrolyte, and acid-base balance in humans, but they also have important endocrine functions, known to include vitamin D metabolism and the production of both renin and erythropoietin.

35. **d. 150 grams.** The normal kidney in the adult male weighs approximately 150 g.

36. **d. is a normal variant.** It is neither unusual nor abnormal to see persistence of some degree of fetal lobation throughout adult life.

37. **d. all of the above.** The diaphragm covers roughly the upper third or upper pole of each kidney. With the diaphragm travels the pleural reflection, and thus any direct approach to the upper portion of the kidney, whether percutaneous or open surgical, risks entering the pleural space. The 12th rib on either side crosses the kidney at approximately the lower extent of the diaphragm.

38. **e. All of the above.** In part as a result of the contour of the psoas muscle, the lower pole of either kidney lies farther from the midline than does the upper pole, so that the upper poles tilt medially at a slight angle (see Fig. 1-25). Similarly, the kidneys do not lie in a simple coronal plane, but the lower pole of the kidney is pushed slightly more anterior than the upper pole. The medial aspect of each kidney is rotated anteriorly on a longitudinal axis at an angle of about 30 degrees from the true coronal plane, with the renal vessels and pelvis exiting the hilum medially in a relatively anterior direction (see Figs. 1-11 and 1-25). Typically, two longitudinal rows of renal pyramids and corresponding minor calyces, roughly perpendicular to one another, extend anteriorly and posteriorly. The anterior calyces extend laterally in a coronal plane, whereas the posterior calyces extend posteriorly in a sagittal plane.

39. **d. Both b and c.** There is typically a peritoneal extension between the perirenal fascia covering the upper pole of the left kidney and the inferior splenic capsule, called the splenorenal, or lienorenal, ligament. Just as with the adjacent and often contiguous splenocolic ligamentous attachment, care must be taken not to exert undue tension on the splenorenal ligament during operative procedures on the left kidney, to avoid inadvertent tearing of the spleen.

40. **e. all of the above.** The kidneys and associated adrenal glands are surrounded by varying degrees of perirenal or perinephric fat, and these together are loosely enclosed by the perirenal fascia, commonly called Gerota's fascia (see Figs. 1-7, 1-11, and 1-26 to 1-28.) Inferiorly, Gerota's fascia remains an open potential space, containing the ureter and gonadal vessels on either side.

41. **b. downward into the pelvis.** When very large, such collections can and do extend into the pelvis, following the potential space where Gerota's fascia does not fuse inferiorly.

42. **b. renal pelvis, renal artery, and renal vein.** The renal vein lies most anteriorly, and behind it lies the artery. Both normally lie anterior to the urinary collecting system, that is, the renal pelvis.

43. **c. the posterior segmental artery.** The main renal artery typically divides into four or more segmental vessels, with five branches most commonly described (see Figs. 1-29 and 1-30). The first and most constant segmental division is a posterior branch.

44. **b. ischemic loss of a large posterior segment of the renal parenchyma.** The posterior segmental artery usually exits the main renal artery before it enters the renal hilum and proceeds posteriorly to the renal pelvis to supply a large posterior segment of the kidney. The main renal artery and each segmental artery, as well as their multiple succeeding branch arteries, are all "end arteries," without anastomosis or collateral circulation; and occlusion of any of these vessels produces ischemia and infarction of the corresponding renal parenchyma that it supplies.

45. **a. segmental, interlobar, arcuate, interlobular, and afferent arteriole.** The segmental arteries course through the renal sinus and branch further into lobar arteries, which divide again and enter the renal parenchyma as interlobar arteries (see Fig. 1-31). The interlobar arteries branch into arcuate arteries, which arc parallel to the renal contour along the corticomedullary junction. The arcuate arteries, in turn, produce multiple radial arterial branches, the interlobular arteries. These have multiple side branches, which are the afferent arterioles to the glomeruli.

46. **a. no effect on the kidney.** Unlike the renal arteries, none of which communicate, the renal parenchymal veins anastomose freely.

47. **e. None of the above**. The right renal vein is short (2 to 4 cm) and enters the right lateral aspect of the inferior vena cava directly, usually without receiving other venous branches.

48. **a. a supernumerary left renal artery.** The most common variation is the occurrence of supernumerary renal arteries. These supernumerary arteries usually arise from the lateral aorta, occur perhaps slightly more often on the left than on the right, and may enter the renal hilum or directly into the parenchyma of one of the poles of the kidney.

49. **a. left lateral para-aortic lymph nodes.** From the left kidney (see Fig. 1-34), the lymphatic trunks then drain primarily into the left lateral para-aortic lymph nodes, including nodes anterior and posterior to the aorta, from a level below the inferior mesenteric artery to the diaphragm.

50. **b. 7 to 9.** The renal papillae may number as few as 4 or as many as 18, but 7 to 9 are present in the typical kidney.

51. **e. none of the above.** A compound renal papilla and calyx often occurs at the renal poles. The compound papillae are of physiologic significance in that their configuration permits urinary reflux into the renal parenchyma with sufficient back pressure, also allowing bacterial reflux into the kidney in the presence of infected urine (see Fig. 1-39). Renal parenchymal scarring secondary to infection is typically most severe overlying such compound papillae.

52. **d. two layers—an inner layer of longitudinal muscle and an outer layer of circular and oblique muscle.** Smooth muscle covers the renal calyces, renal pelvis, and ureter. In the ureter, this muscle can usually be divided into an inner layer of longitudinally coursing muscle bundles and an outer layer of circular and oblique muscle.

53. **e. all of the above.** The ureter receives its blood supply from multiple feeding arterial branches along its course (see Fig. 1-46). In the retroperitoneum, the ureter may receive branches from the renal artery, gonadal artery, abdominal aorta, and common iliac artery.

54. **a. left para-aortic lymph nodes.** In the abdomen, the left para-aortic lymph nodes form the primary drainage sites for the left ureter.

55. **c. crossing the common iliac artery at the branching of the internal iliac artery.** The ureter is related posteriorly to the psoas muscle throughout its retroperitoneal course, crossing the iliac vessels to enter the pelvis at approximately the bifurcation of the common iliac artery into internal and external iliac arteries (see Fig. 1-1).

56. **d. All of the above.** Anteriorly, the right ureter is related to the terminal ileum, cecum, appendix, and ascending colon and their mesenteries.

57. **d. all of the above.** The ureter is not of uniform caliber, with three distinct narrowings normally present along its course (see Fig. 1-44). The first of these is the ureteropelvic junction, the second is the crossing of the iliac vessels, and the third is the ureterovesical junction in the pelvis.

58. **a. celiac plexus.** The kidneys receive preganglionic sympathetic input from the eighth thoracic through the first lumbar spinal segments. Postganglionic fibers arise primarily from the celiac and aorticorenal ganglia.

59. **e. intrinsic smooth muscle pacemakers in the renal collecting system.** Normal ureteral peristalsis does not require outside autonomic input but rather originates and is propagated from intrinsic smooth muscle pacemaker sites located in the minor calyces of the renal collecting system.

60. **e. all of the above.** Pain fibers leave the kidney, renal pelvis, and ureter, traveling with the sympathetic nerves. They are primarily stimulated by nociceptors sensitive to increased tension (distention) in the renal capsule, renal collecting system, or ureter. The resulting visceral pain is felt directly and is referred to somatic distributions that correspond to the spinal segments providing the sympathetic distribution to the kidney and ureter (eighth thoracic through second lumbar segments). Pain and reflex muscle spasm are typically produced over the distributions of the subcostal, iliohypogastric, ilioinguinal, and/or genitofemoral nerves.

2

Anatomy of the Lower Urinary Tract and Male Genitalia

JAMES D. BROOKS

QUESTIONS

1. The greater and lesser sciatic foramina are separated by the:
   a. sacrotuberous ligament.
   b. Cooper's (pectineal) ligament.
   c. arcuate line.
   d. sacrospinous ligament.
   e. piriformis muscle.
2. During inguinal incisions, the vessels invariably encountered in Camper's fascia are the:
   a. superficial inferior epigastric artery and vein.
   b. superficial circumflex iliac artery and vein.
   c. external pudendal artery and vein.
   d. gonadal artery and veins.
   e. accessory obturator vein.
3. Rupture of the penile urethra at the junction of the penis and scrotum can result in urinary extravasation into all of the following structures EXCEPT the:
   a. anterior abdominal wall up to the clavicles.
   b. scrotum.
   c. penis, deep to the dartos fascia.
   d. perineum in a "butterfly" pattern.
   e. buttock.
4. During inguinal hernia repair in a male patient, the ilioinguinal nerve is injured in the canal, which will most likely produce:
   a. anesthesia over the dorsum of the penis.
   b. anesthesia over the pubis and scrotum and loss of cremasteric contraction.
   c. anesthesia over the pubis and anterior scrotum only.
   d. anesthesia over the anterior and medial thigh.
   e. anesthesia over the pubis only.
5. A child has dense scarring after failed extravesical reimplantation. The landmark that can assist in locating the ureter in the pelvis is the:
   a. obturator nerve; the ureter will be medial to it.
   b. obliterated umbilical artery; the ureter will be found lateral to it.
   c. obliterated umbilical artery; the ureter will be found medial to it.
   d. external iliac artery; the ureter crosses it to reach the pelvis.
   e. vas deferens; the ureter will pass anterior to it.
6. The levator ani attaches to all of the following EXCEPT the:
   a. perineal body.
   b. pubis.
   c. coccyx.
   d. vagina.
   e. arcus tendineus fascia pelvis.
7. Accessory obturator veins (from the external iliac artery) and accessory obturator arteries (from the inferior epigastric artery) are encountered in:
   a. 50% and 25% of patients, respectively.
   b. 5% and 50% of patients, respectively.
   c. 50% and 75% of patients, respectively.
   d. 25% and 50% of patients, respectively.
   e. 25% and 5% of patients, respectively.
8. A retractor blade has rested on the psoas muscle during a prolonged procedure, resulting in a femoral nerve palsy. Postoperatively, the patient will experience:
   a. inability to flex the hip and numbness over the anterior thigh.
   b. inability to flex the knee and numbness over the thigh.
   c. numbness over the anterior thigh only.
   d. inability to extend the knee and numbness over the anterior thigh.
   e. inability to flex the knee only.
9. Autonomic nerves contributing to the pelvic plexus include the:
   a. superior hypogastric nerves from the para-aortic plexuses.
   b. pelvic sympathetic trunks.
   c. pelvic parasympathetic neurons from the sacral spinal cord.
   d. a and c only.
   e. a, b, and c.
10. To preserve the vascular supply to the ureter, incisions in the peritoneum should be made:
    a. medially in the abdomen and laterally in the pelvis.
    b. laterally in the abdomen and medially in the pelvis.
    c. always medial to the ureter.
    d. always lateral to the ureter.
    e. directly over the ureter.

11. Relative to the ureter, the uterine vessels are found:
    a. laterally.
    b. posteriorly.
    c. anteriorly.
    d. medially.
    e. running together in a common sheath.
12. All of the following features of the ureterovesical junction cooperate to prevent vesicoureteral reflux EXCEPT:
    a. fixation of the ureter to the superficial trigone.
    b. sphincteric closure of the ureteral orifice.
    c. detrusor backing.
    d. telescoping of the bladder outward over the ureter.
    e. passive closure of the intramural ureter caused by bladder filling.
13. In contrast to that of the male, the female bladder neck:
    a. has extensive adrenergic innervation.
    b. has a thickened middle smooth muscle layer.
    c. is largely responsible for urinary continence.
    d. is surrounded by type I (slow-twitch) fibers.
    e. has longitudinal smooth muscle fibers that extend to the external meatus.
14. Which of the following statements about the trigone is true?
    a. Epithelium is thicker than the rest of the bladder and densely adherent.
    b. Superficial smooth muscle is a continuation of Waldeyer's sheath.
    c. Smooth muscle enlarges to form thick fascicles.
    d. Smooth muscle of the ureter forms the interureteric ridge (Mercier's bar).
    e. When the bladder empties, the trigone is thrown into thick folds.
15. During a perineal prostatectomy, the muscle that must be divided to gain access to the apex of the prostate is the:
    a. rectourethralis.
    b. internal anal sphincter.
    c. perineal body.
    d. external anal sphincter.
    e. puboanalis.
16. Arterial supply to the bladder includes the:
    a. superior vesical artery.
    b. inferior vesical artery.
    c. obturator artery
    d. uterine artery.
    e. all of the above.
17. The ducts of which of the following prostatic zones drain into the preprostatic urethra?
    a. Periurethral glands
    b. Central zone
    c. Transition zone
    d. Peripheral zone
    e. a and c
18. Benign prostatic hyperplasia (BPH) may arise from the:
    a. periurethral glands.
    b. central zone.
    c. transition zone.
    d. peripheral zone.
    e. a and c.
19. In BPH, blood supply to the adenoma arises from the:
    a. superior vesical artery.
    b. urethral arteries extending down the urethra from the bladder neck.
    c. capsular arteries that arise laterally.
    d. dorsal venous complex.
    e. neurovascular bundle.
20. Which of the following statements concerning the striated urethral sphincter is TRUE?
    a. It is composed of type I (slow-twitch) and type II (fast-twitch) fibers.
    b. It is bounded above by the superior fascia.
    c. It receives motor blanches from the dorsal nerve of the penis.
    d. It is shaped like a signet ring and is 2 to 2.5 cm in length.
    e. It is densely supplied with proprioceptive muscle spindles.
21. The seminal vesicle:
    a. is normally palpable in a rectal examination.
    b. is a lateral outpouching of the prostate (central zone).
    c. contracts in response to excitatory efferents from the sacral parasympathetic nerves.
    d. is medial to the vas deferens.
    e. stores sperm.
22. From medial to lateral, the segments of the fallopian tube are:
    a. uterine, ampulla, infundibulum, isthmus, fimbriae.
    b. uterine, ampulla, isthmus, infundibulum, fimbriae.
    c. uterine, isthmus, ampulla, infundibulum, fimbriae.
    d. uterine, infundibulum, ampulla, isthmus, fimbriae.
    e. uterine, isthmus, infundibulum, ampulla, fimbriae.
23. The peritoneum may be accessed transvaginally through the:
    a. posterior fornix.
    b. anterior fornix.
    c. rectovaginal septum.
    d. lateral fornices.
    e. vesicovaginal space.
24. To avoid denervation of the striated urethral sphincter, incisions through the vaginal wall to enter the retropubic space should be made:
    a. perpendicular to the urethra.
    b. over the urethra.
    c. close to the lateral margins of the urethra.
    d. cephalad to the bladder neck.
    e. far lateral in the vaginal wall, parallel to the urethra.
25. When the endopelvic fascia lateral to the prostate and puboprostatic ligaments is opened, vessels are commonly encountered that pierce the levator ani to join the periprostatic plexus laterally. These vessels are communicating branches from the:
    a. pampiniform plexus of veins.
    b. dorsal vein of the penis.
    c. internal pudendal veins.
    d. external pudendal veins.
    e. accessory obturator veins.
26. Lymphatic drainage from the prostate flows to the:
    a. external iliac and common iliac nodes.
    b. internal iliac and obturator nodes.
    c. para-aortic nodes.
    d. internal iliac and inguinal nodes.
    e. perirectal and common iliac nodes.

27. The first branch of the pudendal nerve in the perineum is the:
    a. dorsal nerve of the penis.
    b. inferior rectal nerve(s).
    c. perineal nerve.
    d. posterior femoral cutaneous branches.
    e. posterior scrotal branches.

28. After fracture of the penis (disruption of the tunica albuginea), if Buck's fascia remains intact, the hematoma will be visible in the:
    a. perineum in a butterfly pattern.
    b. penis and scrotum only.
    c. penis, scrotum, and perineum and tracking up the anterior abdominal wall.
    d. shaft of the penis only.
    e. shaft and glans of the penis.

29. The skin of the penile shaft and foreskin can be elevated as a rotational flap supplied by the:
    a. dorsal artery of the penis.
    b. superficial inferior epigastric vessels.
    c. gonadal vessels.
    d. external pudendal vessels.
    e. several branches of the perineal vessels.

30. The dartos layer of smooth muscle and fascia in the scrotum is continuous with:
    a. the dartos layer of the penis.
    b. Colles' fascia.
    c. Scarpa's fascia.
    d. Buck's fascia.
    e. a, b, and c.

31. The cremaster muscle is supplied by the:
    a. ilioinguinal nerve.
    b. genital branch of the genitofemoral nerve.
    c. femoral branch of the genitofemoral nerve.
    d. terminal branches of the subcostal nerve (T12).
    e. iliohypogastric nerve.

32. Lymphatic drainage from the bulbar urethra travels:
    a. through perianal nodes to reach the pelvis.
    b. directly to the deep pelvic lymph nodes.
    c. through the superficial and deep inguinal lymph nodes.
    d. to pre-pubic nodes.
    e. to para-aortic lymph nodes along with testicular drainage.

33. In their course from the seminiferous tubule to the epididymis, sperm pass through, in order:
    a. straight tubules, efferent ductules, rete testis.
    b. rete testis, straight tubules, efferent ductules.
    c. efferent ductules, rete testis, straight tubules.
    d. straight tubules, rete testis, efferent ductules.
    e. rete testis, efferent ductules, straight tubules.

34. The testicular artery may be ligated without sacrificing the testis because of collateral circulation from:
    a. vasal and cremasteric arteries.
    b. external pudendal and vasal arteries.
    c. external pudendal, vasal, and cremasteric arteries.
    d. numerous anastomotic branches from the scrotal arteries.
    e. cremasteric and external pudendal arteries.

35. To avoid damage to subtunical testicular vessels, biopsy of the testis should be performed at the:
    a. lower pole of the testis.
    b. anterior upper pole directly opposite the testicular mesentery.
    c. medial surface of the lower pole.
    d. lateral surface of the lower pole.
    e. lateral or medial surface of the upper pole.

36. Which layers of the scrotum and testicular tunics usually need to be débrided in patients with Fournier's gangrene?
    a. The scrotal skin only
    b. The scrotal skin and dartos layer
    c. The scrotal skin, dartos layer, and external spermatic fascia
    d. The scrotal skin, dartos layer, and external cremasteric and internal spermatic fasciae, leaving the tunica vaginalis intact
    e. All tissues including the tunica vaginalis

37. A Martius (labial fat pad) rotational flap used in the repair of a vesicovaginal fistula receives blood supply from the:
    a. terminal branches of the internal pudendal artery and vein.
    b. superficial inferior epigastric vessels.
    c. inferior epigastric vessels.
    d. accessory pudendal vessels.
    e. external pudendal vessels.

38. Lymphatic drainage from the bladder passes through the:
    a. external iliac lymph nodes.
    b. obturator and internal iliac lymph nodes.
    c. internal and common iliac lymph nodes.
    d. common iliac, periureteral, and para-aortic lymph nodes.
    e. a, b, and c.

39. To preserve potency during a radical cystectomy, ligation of the lateral and posterior vascular pedicles is best carried out:
    a. close to their origin from the internal iliac vessels.
    b. near the bladder.
    c. from beneath the bladder after rotating the prostate cephalad.
    d. as they cross the ureter.
    e. lateral to the rectum.

ANSWERS

1. **d. sacrospinous ligament.** The sacrospinous ligament separates the greater and lesser sciatic foramina.

2. **a. superficial inferior epigastric artery and vein.** The superficial inferior epigastric vessels are encountered during inguinal incisions and can cause troublesome bleeding during placement of pelvic laparoscopic ports.

3. **e. buttock.** Blood and urine can accumulate in the scrotum and penis deep to the Dartos fascia after an anterior urethral injury. In the perineum, their spread is limited by the fusions of Colles' fascia to the ischiopubic rami laterally and to the posterior edge of the perineal membrane; the resulting hematoma is therefore butterfly shaped. These processes will not extend down the leg or into the buttock, but they can freely travel up the anterior abdominal wall deep to Scarpa's fascia to the clavicles and around the flank to the back.

4. **c. anesthesia over the pubis and anterior scrotum only.** The ilioinguinal nerve (L1) passes through the internal oblique muscle to enter the inguinal canal laterally. It travels anterior to the cord and exits the external ring to provide sensation to the mons pubis and anterior scrotum or labia majora.

5. **c. obliterated umbilical artery; the ureter will be found medial to it.** The obliterated umbilical artery in the medial umbilical fold serves as an important landmark for the surgeon. It can be traced to its origin from the internal iliac artery to locate the ureter, which lies on its medial side.

6. **e. arcus tendineus fascia pelvis.** The tendinous arc of the levator ani serves as the origin of the muscles of the pelvic diaphragm: pubococcygeus and iliococcygeus. The muscle bordering this hiatus has been referred to as "pubovisceral" because it provides a sling for (pubourethralis, puborectalis), inserts directly into (pubovaginalis, puboanalis, levator prostatae), or inserts into a structure intimately associated with the pelvic viscera. The coccygeus muscle extends from the sacrospinous ligament to the lateral border of the sacrum and coccyx to complete the pelvic diaphragm.

7. **a. 50% and 25% of patients, respectively.** In half of patients, one or more accessory obturator veins drain into the underside of the external iliac vein and can easily be torn during lymphadenectomy. In 25% of people, an accessory obturator artery arises from the inferior epigastric artery and runs medial to the femoral vein to reach the obturator canal.

8. **d. inability to extend the knee and numbness over the anterior thigh.** The femoral nerve (L2, L3, L4) supplies sensation to the anterior thigh and motor innervation to the extensors of the knee.

9. **e. a, b, and c.** The presynaptic sympathetic cell bodies reach the pelvic plexus by two pathways: (1) the superior hypogastric plexus and (2) the pelvic continuation of the sympathetic trunks. Presynaptic parasympathetic innervation arises from the intermediolateral cell column of the sacral cord.

10. **b. laterally in the abdomen and medially in the pelvis.** Blood supply to the pelvic ureter enters laterally; thus, the pelvic peritoneum should be incised only medial to the ureter.

11. **c. anteriorly.** In women, the ureter first runs posterior to the ovary, then turns medially to run deep to the base of the broad ligament before entering a loose connective tissue tunnel through the substance of the cardinal ligament.

12. **b. sphincteric closure of the ureteral orifice.** The intravesical portion of the ureter lies immediately beneath the bladder urothelium and is therefore quite pliant; it is backed by a strong plate of detrusor muscle. With bladder filling, this arrangement is thought to result in passive occlusion of the ureter, like a flap valve.

13. **e. has longitudinal smooth muscle fibers that extend to the external meatus.** At the female bladder neck, the inner longitudinal fibers converge radially to pass downward as the inner longitudinal layer of the urethra. The middle circular layer does not appear to be as robust as that of the male. The female bladder neck differs strikingly from the male in possessing little adrenergic innervation.

14. **d. smooth muscle of the ureter forms the interureteric ridge (Mercier's bar).** Fibers from each ureter meet to form a triangular sheet of muscle that extends from the two ureteral orifices to the internal urethra meatus. The edges of this muscular sheet are thickened between the ureteral orifices (the interureteric crest, or Mercier's bar) and between the ureters and the internal urethral meatus (Bell's muscle).

15. **a. rectourethralis.** When approached from below, these fibers, the rectourethralis muscle, are 2 to 10 mm thick and must be divided to gain access to the prostate.

16. **e. all of the above.** In addition to the vesical branches, the bladder may be supplied by any adjacent artery arising from the internal iliac artery.

17. **a. Periurethral glands.** At its midpoint, the urethra turns approximately 35 degrees anteriorly, but this angulation can vary from 0 to 90 degrees (see Figs. 2-23, 2-25, and 2-28). This angle divides the prostatic urethra into proximal (preprostatic) and distal (prostatic) segments, which are functionally and anatomically discrete. Small periurethral glands, lacking periglandular smooth muscle, extend between the fibers of the longitudinal smooth muscle to be enclosed by the preprostatic sphincter.

18. **e. a and c.** The periurethral glands can contribute significantly to prostatic volume in older men as one of the sites of origin of BPH. The transition zone commonly gives rise to BPH.

19. **b. urethral arteries extending down the urethra from the bladder neck.** The urethral arteries penetrate the prostatovesical junction posterolaterally and travel inward, perpendicular to the urethra. They approach the bladder neck in the 1- to 5-o'clock and 7- to 11-o'clock positions, with the largest branches located posteriorly. They then turn caudally, parallel to the urethra, to supply it, the periurethral glands, and the transition zone. Thus, in BPH, these arteries provide the principal blood supply of the adenoma.

20. **d. It is shaped like a signet ring and is 2 to 2.5 cm in length.** The membranous urethra spans on average 2.0 to 2.5 cm (range: 1.2 to 5.0 cm). It is surrounded by the striated (external) urethral sphincter, which is often incorrectly depicted as a flat sheet of muscle sandwiched between two layers of fascia. The striated sphincter is actually shaped like a signet ring, broad at its base and narrowing as it passes through the urogenital hiatus of the levator ani to meet the apex of the prostate.

21. **c. contracts in response to excitatory efferents from the sacral parasympathetic nerves.** Innervation arises from the pelvic plexus, with major excitatory efferents contributed by the (sympathetic) hypogastric nerves.

22. **c. uterine, isthmus, ampulla, infundibulum, fimbriae.** The tubes are divided into four segments: uterine, isthmus, ampulla, and infundibulum, which is crowned by the fimbriae.

23. **a. posterior fornix.** Because the apex of the vagina is covered with the peritoneum of the rectouterine pouch, the peritoneal cavity may be accessed through the posterior fornix.

24. **e. far lateral in the vaginal wall, parallel to the urethra.** Somatic and autonomic nerves to the urethra travel on the lateral walls of the vagina near the urethra. During transvaginal incontinence surgery, the anterior vaginal wall should be incised laterally to avoid these nerves and prevent type III urinary incontinence.

25. **c. internal pudendal veins.** The internal pudendal veins communicate freely with the dorsal vein complex by piercing the levator ani. These communicating vessels enter the pelvic venous plexus on the lateral surface of the prostate and are a common, often unexpected, source of bleeding during apical dissection of the prostate.

26. **b. internal iliac and obturator nodes.** Lymphatic drainage is primarily to the obturator and internal iliac nodes.

27. **a. dorsal nerve of the penis.** The pudendal nerve follows the vessels in their course through the perineum (see Fig. 2-37). Its first branch, the dorsal nerve of the penis, travels ventral to the main pudendal trunk in Alcock's canal.

28. **d. shaft of the penis only.** Bleeding from a tear in the corporal bodies (e.g., penile fracture) is usually contained within Buck's fascia, and ecchymosis is limited to the penile shaft.

29. **d. external pudendal vessels.** The blood supply of the skin of the penile shaft is independent of the erectile bodies and is

derived from the external pudendal branches of the femoral vessels.

30. **e. a, b, and c.** The dartos layer of smooth muscle is continuous with Colles' fascia, Scarpa's fascia, and the dartos fascia of the penis.

31. **b. genital branch of the genitofemoral nerve.** The genital branch of the genitofemoral nerve follows the cord through the inguinal canal, supplies the cremaster muscle, and supplies sensation to the anterior scrotum.

32. **c. through the superficial and deep inguinal lymph nodes.** The penis, scrotum, and perineum drain into the inguinal lymph nodes. These nodes can be divided into a superficial groups and deep groups.

33. **d. straight tubules, rete testis, efferent ductules.** Septa form 200 to 300 cone-shaped lobules, each containing one or more convoluted seminiferous tubules. Each tubule is U-shaped and has a stretched length of nearly 1 m. Interstitial (Leydig) cells lie in the loose tissue surrounding the tubules and are responsible for testosterone production. Toward the apices of the lobules, the seminiferous tubules become straight (tubuli recti) and enter the mediastinum testis to form an anastomosing network of tubules lined by flattened epithelium. This network, known as the rete testis, forms 12 to 20 efferent ductules and passes into the largest portion of epididymis, the caput.

34. **a. vasal and cremasteric arteries.** A rich arterial anastomosis occurs at the head of the epididymis, between the testicular and capital arteries, and at the tail between the testicular, epididymal, cremasteric, and vasal arteries.

35. **e. lateral or medial surface of the upper pole.** The testicular arteries enter the mediastinum and ramify in the tunica vasculosa, principally in the anterior, medial, and lateral portions of the lower pole and the anterior segment of the upper pole (see Fig. 2-45). Thus, placement of a traction suture through the lower pole tunica albuginea risks damaging these important superficial vessels and devascularizing the testis. Testicular biopsy should be carried out in the medial or lateral surface of the upper pole, where the risk of vascular injury is minimal.

36. **b. The scrotal skin and dartos layer.** The external, cremasteric, and internal spermatic fasciae are embryologically distinct from the scrotal and dartos layers and have their own blood and nerve supplies. It is very uncommon for them to be involved in the necrotic process in Fournier's gangrene and can therefore be spared.

37. **e. external pudendal vessels.** The labial fat pads receive blood supply from the external pudendal braches of the femoral vessels.

38. **e. a, b, and c.** The bulk of the lymphatic drainage passes to the external iliac lymph nodes. Some anterior and lateral drainage may go through the obturator and internal iliac nodes, and portions of the bladder base and trigone may drain into the internal and common iliac groups. Complete lymph node dissection during radical cystectomy should encompass all of these lymph node groups.

39. **b. near the bladder.** The bladder vasculature pierces the pelvic autonomic plexuses near the origin of the arteries from the internal iliac arteries. Ligation of these vessels proximally will injure the pelvic autonomic nervous plexuses. Ligation is best carried out near the bladder to avoid nerve damage.

SECTION II

CLINICAL DECISION-MAKING

3

Evaluation of the Urologic Patient: History, Physical Examination, and Urinalysis

GLENN S. GERBER • CHARLES B. BRENDLER

QUESTIONS

1. What causes the pain associated with a stone in the ureter?
   a. Obstruction of urine flow with distention of the renal capsule
   b. Irritation of the ureteral mucosa by the stone
   c. Excessive ureteral peristalsis in response to the obstructing stone
   d. Irritation of the intramural ureter
   e. Urinary extravasation from a ruptured calyceal fornix
2. What is the most common cause of gross hematuria in a patient older than 50 years of age?
   a. Renal calculi
   b. Infection
   c. Bladder cancer
   d. Benign prostatic hyperplasia
   e. Trauma
3. What is the most common cause of pain associated with gross hematuria?
   a. Simultaneous passage of a kidney stone
   b. Ureteral obstruction due to blood clots
   c. Urinary tract malignancy
   d. Prostatic inflammation
   e. Prostatic enlargement
4. All of the following are typical lower urinary tract symptoms associated with benign prostatic hyperplasia EXCEPT:
   a. urgency.
   b. frequency.
   c. nocturia.
   d. dysuria.
   e. weak urinary stream.
5. What is the most common cause of continuous incontinence (loss of urine at all times and in all positions)?
   a. Enterovesical fistula
   b. Noncompliant bladder
   c. Detrusor hyperreflexia
   d. Vesicovaginal fistula
   e. Sphincteric incompetence
6. All of the following are potential causes of anejaculation EXCEPT:
   a. sympathetic denervation.
   b. pharmacologic agents.
   c. bladder neck and prostatic surgery.
   d. androgen deficiency.
   e. cerebrovascular accidents.
7. What percentage of patients with multiple sclerosis will present with urinary symptoms as the first manifestation of the disease?
   a. 1%
   b. 5%
   c. 10%
   d. 15%
   e. 20%
8. What important information is gained from pelvic bimanual examination that cannot be obtained from radiologic evaluation?
   a. Presence of bladder mass
   b. Invasion of bladder cancer into perivesical fat
   c. Presence of bladder calculi
   d. Presence of associated pathologic lesion in female adnexal structures
   e. Mobility/fixation of pelvic organs

9. With what disease is priapism primarily associated?
   a. Peyronie's disease
   b. Sickle cell anemia
   c. Parkinson's disease
   d. Organic depression
   e. Leukemia

10. What is the most common cause of cloudy urine?
   a. Bacterial cystitis
   b. Urine overgrowth with yeast
   c. Phosphaturia
   d. Alkaline urine
   e. Significant proteinuria

11. Conditions that decrease urine specific gravity include all of the following EXCEPT:
   a. increased fluid intake.
   b. use of diuretics.
   c. decreased renal concentrating ability.
   d. dehydration.
   e. diabetes insipidus.

12. Urine osmolality usually varies between:
   a. 10 and 200 mOsm/L.
   b. 50 and 500 mOsm/L.
   c. 50 and 1200 mOsm/L.
   d. 100 and 1000 mOsm/L.
   e. 100 and 1500 mOsm/L.

13. Elevated ascorbic acid levels in the urine may lead to false-negative results on a urine dipstick test for which of the following?
   a. Glucose
   b. Hemoglobin
   c. Myoglobin
   d. Red blood cells
   e. Leukocytes

14. Hematuria is distinguished from hemoglobinuria or myoglobinuria by:
   a. dipstick testing.
   b. the simultaneous presence of significant leukocytes.
   c. microscopic presence of erythrocytes.
   d. examination of serum.
   e. evaluation of hematocrit.

15. The presence of one positive dipstick reading for hematuria is associated with significant urologic pathologic findings on subsequent testing in what percentage of patients?
   a. 2%
   b. 10%
   c. 25%
   d. 50%
   e. 75%

16. The most common cause of glomerular hematuria is:
   a. transitional cell carcinoma.
   b. nephritic syndrome.
   c. Berger's disease (IgA nephropathy).
   d. poststreptococcal glomerulonephritis.
   e. Goodpasture's syndrome.

17. The most common cause of proteinuria is:
   a. Fanconi's syndrome.
   b. excessive glomerular permeability due to primary glomerular disease.
   c. failure of adequate tubular reabsorption.
   d. overflow proteinuria due to increased plasma concentration of immunoglobulins.
   e. diabetes.

18. Transient proteinuria may be due to all of the following EXCEPT:
   a. exercise.
   b. fever.
   c. emotional stress.
   d. congestive heart failure.
   e. ureteroscopy.

19. Glucose will be detected in the urine when the serum level is above:
   a. 75 mg/dL.
   b. 100 mg/dL.
   c. 150 mg/dL.
   d. 180 mg/dL.
   e. 225 mg/dL.

20. The specificity of dipstick nitrite testing for bacteriuria is:
   a. 20%.
   b. 40%.
   c. 60%.
   d. 80%.
   e. >90%.

21. All of the following are microscopic features of squamous epithelial cells EXCEPT:
   a. large size.
   b. small central nucleus.
   c. irregular cytoplasm.
   d. presence in clumps.
   e. fine granularity in the cytoplasm.

22. The number of bacteria per high-power microscopic field that correspond to colony counts of 100,000/mL is:
   a. 1.
   b. 3.
   c. 5.
   d. 10.
   e. 20.

23. Pain in the flaccid penis is usually due to:
   a. Peyronie's disease.
   b. bladder or urethral inflammation.
   c. priapism.
   d. calculi impacted in the distal ureter.
   e. hydrocele.

24. Chronic scrotal pain is most often due to:
   a. testicular torsion.
   b. trauma.
   c. cryptorchidism.
   d. hydrocele.
   e. orchitis.

25. Terminal hematuria (at the end of the urinary stream) is usually due to:
   a. bladder neck or prostatic inflammation.
   b. bladder cancer.
   c. kidney stones.
   d. bladder calculi.
   e. urethral stricture disease.

26. Enuresis is present in what percentage of children at age 5 years?
    a. 5%
    b. 15%
    c. 25%
    d. 50%
    e. 75%
27. All of the following in the medical history suggest that erectile dysfunction is more likely due to organic rather than psychogenic causes EXCEPT:
    a. sudden onset.
    b. peripheral vascular disease.
    c. absence of nocturnal erections.
    d. diabetes mellitus.
    e. inability to achieve adequate erections in a variety of circumstances.
28. All of the following should be routinely performed in men with hematospermia EXCEPT:
    a. cystoscopy.
    b. digital rectal examination.
    c. serum prostate-specific antigen (PSA) level.
    d. genital examination.
    e. urinalysis.
29. Pneumaturia may be due to all of the following EXCEPT:
    a. diverticulitis.
    b. colon cancer.
    c. recent urinary tract instrumentation.
    d. inflammatory bowel disease.
    e. ectopic ureter.
30. Which of the following disorders may commonly lead to irritative voiding symptoms?
    a. Parkinson's disease
    b. Renal cell carcinoma
    c. Bladder diverticula
    d. Prostate cancer
    e. Testicular torsion

ANSWERS

1. **a. Obstruction of urine flow with distention of the renal capsule.** Pain is usually caused by acute distention of the renal capsule, usually from inflammation or obstruction.
2. **c. Bladder cancer.** The most common cause of gross hematuria in a patient older than age 50 years is bladder cancer.
3. **b. Ureteral obstruction due to blood clots.** Pain in association with hematuria usually results from upper urinary tract hematuria with obstruction of the ureters with clots.
4. **d. dysuria.** Dysuria is painful urination that is usually caused by inflammation.
5. **d. Vesicovaginal fistula.** Continuous incontinence is most commonly due to a urinary tract fistula that bypasses the urethral sphincter.
6. **e. cerebrovascular accidents.** Anejaculation may result from several causes: (1) androgen deficiency, (2) sympathetic denervation, (3) pharmacologic agents, and (4) bladder neck and prostatic surgery.
7. **b. 5%.** In fact, 5% of patients with previously undiagnosed multiple sclerosis present with urinary symptoms as the first manifestation of the disease.
8. **e. Mobility/fixation of pelvic organs.** In addition to defining areas of induration, the bimanual examination allows the examiner to assess the mobility of the bladder; such information cannot be obtained by radiologic techniques such as CT and MRI, which convey static images.
9. **b. Sickle cell anemia.** Priapism occurs most commonly in patients with sickle cell disease but can also occur in those with advanced malignancy, coagulation disorders, and pulmonary disease, and in many patients without an obvious cause.
10. **c. Phosphaturia.** Cloudy urine is most commonly caused by phosphaturia.
11. **d. dehydration.** Conditions that decrease specific gravity include (1) increased fluid intake, (2) diuretics, (3) decreased renal concentrating ability, and (4) diabetes insipidus.
12. **c. 50 and 1200 mOsm/L.** Osmolality is a measure of the amount of material dissolved in the urine and usually varies between 50 and 1200 mOsm/L.
13. **a. Glucose.** False-negative results for glucose and bilirubin may be seen in the presence of elevated ascorbic acid concentrations in the urine.
14. **c. microscopic presence of erythrocytes.** Hematuria can be distinguished from hemoglobinuria and myoglobinuria by microscopic examination of the centrifuged urine; the presence of a large number of erythrocytes establishes the diagnosis of hematuria.
15. **c. 25%.** Investigators at the University of Wisconsin found that 26% of adults who had at least one positive dipstick reading for hematuria were subsequently found to have significant urologic pathologic findings.
16. **c. Berger's disease (IgA nephropathy).** IgA nephropathy, or Berger's disease, is the most common cause of glomerular hematuria, accounting for about 30% of cases.
17. **b. excessive glomerular permeability due to primary glomerular disease.** Glomerular proteinuria is the most common type of proteinuria and results from increased glomerular capillary permeability to protein, especially albumin. Glomerular proteinuria occurs in any of the primary glomerular diseases such as IgA nephropathy or in glomerulopathy associated with systemic illness such as diabetes mellitus.
18. **e. ureteroscopy.** Transient proteinuria occurs commonly, especially in the pediatric population, and usually resolves spontaneously within a few days. It may result from fever, exercise, or emotional stress. In older patients, transient proteinuria may be due to congestive heart failure.
19. **d. 180 mg/dL.** This so-called renal threshold corresponds to a serum glucose level of about 180 mg/dL; above this level, glucose will be detected in the urine.

20. **e. >90%.** The specificity of the nitrite dipstick test for detecting bacteriuria is over 90%.

21. **d. presence in clumps.** Squamous epithelial cells are large, have a central small nucleus about the size of an erythrocyte, and have an irregular cytoplasm with fine granularity.

22. **c. 5.** Therefore, 5 bacteria per high-power field reflect colony counts of about 100,000/mL.

23. **b. bladder or urethral inflammation.** Pain in the flaccid penis is usually secondary to inflammation in the bladder or urethra, with referred pain that is experienced maximally at the urethral meatus.

24. **d. hydrocele.** Chronic scrotal pain is usually related to noninflammatory conditions such as a hydrocele or varicocele, and the pain is usually characterized as a dull, heavy sensation that does not radiate.

25. **a. bladder neck or prostatic inflammation.** Terminal hematuria occurs at the end of micturition and is usually secondary to inflammation in the area of the bladder neck or prostatic urethra.

26. **b. 15%.** Enuresis refers to urinary incontinence that occurs during sleep. It occurs normally in children up to 3 years of age but persists in about 15% of children at age 5 and about 1% of children at age 15.

27. **a. sudden onset.** A careful history will often determine whether the problem is primarily psychogenic or organic. In men with psychogenic impotence, the condition frequently develops rather quickly secondary to a precipitating event such as marital stress or change or loss of a sexual partner.

28. **a. cystoscopy.** A genital and rectal examination should be done to exclude the presence of tuberculosis, a PSA assessment and digital rectal examination should be done to exclude prostatic carcinoma, and a urinary cytologic assessment should be done to exclude the possibility of transitional cell carcinoma of the prostate.

29. **e. ectopic ureter.** Pneumaturia is the passage of gas in the urine. In patients who have not recently had urinary tract instrumentation or a urethral catheter placed, this is almost always due to a fistula between the intestine and bladder. Common causes include diverticulitis, carcinoma of the sigmoid colon, and regional enteritis (Crohn's disease).

30. **a. Parkinson's disease.** The second important example of nonspecific lower urinary tract symptoms that may occur secondary to a variety of neurologic conditions is irritative symptoms resulting from neurologic disease, such as cerebrovascular accident, diabetes mellitus, and Parkinson's disease.

4

Urinary Tract Imaging: Basic Principles

SAM B. BHAYANI • CARY L. SIEGEL

QUESTIONS

1. Calculi composed of which of the following are not seen on plain radiographs?
   a. Calcium oxalate dihydrate
   b. Cystine
   c. Uric acid
   d. Calcium oxalate monohydrate
   e. Calcium phosphate
2. Contrast reactions such as urticaria and edema are classified as:
   a. anaphylactoid.
   b. delayed type hypersensitivity.
   c. IgG mediated.
   d. IgE mediated.
   e. cell mediated.
3. Treatment of anaphylactoid reactions does not include:
   a. antihistamines.
   b. transfusion.
   c. β-adrenergic agonists.
   d. epinephrine.
4. During an intravenous urogram, which view may distend the ureters to allow better distal ureteral imaging?
   a. Supine
   b. Oblique
   c. Upright
   d. Prone
   e. Nephrographic
5. What general formula is used to assess the volume in milliliters of the bladder in the pediatric population?
   a. [(age in years) +5] × 20
   b. [(age in years)+4] × 20
   c. [(age in years)+2] × 30
   d. [(age in years)+1] × 40
   e. [(age in years)+3] × 50
6. When performing ultrasonography, as the frequency of the transducer increases, what decreases?
   a. Resolution
   b. Visualization
   c. Size of the field
   d. Depth of penetration
   e. Doppler waveforms
7. What technique is the imaging study of choice in evaluating scrotal pathology?
   a. Plain films
   b. Ultrasound
   c. Computed tomography
   d. Magnetic resonance imaging
   e. Nuclear scintigraphy
8. How do adrenal adenomas usually measure on CT?
   a. Less than 50 HU
   b. Less than 30 HU
   c. Less than 0 HU
   d. Less than −30 HU
   e. Less than −50 HU
9. On T2-weighted MRI images, fluid is:
   a. dark.
   b. bright.
   c. not seen.
   d. variable.
   e. gray.
10. Which of the following techniques is most useful in evaluating invasion of the bladder wall by transitional cell carcinoma?
    a. IVU
    b. Nephrostogram
    c. CT
    d. MRI
    e. Cystourethrography
11. MRI of the prostate can be used to visualize:
    a. peripheral zone.
    b. neurovascular bundles.
    c. seminal vesicles.
    d. dorsal venous complex.
    e. all of the above.

12. MRI and MR-urography have difficulty imaging:
    a. renal masses.
    b. prostate.
    c. hydronephrosis.
    d. renal vasculature.
    e. urolithiasis.

13. Which ^{99m}Tc nuclear agent is best used for renal cortical imaging?
    a. DMSA
    b. MAG3
    c. DTPA
    d. Glucoheptonate
    e. Pertechnetate

ANSWERS

1. **c. Uric acid.** Uric acid calculi are radiolucent and will not be seen on plain radiographs.
2. **a. anaphylactoid.** These reactions are thought to be allergic or anaphylactoid.
3. **b. transfusion.** Anaphylactoid reactions including bronchospasm are treated with medicines to reverse the allergic mediated response. Transfusion may increase allergic responses.
4. **d. Prone.** The prone view places the ureters in a dependent position, allowing better visualization.
5. **c. [(age in years)+2] × 30.** This formula is useful when evaluating the pediatric patient with cystography.
6. **d. Depth of penetration.** Increasing frequencies give better resolution, but at lower depths.
7. **b. Ultrasound.** Ultrasound allows excellent visualization of the scrotum and testes, and Doppler studies can be used to assess for flow at the time of the study.
8. **c. Less than 0 HU.** When such an adrenal finding is discovered, further workup is unnecessary because adenomas measure less than 0 HU.
9. **b. bright.** Fluid is dark on T1-weighted images and bright on T2-weighted images.
10. **d. MRI.** MRI is a highly effective technique for imaging the bladder wall, and muscle invasion can be suspected with its use.
11. **e. all of the above.** T2-weighted MRI of the prostate can evaluate virtually all aspects of prostatic anatomy.
12. **e. urolithiasis.** Stones are not well visualized on MRI, and noncontrast CT is the preferred modality.
13. **a. DMSA.** DMSA is cleared in a complex fashion but does bind to parenchymal tissues. It is best used for the evaluation of cortical scars.

5

Outcomes Research

MARK S. LITWIN

QUESTIONS

1. Barriers to health care access may include which of the following?
   a. Lack of health insurance
   b. Lack of transportation
   c. Beliefs about the health care system
   d. All of the above
2. Costs of hospital care are best approximated by measuring:
   a. charges.
   b. collections.
   c. resources used.
   d. all of the above.
3. A true assessment of health care costs must include the amount of money spent on:
   a. facilities and equipment.
   b. disposable supplies.
   c. personnel.
   d. all of the above.
4. The introduction of diagnosis-related groups (DRGs) in the 1980s led to:
   a. longer hospital stays for most patients.
   b. shorter hospital stays for most patients.
   c. higher reimbursements for hospitals.
   d. higher reimbursements for physicians.
5. Quality-adjusted life-years (QALYs) are a metric used in:
   a. basic quality-of-life analysis in individual patients.
   b. cost-effectiveness analysis for populations of patients.
   c. patient satisfaction analysis for individual patients.
   d. cost-benefit analysis for individual patients.
6. Case mix is a metric that may be used in the study of medical outcomes to adjust for:
   a. comorbidity of a population cared for by a given provider.
   b. severity of illness in a population cared for by a given provider.
   c. both.
   d. neither.
7. In the Donabedian model of quality-of-care, measures of structure include:
   a. interpersonal skill with which a physician interacts with patients.
   b. perioperative mortality rates.
   c. patient satisfaction.
   d. board certification of physicians in a provider group.
8. In the Donabedian model of quality-of-care, measures of outcome include:
   a. patient satisfaction.
   b. health-related quality of life.
   c. survival.
   d. all of the above.
9. Health-related quality of life is best assessed by:
   a. patients themselves.
   b. spouses or immediate family members of patients.
   c. primary care physicians caring for patients.
   d. specialists caring for patients.
10. Dysfunction and its related distress (also called “bother”) are generally:
    a. perfectly correlated.
    b. completely independent.
    c. related but imperfectly correlated.
    d. measures of the same phenomenon.
11. Disease-specific health-related quality of life domains in patients with urologic cancer include:
    a. physical function.
    b. emotional well-being.
    c. social function.
    d. sexual dysfunction.
12. In psychometric terms, reliability refers to how free an instrument is of:
    a. missing data.
    b. measurement error.
    c. grammatical or typographical errors.
    d. invalid data.
13. When a scale has a coefficient alpha of 0.90, the scale is a high degree of:
    a. alternate form reliability.
    b. test-retest reliability.
    c. internal consistency reliability.
    d. concurrent validity.

ANSWERS

1. **d. All of the above.** Barriers to access may be financial or nonfinancial and include any factor that decreases the likelihood that an individual in need will receive medical services.
2. **c. resources used.** Charges are notoriously poor proxies for actual medical costs because of the way in which hospital budgets are calculated; actual collections do not account for deductibles, copayments, and opportunity costs.
3. **d. all of the above.** Each of the factors mentioned contributes to the total cost of health care.
4. **b. shorter hospital stays for most patients.** DRGs allow for the calculation of prospective payments to hospitals and as such have led to shorter lengths of stay; they have also led to decreased reimbursements to hospitals.
5. **b. cost-effectiveness analysis for populations of patients.** QALYs are used in population analysis and not for individual patients.
6. **c. both.** Measuring case mix allows for outcomes to be controlled for both the underlying medical diseases and the severity of the disease of interest among groups of patients under the care of a provider.
7. **d. board certification of physicians in a provider group.** Structural attributes of health care include clinician characteristics, such as board certification but not measures of process, such as interpersonal style or outcome measures, such as mortality and patient satisfaction.
8. **d. all of the above.** Each of these factors may be considered a valid measure of medical outcomes.
9. **a. patients themselves.** It is axiomatic that health-related quality of life outcomes be reported by patients themselves, as they perceive them.
10. **c. related but imperfectly correlated.** In the various domains of disease-specific health-related quality of life, function and bother are loosely associated with each other but measure discrete phenomena.
11. **d. sexual dysfunction.** Disease-specific health-related quality of life instruments focus on domains that are directly relevant to the specific disease or treatment.
12. **b. measurement error.** Reliability refers to what proportion of a test score is true and what proportion is due to chance variation (or measurement error).
13. **c. internal consistency reliability.** Cronbach's coefficient alpha is a well-established measure of internal consistency reliability.

SECTION III

BASICS OF UROLOGIC SURGERY

6

Basic Instrumentation and Cystoscopy

H. BALLENTINE CARTER • DAVID Y. CHAN

QUESTIONS

1. The measurement system most often used when referring to catheter and instrument size is:

   a. English.
   b. French (Fr).
   c. metric.
   d. U.S.
   e. conventional.

2. A millimeter in diameter is approximately how many French?

   a. 1 French.
   b. 1.5 French.
   c. 3 French.
   d. 3.5 French.
   e. 5 French.

3. The size of a catheter or instrument refers to the:

   a. inside circumference.
   b. inside diameter.
   c. outside circumference.
   d. outside diameter.
   e. none of the above.

4. The catheter designed to help negotiate the male urethra when catheterization is difficult is the:

   a. Foley.
   b. Malecot.
   c. Pezzer.
   d. coudé.
   e. Councill.

5. The catheter with the largest luminal size is the:

   a. No. 20 Fr Foley.
   b. No. 20 Fr three-way irrigation catheter.
   c. No. 20 Fr coudé Foley.
   d. No. 20 Fr Malecot.
   e. No. 18 Fr Malecot.

6. The catheter material best suited for long-term urethral catheterization is:

   a. latex.
   b. silicone.
   c. rubber.
   d. Dacron.
   e. polyurethane.

7. When multiple attempts to gently bypass a urethral obstruction are unsuccessful, the next best step is:

   a. a more vigorous attempt with stiffer catheters.
   b. balloon dilatation of the obstruction under direct vision.
   c. incision of the obstruction under direct vision.
   d. placement of percutaneous cystostomy.
   e. perineal urethrostomy.

8. When cystoscopic electrocoagulation is planned, the irrigant solution that should be avoided is:

   a. sorbitol.
   b. normal saline.
   c. sterile water.
   d. glycine.
   e. mannitol.

ANSWERS

1. **b. French (Fr).** Catheter size is usually referred to using the French (Fr) scale (circumference is in millimeters), in which 1 Fr = 0.33 mm in diameter.
2. **c. 3 French.** For conversion from one scale to the other, it is easier to remember that each millimeter in diameter is approximately 3 Fr; thus, an 18-Fr catheter is about 6 mm in diameter.
3. **c. outside circumference.** Catheter sizes refer to the outside circumference of the catheter, not the luminal diameter.
4. **d. coudé.** Catheters with a curved tip (e.g., coudé catheters; see Fig. 4-1D) are specifically designed to help bypass areas of the male urethra that are difficult to negotiate with a straight catheter.
5. **d. No. 20 Fr Malecot.** Catheters without a lumen for balloon inflation (e.g., Malecot) have a larger luminal size for bladder drainage than do Foley catheters of the same outer circumference. Likewise, for a given outer circumference, two-way catheters (with a balloon port) have a larger luminal size for urinary drainage than do three-way catheters (with a balloon port and fluid instillation port).
6. **b. silicone.** If long-term catheterization is anticipated (more than 1 week), it is advisable to use a Foley catheter made of the most biocompatible material. Catheters made of silicone in general are better tolerated over the long term than those made of materials such as latex and polyurethane.
7. **d. placement of percutaneous cystostomy.** When it is not possible to gently bypass a bladder neck contracture by using other approaches (e.g., use of a guidewire to introduce a ureteral catheter or to guide passage of an Amplatz semirigid dilator), placement of a cystostomy tube is preferable to continued attempts at catheterization, to avoid urethral trauma.
8. **b. normal saline.** If electrocoagulation is planned, it is necessary to avoid solutions containing electrolytes.

7

Basics of Laparoscopic Urologic Surgery

LOUIS EICHEL • ELSPETH M. MCDOUGALL • RALPH V. CLAYMAN

QUESTIONS

1. Absolute contraindications to laparoscopic surgery include all of the following EXCEPT:
   a. uncorrectable coagulopathy.
   b. intestinal obstruction.
   c. abdominal wall infection.
   d. suspected malignant ascites.
   e. extensive prior abdominal or pelvic surgery.
2. Of the following, which is considered a relative contraindication to laparoscopic surgery?
   a. Generalized peritonitis
   b. Hemoperitoneum
   c. Intestinal obstruction
   d. Extensive prior abdominal or pelvic surgery
   e. Abdominal wall infection
3. Which of the following is TRUE regarding preoperative preparation of patients undergoing laparoscopic renal surgery?
   a. A mechanical bowel preparation is mandatory if an extraperitoneal or retroperitoneoscopy approach is anticipated.
   b. A full mechanical bowel preparation and antibiotic preparation with neomycin and metronidazole should be given to all patients undergoing transperitoneal laparoscopy.
   c. For most uncomplicated patients undergoing laparoscopic renal surgery, a clear liquid diet and a light mechanical bowel preparation the day before surgery is satisfactory.
   d. In patients who have had previous abdominal surgery and one anticipates encountering dense intraabdominal adhesions, the laparoscopic approach should not be undertaken.
   e. If the surgery involves entering the bowel such as in enteric augmentation of the bladder, then a light mechanical bowel preparation is all that is required.
4. Which of the statements regarding pneumoperitoneum is TRUE?
   a. CO_2 as an insufflant can be dangerous as it can support combustion.
   b. CO_2 is most commonly used because it is insoluble in the blood.
   c. In patients with chronic respiratory disease, CO_2 is advantageous because it does not accumulate in the blood stream.
   d. Argon gas would be an ideal insufflant due to its low cost and poor solubility in blood.
   e. Nitrous oxide has previously been used for insufflation; however, it is no longer routinely used because of the potential for intra-abdominal explosion.
5. Studies have shown that during insufflation of the abdomen, 94% of the maximal intraperitoneal volume is achieved at an insufflation pressure of:
   a. 5 mm Hg.
   b. 10 mm Hg.
   c. 15 mm Hg.
   d. 20 mm Hg.
   e. 25 mmHg.
6. Which of the following access techniques is considered to be the safest when obtaining a pneumoperitoneum and access to the abdomen for laparoscopy?
   a. Closed technique with Veress needle
   b. Closed technique with blind trocar insertion
   c. Open access technique
   d. Hand-port access
   e. Gasless technique
7. Which of the following hemostatic devices would be considered appropriate for control of a 6-mm vessel?
   a. Monopolar hook electrode
   b. Bipolar scissors
   c. Harmonic shears
   d. Ligasure device
   e. Tissuelink device

8. Which of the following can be used to secure the renal vein?
   a. Titanium clips
   b. Hem-o-Lok plastic clips
   c. Endo GIA with 2.5-mm staples
   d. Endo GIA with 4.8-mm staples
   e. 5-mm Ligasure

9. For morcellation purposes, if the specimen is entrapped in a nylon impermeable sac (e.g., LapSac, Cook Urological, Spence, IN) what is the recommended safest way to proceed?
   a. High speed morcellator
   b. Ring forceps
   c. Scissors morcellation
   d. Kelly clamp
   e. Ultrasonic tissuetripsy

10. Which of the following port sites most often may require formal closure with a fascial and peritoneal suture?
    a. 5-mm nonbladed ports
    b. 5-mm bladed ports
    c. 10- to 12-mm nonbladed ports placed on the midline
    d. 10- to 12-mm nonbladed ports placed on the midclavicular line
    e. 10- to 12-mm nonbladed ports placed on the anterior axillary line

11. Which of the following pneumoperitoneum pressures is associated with the least perturbation in cardiac parameters, that is, change in stroke volume?
    a. 12 mm Hg
    b. 15 mm Hg
    c. 18 mm Hg
    d. 21 mm Hg
    e. 24 mm Hg

12. Which of the following physiologic effects has been noted with establishment of pneumoperitoneum?
    a. Increase in diaphragmatic motion
    b. Increase in disturbances of gastrointestinal motility
    c. Alkalosis
    d. Decrease in urinary output
    e. Increase in mesenteric vessel blood flow

13. Which of the following combinations is the most correct, from review of the current literature, for the morbidity and mortality related to laparoscopic urology?
    a. 2% morbidity, 0.8% mortality
    b. 13% morbidity, 0.2% mortality
    c. 20% morbidity, 0.5% mortality
    d. 20% morbidity, 0.8% mortality
    e. 25% morbidity, 0.8% mortality

14. What is the most common intra-abdominal site of injury associated with laparoscopic surgery?
    a. Bowel injury
    b. Vascular injury
    c. Liver injury
    d. Splenic laceration
    e. Bladder injury

15. What is a characteristic of a blunt trocar, as compared with a bladed trocar?
    a. The blunt trocar requires formal closure of the port site regardless of its size.
    b. The blunt trocar takes less force to insert than the bladed trocar.
    c. The blunt trocar decreases the chance of injury to the epigastric vessels.
    d. The blunt trocar requires more force to insert than the bladed trocar.
    e. The blunt trocar eliminates possible trocar injury to the bowel.

16. Which of the following options for treatment of a gas embolism during laparoscopy is FALSE?
    a. Hyperventilate the patient with 100% oxygen.
    b. Immediately cease insufflation.
    c. Place the patient in a head-down position.
    d. Advance a central venous line into the right side of the heart.
    e. Place the patient in a right lateral decubitus position with the left side up.

17. Pneumomediastinum, pneumothorax, and pneumopericardium associated with laparoscopy is a result of:
    a. gas leaking along major blood vessels through congenital defects in the diaphragm.
    b. gas passing through secondary enlargement of openings in the diaphragm.
    c. diffusion of gas across the peritoneum and diaphragm.
    d. A and B.
    e. A and C.

18. If during insufflation of the abdomen, the Veress needle is determined to have been placed into the iliac artery, which of the following is the best course of action?
    a. Remove the Veress needle and proceed to open the abdomen.
    b. Remove the Veress needle and then proceed with insufflating at a different location.
    c. Leave the Veress needle in place and open the abdomen.
    d. Leave the Veress needle in place and proceed with insufflation of the abdomen at a different location.
    e. Call for a vascular surgery consult.

19. What is the best management option if trocar injury to the iliac artery should occur during the placement of the first trocar?
    a. Remove the trocar and open the abdomen immediately.
    b. Remove the trocar immediately and proceed with re-insufflation of the abdomen and placement of the trocar at an alternate site.
    c. Leave the trocar in place, consult a vascular surgeon, and convert to open laparotomy.
    d. Leave the trocar in place and proceed with insufflation of the abdomen and placement of another port at an alternate site.
    e. Remove the obturator and immediately flush the port with fibrin glue.

20. Which of the following clinical presentations is commonly seen with a postoperative bowel injury following laparoscopy?
    a. Abdominal distension and leukocytosis
    b. Clinical signs of peritonitis and a high fever
    c. Leukopenia, low-grade fever, and pain at one port site
    d. High fever, abdominal distention, and leukocytosis
    e. Low-grade fever, clinical findings of peritonitis, and abdominal distention

21. When a bladder injury is diagnosed postoperatively after a laparoscopic procedure, what is the best treatment?
    a. Transurethral indwelling Foley catheter if it is an intraperitoneal injury of the bladder
    b. Open repair if it is an extraperitoneal injury of the bladder
    c. Laparoscopic or open repair if it is an intraperitoneal injury to the bladder
    d. Laparoscopic repair if it is an extraperitoneal injury to the bladder
    e. Transurethral injection of fibrin glue into the bladder injury site if it is an extraperitoneal injury to the bladder
22. During retroperitoneal renal laparoscopy, balloon dilatation should be preformed in which of the following compartments?
    a. Anterior pararenal space
    b. Posterior pararenal space
    c. Lateral pararenal space
    d. Medial pararenal space
    e. All of the above
23. Hypercarbia during laparoscopy may be related to all of the following EXCEPT:
    a. severe chronic respiratory disease.
    b. subcutaneous emphysema.
    c. increased insufflation pressures.
    d. prolonged operative time.
    e. radical nephrectomy.
24. Possible advantages of retroperitoneal laparoscopy include all of the following EXCEPT:
    a. less need for adhesiolysis.
    b. decreased risk of paralytic ileus.
    c. decreased risk of port site hernias.
    d. direct rapid access to the renal hilum.
    e. technically easier to learn.
25. After extraperitoneal pelvic lymph node dissection, the incidence of which one of the following is higher than with transperitoneal pelvic node dissection?
    a. Urinoma
    b. Lymphocele
    c. Bowel injury
    d. Laparoscopic repair if it is an extraperitoneal injury to the bladder
    e. Shoulder/hip pain
26. All of the following instruments might be part of a hemorrhage control tray EXCEPT:
    a. laparoscopic needle drivers.
    b. laparoscopic Satinsky clamp and accompanying trocar.
    c. Lapra-Ty clip applier and 6-inch length of 3.0 absorbable suture.
    d. hemostatic agents (fibrin glue, gelatin matrix thrombin, etc.) plus laparoscopic applicators.
    e. laparoscopic renal biopsy forceps.
27. Which of the following hemostatic agents requires a 20-minute setup time before use?
    a. Tisseel
    b. FloSeal
    c. CrossSeal
    d. BioGlue
    e. CoSeal

ANSWERS

1. **e. extensive prior abdominal or pelvic surgery.** Absolute contraindications for laparoscopic surgery include uncorrectable coagulopathy, intestinal obstruction, abdominal wall infection, massive hemoperitoneum or hemoretroperitoneum, generalized peritonitis or retroperitoneal abscess, and suspected malignant ascites.
2. **d. Extensive prior abdominal or pelvic surgery.** When extensive intra-abdominal or pelvic adhesions are suspected, close attention must be given to access into the abdomen whether this is by Veress needle or some open access technique. Alternatively, in these patients, a retroperitoneal approach may be preferable to a transperitoneal approach, but this is only a relative contraindication to performing laparoscopic surgery. All of the other options listed are absolute contraindications to laparoscopic surgery.
3. **c. For most uncomplicated patients undergoing laparoscopic renal surgery, a clear liquid diet and a light mechanical bowel preparation the day before surgery is satisfactory.** For extraperitonoscopy or retroperitonoscopy, no bowel preparation is needed. For transperitoneal laparoscopic procedures, a light mechanical bowel preparation can be given in an effort to decompress the bowel. This usually consists of clear liquid diet and a Dulcolax suppository or half bottle of magnesium citrate the day before the procedure.
4. **e. Nitrous oxide has previously been used for insufflation; however, it is no longer routinely used because of the potential for intra-abdominal explosion.** Most commonly, CO_2 is used as the insufflant because it does not support combustion and is very soluble in blood. However, in patients with chronic respiratory disease, CO_2 may accumulate in the bloodstream to dangerous levels. In these patients, helium may be used for insufflation once the initial pneumoperitoneum has been established with CO_2. The drawback of helium is that, like air, it is much less soluble in the blood than CO_2. However, its use precludes problems with hypercarbia. Other gases that were once used for insufflation, including room air, oxygen, and nitrous oxide, are no longer routinely used because of their potential side effects, such as air embolus or intra-abdominal explosion and potential to support combustion.
5. **c. 15 mm Hg.** During prospectively performed pressure volume analysis in patients undergoing transperitoneal laparoscopic procedures, it was found that 94% of maximal intraperitoneal volume is achieved with an insufflation pressure of 15 mm Hg. Additional pressure did not significantly increase the volume. Furthermore, in a porcine study, elevation of the pneumoperitoneum pressure above 15 mm Hg did not significantly ease bladed trocar insertion.
6. **c. Open access technique.** A pneumoperitoneum can be more easily and, in one's early experience, more safely established using an open technique. However, its use involves making a larger incision and increases the chances of port site gas leakage during the procedure. Studies in general surgery have shown the open technique to be as efficient as a closed approach and slightly more or equally safe.

7. **d. Ligasure device.** The Ligasure vessel-sealing system consists of a 5- or 10-mm grasper/dissector connected to a bipolar radiofrequency generator. When the vascular structure is grasped by the instrument, the tissue is evaluated by a feedback response system that subsequently delivers the optimal energy required to seal it more effectively. Therefore, up to and including 7-mm veins and 5-mm arteries can be effectively secured with this device.
8. **c. Endo GIA with 2.5-mm staples.** The Universal 12-mm stapler can be loaded with a variety of 30-, 45-, or 60-mm loads. Each staple load cartridge is color coded depending on the size of the staples: 2.0-mm staples (gray) or 2.5-mm staples (white) are preferred for vascular (renal vein) stapling, whereas 3.8-mm (blue) and 4.8-mm (green) staples are used in thicker tissues (ureter, bowel, bladder). The other choices are not appropriate for control of the renal vein.
9. **b. Ring forceps.** The LapSac, which is made of nylon with a polyurethane inner coating and a polypropylene drawstring, is the least susceptible to tearing or leakage of cells. Currently available, high-speed morcellators shred the sack scissors, and a Kelly clamp is more likely to damage the sack than ring forceps.
10. **c. 10- to 12-mm nonbladed ports placed on the midline.** Currently, the shift from bladed to nonbladed trocars has resulted in a reduced need for port closure for even the 12-mm ports. The 12-mm ports that are not located on the midline do not require fascial closure. However, those on the midline are still considered to be at some risk for possible herniation and therefore most surgeons will close 10- to 12-mm nonbladed ports on the midline. All bladed port sites that are greater than 5 mm should be formally closed. Indeed, postoperative hernia rates with bladed trocars are reported at a frequency of 1.8% vs. only 0.19% for the nonbladed trocars.
11. **a. 12 mm Hg.** Recent studies support a pneumoperitoneum pressure of 12 mm Hg, because this results in no perturbation in cardiac parameters, that is, no change in stroke volume, versus a pressure of 15 mm Hg. Working at lower pneumoperitoneum pressures has also been found to reduce postoperative pain. Also, a marked reduction in oliguria has been associated with working at 10-mm Hg pressure.
12. **d. Decrease in urinary output.** Because of increased intra-abdominal pressure from the pneumoperitoneum, diaphragmatic motion is limited. Laparoscopic surgery causes less significant disturbances of the gastrointestinal motility pattern compared with open surgery. Insufflation with CO_2 results in variable amounts of gas absorption, thereby raising the PCO_2 in the blood and creating an acidosis. Increased intra-abdominal pressure was found to be associated with a significant decrease in urinary output secondary to decreased blood flow to the renal cortex with an associated decrease in renal vein blood flow of up to 90% at 15 mm Hg.
13. **b. 13% morbidity, 0.2% mortality.** Historically, in large series, the overall incidence of laparoscopic complications in urology was in the range of 4%. Mortality was distinctly unusual, with a rate of 0.03% to 0.08%. However, a recent update from Johns Hopkins University reported a 0.2% mortality rate and a 12% overall complication rate.
14. **b. Vascular injury.** The most common site of injury, during laparoscopic surgery, in reports in the literature, is vascular in origin, occurring in 2.8% of patients, followed by bowel injury at 1.1%. The most often injured intra-abdominal organ was bowel at an incidence of 1.2%.
15. **c. The blunt trocar decreases the chance of injury to the epigastric vessels.** The use of only blunt trocars decreases the chance of injury to the epigastric vessels by fivefold.
16. **e. Place the patient in a right lateral decubitus position with the left side up.** The treatment for a suspected gas embolism is immediate cessation of insufflation and prompt desufflation of the peritoneal cavity. The patient is turned into a left lateral decubitus head-down position (i.e., right side up) to minimize right ventricular outflow problems. The patient is hyperventilated with 100% oxygen. Advancement of a central venous line into the right side of the heart with subsequent attempts to aspirate the gas may rarely be helpful. The use of hyperbaric oxygen and cardiopulmonary bypass has also been reported.
17. **d. a and b.** Gas leaking along major blood vessels through congenital defects or secondary enlargement of openings in the diaphragm may lead to pneumomediastinum, pneumopericardium, and pneumothorax.
18. **d. Leave the Veress needle in place and proceed with insufflation of the abdomen at a different location.** If vascular injury should occur with the Veress needle, the needle should be left in place to identify the area of injury and insufflation of the abdomen can be re-performed at an alternate site and then the laparoscope inserted to identify the area of injury and to observe this as the Veress needle is removed in order to control any hemorrhage that may occur from the site.
19. **c. Leave the trocar in place, consult a vascular surgeon, and convert to open laparotomy.** A trocar injury to a major arterial vessel is a potentially life-threatening complication. The trocar should remain in place to tamponade the bleeding and also identify the area of injury once the abdomen is opened. The patient should be typed and crossed for blood and immediate laparotomy should be performed and the site of vascular injury identified. A vascular surgery consultation should be obtained.
20. **c. Leukopenia, low-grade fever, and pain at one port site.** Postoperative bowel injury should be suspected in any patient who complains of increasing abdominal discomfort particularly at one port site and low-grade fever associated not uncommonly with a leukopenia, although there usually will be a left shift in the differential white cell count. If unrecognized by these subtle clinical findings, the patient may succumb to the bowel injury in a matter of 1 to 2 days. The diagnosis is made with a CT scan of the abdomen with oral contrast; it is recommended to obtain a repeat plan CT 4 to 6 hours later to best identify any small bowel leakage.
21. **c. Laparoscopic or open repair if it is an intraperitoneal injury to the bladder.** When bladder injury is diagnosed postoperatively, the surgeon must determine whether the perforation is extraperitoneal or intraperitoneal. Extraperitoneal injury, without any complicating additional problems, may be treated by simple placement of a transurethral indwelling Foley catheter. Intraperitoneal injury is an indication for subsequent laparoscopic or open repair.
22. **b. Posterior pararenal space.** The space dorsolateral to Gerota's fascia is the posterior pararenal space. This is the space dilated during retroperitoneoscopy.
23. **e. radical nephrectomy.** The potential for developing hypercarbia exists during both transperitoneal and preperitoneal laparoscopic procedures. Conceivably, this assumes greater importance in patients with preexisting airway and cardiovascular compliance. Vigilant perioperative anesthetic management is essential to prevent the development

of potential complications related to CO_2 buildup. A rise in end-tidal CO_2 should prompt the anesthesiologist to adjust the respiratory rate and tidal volume to enhance CO_2 elimination. Simultaneously, the insufflation pressure of CO_2 should be decreased by the surgeon or, if need be, the operation should be halted and the abdomen desufflated until the end-tidal CO_2 returns to an acceptable level.

24. **e. technically easier to learn.** Retroperitoneoscopy is associated with unique anatomic orientation and a relatively restricted initial working area compared with transperitoneal laparoscopy. This results in a steeper learning curve.
25. **b. Lymphocele.** Absence of the peritoneal absorptive surface after extraperitoneaoscopic lymphadenectomy may increase the risk of development of postoperative lymphocele.
26. **e. laparoscopic renal biopsy forceps.** *Contents of hemorrhage tray for laparoscopic surgery:*

    Laparoscopic Satinsky clamp
    10-mm suction/irrigation tip
    Endostitch device with a 4-0 absorbable suture
    Lapra-Ty clip Applier and a packet of Lapra-Ty clips
    6-inch length of 4-0 vascular suture on an SH needle with a Lapra-Ty clip preplaced on the end
    2 laparoscopic needle drivers
    Topical hemostatic agent of choice
27. **a. Tisseel.** Tisseel (Baxter, Glendale, CA) is a form of fibrin glue containing fibrinogen calcium chloride, aprotinin, and thrombin. It is useful as a topical hemostatic agent as well as a tissue glue, but it has a 20-minute setup time and thus must be prepared well in advance of potential use.

SECTION IV

INFECTIONS AND INFLAMMATION

8

Infections of the Urinary Tract

ANTHONY J. SCHAEFFER • EDWARD M. SCHAEFFER

QUESTIONS

1. Acute pyelonephritis is best diagnosed by:
   a. chills, fever, and flank pain.
   b. bacteria and pyuria.
   c. focal scar in renal cortex.
   d. delayed renal function.
   e. vesicoureteral reflux.
2. Bacteriuria without pyuria is indicative of:
   a. infection.
   b. colonization.
   c. tuberculosis.
   d. contamination.
   e. stones.
3. Which one of the following statements is true of nosocomial health care-associated UTIs?
   a. They occur in patients who are hospitalized or institutionalized.
   b. They are caused by common bowel bacteria that are susceptible to most antimicrobials.
   c. They can be suppressed by low-dose antimicrobial therapy.
   d. They are due to reinfection.
   e. They are due to bacterial persistence.
4. Most recurrent infections in female patients are:
   a. complicated.
   b. reinfections.
   c. due to bacterial resistance.
   d. hereditary.
   e. surgically correctable.
5. Rates of reinfection (i.e., time to recurrence) are influenced by:
   a. bladder dysfunction.
   b. renal scarring.
   c. vesicoureteral reflux.
   d. antimicrobial treatment.
   e. age.
6. The long-term effect of uncomplicated recurrent UTIs is:
   a. renal scarring.
   b. hypertension.
   c. azotemia.
   d. ureteral vesical reflux.
   e. nothing.
7. The ascending route of infection is *not* enhanced by:
   a. catheterization.
   b. spermicidal agents.
   c. indwelling catheter.
   d. fecal soilage of perineum.
   e. frequent voiding.
8. Approximately 10% of symptomatic lower UTIs in young, sexually active female patients are caused by:
   a. *Escherichia coli.*
   b. *Staphylococcus saprophyticus.*
   c. *Pseudomonas.*
   d. *Proteus mirabilis.*
   e. *Staphylococcus epidermidis.*
9. The virulence factor that is most important for adherence is:
   a. hemolysin.
   b. K antigen.
   c. pili.
   d. colicin production.
   e. O serogroup.
10. Phase variation of bacterial pili:
    a. occurs only in vitro.
    b. affects bacterial virulence.
    c. is characteristic of pyelonephritic *E. coli.*
    d. is irreversible.
    e. refers to change in pili length.

11. The first demonstrable biologic difference that has been shown in women susceptible to UTIs is:
    a. increased adherence of bacteria to vaginal cells.
    b. decreased estrogen concentration in vaginal cells.
    c. elevated vaginal pH.
    d. nonsecretor status.
    e. postmenopausal status.

12. Increased susceptibility of women to recurrent UTIs has NOT been associated with increased bacterial adherence to:
    a. introital mucosa.
    b. urethral mucosa.
    c. buccal mucosa.
    d. vaginal fluid.
    e. bladder mucosa.

13. The primary bladder defense is:
    a. low urine pH.
    b. low urine osmolarity.
    c. voiding.
    d. Tamm-Horsfall protein (uromucoid).
    e. vaginal mucus.

14. The most significant sequela of renal papillary necrosis is renal:
    a. failure.
    b. abscess.
    c. obstruction.
    d. stone.
    e. cancer.

15. Severity and morbidity of bacteriuria is worst in patients with:
    a. spinal cord injuries.
    b. pregnancy.
    c. reflux.
    d. diabetes mellitus.
    e. HIV.

16. The most reliable urine specimen is obtained by:
    a. urethral catheterization.
    b. catheter aspiration.
    c. midstream voiding.
    d. suprapubic aspiration.
    e. antiseptic periurethral preparation.

17. The validity of a midstream urine specimen should be questioned if microscopy reveals:
    a. squamous epithelial cells.
    b. red blood cells.
    c. bacteria.
    d. white blood cells.
    e. casts.

18. Rapid screening methods for detecting UTIs should be used primarily for:
    a. low-risk asymptomatic patients.
    b. pregnant women.
    c. children.
    d. catheterized patients.
    e. elderly patients.

19. The most accurate test for evaluation of infection in the kidney is:
    a. the Fairley bladder washout test.
    b. ureteral catheterization.
    c. gallium scanning.
    d. CT.
    e. the antibody-coated bacteria test.

20. Urinary tract imaging is NOT usually indicated for recurrent UTIs in:
    a. women.
    b. girls.
    c. men.
    d. boys.
    e. spinal cord–injured patients.

21. The most sensitive imaging modality for diagnosing renal abscess is:
    a. ultrasonography.
    b. indium scanning.
    c. gallium scanning.
    d. excretory urography.
    e. CT.

22. Cure of UTIs depends most on antimicrobial:
    a. serum half-life.
    b. serum level.
    c. urine level.
    d. duration of therapy.
    e. frequency of therapy.

23. During the past 5 years, the least development of antimicrobial resistance has been observed for:
    a. ampicillin.
    b. cephalosporins.
    c. nitrofurantoin.
    d. fluoroquinolones.
    e. trimethoprim-sulfamethoxazole (TMP-SMX).

24. The ideal class of drugs for empirical treatment of uncomplicated UTIs is:
    a. aminopenicillins.
    b. aminoglycosides.
    c. fluoroquinolones.
    d. cephalosporins.
    e. nitrofurantoins.

25. Antimicrobial prophylaxis is characterized as:
    a. administration of an antimicrobial within 4 to 6 hours of the procedure.
    b. administration of an antimicrobial for a period of time covering the first 48 hours after the procedure.
    c. administration of an antimicrobial within 30 minutes of the initiation of a procedure and for a period of time covering the first 48 hours after the procedure.
    d. administration of an antimicrobial within 30 minutes of the initiation of a procedure and for a period of time that covers the duration of the procedure.
    e. administration of an antimicrobial the night before the initiation of a procedure and for a period of time that covers the duration of the procedure.

26. Antimicrobial prophylaxis for transurethral resection of the prostate is not indicated for patients with:
    a. valvular heart disease.
    b. prosthetic valves.
    c. unknown urine culture.
    d. sterile urine.
    e. indwelling catheter.

27. A risk of endocarditis is not associated with:
    a. a history of childhood heart murmurs.
    b. heart valves inserted more than 5 years ago.
    c. calcified heart valves associated with a murmur.
    d. all synthetic heart valves.
    e. cadaveric heart valves.

28. This host factor is not associated with an increased risk of infection:
    a. advanced age.
    b. a history of previous infection in the site/organ of interest.
    c. residence in a chronic care facility.
    d. indwelling orthopedic pins.
    e. coexistent infection.
29. Urine culture is not routinely recommended for the clinical diagnosis of acute cystitis in:
    a. young women.
    b. elderly women.
    c. children.
    d. men.
    e. patients with hematuria.
30. The drug of choice for uncomplicated cystitis in most young women is:
    a. TMP-SMX.
    b. fluoroquinolone.
    c. penicillin.
    d. cephalosporin.
    e. nitrofurantoin.
31. The optimal duration of antimicrobial therapy for symptomatic acute uncomplicated cystitis in women is:
    a. 1 day.
    b. 3 days.
    c. 7 days.
    d. 14 days.
    e. 21 days.
32. Treatment of asymptomatic bacteriuria is indicated for patients who are:
    a. elderly.
    b. catheterized.
    c. pregnant.
    d. confused.
    e. incontinent.
33. Screening for bacteriuria is beneficial in:
    a. pregnant women.
    b. elderly patients.
    c. men.
    d. children.
    e. spinal cord–injured patients.
34. The most common cause of unresolved bacteriuria during antimicrobial therapy is:
    a. development of bacterial resistance.
    b. rapid reinfections.
    c. azotemia.
    d. giant staghorn calculi.
    e. initial bacterial resistance.
35. Nitrofurantoin prophylaxis is effective because of the concentration of the drug in the:
    a. urine.
    b. vaginal mucus.
    c. bowel.
    d. serum.
    e. bladder.
36. The ideal antimicrobial for self-start therapy for a UTI is:
    a. a fluoroquinolone.
    b. a cephalosporin.
    c. nitrofurantoin.
    d. TMP-SMX.
    e. tetracycline.
37. The most common cause of acute pyelonephritis in young women is:
    a. vesicoureteral reflux.
    b. P-piliated bacteria.
    c. type 1 piliated bacteria.
    d. recurrent UTIs.
    e. bacterial endotoxin.
38. The optimal antimicrobial for treatment of acute uncomplicated pyelonephritis in women is:
    a. TMP-SMX.
    b. a cephalosporin.
    c. an aminoglycoside.
    d. a fluoroquinolone.
    e. nitrofurantoin.
39. A patient with acute pyelonephritis, persistent fever, and flank pain for 24 hours warrants:
    a. observation.
    b. CT.
    c. change in antimicrobial therapy.
    d. ultrasonography.
    e. blood cultures.
40. The overall mortality rate in emphysematous pyelonephritis is approximately:
    a. 5%.
    b. 10%.
    c. 20%.
    d. 40%.
    e. 60%.
41. In chronic renal abscess, the predominant urographic abnormality is:
    a. calyceal distortion.
    b. renal mass.
    c. calculi.
    d. hydronephrosis.
    e. calyceal amputation.
42. The high mortality rate associated with perinephric abscess is primarily attributed to:
    a. bacterial hemolysis.
    b. diabetes mellitus.
    c. delay in diagnosis.
    d. inappropriate antimicrobial therapy.
    e. inadequate drainage.
43. The primary treatment for a small perirenal abscess in a functioning kidney is:
    a. nephrectomy.
    b. partial nephrectomy.
    c. open surgical drainage.
    d. percutaneous drainage.
    e. retrograde ureteral drainage.
44. Most patients with chronic pyelonephritis present with:
    a. hypertension.
    b. renal failure.
    c. chronic infection.
    d. flank pain.
    e. no symptoms.
45. The most common bacterial cause of xanthogranulomatous pyelonephritis is:
    a. *Escherichia coli.*
    b. *Pseudomonas.*
    c. *Klebsiella.*
    d. *Proteus mirabilis.*
    e. *Staphylococcus.*

46. It is hypothesized that the nidus for the Michaelis-Gutmann body is:
    a. renal papillae.
    b. bacterial fragments.
    c. calcium crystals.
    d. macrophages.
    e. uric acid stones.

47. Echinococcosis is rare in/among:
    a. the former Soviet Union.
    b. Eskimos.
    c. Native Americans.
    d. the United States.
    e. Eastern Europe.

48. The most reliable early clinical indicator of septicemia is:
    a. chills.
    b. fever.
    c. hyperventilation.
    d. lethargy.
    e. change in mental status.

49. Compared with nonpregnant women, pregnant women have a higher prevalence and increased risk from:
    a. asymptomatic bacteriuria.
    b. acute cystitis.
    c. acute pyelonephritis.
    d. recurrent cystitis.
    e. bacterial persistence.

50. Clinical pyelonephritis during pregnancy is most commonly linked to:
    a. maternal sepsis.
    b. maternal anemia.
    c. maternal hypertension.
    d. eclampsia.
    e. congenital malformations.

51. The drug thought to be safe in any phase of pregnancy is:
    a. a fluoroquinolone.
    b. nitrofurantoin.
    c. a sulfonamide.
    d. penicillin.
    e. tetracycline.

52. The majority of elderly patients with bacteriuria are:
    a. asymptomatic.
    b. febrile.
    c. incontinent.
    d. confused.
    e. dysuric.

53. In the absence of obstruction, treatment of asymptomatic bacteriuria in the elderly:
    a. is cost effective.
    b. prevents renal failure.
    c. reduces mortality.
    d. reduces morbidity.
    e. is unnecessary.

54. The most common predisposing factor for hospital-acquired UTIs is:
    a. surgery.
    b. antimicrobial use.
    c. age.
    d. catheterization.
    e. diabetes mellitus.

55. The most effective measure for reducing catheter-associated UTI is:
    a. closed drainage.
    b. antimicrobial prophylaxis.
    c. catheter irrigation.
    d. intermittent catheterization.
    e. daily meatal care.

56. In spinal cord–injured patients, the bladder drainage technique with the lowest complication rate is:
    a. clean intermittent catheterization (CIC).
    b. suprapubic drainage.
    c. indwelling catheter.
    d. condom catheter.
    e. suprapubic pressure.

57. Fournier's gangrene is not associated with scrotal:
    a. pain.
    b. discharge.
    c. crepitation.
    d. erythema.
    e. swelling.

ANSWERS

1. **a. chills, fever, and flank pain.** Acute pyelonephritis is a clinical syndrome of chills, fever, and flank pain that is accompanied by bacteriuria and pyuria, a combination that is reasonably specific for an acute bacterial infection of the kidney.

2. **b. colonization.** Bacteriuria without pyuria is generally indicative of bacterial colonization without infection of the urinary tract.

3. **a. They occur in patients who are hospitalized or institutionalized.** Nosocomial or health care–associated UTIs occur in patients who are hospitalized or institutionalized and are caused by *Pseudomonas* and other more antimicrobial-resistant strains.

4. **b. reinfections.** Of these recurrent infections, 71% to 73% are caused by reinfection with different organisms, rather than recurrence with the same organism.

5. **d. antimicrobial treatment.** Whether a patient receives no treatment or short-term, long-term, or prophylactic antimicrobial treatment, the risk of recurrent bacteriuria remains the same; antimicrobial treatment appears to alter only the time until recurrence.

6. **e. nothing.** The long-term effects of uncomplicated recurrent UTIs are not completely known, but, so far, no association between recurrent infections and renal scarring, hypertension, or progressive renal azotemia has been established.

7. **e. frequent voiding.** This route is further enhanced in individuals with significant soilage of the perineum with feces, women using spermicidal agents, and patients with intermittent or indwelling catheters.

8. **b. *Staphylococcus saprophyticus.*** *S. saprophyticus* is now recognized as causing approximately 10% of symptomatic lower UTIs in young, sexually active females, whereas it rarely causes infection in males and elderly individuals.

9. **c. pili.** Studies have demonstrated that interactions between FimH and receptors expressed on the luminal surface of the

bladder epithelium are critical to the ability of many uropathogenic *E. coli* strains to colonize the bladder and cause disease.

10. **b. affects bacterial virulence.** This process is called phase variation and has obvious biologic and clinical implications. For example, the presence of type 1 pili may be advantageous to the bacteria for adhering to and colonizing the bladder mucosa but disadvantageous because the pili enhance phagocytosis and killing by neutrophils.
11. **a. increased adherence of bacteria to vaginal cells.** These studies established increased adherence of pathogenic bacteria to vaginal epithelial cells as the first demonstrable biologic difference that could be shown in women susceptible to UTI.
12. **e. bladder mucosa.** These studies individually and collectively support the concept that there is an increased epithelial receptivity for *E. coli* on the introital, urethral, and buccal mucosa that is characteristic of women susceptible to recurrent UTIs and may be a genotypic trait. Thus the vaginal fluid appears to influence adherence to cells and presumably vaginal mucosal colonization.
13. **c. voiding.** Bacteria presumably make their way into the bladder fairly often. Whether small inocula of bacteria persist, multiply, and infect the host depends in part on the ability of the bladder to empty.
14. **c. obstruction.** A patient who suffers from an acute ureteral obstruction caused by a sloughed papilla and who has a concomitant UTI is a urologic emergency.
15. **a. spinal cord injuries.** Of all patients with bacteriuria, no group compares in severity and morbidity with those who have spinal cord injury.
16. **d. suprapubic aspiration.** A single aspirated specimen reveals the bacteriologic status of the bladder urine without introducing urethral bacteria, which can start a new infection.
17. **a. squamous epithelial cells.** The validation of the midstream urine specimen can be questioned if numerous squamous epithelial cells (indicative of preputial, vaginal, or urethral contaminants) are present.
18. **a. low-risk asymptomatic patients.** The main role of rapid screening methods for UTIs is in screening asymptomatic patients.
19. **b. ureteral catheterization.** Ureteral catheterization allows not only separation of bacterial persistence into upper and lower urinary tracts but also separation of the infection between one kidney and the other.
20. **a. women.** Several reports of women patients with recurrent UTIs show that excretory urograms are unnecessary for routine evaluation if women who have special risk factors are excluded.
21. **e. CT.** CT and MRI are more sensitive than excretory urography or ultrasonography in the diagnosis of acute focal bacterial nephritis, renal and perirenal abscesses, and radiolucent calculi.
22. **c. urine level.** Efficacy of the antimicrobial therapy is critically dependent on the antimicrobial levels in the urine and the duration that this level remains above the minimum inhibitory concentration of the infecting organism. Hence, resolution of infection is closely associated with the susceptibility of the bacteria to the concentration of the antimicrobial agent achieved in the urine.
23. **c. nitrofurantoin.** Over a 5-year period, the prevalence of resistance to trimethoprim/sulfamethoxazole, ampicillin, and cephalothin increased significantly, whereas resistance to nitrofurantoin and ciprofloxacin remained uncommon.
24. **c. fluoroquinolones.** The fluoroquinolones have a broad spectrum of activity that makes them ideal for the empirical treatment of UTIs.
25. **d. administration of an antimicrobial within 30 minutes of the initiation of a procedure and for a period of time that covers the duration of the procedure.** Surgical antimicrobial prophylaxis entails treatment with an antimicrobial before and for a *limited* time after a procedure to prevent local or systemic postprocedural infections.
26. **e. indwelling catheter.** Prolonged use of an indwelling urethral catheter is common in hospitalized patients and is associated with an increased risk of bacterial colonization with a 3% to 10% incidence of bacteriuria per catheter day in one study and 100% incidence of bacteriuria with long-term catheterization (>30 days). Prophylactic antimicrobials during catheterization are not generally recommended because bacterial resistance can develop rapidly. For chronically catheterized patients, preoperative antimicrobial agents are therapeutic not prophylactic.
27. **a. a history of childhood heart murmurs.** The American Heart Association's recommendations on the prevention of bacterial endocarditis are based on the patient's risk of developing endocarditis and the likelihood that a procedure will cause bacteremia with an organism that can cause endocarditis. Prophylaxis is recommended for both high- and moderate-risk patients. High-risk patients include individuals with prosthetic heart valves, previous bacterial endocarditis, cyanotic congenital heart disease, and systemic-pulmonary shunts or conduits. Moderate-risk patients include other congenital malformations (excluding isolated secundum atrial septal defects, surgically repaired ASD, ventricular septal defects, or patent ductus arteriosus), acquired valvular dysfunction, hypertrophic cardiomyopathy, and mitral valve prolapse with valvular regurgitation and/or thickened leaflets. Antimicrobial prophylaxis is not recommended for patients with congenital malformations including isolated secundum atrial septal defects, surgically repaired ASD, ventricular septal defects or patent ductus arteriosus, previous coronary artery bypass graft surgery, benign heart murmurs, previous Kawasaki disease or rheumatic fever without valvular dysfunction, or implanted pacemakers or defibrillators.
28. **d. indwelling orthopedic pins.** Bacterial seeding of implanted orthopedic hardware is a rare but morbid event. A joint commission of the American Urological Association, the American Academy of Orthopaedic Surgeons, and infectious disease specialists convened in 2003 and released an advisory statement on antibiotic prophylaxis for urologic patients with total joint replacement. In general, antimicrobial prophylaxis for urologic patients with total joint replacements, pins, plates, or screws is not indicated. Prophylaxis is advised for individuals at higher risk of seeding a prosthetic joint and include those with recently inserted implants (within 2 years).
29. **a. young women.** Thus, in women with recent onset of symptoms and signs suggesting acute cystitis and in whom factors associated with upper tract or complicated infection are absent, a urinalysis that is positive for pyuria, hematuria, or bacteriuria or a combination should provide sufficient documentation of UTI, and a urine culture may be omitted.
30. **a. TMP-SMX.** TMP and TMP-SMX are recommended in areas where the prevalence of resistance to these drugs among *E. coli* strains causing cystitis is less than 20%.
31. **b. 3 days.** Three-day therapy is the preferred regimen for uncomplicated cystitis in women.
32. **c. pregnant.** Thus, in populations other than those for whom treatment has been documented to be beneficial (e.g., pregnant women and patients undergoing urologic interventions),

screening for or treatment of asymptomatic bacteriuria is not appropriate and should be discouraged.

33. **a. pregnant women.** Thus, in populations other than those for whom treatment has been documented to be beneficial (e.g., pregnant women and patients undergoing urologic interventions), screening for or treatment of asymptomatic bacteriuria is not appropriate and should be discouraged.

34. **e. initial bacterial resistance.** Most commonly, the bacteria are resistant to the antimicrobial agent selected to treat the infection.

35. **a. urine.** Nitrofurantoin, which does not alter the bowel flora, is present for brief periods at high concentrations in the urine and leads to repeated elimination of bacteria from the urine, presumably by interfering with bacterial initiation of infection.

36. **a. a fluoroquinolone.** Fluoroquinolones are ideal for self-start therapy because they have a spectrum of activity broader than that of any of the other oral agents and are superior to many parenteral antimicrobials, including aminoglycosides.

37. **b. P-piliated bacteria.** If VUR is absent, a patient bearing the P blood group phenotype may have special susceptibility to recurrent pyelonephritis caused by *E. coli* that have P pili and bind to the P blood group antigen receptors.

38. **d. a fluoroquinolone.** For patients who will be managed as outpatients, single-drug oral therapy with a fluoroquinolone is more effective than TMP-SMX for patients with domiciliary infections.

39. **a. observation.** Even though the urine usually becomes sterile within a few hours of starting antimicrobial therapy, patients with acute uncomplicated pyelonephritis may continue to have fever, chills, and flank pain for several more days after initiation of successful antimicrobial therapy. They should be observed.

40. **d. 40%.** Emphysematous pyelonephritis should be considered a complication of severe pyelonephritis rather than a distinct entity. The overall mortality rate is 43%.

41. **b. renal mass.** In a more chronic abscess, the predominant urographic abnormalities are those of a renal mass lesion.

42. **c. delay in diagnosis.** Although 71% of all the patients had eventual surgical treatment of their perinephric abscesses, the diagnostic delay of those patients admitted to medical services postponed definitive treatment and consequently caused higher mortality.

43. **d. percutaneous drainage.** Although surgical drainage, or nephrectomy if the kidney is nonfunctioning or severely infected, is the classic treatment for perinephric abscesses, renal sonography and CT make percutaneous aspiration and drainage of small perirenal collections possible.

44. **e. no symptoms.** There are no symptoms of chronic pyelonephritis until it produces renal insufficiency, and then the symptoms are similar to those of any other form of chronic renal failure.

45. **d. *P. mirabilis*.** Although review of the literature shows *Proteus* to be the most common organism involved with xanthogranulomatous pyelonephritis, *E. coli* is also common.

46. **b. bacterial fragments.** It is hypothesized that bacteria or bacterial fragments form the nidus for the calcium phosphate crystals that laminate the Michaelis-Gutmann bodies.

47. **d. the United States.** In the United States, the disease is rare but it is found in immigrants from Eastern Europe or other foreign endemic areas, or as an indigenous infection among Native Americans in the Southwest United States and in Eskimos.

48. **c. hyperventilation.** Even before temperature extremes and the onset of chills, bacteremic patients often begin to hyperventilate. Thus, the earliest metabolic change in septicemia is a resultant respiratory alkalosis.

49. **c. acute pyelonephritis.** Pyelonephritis develops in 1% to 4% of all pregnant women and in 20% to 40% of pregnant women with untreated bacteriuria.

50. **a. maternal sepsis.** However, because women with asymptomatic bacteriuria are at higher risk for developing a symptomatic UTI that results in adverse fetal sequelae, complications associated with bacteriuria during pregnancy, and pyelonephritis and its possible sequelae, such as sepsis in the mother, all women with asymptomatic bacteriuria should be treated.

51. **d. penicillin.** The aminopenicillins and cephalosporins are considered safe and generally effective throughout pregnancy. In patients with penicillin allergy, nitrofurantoin is a reasonable alternative.

52. **a. asymptomatic.** Most elderly patients with bacteriuria are asymptomatic; estimates among women living in nursing homes range from 17% to 55%, as compared with 15% to 31% for their male cohorts.

53. **e. is unnecessary.** Prospective randomized comparative trials of antimicrobial or no therapy in elderly male and female nursing home residents with asymptomatic bacteriuria consistently document no benefit of antimicrobial therapy. There was no decrease in symptomatic episodes and no improvement in survival. In fact, treatment with antimicrobial therapy increases the occurrence of adverse drug effects and reinfection with resistant organisms and increases the cost of treatment. Therefore, asymptomatic bacteriuria in elderly residents of long-term care facilities should not be treated with antimicrobials.

54. **d. catheterization.** Catheter-associated bacteriuria is the most common hospital-acquired infection, accounting for up to 40% of such infections and more than 1 million per year.

55. **a. closed drainage.** Careful aseptic insertion of the catheter and maintenance of a closed dependent drainage system are essential to minimize development of bacteriuria.

56. **a. clean intermittent catheterization.** Although never rigorously compared with indwelling urethral catheterization, CIC has been shown to decrease lower urinary tract complications by maintaining low intravesical pressure and reducing the incidence of stones.

57. **b. discharge.** Early on, the involved area is swollen, erythematous, and tender as the infection begins to involve the deep fascia. Pain is prominent, and fever and systemic toxicity are marked. The swelling and crepitus of the scrotum quickly increase, and dark purple areas develop and progress to extensive gangrene.

9

Inflammatory Conditions of the Male Genitourinary Tract: Prostatitis and Related Conditions, Orchitis, and Epididymitis

J. CURTIS NICKEL

QUESTIONS

1. The prevalence of chronic prostatitis (diagnoses/symptoms) in population-based studies is:
   a. <1%.
   b. 2% to 10%.
   c. >20%.
   d. 50%.
   e. unknown.
2. Which of the following etiologic agents or mechanisms has been unequivocally confirmed to be associated with prostatic inflammation?
   a. Intraprostatic ductal reflux
   b. Enterobacteriaceae
   c. *Chlamydia* species
   d. *Ureaplasma* species
   e. *Corynebacterium* species
3. The most likely candidate for cryptic infection in category III prostatitis is:
   a. *Chlamydia*.
   b. *Ureaplasma*.
   c. Nanobacteria.
   d. Corynebacteria.
   e. unknown.
4. The presence of white blood cells (WBCs) in the expressed prostatic secretion (EPS) of patients with category III chronic pelvic pain syndrome (CPPS):
   a. confirms significant prostatic inflammation.
   b. correlates with severity of symptoms.
   c. differentiates CPPS patients from control patients.
   d. differentiates CPPS Cat IIIA patients from Cat IIIB patients.
   e. differentiates CP Cat II patients from CPPS Cat III patients.
5. What is the National Institutes of Health (NIH) Chronic Prostatitis Symptom Index?
   a. A research tool that is useful only in clinical trials
   b. A research tool that is useful in clinical practice
   c. Another invalidated and unreliable clinical symptom index
   d. An index that has been validated only in English
   e. A simple pain questionnaire that can be applied to prostatitis patients
6. An obese 26-year-old man has an 8-hour history of severe dysuria, stranguria, and suprapubic and perineal pain with fever. On examination, he has suprapubic tenderness and his prostate is enlarged, boggy, and exquisitely tender. Urinalysis shows pyuria. He continues to complain of symptoms despite insertion of a Foley catheter and has persistent fever after 30 hours of intravenous gentamicin and ampicillin. Culture grew *Escherichia coli*. What is the best next step?
   a. Change antibiotic to a third-generation cephalosporin
   b. Perform a transrectal ultrasonographic examination
   c. Perform a cystoscopic examination
   d. Perform a bladder scan ultrasonographic examination
   e. Perform an intravenous pyelogram examination
7. A 36-year-old man has a 4-month history of dull perineal and suprapubic discomfort, postejaculatory pain, and moderate obstructive voiding symptoms. A preprostatic massage urine sample was sterile, and microscopic evaluation of the sediment showed 2 WBC/HPF. No EPS was obtained during an uncomfortable digital rectal examination. A postprostatic massage urine sample grew 10^2 *Staphylococcus epidermidis* organisms per milliliter, and microscopy of the sediment showed 10 to 12 WBC/HPF. What is the NIH chronic prostatitis (CP)/CPPS classification?
   a. Category I
   b. Category II
   c. Category IIIA
   d. Category IIIB
   e. Category IV

8. A 24-year-old man has an 8-month history of obstructive voiding symptoms and perineal and ejaculatory discomfort. A preprostatic massage urine sample was sterile, and microscopic evaluation of sediment showed 1 WBC/HPF. Microscopy of a minute amount of EPS showed 3 WBC/HPF. A postprostatic massage urine sample was sterile, and microscopy of the sediment showed 2 WBC/HPF. What is the CP/CPPS classification?

   a. Category I
   b. Category II
   c. Category IIIA
   d. Category IIIB
   e. Category IV

9. A 42-year-old man was treated for cystitis but continued to have dysuria, ejaculatory pain, and perineal/testicular discomfort after 7 days of antibiotics. The prostate examination was unremarkable. A midstream urine sample was sterile, but culture of a drop of EPS produced moderate growth of *Enterococcus faecalis*. A postprostatic massage urine sample grew 10^2 *E. faecalis* organisms, and microscopic examination of the sediment showed 12 WBC/HPF. What is the CP/CPPS classification?

   a. Category I
   b. Category II
   c. Category IIIA
   d. Category IIIB
   e. Category IV

10. A 32-year-old man had been successfully treated for an *E. coli* cystitis with trimethoprim-sulfamethoxazole (7-day course) 4 months previously. A recurrence of similar symptoms was again successfully treated with ciprofloxacin (3 days), but no culture was done at this time. Three days after antibiotics were discontinued, the patient presents with continued perineal discomfort, ejaculatory pain and mild dysuria. Preprostatic and postprostatic massage urine and EPS samples were sterile. Evaluation of the EPS showed 20 WBC/HPF. The prostate felt normal. What is the next best step?

    a. Treat with anti-inflammatory agents
    b. Do a standard Meares-Stamey 4-glass test
    c. Wait for 3 days and do standard Meares-Stamey 4-glass test
    d. Restart trimethoprim-sulfamethoxazole
    e. Restart fluoroquinolone antibiotics

11. A 47-year-old man has a 5-year history of perineal and suprapubic pain/discomfort and obstructive voiding symptoms that has not responded to multiple courses of antibiotics, α- blockers, anti-inflammatory agents, repetitive prostatic massage, or phytotherapy. The prostate is tender, and the postprostatic massage urine sample was sterile and showed 20 WBC/HPF. The prostate-specific antigen (PSA) value was 1.2 mg/mL. What is the next best step?

    a. Incision of bladder neck
    b. Flow rate and bladder scan for residual urine
    c. Video-urodynamics
    d. CT scan of pelvis
    e. Cystoscopy and transrectal ultrasound

12. A 28-year-old man has been successfully treated for three episodes of cystitis (cultures not performed). He now presents with a 3-day history of frequency, urgency, dysuria, and suprapubic discomfort. The prostate feels normal and is nontender. An abdominal and pelvic ultrasonographic study had normal results. A midstream culture done 24 hours earlier by his family physician grew 10^5 *E. coli* organisms per milliliter. What is the next best step?

    a. A lower urinary tract localization test (2- or 4-glass test)
    b. Several days of nitrofurantoin therapy followed by a lower urinary tract localization test
    c. 4 weeks of fluoroquinolone antibiotics therapy
    d. Cystoscopy
    e. Transrectal ultrasonography

13. A 37-year-old man has a 3-month history of urinary frequency and urgency and discomfort localized to the perineum, suprapubic area, testes, and penis. A sterile post-prostatic massage urine sample showed 15 WBC/HPF on microscopy. A year earlier, the patient had been successfully treated for moderately severe symptoms with an unspecified antibiotic. He is allergic to many medications, including ciprofloxacin. The symptoms are now a significant bother and affecting his quality of life. The best initial treatment is a trial of:

    a. anti-inflammatory agents.
    b. tetracycline.
    c. trimethoprim-sulfamethoxazole.
    d. trimethoprim.
    e. carbenicillin.

14. A 58-year-old man with a 2-year history of symptomatic recurrent urinary tract infections with *Pseudomonas* (6 to 8 per year) is asymptomatic between treated episodes. *Pseudomonas aeruginosa* is localized to the EPS and postprostatic massage (voided bladder 3 [VB3]) samples (but not the midstream urine sample, or VB2) during a period when he was asymptomatic. The EPS shows severe pyuria with WBC plugs or aggregates on microscopy. Transrectal ultrasonography shows extensive prostatic calcifications. Cystoscopy results are normal, residual urine is negligible, and the PSA value is 1.0 mg/mL. What is the best treatment?

    a. Low-dose prophylactic antibiotics
    b. Intraprostatic antibiotic injection
    c. Radical TURP
    d. Radical prostatectomy
    e. Transurethral microwave thermotherapy

15. A 24-year-old man with a 6-year history of severe perineal pain with irritative and obstructive voiding symptoms has no significant benefits with 4 weeks of therapy with trimethoprim-sulfamethoxazole, anti-inflammatory agents, α-adrenergic blockers, or phytotherapy, respectively. Prostate-specific specimens were sterile, and no WBCs were noted on microscopy. The physical examination had normal findings except for anal sphincter spasm and a tender but normal-feeling prostate gland. Video-urodynamics showed a bladder neck/proximal urethra region that opened minimally with detrusor voiding pressure. What is the next best step?

    a. 4 weeks of fluoroquinolone therapy
    b. Muscle relaxant therapy
    c. Bladder neck incision
    d. Biofeedback
    e. Transurethral microwave thermotherapy

ear-old man continues to have high, spiking fever despite pubic catheterization and 36 hours of treatment with -spectrum intravenous antibiotics. Transrectal ısonography confirms a large prostatic abscess. What is the t best step?

Transperineal drainage
Transrectal aspiration
. Transurethral drainage
d. Open drainage
e. Suprapubic aspiration

Clinical improvement has been demonstrated with α-adrenergic blocker therapy in which of the following NIH categories of CP/CPPS?

a. Category I
b. Category II
c. Categories II and IIIA
d. Categories II and IIIB
e. Categories II and III

18. Which of the following is the only therapy that has NOT been evaluated against placebo in a randomized controlled trial for chronic prostatitis?

a. 5α-Reductase inhibitors
b. α-Adrenergic blockers
c. Antibiotics
d. Neuromodulators
e. Anti-inflammatory agents

19. An asymptomatic 65-year-old man undergoes a prostate biopsy because of an indistinct prostate asymmetry on digital rectal examination. The PSA value is 2.2 ng/mL. Pathology reveals extensive glandular and periglandular infiltration with acute and chronic inflammatory cells. What is the next best step?

a. Observation
b. 4 weeks of antibiotics and then reassess
c. 4 weeks of antibiotics and anti-inflammatory agents and then reassess
d. Repeat biopsy
e. Cystoscopy

20. Which of the following invasive procedures has been shown to have efficacy compared with placebo-sham therapy in CP/CPPS?

a. Radical transurethral resection of the prostate
b. Transurethral balloon dilatation of prostate/bladder neck
c. Transurethral incision of the bladder neck
d. Microwave heat therapy
e. Transurethral needle ablation

ANSWERS

1. **b. 2% to 10%.** Population-based studies employing the validated National Institutes of Health Chronic Prostatitis Symptom Index (NIH-CPSI) showed that the prevalence of prostatitis-like symptoms in the general population of men was between 2% and 10% (8.0% in Malaysia, 6.6% in Canada, 2.7% in Singapore, and approximately 2.2% in older men in Olmsted County, Minnesota.
2. **b. Enterobacteriaceae.** The most common cause of bacterial prostatitis is the Enterobacteriaceae family of gram-negative bacteria.
3. **e. unknown.** A careful review of the evidence for and against the role of microorganisms—culturable, fastidious, or nonculturable—leaves the reviewer undecided, and etiologic mechanisms other than microorganisms must be considered.
4. **d. differentiates CPPS Category IIIA from Category IIIB.** The differentiation of the two subtypes of category III CPPS is dependent on cytologic examination of the urine and/or EPS.
5. **b. A research tool that is useful in clinical practice.** The National Institutes of Health Chronic Prostatitis Collaborative Research Network developed a reproducible and valid instrument to measure the symptoms and quality of life/impact of chronic prostatitis for use in research protocols as well as in clinical practice. The symptom index has also proved its usefulness in the evaluation and follow-up of patients in general clinical urologic practice.
6. **b. Perform a transrectal ultrasonographic examination.** Development of a prostate abscess is best detected with transrectal ultrasonography. Patients with acute bacterial prostatitis are easily diagnosed and successfully treated with appropriate antibiotic therapy, as long as the clinician keeps a high index of suspicion for prostate abscess in patients who fail to respond quickly to the antibiotics.
7. **c. Category IIIA.** Diagnosis of category IIIA CP/CPPS, or inflammatory CPPS, is based on the presence of excessive leukocytes in EPS, a post-prostatic massage urine sample, or semen.
8. **d. Category IIIB.** Diagnosis of category IIIB CP/CPPS, or noninflammatory CPPS, rests on no significant leukocytes being found in similar specimens.
9. **b. Category II.** Category I is identical to the acute bacterial prostatitis category of the traditional classification system. Category II is identical to the traditional chronic bacterial prostatitis classification.
10. **e. Restart fluoroquinolone antibiotics.** The most important clue in the diagnosis of category II, chronic bacterial prostatitis, is a history of documented recurrent urinary tract infections. The fluoroquinolone should be continued for a minimum of 4 weeks.
11. **c. Video-urodynamics.** A wide constellation of irritative and obstructive voiding symptoms is associated with CP/CPPS. Proposed etiologies to account for the persistent irritative and obstructive voiding symptoms include detrusor vesical neck or external sphincter dyssynergia, proximal or distal urethral obstruction, and fibrosis or hypertrophy of the vesical neck. Whereas flow rate and bladder scan can be done to further delineate these conditions, these abnormalities can be clarified and diagnosed best by urodynamics, particularly video-urodynamics.
12. **b. Several days of nitrofurantoin therapy followed by a lower urinary tract localization test.** In a patient who has acute cystitis, the localization of bacteria in the EPS or VB3 specimen (postprostatic massage sample) is impossible, and, in this case, the patient can be treated with a short course (1 to 3 days) of antibiotics such as nitrofurantoin, which penetrates the prostate poorly but eradicates the bladder bacteriuria.

Subsequent localization of bacteria in the postprostatic massage urine sample or EPS sample is then diagnostic of category II prostatitis.

13. **d. trimethoprim.** Studies of animals with and without infection showed that trimethoprim concentrated in prostatic secretion and prostatic interstitial fluid (exceeding plasma levels) whereas sulfamethoxazole and ampicillin did not. It would be appropriate, therefore, to not prescribe the combination trimethoprim-sulfamethoxazole in a patient with multiple allergies.

14. **a. Low-dose prophylactic antibiotics.** Prolonged therapy with low-dose prophylactic or suppressive antimicrobial agents can be considered for recurrent or refractory prostatitis, respectively.

15. **d. Biofeedback.** On the basis of the possibility that the voiding and pain symptoms associated with CPPS may be secondary to some form of pseudodyssynergia during voiding or repetitive perineal muscle spasm, biofeedback has the potential to improve this process. Bladder neck incision in a young man should be avoided until after he has his family because of the possibility of retrograde ejaculation.

16. **c. Transurethral drainage.** In patients who fail to respond quickly to antibiotics, a prostatic abscess is optimally drained by the transurethral incision route, although ultraso percutaneous aspiration (via any route) could be d

17. **e. Categories II and III.** After 1 month of therapy irst. category II patients, 47% of category IIIA patients category IIIB patients had resolution of their sympt Randomized placebo-controlled trials have shown terazosin, alfuzosin, and tamsulosin in patients with

18. **d. Neuromodulators.** While there is considerable exc about the possibility of neuromodulatory therapy pro significant benefit for CPPS patients, there have been randomized placebo controlled trials to confirm this. controlled trials have examined the efficacy of antibioti α-adrenergic blockers, anti-inflammatory agents, horm therapies, and phytotherapies.

19. **a. Observation.** Asymptomatic inflammatory prostatitis (category IV) by definition does not require symptomatic therapy.

20. **d. Microwave heat therapy.** Although many uncontrolled t employing heat therapy have shown benefit, three published studies have used sham controls.

10

Painful Bladder Syndrome/Interstitial Cystitis and Related Disorders

PHILIP M. HANNO

QUESTIONS

1. Essential for the diagnosis of painful bladder syndrome/ interstitial cystitis (PBS/IC) is the presence of:
   a. urinary urgency.
   b. pain or discomfort related to the bladder.
   c. glomerulations on cystoscopy.
   d. Hunner's ulcer.
   e. urinary frequency.
2. The definition of interstitial cystitis proposed by the National Institute of Diabetes, Digestive and Kidney Diseases (NIDDK) is best considered a:
   a. de facto definition of the disease.
   b. diagnostic pathway.
   c. definition applicable mainly to clinical research studies.
   d. historic document of no current value.
   e. purely symptom-based description of PBS/IC.
3. The best circumstantial evidence for a urine abnormality in IC comes from what finding?
   a. The absence of pain when a Foley catheter is left indwelling
   b. Relief of symptoms as a result of using narcotic analgesics
   c. Failure of conduit diversion to relieve symptoms
   d. Late occurrence of pain and bowel segment contraction after substitution cystoplasty and continent diversion
   e. Symptom relief associated with urinary alkalinization
4. IC symptom and problem indices have been validated to:
   a. monitor disease progression or regression with or without treatment.
   b. correctly choose who should undergo cystectomy and diversion.
   c. determine on whom to perform diagnostic testing.
   d. accurately diagnose PBS/IC.
   e. determine appropriate candidates for clinical research.
5. Which of the following statements best categorizes the natural history of PBS/IC?
   a. The onset is generally insidious, occurring gradually over many years.
   b. Major deterioration in symptom severity is the rule.
   c. Symptoms follow a culture-documented urinary tract infection.
   d. Symptom resolution occurs regardless of treatment after 1 to 2 years.
   e. Subacute onset with full development of the symptom-complex occurs over a relatively short time span.
6. Which statement best describes the relationship of PBS/IC to bladder cancer?
   a. PBS/IC is a premalignant lesion.
   b. PBS/IC is often associated with bladder cancer.
   c. A positive urine cytology can safely be ignored in patients with PBS/IC.
   d. No reports have documented an association of PBS/IC with subsequent development of bladder cancer.
   e. Dysplasia is a typical pathologic finding on bladder biopsy in PBS/IC patients.
7. The only animal with a known syndrome that appears to mimic IC is the:
   a. cat.
   b. rabbit.
   c. dog.
   d. goat.
   e. rat.
8. The antibiotic of choice in IC is:
   a. doxycycline.
   b. none.
   c. gentamicin.
   d. ciprofloxacin.
   e. amoxicillin.
9. The cell most likely to play a central role in the pathogenesis of IC is the:
   a. granulocyte.
   b. lymphocyte.
   c. mast cell.
   d. platelet.
   e. eosinophil.
10. Which statement best categorizes the potassium chloride test?
    a. It is soothing and calming to the painful bladder.
    b. It has high sensitivity and specificity for diagnosing PBS/IC.
    c. It is an important element in choosing effective therapy.
    d. It provides proof of abnormal mucosal permeability.
    e. None of the above.

11. Bladder ulceration:
    a. is required to make a diagnosis of PBS/IC.
    b. is generally found in less than 10% of IC patients.
    c. was not considered a part of the syndrome when it was initially described by Hunner.
    d. is synonymous with glomerulation.
    e. is pathognomonic of PBS/IC even in the absence of symptoms.
12. Exclusive use of the NIDDK criteria to diagnose PBS/IC would result in:
    a. an accurate depiction of the true prevalence of the condition.
    b. an improved treatment algorithm.
    c. increased diagnostic specificity.
    d. increased diagnostic sensitivity.
    e. a minimum of diagnostic testing and significant cost savings.
13. The disorder most commonly associated with PBS/IC is
    a. irritable bowel syndrome.
    b. incontinence.
    c. lupus.
    d. allergy.
    e. fibromyalgia.
14. Where is the antiproliferative factor (APF) produced?
    a. Bladder urothelial cells
    b. Glomeruli
    c. Transitional urothelial cells in the upper tracts
    d. Mast cells
    e. Neutrophils
15. The postulated direct effect of antiproliferative factor is to:
    a. increase afferent neuron sensitivity.
    b. increase potassium efflux into urothelial cells.
    c. protect the surface glycosaminoglycan layer.
    d. elevate leukotriene levels.
    e. regulate growth factor production by bladder epithelial cells.
16. The central role of histopathology in IC is to:
    a. determine whether the patient has ulcerative or nonulcerative IC.
    b. help determine the most efficacious treatment modality.
    c. predict prognosis.
    d. rule out other disorders that might be responsible for the symptoms.
    e. confirm the diagnosis with pathologic criteria.
17. Which of the following has the least in common with PBS/IC?
    a. Vulvodynia
    b. Chronic bacterial prostatitis
    c. Orchialgia
    d. Penile pain
    e. Perineal and scrotal pain
18. Urodynamic findings typical of IC include:
    a. uninhibited detrusor contractions.
    b. obstructed flow patterns.
    c. abnormal bladder compliance.
    d. decreased capacity and hypersensitivity.
    e. increased volume at first urge to void.
19. The finding of glomerulations:
    a. is significant only when cystoscopy is performed with the patient under anesthesia.
    b. is of no consequence in an asymptomatic patient.
    c. indicates a likelihood of response to laser fulguration of the bladder.
    d. is present only in patients with PBS/IC.
    e. is sufficient to make a diagnosis of PBS/IC.
20. The incidence of short-term spontaneous remission in IC approaches:
    a. 50%.
    b. 100%.
    c. 30%.
    d. 10%.
    e. 75%.
21. Which test is potentially helpful for diagnosis, prognosis, and therapy?
    a. Potassium chloride test
    b. Intravesical heparin
    c. Bladder hydrodistention
    d. Bladder biopsy
    e. Urodynamics
22. Which of the following treatments is targeted to the glycosaminoglycan layer of the bladder?
    a. Sodium pentosan polysulfate
    b. Amitriptyline
    c. Hydroxyzine
    d. L-Arginine
    e. None of the above
23. Which of the following intravesical treatments has shown proven efficacy for PBS/IC in pivotal U. S. Food and Drug Administration trials?
    a. BCG (bacillus Calmette-Guérin)
    b. Hyaluronic acid
    c. Botulinum toxin
    d. Heparin
    e. None of the above
24. Which of the following statements is true of narcotic analgesics?
    a. They have no place in the treatment of a chronic, nonmalignant condition such as IC.
    b. They make patients physically dependent on them.
    c. They generally result in drug addiction when used for chronic pain.
    d. They tend to cause diarrhea and sleeplessness.
    e. All of the above.
25. Which of the following is a reasonable surgical procedure to relieve the pain of IC?
    a. Transurethral fulguration of Hunner's ulcer
    b. Reduction cystoplasty
    c. Sympathectomy and intraspinal alcohol injections
    d. Cystolysis
    e. Transvesical infiltration of the pelvic plexuses with phenol
26. The most important early step in the management of PBS/IC is:
    a. beginning intravesical treatment.
    b. patient education.
    c. initiating pentosan polysulfate therapy.
    d. physical therapy.
    e. strict adherence to "IC" diet.

27. The chronic urethral syndrome and IC can be differentiated by:
    a. symptom-complex.
    b. response to antibiotic treatment.
    c. natural history.
    d. name only.
    e. response to urethral dilatation.
28. A finding of detrusor overactivity on urodynamics in a patient with bladder pain in the absence of urinary frequency or urgency indicates:
    a. treatment is antimuscarinic medication.
    b. PBS/IC is not present.
    c. urinary tract infection is likely.
    d. neuromodulation is the most effective treatment.
    e. none of the above.
29. Men with irritative voiding symptoms and pelvic pain should be evaluated for:
    a. chronic pelvic pain syndrome.
    b. bacterial prostatitis.
    c. PBS/IC.
    d. bladder carcinoma in situ.
    e. all of the above.
30. The symptoms of PBS/IC are mostly allodynic. This implies that:
    a. they are related to fluid intake.
    b. they do not affect life expectancy.
    c. they have pain as the primary component.
    d. they do not respond to therapy.
    e. they are an exaggeration of normal sensations.
31. The most common endoscopic finding in PBS/IC is:
    a. glomerulations with distention under regional or general anesthesia.
    b. glomerulations under local cystoscopy.
    c. Hunner's ulceration with distention under regional or general anesthesia.
    d. normal mucosa appearance with distention under regional or local anesthesia.
    e. diffuse mucosal hemorrhage under local anesthesia.
32. The urgency of PBS/IC is driven by a fear of:
    a. incontinence.
    b. frequency.
    c. hematuria.
    d. pain.
    e. dysuria.
33. Population studies comparing disease prevalence by country are unreliable because:
    a. there is a lack of an accepted definition of the syndrome being studied.
    b. there is no validated diagnostic marker of the PBS/IC syndrome.
    c. methodology differs among studies.
    d. pathophysiology and etiology are unclear.
    e. all of the above.
34. The extraordinary urinary frequency syndrome of childhood can be differentiated from PBS/IC by:
    a. cystoscopy.
    b. duration of symptoms.
    c. urodynamics.
    d. pathologic findings on bladder biopsy.
    e. family history.
35. Which of the following is not a glycosaminoglycan?
    a. Heparin sulfate
    b. Hyaluronic acid
    c. Hydrogen sulfate
    d. Dermatan sulfate
    e. Chondroitin-4-sulfate
36. The relationship of stress to PBS/IC is best categorized as:
    a. stress initiates the pathologic cascade that results in the syndrome.
    b. stress plays no role in the syndrome.
    c. stress can increase severity of symptoms.
    d. anxiolytics are a mainstay of treatment.
    e. surgical stress often is responsible for initial disease onset.
37. The transition of nonulcerative to ulcerative PBS/IC is:
    a. a common occurrence.
    b. a rare event.
    c. a response to treatment.
    d. a primary reason for cystoscopic surveillance.
    e. a result of intravesical therapy.
38. Electron microscopy in the definitive diagnosis of PBS/IC is:
    a. essential for proper diagnosis and therapy.
    b. for clinical research studies only, where definitive diagnosis is necessary.
    c. a useful but extremely expensive adjunct to diagnosis.
    d. effective because of its ability to accurately assess the glycosaminoglycan layer of the bladder.
    e. not of use.
39. In a patient who presents with a history of bladder pain, frequency, and urgency with urge incontinence, the first step in evaluation should include:
    a. empirical treatment with sodium pentosan polysulfate for 6 months.
    b. bladder distention using anesthesia.
    c. dietary modification.
    d. imaging studies of the urinary tract.
    e. pressure-flow urodynamics.

ANSWERS

1. **b. pain or discomfort related to the bladder.** Urgency, frequency, and the presence of glomerulations or Hunner's ulcer on endoscopy are often associated with PBS/IC, but the presence of pain or discomfort is the primary component. IC may form a subgroup of the painful bladder group, but the criteria are not clear, and at this point the terms can be used interchangeably.
2. **c. definition applicable mainly to clinical research studies.** It was never meant to define the disease but rather was developed to ensure that patients included in basic and clinical research studies were homogeneous enough that experts could agree on the diagnosis.
3. **d. Late occurrence of pain and bowel segment contraction after substitution cystoplasty and continent diversion.** Substitution cystoplasty and continent diversion both fail in some IC patients because of the development of pain in the bowel segment used or contraction of the bowel segment. Some studies have shown histologic changes in bowel segments used in IC patients similar to those that occur in the IC bladder. Both of these findings provide circumstantial evidence that the

urine of IC patients may have toxicity associated with the symptomatic expression of the disorder. However, recent data with regard to antiproliferative factor make this evidence suspect.

4. **a. monitor disease progression or regression with or without treatment.** IC symptom and problem indices like the one developed by O'Leary and Sant are not intended to diagnose IC. Like the American Urologic Association Symptom Score for benign prostatic hypertrophy, these indices are designed to evaluate the severity of symptoms and to monitor disease progression or regression and response to treatment.

5. **e. Subacute onset with full development of the symptom-complex over a relatively short time span.** Several epidemiologic studies have concluded that the onset of IC is commonly subacute rather than insidious. It presents more like one would expect an infectious disorder to present, rather than like a chronic disease process. Full development of the classic symptom-complex takes place over a relatively short period of time. In the majority of cases, it does not progress continuously but reaches its final stage rapidly and then continues without significant change in overall symptoms.

6. **d. No reports have documented an association of PBS/IC with subsequent development of bladder cancer.** In the 1970s, the Mayo Clinic documented bladder cancer in 12 of 53 men who had been treated for IC but the association was the result of incorrect diagnosis rather than progression. Peters and others have noted that patients with bladder cancer can be misdiagnosed as having PBS/IC.

7. **a. cat.** The feline urologic syndrome may represent the animal equivalent of IC. Approximately two thirds of cats with lower urinary tract disease have sterile urine and no evidence of other urinary tract disorders. A portion of these cats experience frequency and urgency of urination, pain, and bladder inflammation. Glomerulations have been found in some of these cat bladders. Other findings similar to IC include bladder mastocytosis, increased histamine excretion, and increased bladder permeability.

8. **b. none.** Antibiotics are not indicated for the treatment of IC, nor have they been implicated as a causative factor. Numerous studies have concluded that it is unlikely that active infection is involved in the ongoing pathologic process or that antibiotics have a role to play in treatment.

9. **c. mast cell.** Mast cells are strategically localized in the urinary bladder close to blood vessels, lymphatics, nerves, and detrusor smooth muscle. IC appears to be a syndrome with neural, immune, and endocrine components in which activated mast cells play a central, although not primary, role in many patients.

10. **e. None of the above.** Up to 25% of patients meeting the NIDDK criteria for IC will have a negative KCl test. It is positive in the majority of patients with radiation cystitis, urinary tract infection, and nonbacterial prostatitis and in women with pelvic pain. It is neither sensitive nor specific for PBS/IC, is uncomfortable for the patients, and does not help to guide therapeutic decisions.

11. **b. is generally found in less than 10% of IC patients.** Bladder ulceration (so-called Hunner's ulcer) is more appropriately referred to as Hunner's patch and is found in only a small proportion of patients with symptoms of IC, certainly less than 10%. A circumscribed red patch that cracks and bleeds with distention is best appreciated with the patient under anesthesia.

12. **c. increased diagnostic specificity.** Ninety percent of expert clinicians in the NIDDK database study agreed that patients diagnosed with IC by those criteria had IC. However, 60% of patients diagnosed by these clinicians as having IC did not fulfill the NIDDK criteria. Using the criteria as a basis for diagnosis would probably exclude the majority of patients with this symptom-complex from the correct diagnosis.

13. **d. allergy.** Forty-one percent of IC patients have been diagnosed with allergies, and 45% suffer from allergic symptoms. Fibromyalgia and irritable bowel syndrome are also overrepresented in the IC population. Vulvodynia, migraine headaches, endometriosis, chronic fatigue syndrome, incontinence, and asthma have prevalence similar to that in the general population. Systemic lupus erythematosus can cause bladder symptoms that are difficult to distinguish from IC.

14. **a. Bladder urothelial cells.** APF can be obtained from cultured uroepithelial cells and is not present in renal pelvic urine. It is associated with decreased production of heparin-binding epidermal growth factor–like growth factor.

15. **e. regulate growth factor production by bladder epithelial cells.** It has been postulated that any of a variety of injuries to the bladder (infection, trauma, overdistention) in a susceptible individual may result in PBS/IC if APF is present and suppresses production of heparin-binding epidermal growth factor–like growth factor.

16. **d. rule out other disorders that might be responsible for the symptoms.** The differentiation between ulcerative and nonulcerative IC is based on endoscopic features. There is no pathognomonic histologic finding for the disorder, nor can histology predict prognosis. Even a severely abnormal microscopic picture does not necessarily indicate a poor prognosis. At this time, no data suggest that the treatment algorithm can be rationally predicated on the basis of the histologic findings.

17. **b. Chronic bacterial prostatitis.** IC can be considered one of the pain syndromes of the urogenital and rectal area, all of which are well described but poorly understood. These include vulvodynia, orchialgia, perineal pain, penile pain, and rectal pain. Bacterial prostatitis is a well-understood entity with a known etiology and generally responds to treatment directed at the offending organism. It has no relationship to IC.

18. **d. decreased capacity and hypersensitivity.** Cystometry in conscious IC patients generally demonstrates normal function, the exception being decreased bladder capacity and hypersensitivity, perhaps exaggerated by the use of carbon dioxide as a medium. Pain on bladder filling, which reproduces the patient's symptoms, is very suggestive of IC. Bladder compliance in patients with IC is normal, as hypersensitivity would prevent the bladder from filling to the point of noncompliance.

19. **b. is of no consequence in an asymptomatic patient.** Glomerulations are not specific for IC, and only when seen in conjunction with the clinical criteria of pain and frequency can the presence of glomerulations be viewed as significant. Glomerulations can be seen after radiation therapy, in patients with bladder carcinoma, after exposure to toxic chemicals or chemotherapeutic agents, and in patients undergoing dialysis or after urinary diversion when the bladder has not filled for extended periods. They have also been reported in the majority of men with prostate pain syndromes.

20. **a. 50%.** There is a 50% incidence of temporary remission unrelated to therapy, with a mean duration of 8 months. The clinical course of IC is extremely variable, and it can be difficult to differentiate the effects of treatment from the natural history of the disease.

21. **c. Bladder hydrodistention.** Bladder hydrodistention with the patient under anesthesia is often the first therapeutic modality employed for IC, frequently as part of the diagnostic

evaluation. Between 30% and 50% of patients experience some short-term relief in symptoms after the procedure. About 30% will note a brief exacerbation in their symptoms. A bladder capacity under anesthesia of less than 200 mL is a sign of poor prognosis.

22. **a. Sodium pentosan polysulfate.** The target of sodium pentosan polysulfate therapy is the GAG layer of the urothelium. This agent is an oral analogue of heparin. About 6% of an ingested dose is excreted in the urine. The proposed mechanism of action is the correction of a GAG dysfunction, thus presumably reversing the abnormal epithelial permeability in about 30% of patients in placebo-controlled trials.

23. **e. None of the above.** None of these treatments has been proven efficacious for PBS/IC in double-blind placebo-controlled trials. Hyaluronic acid in both high and low concentrations and BCG have recently failed to show significant efficacy in large, multicenter American trials.

24. **b. They make patient physically dependent on them.** Narcotic analgesics can be very useful in a subset of IC patients with severe disease. Unlike other classes of analgesics, they have no therapeutic ceiling, dosing being limited by tolerance of side effects. They tend to cause constipation and can cause some sedation. Physical dependence is unavoidable, but physical addiction, a chronic disorder characterized by the compulsive use of a substance resulting in physical, psychological, or social harm to the user and the continued use despite that harm, is rare.

25. **a. Transurethral fulguration of Hunner's ulcer.** Transurethral fulguration or laser irradiation of Hunner's ulcer can provide symptomatic relief. None of the other procedures listed has any place in the treatment of IC.

26. **b. patient education.** This condition is incurable, the symptoms wax and wane, and remissions are not uncommon. It lends itself to practitioner abuse, and the uninformed, desperate patient is easy prey. Treatment is symptom-driven, and an informed patient makes the best decisions.

27. **d. name only.** The symptomatic manifestations of IC and those of chronic urethral syndrome are indistinguishable. *Chronic urethral syndrome* is a historical term no longer used in the medical literature.

28. **e. none of the above.** Clinically insignificant detrusor overactivity may be seen in 14% of patients with PBS/IC, a rate of involuntary contractions that has been reported in normal individuals undergoing ambulatory urodynamics. The finding does not rule out the diagnosis of PBS/IC, and treatment of this finding would be unlikely to result in improvement of the patient's bladder pain.

29. **e. all of the above.** IC should be considered in the differential diagnosis of voiding disorders in men accompanied by irritative symptoms and pelvic pain. A rigorous IC evaluation can be useful in differentiating IC from bladder carcinoma in situ, functional or anatomic bladder outlet obstruction, and bacterial prostatitis. Many men with IC have undergone what has proved to be unnecessary and ill-founded bladder neck surgery.

30. **e. they are an exaggeration of normal sensations.** Allodynia is defined as "Pain from stimuli which are not normally painful. The pain may occur other than in the area stimulated." When referring to PBS/IC it suggests that the normal sensations of bladder filling and urgency have become pathologic in intensity and may no longer be directly related to the area stimulated.

31. **a. glomerulations with distention under regional or general anesthesia.** Although glomerulations are not specific for PBS/IC, they are often found in patients undergoing cystoscopy with bladder distention under anesthesia. Their presence or absence is not necessary to make a diagnosis.

32. **d. pain.** Pain and pressure are more involved in the frequency of PBS/IC and fear of incontinence drives the urgency of overactive bladder syndrome.

33. **e. all of the above.** Variations in prevalence range from 1.2 per 100,000 in Japan to 20% of the American population. A new paradigm is needed to study the epidemiology of PBS/IC.

34. **b. duration of symptoms.** The extraordinary urinary frequency syndrome of childhood is a self-limited condition of unknown etiology.

35. **c. Hydrogen sulfate.** A defect in the epithelial permeability barrier of the bladder surface glycosaminoglycans may play a role in PBS/IC.

36. **c. stress can increase severity of symptoms.** There are no data to suggest that stress initiates the chronic syndrome of IC, although it certainly can increase symptom severity.

37. **b. a rare event.** Transition from nonulcerative to ulcerative PBS/IC is a rare event, and pathologically the two types of IC may be completely separate entities.

38. **e. not of use.** Attempts to definitively diagnose IC by electron microscopy have been unsuccessful.

39. **e. pressure-flow urodynamics.** This case is complex and will require urodynamics to help determine the presence of detrusor overactivity and its role in the patient's symptoms. A new onset of detrusor overactivity and incontinence may suggest the need for neurologic consultation.

11

Sexually Transmitted Diseases

TARA FRENKL • JEANNETTE POTTS

QUESTIONS

1. The lifetime prevalence of HPV among sexually active women is approximately:
   a. 90%.
   b. 60% to 80%.
   c. 50%.
   d. 20% to 40%.
   e. less than 10%.
2. A very uncomfortable 36-year-old businessman returning from Thailand presents to his urologist with a 4-day history of worsening testicular swelling and pain. He has also noted dysuria but no penile discharge. The best empirical therapy is:
   a. ciprofloxacin, 500 mg PO, plus doxycycline BID times 7 days.
   b. ciprofloxacin, 500 mg PO, plus azithromycin, 1 g PO.
   c. ceftriaxone, 125 mg IM.
   d. Achromycin, 2 g PO.
   e. ceftriaxone, 125 mg IM, plus azithromycin, 1 g PO.
3. Trichomoniasis:
   a. can be treated using metronidazole in pregnant women during the second trimester.
   b. responds to a single dose of 500 mg of metronidazole.
   c. like many sexually transmitted diseases is more likely to be asymptomatic in women than in men.
   d. can be treated twice daily with metronidazole for 7 days but with greater gastrointestinal side effects than the single dose therapy.
   e. can be harbored in the mouth and rectum.
4. A 62-year-old widower presents to his urologist concerned about a large painless, exfoliating lesion on his glans. He has no inguinal lymphadenopathy. He has been sexually active with one partner for the past 4 months. He has chronic bacterial prostatitis, and his urologist had recently initiated daily suppressive therapy with trimethoprim-sulfamethoxazole. The most likely diagnosis is:
   a. chancroid.
   b. amebiasis.
   c. lichen planus.
   d. drug reaction.
   e. primary syphilis.
5. A 32-year-old married man seeks counsel because his wife has been recently diagnosed with HPV on her annual cervical Papanicolaou smear. The couple has been married 8 years. Patient consumes alcohol in moderation and smokes half a pack of cigarettes per day. His history reveals no lower urinary tract symptoms, and his genital examination is normal. A microscopic urinalysis is acellular. His urologist should advise him to:
   a. undergo androscopy.
   b. use condoms indefinitely.
   c. apply one course of 5-FU empirically.
   d. quit smoking.
   e. seek marriage counseling.
6. HIV testing should always be a consideration in any patient with possible STD exposure; however, which one of the following scenarios is least worrisome for HIV exposure or transmission?
   a. A patient suspected to have syphilis
   b. A patient with several umbilicated papules consistent with MCV in the groin and lower abdomen
   c. A woman with recurrent vaginal yeast infections
   d. A man who has a small papillomatous lesion on his shaft
   e. A person who had polymerase chain reaction–proven chancroid, treated 5 years ago
7. Which one of the following statements about women and STDs is TRUE?
   a. Chancroid affects more women than it does men.
   b. Women with HSV are usually easily identified by the presence of vesicular eruptions in the perivaginal area.
   c. Cervical cancer may be considered an AIDS-defining illness.
   d. Women tend to seek prompt medical attention due to the high probability of symptomatology attributed to STDs.
   e. Urologists can easily differentiate women with UTIs from those with vaginal infections by taking a thorough history of their lower urinary tract symptoms.
8. Of the antibiotics listed below the only group that is safe during pregnancy is:
   a. erythromycin, azithromycin, ceftriaxone.
   b. erythromycin, penicillin, tetracycline.
   c. metronidazole, tetracycline, amoxicillin.
   d. doxycycline, azithromycin, trimethoprim-sulfamethoxazole.
   e. ciprofloxacin, cefixime, erythromycin.

9. A patient diagnosed with a primary infection due to HSV 2:
   a. has probably had HSV 1 in the past.
   b. can expect to have fewer recurrences than patients with HSV 1.
   c. can expect to engage in intercourse safely without risk of transmission as soon as the lesions heal.
   d. may have buccal lesions as well as genital ulcers.
   e. should immediately begin suppression therapy.
10. If a patient presents with a history or signs suspicious for syphilis, a urologist should consider all of these facts, EXCEPT:
   a. sensitivity for RPR and VDRL combined is 100% in secondary syphilis.
   b. RPR and VDRL decrease and normalize with successful therapy.
   c. positive HIV status may lead to higher false-negative serologic studies.
   d. RPR and VDRL have a high rate of false-positive results.
   e. fluorescent treponemal antibody (FTA) should be the initial screening test.
11. A 24-year-old female graduate student who "always" uses condoms, presents with her first ever vesicular eruption on her labia, which appeared 2 days ago. Bilateral inguinal adenopathy is appreciated on examination, and the area is somewhat tender. The most important confirmatory test for this patient at this time is:
   a. darkfield microscopy of the specimen scraped from the wound.
   b. vaginal swabs for *Chlamydia* L1, L2, L3.
   c. viral cultures for HSV.
   d. PCR assay for *Haemophilus ducreyi.*
   e. serum RPR or VDRL
12. A 29-year-old homosexual male notices mild dysuria with a mucopurulent discharge within 2 weeks of the most recent sexual encounter. After obtaining cultures, you initiate empirical therapy using a single dose of:
   a. azithromycin, 1 g PO.
   b. ciprofloxacin, 500 mg PO.
   c. ciprofloxacin, 1000 mg PO.
   d. ceftriaxone, 125 mg IM.
   e. Levofloxacin, 250 mg PO.
13. A patient is concerned about the sudden appearance of a single 1.5-cm ulcer with irregular borders. It is located on the distal part of his shaft and part of the proximal portion of his glands. The urologist recognizes the following facts EXCEPT:
   a. genital ulcers can also result from noninfectious causes.
   b. sensitivity for identification based on appearance alone is 31% to 35%.
   c. co-infection of STDs occurs in approximately 10% of patients.
   d. diagnosis can be reliably made by combining the appearance of the ulcer with the characteristic of inguinal adenopathy.
   e. confirmatory cultures and serologic studies should be performed whenever possible.

ANSWERS

1. **b. 60% to 80%.** Epidemiologic studies indicate that this virus is extremely prevalent among sexually active women.
2. **e. ceftriaxone, 125 mg IM, plus azithromycin, 1 g PO.** Although ciprofloxacin is highly effective for the treatment of gonococcus, a quinolone-resistant strain has emerged in eastern Asia and the South Pacific. Either doxycycline or azithromycin would be appropriate to treat possible co-infection with *Chlamydia.*
3. **a. can be treated using metronidazole in pregnant women during the second trimester.** Metronidazole is safe during the second trimester of pregnancy, and as a single 2-g dose or a better-tolerated regimen of 500 mg BID × 7 days can be administered to nonpregnant patients as well.
4. **d. drug reaction.** While it would not be incorrect to suspect and test for an STD, a fixed drug reaction is the most probable condition in this setting.
5. **d. quit smoking.** An abnormal Papanicolaou smear does not imply infidelity given the long and variable latency of HPV. The only meaningful and practical suggestion is to recommend smoking cessation, because smoking in either partner is associated with higher rates of progression and malignancy.
6. **d. A man who has a small papillomatous lesion on his shaft.** Because of the ubiquitous nature of papillomatous lesions, it would be inappropriate to screen such patients for HIV, in the absence of any other risk factors.
7. **c. Cervical cancer may be considered an AIDS-defining illness.** Women are likely to contract STDs and suffer more from the consequences due to late diagnosis and prolonged asymptomatic periods. Because a woman's immune status can influence the behavior of HPV, cervical cancer is considered an AIDS-defining illness in patients who are HIV positive, similar to the way in which AIDS is defined in HIV-positive patients who are newly diagnosed with *Pneumocystis carinii.*
8. **a. erythromycin, azithromycin, ceftriaxone.**
9. **d. may have buccal lesions as well as genital ulcers.** Patients diagnosed with primary infection due to HSV 2 may expect more recurrences than in setting of type 1 infection, can have buccal lesions, and will have asymptomatic shedding for up to 3 months after the first outbreak.
10. **e. fluorescent treponemal antibody (FTA) should be the initial screening test.** Because of decreased sensitivity in the setting of primary syphilis, FTA should not be part of initial screening. However, the physician must be aware of false-positive VDRL and RPR, as well as the better sensitivity.
11. **c. viral cultures for HSV.** The most likely diagnosis is herpes simplex virus, given the latency period and tender, bilateral inguinal adenopathy and patient demographics. The most important point about this question, however, is the fact that condoms are not effective in preventing all infections.
12. **d. ceftriaxone, 125 mg IM.** Not only have quinolone-resistant strains of gonococcus affected Asia, but they have also become more frequently detected in homosexual males in the United States. Therefore, ceftriaxone would remain the most appropriate first choice for treatment.
13. **d. diagnosis can be reliably made by combining the appearance of the ulcer with the characteristic of inguinal adenopathy.**

12

Urologic Implications of AIDS and HIV Infection

JOHN N. KRIEGER

QUESTIONS

1. Life expectancy in the countries most affected by HIV infection was:
   a. reduced as much as 15 years by the year 2000.
   b. reduced as much as 5 years by the year 2003.
   c. unchanged.
   d. reduced as much as 10 years by the year 2004.
   e. increased by 5 years.
2. With the availability of antiretroviral therapy, blood screening, and treatment of sexually transmitted infections, the number of new HIV infections in the United States has:
   a. decreased dramatically.
   b. decreased to less than 10,000 per year.
   c. remained at a plateau of 40,000 infections per year.
   d. increased, but at a slower rate of 100,000 per year.
   e. increased to 75,000 per year.
3. Factors that influence sexual transmission of HIV include all of the following EXCEPT:
   a. sexually transmitted infections.
   b. antiretroviral therapy.
   c. circumcision status.
   d. anti-inflammatory therapy.
   e. gynecologic factors.
4. The typical course of untreated HIV infection includes all of the following EXCEPT:
   a. takes 8 to 12 years from infection to death in the absence of treatment.
   b. has three, distinct phases.
   c. occurs in 60% to 70% of patients.
   d. takes more than 15 years from infection to death in the absence of treatment.
   e. is determined largely during the initial phase of infection.
5. The virologic set point indicates:
   a. response to antiretroviral therapy.
   b. risk for disease progression.
   c. prospects for HIV eradication.
   d. effect of HAART on the viral reservoirs in lymphoid tissue.
   e. time from infection.
6. With complete and sustained suppression of HIV replication by antiretroviral therapy, it is estimated that HIV could be eliminated from an infected person in what time period?
   a. 2 to 3 years
   b. 3 to 6 months
   c. 5 years
   d. 10 years or more
7. Herpetic lesions in an HIV-infected patient are not responding well to oral acyclovir. Which of the following should be done?
   a. Obtain genital herpes culture and sensitivity testing
   b. Determine the patient's HIV viral load and CD4 count
   c. Change to an alternative oral drug
   d. Change to IV acyclovir
   e. Add photodynamic therapy
8. The optimal approach to suspected voiding dysfunction in an HIV-infected patient begins with:
   a. urodynamic testing.
   b. standard pharmacologic measures.
   c. antiviral therapy.
   d. checking viral load.
   e. clean intermittent catheterization.
9. Most patients with presumed indinavir-containing urinary calculi require:
   a. ESWL.
   b. ureteroscopy.
   c. noncontrast CT for diagnosis.
   d. hydration, analgesics, and temporary cessation of indinavir.
   e. Changing to an alternative protease inhibitor.
10. Which statement about HIVAN is incorrect?
    a. It is more common in black patients.
    b. It seldom presents as renal insufficiency.
    c. It may present with proteinuria.
    d. It often responds to HAART.
    e. Ultrasound shows echogenic kidneys with preserved size.
11. Kaposi's sarcoma:
    a. usually presents as renal disease.
    b. has an incidence that has changed little since the advent of HAART.
    c. is related to co-infection with both HIV and a herpesvirus.
    d. is related to activation of epithelial cells.
    e. is most common in patients who use IV drugs.

ANSWERS

1. **a. reduced as much as 15 years by the year 2000.** Life expectancy in the most affected sub-Saharan countries was reduced as much as 15 years by the year 2000, compared with projections without HIV.
2. **c. remained at a plateau of 40,000 infections per year.** Despite antiretroviral therapy, blood screening, and treatment of sexually transmitted infections, the number of infections has remained at a plateau of 40,000 new HIV infections/year in the United States over the past decade.
3. **d. anti-inflammatory therapy.** Anti-inflammatory therapy is the only factor that has NOT been implicated as an epidemiologic risk factor for sexual transmission of HIV. Sexually transmitted diseases, antiretroviral therapy, circumcision status, and gynecologic factors have all been shown to influence the risk for sexual transmission of HIV.
4. **d. takes more than 15 years from infection to death in the absence of treatment.** This is the only statement that is NOT supported by current data. Current data support each of the other statements.
5. **b. risk for disease progression.** During the transition from primary to chronic infection, HIV plasma RNA levels reach a virologic set point that predicts the rate of disease progression. The virologic set point varies among HIV-infected individuals and tends to remain stable in the same person during the chronic phase. The virologic set point that a person attains is determined by both the mechanisms involved in the establishment of chronic infection and by host factors that can modulate the course of HIV disease.
6. **d. 10 years or more.** Current estimates are that it may take 5 to 10 years or more to eliminate HIV, considering a half-life of 4 months for the long-lived infected CD4+ cells and provided that effective and durable suppression of viral replication is achieved by HAART.
7. **a. Obtain genital herpes culture and sensitivity testing.** HSV-resistance should be suspected if lesions persist or recur despite antiviral therapy. Viral culture and resistance testing should be obtained, if possible.
8. **b. standard pharmacologic measures.** Standard pharmacologic measures are preferred for patients with mild dysfunction, and routine urodynamic investigation has proven to be of low yield.
9. **d. hydration, analgesics, and temporary cessation of indinavir.** Our experience is consistent with recommendations for conservative treatment in most cases, consisting of hydration, analgesics, and temporary cessation of indinavir.
10. **b. It seldom presents as renal insufficiency.** HIVAN typically presents as proteinuria in the nephrotic range (and often massive) and renal insufficiency.
11. **c. is related to co-infection with both HIV and a herpesvirus.** Co-infection with HIV and Kaposi's sarcoma (KS)–associated herpesvirus increases the risk of developing KS 10,000-fold compared with KS-associated herpesvirus infection alone. The probability of developing KS after co-infection with both KS-associated herpes virus and HIV approaches 50% over 10 years.

13

Cutaneous Diseases of the External Genitalia

RICHARD E. LINK

QUESTIONS

1. Which of the following is classified as a secondary skin lesion?
   a. Macule
   b. Papule
   c. Ulcer
   d. Vesicle
2. The periodic acid–Schiff stain is used to identify what organism in scraped or touched skin preparations?
   a. *Pseudomonas* species
   b. *Candida*
   c. Herpes simplex
   d. *Molluscum contagiosum*
3. Oral glucocorticosteroids are often used to treat dermatologic conditions and have a duration of effect lasting:
   a. 30 to 90 minutes.
   b. 1 to 5 hours.
   c. 8 to 48 hours.
   d. 5 to 7 days.
4. The preferred dosage schedule for a short course of oral glucocorticosteroids used to treat a cutaneous disorder is:
   a. a single morning dose.
   b. a single evening dose.
   c. doses in the morning and evening.
   d. re-dosing every 8 hours.
5. A 12-year-old boy has a long-standing history of asthma and occasional outbreaks of erythematous, pruritic papules on his scrotum and lower extremities. Which of the following options represents a rational approach to treating this condition?
   a. Long-term suppressive topical corticosteroids
   b. Frequent soaking in warm water to prevent the development of lesions
   c. Low-dose systemic corticosteroids
   d. Frequent application of emollients
6. Patch testing is a useful diagnostic test to identify:
   a. psoriasis.
   b. contact dermatitis.
   c. erythema gangrenosum.
   d. atopic dermatitis.
7. The North American Contact Dermatitis Group identified a series of common allergens that were associated with contact dermatitis. Which allergen was the most common offending agent in contact dermatitis cases?
   a. Silver
   b. Textile dyes
   c. Ragweed
   d. Nickel sulfate
8. A 35-year-old textile worker spills a small amount of green dye onto her left thigh. By the end of the workday, she is complaining of pain and burning over a 5-cm irregular patch of skin on her left thigh. What is the most likely diagnosis?
   a. Allergic contact dermatitis
   b. Hailey-Hailey disease
   c. Irritant contact dermatitis
   d. Koebner phenomenon
9. After a recent exacerbation of genital herpes, a 22-year-old man notes the development of erythematous papules and targetoid lesions on his thighs, scrotum, and oral mucosa. The best next course of action is:
   a. oral antihistamines.
   b. systemic corticosteroids.
   c. observation.
   d. oral acyclovir.
10. A 19-year-old woman is 2 days into a course of sulfonamides for an *E. coli* urinary tract infection. She develops painful labial erosions that progress to a generalized rash with the formation of blisters. The most likely diagnosis is:
   a. erythema multiforme minor.
   b. Stevens-Johnson syndrome.
   c. pyoderma gangrenosum.
   d. Sézary syndrome.

11. A 42-year-old circumcised man has a history of widely distributed erythematous plaques most severe on his knees, elbows, inguinal folds, and glans penis. The condition has waxed and waned since he was in his early 20s. What is an appropriate therapy during an exacerbation?
    a. Topical 3% liquor carbonis detergens in 1% hydrocortisone cream
    b. Oral psoralen combined with ultraviolet radiation (PUVA)
    c. Topical 5-fluorouracil cream
    d. Oral azathioprine
12. A 21-year-old man presents with dysuria, blurred vision, oral ulcers. and erythematous plaques in his genitalia. He has mild soreness in his knees and ankles. He is HIV negative and has had no prior history of sexually transmitted disease. What is a likely risk factor for development of this disorder?
    a. Genital herpes simplex
    b. HLA-B27 haplotype
    c. Exposure to benzene-containing chemicals
    d. Family history of psoriasis
13. Which of the following statements is true about the treatment of symptomatic genital lichen planus?
    a. Systemic corticosteroids can prevent the development of lesions.
    b. In clinical trials, the most effective agent for treating lichen planus is systemic acitretin.
    c. Systemic corticosteroids can shorten the time to clearance of existing lesions from 29 to 18 weeks.
    d. Phytotherapy is the therapeutic modality of choice for treating lichen planus.
14. The late stage of lichen sclerosus involving the glans penis is termed:
    a. keratinizing balanoposthitis.
    b. pseudoepitheliomatous, keratotic, and micaceous balanitis.
    c. bowenoid papulosis.
    d. balanitis xerotica obliterans.
15. Which of the following cutaneous conditions has been associated with an increased risk of squamous cell carcinoma?
    a. Lichen sclerosus et atrophicus
    b. Lichen planus
    c. Psoriasis
    d. Bullous pemphigoid
16. An 18-year-old man has a history of seizures after an automobile accident 2 weeks ago. He was sexually active before the accident. Today, he presents with a solitary, painful erosion on the penis. What course of action is appropriate at this time?
    a. Urethra swab for gonorrhea and chlamydia
    b. Consultation with neurology to alter antiseizure medication regimen
    c. Start oral acyclovir
    d. Start oral doxycycline
17. A 35-year-old previously healthy woman notes the rapid development of sharply demarcated, pruritic red-brown plaques over a large extent of her skin surface. The plaques are particularly dense in her nasolabial folds and perianal area and the nails are spared. What is the next step?
    a. Systemic corticosteroids
    b. HIV test
    c. Skin culture for *Malassezia furfur*
    d. Biopsy of the lesions
18. In patients with pemphigus vulgaris, the characteristic clinical sign showing loss of epidermal cohesion is the:
    a. dimple sign.
    b. Asboe-Hansen sign.
    c. Leser-Trélat sign.
    d. bullous blanching sign.
19. Which of the following statements is FALSE concerning pemphigus vulgaris?
    a. Majority of pemphigus patients have painful oral mucosal erosions.
    b. Pemphigus appears to have an autoimmune pathogenesis.
    c. Treatment of pemphigus relies on systemic corticosteroids.
    d. Given enough time, even advanced cases of pemphigus generally resolve spontaneously without sequelae.
20. Which of the following dermatoses has an association with celiac disease?
    a. Dermatitis herpetiformis
    b. Hailey-Hailey disease
    c. Bullous pemphigoid
    d. Psoriasis
21. Which of the following is not a vesicobullous dermatosis?
    a. Hailey-Hailey disease
    b. Pyoderma gangrenosum
    c. Pemphigus vulgaris
    d. Linear IgA bullous dermatoses
22. Which agent has been shown to be effective in treating linear IgA bullous dermatoses?
    a. Azathioprine
    b. Cyclosporine
    c. Dapsone
    d. Sulfonylureas
23. A 45-year-old woman has pruritic, foul-smelling blistering in the inframammary folds and groin. The skin findings are confluent areas of vesicles with fragile blisters. Which of the following statements is FALSE concerning this condition?
    a. The condition is usually worse during the summer months.
    b. Intralesional corticosteroids may be effective for treatment.
    c. Involvement of the vulva is common in women.
    d. Laser vaporization has been applied successfully to this condition.
24. A 35-year-old man presents with painful ulcerations in his mouth and on his penis as well as blurred vision and a history of recurrent epididymitis. What is the likely diagnosis?
    a. Behçet's disease
    b. Oculocutaneous aphthous ulcer syndrome
    c. Epidermolysis bullosa
    d. Fabry's disease
25. Which of the following statements is FALSE concerning pyoderma gangrenosum?
    a. Pyoderma gangrenosum most likely has an autoimmune mechanism of pathogenesis.
    b. There is an association with collagen vascular disease.
    c. The presence of vacuolated keratinocytes in an inflammatory background is pathognomonic for this condition.
    d. This condition is more common in women than in men.

26. Which of the following cutaneous conditions has an association with borderline personality disorder?
    a. Factitial dermatitis
    b. "Innocent" traumatic dermatitis
    c. Munchausen syndrome by proxy
    d. Behçet's disease

27. The most common organisms causing erysipelas are:
    a. dermatophytes.
    b. *Staphylococcus aureus.*
    c. *Streptococcus pyogenes.*
    d. *Pseudomonas* species.

28. Which of the following statements is FALSE concerning Fournier's gangrene?
    a. The mortality rate even with modern treatment may be > 15%.
    b. Most of the cases of Fournier's gangrene are caused by *Streptococcus pyogenes.*
    c. In severe cases, débridement may need to extend into the chest wall.
    d. Fournier's gangrene can be caused by either a cutaneous, urethral, or perirectal source of infection.

29. An 18-year-old woman develops a pruritic rash over her thighs and buttocks after using a whirlpool spa. Her face and upper extremities are spared. What is the likely diagnosis?
    a. Candidal intertrigo
    b. Pseudomonal folliculitis
    c. Contact dermatitis
    d. Herpes simplex

30. Which of the following conditions has an association with hyperhidrosis?
    a. Trichomycosis axillaris
    b. Hidradenitis suppurativa
    c. Psoriasis
    d. Genital lichen planus

31. A patient being treated for tinea cruris has significant scrotal involvement. What alternative diagnosis does this suggest?
    a. Seborrheic dermatitis
    b. Erythrasma
    c. Cutaneous candidiasis
    d. Contact dermatitis

32. The following treatment for scabies is contraindicated in pediatric patients:
    a. lindane.
    b. permethrin.
    c. ivermectin.
    d. doxycycline.

33. Which of the following statements concerning Bowen's disease is incorrect?
    a. Bowen's disease and squamous cell carcinoma in situ are the same condition.
    b. Bowen's disease involving the glans penis is termed *erythroplasia of Queyrat.*
    c. Bowen's disease may be treated with topical imiquimod.
    d. Bowen's disease is associated with human papillomavirus types 6 and 11.

34. Which of the following statements concerning verrucous carcinoma is correct?
    a. Verrucous carcinoma has a high propensity to metastasize.
    b. Verrucous carcinoma should not be treated with primary radiation therapy because of the risk of anaplastic transformation.
    c. Verrucous carcinoma is an exceedingly rare malignancy on the genitalia.
    d. Verrucous carcinoma is associated with human papillomavirus types 16 and 18.

35. What is the most common site of presentation for Kaposi sarcoma in immunocompetent individuals?
    a. Chest
    b. Face
    c. Lower extremities
    d. Genitalia

36. The following malignancy has been found concurrently in lesions of pseudoepitheliomatous, keratotic, and micaceous balanitis:
    a. basal cell carcinoma.
    b. cutaneous T-cell lymphoma.
    c. squamous cell carcinoma.
    d. verrucous carcinoma.

37. Which of the following statements about extramammary Paget's disease (EPD) is FALSE?
    a. EPD is an adenocarcinoma.
    b. EPD is associated with another underlying malignancy in more than 60% of cases.
    c. EPD has been associated with malignancies of the urethra and bladder.
    d. EPD lesions show vacuolated Paget's cells on histopathologic examination.

38. Patients with cutaneous T-cell lymphoma who develop hematologic involvement are given the diagnosis of:
    a. lymphoid papulosis.
    b. mycosis fungoides.
    c. pagetoid reticulosis.
    d. Sézary syndrome.

39. Which of the following conditions has the most in common histologically with pearly penile papules?
    a. Tuberous sclerosis
    b. Molluscum contagiosum
    c. Herpes simplex
    d. Angiokeratoma of Fordyce

40. The most effective treatment for Zoon's balanitis is:
    a. topical 5-fluorouracil.
    b. topical corticosteroids.
    c. circumcision.
    d. laser therapy.

41. Skin tags are also termed:
    a. fibrofolliculomas.
    b. angiokeratomas.
    c. hamartomas.
    d. acrochordons.

42. The Leser-Trélat syndrome refers to:
    a. rapid progression of lichen planus associated with the HLA-B27 haplotype.
    b. abrupt increase in the size and number of seborrheic keratoses, suggesting internal malignancy.
    c. combination of hand, foot, and genital psoriasis.
    d. development of brown macules on the genitalia, unrelated to sun exposure.

ANSWERS

1. **c. Ulcer.** Secondary skin lesions develop as the skin condition evolves or are caused by scratching or superinfection.
   A secondary skin lesion is classified morphologically as a scale, crust, erosion, ulcer, atrophy, or scar.

2. **b. *Candida.*** To identify cutaneous fungi such as dermatophytes and *Candida* species, periodic acid–Schiff (PAS) staining may be applied to scraped or touched skin specimens.

3. **c. 8 to 48 hours.** Oral glucocorticosteroids (GCS) are absorbed in the jejunum with peak plasma concentrations occurring in 30 to 90 minutes. Despite short plasma half-lives of 1 to 5 hours, the duration of effect of GCS lasts between 8 and 48 hours, depending on the agent.

4. **a. a single morning dose.** For short-term (= 3 weeks) treatment of dermatologic conditions such as allergic contact dermatitis, a single morning dose of oral glucocorticosteroids is given to minimize suppression of the hypothalamic-pituitary-adrenal axis.

5. **d. Frequent application of emollients.** The condition described is atopic dermatitis (AD or eczema), which is associated with susceptibility to irritants and proteins as well as the tendency to develop asthma and allergic rhinitis. Intense pruritus is the hallmark of AD, and controlling the patient's urge to scratch is critical for successful treatment. Removal of various "trigger factors" from the environment (e.g., chemicals, detergents, and household dust mites) may be beneficial in some cases. The mainstay of treatment for AD includes gentle cleaning with nonalkali soaps and the frequent use of emollients.

6. **b. contact dermatitis.** Patch testing is a simple technique of exposing an area of skin to a variety of potential allergens in a grid template. Generally performed by dermatologists, patch testing can help to confirm the diagnosis of allergic contact dermatitis and the allergen involved.

7. **d. Nickel sulfate.** In 2003, the North American Contact Dermatitis Group (NACDG) reported a long list of common allergens implicated in allergic contact dermatitis based on patch testing results. The most common sensitizing allergen identified was nickel sulfate, which is a common component of costume jewelry and belt buckles.

8. **c. Irritant contact dermatitis.** Irritant contact dermatitis results from a direct cytotoxic effect of an irritant chemical touching the skin and is responsible for approximately 80% of contact dermatitis cases. Occupational exposure is also common. Examples of offending agents include soaps, metal salts, acid or alkali-containing compounds, and industrial solvents.

9. **c. observation.** Erythema multiforme (EM) minor is an acute, self-limited skin disease characterized by the abrupt onset of symmetrical fixed red papules that may evolve into target lesions. The majority of cases are precipitated by herpesvirus type I and II, with herpetic lesions usually preceding the development of target lesions by 10 to 14 days. Although continuous suppressive acyclovir may prevent EM episodes in patients with herpes infection, administration of the drug after development of target lesions is of no benefit. With observation alone, the natural history of EM minor is spontaneous resolution after several weeks without sequelae, although recurrences are common.

10. **b. Stevens-Johnson syndrome.** Stevens-Johnson syndrome (SJS) is a life-threatening severe allergic reaction with features similar to extensive skin burns. A vast array of inciting factors has been implicated in the development of SJS, with drug exposures being the most commonly identified. Nonsteroidal anti-inflammatory agents are the most frequent offending agents followed by sulfonamides, tetracycline, penicillin, doxycycline, and anticonvulsants.

11. **a. Topical 3% liquor carbonis detergens in 1% hydrocortisone cream.** Psoriasis is a papulosquamous disorder affecting up to 2% of the population with a relapsing and remitting course. For genital psoriasis, the mainstay of therapy is the use of low-potency topical corticosteroid creams for short courses. Photochemotherapy combining an ingested psoralen with ultraviolet radiation (PUVA) has been used extensively to treat psoriasis. However, a dose-dependent increase in the risk of genital squamous cell carcinoma has been associated with high-dose PUVA therapy for psoriasis elsewhere on the body. Genital shielding during PUVA therapy is strongly recommended; therefore, this modality is contraindicated for treating psoriatic lesions localized to genital skin.

12. **b. The HLA-B27 haplotype.** Reiter's syndrome is a syndrome composed of urethritis, arthritis, ocular findings, oral ulcers, and skin lesions. It is generally preceded by an episode of either urethritis (*Chlamydia*, *Gonococcus*) or gastrointestinal infection (*Yersinia*, *Salmonella*, *Shigella*, *Campylobacter*, *Neisseria*, or *Ureaplasma* species) and is more common in HIV-positive patients. There is a strong genetic association with the HLA-B27 haplotype.

13. **c. Systemic corticosteroids can shorten the time to clearance of existing lesions from 29 to 18 weeks.** Although bothersome pruritus is common with lichen planus (LP), asymptomatic lesions on the genitalia do not require treatment. The primary modality of treatment for symptomatic lesions is topical corticosteroids, although for severe cases, systemic corticosteroids have been shown to shorten the time course to clearance of LP lesions from 29 weeks to 18 weeks.

14. **d. balanitis xerotica obliterans.** Lichen sclerosis (LS) is a scarring disorder, with a predilection for the external genitalia of both sexes, characterized by tissue pallor, loss of architecture, and hyperkeratosis. The late stage of this disease is called balanitis xerotica obliterans, which can involve the penile urethra and result in troublesome urethral stricture disease.

15. **a. Lichen sclerosus et atrophicus.** Despite the similarities in name, lichen sclerosis (LS) shares little in common with lichen planus and lichen nitidus other than pruritus and a predilection for the genital region. Another critical distinction is that LS has been associated with squamous cell carcinoma of the penis, particularly those variants not associated with human papillomavirus, and may represent a premalignant condition. Biopsy is worthwhile both to confirm the diagnosis and exclude malignant change.

16. **b. Consultation with neurology to alter antiseizure medication regimen.** The association of epileptic seizures and a solitary painful genital lesion is suggestive of a diagnosis of Behçet's disease (BD). Other causes for genital ulceration, however, including aphthous ulcers, syphilis, herpes simplex, and chancroid must be considered before a diagnosis of BD is made. In this case, the patient's neurologic issues should take priority over treatment for his genital ulcer.

17. **b. HIV test.** Seborrheic dermatitis (SD) is a common skin disease characterized by the presence of sharply demarcated pink-yellow to red-brown plaques with a flaky scale. Particularly in immunosuppressed individuals, SD may involve a significant proportion of the body surface area. Extensive and/or severe SD should raise concerns for possible underlying HIV infection.

18. **b. The Asboe-Hansen sign.** The loss of epidermal cohesion seen in pemphigus vulgaris leads to the characteristic Asboe-Hansen sign: spreading of fluid under the adjacent normal appearing skin away from the direction of pressure on a blister.

19. **d. Given enough time, even advanced cases of pemphigus generally resolve spontaneously without sequelae.** Severe cases of pemphigus vulgaris without appropriate treatment may be fatal due to the loss of the epidermal barrier function of large areas of affected skin. Treatment usually depends on systemic corticosteroids, although minimization of steroid dose is an important goal to limit side effects. The addition of immunosuppressive agents such as azathioprine and cyclophosphamide may be beneficial owing to their corticosteroid-sparing effect.

20. **a. Dermatitis herpetiformis.** Dermatitis herpetiformis (DH) is a cutaneous manifestation of celiac disease and is generally associated with gluten sensitivity. Diagnosis can be confirmed by biopsy and direct immunofluorescence, which shows a granular pattern of IgA deposition at the basement membrane. Treatment includes the use of dapsone and a strict gluten-restricted diet.

21. **b. Pyoderma gangrenosum.** Pyoderma gangrenosum (PG) is a ulcerative skin disease associated with systemic illnesses including inflammatory bowel disease, arthritis, collagen vascular disease, and myeloproliferative disorders. The classic morphologic presentation of PG is painful cutaneous and mucous membrane ulceration, often with extensive loss of tissue and a purulent base.

22. **c. Dapsone.** Characteristic clinical features of linear IgA bullous dermatosis (LABD) include vesicles and bullae arranged in a combination of circumferential and linear orientations. Treatment with either sulfapyridine or dapsone is usually effective in controlling LABD, and long-term spontaneous remission rates of 30% to 60% have been described.

23. **c. Involvement of the vulva is common in women.** Hailey-Hailey disease (HH) is an autosomal dominant blistering dermatosis that has a predilection for the intertriginous areas including the groin and perianal region. Symptoms include an unfortunate combination of pruritus, pain, and a foul odor. As heat and sweating exacerbate the condition, HH tends to worsen during the summer. In women, disease in the inframammary folds is common although vulvar disease is unusual. For disease resistant to medical therapy, wide excision and skin grafting have been effective, as have local ablative techniques such as dermabrasion and laser vaporization.

24. **a. Behçet's disease.** When oral and genital aphthous ulcers coexist, the clinician should consider the diagnosis of Behçet's disease, which is a generalized relapsing and remitting ulcerative mucocutaneous disease that likely involves a genetic predisposition and an autoimmune mode of pathogenesis. Affected individuals may also suffer from epididymitis, thrombophlebitis, aneurysms, and gastrointestinal, neurologic, and arthritic problems.

25. **c. The presence of vacuolated keratinocytes in an inflammatory background is pathognomonic for this condition.** Pyoderma gangrenosum (PG) is a ulcerative skin disease associated with systemic illnesses, including inflammatory bowel disease, arthritis, collagen vascular disease, and myeloproliferative disorders. It most commonly affects women between the 2nd and 5th decades of life and likely has an autoimmune pathogenesis given its association with other autoimmune diseases. As was the case in Behçet's disease, no specific diagnostic laboratory test or histopathologic feature is pathognomonic for PG, although a history of underlying systemic disease may raise suspicion.

26. **a. Factitial dermatitis.** Factitial dermatitis is a psychocutaneous disorder in which the individual self-inflicts cutaneous lesions usually for an unconscious motive. An association between factitial dermatitis and borderline personality disorder appears to exist.

27. **c. *Streptococcus pyogenes*.** Erysipelas is a superficial bacterial skin infection limited to the dermis with lymphatic involvement. In contrast to the cutaneous lesion of cellulitis, erysipelas generally has a raised and distinct border at the interface with normal skin. The causative organism is usually *S. pyogenes*.

28. **b. Most of the cases of Fournier's gangrene are caused by *Streptococcus pyogenes*.** Fournier's gangrene (FG) is a potentially life-threatening progressive infection of the perineum and genitalia. In the genital region, most cases of FG are caused by mixed bacterial flora, which include gram-positive, gram-negative, and anaerobic bacteria.

29. **b. Pseudomonal folliculitis.** Folliculitis is a common disorder characterized by perifollicular pustules on an erythematous base. It occurs most frequently in heavily hair-bearing areas such as the scalp, beard, axilla, groin, and buttocks and can be exacerbated by local trauma from shaving, rubbing, or clothing irritation. Folliculitis has also been associated with the use of contaminated hot tubs and swimming pools, with the offending organism usually *Pseudomonas aeruginosa*.

30. **a. Trichomycosis axillaris.** Trichomycosis axillaris (TA) is a superficial bacterial infection of axillary and pubic hair caused by *Corynebacterium*, which is associated with hyperhidrosis. Shaving can provide immediate improvement and antibacterial soaps may prevent further infection. For pubic TA, clindamycin gel, bacitracin, and oral erythromycin have also proven effective.

31. **c. Cutaneous candidiasis.** *Tinea cruris* is the term given to dermatophyte infection of the groin and genital area and is commonly known as "jock itch." The inner thighs and inguinal region are the most commonly affected areas, and the scrotum and penis are usually spared in men. Significant scrotal involvement should raise suspicion for cutaneous candidiasis as an alternative diagnosis.

32. **a. Lindane.** As in the case of pediculosis pubis, the treatment of choice for scabies is 5% permethrin cream applied to the entire body overnight with a second application 1 week later. An alternative scabicide, lindane, is not favored owing to both CNS toxicity in children and a rising rate of resistance among mites.

33. **d. Bowen's disease is associated with human papillomavirus types 6 and 11.** Bowen's disease occurring on the mucosal surfaces of the male genitalia is referred to as erythroplasia of Queyrat. In that location, co-infection with human papillomavirus types 8, 16, 39, and 51 has been identified. In contrast, the variant of squamous cell carcinoma termed *verrucous carcinoma* has been associated with human papillomavirus types 6 and 11 infection but not with the more classically oncogenic types 16 and 18.

34. **b. Verrucous carcinoma should not be treated with primary radiation therapy because of the risk of anaplastic transformation.** Verrucous carcinoma (VC) is a locally aggressive, exophytic, low-grade variant of squamous cell carcinoma that has little metastatic potential. It most commonly occurs in uncircumcised men on the glans or prepuce, although similar lesions can be found on the vulva, vagina, cervix, or anus. Treatment is preferably by local excision. Primary radiation therapy is relatively contraindicated due to the potential for anaplastic transformation with a subsequent increase in metastatic potential.

35. **c. Lower extremities.** Kaposi's sarcoma (KS) in immunocompetent individuals presents as slowly growing blue-red pigmented macules on the lower extremities. Although oral and gastrointestinal lesions may occur, the genitalia are seldom involved. This is in contrast to the case with AIDS in which a solitary genital lesion may be the first manifestation of KS. The clinical features of KS in AIDS patients are diverse, ranging from a single lesion to disseminated cutaneous and visceral disease.

36. **d. verrucous carcinoma.** Pseudoepitheliomatous, keratotic, and micaceous balanitis (PEKMB) is a rare entity characterized by the development of a thick, hyperkeratotic plaque on the glans penis of older men. There remains controversy as to whether PEKMB is a premalignant condition. PEKMB was originally thought to be a purely benign process, although several case reports have documented the presence of concurrent verrucous carcinoma associated with this lesion.

37. **b. EPD is associated with another underlying malignancy in more than 60% of cases.** Extramammary Paget's disease (EPD) is an uncommon intraepithelial adenocarcinoma of sites bearing apocrine glands. There is an important association between EPD and another underlying malignancy in 10% to 30% of cases. In the male, associations between urethral, bladder, rectal, and apocrine malignancies with EPD have been described.

38. **d. Sézary syndrome.** Cutaneous T-cell lymphoma (CTCL) represents a group of related neoplasms derived from T cells that affect the skin. CTCL generally presents with pruritus, which must be differentiated from a variety of benign dermatoses, including psoriasis, eczema, superficial fungal infections, and drug reactions. Patients may subsequently develop hematologic involvement (Sézary syndrome) and cutaneous plaques, erosions, ulcers, or frank skin tumors.

39. **a. Tuberous sclerosis.** Pearly penile papules (PPP) are white, dome-shaped, closely spaced small papules located on the glans penis. Histologically, these lesions are angiofibromas similar to the lesions seen on the face in tuberous sclerosis.

40. **c. circumcision.** Zoon's balanitis, also called plasma cell balanitis, occurs in uncircumcised men from the third decade onward. Squamous cell carcinoma and extramammary Paget's disease should be excluded, often by biopsy. Circumcision appears to be proof against development of the disease and can be performed to cure the majority of cases. For patients averse to circumcision, topical corticosteroids may provide symptomatic relief and laser therapy may also have a role.

41. **d. acrochordons.** Skin tags (acrochordons, fibroepithelial polyps) are soft, skin-colored, pedunculated lesions that can be present anywhere on the body. It is important to distinguish these lesions from the hamartomatous skin lesions (multiple fibrofolliculomas) associated with Birt-Hogg-Dubé syndrome, which are histologically distinct from common skin tags.

42. **b. abrupt increase in the size and number of seborrheic keratoses, suggesting internal malignancy.** The presence of brown macules unrelated to sun exposure suggests a diagnosis of seborrheic keratoses (SK). This condition may commonly involve the genitalia but generally spares the mucous membranes, palms, and soles of the feet. An abrupt increase in the size and number of multiple seborrheic keratoses (SK) has been termed Leser-Trélat syndrome and has been implicated as a cutaneous marker of internal malignancy. The HLA-B27 haplotype is associated with Reiter's syndrome, not rapidly progressive lichen planus.

14

Tuberculosis and Parasitic and Fungal Infections of the Genitourinary System

SARAH J. MCALEER • CHRISTOPHER W. JOHNSON • WARREN D. JOHNSON, JR.

QUESTIONS

1. Which of the following statements about the epidemiology of tuberculosis is TRUE?
   a. Tuberculosis (TB) incidence has increased in the United States since the 1990s.
   b. Tuberculosis incidence among Asian immigrants is comparable to that for persons born in the United States.
   c. Tuberculosis incidence is decreasing worldwide.
   d. Tuberculosis occurs predominantly in patients with acquired immunodeficiency syndrome (AIDS) late in the course of their disease (CD4+ T-cell count of <200 cells/mm^3).
   e. Globally, tuberculosis is the most common opportunistic infection in AIDS patients.
2. The spread of *Mycobacterium tuberculosis* is least dependent on which of the following?
   a. Size of the bacillary inoculum inhaled
   b. Infectivity of the mycobacterial strain
   c. Duration of exposure to the source case
   d. Immune status of the source case
   e. Immune status of the exposed individual
3. Which of the following statements regarding tuberculosis is correct?
   a. Humans are not the only reservoir for *M. tuberculosis*.
   b. Renal tuberculosis is usually the result of activation of prior bloodborne metastatic renal infection.
   c. Epididymitis is a rare presenting symptom of genitourinary tuberculosis.
   d. Transmission of genitourinary tuberculosis from male to female is common.
   e. Renal tuberculosis is most common in children younger than 5 years of age.
4. Which one of the following conditions is most likely to reactivate a dormant *M. tuberculosis* infection?
   a. Human immunodeficiency virus (HIV) infection
   b. Pulmonary hypertension
   c. Emphysema
   d. Allergic asthma
   e. Osteoarthritis
5. The Centers for Disease Control and Prevention (CDC) has recommended defining a tuberculin reaction of 5 mm of induration as positive for which of the following?
   a. Infants
   b. Intravenous drug abusers
   c. Homeless individuals
   d. Diabetics
   e. HIV positive individuals
6. The radiologic test that is most useful for evaluating the anatomic manifestations of genitourinary tuberculosis is:
   a. ultrasonography.
   b. intravenous pyelography.
   c. computed tomography.
   d. magnetic resonance imaging.
   e. retrograde pyelography.
7. All of the following features of genitourinary tuberculosis can be seen on an intravenous urogram EXCEPT:
   a. infundibular stenosis.
   b. renal calcifications.
   c. ureteral stricture.
   d. "thimble" bladder.
   e. vesicoureteral reflux.
8. Which of the following antituberculous drugs can cause visual changes?
   a. Isoniazid
   b. Streptomycin
   c. Rifampicin
   d. Pyrazinamide
   e. Ethambutol
9. Which form of tuberculosis is usually treated for more than 6 months?
   a. Pulmonary
   b. Genitourinary
   c. Osteomyelitis
   d. Nodal
   e. Concomitant pulmonary and genitourinary

10. Hepatic toxicity from INH is:
    a. preventable with vitamin B_6.
    b. irreversible.
    c. evident almost immediately after initiation of therapy.
    d. manifested as hyperbilirubinemia.
    e. often normalizes after several months of continued therapy.

11. Which of the following statements regarding surgery for genitourinary tuberculosis is correct?
    a. Patients should have at least 4 to 6 weeks of extensive chemotherapy before surgery.
    b. Lack of renal calcification is not a contraindication to partial nephrectomy.
    c. Open surgical drainage of an abscess is usually required.
    d. There is no indication for an epididymectomy in the modern era of chemotherapy.
    e. Strictures at the ureteropelvic junction are common and frequently require endopyelotomy.

12. Which of the following statements regarding intravesical BCG treatment is FALSE?
    a. Mechanism of action is unknown.
    b. Administered immediately after a transurethral resection.
    c. Serious side effects are common.
    d. BCG sepsis treatment begins with isoniazid.
    e. BCG is commonly used to reduce recurrence rates of superficial urothelial carcinoma.

13. Which of the following statements about *Schistosoma haematobium* and its life cycle is TRUE?
    a. Worm pairs are principally located in the hepatic vasculature in humans.
    b. It is common in South America.
    c. Human infection is acquired by exposure to fresh water that harbors infected snails.
    d. Worm pairs have life spans estimated between 3 and 6 months.
    e. Sexual reproductive phase occurs in snails.

14. When one evaluates a patient for *S. haematobium* infection, which one of the following statements is TRUE?
    a. An active infection can be diagnosed by the presence of laterally spined eggs in the urine.
    b. An active infection has the full complement of egg stages present.
    c. A history of living or traveling in Africa means that the patient has been to endemic areas.
    d. The intensity of infection is inversely related to the egg burden found in tissues or body fluids.
    e. Calculating the number of eggs per 10 mL of urine is not an indication of the intensity of the infection.

15. The human host response to *S. haematobium* is characterized by which one of the following?
    a. T cell–dependent host responses modulate granuloma formation.
    b. Granulomatous host response to the schistosome eggs does not cause the pathologic tissue changes.
    c. Eosinophil-mediated killing is effective against adult worms.
    d. HIV-positive patients with lower CD4+ T-cell counts have higher egg burdens than patients with normal CD4+ T-cell counts.
    e. A "sandy patch" is a granulomatous ulcer.

16. Which one of the following is the most common presentation of acute *S. haematobium* disease?
    a. Katayama fever
    b. Swimmer's itch
    c. Renal failure
    d. Calcified bladder
    e. Hematuria

17. Bilharzial bladder cancer is a known sequela of *S. haematobium* infection. Which of the following statements is TRUE?
    a. Bladder cancer is often manifested at 20 to 30 years of age.
    b. Squamous cell carcinoma accounts for 30% to 40% of the cancers.
    c. Nitrates, nitrite, *N*-nitroso compounds, and tryptophan metabolites have been identified in elevated amounts in the urine of patients with bilharzial bladder cancer.
    d. More than about 45% of the squamous cell carcinomas are well differentiated.
    e. Patients are frequently treated with partial cystectomy.

18. A 43-year-old woman from Madagascar has schistosomal obstructive uropathy (SOU). What might you expect to find at workup?
    a. The SOU usually obstructs the ureters symmetrically.
    b. The egg burden would be highest at the distal end of the ureter.
    c. The obstruction would likely be at her UPJ.
    d. If untreated, hydronephrosis remains stable.
    e. There is no change in ureteral function until radiologically demonstrable disease is noted.

19. A 24-year-old man who had recently come from Syria had been previously diagnosed with urinary schistosomiasis. He had not received any treatment. His medical records from Syria noted that he had *S. haematobium* infection, and an intravenous pyelogram had demonstrated severe hydroureter on the left with a segmental distal ureteral lesion and delayed excretion. He has a normal creatinine level. He should be initially managed with:
    a. cystoscopy with ureteral stent placement.
    b. cystoscopy with ureteral stent placement and intravesical medical therapy.
    c. medical management with oral praziquantel.
    d. percutaneous nephrostomy tube placement followed by medical therapy.
    e. distal ureterectomy and primary reimplantation into the bladder.

20. Filarial disease can be characterized by all of the following EXCEPT:
    a. Elephantiasis of the limbs, chyluria, fever, localized lymphangitis, and hydrocele formation are seen.
    b. Biopsy and removal of involved lymph nodes are often necessary.
    c. Obstructive lymphatic disease occurs in patients who are repeatedly infected.
    d. Female mosquito *(Culex pipiens)* is the vector.
    e. After inoculation, larvae travel through the lungs via blood before settling in their ultimate destination, large lymphatic vessels.

21. A 34-year-old shepherd from Spain has dull bilateral flank pain and intermittent microscopic hematuria. You suspect that a parasite may be responsible for the patient's complaints. If you are correct, which of the following statements would be valid?
    a. Hanging groin, or scrotal elephantiasis, may ultimately develop.
    b. Ivermectin is a first-line treatment option.
    c. Needle aspiration of any lesion is indicated before initiating therapy.
    d. Thick walled fluid-filled cysts with calcified walls are diagnostic.
    e. Metronidazole is a first-line treatment option.
22. Which fungus is the most common cause of systemic fungal infection in severely immunocompromised patients?
    a. *Aspergillus*
    b. *Cryptococcus neoformans*
    c. *Blastomyces*
    d. *Histoplasma*
    e. *Mucor*
23. What is the most prevalent underlying disease associated with a single episode of candiduria?
    a. Malignancy
    b. Diabetes
    c. Collagen disease
    d. Neurogenic bladder
    e. Concomitant antibiotic administration
24. The recommended treatment for vulvovaginal candidiasis is:
    a. vinegar douches.
    b. intravaginal amphotericin lavage.
    c. one week of oral therapy with fluconazole.
    d. single oral dose of fluconazole.
    e. saline vaginal irrigations.
25. Which of the following statements is FALSE regarding genitourinary candidiasis?
    a. The bladder may have a "snow effect" appearance on cystoscopy.
    b. The patient rarely develops urinary obstruction.
    c. The patient with candiduria is usually asymptomatic.
    d. Foley catheters in the postsurgical patient increases the risk for acquiring candiduria.
    e. The patient may need the placement of various drains to clear infections.
26. All of the following are major predisposing factors for renal candidal infection in pediatric patients EXCEPT:
    a. indwelling intravascular catheters.
    b. maternal diabetes mellitus.
    c. low birth weight.
    d. prematurity.
    e. broad-spectrum antibiotics.
27. The best treatment for systemic candidal infection is:
    a. ketoconazole.
    b. fluconazole.
    c. miconazole.
    d. flucytosine.
    e. itraconazole.
28. When treating candiduria which of the following apply?
    a. Foley catheters or intravenous lines are not risk factors.
    b. Treat with topical agents.
    c. Not all patients with candiduria need treatment.
    d. Fungal balls resolve with medical therapy.
    e. Patients undergoing urologic procedures may be observed.
29. Aspergillosis outbreaks can be seen in:
    a. shepherds.
    b. aviaries.
    c. the central United States.
    d. dialysis centers.
    e. the western United States.
30. In AIDS patients, which genitourinary organ becomes the "reservoir" for *Cryptococcus* after treatment of cryptococcal meningitis?
    a. Kidney
    b. Bladder
    c. Epididymis
    d. Kidney
    e. Prostate
31. Radiographic findings may be similar to those of tuberculosis in which genitourinary fungal infection?
    a. Candidiasis
    b. Hydatid disease
    c. Schistosomiasis
    d. Coccidioidomycosis
    e. Phycomycosis
32. *Candida krusei and C. glabrata* are resistant to which drug?
    a. Amphotericin B
    b. Fluconazole
    c. Itraconazole
    d. Flucytosine
    e. Ketoconazole

ANSWERS

1. **e. Globally, tuberculosis is the most common opportunistic infection in AIDS patients.**
2. **d. Immune status of the source case.** The probability that a person will become infected depends on the duration of exposure to the source case, the size of the bacillary inoculum inhaled, and the infectivity of the mycobacterial strain. Virtually all AIDS patients with a positive purified protein derivative (PPD) test develop active TB during their lifetime unless antituberculous prophylaxis is offered.
3. **b. Renal tuberculosis is usually the result of activation of prior bloodborne metastatic renal infection.** Genitourinary TB is caused by metastatic spread of the organism through the bloodstream during the initial infection. The kidney is usually the primary organ infected in urinary disease, and other parts of the urinary tract become involved by direct extension.
4. **a. Human immunodeficiency virus (HIV) infection.** Most persons control the initial infection and develop no clinical illness. They have dormant bacilli, which may begin to produce disease years later after debilitating disease, trauma, corticosteroids, immunosuppressive therapy, diabetes, or AIDS.

5. **e. HIV positive individuals.**
6. **c. computed tomography.** CT has become more widely available and has arguably replaced IVU as the imaging modality of choice for the diagnosis and evaluation of genitourinary TB. The latest CT software allows for the creation of three-dimensional reconstructed images, adding another dimension to the images that a CT scan can produce. It is at least the equal of IVU in identifying caliceal abnormalities, hydronephrosis or hydroureter, autonephrectomy, amputated infundibulum, urinary tract calcifications, and renal parenchymal cavities.
7. **e. vesicoureteral reflux.** Renal lesions can be visualized on IVU. They may appear as a distortion of a calyx, as a calyx that is fibrosed and completely occluded (lost calyx from infundibular stenosis), as multiple small calyceal deformities, or as severe calyceal and parenchymal destruction. Other manifestations of genitourinary TB that can be visualized on IVU include ureteral dilatation above an ureterovesical junction (UVJ) stricture or a rigid fibrotic ureter with multiple strictures. The cystographic phase of the IVU can give valuable information about the condition of the bladder, which may be small and contracted (thimble bladder) or irregular, with filling defects and bladder asymmetry.
8. **e. Ethambutol.** Ethambutol rarely causes retrobulbar neuritis and should be discontinued if ocular changes occur. Changes in visual acuity and red-green color perception are early findings, and these parameters should be tested at baseline and every 4 to 6 weeks.
9. **c. Osteomyelitis.** Six-month regimens are effective for most forms of TB, including genitourinary TB, with the exception of disseminated TB, TB osteomyelitis, and TB meningitis.
10. **e. often normalizes after several months of continued therapy.** INH is associated with hepatic "toxicity" in 10% to 20% of patients, usually in the form of asymptomatic elevations in transaminase levels. This occurs after 6 to 8 weeks of therapy and may normalize with continued INH treatment.
11. **a. Patients should have at least 4 to 6 weeks of extensive chemotherapy before surgery.**
12. **b. Administered immediately after a transurethral resection.** To avoid systemic absorption and therefore reduce the risk of major adverse reactions, one should wait 1 to 3 weeks after transurethral resection before starting BCG treatment.
13. **c. Human infection is acquired by exposure to fresh water that harbors infected snails.** On deposition into fresh water (not salt), the miracidia emerge as short-lived, ciliated larvae that swim and seek hosts.
14. **c. A history of living or traveling in Africa means that the patient has been to endemic areas.** Transmission of *S. haematobium* occurs in 53 countries in the Middle East and in most of the African continent. In Southwest Asia, it is found in Southern Yemen, Yemen, Saudi Arabia, Lebanon, Syria, Turkey, Iraq, and Iran (World Health Organization, 1998).
15. **a. T cell–dependent host responses modulate granuloma formation.** The host responds to egg antigens by forming granulomas around the egg, which is a T cell–dependent host response.
16. **e. Hematuria.**
17. **d. More than about 45% of the squamous cell carcinomas are well differentiated.**
18. **b. The egg burden would be highest at the distal end of the ureter.** Ureteral obstruction seen during active schistosomiasis is most often caused by concentric or hemiconcentric polypoid lesions that "girdle" the ureteral muscle in the intramural and adjacent extravesical ureter.
19. **c. medical management with oral praziquantel.** In general, surgery is reserved for complications that have not responded to adequate medical treatment within a reasonable follow-up time (e.g., obstructive uropathy) or for those mandating immediate intervention such as intractable bladder hemorrhage.
20. **b. Biopsy and removal of involved lymph nodes is often necessary.**
21. **d. Thick walled fluid-filled cysts with calcified walls are diagnostic.** Diagnosis can be made by plain film radiography, ultrasonography, or CT, which shows a thick-walled, fluid-filled spherical cyst, often with a calcific cyst wall.
22. **a. *Aspergillus*.** Disseminated *Aspergillus* is a major opportunistic fungus in patients compromised by malignancy, diabetes mellitus, AIDS, immunosuppressive agents, and organ transplantation.
23. **b. Diabetes.** In a documented single episode of candiduria, the major associated illnesses included diabetes mellitus (39%), urinary tract disease (37.7%), malignancy (22.2%), and malnutrition (17%).
24. **d. a single oral dose of fluconazole.** Treatment with oral fluconazole (a single 150-mg dose) is as effective as topical intravaginal therapy in the treatment of vulvovaginal candidiasis.
25. **b. The patient rarely develops urinary obstruction.**
26. **b. maternal diabetes mellitus.**
27. **b. fluconazole.** Fluconazole administered by mouth or by the IV route achieves high urine levels.
28. **c. Not all patients with candiduria need treatment.** It should be emphasized that *Candida* species in the urine may represent contamination of the specimen during collection or colonization, without true infection. However, the persistence of candiduria requires evaluation and consideration of treatment.
29. **d. dialysis centers.** Outbreaks of disease have been attributed to contaminated air conditioning systems, surgical theaters, dialysis fluid, and construction dust.
30. **e. Prostate.**
31. **d. Coccidioidomycosis.**
32. **b. Fluconazole.**

SECTION V

MOLECULAR AND CELLULAR BIOLOGY

15

Basic Principles of Immunology

STUART M. FLECHNER • JAMES H. FINKE • ROBERT L. FAIRCHILD

QUESTIONS

1. Antigen presentation involves both uptake of foreign proteins and processing to form peptide/MHC complexes. Each of the following immune responsive cell types can carry out this function EXCEPT:

   a. Granulocytes
   b. Vascular endothelial cells
   c. Monocytes
   d. Macrophages
   e. Dendritic cells

2. Transplants between two siblings who are HLA identical (perfect class I and II match) can be rejected. This is primarily a consequence of:

   a. Direct antigen presentation
   b. Differences in complement proteins
   c. Indirect antigen presentation
   d. Differences in childhood antimicrobial vaccination
   e. Differences in numbers of circulating platelets

3. Lymphocyte activation depends on complex interactions between many intracellular enzymes, transcription factors, and electrolytes. The influx of which electrolyte is most important for T-cell activation:

   a. Sodium
   b. Magnesium
   c. Potassium
   d. Phosphorus
   e. Calcium

4. Anergy describes a state of immune nonresponsiveness to antigenic stimulation. The most effective way to induce a state of anergy is by:

   a. Splenic irradiation
   b. Delivery of signal 1 and signal 2
   c. Depletion of complement proteins
   d. Delivery of signal 1 without signal 2
   e. Depletion of helper CD4+ T cells

5. Each of the following characteristics describes the utility and adaptability of the immune system EXCEPT:

   a. Memory
   b. Rapid amplification
   c. Identification of self
   d. Antigen restriction

6. Innate immune responses are nonspecific and include all of the following EXCEPT:

   a. Natural killer cells
   b. Antibody-dependent cell-mediated cellular cytotoxicity
   c. Complement
   d. Acute phase proteins
   e. Physical and mucosal barriers

7. Which cell surface glycoprotein is commonly referred to as the "pan T cell marker" due to its presence on all T lymphocytes?

   a. CD3
   b. CD4
   c. CD8
   d. CD28
   e. CD45

8. The part of an IgG antibody molecule that interacts with cell surface receptors on other immune reactive cells such as NK cells is the:

   a. Hypervariable region
   b. Disulfide bonds
   c. Amino terminal end of the antibody
   d. Fc fragment
   e. Fab fragment

9. The family of transcription factors termed nuclear factor of activated T cells (NFAT) are essential for T-cell activation and clonal expansion through the expression of the gene for:

   a. Interferon γ
   b. Transferrin
   c. Tumor necrosis factor
   d. Interleukin-2
   e. Interleukin-10

10. The receptor on B cells that recognizes antigen and transmits signals to the nucleus for gene expression is:

    a. T-cell receptor.
    b. surface IgD molecule.
    c. surface IgM molecule.
    d. CD40.
    e. CD28.

11. The Jak/STAT signaling pathways are critical in regulating cytokine expression. Inborn deficiencies in these pathways may lead to diseases such as:

    a. Burkitt's lymphoma.
    b. Wilms' tumor.
    c. neuroblastoma.
    d. retinoblastoma.
    e. severe combined immunodeficiency.

12. The initial contact of host immunoresponsive cells with foreign antigen or transplanted donor tissue takes place in the:

    a. peripheral lymph nodes.
    b. thymus gland.
    c. spleen.
    d. bursa of Fabricius.
    e. bone marrow.

13. Programmed cell death, apoptosis, is a mechanism responsible for the elimination of aged, damaged, autoimmune, or redundant cells. Caspase proteins are responsible for executing the suicide program by:

    a. release of granzyme B.
    b. activating the alternative complement pathway.
    c. activating natural killer cells.
    d. mediating DNA fragmentation and condensation.
    e. release of perforin.

14. Tolerance describes the absence of lymphocyte reactivity to specific antigens that have been previously encountered by the immune system. Known mechanisms of tolerance include each of the following EXCEPT:

    a. deletion of reactive T cells.
    b. deletion of reactive B cells.
    c. blocking by antigen-antibody complexes.
    d. clonal anergy by delivery of signal 1 without co-stimulation.
    e. suppression of immune responses by regulatory cells.

15. Chemokines are chemoattractant cytokines that localize various cell populations to tissue sites of inflammation. Each of the following cell types respond to chemokines EXCEPT:

    a. erythrocytes.
    b. granulocytes.
    c. natural killer cells.
    d. dendritic cells.
    e. monocytes.

16. Although most human tumors are antigenic, the immune system is often not a significant barrier to tumor growth and metastasis. A major reason for the relative weakness of the immune system to eradicate tumors is:

    a. absence of co-stimulation by tumors leading to anergy.
    b. tumor-induced alterations of immune function.
    c. impaired function of tumor neovasculature.
    d. rapid tumor cell proliferation.
    e. lack of tumor cell Fc receptors.

17. Tumor cell destruction by the immune system often is weak due to tumor cell escape mechanisms, which include all of the following EXCEPT:

    a. tumor cell release of IL-2.
    b. reduced expression of MHC class I and II molecules on tumor cells.
    c. tumor cell and local release of IL-10.
    d. ligation of tumor cell Fas by Fas ligand to induce apoptosis of host T cells.
    e. tumor cell and local release of transforming growth factor-β.

18. Immunotherapy for metastatic renal cell carcinoma in humans has included the use of cytokines such as interferon γ and interleukin-2. The objective response rate (both complete and partial responses) has been demonstrated in what percentage of patients?

    a. 95%
    b. 75%
    c. 55%
    d. 35%
    e. 15%

19. Extracellular bacteria are susceptible to killing by phagocytosis and complement, but some have developed capsules to block these mechanisms. The most effective immune counter measure for bacterial encapsulation is the:

    a. classical complement pathway.
    b. alternative complement pathway.
    c. opsonization of bacteria by circulating antibodies.
    d. increased secretion of TGF-β in tears.
    e. increased beating of bronchial cilia.

20. Clearance of intracellular bacteria is most dependent on which immune cell population?

    a. Macrophages
    b. Plasma cells
    c. Natural killer cells
    d. Dendritic cells
    e. Primed T lymphocytes

21. Passive immune therapy may be particularly useful for patients with immunodeficiency. Passive therapy is delivered via:

    a. attenuated viral organisms.
    b. lyophilized vaccines.
    c. heterologous serum.
    d. live viral organisms.
    e. cow's milk.

22. Toll-like receptors can be engaged by all of the following EXCEPT:

    a. bacterial flagellin.
    b. bacterial lipopolysaccharides.
    c. calcium.
    d. double-stranded viral RNA.
    e. paclitaxel.

23. Recognition of Toll-like receptors by microbial products can activate all of the following immune mechanisms EXCEPT:
   a. adaptive immunity.
   b. intracellular microbial killing.
   c. innate immunity.
   d. IgE antibody formation.
   e. expression of co-stimulatory molecules.

24. DNA microarrays depend on the ability of target nucleic acid sequences to:
   a. bind to the surface of activated lymphocytes.
   b. hybridize to complementary oligonucleotides or PCR products.
   c. engage the T-cell receptor.
   d. bind to antibody fixed to a glass slide.
   e. fix complement.

25. Gene expression profiling using DNA microarrays can be used to distinguish the following characteristics of urologic cancers EXCEPT:
   a. pathologic stage of the malignancy.
   b. diagnosis and classification of the malignancy.
   c. monitoring the host response to the malignancy.
   d. discovery of targets for treatment of the malignancy.
   e. definition of the clinical prognosis of the malignancy.

26. Which of the following events do not play a role in the initiation of TCR signaling after engagement with antigen and MHC class II molecules?
   a. TCR interaction with CD4 co-receptor
   b. TCR interaction with CD8 co-receptor
   c. Phosphorylation of TCR and -CD3 ITAMs by Lck and Fyn kinases
   d. Recruitment of ZAP-70 to TCR and its activation
   e. Activation of adaptor molecule, LAT

27. Which of the following is a FALSE statement regarding the Janus family of kinases?
   a. The 4 Jak kinases are not constitutively associated with various cytokine receptors.
   b. The Jak kinases regulate different cytokine receptors.
   c. The cytokine-receptor binding causes dimerization of receptor chains resulting in Jak activation and phosphorylation of receptors.
   d. The STATs are recruited to receptors and phosphorylated by Jak kinases.
   e. Mutation in Jak3 results in severe combined immunodeficiency.

28. Which of the following statements is TRUE regarding programmed cell death (apoptosis)?
   a. It is a mechanism for the elimination of aged, damaged, and autoimmune cells or cells no longer needed for differentiation.
   b. It is a mechanism for inducing a primary immune response.
   c. The proteins responsible for executing apoptosis, caspases, are Jak kinases.
   d. Caspase-8 is the initiator caspase for apoptosis initiated by Fas and the T-cell receptor.
   e. Bcl-2 and Bcl-xl are anti-apoptotic proteins that protect the nucleus from damage.

29. The development of an effective immune response to cancer cells is dependent on appropriate antigen presentation by dendritic cells and the subsequent activation of CD4+ and CD8+ T cells. Which of the statements listed below are TRUE?
   a. Many human tumors express antigenic epitopes that can be recognized by either CD4+ T cells or by CD8+ T cells.
   b. T cells can destroy tumor cells by several mechanisms, which include the elaboration of granules containing pore forming proteins, the upregulation of FasL that can bind Fas receptors, and the activation of macrophages.
   c. IFN-γ production by lymphocytes is necessary but not sufficient for promoting antitumor immune response.
   d. Tumors may evade T-cell detection because of a loss of MHC class I /II molecules or because of a decrease in expression of transporter proteins associated with antigen processing.
   e. T-reg cells, TGF-β, IL-10, gangliosides, and prostaglandin represent potential immune suppressive mechanisms within the tumor microenvironment.

ANSWERS

1. **a. Granulocytes.** Macrophages, monocytes, some B cells, Langerhans cells of the skin, dendritic reticulum cells, and vascular endothelial cells can process and present antigen.

2. **c. Indirect antigen presentation.** The evidence for an indirect recognition pathway for alloantigens comes from observations that rejection can take place even if donor and recipient share most, if not all, MHC antigens.

3. **e. Calcium.** This event also leads to the opening of the calcium channels in the plasma membrane, which further increases Ca^{2+} levels. Elevated intracellular Ca^{2+} results in the activation of the enzyme calcineurin, which is a cytosolic serine/threonine protein phosphatase that regulates the activation of a family of transcription factors termed nuclear factor of activated T cells (NFAT).

4. **d. Delivery of signal 1 without signal 2.** In fact, stimulation by signal 1 alone leads to a state of anergy, whereby the T cell becomes unresponsive to further stimulation by antigen.

5. **d. Antigen restriction.** Unique characteristics that help explain the utility and adaptability of the immune system against many different foreign invaders include (1) the ability to identify self from non-self, (2) specificity, (3) memory, and (4) rapid amplification.

6. **b. Antibody-dependent cell-mediated cellular cytotoxicity.** Innate defense mechanisms represent nonspecific barriers to invaders, which rely primarily on physical barriers, phagocytic cells, natural killer cells, complement, acute phase proteins, lysozyme, and the interferons.

7. **a. CD3.** Each T-cell precursor retains the pan–T-cell CD3 marker, which is the signal-transducing complex closely linked to the T cell receptor.

8. **d. Fc fragment.** The Fc fragment does not bind antibody but is responsible for fixation to complement and attachment of the molecule to the cell surface.

9. **d. Interleukin-2.** NFAT along with other transcription factors plays a critical role in T-cell activation and clonal expansion through activation of the IL-2 gene.

10. **b. the surface IgD molecule.** The receptor on B cells that recognizes antigen and transmits signals to the nucleus for gene expression is composed of a cell surface immunoglobulin containing heavy and light chains with variable regions.

11. **e. severe combined immunodeficiency.** The biologic importance of different Jaks and STATs has been revealed by deficiencies of these proteins both in humans and in

animal models. Mutations in Jak3 have resulted in patients' having severe combined immunodeficiency (SCID) that is similar to X-linked SCID, which occurs because of a mutation in the common cytokine receptor γ chain.

12. **a. peripheral lymph nodes.** Activation of specific T cells and the generation of an immune response require transport of antigenic components to the lymphoid tissue. For the induction of most T cell–mediated immune responses, the crucial antigen-presenting cell is the dendritic cell, which is interspersed throughout peripheral tissues.

13. **d. mediating DNA fragmentation and condensation.** The proteins responsible for executing the suicide program, the caspases, are essentially common to all the stimuli and pathways and mediate the nuclear and cytoplasmic alterations characteristic of apoptotic cell death. The specific roles of each member of the caspase cascade are gradually becoming defined, whereby caspases 3, 6, and 7 have been identified as the terminal effectors mediating DNA fragmentation and chromatin condensation.

14. **c. blocking by antigen-antibody complexes.** An important mechanism mediating tolerance to self-proteins is the deletion of self-reactive T cells and B cells during maturation. Clonal anergy of T cells is induced by T-cell receptor engagement of peptide/MHC complexes in the absence of co-stimulatory signals. An active mechanism of tolerance mediated by T cells with suppressive or downregulatory activities may also be induced to inhibit immune responses to self and exogenous antigens.

15. **a. erythrocytes.** Cytokines with chemoattractant properties, chemokines, are also crucial in mediating localization and trafficking of leukocytes to tissue sites during physiologic processes, including inflammation and homeostasis.

16. **b. tumor-induced alterations of immune function.** Tumor-induced alterations in the functional status of immune cells may be responsible for the poor development of antitumor immunity in many cancer patients.

17. **a. tumor cell release of IL-2.** Natural killer cells can recognize and destroy some tumors, particularly those of lymphoid origin, without any exogenous activation. Reduction in or loss of MHC class I and class II expression by tumors, including renal cell carcinoma, has been well documented. In some tumors, there is also decreased expression of transporter proteins associated with antigen processing (TAP proteins). Among the best studied immunosuppressive molecules overexpressed in the tumor microenvironment is the TH2 cytokine interleukin-10. TGF-β is also thought to contribute to the suppression of tumor immunity. Evidence suggests that the downregulation of antitumor immunity may be due in part to the induction of the Fas apoptotic pathway in T cells.

18. **e. 15%.** It is clear from these and other studies that a subset of individuals with metastatic renal cancer does respond favorably to cytokine therapy; however, they represent a minority of patients (<15% response rate).

19. **c. opsonization of bacteria by circulating antibodies.** Many of these bacterial mechanisms can be overridden by host antibodies, which are soluble or secreted on external mucosal surfaces. Circulating antibodies can directly bind to bacterial exotoxins and "neutralize" them. They can also bind to the encapsulated bacteria, which will permit ingestion by polymorphs and macrophages.

20. **e. Primed T lymphocytes.** Clearance of these intracellular microbes depends directly on T cells, which in turn must activate the infected macrophages. Specifically primed T cells react with processed antigen derived from the intracellular bacteria in association with MHC class II molecules on the macrophage surface.

21. **c. heterologous serum.** Protection against a specific infection can be passively transferred from one individual to another via serum containing preformed antibodies. This type of passive immunity is generally short-lived, because the half-life of immunoglobulins is 1 to 2 weeks. Patients with immunodeficiency diseases may actually be sustained by regular treatments with pooled nonspecific human immune globulin treatments.

22. **c. calcium.** Toll-like receptors are cell surface glycoproteins that need physical contact with other macromolecules such as bacterial flagellins, lipopolysaccharides, phytins, or nucleic acids. Minerals such as calcium are too small.

23. **d. IgE antibody formation.** Engagement of Toll-like receptors activates various cellular immune responses. IgE antibody on the surface of mast cells promotes degranulation and allergy. IgE antibody is constitutively expressed on basophils/mast cells.

24. **b. hybridize to complementary oligonucleotides or PCR products.** DNA microarrays or gene chips are tests performed in a laboratory. They depend on the natural ability of two complementary strands of nucleic acids to hybridize to each other. The others are in-vivo biologic processes.

25. **a. pathologic stage of the malignancy.** DNA microarrays can identify a unique molecular signature of a cancer, which represents the sum of genes upregulated or downregulated by the tumor. This can help classify the specific cancer, aid in identifying potential molecular targets for therapy, or possibly predict outcome of therapy. The pathologic stage of the cancer is a description of its extent in the host. It is usually defined clinically, often aided by radiologic and histologic evaluation.

26. **b. TCR interaction with CD8 co-receptor.** The interaction of the TCR and class II HLA antigens requires the stabilization of CD4 on T cells. Class I antigen would be required to engage the CD8 molecules. The initiation of further downstream intracellular events is dependent on the cell surface engagement of class II antigen and CD4.

27. **a. The 4 Jak kinases are not constitutively associated with various cytokine receptors.** The Janus family of kinases are constitutively expressed and are associated with various cell surface cytokine receptors. Once these receptors are engaged the Jak kinases become activated and promote cytokine gene expression.

28. **a. It is a mechanism for the elimination of aged, damaged, and autoimmune cells or cells no longer needed for differentiation.** The proteins responsible for executing the suicide program are the caspases, and they can be triggered by a number of mechanisms such as Fas and TNFR but not the T cell receptor or Jak kinases.

29. **All of the statements are true.**
    a. **Many human tumors express antigenic epitopes that can be recognized by either CD4+ T cells or by CD8+ T cells.**
    b. **T cells can destroy tumor cells by several mechanisms, which include the elaboration of granules containing pore forming proteins, the upregulation of FasL that can bind Fas receptors, and the activation of macrophages.**
    c. **IFN-γ production by lymphocytes is necessary but not sufficient for promoting antitumor immune response.**
    d. **Tumors may evade T-cell detection because of a loss of MHC class I /II molecules or because of a decrease in expression of transporter proteins associated with antigen processing.**
    e. **T-reg cells, TGF-β, IL-10, gangliosides, and prostaglandin represent potential immune suppressive mechanisms within the tumor microenvironment.**

16

Molecular Genetics and Cancer Biology

ADAM S. KIBEL

QUESTIONS

1. DNA is composed of all of the following elements EXCEPT:
   a. a base, either a purine or a pyrimidine.
   b. a sugar, called ribose.
   c. a phosphate.
   d. two complementary strands.
   e. hydrogen bonds.
2. The physical chemistry of DNA bases requires:
   a. uracil to form a hydrogen bond with guanine.
   b. purine to form a hydrogen bond with another purine.
   c. pyrimidine to form a hydrogen bond with a purine.
   d. adenine to form a hydrogen bond with cytosine.
   e. thymine to form a hydrogen bond with guanine.
3. Which of the following does DNA expression require?
   a. Linear DNA to be converted into linear RNA, a process called translation
   b. Conversion of linear RNA into a linear set of amino acids, a process called transcription
   c. Protein synthesis exclusively within the nucleus
   d. Mitosis
   e. A mechanism to bridge the gap between the genetic code and protein synthesis
4. Which of the following statements about transcriptional regulation is NOT true?
   a. Two general components involved in transcriptional regulation are specific sequences in the RNA and proteins that interact with those sequences.
   b. In addition to the genetic information carried within the nucleotide sequence of DNA, it provides specific docking sites for proteins that enhance the activity of the transcriptional machinery.
   c. Specific sequences within the promoter or enhancer region of a gene are called response elements.
   d. DNA sequences, often referred to as consensus sequences, are found in many genes and respond in a coordinated manner to a specific signal.
   e. It is an important mechanism to ensure coordinated gene expression.
5. What is alternative splicing?
   a. A form of protein modification occurring after a mature polypeptide is produced
   b. A modification to DNA during meiosis
   c. A process of including or excluding certain exons in an mRNA transcript
   d. A process in which novel RNA sequences are randomly inserted into a transcript
   e. A method of RNA degradation
6. Which of the following statements is TRUE regarding the nuclear matrix?
   a. It has the same protein composition in every tissue type.
   b. It is the site of mRNA transcription.
   c. It has the same protein composition whether a cell is proliferating or undergoing differentiation.
   d. It provides a mechanism to trace the cell type of origin for a cancer, because the nuclear matrix is identical within tissue types.
   e. It is a form of DNA.
7. What happens in the process of translation?
   a. The RNA message of four parts (the nucleotides A, U, C, G) is converted into 20 amino acids by using a functional group of three adjacent nucleotides called a codon.
   b. Each amino acid is encoded by only one codon.
   c. Shifts in the reading frame are of no consequence in the production of the polypeptide chain because of the fidelity of template DNA.
   d. Single-base substitutions always encode for the identical amino acid, known as a polymorphism.
   e. Transfer of genetic information from the DNA to the RNA occurs.
8. Which of the following statements about ubiquitization is NOT true?
   a. Ubiquitization is an important regulatory mechanism of a cell, used in the efficient disposal of proteins.
   b. A small protein called ubiquitin is linked to a protein, tagging it for destruction.
   c. The proteosome is the site of protein-ubiquitin complex degradation.
   d. The proteosome has a cylindrical shape.
   e. The targeted inhibition of proteosome function appears to enhance cancer progression.

9. Which of the following statements about oncogenes is TRUE?
   a. They are mutated forms of abnormal genes, known as proto-oncogenes.
   b. They can be produced by an inactivating mutation of a proto-oncogene, resulting in the silencing of the gene.
   c. They can be produced by gene amplification, resulting in many copies of the gene, or by chromosomal rearrangement.
   d. They are always due to retroviruses, capable of inducing malignant transformation of normal cells.
   e. They are endogenous cancer-fighting genes.
10. Which of the following statements about hypermethylation is TRUE?
   a. It is a direct change to the DNA sequence, similar to a mutation.
   b. It occurs exclusively on cytosine nucleotides in the dinucleotide sequence CG.
   c. Somatic methylation of CpG dinucleotides in the regulatory regions of genes is very often associated with increased transcriptional activity, leading to increased expression of that gene.
   d. In cancer, hypermethylation is associated with enhanced activity of oncogenes, and demethylation may be an effective strategy for the treatment of cancer.
   e. It marks cells for ubiquitinization.
11. Von Hippel-Lindau disease predisposes patients to:
   a. Epididymal carcinoma
   b. Clear cell renal carcinoma
   c. Papillary renal cell carcinoma
   d. Adrenocortical carcinoma
   e. All of the above
12. Hereditary prostate carcinoma is estimated to account for what percentage of patients diagnosed with prostate cancer before 55 years of age?
   a. 0% to 20%
   b. 21% to 40%
   c. 41% to 60%
   d. 61% to 80%
   e. 81% to 100%
13. Hereditary prostate cancer genes that have been proven to cause prostate carcinoma include:
   a. *ELAC2*
   b. *MSR1*
   c. *RNASEL*
   d. None of the above
   e. All of the above
14. Wilms' tumor has been linked to which of the following hereditary tumor syndromes?
   a. WAGR syndrome
   b. Denys-Drash syndrome
   c. Beckwith-Wiedemann syndrome
   d. None of the above
   e. All of the above
15. Polymorphism with which of the following genes has been linked to prostate cancer?
   a. Vitamin D receptor
   b. 5α-Reductase type II
   c. Androgen receptor
   d. None of the above
   e. All of the above
16. Polymorphisms:
   a. are mutations.
   b. usually have functional significance.
   c. can alter expression of genes.
   d. occur rarely in normal population.
   e. All of the above.
17. The two main points of control in the cell cycle are:
   a. S and G_0
   b. S and G_2M
   c. M and G_1S
   d. G_1S and G_2M
   e. G_2 and M
18. The *TP53* tumor suppressor gene plays a critical role in which of the following processes?
   a. Apoptosis
   b. Angiogenesis
   c. DNA replication
   d. Signal transduction
   e. All of the above
19. Which of the following is an alternative splice variant of $p16^{INK4a}$?
   a. $p27^{kip1}$
   b. $p57^{kip2}$
   c. $p15^{INK4b}$
   d. $p14^{ARF}$
   e. $p21^{cip1}$
20. INK4 family members inhibit the activity of:
   a. cyclin D/cdk4.
   b. cyclin E/cdk2.
   c. cyclin A/cdk2.
   d. cyclin B/cdc2.
   e. all of the above.
21. Cyclin-cdk complexes primarily function at the G_1S boundary by:
   a. dephosphorylation of RB.
   b. phosphorylation of mdm2.
   c. dephosphorylation of E2F.
   d. phosphorylation of E2F.
   e. phosphorylation of RB.
22. The regulatory proteins at the G_2M checkpoint primarily respond to:
   a. hypoxia.
   b. nutrient poor environment.
   c. DNA damage.
   d. cytokines.
   e. all of the above.
23. Nucleotide excision repair primarily protects the cell from DNA damage caused by:
   a. reactive oxygen species.
   b. DNA polymerase errors.
   c. double-stranded breaks.
   d. ultraviolet light.
   e. all of the above.
24. The mismatch repair pathway heterodimers responsible for single nucleotide mismatches are:
   a. MSH2/MSH6.
   b. MSH2/MSH3.
   c. MSH3/MSH6.
   d. MLH1/PMS2.
   e. PMS2/MSH6.

25. Which of the following genes has been linked to double strand break repair?
   a. *TP53*
   b. *VHL*
   c. *BRCA1*
   d. *RB*
   e. *PTEN*

26. Which of the following is a procaspase?
   a. TRAIL
   b. FLICE
   c. FAS
   d. TRID
   e. *bcl-2*

27. Ligand-dependent apoptosis is an attractive therapeutic target because activation is:
   a. independent of *p53*.
   b. dependent on *p53*.
   c. independent of caspases.
   d. dependent on caspases.
   e. dependent on Rb.

28. The *p53*-induced apoptosis is mediated through:
   a. APAF-1/caspase 9.
   b. CD95 receptor.
   c. TRAIL.
   d. Bcl-2.
   e. $p21^{cip}$.

29. How do proapoptotic *bcl-2* family members function? By:
   a. digesting the mitochondria.
   b. increasing the cellular membrane permeability.
   c. increasing the mitochondrial membrane permeability.
   d. directly activating executioner caspases.
   e. increasing nuclear membrane permeability.

30. Telomerase immortalizes cells by:
   a. protecting the cells from DNA damage.
   b. stabilizing *p53*.
   c. allowing the cell to grow in a nutrient poor environment.
   d. inhibiting apoptosis.
   e. maintaining chromosomal length.

31. Hepatitis B and papilloma viruses are responsible for what percentage of virus-induced malignancies?
   a. 20%
   b. 40%
   c. 60%
   d. 80%
   e. 100%

32. The viral protein E6 functions by inactivating:
   a. VHL.
   b. Rb.
   c. $p16^{INK4a}$.
   d. *p53*.
   e. E2F.

33. Human papillomavirus has been most convincingly linked to which one of the following genitourinary carcinomas?
   a. Testis
   b. Prostate
   c. Renal
   d. Bladder
   e. Penile

34. High-risk human papillomavirus subtypes include:
   a. HPV-11.
   b. HPV-16.
   c. HPV-18.
   d. HPV-33.
   e. All of the above.

35. Conditional knockout mice are useful genetic tools because they:
   a. exactly recapitulate tumor syndromes in humans.
   b. allow induction of tumor formation in the adult.
   c. have organ systems that can be selectively targeted.
   d. have none of the above.
   e. have all of the above.

36. Immunohistochemistry is useful to identify:
   a. tumors of uncertain origin
   b. prognostic markers in tumors
   c. molecular targets for therapy
   d. all of the above
   e. none of the above

37. An isochromosome of 12p has been identified in which genitourinary carcinoma?
   a. Testis
   b. Prostate
   c. Renal
   d. Bladder
   e. Penile

ANSWERS

1. **b. a sugar, called ribose.** Ribose is an element of RNA, not DNA. In a rudimentary form, DNA is the fusion of three different elements: a base (either a pyrimidine or a purine), a sugar (in the case of DNA called 2-deoxyribose; for RNA called ribose), and a phosphate (which links individual nucleotides together). The repeating connections between the phosphates and the sugars provide the backbone from which the information-carrying bases protrude. In its "resting" or nonreplicating form, this chain of elements forms a helix of two complementary strands; this double helix is held together by the hydrogen bonds.

2. **c. a pyrimidine to form a hydrogen bond with a purine.** The double helix is held together by the formation of a hydrogen bond between the pyrimidine on one strand and the purine base on the other. Uracil is in RNA not DNA. Purines do not form bases with purines. The purine adenine (A) always forms a hydrogen bond to the pyrimidine thymine (T), and the purine guanine (G) always forms a hydrogen bond to the pyrimidine cytosine (C).

3. **e. a mechanism to bridge the gap between the genetic code and protein synthesis.** The physical locations of DNA and its genetic code and protein synthesis and the manifestation of that code

are separate: DNA is in the nucleus, and protein synthesis is cytoplasmic. DNA message must be converted into mRNA by a process called transcription in the nucleus. The mRNA is transferred into the cytoplasm where the mRNA is converted into a protein by a process called translation.

4. **a. The two general components involved in transcriptional regulation are specific sequences in the RNA and proteins that interact with those sequences.** Specific sequences in the DNA called response elements bind to the nuclear proteins that control transcription. Importantly, this provides a mechanism to coordinate gene expression by providing similar docking sites for genes that need to be expressed at specific time points. Whereas mRNA transcription, stability, transport, and translation are all highly regulated, they are not controlled by the transcriptional machinery binding to specific mRNA sequences.

5. **c. a process of including or excluding certain exons in an mRNA transcript.** A specific gene may have multiple similar (not identical) forms (isoforms). This is accomplished by having specific exons included or excluded from the final mRNA transcript. This allows one DNA sequence to produce several protein products that have different functions. It is not a random process but is very tightly regulated to ensure that the correct mRNA transcript is produced in the correct cell at the correct point in time.

6. **b. It is the site of mRNA transcription.**

7. **a. The RNA message of four parts (the nucleotides A, U, C, G) is converted into 20 amino acids by using a functional group of three adjacent nucleotides called a codon.** There is significant redundancy with several codons encoding for each amino acid. As a result, the RNA sequence between individuals *can* be different and yet still encode the same amino acid sequence (a polymorphism). However, some polymorphisms do result in amino acid changes. Shifts in reading frame are the most deleterious mutations because they result in a change in all the codons after the insertion/deletion and as a result a dramatic change in the amino acid sequence.

8. **e. The targeted inhibition of proteosome function appears to enhance cancer progression.** Degradation of proteins in the cell is an active, not passive, process. Ubiquitinization is the process by which proteins are tagged for transport to the proteosome for destruction. Perturbation of this process is often found in cancer and therefore inhibition of ubiquitinization is a promising therapy for cancer.

9. **c. They can be produced by gene amplification, resulting in many copies of the gene, or by chromosomal rearrangement.** There are at least three ways a proto-oncogene can be converted into an oncogene. First, a mutation can occur within the coding sequence, producing a permanently activated form of the gene. A second mechanism converting a proto-oncogene into an oncogene is through gene amplification. A third mechanism of oncogene formation is through chromosomal rearrangement.

10. **b. It occurs exclusively on cytosine nucleotides in the dinucleotide sequence CG.** Hypermethylation is a normal process by which DNA is modified by the addition of a methyl group to a cytosine nucleotide in a CpG DNA sequence. There is no change in DNA sequence. Methylation results in gene silencing, that is, decreased expression of the gene. As a result, hypermethylation in cancer is associated with decreased transcription and, therefore, expression of a tumor suppressor gene. Ubiquitinization decreases levels of proteins but does so by increasing the degradation of the protein. Whereas alterations in ubiquitinization occur in cancer, they are not directly related to methylation.

11. **b. Clear cell renal carcinoma.** VHL is a hereditary tumor syndrome that predisposes patients to clear cell renal carcinoma, retinal angiomas, pheochromocytomas, hemangiomas of the CNS, epididymal cystadenomas, and pancreatic islet cell tumors. It is not associated with epididymal, papillary renal cell, or adrenocortical carcinomas.

12. **c. 41% to 60%.** Although the inherited form of prostate cancer is estimated to be responsible for only 9% of all prostate cancer, it is implicated in 43% of cases of disease diagnosed before 55 years of age.

13. **d. none of the above.** All of the genes above have been linked to prostate cancer by both linkage studies examining families with a strong predisposition to prostate cancer and in some cases by case control studies examining polymorphisms within these genes. However, no data have demonstrated that these genes cause prostate cancer.

14. **e. All of the above.** Hereditary Wilms' tumor accounts for approximately 1% of Wilms' tumor cases. The classic disease was first described by Fitzgerald and Hardin in 1955 and is characterized by bilateral and multicentric tumors. Wilms' tumor can also occur as part of the more complex tumor syndromes WAGR and Denys-Drash syndrome. WAGR syndrome is characterized by Wilms' tumor, aniridia, genitourinary abnormalities, gonadoblastoma, and mental retardation and was first described by Miller and colleagues in 1964. Denys-Drash syndrome is characterized by Wilms' tumor, genitourinary abnormalities, pseudohermaphroditism, and nephropathy and was first described in 1967. All three syndromes are caused, at least in part, by genetic abnormalities in the same gene, *WT1*. Wilms' tumor is also associated with Beckwith-Wiedemann syndrome and is characterized by exomphalos, macroglossia, and gigantism in the neonate. However, Beckwith-Wiedemann syndrome has not been linked to *WT1*.

15. **e. All of the above.** The link between prostate cancer and polymorphisms within genes important in steroid metabolism or function provides one of the best examples in genitourinary malignancies. The relationship between androgens and prostate cancer is well known. Although the androgen receptor has been targeted for the treatment of advanced prostate cancer for many years, it is only recently that the association between androgen receptor polymorphisms and prostate cancer has been identified. Shorter CAG repeat variants within the open reading frame have been linked to not only localized prostate cancer but also advanced and even lethal disease. Polymorphisms within the 5α-reductase type II gene have also been linked to aggressive prostate carcinoma. The known association between prostate cancer and vitamin D, coupled with the discovery that certain vitamin D receptor genotypes have altered activity, has stimulated interest in the effect of vitamin D receptor genotype on prostate cancer risk, and an association between the less active receptor variant and prostate cancer has been demonstrated.

16. c. **can alter expression of genes.** With the cloning of the human genome it has become apparent that genetic anomalies are not limited to high-risk individuals; over 10 million common genetic variants exist. These are not mutations but are normal differences in the human genome. Although the majority have no functional significance, variants within the reading frame of the gene can change the amino acid sequence, variants within the promoter can alter transcription of a gene, and variants in close proximity to intron-exon boundaries can alter splicing.

17. **d. G_1S and G_2M.**

18. **a. Apoptosis.** Active *TP53* binds to the promoter region of *TP53*-responsive genes and stimulates the transcription of genes responsible for cell cycle arrest, repair of DNA damage, and apoptosis. *TP53* responds to DNA damage by inducing cell cycle arrest through p21cip1 and then transcriptionally activating DNA repair enzymes. If the cell cannot arrest growth and/or repair the DNA, *TP53* induces apoptosis. Whereas angiogenesis, DNA replication, and signal transduction are all critical cellular processes, *TP53* does not directly influence any of them.

19. **d. p14^{ARF}.** p14ARF was originally identified as an alternative splice variant of the cdk inhibitor p16INK4a. It has been demonstrated that p14^{ARF} functions not by acting as a cdk inhibitor but by degrading mdm2.

20. **a. cyclin D/cdk4.** The INK4 family of cdk inhibitors directly inhibits the assembly of cyclin D with cdk4 and cdk6 by blocking the phosphorylation of the cyclin D-cdk4/6 complex. This phosphorylation is necessary for activation of the complex.

21. **e. phosphorylation of RB.** Phosphorylation is the attachment of a phosphate to a protein. It alters the conformation of the protein and therefore is an excellent method of regulating gene function. Cyclin-cdk complexes phosphorylate RB or its family members, p107 and p130. Phosphorylated RB can no longer bind to members of the E2F family of transcription factors. Free E2F heterodimerizes with DP1 or DP2 and transcriptionally activates genes important in DNA replication, such as DNA polymerase-A and the cell cycle, such as E2F-1. Dephosphorylation of RB has the opposite effect.
E2F regulation does not occur directly though phosphorylation or dephosphorylation. Mdm2 regulates p53 and is not directly affected by cyclin-cdk complexes.

22. **c. DNA damage.** Hypoxia, nutrient-poor environment, and cytokines are all signals to the cell that it is not in an environment that is conducive to cellular division. These signals influence the cell BEFORE it invests its energy in replicating the DNA, that is, it is a G1S checkpoint. If DNA damage occurs, it is critical the errors are repaired before cellular division. Therefore, DNA damage can lead to cell cycle arrest at both the G_1S and G_2M checkpoints.

23. **d. ultraviolet light.** Nucleotide excision repair (NER) is a major defense against DNA damage caused by ultraviolet radiation and chemical exposure. NER acts on a wide range of alterations that result in large local distortions in DNA by recognizing distortions in the DNA helix, excising the damaged DNA, and replacing it with the correct sequence. Base excision repair is the primary mechanism for repairing damage caused by reactive oxygen species. Mismatch repair is the primary mechanism for polymerase errors. Double-strand break repair is the primary mechanism for repairing double-strand breaks.

24. **a. MSH2/MSH6.** Mismatch repair (MMR) removes nucleotides mispaired by DNA polymerases and insertion/deletion loops (ranging from one to ten or more bases) that result from slippage during replication of repetitive sequences or during recombination. The MMR proteins form heterodimers, each of which is responsible for detecting specific DNA replication errors. The MSH2/MSH3 heterodimer (MutSβ) mediates repair of insertions and deletions whereas the MSH2/MSH6 heterodimer (MutSα) recognizes the single nucleotide mismatches in addition to insertions and deletions.

25. **c. *BRCA1*.** *BRCA1* is associated with familial breast and ovarian cancer. It is believed that the breast cancer susceptibility gene *BRCA1* (as well as *BRCA2*) play an important role in homologous recombination as well as sensing DNA damage. Both *BRCA1* and *BRCA2* are part of an enzymatic complex with *RAD51*- and *BRCA1*-associated RING domain 1 (BARD1). This complex is recruited by proliferating cell nuclear antigen (PCNA) to regions that have undergone DNA damage to repair DNA breaks.

26. **b. FLICE.** In turn, procaspase 8, or FLICE, binds to FADD via the death effector domain. Procaspase 8 oligomerization promotes autoactivation to caspase 8.

27. **a. independent of *p53*.** The identification of ligand-dependent apoptosis receptors may have a profound impact on therapy. Most cancer therapies (e.g., chemotherapy and external beam radiotherapy) depend on *p53* to induce apoptosis in the cancer cell. Because *p53* is mutated in more than half of malignancies, *p53*-independent pathways for apoptosis are of great clinical interest. Because ligand-dependent apoptosis is independent of *p53*, these receptors and ligands are attractive and novel treatment targets.

28. **a. APAF-1/caspase 9.** The *p53*-induced apoptosis is dependent on the APAF-1/caspase 9 activation pathway.

29. **c. increasing the mitochondrial membrane permeability.** Although each proapoptotic *bcl-2* family member responds to different stimuli, the principal mechanism by which these family members induce cell death is by increasing mitochondrial membrane permeability.

30. **e. maintaining chromosomal length.** Telomerase immortalizes cells by maintaining the ends of the chromosomes, or telomeres, which normally shorten with each cell division.

31. **d. 80%.** DNA viruses are believed to play much more of a role in human tumorigenesis than RNA viruses, with hepatitis B virus and papillomaviruses responsible for 80% of virus-induced malignancies.

32. **d. *p53*.** E6 appears to primarily function by targeting *p53* for ubiquitin-mediated degradation. Inactivation of *p53* blocks both cell cycle arrest and apoptosis and in doing so promotes the malignant phenotype.

33. **e. Penile.** Human papillomavirus infection with high-risk subtypes has been linked to penile carcinoma. This virus has been detected in 15% to 80% of penile lesions.

34. **e. All of the above.** HPV-16 appears to be the dominant subtype and has been identified in up to 90% of human papillomavirus-positive lesions. HPV-11, HPV-18, and HPV-33 have also been identified in penile tumors.

35. **c. have organ systems that can be selectively targeted.** Selective deletion of genes, once the mouse reached maturity, became possible in 1988 when Sauer and Henderson demonstrated that the Cre protein isolated from bacteriophage could be used to induce recombination events in mammalian cells at genetically engineered sites. This allowed the mouse to develop normally until exposed to the protein, at which point the cells exposed would delete the gene of interest. Conditional knockouts of the *apc* gene are allowed to develop normally until adulthood. Exposure of the colonic mucosa to Cre leads to loss of the *apc* gene in some cells and the development of colon carcinoma. This more closely recapitulates the chain of events that leads to colon carcinoma. In the near future, additional conditional knockouts will be developed.

36. **d. all of the above.** Immunohistochemistry has several important uses in oncology. Immunohistochemistry is crucial to the accurate identification of tumors of uncertain origin, if conventional light microscopy cannot identify the tumor. This can be crucial for instituting proper therapy. For example, prostate-specific antigen staining has proved to be a useful adjunct in identifying adenocarcinomas of uncertain origin as in the prostate. Cancer markers have also proved useful for identifying bladder tumors from metastatic lesions. A second use of immunohistochemistry is to stain for prognostic biomarkers. The subclassification of

tumors into aggressive and indolent on the basis of the molecular profile has the potential to radically change practice. Prostate cancers of identical stage and grade can have variable clinical courses. The ability to identify patients with poor prognoses and those with a good prognoses or who will respond to a particular treatment independent of grade and stage would be of significant clinical utility. Although still experimental, *p53* in bladder cancer is emerging as a potential independent indicator of aggressive disease and may prove useful for stratifying cases for neoadjuvant chemotherapy. Molecular identification of tumor targets for therapy will become increasingly prevalent in the near future. The best example of this is the use of immunohistochemistry to identify the presence of her-2/neu receptor in breast cancer. Not only does her-2/neu receptor provide prognostic information in breast cancer, but if the receptor is present it provides a molecular target for antibody therapy. Preliminary data have demonstrated that the antibody herceptin is effective in treating patients whose tumors express the receptor.

37. a. **Testis.** The urologic malignancy most closely linked to a karyotypic abnormality is a testis tumor. A 12p isochromosome was first identified in a testis tumor in the 1980s, and experimentally this cytogenetic hallmark of testicular tumors has diagnostic and prognostic value.

17

Tissue Engineering and Cell Therapy: Perspectives for Urology

ANTHONY ATALA

QUESTIONS

1. Currently, possible tissue replacements for reconstruction include which of the following?
   a. Native nonurologic tissues
   b. Homologous tissues
   c. Heterologous tissues
   d. Artificial biomaterials
   e. All of the above
2. What are the most common types of synthetic prostheses for urologic use made of?
   a. Latex
   b. Silicone
   c. Urethane
   d. Biodegradable polymers
   e. Polyvinyl
3. What does tissue engineering involve?
   a. The principles of cell transplantation
   b. The principles of materials science
   c. The use of matrices alone
   d. The use of matrices with cells
   e. All of the above
4. In tissue engineering, when autologous cells are used:
   a. donor tissue is dissociated into individual cells.
   b. cells are either implanted directly into the host or expanded in culture.
   c. cells are attached to a support matrix.
   d. cells and matrix are implanted in vivo.
   e. all of the above.
5. Which of the following statements is true regarding biomaterials?
   a. They facilitate the localization and delivery of cells.
   b. They facilitate the localization and delivery of bioactive factors.
   c. They define a three-dimensional space for the formation of new tissues.
   d. They guide the development of new tissues with appropriate function.
   e. All of the above.
6. Types of biomaterials that have been utilized for engineering genitourinary tissues include which of the following?
   a. Naturally derived materials
   b. Acellular tissue matrices
   c. Synthetic polymers
   d. All of the above
   e. None of the above
7. Procedures and techniques that allow for the exclusion of nonurologic tissues during augmentation cystoplasty include which of the following?
   a. Autoaugmentation
   b. Ureterocystoplasty
   c. Tissue expansion
   d. Tissue engineering
   e. All of the above
8. In demucosalized intestinal segments for urinary reconstruction, removal of the mucosa and submucosa may lead to:
   a. contraction of the intestinal patch.
   b. mucosal regrowth.
   c. tissue necrosis.
   d. decreased vascularity.
   e. angiogenesis.
9. Permanent synthetic materials, when used in continuity with the urinary tract, have been associated with:
   a. mechanical failure.
   b. emboli.
   c. calculus formation.
   d. a and c.
   e. none of the above.
10. Urothelium is associated with:
    a. high reparative capacity.
    b. inherent capacity for artificial extracellular matrix attachment.
    c. frequent malignant differentiation.
    d. poor growth parameters.
    e. none of the above.

11. Major limitations in phallic reconstructive surgery include which of the following?
    a. The availability of adequate growth factors
    b. The availability of sufficient autologous tissue
    c. The availability of adequate surgical techniques
    d. All of the above
    e. None of the above

12. What is the most prevalent form of renal replacement therapy?
    a. Organ transplantation
    b. Dialysis
    c. Bioartificial hemofilters
    d. Bioartificial renal tubules
    e. Engineered functional renal structures

13. The ideal bulking substance for the endoscopic treatment of reflux and incontinence should have what characteristic?
    a. Easily injectable
    b. Nonantigenic
    c. Nonmigratory
    d. Volume stable
    e. All of the above

14. Which of the following statements regarding microencapsulated cells is TRUE?
    a. They have a semipermeable barrier.
    b. They are protected from the host's immune system.
    c. They allow for physiologic release of substances.
    d. They provide a long-term delivery system of by-products.
    e. All of the above.

15. What are the most common cell sources for tissue engineering today?
    a. Embryonic stem cells
    b. Adult unipotent stem cells
    c. Autologous primary cells
    d. Stem cells derived from nuclear transfer techniques
    e. None of the above

ANSWERS

1. **e. All of the above.** Whenever there is a lack of native urologic tissue, reconstruction may be performed with native nonurologic tissues (skin, gastrointestinal segments, or mucosa from multiple body sites), homologous tissues (cadaver fascia, cadaver or donor kidney), heterologous tissues (bovine collagen), or artificial materials (silicone, polyurethane, Teflon).

2. **b. Silicone.** The most common type of synthetic prostheses for urologic use is made of silicone.

3. **e. All of the above.** Tissue engineering follows the principles of cell transplantation, materials science, and engineering toward the development of biologic substitutes that would restore and maintain normal function. Tissue engineering may involve matrices alone, wherein the body's natural ability to regenerate is used to orient or direct new tissue growth, or the use of matrices with cells.

4. **e. all of the above.** When cells are used for tissue engineering, donor tissue is dissociated into individual cells, which either are implanted directly into the host or are expanded in culture, attached to a support matrix, and reimplanted after expansion. The implanted tissue can be heterologous, allogeneic, or autologous.

5. **e. All of the above.** Biomaterials facilitate the localization and delivery of cells and/or bioactive factors (e.g., cell adhesion peptides and growth factors) to desired sites in the body, define a three-dimensional space for the formation of new tissues with appropriate structure, and guide the development of new tissues with appropriate function.

6. **d. All of the above.** Generally, three classes of biomaterials have been used for engineering genitourinary tissues: naturally derived materials (e.g., collagen and alginate), acellular tissue matrices (e.g., bladder submucosa and small intestinal submucosa), and synthetic polymers (e.g., polyglycolic acid [PGA], polylactic acid [PLA], and poly(lactic-co-glycolic acid) [PLGA]).

7. **e. All of the above.** Because of the problems encountered with the use of gastrointestinal segments, numerous investigators have attempted alternative methods, materials, and tissues for bladder replacement or repair. These include autoaugmentation, ureterocystoplasty, methods for tissue expansion, seromuscular grafts, matrices for tissue regeneration, and tissue engineering using cell transplantation.

8. **a. contraction of the intestinal patch.** It has been noted that removal of only the mucosa may lead to mucosal regrowth whereas removal of the mucosa and submucosa may lead to retraction of the intestinal patch.

9. **d. a and c.** Usually, permanent synthetic materials used for bladder reconstruction succumb to mechanical failure and urinary stone formation, and degradable materials lead to fibroblast deposition, scarring, graft contracture, and a reduced reservoir volume over time.

10. **a. a high reparative capacity.** It has been well established for decades that the bladder is able to regenerate generously over free grafts. Urothelium is associated with a high reparative capacity. Bladder muscle tissue is less likely to regenerate in a normal manner.

11. **b. The availability of sufficient autologous tissue.** One of the major limitations of phallic reconstructive surgery is the availability of sufficient autologous tissue.

12. **b. Dialysis.** Although dialysis therapy is currently the most prevalent form of renal replacement therapy, the relatively high morbidity and mortality rates have prompted investigators to seek alternative solutions involving ex-vivo systems.

13. **e. All of the above.** The ideal substance for the endoscopic treatment of reflux and incontinence should be injectable, nonantigenic, nonmigratory, volume stable, and safe for human use.

14. **e. All of the above.** Microencapsulated Leydig cells offer several advantages, such as serving as a semipermeable barrier between the transplanted cells and the host's immune system, as well as allowing for the long-term physiologic release of testosterone.

15. **c. Autologous primary cells.** Most current strategies for engineering urologic tissues involve harvesting of autologous cells from the host diseased organ. However, in situations in which extensive end-stage organ failure is present, a tissue biopsy may not yield enough normal cells for expansion. Under these circumstances, the availability of pluripotent stem cells may be beneficial.

SECTION VI

REPRODUCTIVE AND SEXUAL FUNCTION

18

Male Reproductive Physiology

PETER N. SCHLEGEL • MATTHEW P. HARDY • MARC GOLDSTEIN

QUESTIONS

1. The proportion of testicular volume comprised of seminiferous tubules in the human testis is:
   a. 5%.
   b. 10% to 20%.
   c. 50% to 60%.
   d. 70% to 80%.
   e. 90% to 95%.
2. Testicular blood supply is derived from all of the following sources EXCEPT:
   a. internal spermatic artery.
   b. deferential artery.
   c. external spermatic artery.
   d. cremasteric artery.
   e. pudendal artery.
3. How often is more than one artery identifiable in the spermatic cord during inguinal dissection?
   a. 10%
   b. 20%
   c. 50%
   d. 80%
   e. 95%
4. What is the temperature differential (in °C) between the testes and rectal temperature in a normal man?
   a. 0
   b. 0 to 1
   c. 1 to 2
   d. 2 to 3
   e. 4 to 5
5. Primary, acute regulation of testosterone is dependent on which of the following hormones?
   a. LH
   b. StAR
   c. FSH
   d. Estradiol
   e. Inhibin
6. When does a testosterone peak occur during a human male's life?
   a. 2 months
   b. 6 to 9 months
   c. 30 to 40 years
   d. 50 to 60 years
   e. >70 years
7. Which hormones play a central role in regulation of Sertoli cell function?
   a. LH, FSH
   b. FSH, estradiol
   c. Prolactin, LH
   d. FSH, testosterone
   e. ABP, testosterone
8. Structural components of the blood-testis barrier are seen at what levels?
   a. Sertoli-Sertoli cell junctions
   b. Leydig cells
   c. Basement membrane
   d. Desmosomes between spermatocytes
   e. Spermatids
9. What is the normal developmental pattern of spermatogenic cells?
   a. Sertoli→spermatogonia→spermatocyte.
   b. Spermatocyte→spermatogonia→spermatid.
   c. Spermatid→Sertoli→spermatocytes.
   d. Spermatogonia→spermatid→spermatocyte.
   e. Spermatogonia→spermatocyte→spermatid.

10. When does mitotic activity of gonocytes end?
    a. Week 36 of gestation
    b. 3 months
    c. 2 years
    d. 9 years
    e. 14 years
11. Development of type A spermatogonia to type B spermatogonia is dependent on:
    a. c-*kit*
    b. Fas
    c. DBY
    d. SRY
    e. ABP
12. Spermiogenesis includes all of the following processes EXCEPT:
    a. loss of cytoplasm.
    b. formation of the acrosome.
    c. flagellar formation.
    d. migration of cytoplasmic organelles.
    e. cell division.
13. The hormone needed for maintenance of spermatogenesis is:
    a. testosterone.
    b. dihydrotestosterone.
    c. estradiol.
    d. oxytocin.
    e. inhibin.
14. The proportion of men with nonobstructive azoospermia who have microdeletions of the Y chromosome is:
    a. <1%.
    b. 2% to 5%.
    c. 5% to 10%.
    d. 20% to 30%.
    e. 50%.
15. Major components of the epididymis include:
    a. caput, corpus, cauda.
    b. globus minor, ductus deferens, cauda.
    c. rete testis, efferent ductules, caput.
    d. efferent ductules, caput, cauda.
    e. septa, efferent ductules, corpus.
16. The progenitors of basal cells in the epididymis are:
    a. goblet cells.
    b. pyramidal cells.
    c. neutrophils.
    d. macrophages.
    e. stromal cells.
17. With chronic obstruction, optimal sperm quality is found in what region of the epididymis?
    a. Rete testis
    b. Efferent ducts
    c. Proximal epididymis
    d. Mid epididymis
    e. Distal epididymis
18. Changes in sperm characteristics during epididymal transit include:
    a. increased positive charge.
    b. sulfhydryl reduction.
    c. decreased phospholipid content.
    d. reduced membrane rigidity.
    e. increased capacity for glycolysis.
19. The spermatozoal region containing mitochondria is the:
    a. tail.
    b. head.
    c. acrosome.
    d. mid-piece.
    e. dynein cross-arms.
20. Human embryonic mitotic activity is controlled by sperm:
    a. DNA.
    b. RNA.
    c. acrosome.
    d. centrosome.
    e. mitochondria.
21. After ejaculation the contents of the vas deferens are:
    a. returned to the seminal vesicles.
    b. maintained in the ampulla.
    c. released into the ejaculatory ducts.
    d. propelled back into the epididymis.
    e. released into the bladder.

ANSWERS

1. **d. 70% to 80%.** In humans, interstitial tissue takes up 20% to 30% of the total testicular volume.
2. **e. pudendal artery.** The arterial supply to the human testis and epididymis is derived from three sources: the internal spermatic artery, the deferential artery, and the external spermatic or cremasteric artery.
3. **c. 50%.** An intraoperative dissection study of more than 100 spermatic cords identified a single internal spermatic artery in 50% of cases, with two arteries in 30% of spermatic cords and three arteries in 20%.
4. **d. 2 to 3.** The countercurrent exchange of heat in the spermatic cord provides blood to the testis that is 2°C to 3°C cooler than the rectal temperature in the normal individual.
5. **a. LH.** LH stimulates Leydig cells to secrete testosterone.
6. **a. 2 months.** A testosterone peak occurs at approximately 2 months of age.
7. **d. FSH, testosterone.** The consensus is that FSH and testosterone play an important role in the regulation of Sertoli cell function, including ABP production.
8. **a. Sertoli-Sertoli cell junctions.** Sertoli-Sertoli tight junctions prevent the deep penetration of electron-opaque tracers into the seminiferous epithelium from the testicular interstitium. The blood-testis barrier appears to have three different levels within the testis. The primary level is formed by tight junctions between Sertoli cells and segregates premeiotic germ cells (spermatogonia) from other germ cells.
9. **e. Spermatogonia→spermatocyte→spermatid.** Proceeding from the least to the most differentiated, they were named dark type A spermatogonia (Ad); pale type A spermatogonia (Ap); type B spermatogonia (B); preleptotene primary spermatocytes (R); leptotene primary spermatocytes (L); zygotene primary spermatocytes (z); pachytene primary spermatocytes (p); secondary spermatocytes (II); and Sa, Sb1, Sb2, Sc, Sd1, and Sd2 spermatids.
10. **d. 9 years.** From 7 to 9 years of life, mitotic activity of gonocytes is detectable, with spermatogonia populating the base of the seminiferous tubule in numbers equal to those of the Sertoli cells.

11. **a. c-*kit*.** Evidence has suggested that a growth factor/receptor called the *kit* ligand/c-*kit* receptor system is involved in spermatagonial stem cell self-renewal. In fact, the c-*kit* receptor is a marker for type A cells in rats. The result of this process is that some type A_4 spermatogonia differentiate into intermediate and then type B spermatogonia that proceed through spermatogenesis, in a c-*kit*–dependent process, whereas other A_4 spermatogonia renew the stem cell population of type A_1 spermatogonia.

12. **e. cell division.** During spermiogenesis, the products of meiosis, the round Sa spermatids, metamorphose into mature spermatids (see Fig. 18-13). During this metamorphosis, extensive changes occur in both the spermatid cytoplasm and the nucleus but cell division is not required. These changes have been described in detail and include loss of cytoplasm, formation of the acrosome, formation of the flagellum, and migration of cytoplasmic organelles to positions characteristic of the mature spermatozoon.

13. **a. testosterone.** Testosterone will initiate and qualitatively maintain spermatogenesis in humans.

14. **c. 5% to 10%.** The detection of microdeletions of a region of the Y chromosome referred to as interval 6 in 5% to 10% of azoospermic men has focused attention on this area as the site for a critical factor (azoospermic factor) important for spermatogenesis.

15. **a. caput, corpus, cauda.** Anatomically, the epididymis is divided into three regions: the caput, the corpus, and the cauda epididymis (see Fig. 18-16). On the basis of histologic criteria, each of these regions can be subdivided into distinct zones separated by transition segments. The human caput epididymis consists of 8 to 12 ductuli efferentes and the proximal segment of the ductus epididymis. The lumen of the ductuli efferentes is large and somewhat irregular near the testis and becomes narrow and oval near the junction with the ductus epididymis. Distal to this junction, the diameter of the duct increases slightly and thereafter remains relatively constant throughout the corpus, or body, of the epididymis. In the bulky cauda epididymis, the diameter of the duct enlarges substantially and the lumen acquires an irregular shape.

16. **d. macrophages.** Basal cells are thought to be derived from macrophages.

17. **c. Proximal epididymis.** Data from studies of patients with congenital absence of the vas deferens or with epididymal obstruction frequently report poor motility in spermatozoa aspirated from the distal epididymis, with optimal sperm quality in the proximal epididymis.

18. **e. increased capacity for glycolysis.** Spermatozoa undergo numerous metabolic changes during epididymal transit. Studies using experimental animals described the acquisition of an increased capacity for glycolysis, changes in intracellular pH and calcium content, modification of adenylate cyclase activity, and alterations in cellular phospholipid and phospholipid-like fatty acid content.

19. **d. mid-piece.** The middle piece of the spermatozoon is a highly organized segment consisting of helically arranged mitochondria surrounding a set of outer dense fibers and the characteristic 9 + 2 microtubular structure of the sperm axoneme.

20. **d. centrosome.** In humans, the mitotic activity of embryos appears to be organized normally by the paternally derived centrosome.

21. **d. propelled back into the epididymis.** Studies have shown that after sexual stimulation and/or ejaculation, an interesting phenomenon occurred. The contents of the ductus deferens were propelled back toward the proximal epididymis and even into the cauda epididymis, because the distal portion of the ductus deferens contracted with greater amplitude, frequency, and duration than did the proximal portion of the ductus deferens.

19

Male Infertility

MARK SIGMAN • JONATHAN P. JAROW

QUESTIONS

1. The baseline pregnancy rates by intercourse for normal and infertile couples are:
   a. 50% per month for normal couples and 30% per month for infertile couples.
   b. the same for both fertile and infertile couples.
   c. 10% per month for normal couples and 3% per month for infertile couples.
   d. 20% to 25% per month for normal couples and 1% to 3% per month for infertile couples.
   e. 50% per month for normal couples and 25% per month for infertile couples.
2. How many days does the average sperm remain viable within the normal female reproductive tract?
   a. 1
   b. 3
   c. 5
   d. 7
   e. 10
3. How many days does the average egg remain receptive to fertilization after ovulation?
   a. 1
   b. 2
   c. 4
   d. 6
   e. 10
4. Which of the following lubricants is least likely to adversely affect sperm motility?
   a. KY jelly
   b. Astroglide
   c. Saliva
   d. Surgilube
   e. Peanut oil
5. After an acute toxic event such as a febrile illness, how long would you expect sperm counts to be depressed?
   a. 1 week
   b. 3 weeks
   c. 3 months
   d. 6 months
   e. 1 year
6. In couples in which the female is approaching 40:
   a. pregnancy rates are the same as when the female is 25 years old.
   b. treatment is often more aggressive than when the female is younger.
   c. infertility is treated in a slow stepwise fashion.
   d. treatment approaches never include in-vitro fertilization (IVF).
   e. insemination with donor sperm is encouraged.
7. What percentage of testicular volume is directly involved in producing sperm?
   a. 20%
   b. 40%
   c. 50%
   d. 80%
   e. 100%
8. The evaluation of the infertile male:
   a. should always include at least two semen analyses.
   b. should include semen analysis only if the female evaluation is normal.
   c. should include semen analyses, the results of which will determine whether the patient is fertile or sterile.
   d. should be performed only if the couple does not conceive after in-vitro fertilization.
   e. should usually include the analysis of semen samples collected by coitus interruptus rather than by masturbation.
9. Low-volume ejaculates may be due to all of the following EXCEPT:
   a. varicocele.
   b. ejaculatory duct obstruction.
   c. partial retrograde ejaculation.
   d. androgen deficiency.
   e. sympathetic denervation.
10. Couples in which the semen demonstrates low (<4%) sperm morphology as measured by rigid criteria:
    a. should use donor sperm.
    b. have low fertilization rates during standard in-vitro fertilization.
    c. likely have infertility due to a varicocele in the male.
    d. have the same fertilization rate during in-vitro fertilization as couples with normal morphology scores.
    e. cannot conceive by any method.

11. Semen pH is normally:
    a. below 7 due to prostatic secretions.
    b. 7 or more due to alkaline secretions from the seminal vesicles.
    c. 7 or more due to alkaline secretions from the prostate.
    d. alkaline with ejaculatory duct obstruction.
    e. never acidic.
12. Couples in which the male has sperm densities:
    a. below 70 to 100 million sperm/mL are likely to be infertile.
    b. of 70 to 100 million sperm/mL are always fertile.
    c. below 20 million sperm/mL are more likely to have a male infertility factor than those cases in which the sperm density is greater than this.
    d. above 5 million sperm/mL have normal fertility as long as the motility is normal.
    e. below the average of the normal male population are likely be sterile.
13. What percent of infertile men have endocrine disorders?
    a. 2%
    b. 10%
    c. 20%
    d. 40%
    e. 50%
14. Initial hormonal evaluation of an infertile man with a sperm count of 5 million/mL should include a testosterone level and:
    a. prolactin level.
    b. FSH level.
    c. FSH, LH, and prolactin levels.
    d. FSH level and thyroid function studies.
    e. SHBG level.
15. The next step in the management of an infertile man with low serum testosterone and LH levels associated with a normal prolactin is:
    a. cranial MRI.
    b. testosterone therapy.
    c. thyroid function studies.
    d. GnRH stimulation test.
    e. gonadotropin therapy.
16. The most common cause of low ejaculate volume is:
    a. retrograde ejaculation.
    b. hypogonadism.
    c. incomplete collection.
    d. ejaculatory duct obstruction.
    e. failure of emission.
17. Patients with cystic fibrosis have infertility due to:
    a. immotile sperm.
    b. obstruction secondary to inspissated secretions.
    c. obstruction due to absence of the vasa.
    d. abnormal spermatogenesis.
    e. hypogonadism.
18. Vasal agenesis is best diagnosed by:
    a. palpation.
    b. scrotal ultrasonography.
    c. vasography.
    d. surgical exploration.
    e. transrectal ultrasonography.
19. The best next step in the management of an azoospermic man with normal serum testosterone and FSH, normal testicular volume, and palpable vasa is:
    a. vasography.
    b. transrectal ultrasonography.
    c. testis biopsy.
    d. cranial MRI.
    e. donor insemination.
20. Isolated asthenospermia may be due all of the following EXCEPT:
    a. antisperm antibodies.
    b. lack of dynein arms in the axoneme.
    c. genital tract infection.
    d. varicocele.
    e. prolactinoma.
21. Potential risk factors for the presence of antisperm antibodies include all of the following EXCEPT:
    a. vasectomy.
    b. Kartagener's syndrome.
    c. cryptorchidism.
    d. genital trauma.
    e. sperm agglutination.
22. Direct antisperm antibody assays:
    a. detect antisperm antibodies in serum.
    b. are only performed in females.
    c. determine antibody titers.
    d. detect antisperm antibodies on the sperm surface.
    e. are positive in 30% of infertile men.
23. Round cells in semen:
    a. may be white blood cells or immature germ cells.
    b. are most often white blood cells.
    c. always indicate the presence of a genital tract infection.
    d. are normally present in numbers greater than 5 million/mL.
    e. indicate the presence of antisperm antibodies.
24. Semen cultures:
    a. are obtained in most men as part of the infertility evaluation.
    b. often demonstrate distal urethral organisms.
    c. if positive for any bacteria, indicate a need to treat the male with antibiotics.
    d. are only necessary in the absence of pyospermia.
    e. are obtained in all patients with increased numbers of immature germ cells in the semen.
25. Color Doppler scrotal ultrasonography to detect varicoceles should be obtained on which of the following patient groups?
    a. All infertile men
    b. All infertile men with clinical varicoceles
    c. Infertile men with equivocal examinations
    d. Infertile men with low testosterone levels
    e. Men following varicocele repair
26. What percentage of patients with unilateral vasal agenesis have upper tract abnormalities?
    a. 10%
    b. 30%
    c. 50%
    d. 80%
    e. 95%

27. The post-coital test:
    a. need not be performed in couples in which the male's sperm demonstrates poor motility.
    b. if abnormal always indicates a significant infertility factor.
    c. is rarely abnormal because of poor timing relative to ovulation.
    d. has results that depend on the sperm quality but are independent of the cervical mucus quality.
    e. if normal rules out the presence of a male factor.
28. Genetic causes of defects in spermatogenesis:
    a. occur with the same frequency in all infertile men regardless of the sperm count.
    b. are all detected by karyotype analysis.
    c. include karyotypic abnormalities and Y chromosome microdeletions.
    d. result in a strict correlation between the genetic findings and testicular histology.
    e. always result in azoospermia.
29. Differentiation between late maturation arrest and normal spermatogenesis on testicular biopsy is best accomplished by:
    a. spermatid count per tubule.
    b. Sertoli cell count per tubule.
    c. touch preparation.
    d. ratio of spermatids to Sertoli cells.
    e. absolute spermatid count.
30. An azoospermic patient has anosmia, bilateral atrophic testes, and low serum testosterone and LH. The best treatment for his infertility is:
    a. gonadotropins.
    b. testosterone.
    c. anti-estrogens.
    d. bromocriptine.
    e. cabergoline.
31. The best initial therapy of a patient with low serum testosterone and gonadotropin levels and an elevated 17-hydroxyprogesterone level is:
    a. GnRH.
    b. gonadotropins.
    c. testosterone.
    d. cabergoline.
    e. corticosteroids.
32. An infertile man has low testosterone and LH levels and elevated prolactin levels. Cranial MRI reveals a 4-cm pituitary tumor. The best next step in management is:
    a. pituitary radiation.
    b. cabergoline.
    c. hypophysectomy.
    d. gonadotropins.
    e. testosterone.
33. Which of the following hormone patterns are suggestive of androgen insensitivity?
    a. High testosterone, high LH, normal FSH
    b. High testosterone, normal LH, normal FSH
    c. High testosterone, low LH, low FSH
    d. Low testosterone, high LH, high FSH
    e. Low testosterone, low LH, low FSH
34. An extra X chromosome in the male:
    a. leads to a higher risk of testicular cancer.
    b. is the hallmark of Klinefelter's syndrome.
    c. means that sperm cannot be recovered from the testes through attempts at testicular sperm retrieval.
    d. is found in sex reversal syndrome.
    e. has no effect on spermatogenesis.
35. Genes involved in spermatogenesis:
    a. are located on the short arm of the Y chromosome.
    b. when absent, result in intersex phenotypes.
    c. are rarely present in infertile men.
    d. include *DAZ*.
    e. are absent only when the karyotype is abnormal.
36. What percentage of patients with a history of unilateral cryptorchidism have abnormal semen analyses?
    a. 10%
    b. 25%
    c. 50%
    d. 75%
    e. 100%
37. Varicoceles:
    a. should be examined for with the patient supine.
    b. usually result in infertility.
    c. may affect sperm motility and sperm count.
    d. result in lower testicular temperatures.
    e. should always be repaired if identified.
38. Sertoli-cell-only syndrome:
    a. is diagnosed by examination of testicular histology.
    b. is caused by a specific deletion on the X chromosome.
    c. is associated with the absence of Leydig cells.
    d. is found exclusively in patients with abnormal androgenization.
    e. if present precludes finding sperm in testicular tissue.
39. After chemotherapy:
    a. patients should immediately try to conceive.
    b. spermatogenesis returns within one spermatogenic cycle.
    c. FSH levels are rarely elevated.
    d. patients who develop azoospermia never regain spermatogenesis.
    e. there is no increased risk of congenital abnormalities in children conceived by these patients.
40. Radiation therapy directed at the retroperitoneum, as given to patients with testicular seminoma:
    a. results in an increase in congenital abnormalities in children born to these patients.
    b. results in erectile dysfunction in most patients.
    c. has no effect on spermatogenesis if gonadal shielding is used.
    d. should be delayed until after the patient desires no more children.
    e. may temporarily depress spermatogenesis.
41. What is the background spontaneous pregnancy rate for couples with infertility due to idiopathic oligospermia?
    a. 10%
    b. 25%
    c. 40%
    d. 60%
    e. 75%
42. What is the purported mechanism of action of anti-estrogens when used to treat idiopathic oligospermia?
    a. Reducing of estradiol in the testis
    b. Blocking of conversion of testosterone to estradiol
    c. Enhancing gonadotropin action in the testis
    d. Blocking feedback inhibition in the pituitary
    e. Blocking inhibin

43. Exogenous testosterone administration has a contraceptive effect in the male by:
    a. lowering intratesticular testosterone concentration.
    b. causing testosterone toxicity.
    c. increasing hepatic production of SHBG.
    d. altering testosterone-estradiol ratio.
    e. increasing testicular production of ABP.
44. The currently recommended management of a couple with infertility due to bilateral absence of the vasa deferentia is:
    a. alloplastic spermatocele.
    b. vasal reconstruction.
    c. sperm harvesting and IVF.
    d. donor insemination.
    e. adoption.
45. A patient with retrograde ejaculation secondary to prior bladder neck incision is best managed with:
    a. donor insemination.
    b. imipramine.
    c. epididymal sperm aspiration and IVF.
    d. bladder wash and IUI.
    e. pseudoephedrine.
46. The initial management of aspermia in a man with a T6 spinal cord injury should be:
    a. vibratory stimulation.
    b. electroejaculation.
    c. seminal vesicle sperm aspiration and IVF.
    d. vasal sperm aspiration and IVF.
    e. epididymal sperm aspiration and IVF.
47. Which of the following management options is inappropriate for the couple in which the male has antisperm antibodies?
    a. In-vitro fertilization with intracytoplasmic sperm injection
    b. Clomiphene therapy for the man
    c. Intrauterine insemination
    d. Donor insemination
    e. Immunosuppressive therapy of the man
48. Ultrastructural spermatozoal defects:
    a. are best detected by 400 × microscopic examination of live sperm.
    b. improve with hormone therapy of the male.
    c. may be associated with abnormalities of other organ systems.
    d. result in total necrospermia (dead sperm).
    e. should be suspected in patients with sperm counts of less than 10 million sperm/mL.
49. Controlled ovarian hyperstimulation:
    a. is commonly used in conjunction with IUI and IVF.
    b. is used only when the female is anovulatory.
    c. does not increase the risk of multiple gestations with IUI.
    d. should routinely be employed with therapeutic donor insemination.
    e. when combined with IUI, does not increase pregnancy rates as compared with intercourse alone for couples in which the male has sperm counts of less than 20 million/mL.
50. Intracytoplasmic sperm injection:
    a. is used in conjunction with IUI.
    b. involves the injection of spermatogonia into oocytes.
    c. is now the accepted treatment for all men who desire fertility after vasectomy.
    d. is an appropriate option for couples in which the male has idiopathic oligospermia.
    e. should be employed only after therapeutic donor insemination has failed.
51. Epididymal sperm aspiration:
    a. is the retrieval technique of choice for patients with nonobstructive azoospermia.
    b. should be reserved for oligospermic patients.
    c. is usually combined with IUI.
    d. is utilized for retrieving sperm from men with Klinefelter syndrome.
    e. is an appropriate option for men with congenital bilateral absence of the vas deferens.

ANSWERS

1. **d. 20% to 25% per month for normal couples and 1% to 3% per month for infertile couples.** The chance of a fertile couple conceiving is estimated to be 20% to 25% per month, 75% by 6 months, and 90% by 1 year. Of infertile couples without treatment, 25% to 35% will conceive at some time by intercourse alone. Within the first 2 years, 23% will conceive, whereas an additional 10% will do so within 2 more years.
   This baseline pregnancy rate of 1% to 3% per month (in nonazoospermic couples) must be kept in mind while managing infertile couples and evaluating the results of therapy.
2. **c. 5.** Studies have shown that conception may occur when sexual relations take place up to 5 days before ovulation but, owing to the short life span of oocytes, will not occur if intercourse is performed the day after ovulation.
3. **a. 1.** There is a 12- to 24-hour period in which the oocyte is within the fallopian tube and is capable of being fertilized.
4. **e. Peanut oil.** Most of the commonly used lubricants, such as Astroglide, Lubafax, K-Y jelly, Keri lotion, Surgilube, and saliva, adversely affect sperm motility. Lubricants that do not impair in vitro sperm motility include peanut oil, safflower oil, vegetable oil, and raw egg white. In general, a couple should be advised to use a lubricant only if necessary and to use a minimal amount of one that does not impair sperm function.
5. **c. 3 months.** After a febrile illness, spermatogenesis may be impaired for 1 to 3 months.
6. **b. treatment is often more aggressive than when the female is younger.** It is common to recommend more aggressive therapy in couples in which the woman is approaching 40 years old and to take a slower, stepwise approach in younger couples.
7. **d. 80%.** Because the majority of the testicular volume (~80%) consists of seminiferous tubules and germinal elements, a reduction in the number of these cells is typically manifested by a reduction in testicular volume or testicular atrophy.
8. **a. should always include at least two semen analyses.** All patients should have at least two semen analyses.
9. **a. varicocele.** Small-volume ejaculates may be produced in patients with obstruction of the ejaculatory ducts, androgen deficiency, retrograde ejaculation, sympathetic denervation, absence of the vas deferens and seminal vesicles, drug therapy, or bladder neck surgery.
10. **b. have low fertilization rates during standard in-vitro fertilization.** Using these criteria, Kruger and associates found that in a group of men with sperm densities greater than 20 million sperm/mL and motility greater than 30%, fertilization rates during IVF were 37% for those with less than 14% normal

sperm by strict criteria and 91% for those with greater than 14% normal sperm.

11. **b. 7 or more due to alkaline secretions from the seminal vesicles.**
12. **c. below 20 million sperm/mL are more likely to have a male infertility factor than those cases in which the sperm density is greater than this.** The World Health Organization defines the following reference values: volume of 2.0 mL or more; pH of 7.2 or more; sperm concentration of 20×10^6 or more spermatozoa per milliliter; total sperm number of 40×10^6 or more spermatozoa per ejaculate; motility of 50% or more with grade "a + b" motility or 25% or more with grade "a" motility; morphology of 15% or more by strict criteria; viability of 75% or more; white blood cells of less than 1 million/mL. The finding of parameters below these levels is suggestive of infertility, whereas the finding of parameters above these levels is suggestive of fertility.
13. **a. 2%.** Although male reproductive function is critically dependent on endocrinologic control, less than 3% of infertile men have a primary hormonal cause.
14. **b. FSH level.** We recommend that all men with an indication in the history or physical examination or a sperm density of less than 10 million/mL have serum FSH and testosterone levels measured because endocrine abnormalities are rarely present when the sperm concentration is greater than 10 million/mL.
15. **a. cranial MRI.** If the testosterone level remains low, a serum prolactin assay and pituitary MRI should be performed.
16. **c. incomplete collection.** Low ejaculate volume in the nonazoospermic patient is most often due to collection problems, which warrants repeated collection.
17. **c. obstruction due to absence of the vasa.** Congenital bilateral absence of the vasa deferentia (CBAVD) is due to an abnormality in the cystic fibrosis transmembrane conductance regulator (CFTR) gene.
18. **a. palpation.** CBAVD is a clinical diagnosis based on physical examination, and further radiologic imaging is not routinely necessary, although a small percentage of these patients have upper tract abnormalities. An abdominal ultrasonographic scan may be obtained.
19. **c. testis biopsy.** Patients with vasa present, normal testicular volume, and normal serum FSH levels require testicular biopsy to differentiate between spermatogenic abnormalities and ductal obstruction.
20. **e. prolactinoma.** Spermatozoal structural defects, prolonged abstinence periods, genital tract infection, antisperm antibodies, partial ductal obstruction, varicoceles, and idiopathic causes may be responsible for cases of asthenospermia.
21. **b. Kartagener's syndrome.** Risk factors for the development of antisperm antibodies include conditions that may disrupt the blood-testis barrier.
22. **d. detect antisperm antibodies on the sperm surface sperm.** Direct assays detect the presence of antisperm antibodies on the patient's sperm.
23. **a. may be white blood cells or immature germ cells.** Under wet mount microscopy, immature germ cells and leukocytes appear similar and are known as round cells.
24. **b. often demonstrate distal urethral organisms.** Semen may be cultured for bacterial organisms; however, these cultures frequently yield low concentrations of multiple organisms because of distal urethral contamination.
25. **c. Infertile men with equivocal examinations.** Color duplex scrotal ultrasonography should be reserved for those patients with an inadequate physical examination because of either obesity or testicular sensitivity.
26. **d. 80%.** Ipsilateral renal anomalies are present in up to 80% of men with unilateral absence of the vas deferens, with the most common anomaly being renal agenesis.
27. **a. need not be performed in couples in which the male's sperm demonstrates poor motility.** Because patients with very poor quality semen invariably have poor postcoital test results, it is not necessary to perform this test in this group of patients.
28. **c. include karyotypic abnormalities and Y chromosome microdeletions.** Genetic causes for male infertility include karyotypic abnormalities (structural or numerical chromosomal abnormalities), Y chromosome microdeletions, and autosomal gene mutations.
29. **c. touch preparation.** Cases of late maturation arrest are often difficult to differentiate from normal spermatogenesis without the use of a testicular touch preparation.
30. **a. gonadotropins.** Gonadotropin therapy is required for the initiation of spermatogenesis.
31. **e. corticosteroids.** Glucocorticoid therapy results in a reduction of adrenocorticotropic hormone levels, which induces a decrease in peripheral adrenal androgens, thus stimulating endogenous gonadotropin secretion and testicular steroidogenesis.
32. **b. cabergoline.** Although surgery and radiation therapy were used in the past to treat patients with prolactin-secreting pituitary tumors, the vast majority of patients respond to medical therapy. The two most commonly used agents today are bromocriptine and cabergoline. Cabergoline has the advantages of fewer side effects and less frequent dosing required.
33. **a. High testosterone, high LH, normal FSH.** Patients with partial androgen insensitivity have elevated serum testosterone and LH levels.
34. **b. is the hallmark of Klinefelter's syndrome.** The presence of an extra X chromosome is the genetic hallmark of Klinefelter's syndrome.
35. **d. include *DAZ*.** The gene deleted in azoospermia *(DAZ)* is one of the genes thought to be responsible for spermatogenic defects in patients with deletions in this interval.
36. **b. 25%.** Sperm concentrations below 12 to 20 million/mL are found in 50% of patients with bilateral cryptorchidism and in approximately 25% of patients with unilateral cryptorchidism.
37. **c. may affect sperm motility and sperm count.** Semen samples from men with varicoceles have demonstrated decreased motility in 90% of patients and sperm concentrations of less than 20 million sperm/mL in 65% of patients.
38. **a. is diagnosed by examination of testicular histology.** Sertoli-cell-only syndrome is a histologic diagnosis.
39. **e. there is no increased risk of congenital abnormalities in children conceived by these patients.** There appears to be no increased risk of birth defects in children born to patients who have received chemotherapy.
40. **e. may temporarily depress spermatogenesis.** Semen quality will usually return to baseline within 2 years after radiation therapy for seminoma.
41. **b. 25%.** There is a significant background pregnancy rate (26%) for untreated couples with abnormal semen parameters.
42. **d. Blocking feedback inhibition in the pituitary.** They increase pituitary gonadotropin secretion by blocking feedback

inhibition, thus increasing serum FSH and LH levels as well as the testicular production of testosterone.

43. **a. lowering intratesticular testosterone concentration.** Continuous androgen administration has a contraceptive effect on men by lowering intratesticular testosterone concentration and should never be used in the treatment of infertility.

44. **c. sperm harvesting and IVF.** The currently recommended management of couples with infertility due to CBAVD is sperm retrieval combined with IVF using intracytoplasmic sperm injection after appropriate genetic testing and counseling of the couple regarding the risk of cystic fibrosis.

45. **d. bladder wash and IUI.** Those patients with retrograde ejaculation unresponsive to medical therapy or due to ablation of the bladder neck may be treated by recovery of sperm from the bladder urine combined with intrauterine insemination.

46. **a. vibratory stimulation.** Penile vibratory stimulation results in ejaculation in approximately 70% of spinal cord–injured men. Although specially designed equipment with specific vibration frequency and amplitudes is available, many practitioners have had good results using readily available vibrators intended for general use. This approach should be used in patients with upper motor neuron lesions such as spinal cord injuries above T10.

47. **b. Clomiphene therapy for the man.** Although we present the patient with the option of corticosteroid treatment, we encourage couples to consider intrauterine insemination or IVF with intracytoplasmic sperm injection if the semen is of adequate quality. For couples wishing to proceed with immunosuppressive therapy, we recommend an intermediate cyclic steroid regimen such as the one used by Hendry and colleagues.

48. **c. may be associated with abnormalities of other organ systems.** When these clinical findings are combined with situs inversus, which is present in 50% of these cases, the patient has Kartagener's syndrome.

49. **a. is commonly used in conjunction with IUI and IVF.** Controlled ovarian hyperstimulation, hormonal stimulation of superovulation using gonadotropins, plays a crucial part in most forms of assisted reproductive techniques.

50. **d. is an appropriate option for couples in which the man has idiopathic oligospermia.** IVF with intracytoplasmic sperm injection is indicated in cases of severe male factor infertility, in couples with prior failed or poor fertilization during regular IVF cycles, or in cases in which the sperm demonstrate significant fertilizing ability defects (e.g., with rounded-head sperm).

51. **e. is an appropriate option for men with congenital bilateral absence of the vas deferens.** Microsurgical epididymal sperm aspiration is commonly employed to retrieve sperm out of the ductal system in cases with obstructive azoospermia such as congenital bilateral absence of the vasa deferentia.

20

Surgical Management of Male Infertility

LARRY I. LIPSHULTZ • ANTHONY J. THOMAS, JR. • MOHIT KHERA

QUESTIONS

1. In which of the following scenarios is a testis biopsy (diagnostic or therapeutic) least helpful?
   a. Failure to retrieve motile sperm from the epididymis
   b. Sperm retrieval for nonobstructive azoospermia
   c. Diagnostic evaluation of congenital absence of vas but normal FSH level
   d. Diagnostic evaluation of azoospermic men with normal findings on scrotal examination and normal serum testosterone and FSH levels
   e. Sperm retrieval for men diagnosed with a Sertoli-cell-only pattern in the testes
2. A 30-year-old man presenting with primary infertility was found to be azoospermic on two semen analyses. Which of the following findings would contraindicate a testicular biopsy for diagnostic purposes?
   a. Ejaculate volume below 2.0 mL
   b. Semen pH less than 7.2
   c. Semen negative for fructose
   d. Serum FSH greater than 25 IU/L
   e. Absence of vasa deferentia and normal serum FSH level
3. In which of the following cases would a diagnostic testicular biopsy provide valuable clinical information?
   a. Men with azoospermia and an FSH level of 25 IU/L
   b. Men with a 47,XXY karyotype
   c. Men with a fecundity history who seek vasectomy reversal
   d. Men with primary infertility, azoospermia, normal physical examination findings, and normal serum FSH level
   e. Men with anejaculation caused by high spinal cord injury
4. When performing a testicular biopsy, which of the following is FALSE?
   a. If there is a discrepancy in size, biopsy the larger, more normal testis first because it is most likely to reveal the most favorable histology.
   b. It is best to choose the least vascular site possible, such as the upper medial portion of the testis.
   c. Several studies have found no correlation between testicular size and the presence or absence of sperm on a testicular biopsy.
   d. The specimen is placed in either Zenker's, Bouin's, or buffered glutaraldehyde solution.
   e. All are true.
5. Which of the following venous structures are intentionally preserved during varicocelectomy?
   a. External spermatic veins
   b. Internal spermatic veins
   c. Gubernacular veins
   d. Vasal veins
   e. Cremasteric veins
6. Which of the following are TRUE regarding varicocele?
   a. Treatment in infertile men rarely results in improved semen parameters.
   b. Severity of testicular insult is related to the size of the varicoceles.
   c. Severity of testicular insult from varicocele is worse when the varicocele is on the left side.
   d. Because of the severity of testicular insult, repair of large varicoceles is not warranted.
   e. Surgical treatment of subclinical varicoceles results in greater improvement in semen quality than treatment of large varicoceles.
7. All of the following are expected outcomes of varicocele repair EXCEPT:
   a. improved sperm motility.
   b. increased risk of multiple gestation.
   c. improved sperm counts.
   d. elevated serum testosterone levels.
   e. return of sperm to the ejaculate in azoospermic men.
8. What is the most common complication of nonmicrosurgical varicocelectomy?
   a. Vasal obstruction
   b. Testicular atrophy
   c. Varicocele recurrence
   d. Epididymal injury
   e. Hydrocele
9. Which of the following techniques of varicocele repair is associated with the highest recurrence rate?
   a. Retroperitoneal ligation
   b. Laparoscopic ligation
   c. Microsurgical ligation
   d. Nonmicrosurgical ligation
   e. Radiographic embolization

10. Before varicocele repair is initiated in adults, which of the following criteria should be met?
    a. The couple has a known history of infertility.
    b. The female partner has normal fertility or a potentially treatable cause of infertility.
    c. The varicocele is palpable on physical examination or, if suspected, is corroborated by ultrasound.
    d. The male partner has an abnormal semen analysis.
    e. All of the above criteria should be met before varicocele repair.
11. If at the first postvasectomy visit after 30 ejaculations, a patient's semen sample revealed a rare nonmotile sperm, the following advice would be most appropriate:
    a. Nothing further needs to be done. The patient is considered sterile.
    b. Repeat the semen examination after 12 to 20 more ejaculations.
    c. Redo the vasectomy.
    d. Use some method of birth control for 3 more months, then discontinue.
    e. Tell the man he is probably sterile, because nonmotile sperm do not cause pregnancies.
12. If the semen of men who have had successful vasectomies is centrifuged and stained:
    a. none will have sperm in the semen.
    b. macrophages will be found in almost all of their semen samples.
    c. 1% will have rare sperm present.
    d. 10% will have rare sperm present (probably >10%!).
    e. 5% will have rare sperm present.
13. Mr. Jones underwent a vasectomy without complication 1 year ago. He had a single semen analysis afterward that indicated azoospermia. Now his wife of 15 years reports she is pregnant. He returns to his urologist who requests a semen sample. No sperm are found. What course of action should be recommended?
    a. Repeat the semen analysis in 3 months.
    b. Redo the vasectomy as soon as possible.
    c. Divorce his wife.
    d. Wait for DNA testing of the infant and, if it is the patient's child, redo vasectomy.
    e. Centrifuge and stain the semen sample to look for sperm.
14. Pregnancy after vasectomy reversal is most closely related to:
    a. years of obstruction and age of female partner.
    b. method of vasectomy.
    c. presence or absence of a sperm granuloma.
    d. age and number of children of the man at the time of vasectomy.
    e. performance of a multilayer anastomosis as opposed to a modified single-layer procedure.
15. Vasoepididymostomy should be considered at the time of vasectomy reversal when:
    a. the fluid from the proximal vas is clear and copious but without sperm.
    b. it has been more than 15 years since the vasectomy.
    c. if only nonmotile sperm are found coming from the proximal (testicular) vas.
    d. if the fluid from the proximal vas is creamy and devoid of sperm.
    e. if the fluid is creamy and contains sperm heads and sperm with broken tails.
16. A patient is seen with an undescended *left* testis brought into the scrotum when he was 8 years old. He and his wife had a child without difficulty but have been unable to have another since the patient had an uneventful laparoscopic *right* inguinal hernia repair using mesh. He is found to be azoospermic, and vasography indicates that the right vas is obstructed in the groin. The couple does not want IVF. The best treatment to help them have another child is:
    a. epididymal sperm extraction and insemination.
    b. exploration of the right groin and vasovasostomy.
    c. vasogram of the left vas and, if patent, performance of a scrotal crossover vasovasostomy.
    d. right-sided laparoscopic vasovasostomy staying away from the mesh area.
    e. testicular sperm extraction and insemination.
17. The diagnosis of congenital bilateral absence of the vas deferens can best be ascertained by:
    a. bilateral surgical scrotal exploration.
    b. physical examination.
    c. cystic fibrosis transmembrane receptor gene mutation testing.
    d. transrectal ultrasound.
    e. testicular biopsy.
18. The characteristics suggestive of a surgically correctable epididymal obstruction in an azoospermic male are:
    a. testes of normal size, soft epididymides, and palpable vas deferens.
    b. semen pH of less than 6.5 with palpable vasa.
    c. full or indurated epididymides with a negative fructose test and nonpalpable vasa.
    d. full epididymides and vasa that feel normal.
    e. a semen volume of less than 1 mL, testes of normal size, and full epididymides.
19. A 30-year-old man presents with normal volume oligospermia (<3 million sperm/mL). Testes are small, and the serum FSH level is elevated more than two times the upper limits of normal. Testosterone level is in the low-normal range. The following tests are indicated before he and his partner embark on a course of IVF/ICSI:
    a. Serum LH, prolactin, and Y chromosome deletion study
    b. Y-chromosome deletion study and karyotype
    c. Sweat test and cystic fibrosis transmembrane receptor gene mutation test
    d. Cystic fibrosis transmembrane receptor gene mutation test and karyotype
    e. Y-chromosome deletion study and cystic fibrosis transmembrane receptor gene mutation test
20. The most appropriate first means of obtaining sperm from a spinal cord–injured man unable to ejaculate is:
    a. seminal vesicle aspiration.
    b. electroejaculation.
    c. vasal aspiration of sperm.
    d. testicular sperm extraction.
    e. vibratory stimulation of penis.
21. The following is used in an attempt to obtain sperm from men with nonobstructive azoospermia:
    a. percutaneous epididymal sperm aspiration.
    b. microsurgical epididymal sperm aspiration.
    c. electroejaculation.
    d. testicular sperm extraction.
    e. vasal aspiration of sperm.

22. In the evaluation for azoospermia, all of the following tests should be considered in making the diagnosis of obstructive azoospermia EXCEPT:
    a. transrectal ultrasonography.
    b. testicular biopsy.
    c. antisperm antibody assay.
    d. epididymal biopsy.
    e. serum testosterone and FSH assay.
23. Which of the following is the best diagnostic study to determine whether an azoospermic man has an ejaculatory duct obstruction?
    a. Semen fructose test
    b. Complete semen analysis
    c. Antisperm antibody assay
    d. Transrectal ultrasonography
    e. Cystoscopy
24. All of the following are potential complications of transurethral resection of the ejaculatory ducts EXCEPT:
    a. urinary incontinence.
    b. retrograde ejaculation.
    c. recurrent epididymitis.
    d. testicular atrophy.
    e. rectourethral injury.
25. A midline cyst compressing the ejaculatory duct is found on a transrectal ultrasonographic scan. What does the presence of sperm in the cyst aspirate suggest?
    a. Congenital absence of vas on at least one side
    b. Nonobstructive azoospermia
    c. Bilateral epididymal obstruction
    d. The possibility of XXY karyotype
    e. Patency of a vas deferens and epididymis on at least one side
26. Which of the following is associated with a higher rate of success after TURED?
    a. Treatment of a patient with congenital, as opposed to acquired, ejaculatory duct obstruction
    b. Treatment of a patient with partial, as opposed to complete, ejaculatory duct obstruction
    c. Treatment of a patient with a midline cyst
    d. All of the above
    e. None of the above
27. All of the following *reduce* the potential complications of vasography EXCEPT:
    a. using water-soluble, low-ionic contrast medium.
    b. diluting the contrast medium.
    c. flushing with saline or lactated Ringer's solution after contrast medium infusion.
    d. performing vasography as an isolated diagnostic procedure.
    e. using low injection pressure.
28. In which of the following scenarios is a vasogram indicated?
    a. Azoospermia, Sertoli-cell-only on testis biopsy
    b. Azoospermia, testicular volume of 10 mL, FSH value 25 IU/L
    c. Azoospermia, normal testicular volume, and biopsy
    d. Azoospermia, no palpable vasa deferentia
    e. Sperm count 5.0 × 106/mL, 5% motility, grade II varicoceles bilaterally
29. All of the following diagnoses can be made from a radiocontrast vasogram EXCEPT:
    a. inguinal vasal obstruction.
    b. ejaculatory duct obstruction.
    c. seminal vesicle agenesis.
    d. spermatogenic failure.
    e. partial agenesis of vasa deferentia.
30. All of the following are potential complications of vasography EXCEPT:
    a. vasal obstruction at the site of vasography.
    b. perivasal hematoma.
    c. sperm granuloma at the site of vasography.
    d. injury to the vasal artery.
    e. retrograde ejaculation.
31. Which of the following is FALSE in terms of vasography?
    a. Blind insertion of a needle into the vas not only is technically challenging but also is associated with potential complications such as perivasal bleeding and vasal injury with subsequent vasal obstruction.
    b. It is often difficult to obtain sufficient vasal sperm for cryopreservation using fine-needle vasography.
    c. Contrast medium should not be injected in the direction of the epididymis because of the risk of epididymal injury associated with this procedure.
    d. Methylene blue should be used instead of indigo carmine because indigo carmine has been shown to significantly impair sperm motility.
    e. All of the above are true.
32. Which of the following is FALSE with regard to Peyronie's disease?
    a. Peyronie's disease initially is managed conservatively with nonsurgical treatments.
    b. The surgical treatment of Peyronie's disease can be divided into three main categories: penile shortening procedures, penile lengthening procedures, and penile prosthesis implantation.
    c. Peyronie's disease has a prevalence of 10% and occurs in men between 40 and 70 years of age.
    d. Peyronie's disease can be treated by insertion of a penile prosthesis and modeling.
    e. Peyronie's disease is associated with Dupuytren's contracture.
33. Which of the following is FALSE with regard to anejaculation?
    a. Anejaculation should be suspected in patients with complete absence of antegrade ejaculation as well as a fructose-negative, sperm-negative, nonviscous postorgasmic urinalysis.
    b. The most common cause of anejaculation is retroperitoneal surgery.
    c. Anejaculation can be treated medically, using penile vibratory stimulation (PVS) or with electroejaculation (EEJ).
    d. Spinal cord-injured patients with lesions above T10 are more likely to benefit from vibratory stimulation whereas those with lesions below T10 are less likely to benefit from this procedure.
    e. Bupropion (Wellbutrin) has been shown to be effective in treating anejaculation.
34. When electroejaculation (EEJ) is performed:
    a. the patient should be placed in the prone position.
    b. the Foley catheter should be well lubricated with K-Y jelly.
    c. the rectal probe should be inserted with the electrodes facing posteriorly.
    d. the antegrade and retrograde specimens should be processed separately.
    e. the urine should be initially acidified to help preserve the specimen.
35. Patients with cystic fibrosis have infertility caused by:
    a. immotile sperm.
    b. obstruction secondary to inspissated secretions.
    c. obstruction due to absence of the vasa.
    d. abnormal spermatogenesis.
    e. hypogonadism.

36. Genetic causes of defects in spermatogenesis:
    a. occur with the same frequency in all infertile men regardless of the sperm count.
    b. are all detected by karyotype analysis.
    c. include karyotypic abnormalities and Y chromosome microdeletions.
    d. result in a strict correlation between the genetic findings and testicular histology.
    e. always result in azoospermia.
37. Genes involved in spermatogenesis:
    a. are located on the short arm of the Y chromosome.
    b. when absent result in intersex phenotypes.
    c. are rarely present in infertile men.
    d. include *DAZ*.
    e. are absent only when the karyotype is abnormal.
38. Which of the following statements is TRUE regarding controlled ovarian hyperstimulation?
    a. It is commonly used in conjunction with intrauterine insemination and IVF.
    b. It is used only when the female is anovulatory.
    c. It does not increase the risk of multiple gestations with intrauterine insemination.
    d. It should routinely be employed with therapeutic donor insemination.
    e. When combined with intrauterine insemination, it does not result in higher pregnancy rates than intercourse alone for couples in whom the man has sperm counts of less than 20 million/mL.
39. Which of the following is TRUE regarding intracytoplasmic sperm injection?
    a. It is used in conjunction with intrauterine insemination.
    b. It involves the injection of spermatogonia into oocytes.
    c. It is now the accepted treatment for all men who desire fertility after vasectomy.
    d. It is an appropriate option for couples in whom the man has idiopathic oligospermia.
    e. It should be employed only after therapeutic donor insemination has failed.

ANSWERS

1. **c. Diagnostic evaluation of congenital absence of vas but normal FSH level.** Testis biopsy is indicated in azoospermic men with testes of normal size and consistency, palpable vasa deferentia, and normal serum FSH levels. Under these circumstances, biopsy will distinguish obstructive azoospermia from primary seminiferous tubular failure. In the testes of men with congenital absence of vasa, biopsy always reveals normal or at least some spermatogenesis, and biopsy is not necessary before definitive sperm aspiration and IVF with ICSI.
2. **e. Absence of vasa deferentia and normal serum FSH level.** In the testes of men with congenital absence of vasa and normal serum FSH level, biopsy always reveals normal or at least some spermatogenesis, and biopsy is not necessary before definitive sperm aspiration and IVF with ICSI.
3. **d. Men with primary infertility, azoospermia, normal physical examination findings, and normal serum FSH level.** Testis biopsy is indicated in azoospermic men with testes of normal size and consistency, palpable vasa deferentia, and normal serum FSH levels.
4. **e. All are true.** If the testes are normal and equal in size, a single biopsy of one testis should be sufficient to determine if there is active spermatogenesis. If there is a discrepancy in size, the larger, more normal testis should be sampled first, because it is most likely to reveal the most favorable histology. Then, if necessary, the smaller testis can be sampled. An otherwise normal obstructed testis should reveal active spermatogenesis in any randomly chosen site that is sampled. It is best to choose a site that is the least vascular site possible, such as the upper medial portion of the testis. Taking biopsies from multiple sites should be reserved for patients with nonobstructive azoospermia when actively searching for sperm to be cryopreserved or used fresh for IVF/ICSI.
5. **d. Vasal veins.** All veins within the cord, with the exception of the vasal veins, are doubly ligated.
6. **b. Severity of testicular insult is related to the size of the varicoceles.** Larger varicoceles appear to cause more damage than small varicoceles; large varicoceles are associated with greater preoperative impairment in semen quality than are small varicoceles.
7. **b. increased risk of multiple gestation.** Varicocelectomy results in significant improvement in the semen analysis in 60% to 80% of men. Reported pregnancy rates after varicocelectomy vary from 20% to 60%. A randomized controlled trial of surgery versus no surgery in infertile men with varicoceles revealed a pregnancy rate of 44% at 1 year in the surgery group versus 10% in the control group. Microsurgical varicocelectomy results in return of sperm to the ejaculate in 50% of azoospermic men with palpable varicoceles. Repair of large varicoceles results in a significantly greater improvement in semen quality than repair of small varicoceles. In addition, large varicoceles are associated with greater preoperative impairment in semen quality than are small varicoceles, and consequently overall pregnancy rates are similar regardless of varicocele size. Some evidence suggests that the younger the patient is at the time of varicocele repair, the greater the improvement after repair, and the more likely the testis is to recover from varicocele-induced injury. Varicocele recurrence and testicular artery ligation are often associated with poor postoperative results. In infertile men with low serum testosterone levels, microsurgical varicocelectomy alone results in improvement in serum testosterone levels.
8. **e. Hydrocele.** Hydrocele formation is the most common complication reported after nonmicroscopic varicocelectomy. The incidence of this complication varies from 3% to 33%, with an average incidence of about 7%.

9. **a. Retroperitoneal ligation.** A disadvantage of a retroperitoneal approach is the high incidence of varicocele recurrence, especially in children and adolescents, when the testicular artery is intentionally preserved. Recurrence rates after retroperitoneal varicocelectomy are about 15%. Failure is usually due to preservation of the periarterial plexus of fine veins (venae comitantes) along with the artery. These veins have been shown to communicate with larger internal spermatic veins. If left intact, they may dilate with time and cause recurrence.

10. **e. All of the above criteria should be met before varicocele repair.** Infertile adult males with a varicocele should be considered for a varicocele repair if all of the following four conditions are met: (1) the couple has known infertility; (2) the female partner has normal fertility or a potentially treatable cause of infertility; (3) the varicocele is palpable on physical examination or, if suspected, is corroborated by ultrasound; and (4) the male partner has an abnormal semen analysis. Adult males with a varicocele and abnormal semen parameters who may wish to conceive in the future but not now could be considered for a varicocele repair. Adolescent males with varicoceles should be considered for a varicocele repair if there is a reduction in the ipsilateral testicular volume. If there is no reduction in ipsilateral testicular volume, these young men can be followed with annual physical examinations and/or a semen analysis if they are psychosexually mature.

11. **b. Repeat the semen examination after 12 to 20 more ejaculations.** Although there have been "special circumstances" in which some physicians have told men with a few persistent, nonmotile sperm in their semen that nothing further needs to be done, it is better to allow more time because it has been shown that these men will eventually become azoospermic.

12. **d. 10% will have rare sperm present (probably >10%!).** It has been reported that more than 10% of men requesting a vasectomy reversal may have rare nonmotile sperm in their ejaculate, seen in the stained pellet of cells after centrifugation of their semen. (Lemack GE, Goldstein M: Presence of sperm in the pre-vasectomy reversal semen analysis: Incidence and implications. J Urol 155:167-169, 1996.)

13. **b. Redo the vasectomy as soon as possible.** There are a number of issues raised in the situation described, but if it is assumed that the pregnancy was caused by Mr. Jones, he should undergo another vasectomy even if he currently is azoospermic because sperm can be found intermittently in the semen of someone who has recanalized the vas after vasectomy. (Philip T, Guillebaud J, Budd D: Late failure of vasectomy after two documented analyses showing azoospermic semen. BMJ Clin Res Ed 289:77-79, 1984; and Smith JC, Cranston D, O'Brien T, et al: Fatherhood without apparent spermatozoa after vasectomy. Lancet 344:30, 1994.)

14. **a. years of obstruction and age of female partner.** In the presence of normal spermatogenesis and a technically successful reversal, the years of obstruction and female partner's age are the two factors that correlate most with the establishment of a pregnancy. (Belker AM, Thomas AJ Jr, Fuchs EF, et al: Results of 1,469 microsurgical vasectomy reversals by the Vasovasostomy Study Group. J Urol 145:505-511, 1991; and Fuchs EF, Burt RA: Vasectomy reversal performed 15 years or more after vasectomy: Correlation of pregnancy outcome with partner age and with pregnancy results of in vitro fertilization with intracytoplasmic sperm injection. Fertil Steril 77:516-519, 2002.)

15. **d. if the fluid from the proximal vas is creamy and devoid of sperm.** The presence of thick creamy or "pasty" fluid without sperm is generally considered a sign of epididymal obstruction, particularly when related to a longer obstructive period. This material is probably a result of cellular breakdown from the vasal epithelium rather than the debris of old, degenerative sperm. (Anger JR, Goldstein M: Intravasal "toothpaste" in men with obstructive azoospermia is derived from vasal epithelium, not sperm. J Urol 172:634-636, 2004.)

16. **c. vasogram of the left vas and, if patent, performance of a scrotal crossover vasovasostomy.** Once the site of obstruction is identified by vasography as probably related to the earlier hernia repair, the choices to restore sperm to the semen are either to explore the groin cutting through the mesh, an often difficult procedure, or to use the vas of the opposite testis since the cryptorchid testis is not contributing to the patient's sperm output. This "crossover vasovasostomy" is a much simpler procedure for both patient and surgeon and, more importantly, has a higher rate of success than the inguinal exploration. It is important to confirm that the blood supply to the previously undescended testis is intact and not solely based on the vasal vessels.

17. **b. physical examination.** If the vasa cannot be identified on careful examination of the cord structures in a patient with otherwise normal scrotal anatomy, they likely are not present. If the patient has previously had scrotal surgery and scarring makes the examination difficult, exploration may be necessary to prove the vas to be present or absent.

18. **d. full epididymides and vasa that feel normal.** Induration or thickening of the epididymides is the most characteristic physical sign of an obstruction in the excurrent ductal system. When there is a distal (i.e., ejaculatory duct obstruction) the vasa are often thick. In the presence of active spermatogenesis, if the vasa are palpably normal, the semen volume normal, and the epididymis thickened, the obstruction is most likely in the epididymis.

19. **b. Y-chromosome deletion study and karyotype.** Four percent of men with oligospermia have Y chromosome microdeletions. This increases to 14% in men with sperm concentrations less than 5 million/mL and 11% to 18% in men with nonobstructive azoospermia. Whereas approximately 12% of men with nonobstructive azoospermia will have an abnormal karyotype, about half that number of severely oligospermic men will exhibit an abnormal karyotype.

20. **e. vibratory stimulation of penis.** Success in obtaining an ejaculate with penile vibratory stimulation has been reported in approximately 80% of spinal cord–injured men who have an intact ejaculatory reflex above the T10 spinal level.

21. **d. testicular sperm extraction.** Multiple testicular biopsy specimens can be taken at random and examined for the presence of sperm. Using the operating microscope, it has been reported that less tissue can be removed with a higher rate of sperm retrieval. (Schlegel PN: Testicular sperm extraction: Microdissection improves sperm yield with minimal tissue excision. Hum Reprod 14:131-135, 1999.)

22. **d. epididymal biopsy.** Before attempted surgical reconstruction of the reproductive tract, spermatogenesis in the patient should be evident. A testicular biopsy may be indicated to confirm the presence of spermatogenesis. Men with a low semen volume should have a transrectal ultrasonographic scan to address the possibility of an additional ejaculatory duct obstruction. The presence of serum or semen antisperm antibodies corroborates the diagnosis of obstruction and the presence of active spermatogenesis. At present, this test is of unknown prognostic value and is optional. In men with small, soft testes, serum FSH should be measured. An elevated FSH level suggests impaired spermatogenesis and a potentially poorer prognosis.

23. **d. Transrectal ultrasonography.** Transrectal sonography has revolutionized the diagnosis and treatment of ejaculatory duct obstruction. A midline cystic lesion or dilated ejaculatory ducts and seminal vesicles can be visualized sonographically.

24. **d. testicular atrophy.** Reflux of urine into the ejaculatory ducts, vas, and seminal vesicles occurs after a majority of ejaculatory duct resections. This reflux can be documented by voiding cystourethrography or by measuring semen creatinine levels. Reflux can lead to acute and chronic epididymitis. Recurrent epididymitis often results in epididymal obstruction. The incidence of epididymitis after transurethral resection is probably underestimated. Symptomatic chemical epididymitis may occur from refluxing urine. If epididymitis is chronic and recurrent, vasectomy or even epididymectomy may be necessary. Even when care has been taken to spare the bladder neck, retrograde ejaculation can occur after transurethral resection. A rectourethral injury can be seen secondary to a rectal injury.

25. **e. Patency of a vas deferens and epididymis on at least one side.** The fine-needle aspirate is examined for sperm. If sperm are present, it means at least one vas and epididymis are patent.

26. **d. All of the above.** Patients with partial, congenital, and midline cysts causing ejaculatory duct obstruction (EDO) tend to have better surgical outcomes after TURED. Studies have shown that after surgical treatment of EDO, improvement of semen parameters was greater in patients with partial EDO (94%) than in patients with complete EDO (59%). Others have demonstrated that of those patients treated with congenital EDO, 83% had an improved sperm count as opposed to those patients treated for acquired EDO, of whom 37.5% had improved semen quality.

27. **d. performing vasography as an isolated diagnostic procedure.** All other options can reduce the complications of vasography. Vasography should not be performed as an isolated procedure but only when a definitive reconstruction procedure is intended in the same setting.

28. **c. Azoospermia, normal testicular volume, and biopsy.** The absolute indications for vasography are azoospermia, with complete spermatogenesis demonstrating many mature spermatids on testicular biopsy, and at least one palpable vas. Relative indications for vasography are severe oligospermia with normal testicular biopsy; a high concentration of sperm-bound antibodies that may be due to obstruction; low semen volume and very poor sperm motility (partial ejaculatory duct obstruction).

29. **d. spermatogenic failure.** Vasography should answer the questions: Are there sperm in the vasal fluid? Is the vas obstructed? If the testis biopsy reveals many sperm, then the absence of sperm in vasal fluid indicates obstruction proximal to the vasal site examined, most likely an epididymal obstruction. Vasography is done in this case with saline or indigo carmine to confirm the patency of the distal end of the vas before a vasoepididymostomy is performed. Copious vasal fluid containing many sperm indicates vasal or ejaculatory duct obstruction, and formal contrast vasography is performed to document the exact location of the obstruction. Copious thick, white fluid without sperm in a dilated vas indicates secondary epididymal obstruction in addition to a potential vasal or ejaculatory duct obstruction.

30. **e. retrograde ejaculation.** Complications of vasography include stricture, injury to the vasal blood supply, hematoma, and sperm granuloma. Multiple attempts at percutaneous vasography using sharp needles can result in stricture or obstruction at the vasography site. Careless or crude closure of a vasotomy can also result in stricture and obstruction. Non-water-soluble contrast agents may also result in stricture and should not be used for vasography. If the vasal blood supply is injured at the site of vasography, vasovasostomy proximal to the vasography site may result in ischemia, necrosis, and obstruction of the intervening segment of vas. A bipolar cautery should be used for meticulous hemostasis at the time of vasostomy to prevent hematoma in the perivasal sheath. Leaky closure of a vasography site may lead to the development of a sperm granuloma, which can result in stricture or obstruction of the vas.

31. **d. Methylene blue should be used instead of indigo carmine because indigo carmine has been shown to significantly impair sperm motility.** Contrast should not be injected in the direction of the epididymis because of the risk of epididymal injury associated with this procedure. Furthermore, indigo carmine should be used instead of methylene blue because methylene blue has been shown to significantly impair sperm motility. A Foley catheter should be placed in the bladder and the balloon filled with air to help identify the bladder neck on radiography. The presence of blue dye in the catheter confirms the patency of the vas deferens.

32. **c. Peyronie's disease has a prevalence of 10% and occurs in men between 40 and 70 years of age.** Peyronie's disease has a prevalence of 0.4% to 3.2% and occurs in men between 40 and 70 years of age. It is initially managed conservatively with nonsurgical treatments. Studies have shown that 14% of patients have complete, spontaneous resolution of their disease, and 40% of patients experience progression of their disease within 1 year. Insertion of a penile prosthesis is reserved for those patients with Peyronie's disease and concomitant erectile dysfunction. After insertion and inflation of the penile prosthesis, the penis is bent in the opposite direction of the curvature, thus breaking the plaque. This technique, described as modeling, has resulted in long-term satisfaction rates of up to 90%.

33. **b. The most common cause of anejaculation is retroperitoneal surgery.** In a review of 560 patients diagnosed with anejaculation, the most common cause of anejaculation was spinal cord injury, followed by retroperitoneal lymph node dissection. Ejaculation can be induced in many neurologically impaired men with penile vibratory stimulation (PVS), which involves placing a vibrator on the frenulum of the glans penis. For vibratory stimulation to induce ejaculation, the ejaculatory reflex arc in the thoracolumbar spinal cord must be intact. Therefore, spinal cord–injured patients with lesions above T10 are more likely to benefit from vibratory stimulation whereas those with lesions below T10 are less likely to benefit from this procedure.

34. **d. the antegrade and retrograde specimens should be processed separately.** The patient should be placed in the lateral decubitus or lithotomy position and a digital rectal examination performed. Anoscopy is performed before and after the procedure to look for any preexisting or iatrogenic preprocedural rectal trauma. (The patient should be pretreated with Sudafed, 60 mg, Urocit-K, and a Fleet enema.) Initially, the bladder should be catheterized to empty the urine, and 30 mL of an alkalinizing medium (Ham's F-10, 20 mmol of HEPES buffer, and 1% human serum albumin) placed inside the bladder. Mineral oil is used when the Foley catheter is inserted because commonly used lubricants are spermicidal. A rectal probe is inserted with the electrodes facing anteriorly and pressed firmly against the prostate and seminal vesicles.

35. **c. obstruction due to absence of the vasa.** Congenital bilateral absence of the vasa deferentia (CBAVD) is due to an abnormality in the cystic fibrosis transmembrane conductance regulator (CFTR) gene.

36. **c. include karyotypic abnormalities and Y chromosome microdeletions.** Genetic causes for male infertility include karyotypic abnormalities (structural or numerical chromosomal abnormalities), Y chromosome microdeletions, and autosomal gene mutations.

37. **d. include *DAZ*.** The gene deleted in azoospermia *(DAZ)* is one of the genes thought to be responsible for spermatogenic defects in patients with deletions in this interval.

38. **a. It is commonly used in conjunction with intrauterine insemination and IVF.** Controlled ovarian hyperstimulation, hormonal stimulation of superovulation using gonadotropins, plays a crucial part in most forms of assisted reproductive techniques.

39. **d. It is an appropriate option for couples in whom the man has idiopathic oligospermia.** IVF with intracytoplasmic sperm injection is indicated in cases of severe male factor infertility, in couples with prior failed or poor fertilization during regular IVF cycles, or in cases in which the sperm demonstrate significant fertilizing ability defects (e.g., with rounded-head sperm).

21

Physiology of Penile Erection and Pathophysiology of Erectile Dysfunction

TOM F. LUE

QUESTIONS

1. The tunica albuginea of the human penis:
   a. is a single layer of strong fibrous tissue, enclosing both the corpora cavernosa and the corpus spongiosum.
   b. is a bilayered structure in the corpora cavernosa but a single-layered structure in the corpus spongiosum.
   c. is commonly called Buck's fascia of the penis.
   d. consists of collagen, smooth muscle, and elastic fibers.
   e. extends all the way to the glans penis to give the glans penis a strong covering.
2. The thickness of the tunica albuginea:
   a. is the same throughout the entire penis.
   b. is less in the pendulous portion of the penis.
   c. is less at the ventral groove of the penis.
   d. remains the same during both the flaccid and the erect phases of the penis.
   e. determines the girth of the penis.
3. The following statements about the accessory pudendal artery are true EXCEPT which one?
   a. It may arise from the obturator artery.
   b. It may travel anterior to the prostate.
   c. It may be damaged during radical prostatectomy.
   d. It may be the dominant blood supply to the corpus cavernosum.
   e. It may occur in 90% of men.
4. The arterial supply of the corpus cavernosum is usually from the:
   a. external pudendal artery.
   b. accessory pudendal artery.
   c. cavernous artery.
   d. dorsal artery.
   e. inferior epigastric artery.
5. The venous channels draining the corpus cavernosum:
   a. originate in the center of the corpus cavernosum.
   b. originate in the emissary veins.
   c. originate in the subtunical venules.
   d. drain exclusively via the dorsal vein of the penis.
   e. drain exclusively via the cavernous vein.
6. Reduced penile venous outflow during erection is due to:
   a. active constriction of the superficial and deep dorsal veins.
   b. opening of penile arteriovenous shunts.
   c. compression of the subtunical venules and emissary veins by the tunica albuginea.
   d. active constriction of emissary veins.
   e. relaxation of the ischiocavernous muscle.
7. Penile erection involves:
   a. arterial dilation and venous constriction.
   b. relaxation of the ischiocavernous muscle.
   c. arterial dilation, venous compression, and sinusoidal relaxation.
   d. contraction of the smooth muscles within the corpus cavernosum.
   e. filling and expansion of the sinusoidal spaces by nitric oxide.
8. The innervation of the penis comes from:
   a. sacral S2-4 spinal segments.
   b. T10-12 and S2-4 spinal segments.
   c. the dorsal nerve.
   d. the cavernous nerve.
   e. all of the above.
9. The ischiocavernous and bulbocavernous muscles:
   a. are innervated by the pudendal nerve.
   b. are responsible for the rigid phase of erection.
   c. are important in the expulsion of semen during ejaculation.
   d. are striated muscles.
   e. all of the above.
10. Stimulation of which area of the brain has been reported to induce penile erection?
    a. Paraventricular area of the hypothalamus
    b. Midbrain raphe
    c. Substantia nigra
    d. Nucleus paragigantocellularis
    e. A 5-catecholamine cell group and locus ceruleus

11. The principal neurotransmitter mediating penile erection is:
    a. Prostaglandin E_1
    b. Nitric oxide
    c. Norepinephrine
    d. Acetylcholine
    e. Neuropeptide P
12. Of the ion channels identified on the penile smooth muscle, which two have been shown to be involved in penile erection?
    a. Sodium and chloride channels
    b. Calcium and potassium channels
    c. Titanium and potassium channels
    d. Chloride and calcium channel
    e. Gold and silver channels
13. The action of nitric oxide within the penile smooth muscle cell involves:
    a. activation of adenylyl cyclase and elevation of cyclic AMP.
    b. activation of phosphodiesterase type 4.
    c. opening of calcium channels resulting in elevated cytosolic calcium levels.
    d. activation of guanylyl cyclase and elevation of the cyclic GMP level.
    e. closure of potassium channels.
14. Which of the following is involved in detumescence of the penis?
    a. Nitric oxide
    b. Phosphodiesterase type 5
    c. Phosphodiesterase type 3
    d. Acetylcholine
    e. Neuropeptide P
15. A gap junction is:
    a. a communication between the tunica albuginea and the sinusoid space.
    b. a communication between the glans penis and the corpora cavernosa.
    c. a communication between the corpus cavernosum and corpus spongiosum.
    d. a communication between intracavernous muscle cells.
    e. the space between presynaptic neurons and postsynaptic receptors.
16. Neurotransmitters involved in modulating sexual function in the brain include:
    a. epinephrine, testosterone, and prolactin.
    b. dopamine, norepinephrine, serotonin, and oxytocin.
    c. endothelin and calcitonin gene-related peptide.
    d. vasoactive intestinal polypeptide and acetylcholine.
    e. all of the above.
17. Apomorphine:
    a. has a strong analgesic action but is not a narcotic.
    b. is a central-acting dopamine receptor agonist.
    c. produces penile erection when injected into the corpus cavernosum.
    d. is an inhibitor of phosphodiesterase type 5 similar to sildenafil.
    e. is often used as an antiemetic.
18. Central norepinephrine transmission seems to enhance sexual function as evidenced by:
    a. clonidine, an α_2-adrenergic agonist, which enhances sexual function.
    b. yohimbine, an α_2-adrenergic antagonist, which enhances sexual function.
    c. intracavernous injection of phenylephrine, which produces penile erection.
    d. oral phentolamine, which enhances penile erection.
    e. intracavernous injection of papaverine, which produces penile erection.
19. The Massachusetts Male Aging Study (MMAS):
    a. reported the prevalence of erectile dysfunction in the United States is about 50% at age 50, 60% at age 60, and 70% at age 70 (including mild, moderate, and severe ED).
    b. reported the prevalence rate of severe ED remains the same but the prevalence rate of mild ED increases with age.
    c. is a hospital-based, cross-sectional survey of sexual function in men and women in the United States.
    d. surveyed more than 1700 hospitalized patients between 1995 and 1997.
    e. estimated that the incidence rate of ED is about 20 million new cases per year in the United States.
20. A 25-year-old healthy man complained of an inability to maintain an erection since meeting his new partner. He did not experience this problem with prior sexual partners. A nocturnal penile tumescence study revealed that 70% of the recorded erections reached full rigidity. The most likely diagnosis is:
    a. psychogenic erectile dysfunction.
    b. testosterone deficiency.
    c. penile vascular insufficiency.
    d. penile venous leakage.
    e. primary erectile dysfunction.
21. A 58-year-old man complained of impotence after radical prostatectomy for cancer of the prostate. Impotence after radical prostatectomy is frequently a result of injury to which of the following?
    a. The dorsal nerve of the penis
    b. The cavernous nerve
    c. The genitofemoral nerve
    d. The sympathetic ganglion
    e. The ilioinguinal nerve
22. The function of testosterone includes each of the following EXCEPT:
    a. enhances sexual interest.
    b. increases frequency of sexual acts.
    c. increases the frequency of nocturnal erections but has little or no effect on fantasy or visually induced erections.
    d. maintains nitric oxide synthase (NOS) activity in the penis (in rats).
    e. prevents hair loss in men.
23. Cavernosal (Venogenic) erectile dysfunction is a disease of the:
    a. deep dorsal vein.
    b. emissary vein.
    c. preprostatic venous plexus.
    d. tunica albuginea or cavernous smooth muscle.
    e. internal pudendal vein.
24. Which of the following is NOT part of the normal aging process?
    a. Greater latency to erection and loss of forceful ejaculation
    b. Decreased ejaculatory volume and a longer refractory period
    c. Decreased frequency and duration of nocturnal erection
    d. Decrease in penile tactile sensitivity
    e. Complete erectile dysfunction
25. Erectile dysfunction associated with diabetes can be a result of:
    a. psychologic impact.
    b. neurologic deficit.
    c. arterial insufficiency.
    d. endothelial cell dysfunction.
    e. all of the above.

26. The following are proposed molecular mechanisms of diabetic erectile dysfunction EXCEPT:
    a. impaired nitric oxide (NO) synthesis.
    b. increased levels of oxygen free radicals.
    c. increased levels of advanced glycosylation end products that quench NO.
    d. selective degeneration of nitric oxide synthase-containing nerves.
    e. decreased level of phosphodiesterase type 5.
27. The causes of erectile dysfunction in an animal model of hyperlipidemia and hypercholesterolemia include each of the following EXCEPT:
    a. increased production of contractile thromboxane and prostaglandin.
    b. increased production of oxytocin.
    c. contractile effect of oxidized low density lipoprotein.
    d. release of superoxide radicals.
    e. increased production of NOS inhibitors.
28. A 60-year-old hypertensive man complained of erectile dysfunction after taking a calcium channel blocker to lower his blood pressure. The most likely cause is:
    a. direct effect of calcium channel blocker on penile smooth muscle.
    b. arrhythmia caused by calcium channel blocker.
    c. decreased penile perfusion due to a decline in blood pressure of the pudendal artery.
    d. anxiety from taking new medication.
    e. decreased level of testosterone from calcium channel blocker.

ANSWERS

1. **b. is a bilayered structure in the corpora cavernosa but a single-layered structure in the corpus spongiosum.** The tunical covering of the corpora cavernosa is a bilayered structure with multiple sublayers: (1) Inner layer bundles support and contain the cavernous tissue and are oriented circularly. Radiating from this inner layer are intracavernosal pillars, acting as struts, augmenting the septum that provides essential support to the erectile tissue. (2) Outer layer bundles are oriented longitudinally, extending from the coronal sulcus to the proximal crura; they insert into the inferior pubic rami but are absent between the 5- and 7-o'clock positions. In contrast, the corpus spongiosum lacks an outer layer or intracorporeal struts, ensuring a low-pressure structure during erection.
2. **c. is less at the ventral groove of the penis.** The outer tunical layer appears to play an additional role in compression of the emissary veins during erection. It also determines, to a large extent, the variability in tunical thickness and strength. At the 7-o'clock position, the tunical thickness is 0.8 ± 0.1 mm; at 9 o'clock, 1.2 ± 0.2 mm; and at 11 o'clock, 2.2 ± 0.4 mm. At 3, 5, and 1 o'clock, the measurements are nearly identical in mirror-image manner. (Differences at specific locations have been found to be statistically significant.) The stress on the tunica before penetration has been measured as $1.6 \pm 0.2 \times 10^7$ N/m^2 at the 7-o'clock position, $3.0 \pm 0.3 \times 107$ N/m^2 at 9 o'clock, and $4.5 \pm 0.5 \times 107$ N/m^2 at 11 o'clock. The strength and thickness of the tunica correlate in a statistically significant manner with location. The most vulnerable area is located on the ventral groove (between the 5 and 7 o'clock positions), which lacks the longitudinally directed outer layer bundles; most prostheses tend to extrude here.
3. **e. It may occur in up to 90% of men.** The main source of blood supply to the penis is usually via the internal pudendal artery, a branch of the internal iliac artery. In many instances, however, accessory arteries exist, arising from the external iliac, obturator, vesical, and femoral arteries, and may occasionally become the dominant or only arterial supply to the corpus cavernosum. The reported incidence of accessory pudendal artery is from 15% to 60%. Damage to these accessory arteries during radical prostatectomy or cystectomy may result in vasculogenic erectile dysfunction (ED) after surgery.
4. **c. cavernous artery.** The cavernous artery is responsible for tumescence of the corpus cavernosum, and the dorsal artery is responsible for engorgement of the glans penis during erection. The bulbourethral artery supplies the bulb and corpus spongiosum. The cavernous artery enters the corpus cavernosum at the hilum of the penis, where the two crura merge.
5. **c. originate in the subtunical venules.** The venous drainage from the three corpora originates in tiny venules leading from the peripheral sinusoids immediately beneath the tunica albuginea. These venules travel in the trabeculae between the tunica and the peripheral sinusoids to form the subtunical venular plexus before exiting as the emissary veins.
6. **c. compression of the subtunical venules and emissary veins by the tunica albuginea.** Sexual stimulation triggers release of neurotransmitters from the cavernous nerve terminals. This results in relaxation of these smooth muscles and the following events: (1) dilatation of the arterioles and arteries by increased blood flow in both the diastolic and the systolic phases; (2) trapping of the incoming blood by the expanding sinusoids; (3) compression of the subtunical venular plexuses between the tunica albuginea and the peripheral sinusoids, reducing the venous outflow; (4) stretching of the tunica to its capacity, which encloses the emissary veins between the inner circular and the outer longitudinal layers and further decreases the venous outflow to a minimum; (5) an increase in intracavernous pressure (maintained at about 100 mm Hg), which raises the penis from the dependent position to the erect state (the full erection phase); and (6) a further pressure increase (to several hundred mm Hg) with contraction of the ischiocavernous muscles (rigid erection phase).
7. **c. arterial dilation venous compression, and sinusoidal relaxation.** Erection involves sinusoidal relaxation, arterial dilatation, and venous compression. The importance of smooth muscle relaxation has been demonstrated in animal and human studies. To summarize the hemodynamic events of erection and detumescence, seven phases can be observed in animal experiments.
8. **e. all of the above.** The sympathetic pathway originates from the 11th thoracic to the 2nd lumbar spinal segments and passes via the white rami to the sympathetic chain ganglia. Some fibers then travel via the lumbar splanchnic nerves to the inferior mesenteric and superior hypogastric plexuses, from which fibers travel in the hypogastric nerves to the pelvic plexus. In humans, the T10-T12 segments are most often the origin of the sympathetic fibers, and the chain ganglia cells projecting to the penis are located in the

sacral and caudal ganglia. The parasympathetic pathway arises from neurons in the intermediolateral cell columns of the second, third, and fourth sacral spinal cord segments. The preganglionic fibers pass in the pelvic nerves to the pelvic plexus, where they are joined by the sympathetic nerves from the superior hypogastric plexus. The cavernous nerves are branches of the pelvic plexus that innervate the penis. Other branches of the pelvic plexus innervate the rectum, bladder, prostate, and sphincters. The cavernous nerves are easily damaged during radical excision of the rectum, bladder, and prostate. A clear understanding of the course of these nerves is essential to the prevention of iatrogenic ED. Recent human cadaveric dissection revealed medial and lateral branches of the cavernous nerves (the former accompany the urethra and the latter pierce the urogenital diaphragm 4 to 7 mm lateral to the sphincter) and multiple communications between the cavernous and dorsal nerves.

9. **e. all of the above.** Onuf's nucleus in the second to fourth sacral spinal segments is the center of somatomotor penile innervation. These nerves travel in the sacral nerves to the pudendal nerve to innervate the ischiocavernous and bulbocavernous muscles. Contraction of the ischiocavernous muscles produces the rigid erection phase. Rhythmic contraction of the bulbocavernous muscle is necessary for ejaculation.

10. **a. paraventricular area of the hypothalamus.** Studies with animals have identified the medial preoptic area and the paraventricular nucleus of the hypothalamus and the hippocampus as important integration centers for sexual function and penile erection. Electrostimulation of this area induces erection, and lesions at this site limit copulation.

11. **b. Nitric oxide.** Most researchers now agree that NO released from nonadrenergic/noncholinergic neurotransmission and from the endothelium is the principal neurotransmitter mediating penile erection. NO increases the production of cyclic GMP, which in turn relaxes the cavernous smooth muscle.

12. **b. Calcium and potassium channels.** In the penis, the NO that is released from nerve endings or endothelial cells diffuses into smooth muscle cells, where it activates soluble guanylyl cyclase, producing cGMP. The mechanism by which intracellular cGMP promotes smooth muscle relaxation has not been settled. The most likely mechanism is the activation of cGMP-specific protein kinase, resulting in the phosphorylation and inactivation of myosin light chain kinase, thereby causing dissociation of myosin and actin and smooth muscle relaxation. Both cGMP and cGMP-specific protein kinase may also activate potassium channels, causing hyperpolarization and closure of voltage-dependent calcium channels and a decrease in intracellular calcium.

13. **d. activation of guanylyl cyclase and elevation of the cGMP level.** cAMP and cGMP are the second messengers involved in smooth muscle relaxation. They activate cAMP- and cGMP-dependent protein kinases, which in turn phosphorylate certain proteins and ion channels, resulting in (1) opening of the potassium channels and hyperpolarization; (2) sequestration of intracellular calcium by the endoplasmic reticulum; and (3) inhibition of voltage-dependent calcium channels, blocking calcium influx. The consequence is a drop in cytosolic free calcium and smooth muscle relaxation.

14. **b. Phosphodiesterase type 5.** During the return to the flaccid state, cGMP is hydrolyzed to GMP by the highly specific cGMP-binding phosphodiesterase type 5.

15. **d. a communication between the intracavernous muscle cells.** Several studies have demonstrated the presence of gap junctions in the membrane of adjacent muscle cells. These intercellular channels allow exchange of ions such as calcium and second-messenger molecules. The major component of gap junctions is connexin-43, a membrane-sparing protein of less than 0.25 μm that has been identified between smooth muscle cells of human corpus cavernosum. Cell-to-cell communication through these gap junctions most likely explains the synchronized erectile response, although their pathophysiologic impact is still unclear.

16. **b. dopamine, norepinephrine, serotonin, and oxytocin.** A variety of neurotransmitters (dopamine, norepinephrine, serotonin, and oxytocin) and neural hormones (oxytocin and prolactin) have been implicated in the regulation of sexual function. It is suggested that dopaminergic and adrenergic receptors may promote sexual function and that serotonin receptors inhibit it.

17. **b. is a central-acting dopamine receptor agonist.** In men, apomorphine, which stimulates both D1 and D2 receptors, induces penile erection that is unaccompanied by sexual arousal.

18. **b. yohimbine, an α_2-adrenergic antagonist, which enhances sexual function.** Central norepinephrine transmission seems to have a positive effect on sexual function. In both humans and rats, inhibition of norepinephrine release by clonidine, an α_2-adrenergic agonist, is associated with a decrease in sexual behavior, and yohimbine, an α_2-receptor antagonist, has been shown to increase sexual activity.

19. **a. reported the prevalence of erectile dysfunction in the United States is about 50% at age 50, 60% at age 60, and 70% at age 70 (including mild, moderate, and severe ED).** As reported in the MMAS study, between the ages of 40 and 70 years the probability of complete ED increased from 5.1% to 15%, the probability of moderate ED increased from 17% to 34%, and the probability of mild ED remained constant at about 17%.

20. **a. psychogenic erectile dysfunction.** A classification recommended by the International Society of Impotence Research is shown in Table 22-4: organic, which includes vasculogenic (arteriogenic, cavernosal, and mixed), neurogenic, anatomic, and endocrinologic; and psychogenic, which includes the generalized type (generalized unresponsiveness and generalized inhibition) and the situational type (partner related; performance related; and psychological distress or adjustment related).

21. **b. The cavernous nerve.** Because of the close relationship between the cavernous nerves and the pelvic organs, surgery on these organs is a frequent cause of impotence. The incidence of iatrogenic impotence from various procedures has been reported as follows: radical prostatectomy, 43% to 100%; perineal prostatectomy for benign disease, 29%; abdominal perineal resection, 15% to 100%; and external sphincterotomy at the 3- and 9-o'clock positions, 2% to 49%.

22. **e. prevents hair loss in men.** Mulligan and Schmitt, in 1993, concluded the following: (1) testosterone enhances sexual interest; (2) testosterone increases the frequency of sexual acts; and (3) testosterone increases the frequency of nocturnal erections but has little or no effect on fantasy- or visually induced erections. Treatment with flutamide, estradiol, or a gonadotropin-releasing hormone antagonist in addition to castration further depresses the erectile response. Although penile NOS activity is reduced in these animals, the contents of nNOS and eNOS are not significantly reduced by the treatment (Mills et al, 1994; Penson et al, 1996).

23. **d. tunica albuginea or cavernous smooth muscles.** Veno-occlusive dysfunction may result from the following pathophysiologic processes: (1) The presence or development of large venous channels draining the corpora cavernosa. (2) Degenerative changes (Peyronie's disease, aging, and diabetes) or traumatic injury to the tunica albuginea (penile fracture), resulting in inadequate compression of the subtunical

and emissary veins. In Peyronie's disease, the inelastic tunica albuginea may prevent the emissary veins from closing. Iacono and colleagues postulated that a decrease in elastic fibers in the tunica albuginea and an alteration of microarchitecture may contribute to impotence in some men. Changes in the subtunical areolar layer may impair the veno-occlusive mechanism as occasionally seen in patients after surgery for Peyronie's disease. (3) Structural alterations in the fibroelastic components of the trabeculae, cavernous smooth muscle, and endothelium may result in a venous leak. (4) Insufficient trabecular smooth muscle relaxation, causing inadequate sinusoidal expansion and insufficient compression of the subtunical venules, may occur in an anxious individual with excessive adrenergic tone or in a patient with inadequate neurotransmitter release. It has been shown that alteration of α-adrenoceptor or decrease in NO release may heighten the smooth muscle tone and impair the relaxation in response to endogenous muscle relaxant. (5) Acquired venous shunts—the result of operative correction of priapism—may cause persistent glans/cavernosum or cavernosum/spongiosum shunting.

24. **e. Complete erectile dysfunction.** A number of studies have indicated a progressive decline in sexual function in "healthy" aging men. Masters and Johnson, in 1977, noted a number of changes in older men, including greater latency to erection, less turgid erection, loss of forceful ejaculation, decreased ejaculatory volume, and a longer refractory period. Decreased frequency and duration of nocturnal erection with increasing age were reported in a group of men who had regular intercourse. Other research has also indicated a decrease in penile tactile sensitivity with age.

25. **e. all of the above.** ED has been estimated to occur in 35% to 75% of men with diabetes mellitus, with onset occurring at an earlier age than in men without diabetes. Deterioration of sexual function was the first symptom in 12% of diabetic men. The incidence of ED in diabetes has been found to be age dependent: 15% at 30 years of age and 55% at 34 to 60 years. Diabetes may cause ED through its effects on central nervous system and peripheral nerve function, androgen production, psychological factors, vascular integrity, and endothelial and smooth muscle function.

26. **e. decreased level of phosphodiesterase type 5.** The following summarizes the proposed mechanisms of ED in diabetic animals: (1) impaired NO synthesis; (2) increase in endothelin B receptor binding sites and ultrastructural changes; (3) increased levels of oxygen free radicals and oxidative stress injury; and (4) NO-dependent selective nitrergic nerve degeneration.

27. **b. increased production of oxytocin.** In a rabbit model of atherosclerosis and hypercholesterolemia, decreased NO synthase activity and increased production of contractile thromboxane and prostaglandin are thought to be the causes of impaired smooth muscle relaxation in response to electrical stimulation. Others have proposed that the impaired NO-mediated smooth muscle relaxation in hypercholesterolemia may be due to the contractile effect of oxidized low-density lipoprotein, the release of superoxide radicals, and the increased production of NO synthase inhibitors. In addition, ultrastructural studies of cholesterol-fed rabbits have revealed early atherosclerotic changes in the corpus cavernosum.

28. **c. decreased penile perfusion due to a decline in blood pressure of the pudendal artery.** In hypertension, the increased blood pressure itself does not impair erectile function; rather, the associated arterial stenotic lesions are thought to be the cause. One study has demonstrated that NO availability is impaired because of the production of cyclooxygenase-derived vasoconstrictor substances and reduced endothelin B receptor–mediated NO activation. In addition to increased peripheral vascular resistance, alteration in the vessel architecture, resulting in an increased wall-to-lumen ratio and reduced dilatory capacity, may contribute to impotence in hypertensive patients.

22

Evaluation and Nonsurgical Management of Erectile Dysfunction and Premature Ejaculation

TOM F. LUE • GREGORY A. BRODERICK

QUESTIONS

1. Which of the following domains is NOT covered in the International Index of Erectile Function?
   a. Erectile function
   b. Partner satisfaction
   c. Orgasm
   d. Sexual drive
   e. Intercourse satisfaction
2. The urologist's role in the era of effective oral pharmacotherapy for treatment of erectile dysfunction (ED) includes specialized diagnostic testing. ED diagnostic evaluations may be of benefit to each of the following selected patients EXCEPT which group?
   a. Patients with perineal trauma
   b. Patients with complaints of ED present since the onset of sexual maturity
   c. Patients with complicated endocrinopathy
   d. Patients with Peyronie's disease
   e. Patients with long-term diabetes and hypertension
3. Which of the following statements is FALSE regarding self-administered sex questionnaires?
   a. They can distinguish psychogenic ED from organic ED.
   b. They are very useful in clinical trials.
   c. They provide quantifiable efficacy endpoints for drug trials.
   d. They attempt to quantify sexual interest and satisfaction.
   e. They can differentiate various causes of organic ED.
4. In duplex ultrasound study, after intracavernous injection, what is the peak systolic flow value below which the man is highly likely to have cavernous arterial disease?
   a. 75 cm/s
   b. 50 cm/s
   c. 25 cm/s
   d. 10 cm/s
   e. 5 cm/s
5. Which of the following intracorporeal injection agents has the highest incidence of painful erection?
   a. Papaverine
   b. Prostaglandin E_1
   c. Phentolamine
   d. Atropine
   e. Moxisylyte
6. All other factors being equal, which disease state has the highest response rate to intracavernous injection?
   a. Hypertension
   b. Diabetes
   c. Spinal cord injury
   d. End-stage renal disease
   e. Perineal trauma
7. Office intracavernous injection testing consists of a penile injection of a vasoactive agent followed by visual rating of the subsequent erection. Each of the following statements about office pharmacotesting with ICI is true EXCEPT which one?
   a. It is the most commonly performed diagnostic procedure in the evaluation of ED.
   b. To produce an erection, arterial vasodilatation, sinusoidal relaxation, and decreased venous outflow must each occur in response to a vasodilating agent.
   c. It is minimally invasive and requires no monitoring equipment.
   d. A normal erection rules out veno-occlusive dysfunction, although some men with borderline arterial insufficiency will also achieve a rigid erection.
   e. Self-stimulation and audiovisual stimulation are of no additional benefit in ICI testing.
8. Which of the following results would indicate a diagnosis of venogenic impotence during duplex ultrasound evaluation?
   a. Peak systolic velocity (PSV) 40 cm/s, end-diastolic velocity (EDV) 10 cm/s, rigid erection after stimulation
   b. PSV 12 cm/s, EDV 5 cm/s, poor erection after stimulation
   c. PSV 40 cm/s, EDV 8 cm/s, poor erection after stimulation
   d. PSV 25 cm/s, EDV 8 cm/s, rigid erection after stimulation
   e. PSV 12 cm/s, EDV 5 cm/s, rigid erection after stimulation

9. If a cavernosometry is performed on a normal man with complete smooth muscle relaxation, what is the flow rate required to maintain an erection with an intracavernous pressure of 100 mm Hg?

   a. No flow
   b. 5 mL/min
   c. 15 mL/min
   d. 25 mL/min
   e. 35 mL/min

10. Which of the following statements about penile duplex ultrasound study is TRUE?

    a. The average patient with severe vasculogenic ED should have a duplex ultrasound study before a trial of oral pharmacotherapy to ensure that adequate penile blood flow exists.
    b. Detection and quantification of flow in the flaccid penis are highly predictive of erectile responses to intracavernous injection.
    c. Color duplex ultrasound study is helpful in the diagnosis of high-flow priapism.
    d. Measurable blood flow in the deep dorsal vein is strongly suggestive of penile venous leakage.
    e. Penile duplex ultrasound study, like pudendal arteriography, is an invasive third-line diagnostic test that should be reserved for patients who are candidates for arterial bypass.

11. Each of the following statements about dynamic infusion cavernosometry and cavernosography (DICC) is true EXCEPT which one?

    a. It involves infusing saline solution into the corpora at a rate sufficient to raise penile pressures above systolic blood pressure.
    b. Like the duplex ultrasound blood flow study, it is minimally invasive and permits the patient a period of privacy and self-stimulation.
    c. The pressure at which the cavernous arterial flows become detectable is defined as the cavernous artery systolic occlusion pressure (CASOP).
    d. CASOP correlates with peak systolic velocity measurements obtained by penile duplex ultrasound.
    e. Cavernosography involves the infusion of contrast solution into the corpora cavernosa during artificial erection to visualize sites of venous leakage.

12. When measuring testosterone levels, blood should be drawn:

    a. after fasting.
    b. early morning.
    c. before lunch.
    d. early afternoon.
    e. postprandial.

13. Nocturnal penile tumescence (NPT) has been measured with the following EXCEPT:

    a. stamps.
    b. snap gauges.
    c. digital camera.
    d. RigiScan.
    e. electrobioimpedance.

14. Audiovisual sexual stimulation (AVSS) has been noted to increase erectile responses to specific sexual stimuli during clinical testing EXCEPT:

    a. vibration.
    b. intracavernous injection.
    c. intraurethral medication.
    d. oral phosphodiesterase type 5 inhibitors.
    e. erotic music.

15. When ED testing is employed, no single test is likely to reveal the cause in all cases. Heaton and Morales (1997) suggested that RigiScan testing may be of value in all of the following situations EXCEPT:

    a. suspected sleep disorders.
    b. measurement and comparison of drug effects in placebo-controlled trials.
    c. medicolegal cases.
    d. suspected psychogenic ED.
    e. Peyronie's disease.

16. Which antihypertensive agent can interfere with testosterone synthesis?

    a. Angiotensin-converting enzyme inhibitors
    b. Calcium channel blockers
    c. Spironolactone
    d. α-Adrenergic blockers
    e. Carbonic anhydrase inhibitors

17. Which of the following is NOT typically considered a risk of testosterone supplementation?

    a. Infertility
    b. Anemia
    c. Sleep apnea
    d. Gynecomastia
    e. Hepatocellular carcinoma

18. In the patient with documented hypogonadism and ED, it is reasonable to initiate androgen therapy. Which of the following is TRUE?

    a. Intramuscular preparations of testosterone are the least expensive form of treatment and mimic normal circadian levels of testosterone.
    b. Transdermal scrotal testosterone patches result in significant levels of dihydrotestosterone (DHT), because of a high content of 5α-reductase in scrotal skin.
    c. The most common reaction to testosterone patches is contact dermatitis secondary to development of testosterone allergy.
    d. Testosterone gel is rapidly absorbed by men and cannot alter female partners' testosterone levels.
    e. Oral testosterone preparations are the safest, most effective means of delivering therapy.

19. Absolute contraindications to androgen supplementation include:

    a. breast cancer.
    b. lung cancer.
    c. hepatocellular cancer.
    d. leukemia.
    e. melanoma.

20. PDE-5 inhibitors function by:

    a. decreasing cyclic GMP levels.
    b. increasing cyclic GMP levels.
    c. increasing nitric oxide production.
    d. decreasing nitric oxide production.
    e. increasing cytoplasmic calcium levels.

21. Side effects associated with PDE-5 inhibitors include all of the following EXCEPT:

    a. constipation.
    b. nasal stuffiness.
    c. myalgias.
    d. flushing.
    e. headache.

22. Intracavernosal papaverine acts via:
    a. increase in nitric oxide production.
    b. decrease in cyclic GMP levels.
    c. increase in cytoplasmic calcium levels.
    d. inhibition of PDE.
    e. decrease in cyclic AMP levels.
23. Alprostadil is the synthetic form of a naturally occurring unsaturated 20-carbon fatty acid, prostaglandin E_1 (PGE1). Which of the following statements is TRUE?
    a. It causes corporeal smooth muscle relaxation through elevation of intracellular cyclic GMP.
    b. Only two formulations have been approved for penile injection in the United States: Caverject and Edex.
    c. It cannot be combined with other vasoactive agents for penile injection.
    d. Transurethral therapy (MUSE) is an alprostadil gel for intraurethral administration.
    e. Because of better urethral absorption, MUSE is more effective than Caverject in producing penile erection.
24. Regarding a three-drug mixture (papaverine, phentolamine, alprostadil) for ICI pharmacotherapy, which of the following statements is TRUE regarding Tri-Mix?
    a. Tri-Mix is the only FDA-approved combination ICI pharmacotherapy for ED.
    b. Tri-Mix proved to be not as effective as alprostadil alone.
    c. Incidence of penile fibrosis is higher with Tri-Mix than with papaverine plus phentolamine therapy.
    d. Vasoactive intestinal polypeptide (VIP) and phentolamine have the same pharmacologic activity and may be equally substituted as the third ingredient in Tri-Mix.
    e. Tri-Mix is more effective than papaverine plus phentolamine in patients with severe arteriogenic or veno-occlusive ED.
25. A contraindication to intracavernosal therapy includes:
    a. use of nitroglycerin.
    b. poor manual dexterity.
    c. sickle cell anemia.
    d. use of anticoagulants.
    e. vascular disease.
26. The most common adverse side-effect after administration of intraurethral alprostadil (MUSE) is:
    a. hypotension.
    b. syncope.
    c. priapism.
    d. corporeal fibrosis.
    e. penile pain.
27. Use of vacuum erection devices (VEDs) is a noninvasive treatment for ED. Which of the following statements is TRUE?
    a. VEDs require physician prescription.
    b. VEDs may be effective in the patient with a malfunctioning penile implant and after explantation.
    c. Dropout rates for long-term VEDs use are very low.
    d. VEDs induce and maintain erection without a constriction band in men with arterial insufficiency but not in men with venous leakage.
    e. Combining ICI with VEDs does not enhance VEDs responses.
28. Selective serotonin reuptake inhibitor (SSRI)–induced ED can be managed with the following EXCEPT:
    a. substitution with bupropion.
    b. drug holiday.
    c. PDE-5 inhibitor.
    d. dosage reduction.
    e. behavioral therapy.
29. The diagnostic criteria for premature ejaculation include the following EXCEPT:
    a. lack of ejaculatory control.
    b. short latency time.
    c. sexual dissatisfaction.
    d. erectile dysfunction.
    e. intravaginal ejaculatory latency time (IVELT) of 59 seconds.
30. The side effects of SSRIs used in treating premature ejaculation include which of the following?
    a. Fatigue, yawning, mild nausea, loose stools, or perspiration
    b. Headache, flushing, and nasal stuffiness
    c. Constipation and abdominal cramps
    d. Visual disturbance due to inhibition of phosphodiesterase type 6
    e. Erythrocytosis and venous thrombosis

ANSWERS

1. **b. Partner satisfaction.** The IIEF is the most widely used SAQ, and it is statistically validated in many languages. The IIEF is a 15-item SAQ; it addresses and quantifies five domains: erectile function, orgasmic function, sexual desire, intercourse satisfaction, and overall satisfaction (Rosen et al, 1997) (see Table 22-2).
2. **e. Patients with long-term diabetes and hypertension.** Generally accepted indications for specialized evaluation are failure of initial treatment, Peyronie's disease, primary ED, history of pelvic/perineal trauma, cases requiring vascular or neurosurgical intervention, complicated endocrinopathy, complicated psychiatric disorder, complex relationship problems, and medicolegal concerns.
3. **e. They can differentiate various causes of organic ED.** One major drawback of sexual inventories is their reliance on patient's self-assessment. Blander and coworkers (1999) have demonstrated that SAQs do not differentiate among the various causes of ED (arterial, venous, or mixed vascular), and evidence-based assessments (diagnostics tests) are still necessary in the evaluation of patients with complex ED. Therefore, in clinical evaluation, a good case history, preferably taken from both partners, with an adequate physical examination and proper laboratory investigations, is still the cornerstone in the evaluation of ED.
4. **c. 25 cm/s.** Total blood flow is a function of both arterial diameter and blood flow velocity. In patients with nonarteriogenic causes of ED (i.e., neurogenic, psychogenic), it has been found that the PSV of the cavernous arteries consistently exceed 25 cm/s within 5 minutes of ICI (Lue et al, 1985; Mueller and Lue, 1988). Additional studies from different institutions have reported the mean PSV in normal subjects

as 34.8 cm/s (Broderick and Lue, 1991); 40 cm/s (Shabsigh et al, 1990); and 47 cm/s (Benson and Vickers, 1989). In the Mayo Clinic series, PSV less than 25 cm/s had a sensitivity of 100% and a specificity of 95% in patients with abnormal pudendal arteriography (Lewis and King, 1994).

5. **b. Prostaglandin E_1.** For combined injection and stimulation test, several vasodilators have been used, including alprostadil alone (Caverject or Edex, 10 to 20 µg), a combination of papaverine and phentolamine (bimix, 0.3 mL), or a mixture of all three of the above agents (brimix, 0.3 mL). In our practice, 0.3 mL of bimix solution is routinely used because of its lower incidence of painful erections as compared with injection with alprostadil, which is a common complaint in patients after radical prostatectomy or cystectomy. In a review of the published literature, Linet and Neff (1994) found that, in doses of 10 to 20 µg, alprostadil produced full erections in 70% to 80% of patients with ED. The most frequent side effects were pain at the injection site or during erection (occurring in 16.8% of patients), hematoma/ecchymosis (1.5%), and prolonged erection/priapism (1.3%).
6. **c. Spinal cord injury.** In a study by Armstrong and associates (1993), a total of 160 men with erectile failure received treatment with 13,030 intracavernous papaverine and phentolamine injections. An erection sufficient for sexual intercourse was achieved in 115 (72%). The response rates for specific etiologies were as follows: vasculogenic (48%), psychogenic (93%), neurogenic (92%), diabetic (68%), idiopathic (63%), traumatic (60%), alcohol related (80%), and drug related (75%).
7. **e. Self-stimulation and audiovisual stimulation are of no additional benefit in ICI testing.** A CIS test consists of intracavernous injection of a vasodilator or a combination of two or three vasodilators, genital or audiovisual sexual stimulation, and assessment of the erection by an observer. This test is the most commonly performed diagnostic procedure for ED. This screening test allows the clinician to bypass neurologic and hormonal influences and to evaluate the vascular status of the penis directly and objectively. The erectile response is periodically evaluated for both rigidity and duration. Comparison with other hemodynamic tests suggests a normal ICI test is associated with normal veno-occlusion. But this test may be normal (false negative) in as many as 20% of patients with borderline arterial inflow (when normal is defined as more than 35 cm/s peak systolic flow on duplex ultrasound and borderline is defined as 25 to 35 cm/s) (Pescatori et al, 1994). False-positive results occur most commonly because of patient anxiety, needle phobia, or inadequate dosage of medication.
8. **c. PSV 40 cm/s, EDV 8 cm/s, poor erection after stimulation.** Cavernous veno-occlusive dysfunction (CVOD) is defined as the inability to achieve and maintain erection despite adequate arterial inflow. When the Doppler spectral waveform continues to exhibit high systolic flow (>25 cm/s PSV) and persistent diastolic flow velocity (>5 cm/s) accompanied by quick detumescence after self-stimulation, the patient is considered to have venogenic impotence. Among patients with PSVs greater than 25 cm/s, venous leakage on cavernosometry was predicted with a sensitivity of 90% and specificity of 56% when EDV was greater than 5 cm/s.
9. **b. 5 mL/min.** To achieve complete smooth muscle relaxation, one to several intracavernous injections are given, followed by measurement of maintenance flow rate, pressure drop, and CASOP. With complete smooth muscle relaxation, the flow rate required to maintain erection at an intracavernous pressure of more than 100 mm Hg is reported to be less than 3 to 5 mL/min whereas the pressure decrease in 30 seconds from 150 mm Hg is less than 45 mm Hg.
10. **c. Color duplex ultrasound study is helpful in the diagnosis of high-flow priapism.** When further diagnostic testing is indicated in the evaluation of the complex patient, the penile blood flow study (PBFS), which consists of CIS and blood flow measurement by duplex ultrasound, is the most reliable and least invasive evidence-based assessment of ED. In color-coded duplex ultrasound, the direction of the blood flow is assigned with red (toward the probe) or blue (away from the probe) color, making the identification of the vessels and recording of blood flow easier (Broderick and Arger, 1993; Herbner et al, 1994; Landwehr, 1995). Duplex ultrasound consists of a high resolution (7 to 10 MHz) real-time ultrasound and a color pulsed Doppler, which enables the ultrasonographer to visualize the dorsal and cavernous arteries selectively and to perform dynamic blood flow analysis with color Doppler (see Fig. 22-3). It is also the best tool available for the diagnosis of high-flow priapism and localization of a ruptured artery.
11. **b. Like the duplex ultrasound blood flow study, it is minimally invasive and permits the patient a period of privacy and self-stimulation.** Cavernous arterial occlusion pressure involves intracavernous injection of a vasodilator (usually tri-mix solution) followed by infusion of saline into the corpora cavernosa at a rate sufficient to raise the intracavernous pressure above the systolic blood pressure. A pencil Doppler transducer is then applied to the side of the penile base. The saline infusion is stopped, and the intracavernous pressure is allowed to fall. The pressure at which the cavernous arterial flow becomes detectable is defined as the cavernous artery systolic occlusion pressure (CASOP). Pharmacologic cavernosometry involves simultaneous saline infusion and intracavernous pressure monitoring to assess the penile outflow system after intracavernous injection of a strong vasodilating solution such as a high dose of alprostadil or tri-mix. Veno-occlusive dysfunction is indicated by either the inability to increase intracavernous pressure to the level of the mean systolic blood pressure with saline infusion or a rapid drop of intracavernous pressure after cessation of infusion. Pharmacologic cavernosography involves the infusion of radiographic contrast solution into the corpora cavernosa after a vasodilator-induced erection to visualize the site of venous leakage.
12. **b. early morning.** Circadian rhythm of testosterone (T) levels should be considered in measuring serum T; blood should be drawn between 8:00 AM and 11:00 AM. For screening, a total T determination is usually adequate. If the T level is below or at the low limit of normal, it should be confirmed with a second determination together with assessment of luteinizing hormone and prolactin levels.
13. **c. digital camera.** NPT has been measured by a number of methods: stamp test (Barry et al, 1980); snap gauges (Diedrich et al, 1992); sleep laboratory nocturnal penile tumescence and rigidity (NPTR); RigiScan (Endocare, Inc., Irvine, CA); and, most recently, NPT electrobioimpedance (NEVA, American Medical Systems, Inc., Minnetonka, MN).
14. **e. erotic music.** Audiovisual sexual stimulation (AVSS) appears to enhance penile responses to a variety of test stimulants: vibratory, intracavernous injection, and topical and oral pharmacologic agents.
15. **e. Peyronie's disease.** Heaton and Morales (1997) have suggested indications for NPTR as follows: (1) suspected sleep disorder; (2) an obscure etiology; (3) nonresponse to therapy; (4) planned surgical treatment; (5) a legally sensitive case; (6) measurement of drug effects in placebo-controlled drug trials; and (7) suspected psychogenic etiology.
16. **c. Spironolactone.** Thiazide diuretics are commonly associated with the complaint of ED, and spironolactone interferes with testosterone synthesis. Switching patients to newer agents,

such as calcium channel blockers and angiotensin-converting enzyme inhibitors, may reverse ED in some patients.

17. **b. Anemia.** Supraphysiologic levels of testosterone will suppress LH and FSH production and result in infertility; breast tenderness and/or gynecomastia is not uncommon with parenteral testosterone dosing. Long-term androgen therapy requires a commitment from the patient and the specialist for follow-up. Testosterone and its metabolite DHT are growth factors. Erythrocytosis is the most common laboratory alteration noted with long-term therapy. Morley and coworkers (1993) noted that the mean hematocrit increased from 42% to 49% after 3 months of treatment. Androgens may induce or worsen sleep apnea.

18. **b. Transdermal scrotal testosterone patches result in significant levels of DHT, because of a high content of 5α-reductase in scrotal skin.** Injectable depot preparations of testosterone, such as testosterone cypionate and enanthate, are the least expensive form of androgen supplementation. These depot preparations do not replicate the normal circadian rhythm. The initial supraphysiologic testosterone "rush" may be disconcerting to some patients, but others enjoy an improved sense of well-being, aggression, and libido. The subphysiologic phase is reported by many patients as unpleasant, with decreased energy and libido as well as depressed mood. Testoderm was initially available only as a scrotal patch without adhesive (4 to 6 mg). Because of high levels of 5α-reductase activity in scrotal skin, significantly high levels of dihydrotestosterone (DHT) were produced. The most common adverse reactions to transdermal testosterone preparation are itching, chronic skin irritation, and allergic contact dermatitis. Patients should alternate application sites and avoid sun-exposed areas. Local application of cortisone cream may relieve irritated skin. Testosterone gel is applied once daily in the morning to clean, dry skin over the shoulders, upper arms, or abdomen. After the skin begins to dry, patients may dress. They should wash their hands thoroughly, because skin contact can transmit testosterone: in clinical studies, 15 minutes of direct skin contact resulted in doubling the female partner's basal testosterone levels.

    Oral testosterone preparations are largely rendered metabolically inactive during the "first-pass" circulation through the liver. Metabolic inactivation requires oral dosing to exceed 200 mg/day to maintain normal serum levels. Large dosages of testosterone are toxic to the liver and can lead to hepatitis, cholestatic jaundice, hepatomas, hemorrhagic liver cysts, and hepatocarcinoma (Bagatell and Bremner, 1996). Chemical modification to 17α-methyltestosterone or fluoxymesterone reduces the amount of testosterone necessary to reach normal serum levels, but significant patient variability remains.

19. **a. breast cancer.** The presence of prostate or breast cancer is an absolute contraindication to androgen supplementation. While on testosterone therapy, patients should be followed every 6 months with a rectal examination and serum PSA test as long as they are on therapy. Laboratory surveillance should also include periodic hemoglobin/hematocrit levels, liver function tests, cholesterol, and lipid profile. The efficacy of testosterone supplementation is reasonably determined by clinical response rather than by repeating testosterone levels.

20. **b. increasing cyclic GMP levels.** The normal pathway for penile erection is initiated by sexual arousal, which stimulates release of nitric oxide at nerve endings in the penis. Another source of nitric oxide is vascular endothelial cells. Nitric oxide diffuses into vascular and cavernous smooth muscle cells in the corpus cavernosum to cause stimulation of guanylyl cyclase and elevation of cyclic GMP in these cells. This leads to activation of cyclic GMP–dependent protein kinase (PKG), phosphorylation of several proteins, and lowering of cytoplasmic calcium, hyperpolarization that results in smooth muscle relaxation and penile erection. PDE5 inhibitors do not increase the nitric oxide level, but they potentiate the nitric oxide effect to enhance erection. Without sexual stimulation and resultant nitric oxide release, these inhibitors are ineffective.

21. **a. constipation.** Most side effects associated with PDE5 inhibitor therapy are due to inhibition of PDE5 in other tissues or organs. Untoward events observed with the three PDE5 inhibitors include headache, dyspepsia, flushing, myalgia/back pain, and rhinitis. In several studies reported, flushing and visual side effects were more common in patients receiving sildenafil or vardenafil, and back pain/myalgia was more common in those receiving tadalafil. These events were mostly mild and transient, abated with time, and prompted treatment discontinuation in only a small number of patients.

22. **d. inhibition of PDE.** Papaverine is an alkaloid isolated from the opium poppy. Its molecular mechanism of action is through an inhibitory effect on PDE, leading to increased cAMP and cyclic GMP in penile erectile tissue. Papaverine also blocks voltage-dependent calcium channels, thus impairing calcium influx, and it may also impair calcium-activated potassium and chloride currents. The advantages are its low cost and stability at room temperature. The major disadvantages are the higher incidence of priapism (0% to 35%) and corporeal fibrosis (1% to 33%), thought to be a result of low acidity (pH 3 to 4) and occasional elevation of liver enzymes. The clinical dosages of papaverine monotherapy range from 20 to 80 mg. Its general efficacy as a monotherapy is less than 55%.

23. **b. Only two formulations have been approved for penile injection in the United States: Caverject and Edex.** Alprostadil is the synthetic form of a naturally occurring fatty acid (i.e., alprostadil refers to the exogenous form, PGE_1 to the endogenous compound). It causes smooth muscle relaxation, vasodilatation, and inhibition of platelet aggregation through elevation of intracellular cAMP. Alprostadil is available in the United States in two proprietary forms: Caverject (Pfizer) and Edex (Schwarz Pharma). Clinical dosing ranges from 2 to 40 μg. Its advantages are lower incidences of prolonged erection, of systemic side effects, and of fibrosis. The disadvantages include a higher incidence of painful erection and higher cost, and, once reconstituted into liquid from powder, it has a shortened half-life if not refrigerated.

24. **e. Tri-Mix is more effective than papaverine plus phentolamine in patients with severe arteriogenic or veno-occlusive ED.** Bennett and coworkers introduced a three-drug mixture containing 2.5 mL papaverine (30 mg/mL), 0.5 mL phentolamine (5 mg/mL), and 0.05 mL alprostadil (500 μg/mL) for ICI. In their 1991 study, 89% of the patients tested had adequate erection and went on to home injection therapy. Two patients had a prolonged erection that required treatment. In another study (Goldstein et al, 1990), 32 patients in whom alprostadil alone or the dual combination of papaverine/phentolamine had failed achieved adequate erection when the triple combination was used. Eight patients reported painful erection. No prolonged erections or systemic side effects were noted. In a randomized crossover study of 228 patients, the triple-drug combination has been shown to be as effective or more effective than alprostadil alone but has a much lower incidence of painful erection. Generally, tri-mix is reserved for men who have failed PGE_1 or papaverine/phentolamine therapy or who have significant penile pain with PGE_1. Tri-mix has not been approved by the U.S. FDA.

25. **c. sickle cell anemia.** The use of ICI therapy is contraindicated in patients with sickle cell anemia, schizophrenia, a severe psychiatric disorder, or severe systemic disease. In patients

taking an anticoagulant or aspirin, compressing the injection site for 7 to 10 minutes after injection is recommended. In patients with poor manual dexterity, the sexual partner can be instructed to perform the injection.

26. **e. penile pain.** The reported penile pain rate was up to 10.6% in Caverject trials and 33% in MUSE trials. In the latter, hypotension and syncope have been noted in 1% to 5.8%, mandating initial administration be in the office setting.

27. **b. VEDs may be effective in the patient with a malfunctioning penile implant and after explantation.** The vacuum constriction device consists of a plastic cylinder connected directly or by tubing to a vacuum-generating source (manual or battery-operated pump). After the penis is engorged by the negative pressure, a constricting ring is applied to the base to maintain the erection. To avoid injury, the ring should not be left in place for longer than 30 minutes. The penile skin may be cold and dusky, and ejaculation may be trapped by the constricting ring. The ring can be uncomfortable or even painful. However, in many patients, the device can produce an erection that is close to normal and rigidity sufficient for coitus. The device also engorges the glans and is useful for patients with glanular insufficiency. The device can be used successfully by men with a malfunctioning penile prosthesis in place (Sidi et al, 1990; Korenman and Viosca, 1992) and has been used after explantation to prevent shortening. In men with severe vascular insufficiency, combining ICI with the vacuum constriction device may enhance the erection (Marmar et al, 1988).

    The patient's satisfaction rate has been reported to range from 68% to 83% (Cookson and Nadig, 1993). Derouet and coworkers (1999) performed a retrospective review of their patients, finding 20% rejected the device primarily and 30.9% after a period ranging to 16 weeks. They cite a primary dropout rate of 50.9% and a secondary dropout rate of 7.3% after 10 months. Long-term users (41.8%) reported 98% satisfaction, and partner satisfaction was 85%. Dutta and Eid (1999) describe an attrition rate of 65% at a mean of 4 months; in their experience, 35% of patients continued with the vacuum constriction device long term (mean, 37 months).

28. **e. behavioral therapy.** Male sexual dysfunction occurs in many patients experiencing major depression (Nicolosi et al, 2005; Nurnberg, 2002). Selective serotonin reuptake inhibitors (SSRIs) have replaced tricyclic antidepressants and monoamine oxidase inhibitors as primary therapy for depression because of equal or better efficacy and reduced adverse effects. Treatment-related arousal disorders (lubrication and anorgasmia in women; ED and retarded ejaculation in men) secondary to SSRIs have been reported to range as high as 70% (Montejo-Gonzalez et al, 1997). Rosen and colleagues (1999) noted that the incidence of ED with fluoxetine was 1.7%; with sertraline, 2.5%; and with paroxetine, 6.4%. Potential mechanisms of SSRI-induced ED are multiple and include central and peripheral effects. Treatment strategies for SSRI-emergent ED include substitution (bupropion, nefazodone, buspirone, mirtazapine), drug holidays, SSRI dosage reduction, watchful waiting, and PDE5 inhibitors (Rosen et al, 1999; Nurnberg et al, 2000).

29. **d. erectile dysfunction.** Both the *DSM-IV-R* and the *ICD-10* refer to three essential components for the diagnosis of premature ejaculation (PE): short ejaculatory latency, a lack of control, and sexual dissatisfaction. The short ejaculatory latency is typically measured by intravaginal ejaculatory latency time (IVELT), defined by the time between vaginal intromission and ejaculation averaged over a number of sexual encounters. The *ICD-10* indicates that latencies of 15 seconds or less are consistent with a PE diagnosis. Others suggest latencies up to 1 or 2 minutes. IVELTs of 2 minutes or less show minimal overlap with those of men without PE, which typically range from 2 to 10 minutes. Accordingly, any latency under 2 minutes suggests a possible PE diagnosis.

30. **a. Fatigue, yawning, mild nausea, loose stools, or perspiration.** Paroxetine, sertraline, and fluoxetine may give rise to side effects such as fatigue, yawning, mild nausea, loose stools, or perspiration. These side effects often start in the first week after intake and gradually disappear within 2 to 3 weeks.

23

Prosthetic Surgery for Erectile Dysfunction

DROGO K. MONTAGUE

QUESTIONS

1. The three treatments that have had the most impact on the history of erectile dysfunction management are:
   a. inflatable penile prostheses, penile arterial surgery, PDE5 inhibitors.
   b. inflatable penile prostheses, penile venous ligation, PDE5 inhibitors.
   c. inflatable penile prostheses, intracavernous injections, PDE5 inhibitors.
   d. intracavernous injections, penile venous ligation, PDE5 inhibitors.
   e. intracavernous injections, penile arterial surgery, PDE5 inhibitors.
2. The most important difference between a prosthetic erection and a normal erection is that the prosthetic erection:
   a. is usually shorter.
   b. has less girth.
   c. has less sensitivity.
   d. has greater rigidity.
   e. is cooler.
3. The feature that differentiates the AMS 700 Ultrex prosthesis from others is:
   a. penile girth expansion.
   b. penile length expansion.
   c. it has two pieces.
   d. it is preconnected.
   e. it is prefilled.
4. The three most commonly used surgical approaches for penile prosthesis implantation are:
   a. ventral penile, infrapubic, inguinoscrotal.
   b. subcoronal, inguinoscrotal, penoscrotal.
   c. ventral penile, infrapubic, penoscrotal.
   d. inguinoscrotal, infrapubic, penoscrotal.
   e. subcoronal, infrapubic, penoscrotal.
5. Compared with the penoscrotal approach, the infrapubic approach has the following advantage:
   a. it avoids dorsal nerve injury.
   b. it allows scrotal pump anchoring.
   c. it provides better corporeal exposure.
   d. it allows reservoir placement under direct vision.
   e. there is less chance of infection.
6. The traditional method of sizing corpora for cylinders:
   a. sizes them correctly.
   b. undersizes them by 1 cm.
   c. undersizes them by 2 cm.
   d. oversizes them by 1 cm.
   e. oversizes them by 2 cm.
7. Cylinders that are too long for the corpora result in:
   a. S-shaped deformity and premature failure.
   b. S-shaped deformity and poor rigidity.
   c. premature failure and poor rigidity.
   d. premature failure and pain.
   e. S-shaped deformity and pain.
8. For most patients the ideal inflatable penile prosthesis reservoir location is:
   a. the inguinal canal.
   b. the scrotum.
   c. the retropubic space.
   d. between the rectus muscle and the peritoneum.
   e. extraperitoneal, lateral to the rectus muscle.
9. Wearing the penis up on the lower abdomen postoperatively helps to:
   a. prevent upward penile curvature.
   b. prevent downward penile curvature.
   c. minimize pain.
   d. avoid infection.
   e. avoid autoinflation.
10. After penile prosthesis implantation, retarded ejaculation (failure to reach orgasm) is best avoided by:
    a. supplemental testosterone.
    b. using a water-soluble lubricant.
    c. not inflating the device to high cylinder pressures.
    d. having adequate foreplay.
    e. using a rear entry position.
11. Infected penile prostheses are best treated by:
    a. removal of the single infected component.
    b. removal of all prosthetic components.
    c. 12 weeks of broad-spectrum antibiotics.
    d. hyperbaric oxygen.
    e. 12 weeks of broad-spectrum antibiotics + hyperbaric oxygen.

12. Five months after three-piece inflatable penile prosthesis implantation the recipient complains of persistent scrotal pain. Physical examination is normal except for adherence of the scrotal skin to the pump. The most likely cause of this man's symptoms and physical findings is:
   a. allergy to silicone.
   b. mechanical irritation from too much pumping.
   c. overly tight undergarments.
   d. infection with gram-positive organisms.
   e. infection with gram-negative organisms.
13. The following coatings for penile prosthesis are being used in attempts to lower the infection rates:
   a. minocycline, rifampin, polyvinylpyrrolidone.
   b. gentamicin, vancomycin, polyvinylpyrrolidone.
   c. gentamicin, vancomycin, rifampin.
   d. gentamicin, rifampin, Betadine.
   e. minocycline, vancomycin, Betadine.
14. Recently infection rates after penile prosthesis revision surgery have been shown to be equivalent to infection rates after first-time penile prosthesis implantation. This is most likely due to:
   a. 6 weeks of post-revision wide-spectrum intravenous antibiotics.
   b. irrigation with hydrogen peroxide, Betadine, and multiple antibiotic solutions.
   c. hydrophilic-coated devices.
   d. antibiotic-coated devices.
   e. removal of all prosthetic components.
15. During three-piece inflatable penile prosthesis implantation, while the right corpus cavernosum is being dilated the 8-mm dilator comes out the urethral meatus. Management of this intraoperative complication should include:
   a. urethral repair, continue implant, leave urethral catheter as stent for 3 weeks.
   b. urethral repair, continue implant, insert suprapubic tube.
   c. abandon implant, leave urethral catheter for 10 days.
   d. abandon implant, repair urethra, leave urethral catheter as stent for 3 weeks.
   e. abandon implant, repair urethra, insert suprapubic tube.

ANSWERS

1. **c. inflatable penile prostheses, intracavernous injections, PDE5 inhibitors.** In the 1970s and 1980s there was considerable enthusiasm regarding penile arterial revascularization and penile venous ligation surgery. However, long-term results with these two treatment modalities have generally been disappointing and, consequently, these procedures are no longer commonly performed.
2. **a. is usually shorter.** In our experience shortness of the prosthetic erection is the most common cause for patient dissatisfaction. The other difference between a prosthetic erection and a normal erection is the absence of glans tumescence.
3. **b. penile length expansion.** The middle fabric layer of the AMS 700 Ultrex cylinder provides both controlled girth and length expansion.
4. **e. subcoronal, infrapubic, penoscrotal.** The subcoronal incision can only be used to implant malleable or positionable devices.
5. **d. it allows reservoir placement under direct vision.** This is the only advantage of this surgical approach.
6. **e. oversizes them by 2 cm.** The correct cylinder size is one whose length is the same as the length of an imaginary line that runs lengthwise through the center of the corpus cavernosum. Traditional sizing techniques overestimate this length by approximately 2 cm.
7. **a. S-shaped deformity and premature failure.** A malleable prosthesis that is too long may cause pain, but a cylinder that is too long does not. Rigidity is usually not affected.
8. **c. the retropubic space.** When the reservoir is in the retropubic space, autoinflation of the prosthesis is less likely.
9. **b. prevent downward penile curvature.** While healing is taking place, a pseudocapsule forms around the prosthesis. If the cylinders are held down by an undergarment as this capsule is forming, they may develop downward curvature.
10. **d. having adequate foreplay.** If a man inflates his prosthesis, he is able to have coitus. However, unless he is sexually aroused, he may be unable to reach orgasm.
11. **b. removal of all prosthetic components.** Although only the scrotal pump may appear clinically to be infected, all components of the prosthesis are joined by tubing and the entire device should be considered infected.
12. **d. infection with gram-positive organisms.** Organisms such as *Staphylococcus epidermidis* typically cause a low-grade infection manifested by these symptoms and clinical findings. Infections due to gram-negative organisms commonly occur earlier and are associated with erythema and often drainage of pus from the wound.
13. **a. minocycline, rifampin, polyvinylpyrrolidone.** Mentor's three-piece inflatable penile prosthesis is coated with polyvinylpyrrolidone. American Medical System's three-piece inflatable penile prostheses are coated with minocycline and rifampin.
14. **e. removal of all prosthetic components.** Infection rates after repeat penile prosthesis surgery approach the rates seen with first-time penile prosthesis implantation if the entire device is replaced.
15. **c. abandon implant, leave urethral catheter for 10 days.** If the implant is not abandoned, the urethra is likely not to heal and the entire device is at risk of infection.

24

Vascular Surgery for Erectile Dysfunction

RONALD W. LEWIS • RICARDO MUNARRIZ

QUESTIONS

1. Vascular surgical procedures, in particular penile revascularization, are recommended for the following patient:
   a. 55-year-old diabetic man with vascular erectile dysfunction.
   b. 60-year-old man with generalized arterial sclerosis.
   c. 35-year-old man who has suffered pelvic trauma and has an isolated injury to the common penile artery.
   d. 40-year-old man who has proven arterial disease causing his ED and who smokes two packs of cigarettes per day.
   e. a post–radical prostatectomy patient.
2. The best incision for exposure of the penile arterial and venous vessels is a:
   a. peri-penile semicircular incision on the scrotal skin around the base of the penis.
   b. horizontal infrapubic incision.
   c. vertical infrapubic incision.
   d. penile scrotal incision on the ventral shaft of the penis.
   e. lower midline incision.
3. The study that is absolutely mandatory before penile revascularization surgery is:
   a. dynamic infusion cavernosometry and cavernosography.
   b. color duplex Doppler of the penile arteries.
   c. nocturnal penile tumescence study (NPT).
   d. common iliac arteriogram and a selective internal pudendal arteriogram.
   e. injection of a vasoactive agent during an office visit.
4. Aids for penile vascular surgery include all of the following EXCEPT:
   a. an attached table retractor.
   b. surgical loops.
   c. a hand-held Doppler probe.
   d. a lighted suction instrument.
   e. a ring retractor with elastic hooks.
5. All the following types of penile revascularization have been described EXCEPT:
   a. inferior epigastric artery to the dorsal artery in an end-to-end anastomosis.
   b. inferior epigastric artery in an end-to-end anastomosis or an end-to-side anastomosis to the deep dorsal vein of the penis.
   c. side-to-side anastomosis of the dorsal penile artery to the dorsal penile vein, which is then connected to the inferior epigastric artery.
   d. saphenous vein graft from the hypogastric artery to the dorsal penile artery.
   e. reverse saphenous vein graft from the superficial femoral artery to the dorsal artery of the penis.
6. Important points to consider in harvesting of the inferior epigastric artery include:
   a. the artery must be carefully dissected away from its accompanying vein.
   b. the nonligating of small tributaries that come off of the major trunk.
   c. the artery is dissected en bloc with the surrounding veins and fat to preserve the vasa vasora.
   d. the inferior epigastric artery is very difficult to dissect because it lies deep in the rectus muscle.
   e. the artery often trifurcates in its midportion.
7. As regards the adventitia tissue of vessels used in penile revascularization the following is important:
   a. it must remain present on all vessels that are anastomosed.
   b. if it is removed near the site of an anastomosis it may cause thrombosis.
   c. it is of no importance to the vessel wall for providing nutrients and innervation.
   d. it is carefully removed only at the site of the vascular anastomosis such as the distal end of the inferior epigastric artery and the free end of the dorsal artery.
8. Complications of vascular surgery of the penis include the following EXCEPT:
   a. penile edema.
   b. penile numbness or hypoesthesia.
   c. traumatic disruption of the suture line.
   d. glans hypervascularization.
   e. extreme shortening of the penis.

9. A crucial time for measuring success for veno-occlusive surgery on the penis is the following:
   a. first 3 months after surgery.
   b. 6 to 12 months after the surgery.
   c. 12 to 24 months after the surgery.
   d. 5 years after the surgery.
   e. immediately after the surgery.

10. The arterial inflow source most commonly used for penile revascularization surgery is the:
    a. inferior epigastric artery.
    b. superficial perineal artery.
    c. obturator artery.
    d. superior epigastric artery.
    e. epididymal artery.

ANSWERS

1. **c. 35-year-old man who has suffered pelvic trauma and has an isolated injury to the common penile artery.** Those patients with discrete focal arterial lesions found on selective pudendal arteriography, particularly younger patients who have a history of trauma (pelvic fracture or perineal blunt trauma), who do not have diabetes or neurologic disease, and who are not currently users of tobacco are the best candidates for penile revascularization procedures.
2. **a. peri-penile semicircular incision on the scrotal skin around the base of the penis.** The choice of incision for the venous surgery and for preparation of the recipient dorsal penile artery or deep dorsal penile vein revascularization is the anterior scrotal peri-penile incision.
3. **d. common iliac arteriogram and a selective internal pudendal arteriogram.** A common iliac arteriogram and a selective internal pudendal arteriogram are necessary to demonstrate the adequacy of the proposed donor artery such as the inferior epigastric artery and the focal lesion in the artery or arteries supplying the corpora cavernosa.
4. **a. an attached table retractor.** Some surgeons prefer the use of loupes for the early dissection in the arterial cases and for all of the venous surgery cases. A hand-held Doppler probe is an excellent accessory tool for monitoring of the dorsal penile artery and/or checking for runoff into revascularized arteries or arterialized veins. A lighted suction instrument is also useful, particularly for the arterial cases; it is also helpful for any venous dissection near the urethra.
5. **d. saphenous vein graft from the hypogastric artery to the dorsal penile artery.** For penile revascularization the most common donor artery is the inferior epigastric artery, which is connected in an end-to-end or end-to-side anastomosis to the dorsal artery of the penis; or in cases of venous arterialization, the inferior epigastric artery is connected to the dorsal penile vein. A procedure has been described in which the donor artery is the inferior epigastric artery connected side-to-side to an anastomosis of the deep penile artery and the dorsal penile vein. Another donor source for re-arterialization of the dorsal artery of the penis, when the inferior epigastric artery is not present, is a reverse saphenous vein graft that is fed into and connected to the superficial femoral artery.
6. **c. the artery is dissected en bloc with the surrounding veins and fat to preserve the vasa vasora.** It is critical to harvest an inferior epigastric artery of sufficient length to prevent tension on the microvascular anastomosis. The vasa vasora are preserved by dissecting the artery en bloc with the surrounding veins and fat. Branches isolated during the dissection are both artery and vein, which can be commonly ligated or clipped using small vascular clips or cauterized by bipolar cautery. Dissection of the inferior epigastric artery is required from its origin at the level of the external iliac artery to the point at the level of the umbilicus. It is at this point that the artery usually bifurcates.
7. **d. it is carefully removed only at the site of the vascular anastomosis such as the distal end of the inferior epigastric artery and the free end of the dorsal artery.** The only location where the adventitial tissue must be carefully removed is at the site of the microvascular anastomosis, that is, the distal end of the inferior epigastric artery and the free end of the dorsal artery, to avoid causing subsequent thrombosis.
8. **d. glans hypervascularization.** Penile edema is common after vascular surgery of the penis. Two other significant complications of penile vascular surgery are penile numbness (or hypoesthesia) and penile shortening from scar entrapment. Mechanical disruption of the microvascular anastomosis has been reported. Another complication of deep dorsal penile vein arterialization is glans hyperemia, when hypervascularization occurs when the communicating vein from the revascularized deep dorsal vein to the glans in the distal dissection has been missed. Penile shortening is not usually extreme.
9. **c. 12 to 24 months after the surgery.** Results of surgery from veno-occlusive sexual dysfunction in the first year have been much higher by almost double than rates for success after 12 months. Long-term results for which most valid studies are reported require 12 months or more follow-up and show a long-term success of about 25%.
10. **a. inferior epigastric artery.** The most common donor artery for penile revascularization surgery is the inferior epigastric artery.

25

Peyronie's Disease

GERALD H. JORDAN

QUESTIONS

1. Which of the following statements regarding Peyronie's disease is correct?
   a. Most patients with Peyronie's disease understand the effects of their disease and thus require little counseling.
   b. The majority of patients with Peyronie's disease will eventually require surgery.
   c. Surgery, when required, can be viewed as palliation for the effects of the Peyronie's disease process.
   d. In many patients with Peyronie's disease, medical therapy has proved curative.
   e. The vast majority of patients will require prosthetic placement.
2. All of the following are associated, in the literature, with the developments of Peyronie's disease EXCEPT which one?
   a. ACE inhibitor antihypertensives
   b. β-Adrenergic blockers
   c. Paget's disease of the bone
   d. Diabetes mellitus
   e. Phenytoin use
3. Which of the following statements regarding Peyronie's disease is NOT correct?
   a. Smith, using an autopsy study, found the asymptomatic incidence of Peyronie's disease to be 22%.
   b. The symptomatic incidence of Peyronie's disease has risen and now is estimated to be approximately 16%.
   c. The average age at onset of Peyronie's disease is in the middle 50s.
   d. The asymptomatic prevalence of Peyronie's disease is established to be 0.4% to 1.0%.
   e. The vast majority of patients with signs of Peyronie's disease will spontaneously resolve the effects of the disease.
4. With regard to Peyronie's disease, select the correct statement:
   a. PDE5 inhibitor medications and the approved intracavernosal injection agents are contraindicated for use in Peyronie's patients.
   b. PDE5 inhibitors may directly lead to the development of Peyronie's disease.
   c. Prolonged use of papaverine and Regitine has been implicated as a cause of intracorporal fibrosis.
   d. Vacuum erection device (VED) is contraindicated for use in the Peyronie's disease patient.
   e. Constriction rings are directly proven to be associated with the development of Peyronie's disease.
5. With regard to the anatomy of the penis pertinent to Peyronie's disease the:
   a. linear longitudinal layer attenuates at the 12-o'clock position (dorsal midline).
   b. circular lamina of the tunica albuginea attenuates at the 6-o'clock position (ventral midline).
   c. septal fibers interweave with the circular fiber lamina of the tunica albuginea.
   d. longitudinal lamina of the tunica albuginea is thickest at the ventral midline.
   e. midline septal fibers interweave with the thickened periurethral outer lamina.
6. Current theory involving the etiology of Peyronie's includes all of the following factors EXCEPT which one?
   a. The inciting event leading to Peyronie's disease seems to be buckling trauma during erection.
   b. The transforming growth factor-β1 (TGF-β1) has been implicated as a cause of the abnormal disordered healing.
   c. The recent investigations also implicate the down-regulation of factors known to be antifibrotic.
   d. The accumulation of plaque has been associated with other disorders governed by increased cholesterol and lipid levels.
   e. The down-regulation of interfibrotic factors is unique to Peyronie's disease.
7. Series that observe the natural history of Peyronie's disease document which of the following?
   a. The majority of patients present with sudden onset of stable deformity.
   b. Many patients require surgery to resolve their painful erections.
   c. All patients eventually develop stable deformity.
   d. Total resolution of the Peyronie's disease process occurs relatively, frequently.
   e. It is unusual for patients to have curvature without painful erections.

8. With regard to the relationship of erectile dysfunction and Peyronie's disease, select the incorrect response:
   a. In many of the older published series, the stratification of erectile problems, functional versus organic, is not clear. Currently with better validated devices, stratification is included in most series.
   b. The highly emotional aspects of Peyronie's disease are expressed in many men via disordered erectile function.
   c. Many men tend to abandon their sexual activities in response to the emotional trauma of Peyronie's disease.
   d. Surgery to address cavernous veno-occlusive dysfunction is often effective in men with Peyronie's disease.
   e. Often, with corrective surgery, disorders of erectile function seen preoperatively resolve with the surgical process.
9. With regard to the presenting complaints of patients with Peyronie's disease, select the correct statement:
   a. Distal flaccidity occurs because of vascular blockage due to involvement of the spongy erectile tissue of the corpora cavernosa by the plaque.
   b. Migratory penile deformity is usually due to the development of additional plaque.
   c. Pain with intercourse rarely disappears without surgical therapy.
   d. Foreshortening of the penis is a frequent complaint of patients with Peyronie's disease.
   e. Indentation of the corpora cavernosa is usually of cosmetic concern only.
10. With regard to medical management of Peyronie's disease, select the correct response:
    a. Vitamin E has been proven to be highly efficacious for the treatment of Peyronie's disease.
    b. Aminobenzoate potassium (Potaba) has not been proven definitively to be efficacious for the treatment of Peyronie's disease.
    c. Nonsteroidal anti-inflammatory agents have been proven to be efficacious in the treatment of Peyronie's disease.
    d. Colchicine is thought to be efficacious by virtue of effects on purine metabolism.
    e. Tamoxifen, by virtue of its action on tubulin, has proved to be highly efficacious.
11. With regard to intralesional injection protocols for Peyronie's disease, select the incorrect response:
    a. Intralesional corticosteroids are not recommended.
    b. Verapamil injection protocols are logistically laborious, but the injections are well tolerated.
    c. Collagenase injection protocols are available only as a part of study protocols.
    d. Interferon injections are proposed to work by mechanisms similar to those of verapamil but are better tolerated.
    e. Colchicine has been proven to limit plaque "contracture."
12. Surgery is absolutely indicated in patients with Peyronie's disease for which of the following reasons?
    a. Persistent pain with erection
    b. Severe foreshortening of the penis
    c. Erectile dysfunction or curvature that precludes intercourse
    d. Indentation of the penis not related to issues of penetration
    e. All of the above
13. With regard to surgery for Peyronie's disease, select the best response:
    a. Algorithms are the best mechanisms to determine surgical candidacy.
    b. Corporoplasty techniques are technically straightforward and thus are the best for the surgeon who does not operate on Peyronie's patients frequently.
    c. Corporoplasty techniques, in most series, have better results for preservation of erectile function and thus are clearly superior for all Peyronie's patients who are surgical candidates.
    d. Incision and grafting techniques using synthetic "graft" material (e.g., Gore-Tex, Silastic) have been proven, in large series, to be highly effective.
    e. Incision and grafting techniques, in emerging well-stratified studies, have been shown to effectively straighten the penis and preserve erectile function in Peyronie's disease patients.

ANSWERS

1. **c. Surgery, when required, can be viewed as palliation for the effects of the Peyronie's disease process.** Fortunately, however, most patients only require counseling, education, and reassurance. While medical therapy is used, few studies have shown medical therapy to have proven efficacy. A minority of patients will have deformity that precludes their having intercourse, which is one of the indications for surgery. In the patient who is adequately sexually active, performing corrective surgery, just to make things better, cannot be recommended. The vast majority of patients with Peyronie's disease thus do not require surgery, and, in most, prosthetic implantation can be avoided.
2. **a. ACE inhibitor antihypertensives.** Peyronie's disease is associated with Dupuytren's contracture. Thirty to 40 percent of Peyronie's disease patients will also have findings compatible with Dupuytren's contracture. Other associated conditions include plantar fascial contracture (Ledderhose disease) and tympanosclerosis. Peyronie's disease is also reported as associated with external trauma to the penis, diabetes mellitus, Paget's disease of the bone, history of urethral instrumentation, β-adrenergic blocker use, phenytoin use, and now more and more patients are being seen with the only identifiable other association being that of having had a radical prostatectomy.
3. **b. The symptomatic incidence of Peyronie's disease has risen and now is estimated to be approximately 16%.** The symptomatic incidence of Peyronie's disease has previously been estimated at 1%. However, with the advent of pharmacologic treatment for erectile dysfunction, the incidence is clearly rising and can be quite conservatively estimated to be 4% to 5% now. In white men the average age at onset of Peyronie's disease is approximately 53 years of age. The asymptomatic prevalence was estimated at 0.4% to 1%. It is reasonable to suggest that the asymptomatic prevalence of Peyronie's disease was also increasing. An autopsy study of 100 men without a known history of Peyronie's disease found 22 of the 100 men to have lesions histologically compatible with Peyronie's disease.
4. **c. Prolonged use of papaverine and Regitine has been implicated as a cause of intracorporal fibrosis.** The PDE5 inhibitor medication and the approved intracavernosal injection agents are not indicated for Peyronie's disease patients. This is because these patients were excluded during the final phase

studies reviewed for drug approval. There has thus never been any suggestion whatsoever that PDE5 inhibitors are directly causally related to the development of Peyronie's disease. There is emerging data that would suggest that certain endothelial impairment can be preserved with the initiation of PDE5 inhibitor therapy; and, in fact, recent data suggest that the use of PDE5 inhibitors may be therapeutic for Peyronie's disease patients. Cyclic GMP, which is one of the mediators of penile erection, is produced by nitric oxide activation of guanylyl cyclase. Cyclic GMP is also antifibrotic in Peyronie's disease plaques. Long-term administration of sildenafil, a phosphodiesterase inhibitor, impedes cyclic GMP breakdown and has been shown to prevent Peyronie's disease plaque formation in rat models. Intracavernosal injection therapy has not been directly implicated as causative in Peyronie's disease. It has certainly been theorized that repeated trauma from insertion of the needle could stimulate a Peyronie's disease–like process. The prolonged use of papaverine and Regitine has been shown to create intracorporal fibrosis. The vacuum erection device is not contraindicated for use in Peyronie's patients, and in fact there are protocols that are examining the vacuum device as a possible treatment method for patients with Peyronie's disease.

5. **c. septal fibers interweave with the circular fiber lamina of the tunica albuginea.** The tunica albuginea is bilaminar throughout most of its circumference. It is composed of an outer longitudinal layer and an inner circular layer. The tunica albuginea varies in thickness from 1.5 to 3 mm depending on the position on the circumference. The outer longitudinal layer attenuates in the ventral midline, and thus the tunica is monolaminar at that point. The outer longitudinal layer is thickest on the ventrum adjacent to the corpus spongiosum and on the dorsum and thinnest on the lateral aspect.

6. **d. The accumulation of plaque has been associated with other disorders governed by increased cholesterol and lipid levels.** Somers and Dawson have shown that Peyronie's disease most likely begins with buckling trauma causing injury to the septal insertion of the tunica albuginea. It has been proposed that the avascular nature of the tunica albuginea may impede clearance of many tissue growth factors, particularly TGF-β1 growth factors. TGF-β1 has been implicated in a number of cases of soft tissue fibrosis as well as with erectile dysfunction. The TGFs are also capable of autoinducement. Recent investigations have also implicated the failure of down-regulation of matrix metalloproteinase (MMP) in the abnormal scarring process of Peyronie's disease. Failure of down-regulation of MMP also has been implicated in a number of disease processes. MMPs function as antifibrotic factors. α_1-Antitrypsin, which is a proteinase inhibitor, has also been implicated as a possible factor in the development of Peyronie's disease. Recent investigation has not verified that implication; however, it was found that α_1-antitrypsin levels do vary with age.

7. **c. All patients eventually develop stable deformity.** In most cases of Peyronie's disease there are two phases: an active phase that often can be associated with painful erections and migratory deformity of the penis and the quiescent phase, which is characterized by stabilization of the deformity and inevitably with disappearance of painful erections if they were present. Up to one third of patients, however, will present with what appears to be sudden development of painless and stable deformity. A review by Mulhall interestingly shows that in a large cohort of men with Peyronie's disease, one third presented with erectile dysfunction at the time that they presented with Peyronie's disease and a significant percentage of them had erectile dysfunction that preceded their notice of the onset of Peyronie's disease and its diagnosis. This confirms the work of other authors.

8. **e. Often, with corrective surgery, disorders of erectile function seen preoperatively resolve with the surgical process.** In publications concerning the natural history of disease, erectile dysfunction is prominently mentioned. In the older literature, patients were not stratified with regard to the functional issues versus the organic issues as they relate to erectile dysfunction. Jones, in 1977, dealt best with the counseling issues of men with sexual dysfunction and described the counseling of a man with Peyronie's disease as being much the same as counseling a person who has suffered a death and is grieving. Recent data show that most men indicated that the impact of Peyronie's disease on their life was severe. That data verify much of what Jones reported. The emotions expressed by many of the men who were interviewed ranged from anger to frustration to hopelessness. A major point made by Jones in dealing with Peyronie's disease patients is to avoid or limit emotional factors. Patients and their partners need to hear the suggestion that they must "keep sexual expression alive." Recent data show that men with Peyronie's disease, even though not in a steady relationship, do continue to have sex; however, it was usually "very different than it used to be", and most were very concerned that their condition would worsen to the point that they would be unable to have sexual intercourse in the future. Cavernous veno-occlusive disease (CVOD) is seen in patients with Peyronie's disease, and the precise mechanism is not clear. What is clear is that surgery to address CVOD is virtually never effective in Peyronie's disease patients.

9. **d. Foreshortening of the penis is a frequent complaint of patients with Peyronie's disease.** The presenting symptoms of Peyronie's disease include (1) in many cases penile pain with erection, (2) penile deformity, (3) shortening of the penis with and without an erection, (4) notice of a plaque or indurated area in the penis, and (5) in many patients erectile dysfunction. Some patients complain of being awakened in the morning with pain during their erection. Spontaneous improvement in pain with erection virtually always occurs as the inflammation resolves. However, this must not be confused with pain during intercourse. Pain during intercourse often does persist and is due to the mechanical forces of intercourse on the curved penis. Distal flaccidity is frequently noted, but it is believed to be due to the mechanical effects of the plaque, limiting stretching of the midline septal fibers and thus creating a hinge effect at that area. Studies have shown that proximally and distally to the plaque the pressures within the corpora cavernosa are the same.

10. **b. Aminobenzoate potassium (Potaba) has not been proven definitively to be efficacious for the treatment of Peyronie's disease.** Any discussion on the medical management of Peyronie's disease begins with the disclaimer that few medical management regimens have been subjected to double-blind drug testing. Vitamin E has not been subjected to blinded or controlled studies and thus has not been proven to be efficacious. The prolonged use of high dose vitamin E is not recommended because of the anticoagulation effects of high dose vitamin E. Aminobenzoate potassium has been looked at in a small blinded study that showed it to be efficacious, but subsequent studies have not verified those results. Additionally, at therapeutic doses, patients complain of gastrointestinal side effects when taking aminobenzoate potassium. Colchicine binds tubulin and causes it to depolymerize and thus inhibits mobility and adhesion of leukocytes but also inhibits mitosis by disrupting spindle cell fibers and thus functions as a very potent anti-inflammatory. Tubulin is also involved in the process of wound contracture. Colchicine also stimulates collagenases. Nonsteroidal anti-inflammatory drugs and steroids have been used anecdotally; however, no studies support an indication for the use of these drugs. Tamoxifen is thought to facilitate the release of TGF-β

from fibroblasts; however, recent studies have not shown the use of tamoxifen to be effective in Peyronie's disease patients.

11. **d. Interferon injections are proposed to work by mechanisms similar to those of verapamil but are better tolerated.** A number of intralesional injection protocols have been examined. It is the recommendation of the consensus committee on penile curvatures that the use of intralesional steroids be eliminated or at least initiated with extreme caution because of the rather significant local side effects, the inconsistent pattern of improvement in well-established curvature, the lack of studies showing proven efficacy, and reports of patients who believed their condition deteriorated after the injections. A number of nonblinded studies have suggested efficacy with the use of intralesional verapamil, but no blinded studies suggest that the use of verapamil as an intralesional agent is efficacious. Collagenase has been subjected to two double-blind studies, but intralesional collagenase is currently available only on study protocol. The use of interferons as intralesional therapy for Peyronie's disease was reported in 1991. The mechanism of action of interferon is very similar to that proposed for verapamil. Verapamil is well tolerated. Complications are associated only with the injection procedure per se and are minimal. However, almost all patients injected with interferon develop a "flu-like" syndrome.

12. **c. Erectile dysfunction or curvature that precludes intercourse.** For a patient to be a surgical candidate, the patient must have stable and mature disease. Indications for surgery include deformity that precludes intercourse and/or erectile dysfunction that precludes intercourse. Surgery for persistent pain or for foreshortening only rarely provides good results and thus is strongly not recommended.

13. **e. Incision and grafting techniques, in emerging well-stratified studies, have been shown to effectively straighten the penis and preserve erectile function in Peyronie's disease patients.** For a patient to be a surgical candidate, the patient must have mature/quiescent disease. The patient likewise should be significantly disabled with regard to the performance of intercourse by either the curvature and/or the associated erectile dysfunction. A number of corporoplasty techniques have been proposed, and all have been shown to be relatively effective. Corporoplasty techniques are not necessarily straightforward techniques; in some cases achieving an adequately straight penis can be technically quite complex. In past series, corporoplasty techniques have been shown to have a better rate of preservation of preoperative erectile function, as compared with excision and grafting techniques. Well-stratified studies that have been recently performed have shown excellent rates of preservation of erectile function with incision and grafting techniques. Because foreshortening is a cardinal finding for most patients with Peyronie's disease, surgery that further "foreshortens the penis" is often not well accepted by nor palatable to the patient. Thus, in determining candidacy for surgery, and in determining the recommended surgical technique, a number of factors must be taken into account: (1) the patient's current symptoms; (2) the patient's stratification with regard to erectile function; (3) the predominant direction of curvature and location of the plaque; and (4) the patient's goals, after a course of education and counseling. In general, there are no large series that show effective use of synthetic graft materials. Those materials can be useful in patients who are having concomitant insertion of a penile prosthesis. In my experience, however, the use of the synthetic graft materials as "stand alone grafts" usually does not provide adequate results.

Peyronie's disease is not the "terminal/no hope" diagnosis that many patients believe it is, and in some cases have been told that it is. With proper counseling and education, proper stratification, and proper tailoring of the approach to patients, most can be effectively managed.

26

Priapism

ARTHUR L. BURNETT

QUESTIONS

1. Heightened priapism incidence in males 40 years and older is attributed to:
   a. sickle cell disease.
   b. hematologic malignancy.
   c. prostate cancer.
   d. erectile dysfunction pharmacotherapy.
   e. testosterone supplementation.
2. The critical pathologic change occurring in the cavernosal tissue at 4 hours after the onset of ischemic priapism is:
   a. threshold maximal hypoxic conditions begin.
   b. glucopenia begins.
   c. hypercoagulable thrombotic conditions begin.
   d. contractile responses deteriorate.
   e. cavernosal fibrosis begins.
3. The nitric oxide/cGMP signaling pathway is implicated in the pathogenesis of priapism based on scientific work showing:
   a. guanylate cyclase activity upregulation.
   b. guanylate cyclase activity downregulation.
   c. nitric oxide synthase activity upregulation.
   d. phosphodiesterase-5 activity upregulation.
   e. phosphodiesterase-5 activity downregulation.
4. Cavernosal blood gas results are PO_2 30 mm Hg, PCO_2 60 mm Hg, and pH 7.25 in a patient with sickle cell disease presenting with a 6-hour episode of priapism. The next step should be:
   a. oral terbutaline.
   b. oral pseudoephedrine.
   c. intracavernous aspiration.
   d. exchange transfusion.
   e. distal surgical shunt.
5. The characteristic blood flow defect of ischemic priapism found on color duplex ultrasonography is:
   a. normal cavernosal artery inflow.
   b. increased cavernosal artery inflow.
   c. decreased cavernosal artery inflow.
   d. arteriovenous malformation.
   e. sinusoidal fistulization.
6. After initial intracavernous treatment for ischemic priapism, blood gas sampling produces an equivocal mixed-venous blood result. Priapism resolution is best confirmed by:
   a. color duplex ultrasonography.
   b. penile scintigraphy.
   c. corpus cavernosography.
   d. penile arteriography.
   e. pelvic CT scan.
7. After a second session of intracavernous treatment consisting of aspiration/irrigation with phenylephrine administration, the priapic penis remains turgid. Cavernosal blood gas results are PO_2 40 mm Hg, PCO_2 50 mm Hg, and pH 7.35. The next step should be:
   a. observation.
   b. oral sympathomimetic.
   c. repeat intracavernous treatment.
   d. distal surgical shunt.
   e. proximal surgical shunt.
8. Phenylephrine is the preferred sympathomimetic used in the treatment of ischemic priapism because of its:
   a. α_1-selective activity.
   b. α_1 and α_2 activity.
   c. β_1-selective activity.
   d. β_2-selective activity.
   e. combined α and β activities.
9. The best indication for arterial embolization for nonischemic priapism is:
   a. unlikely spontaneous priapism resolution.
   b. failure of sympathomimetic therapy.
   c. reduction of recurrent priapism risk.
   d. reduction of subsequent erectile dysfunction risk.
   e. acquiescence to patient preference.
10. Persistent penile turgidity after a technically successful proximal surgical shunt procedure in a patient who presented with a 72-hour episode of ischemic priapism is an optimal indication for:
    a. observation.
    b. gonadotropin-releasing hormone agonist therapy.
    c. pudendal artery ligation.
    d. distal surgical shunt.
    e. penile prosthesis surgery.

ANSWERS

1. **d. erectile dysfunction pharmacotherapy.** The introduction of intracavernous pharmacotherapy approximately 2 decades ago led to a pronounced increase in the incidence of priapism. Because the majority of men requiring this intervention for erectile dysfunction are middle aged to older men, the heightened priapism incidence in this age range is associated with this etiologic factor.
2. **d. contractile responses deteriorate.** The 4-hour interval after the onset of ischemic priapism indicates a timeline when irreversible cavernosal smooth muscle contractile dysfunction occurs. Various ischemic metabolic changes do occur throughout the episode of penile ischemia, but a sufficient duration of combined hypoxia, acidosis, and glucopenia at a time interval of 4 hours critically affects tissue function. Thrombotic conditions and cavernosal fibrosis typically develop at longer intervals.
3. **e. phosphodiesterase-5 activity downregulation.** Recent scientific advances have shown that priapism is associated with decreased phosphodiesterase-5 functional regulation in the penis. The relative lack of this molecular factor needed for controlling chemical signaling of penile erection accounts for priapism.
4. **c. intracavernous aspiration.** These blood gas results suggest a presentation of ischemic priapism, which warrants immediate decompression of the corpora cavernosa for a duration of the problem exceeding 4 hours irrespective of etiology. In sickle cell disease, while concurrent systemic treatments may be offered, relief of the penile ischemia must be immediately pursued.
5. **c. decreased cavernosal artery inflow.** In presentations of ischemic priapism, minimal or absent blood flow in the cavernosal arteries is found using color duplex ultrasonography. The other findings apply to nonischemic priapism.
6. **a. color duplex ultrasonography.** Color duplex ultrasonography may be used as the most reliable imaging technique to differentiate ischemic from nonischemic priapism and to evaluate for priapism resolution after initial treatment for ischemic priapism.
7. **a. observation.** These blood gas results are consistent with normal mixed venous blood. The turgid penis may reflect pathologic changes such as tissue fibrosis. Observation is appropriate at this time.
8. **a. α_1-selective activity.** Phenylephrine has the property of being a selective α_1-adrenergic agonist, with minimal risk of causing cardiovascular side effects usually associated with a drug having β-adrenergic activity.
9. **e. acquiescence to patient preference.** Nonischemic priapism should generally be managed by observation. However, the patient may be distressed enough about his condition to request intervention such as embolization or surgery.
10. **e. penile prosthesis surgery.** Because it is recognized that ischemic priapism persisting for extended durations produces such erectile tissue damage that complete erectile dysfunction predictably results, some experts have advocated penile prosthesis surgery as an appropriate intervention to address the priapism while treating the expected complication of erectile dysfunction.

27

Androgen Deficiency in the Aging Male

ALVARO MORALES • JOHN MORLEY • JEREMY P. W. HEATON

QUESTIONS

1. The prevalence of new cases per year of androgen deficiency in American men 40 to 69 years old is:
   a. unknown.
   b. 50,000 to 99,000.
   c. 100,000 to 199,000.
   d. 200,000 to 299,000.
   e. more than 300,000.
2. Which of the following statements regarding testosterone (T) production and metabolism is incorrect?
   a. T is produced by the Leydig cells under the control of LH only.
   b. T is produced by brain cells, but this portion is not measurable in serum.
   c. T is produced by conversion from other androgens such as DHEA.
   d. T is produced in decreased amounts in the presence of hyperprolactinemia.
   e. T bound to sex hormone–binding globulin (SHBG) is inactive in the prostate.
3. Which of the following statements regarding the clinical diagnosis of androgen deficiency in aging is correct?
   a. Screening questionnaires (ADAM, AMS) have high (>75%) specificity.
   b. Serum T trigger level for symptoms ranges narrowly among individuals.
   c. Recurrence of symptoms is highly reproducible for each individual's serum T levels, with interruption of therapy.
   d. Signs and symptoms of hypogonadism are specific. Biochemical support is desirable but not mandatory.
   e. Sarcopenia and osteopenia/osteoporosis are fundamental elements for the diagnosis of the condition.
4. Which of the following biochemical assays best reflects tissue available testosterone?
   a. Total testosterone
   b. Free T by direct radioimmune assay using a T analog with low affinity for SHBG
   c. Free testosterone by equilibrium dialysis
   d. Free androgen index
   e. Salivary T
5. Which of the following statements is correct?
   a. Intraindividual variations in serum T levels are insignificant. Repeat measurements for diagnosis, therefore, are not necessary.
   b. Intraindividual variations in serum T levels are less apparent with assays for bioavailable T.
   c. In older men (> 65 years) borderline levels of T with normal gonadotropins rule out the diagnosis of hypogonadism.
   d. Repeatedly borderline serum T levels in the presence of symptomatic Late-onset hypogonadism (LOH) justifies a trial of T supplementation.
   e. Repeatedly borderline serum total T levels in the presence of symptomatic LOH is an indication for ordering a direct RIA of free T using a T analog assay with low affinity for SHBG.
6. Alterations in other hormones, besides sex steroids, occur with aging. Which of the following is not true?
   a. Growth hormone decreases at a rate similar to T.
   b. Melatonin production by the pineal gland decreases with aging.
   c. Prolactin production is not affected by aging.
   d. Leptin increases with aging and more so in the presence of hypogonadism.
   e. SHBG decreases in healthy aging.
7. Which of the following is not a contraindication for T therapy in males?
   a. Breast cancer
   b. Gynecomastia
   c. Angina pectoris
   d. Heart failure
   e. Polycythemia
8. The safety and efficacy of T therapy are not conclusively established. Which of the following is not a recommendation by the Institute of Medicine Committee on Testosterone and Aging?
   a. Focus on populations most likely to benefit
   b. Use T for treatment, not for prevention, of disease
   c. Focus on clinical outcomes with preliminary evidence of benefit
   d. Begin with short-term safety trials
   e. Conduct long-term studies only if short-term efficacy is established

9. A 68-year-old type-2 diabetic, hypertensive man presents with low libido, poor quality erections, and low energy but no depression. His medications include insulin, gemfibrozil, enalapril, and metoclopramide. Examination shows weak dorsalis pedis, moderate muscle wasting, and soft testes. Prostate and penis were normal. Biochemistry: HbA1c: 13% (n = 4 to 6); PSA: 0.8 ng/L (n < 4); total T: 210 ng/dL (n = 300 to 800); prolactin: 60 ng/mL (n < 20). Your next step is:
   a. Measure free T by direct RIA.
   b. Repeat prolactin assessment.
   c. Order MRI of the pituitary.
   d. Initiate T replacement therapy.
   e. Initiate treatment with cabergoline or bromocriptine.

10. A 67-year-old man presents with a history of radical retropubic prostatectomy (RRP) for a Gleason sum 7 adenocarcinoma of the prostate, 6 years previously. He complains of fatigue and markedly decreased sexual desire and quality of erections. PSA: < 0.1; bioavailable T: 1.6 nmL/L (2 to 9); LH: 6.7 (<18). Repeat bioavailable T: 1.4 nmL/L. You would:
   a. not consider him a candidate for supplemental T.
   b. wait for 4 more years (10 since RRP) to consider supplemental T.
   c. consider administration of a weak androgen such as DHEA.
   d. inform him of the risks and, with his consent, administer T.
   e. inform him of the risks and advise him against T therapy.

ANSWERS

1. **e. more than 300,000.** The incidence is 500,000 new cases per year. Traditionally, the prevalence of hypogonadism in the aging male was inferred from population projections. Recently, the Massachusetts Male Aging Study reported a crude incidence of 12.3 per 1000 person-years, leading to a prevalence of 481,000 new cases per year.

2. **a. T is produced by the Leydig cells under the control of LH only.** LH modulates most of the biosynthesis of T by the Leydig cells. However, neural influences from the paraventricular nucleus of the hypothalamus and gherelin actively regulate Leydig cell activity. Small amounts of androgens are produced in the brain. In some tissues such as the prostate, T bound to SHBG can activate SHBG receptors and produce effects within the cell (see Fig. 27-1).

3. **c. Recurrence of symptoms is highly reproducible for each individual's serum T levels, with interruption of therapy.** The sensitivity of the screening questionnaires is high (~80%), but their specificity is low (<50%). There is a wide interindividual variation for the T level, triggering specific symptoms of hypogonadism (probably depending on the number of CAG repeats in the androgen receptor). However, after an adequate response to treatment, discontinuation of T administration triggers symptoms at highly reproducible T levels in each individual. Manifestations of hypogonadism are not specific and are seen in other conditions (healthy aging, depression, hypothyroidism). Neither the clinical picture nor the biochemical assays individually are sufficient for diagnosis and management of late-onset hypogonadism (LOH) (see Fig. 27-2 and Table 27-3).

4. **c. Free testosterone by equilibrium dialysis.** Total T is usually sufficient for the initial diagnosis. It may be misleading in conditions associated with an elevation in SHBG levels (healthy aging, hyperthyroidism, obesity). RIA for free T is imprecise and should never be ordered. The most accurate test in this situation is the free T by equilibrium dialysis or by centrifugal ultrafiltration. These tests are expensive and cumbersome. Free androgen index is also inadequate, and the value of salivary T has not been definitively established. Calculated free and bioavailable T are accurate and simpler alternatives (see Table 27-4).

5. **d. Repeatedly borderline serum T levels in the presence of symptomatic LOH justifies a trial of T supplementation.** Longitudinal studies have shown a significant variation in serum T levels over short periods, in the same individuals with any assays and specifically with measurement of bioavailable T. A repeat measurement is, therefore, advisable. The hypothalamus and the pituitary age together with the gonads. The feedback mechanisms are usually blunted in the elderly, and a decrease in number and function of Leydig cells is infrequently associated with elevation of gonadotropins. In the presence of florid clinical manifestations of hypogonadism but a questionable biochemistry, a short (3 month) trial of T supplementation is justified. The assay that should not be used is a commonly available and frequently ordered one: direct RIA of free T using a labeled T analog with low affinity for SHBG. It has poor accuracy and most closely reflects the measurement of total T (see Fig. 27-3).

6. **e. SHBG decreases in healthy aging.** DHEA, GH, melatonin, and thyroxin decrease with aging; and their deficiency shares many of the manifestations of hypogonadism. Prolactin is not particularly affected by the aging process, but hyperprolactinemia can be induced by medications. SHBG increases with several situations, including healthy aging; a misdiagnosis of hypogonadism may occur when only total T is measured. SHBG-bound T is largely inaccessible to tissues, although there are some notable exceptions, such as the prostate (see Table 27-5).

7. **c. Angina pectoris.** Breast cancer growth is stimulated by estrogen (from peripheral conversion/aromatization of T). The same mechanism is considered responsible for the development of gynecomastia during androgen therapy. T has been shown to be a coronary and peripheral vasodilator (through nongenomic mechanisms). Although rare, fluid retention may occur in the elderly; therefore, the administration of T should be regarded with caution. Modest increases in red blood cell mass are common after T therapy. Occasionally, polycythemia may be significant, particularly in the elderly.

8. **d. Begin with short-term safety trials.** The IOM report includes an extensive review of the literature and a set of recommendations for future research in T therapy. The panel believed that efficacy of T treatment has not yet been demonstrated and recommended, therefore, that efficacy must be established first by clinical trials. Only if efficacy is demonstrated should long-term safety trials similar to the Women's Health Initiative be conducted (see Table 27-7).

9. **d. Initiate T replacement therapy.** The combination of symptoms associated with small, soft testes and a marked decrease in total T levels constitutes a clear indication for T supplementation. There is recent but increasing evidence that insulin resistance is associated with a decrease in Leydig cell T secretion. Initiation of treatment based on the clinical picture and clearly decreased T levels is justified but prudence dictates, at least, confirmation the initial result. Although bioavailable T is a more accurate reflection of androgenicity than total T, in this particular case it is not necessary: bioavailable T testing is more expensive and cumbersome to perform. Assessment of the pituitary is generally recommended but, at this man's age, it would not be surprising to find normal LH levels despite profound hypogonadism. The moderate prolactin elevation is,

most likely drug induced (metoclopramide), and the drug should be discontinued (see Table 27-4 and Fig. 27-3).

10. **d. inform him of the risks and, with his consent, administer T.** T administration is an absolute contraindication in the presence of prostate cancer, but there is no evidence that this patient is harboring it. Recommendations regarding T supplementation in this situation are based on limited and, mostly, anecdotal information. However, when there is profound symptomatic late onset hypogonadism testosterone deficiency (SLOH) with significant interference in the quality of life, a trial of T treatment may be justified. Good clinical judgment plays an important role in a situation like this. If T treatment is initiated, the initial follow-up must be frequent and particularly careful. An elevation of the PSA is a clear indication that prostate cells are present and T administration should then be discontinued. Most likely this will lead to a return of the PSA to the pretreatment levels. Familiarity with the Consensus Recommendations on the use of supplemental T is strongly advised.

28

Urologic Management of Women with Sexual Health Concerns

IRWIN GOLDSTEIN

QUESTIONS

1. The urologist is in a unique position to provide sexual health care delivery to women with sexual heath concerns. Which is most correct?
   a. Urologists have contributed significantly to the basic scientific knowledge and contemporary management strategies of men's sexual health care.
   b. Urologists provide urologic health care to women.
   c. Urologists are in a unique position to understand the specialized female pelvic floor anatomy and physiology.
   d. Urologists are in a unique position to understand the effects of pharmacology and surgical treatments on the bladder and urethra and that female peripheral sexual organs are an essential component of the pelvic floor.
   e. All of the above.
2. Concerning the classification and epidemiology of women's sexual dysfunctions, which of the following is correct?
   a. Discussions concerning the appropriateness of the definitions of the various women's sexual disorders are ongoing at international consensus meetings.
   b. Classification of women's sexual disorders includes desire disorder, arousal disorder, orgasmic disorder, and sexual pain disorder.
   c. Women's sexual arousal disorders includes subjective sexual arousal disorder, genital sexual arousal disorder, combined genital and subjective arousal disorder, and persistent sexual arousal disorder.
   d. Based on population studies, for any sexual problems among adult women, the prevalence is estimated at 43%.
   e. All of the above.
3. History taking for women with sexual dysfunction is crucial because it establishes the diagnostic impressions and forms the basis of search on physical examination. The following is most correct:
   a. History taking should focus on the sexual aspects of the problem.
   b. History taking should focus on the medications used by the patient, the medical conditions of the patient, and the urologic surgeries the patient underwent.
   c. History taking should focus on the sexual, medical, and psychosocial aspects so that the many physical and psychological factors that often contribute to the sexual health difficulty can be characterized.
   d. History taking should focus on the social factors, past sexual beliefs, past sexual abuse and trauma, emotional concerns, and interpersonal relationship matters.
   e. History taking is best achieved by administering validated, reliable, standardized self-rated questionnaires to assist the identification of the presence or absence of a sexual problem.
4. The urologist should perform a physical examination under which of the following circumstances in a woman with a sexual health concern?
   a. If a woman with a sexual health concern is younger than age 50, no physical examination is required.
   b. If a woman with a sexual health concern has sexual pain, do not perform an examination because that may make the woman uncomfortable.
   c. Do not perform the physical examination on the first visit because this may cause embarrassment to a woman with a sexual health concern.
   d. A focused peripheral genital examination is recommended in all women with sexual health concerns.
   e. A focused peripheral genital examination is recommended in women with sexual health concerns for complaints of dyspareunia, vaginismus, genital arousal disorder and combined arousal disorder, orgasmic disorder, pelvic trauma history, and any disorder affecting genital health.

5. Blood testing is an integral part of the diagnostic evaluation of a woman with a sexual health concern. What is the most correct statement?
   a. The "gold standard" is total testosterone taken between 8:00 and 10:00 AM between day 8 and day 20 of the cycle.
   b. Androgen values may be assessed using dehydroepiandrosterone sulfate, androstenedione, and dihydrotestosterone.
   c. Thyroid function may be assessed by measurement of thyroid-stimulating hormone.
   d. Estrogen values may be assessed by estrone and progesterone.
   e. There is no consensus on recommended routine laboratory tests for evaluation of women's sexual health concerns.

6. Premenopausal women on oral contraceptive pills may have which of the following blood test abnormalities?
   a. LH and FSH are low, sex hormone–binding globulin is high, total and free testosterone are low.
   b. LH and FSH are high, sex hormone–binding globulin is low, total and free testosterone are low.
   c. LH and FSH are high, sex hormone–binding globulin is high, total and free testosterone are high.
   d. LH and FSH are low, sex hormone–binding globulin is low, total and free testosterone are low.
   e. LH and FSH are low, sex hormone–binding globulin is high, total and free testosterone are high.

7. Premenopausal women on nonhormonal mechanical barrier methods for contraception (including the intrauterine device) may have which of the following blood test abnormalities?
   a. LH and FSH are low, sex hormone–binding globulin is high, total and free testosterone are low.
   b. LH and FSH are high, sex hormone–binding globulin is low, total and free testosterone are low.
   c. LH and FSH are high, sex hormone–binding globulin is high, total and free testosterone are high.
   d. LH and FSH are low, sex hormone–binding globulin is low, total and free testosterone are low.
   e. No hormonal abnormalities are expected.

8. Premenopausal women on long-term LH-RH agonist therapy (e.g., leuprolide acetate) to shrink uterine fibroids may have which of the following blood test abnormalities?
   a. LH and FSH are low, total testosterone is low, estradiol is high.
   b. LH and FSH are high, total testosterone is low, estradiol is low.
   c. LH and FSH are high, total testosterone are high, estradiol is high.
   d. LH and FSH are low, total testosterone is high, estradiol is low.
   e. LH and FSH are low, total testosterone is low, estradiol is low.

9. Premenopausal women who undergo hysterectomy and bilateral salpingo-oophorectomy for uterine fibroids may have which of the following postoperative blood test abnormalities?
   a. LH and FSH are low, total testosterone is low, estradiol is high.
   b. LH and FSH are high, total testosterone is low, estradiol is low.
   c. LH and FSH are high, total testosterone are high, estradiol is high.
   d. LH and FSH are low, total testosterone is high, estradiol is low.
   e. LH and FSH are low, total testosterone is low, estradiol is low.

10. Postmenopausal women on exogenous hormone replacement therapy with conjugated estrogens/medroxyprogesterone acetate tablets (Prempro) may have which of the following blood test abnormalities?
    a. LH and FSH are low, sex hormone–binding globulin is high, total and free testosterone are low.
    b. LH and FSH are high, sex hormone–binding globulin is low, total and free testosterone are low.
    c. LH and FSH are high, sex hormone–binding globulin is high, total and free testosterone are low.
    d. LH and FSH are low, sex hormone–binding globulin is low, total and free testosterone are low.
    e. LH and FSH are low, sex hormone–binding globulin is high, total and free testosterone are high.

11. Postmenopausal women on selective estrogen receptor modulator (SERM) therapy with tamoxifen for breast cancer may have which of the following blood test abnormalities:
    a. LH and FSH are low, sex hormone–binding globulin is high, total and free testosterone are low.
    b. LH and FSH are high, sex hormone–binding globulin is low, total and free testosterone are low.
    c. LH and FSH are high, sex hormone–binding globulin is high, total and free testosterone are low.
    d. LH and FSH are low, sex hormone–binding globulin is low, total and free testosterone are low.
    e. LH and FSH are low, sex hormone–binding globulin is high, total and free testosterone are high.

12. Premenopausal women who have received aggressive chemotherapy for cancer treatment and subsequently developed drug-induced menopause may have which of the following blood test abnormalities?
    a. LH and FSH are low, total testosterone is low, estradiol is high.
    b. LH and FSH are high, total testosterone is low, estradiol is low.
    c. LH and FSH are high, total testosterone is high, estradiol is high.
    d. LH and FSH are low, total testosterone is high, estradiol is low.
    e. LH and FSH are low, total testosterone is low, estradiol is low.

13. Postmenopausal women who do not take hormone therapy may have a problem with vaginal atrophy. Which of the following is TRUE about estrogens in menopause?
    a. All women in menopause will have vaginal atrophy.
    b. All women in menopause will have cessation of ovarian estradiol production.
    c. Estrogen continues to be synthesized in the periphery through conversion of androstenedione to estrone and testosterone to estradiol, but the amount of estradiol synthesized depends, in part, on the enzymatic activity of desmolase.
    d. Estrogen continues to be synthesized in the periphery through conversion of androstenedione to estrone and testosterone to estradiol, but the amount of estradiol synthesized depends, in part, on the enzymatic activity of 17-20 lyase.
    e. Diminished estrogen synthesis in the vagina, vulva, vestibule, labia, and urethra in menopause renders these genital tissues highly susceptible to atrophy.

14. The urologist may consider use of a dopamine agonist in a woman with sexual health concerns. Which is the most correct?
    a. There are no randomized placebo-controlled data supporting the use of dopamine agonists in women with sexual health concerns.
    b. Women with sexual pain disorders appear to benefit the most by dopamine agonists.
    c. Women with aversion disorders appear to benefit the most by dopamine agonists.
    d. Women with desire and orgasmic disorders appear to benefit the most by dopamine agonists.
    e. Side effects of dopamine agonists include headache, flushing, dyspepsia, and rhinitis.
15. The urologist may consider use of the dopamine agonist cabergoline in a woman with sexual health concerns (low libido). Which is the most correct?
    a. Cabergoline increases dopamine by decreasing thyroid stimulating hormone.
    b. Cabergoline increases dopamine by decreasing central serotonin.
    c. Cabergoline increases dopamine by decreasing oxytocin.
    d. Cabergoline increases dopamine by decreasing prolactin.
    e. Cabergoline increases dopamine by decreasing central nitric oxide.
16. The urologist may consider use of a local or systemic vasodilator in a woman with sexual dysfunction under what circumstances?
    a. There are no randomized placebo-controlled data supporting the use of local or systemic vasodilators in women with sexual health concerns.
    b. Women with sexual pain disorders appear to benefit the most by local or systemic vasodilators.
    c. Women with desire disorders appear to benefit the most by local or systemic vasodilators.
    d. Women with arousal and orgasmic disorders and a normal sex steroid hormonal milieu appear to benefit the most by local or systemic vasodilators.
    e. Side effects of local or systemic vasodilators include nausea, syncope, weight loss, and back pain.
17. Women with sexual pain disorders may be managed effectively by nonsurgical, nonpsychologic interventions. Evidence exists for which of the following therapies as beneficial for women with sexual pain disorders?
    a. Estradiol, progesterone, testosterone
    b. Clobetasol
    c. Physical therapy
    d. Amitriptyline and/or gabapentin
    e. All of the above
18. The urologist may consider surgical intervention when conservative therapies are not effective. Which of the following is TRUE concerning surgical management of sexual pain disorders?
    a. Surgery for vulvar vestibulitis syndrome is based on the hypothesis that the pathophysiology is associated with inflamed, irritated, and hypersensitive vestibular glandular tissue with related increased nerve density in the vestibular mucosa and that surgical success is based on excision of this abnormal glandular and nerve tissue in the vestibule.
    b. Surgery for vulvar vestibulitis syndrome is tailored to the woman's needs and symptoms with sexual pain needs and may consist of complete vulvar vestibulectomy, modified vulvar vestibulectomy or vestibuloplasty—excision of vestibular adenitis.
    c. To reduce complications such as hematoma, wound dehiscence, and vaginal stenosis during surgery for vulvar vestibulitis syndrome, the vaginal advancement flap should be anchored by multiple subcutaneous mattress sutures placed in an anteroposterior direction and should be approximated to the perineum with interrupted sutures.
    d. A dorsal slit procedure of the phimotic prepuce may be indicated to relieve the woman of the closed compartment perpetuating the recurrent fungal clitoral glans infection.
    e. All of the above.

ANSWERS

1. **e. All of the above.** For all these above reasons, the current situation, in which urologists provide sexual health care almost virtually, exclusively to a single gender, is likely only temporary. It would be probable that many academic urology departments will soon have trained faculty members to provide safe and effective, evidence-based sexual health care for women as well as for men.
2. **e. All of the above.** Measurements and inventories used to assess and classify women's sexual problems have varied as new information becomes available. The take-home message is that women's sexual health problems are common and their understanding is dynamic.
3. **c. History taking should focus on the sexual, medical, and psychosocial aspects so that the many physical and psychological factors that often contribute to the sexual health difficulty can be characterized.** The cornerstone of the physical-based diagnosis of women with sexual dysfunction is a detailed history, performed by the biologic-focused health care professional, engaging sexual, medical, and psychosocial aspects. In this fashion, the many physical and psychological factors that often contribute to the sexual health difficulty can be characterized. The more information that is available, the better the opportunity to provide maximal sexual health care.
4. **e. A focused peripheral genital examination is recommended in women with sexual health concerns for complaints of dyspareunia, vaginismus, genital arousal disorder and combined arousal disorder, orgasmic disorder, pelvic trauma history, and any disorder affecting genital health.** The genital-focused examination has a personal character that demands that a rational explanation exist for its inclusion in the diagnostic process. A consensus was reached on the above list of women's sexual health problems at a recent international sexual medicine meeting as being consistent with a "rational explanation for inclusion of the genital physical examination in the diagnostic process."
5. **e. There is no consensus on recommended routine laboratory tests for evaluation of women's sexual health concerns.** For multiple reasons, such as lack of agreement as to what are the normal values of sex steroid hormones, what are the most important sex steroids, that sex steroid hormone actions are quite complex and involve critical enzymes and critical hormone receptors that determine tissue exposure, tissue sensitivity, and tissue responsiveness independent of blood tests values—there is no current consensus on recommended routine laboratory tests for evaluation of women's sexual health concerns.

6. **a. LH and FSH are low, sex hormone–binding globulin is high, total and free testosterone are low.** Oral contraceptives suppress ovarian function, including ovarian androgen synthesis as well as inducing hepatic synthesis of sex hormone–binding globulin.
7. **e. No hormonal abnormalities are expected.** Nonhormonal mechanical barrier contraceptive methods such as the intrauterine device or the condom have no effect on the women's sex steroid levels.
8. **e. LH and FSH are low, total testosterone is low, estradiol is low.** Chronic LH-RH agonist therapy suppresses ovarian function, including ovarian synthesis of androgens and estrogens.
9. **b. LH and FSH are high, total testosterone is low, estradiol is low.** Women who undergo surgical menopause have elevated gonadotropins and diminished values of both androgen and estrogen sex steroids.
10. **c. LH and FSH are high, sex hormone–binding globulin is high, total and free testosterone are low.** Postmenopausal women on synthetic estrogen and synthetic progesterone hormone therapy have high levels of gonadotropins and high levels of sex hormone–binding globulin.
11. **c. LH and FSH are high, sex hormone–binding globulin is high, total and free testosterone are low.** Postmenopausal women on selective estrogen receptor modulator (SERM) therapy with tamoxifen for breast cancer have high levels of gonadotropins and high levels of sex steroid–binding globulin.
12. **b. LH and FSH are high, total testosterone is low, estradiol is low.** Premenopausal women who develop drug-induced menopause have high levels of gonadotropins with suppressed levels of androgens and estrogens.
13. **b. All women in menopause will have cessation of ovarian estradiol production.** The definition of menopause engages the concept that ovarian estrogen levels cease in all women who are in menopause.
14. **d. Women with desire and orgasmic disorders appear to benefit the most by dopamine agonists.** Dopamine appears involved as a central neurotransmitter in the hypothalamus in women's sexual interest and orgasm.
15. **d. Cabergoline increases dopamine by decreasing prolactin.** Cabergoline is a long-acting dopamine agonist that is indicated for the treatment of hyperprolactinemia.
16. **d. Women with arousal and orgasmic disorders and a normal sex steroid hormonal milieu appear to benefit the most by local or systemic vasodilators.** Double-blind, placebo-controlled data reveal that vasodilators improve women's sexual arousal and orgasm when sex steroid hormone values are normal.
17. **e. All of the above.** Sexual pain disorders secondary to dermatologic conditions may be managed by ultrapotent steroids, those secondary to pelvic floor spasm may be managed by physical therapy, those secondary to vaginal atrophy may be managed by systemic estrogens (and systemic progesterone in case of an intact uterus), those secondary to oral contraceptive pill-induced dyspareunia may be managed by androgens, and those secondary to vulvodynia may be managed by pain medications.
18. **e. All of the above.** All these principles are involved in the surgical management of women with sexual pain disorders.

SECTION VII

MALE GENITALIA

29

Neoplasms of the Testis

JEROME P. RICHIE • GRAEME S. STEELE

QUESTIONS

1. A young man presents with a right testicular mass after having undergone bilateral orchiopexy as a child. He then undergoes right inguinal orchiectomy and left testicular biopsy. The testicular mass is a mixed nonseminomatous germ cell tumor (NSGCT) containing embryonal carcinoma with vascular invasion—clinical stage T2N0M0. Chest radiograph and abdominal CT were normal. Biopsy of the left testis reveals intratubular germ cell neoplasia (carcinoma in situ). Appropriate management of this patient includes which of the following?
   a. Three cycles of chemotherapy (BEP) and left radical inguinal orchiectomy
   b. Four cycles of chemotherapy (EP) with another transscrotal biopsy of the left testis in 6 months
   c. Left radical inguinal orchiectomy, androgen replacement therapy, and surveillance protocol for mixed germ cell tumors
   d. Modified (template) right-sided retroperitoneal lymph node dissection (RPLND)
   e. Modified (template) right-sided RPLND with low-dose external beam radiotherapy to the left testis
2. A young man presents with a 7-cm left testicular tumor; the serum α-fetoprotein (AFP) value is elevated (220 ng/mL); the clinical stage of disease is T2N1M0S1. He undergoes radical inguinal orchiectomy. Pathologic study reveals an anaplastic seminoma with vascular invasion. The serum AFP value normalizes after orchiectomy. Further management of this patient should include which of the following?
   a. Low-dose external-beam radiation therapy to abdominal and pelvic lymph nodes
   b. Low-dose external-beam radiation therapy to abdominal, pelvic, and mediastinal lymph nodes
   c. Bilateral RPLND with adjuvant radiotherapy
   d. Bilateral RPLND
   e. Two cycles of chemotherapy (BEP)
3. A young man who lost his right testis at a younger age because of torsion undergoes left radical inguinal orchiectomy for a testis tumor. Pathology reports a 3-cm mixed NSGCT, no vascular invasion, and embryonal component 10%. Serum tumor markers reveal persistently elevated β-human chorionic gonadotropin (βHCG) levels. The clinical stage is T1N0M0. What is the best management of this tumor?
   a. Adjuvant cisplatin-based chemotherapy
   b. Bilateral RPLND with excision of the left spermatic cord
   c. Modified left RPLND with excision of both right and left spermatic cords
   d. Androgen replacement therapy and surveillance protocol for germ cell tumor if the serum βHCG level normalizes
   e. Androgen replacement therapy and low-dose external-beam radiation therapy to abdominal and pelvic lymph nodes
4. In the setting of pathologic stage IIB, mixed NSGCT after bilateral RPLND adjuvant cisplatin-based chemotherapy should be administered to which group of patients?
   a. All patients regardless of the pathologic stage of disease
   b. Only those patients with tumor recurrence outside the retroperitoneum
   c. Patients with microscopic evidence of disease in two lymph nodes
   d. Patients with more than six positive lymph nodes
   e. Any patient with a single involved retroperitoneal lymph node measuring 1 cm in diameter

5. A patient presents with a 6-cm right-sided testicular tumor and abdominal discomfort. He undergoes right radical inguinal orchiectomy; pathologic study reveals mixed germ cell tumor. Serum tumor markers are elevated (AFP, 800 ng/mL; βHCG, 2500 mIU/mL). Abdominal CT reveals a 10-cm retroperitoneal mass. The patient undergoes cisplatin-based chemotherapy with resultant 75% resolution of the retroperitoneal mass and normalization of serum tumor markers. What is the best management at this stage?
   a. Observation with physical examinations every 4 months, serum tumor markers, chest radiograph, and abdominal CT
   b. Fine-needle aspiration of the residual retroperitoneal mass followed by salvage radiotherapy for persistent germ cell tumor
   c. Abdominal exploration, tumorectomy, and bilateral RPLND
   d. Abdominal exploration and tumorectomy
   e. Ifosfamide-based salvage chemotherapy
6. A young man undergoes cisplatin-based chemotherapy for a mixed germ cell tumor, with complete response. Two years later he presents with shortness of breath; recurrent disease is detected in both the retroperitoneum and the mediastinum. He then undergoes high-dose cisplatin-based chemotherapy with 80% resolution of all disease. Abdominal and thoracic exploration is planned. Which of the following statements is correct?
   a. The incidence of viable tumor in a partially resolved mass after salvage chemotherapy is lower than it is after primary adjuvant chemotherapy.
   b. During abdominal exploration, frozen section analysis of the residual mass detects only fibrous tissue and necrosis; thoracic exploration can therefore safely be omitted.
   c. Laparoscopic surgery in this scenario has clearly been shown to be of both diagnostic and therapeutic benefit.
   d. External-beam radiation therapy is appropriate after surgical exploration if teratoma is detected.
   e. Neither abdominal nor thoracic exploration is warranted in this patient.
7. A 45-year-old man is found to have a well-delineated 4-cm retroperitoneal mass after cisplatin-based chemotherapy for clinical stage III seminoma. Which of the following statements is correct?
   a. This mass is likely unresectable and therefore best left alone.
   b. Only diffuse desmoplastic retroperitoneal masses should be resected after chemotherapy in patients with advanced seminoma.
   c. Salvage chemotherapy is the best option at this stage.
   d. Surgical resection with bilateral RPLND is the best management at this stage.
   e. There is no possibility that this mass contains embryonal carcinoma.
8. A 72-year-old man with benign prostatic hyperplasia and bothersome symptoms of bladder outlet obstruction presents with a 6-cm painless right-sided testicular mass with an associated hydrocele confirmed by scrotal ultrasonography. Which of the following statements is TRUE?
   a. This mass is likely a spermatocytic seminoma and should therefore be left alone.
   b. The hydrocele should be aspirated and sclerosed with tetracycline and the fluid sent for cytologic study.
   c. Radical inguinal orchiectomy is indicated to exclude the possibility of a hematologic malignancy.
   d. The testicular mass is most likely metastatic disease from either lung or prostate cancer.
   e. Despite the ultrasonographic findings, chronic epididymitis is the most likely cause of this clinical picture.
9. A young adult man presents with a 7-cm right testicular tumor that is found to be invading the scrotal wall and epididymis on that side. Possible sites of lymph node involvement in this patient include which of the following lymph nodes?
   a. Inguinal
   b. Pelvic
   c. Interaortocaval
   d. Left para-aortic
   e. All of the above
10. The incidence of syncytiotrophoblastic elements in seminoma corresponds to which of the following?
    a. The degree of tumor anaplasia
    b. The βHCG production
    c. The presence of testicular lymphoma
    d. The presence and extent of retroperitoneal metastases
    e. The AFP production by the tumor
11. With respect to anaplastic seminoma, which of the following statements is FALSE?
    a. Morphologically, histiocytic lymphoma and embryonal carcinoma may closely resemble anaplastic seminoma.
    b. Anaplastic seminomas are more aggressive than spermatocytic seminomas.
    c. Anaplastic seminomas have an increased rate of metastatic spread compared with classic seminomas.
    d. Anaplastic seminomas are more likely to elaborate βHCG than are classic seminomas.
    e. Anaplastic seminomas have greater mitotic activity than do spermatocytic seminomas.
12. With respect to choriocarcinoma, which of the following statements is FALSE?
    a. Patients with pure choriocarcinoma may present with evidence of advanced distant metastasis.
    b. Choriocarcinomas may be associated with very elevated serum βHCG values.
    c. Choriocarcinomas are best managed by RPLND.
    d. Choriocarcinomas occur in a younger adult age group.
    e. Choriocarcinomas rarely occur in African males.
13. Which of the following choices regarding mixed germ cell tumors is correct?
    a. Mixed germ cell tumors represent approximately 15% of NSGCTs.
    b. The most frequent combination is seminoma and embryonal cell carcinoma.
    c. Mixed germ cell tumors represent approximately 15% of germ cell tumors.
    d. Mixed germ cell tumors can sometimes be classified as seminomas.
    e. The most frequent combination is embryonal carcinoma, yolk sac tumor, teratoma, and syncytiotrophoblasts.
14. Which of the following choices regarding carcinoma in situ (CIS; intratubular germ cell neoplasia) of the testis is FALSE?
    a. Incidence of CIS in the male population is 0.8%.
    b. Prevalence of CIS in the contralateral testis in a patient with germ cell tumor is 5%.
    c. Testicular CIS develops from fetal gonocytes.
    d. Tumor markers for CIS have not been described.
    e. CIS is not evenly distributed throughout the testis, making diagnosis with a single biopsy difficult.

15. With respect to the epidemiology of testicular tumors, which of the following statements is FALSE?
   a. The age-adjusted incidence in Denmark rose from 3.4 to 6.4 per 100,000 between 1945 and 1970.
   b. Overall, the highest incidence is noted in young adults, which makes these neoplasms the most common solid tumors of men between 20 and 34 years of age.
   c. Spermatocytic seminoma occurs most often in patients between the ages of 45 and 55 years.
   d. The incidence of testicular tumors in black African men is higher than that among African-American men.
   e. Two to 3 percent of testicular tumors are bilateral.

16. With respect to the lymphatic drainage of the testis, which one of the following statements is TRUE?
   a. The primary drainage of the right testis is usually located within the group of lymph nodes in the left para-aortic region.
   b. The spermatic cord contains four to eight lymphatic channels that traverse the inguinal canal and peritoneal space.
   c. The spermatic vessels cross dorsal to the ureter, whereas the testicular lymphatics cross ventrally.
   d. The lymphatic drainage has been shown to cross over from right to left, and therefore cross-metastases occur more commonly in patients with right-sided tumors.
   e. The suprahilar lymph node spread is invariable in stage N1 disease.

17. What is the most common clinical symptom or sign in a young adult man with a germ cell tumor of the testis?
   a. Testicular pain
   b. Testicular swelling on the side of the tumor
   c. Reactive hydrocele, which transilluminates in a darkened room
   d. Bilateral gynecomastia
   e. Chronic cough with hemoptysis

18. With respect to ultrasonography of the testis, which of the following statements is FALSE?
   a. Any hypoechoic area within the tunica albuginea is markedly suspicious for testicular cancer.
   b. Ultrasonography avoids the delay in diagnosis previously attributed to confusion with epididymitis.
   c. Intrascrotal fluid collections make adequate visualization of the testis impossible.
   d. In patients with palpably normal genitalia and evidence of extragonadal germ cell malignancy, sonography has been reported to be successful in identifying occult testicular neoplasms.
   e. Transscrotal ultrasonography has the ability to detect testicular microlithiasis.

19. With respect to clinical staging of germ cell tumors of the testis, which of the following statements is FALSE?
   a. Modern staging techniques have reduced the false-negative staging error in clinical stage T1N0M0 to approximately 20%.
   b. Ten to 15 percent of patients with clinical stage T1N0M0 seminoma harbor occult retroperitoneal metastases.
   c. Five percent of patients with clinical stage 1 germ cell tumors harbor occult disease in extranodal sites.
   d. Abdominal and pelvic MRI have a significant advantage over CT with respect to diagnosing micrometastatic disease.
   e. Spermatic cord involvement increases the likelihood of metastatic disease.

20. Which of the following statements concerning tumor markers in germ cell tumors is FALSE?
   a. Serum AFP elevations do not occur in pure seminomas.
   b. Metabolic half-life of AFP is between 5 and 7 days.
   c. Syncytiotrophoblastic cells are responsible for the production of βHCG.
   d. Five to 10 percent of seminoma patients have detectable levels of βHCG.
   e. Placental alkaline phosphatase (PLAP) is elevated in 40% of patients with testicular CIS.

21. What percentage of patients with advanced NSGCTs have normal tumor markers?
   a. 2%
   b. 5%
   c. 10%
   d. 20%
   e. 30%

22. Approximately what percentage of patients presenting with seminoma have disease confined to the testis?
   a. 35%
   b. 55%
   c. 75%
   d. 95%
   e. 99%

23. The overall cure rate for all stages of seminoma approximates what percentage?
   a. 50%
   b. 60%
   c. 70%
   d. 80%
   e. 90%

24. Management options for clinical stage I seminoma after radical inguinal orchiectomy include all of the following EXCEPT:
   a. surveillance protocol.
   b. para-aortic and pelvic radiotherapy.
   c. modified RPLND.
   d. single-agent chemotherapy.
   e. para-aortic radiotherapy.

25. Reliable prognostic factors for pure seminoma include all the following EXCEPT:
   a. tumor size.
   b. lymphatic invasion.
   c. serum βHCG level.
   d. patient's age.
   e. vascular invasion.

26. The 5-year disease-free survival rate for patients with clinical stage T1N2M0 seminoma approximates what percentage?
   a. 50%
   b. 60%
   c. 70%
   d. 80%
   e. 90%

27. Approximately what percentage of patients with clinical stage T1N3M0 seminoma treated with radiotherapy alone will develop metastatic disease?
   a. 50%
   b. 60%
   c. 70%
   d. 80%
   e. 90%

28. In patients with pure seminoma, combination cisplatin-based chemotherapy is the most appropriate treatment for which of the following clinical stages?
    a. T1N0M0
    b. T2N0M0
    c. T1N2M0
    d. T1N3M0
    e. T2N1M0

29. In NSGCTs, all the following prognostic factors are used to determine risk of metastatic disease EXCEPT:
    a. T stage.
    b. embryonal cell carcinoma (>40%).
    c. teratoma (>50%).
    d. vascular invasion.
    e. absence of yolk sac elements.

30. Surveillance in low-risk (absence of prognostic factors) NSGCT is appropriate in all of the following patients EXCEPT:
    a. a motivated and reliable patient.
    b. a patient with an allergy to radiographic contrast agents.
    c. a diabetic patient.
    d. a patient in whom tumor markers persist after orchiectomy.
    e. a patient who underwent scrotal orchiectomy.

31. A young adult male with clinical stage T1N2M0 NSGCT undergoes induction chemotherapy with near-resolution of a 5-cm left para-aortic mass. At this stage, what is the appropriate management?
    a. Salvage chemotherapy
    b. Tumorectomy and bilateral RPLND
    c. Modified RPLND
    d. Radiation therapy
    e. Surveillance

32. What is the incidence of viable germ cell elements in resected specimens after primary chemotherapy for NSGCT?
    a. 0% to 9%
    b. 10% to 19%
    c. 20% to 29%
    d. 30% to 39%
    e. 40% to 49%

33. The most common sites of origin of extragonadal tumors are all of the following EXCEPT:
    a. mediastinum.
    b. retroperitoneum.
    c. sacrococcygeal region.
    d. liver.
    e. pineal gland.

34. With respect to Leydig cell tumors, all the following statements are correct EXCEPT:
    a. Approximately 10% are malignant.
    b. Undescended testis is an important predisposing factor.
    c. Characteristic intracytoplasmic inclusion bodies (Reinke crystals) are often seen.
    d. No consistent reliable histologic features of malignancy exist.
    e. Clinical presentation may be confused with a virilizing type of adrenogenital syndrome.

35. Which of the following statements regarding patterns of spread of germ cell tumors is FALSE?
    a. Primary drainage of the right testis is usually located within the group of lymph nodes in the interaortocaval region at the level of the second vertebral body.
    b. Lymphatic drainage has not been shown to cross over from right to left.
    c. Suprahilar lymph node spread has been shown to be rare in stage N1 disease.
    d. Lymphatics of the epididymis drain primarily into the obturator lymph nodes.
    e. Distant failure rate despite surgical excision of negative retroperitoneal lymph nodes is approximately 5%.

36. Modified RPLND preserves fertility in most patients by sparing which of the following structures?
    a. Internal iliac arteries
    b. Genitofemoral nerve
    c. Postganglionic sympathetic nerve fibers
    d. Seminal vesicles
    e. Pelvic parasympathetic plexus

37. With respect to the International Germ Cell Classification of advanced disease, which of the following statements is FALSE?
    a. Response of poor-risk disease to chemotherapy is approximately 50%.
    b. Response of good-risk disease to chemotherapy is approximately 90%.
    c. Pretreatment tumor markers are an integral part of this classification.
    d. Pretreatment pulmonary metastases are an integral part of this classification.
    e. Early use of chemotherapy in poor-risk disease is advisable.

ANSWERS

1. **d. Modified (template) right-sided retroperitoneal lymph node dissection (RPLND).** The management of testicular CIS depends on a variety of factors such as patient age, whether the patient has bilateral or unilateral CIS, associated testicular atrophy, and the philosophy of the treating physician. In germ cell tumors, CIS of the contralateral testis is present in 5% of patients and with time probably evolves into invasive cancer in the majority of these patients. Although CIS can easily be cured by radiation therapy, this therapy may have undesirable side effects on both fertility and androgen production. Furthermore, the incidence of CIS in the general population is low and therefore screening programs are generally not recommended.

2. **d. Bilateral RPLND.** The potential advantages of RPLND in the treatment of testicular cancer stem from the fact that retroperitoneal deposits are usually the first and frequently the sole evidence of extragonadal spread. Such therapy is capable of eradicating resectable disease in the majority of patients with stage N1-2 tumors. Thorough excision of the retroperitoneal lymph nodes therefore remains the epitome or gold standard of staging. Although noninvasive staging techniques are somewhat accurate, 20% to 25% of patients with clinical stage T1-3N0M0 disease are understaged by all available modalities of nonsurgical staging. The cure rate for patients with pathologically confirmed stage I disease is roughly 95% with surgery alone. The 5% to 10% of patients who may experience relapse after negative

RPLND for low-stage disease have a high cure rate with chemotherapy.

3. **d. Androgen replacement therapy and surveillance protocol for germ cell tumor if the serum βHCG level normalizes.** There are nonmalignant causes of persistent elevated levels of both AFP and βHCG. Liver damage secondary to drugs (chemotherapy, anesthetics, or antiepileptics), viral hepatitis, and alcohol abuse may all lead to an elevated AFP level. Furthermore, nonmalignant causes of persistent βHCG elevations include hypogonadism and marijuana use. Clearly, every effort should be made to exclude all false-positive causes of tumor marker elevation before subjecting patients to adjuvant therapy.

4. **d. Patients with more than six positive lymph nodes.** In a review of 39 patients who underwent RPLND at the Brigham and Women's Hospital for pathologic stage T1-3N1-2M0 disease, with fewer than six positive nodes and no node larger than 2 cm, only 3 of 39 patients experienced relapse at a median follow-up of 3.5 years. Thus, for patients with minimal retroperitoneal disease, resected completely, careful follow-up is recommended. For patients with more extensive disease, adjuvant chemotherapy with two cycles can be initiated relatively shortly after RPLND and almost always prevents relapse.

5. **c. Abdominal exploration, tumorectomy, and bilateral RPLND.** RPLND after chemotherapy involves both resection of residual disease and full bilateral node dissection. In the best of hands, this procedure is associated with an 18% complication rate, which is contributed to by both the technically demanding nature of the surgery and other factors such as reduced pulmonary reserve due to bleomycin.

6. **b. During abdominal exploration, frozen section analysis of the residual mass detects only fibrous tissue and necrosis; thoracic exploration can therefore safely be omitted.** Herr showed that, at the time of RPLND, if frozen section analysis shows only necrosis, then surgical resection of residual masses followed by only limited RPLND is safe, as opposed to residual mass resection and complete RPLND, which is considered the standard of care. In addition, the histologic finding of necrosis plus fibrosis was shown to be strongly predictive of necrosis-fibrosis in patients with concomitant pulmonary disease; this information can then be used to avoid thoracic exploration in some patients.

7. **d. Surgical resection with bilateral RPLND is the best management at this stage.** Residual disease may be well delineated and distinct from surrounding structures and thus usually resectable. According to the Memorial Sloan-Kettering group, surgery is justifiable in this setting because these masses often represent residual seminoma.

8. **c. Radical inguinal orchiectomy is indicated to exclude the possibility of a hematologic malignancy.** Accounting for about 5% of all testis tumors, lymphomas constitute the most common secondary neoplasms of the testis and the most frequent of all testicular tumors in patients older than 50 years of age. The median age at occurrence is approximately 60 years. Primary lymphoma of the testis may occur in children; eight cases in patients ranging from 2 to 12 years of age were reviewed in one study.

9. **e. All of the above.** Involvement of the epididymis or cord may lead to pelvic and inguinal lymph node metastasis, whereas tumors confined to the testis proper usually spread to retroperitoneal nodes.

10. **b. The βHCG production.** Syncytiotrophoblastic elements occur in 10% to 15% of seminomas, and lymphocytic infiltration occurs in approximately 20%. The incidence of syncytiotrophoblastic elements corresponds to the frequency of βHCG production.

11. **a. Morphologically, histiocytic lymphoma and embryonal carcinoma may closely resemble anaplastic seminoma.**

12. **c. Choriocarcinomas are best managed by RPLND.** Choriocarcinoma may occur as a palpable nodule, the size depending on the extent of local hemorrhage. Patients with pure choriocarcinoma may present with evidence of advanced distant metastasis and what seems a paradoxically small intratesticular lesion that may not distort the normal testicular size or shape.

13. **e. The most frequent combination is embryonal carcinoma, yolk sac tumor, teratoma, and syncytiotrophoblasts.** In classifying more than 6000 testis tumors, one study found that in roughly 60%, more than one histologic pattern was identified. The most frequent combination is embryonal carcinoma, yolk sac tumor, teratoma, and syncytiotrophoblasts.

14. **e. CIS is not evenly distributed throughout the testis, making diagnosis with a single biopsy difficult.** CIS is usually evenly distributed throughout the testis; therefore, open surgical biopsy (3 × 3 × 3 mm) will generally be positive in cases in which CIS exists.

15. **d. The incidence of testicular tumors in black African men is higher than that among African-American men.** Variable incidence rates are noted between different ethnic groups within a given geographic region. The incidence of testicular tumors in American black men is approximately one third that in American whites but 10 times that in African black men.

16. **d. The lymphatic drainage has been shown to cross over from right to left, and therefore cross-metastases occur more commonly in patients with right-sided tumors.** Cross-metastases were reported to occur more commonly in patients with right-sided tumors, because of lymphatic drainage from right to left. These observations obviously have important implications for the surgical management of testis cancer.

17. **b. Testicular swelling on the side of the tumor.** The usual presentation of a testicular tumor is a nodule or painless swelling of one gonad. This may be noted incidentally by the patient or by his sexual partner. The classic description is that of a lump, swelling, or hardness of the testis. Thirty to 40 percent of patients may complain of a dull ache or a heavy sensation in the lower abdomen, anal area, or scrotum. In approximately 10% of patients, acute pain is the presenting symptom. Occasionally, patients with a previously small atrophic testis note enlargement. On rare occasions, infertility may be the presenting complaint. Acute onset of pain is rare unless there is associated epididymitis or bleeding within the tumor.

18. **c. Intrascrotal fluid collections make adequate visualization of the testis impossible.** Ultrasonography of the scrotum is basically an extension of the physical examination. Any hypoechoic area within the tunica albuginea is markedly suspicious for testicular cancer. With the advent of scrotal ultrasonography and its general availability throughout the United States, the delay in diagnosis from confusion with epididymitis should be markedly reduced. Intrascrotal fluid collections are no barrier to the examination of the underlying testicular parenchyma by ultrasonography. In patients with palpably normal genitalia and evidence of extragonadal germ cell malignancy, sonography has been reported to be successful in identifying occult testicular neoplasms.

19. **d. Abdominal and pelvic MRI have a significant advantage over CT with respect to diagnosing micrometastatic disease.** MRI offers no advantage over CT for imaging and staging the retroperitoneum in patients with testis cancer.

20. **e. Placental alkaline phosphatase (PLAP) is elevated in 40% of patients with testicular CIS.** Small studies using enzyme-linked immunosorbent assays indicate that as many as 40% of patients with advanced disease have elevated levels of PLAP.

21. **c. 10%.** The overall sensitivity of any test or marker varies with the amount of tumor burden. Determinations of AFP and HCG, in concert with other staging modalities, have helped reduce the understaging error in germ cell tumors to a level of 10% to 15%. Expressed another way, 10% to 15% of patients with NSGCTs can be expected to have normal marker levels even at advanced stages of disease.

22. **c. 75%.** Seminomas account for 30% to 60% of all germ cell tumors of the testis, depending on the hospital population from which the statistics are being reported. Approximately 75% of seminomas are confined to the testis at the time of clinical presentation. Between 10% and 15% of patients harbor metastatic disease in regional retroperitoneal lymph nodes, and no more than 5% to 10% have advanced to juxtaregional lymph node or visceral metastases, which represents a smaller percentage than among patients with NSGCTs, in whom the incidence of occult metastatic retroperitoneal disease is significantly higher.

23. **e. 90%.** The established treatment for low-stage seminoma has been inguinal orchiectomy followed by therapeutic or adjuvant radiation therapy (see Fig. 29-1). This treatment represents a highly effective method of treating low-stage disease with minimal morbidity; with the advent of multidrug chemotherapy for cure of patients with more disseminated disease, the overall cure rate for all stages exceeds 90%.

24. **c. modified RPLND.** In patients with clinically localized disease, treatment options after orchiectomy include adjuvant radiation therapy to retroperitoneal lymph nodes, single-agent chemotherapy, and surveillance. Currently, adjuvant radiotherapy remains the treatment of choice; however, the success of surveillance protocols for low-stage NSGCT has encouraged the use of surveillance protocols in stage I seminoma patients as well.

25. **d. patient's age.** The surveillance series with the most data on recurrence after surgery is the nationwide Danish study involving 261 patients. Univariate analysis showed tumor size, histologic subtype, presence of necrosis, and invasion of rete testis to be predictive of recurrence, but only tumor size was a statistically significant predictor on multivariate analysis. The 4-year relapse-free survival rate was 6% for tumors smaller than 3 cm, 18% for tumors 3 to 6 cm, and 36% for tumors larger than 6 cm. In this study, tumors larger than 6 cm accounted for approximately 25% of the study population. Other studies have reported that vascular invasion increases the risk for failure in stage I seminoma patients. Therefore, although reliable prognostic factors for seminoma have not been developed, it seems appropriate for patients with tumors smaller than 6 cm in diameter, absence of vascular invasion, and normal βHCG levels to be given the option of surveillance.

26. **e. 90%.** Patients with stage II (N1) disease have enjoyed survival rates above 90%, which statistically does not differ from the rates for patients with stage I disease.

27. **a. 50%.** For patients with stage II (N3) disease treated by radiation therapy alone, approximately one half of patients develop metastatic disease outside the treated fields. One study reported an 11% versus 56% relapse rate when comparing patients with N1-2 and N3 disease who received adjuvant irradiation in a nonrandomized trial.

28. **d. T1N3M0.** Seminoma patients with bulky retroperitoneal disease have traditionally received adjuvant irradiation. More recently, however, adjuvant chemotherapy has been preferred to retroperitoneal irradiation for retroperitoneal tumors greater than 5 cm in diameter. At Brigham and Women's Hospital and Dana Farber Cancer Institute, patients with N1 and N2 disease receive 30 and 35 Gy of radiation, respectively, whereas patients with N3 disease are treated with primary cisplatin-based chemotherapy.

29. **c. teratoma (>50%).** Six factors have been analyzed in many of these studies and include stage of the primary tumor ($pT \leq 2$); vascular (including lymphatic) invasion; presence of embryonal carcinoma; absence of yolk sac elements; and elevated preorchiectomy markers. In the Medical Research Council series, four features were independently predictive of relapse: invasion of testicular veins or lymphatics, absence of yolk sac elements, and presence of embryonal cell carcinoma. Of the 259 patients, 55 patients had three or four factors and a relapse rate of 58%; 89 patients had two factors and a relapse rate of 24%; 81 patients had one factor and a relapse rate of 10%; and 8 patients had no factors and no relapses.

30. **d. a patient in whom tumor markers persist after orchiectomy.** Surveillance is appropriate only for patients with clinical stage T1-3N0M0 disease, without any risk factors for relapse, who are motivated to rigidly adhere to a surveillance protocol and who fully understand the risks of failure to comply with the follow-up schedule. These patients require meticulous evaluation before entering a well-designed and well-managed surveillance protocol. Tumor staging should be carried out compulsively in this selected group of patients with no evidence of suspicious nodes or pulmonary masses.

31. **b. Tumorectomy and bilateral RPLND.** The recognition of teratoma within surgically excised residual masses after combination chemotherapy for advanced disease is a relatively recent phenomenon. The rationale to resect residual teratoma is multifactorial. Indolent teratoma growth, known as the growing teratoma syndrome, may compromise vital organ function; malignant transformation of mature teratoma to sarcoma and adenocarcinoma, which is resistant to chemotherapy, has been well described; chemotherapy and radiotherapy are relatively ineffective against benign or malignant teratoma; and expansion of benign solid and cystic teratomatous elements may compromise vital organ function.

32. **b. 10% to 19%.** Early retrospective studies revealed that RPLND defines three subsets of patients based on histopathologic analysis of the resected specimen: 40%, necrosis/fibrosis; 40%, adult teratoma; 20%, residual NSGCT. Therefore, approximately 60% of patients with evidence of a residual mass on postchemotherapy imaging studies will have either viable cancer or teratoma. More recently, however, the Memorial Sloan-Kettering group reported that the likelihood of malignancy in postchemotherapy resected tumor was 13%, with the remainder of tumor specimens containing teratoma or necrosis. In addition, the Indiana group reported that of 417 patients who underwent postchemotherapy RPLND for residual disease, only 10% were found to have viable germ cell tumor in their pathologic specimens.

33. **d. liver.** The most common sites of origin are, in decreasing order of frequency, the mediastinum, retroperitoneum, sacrococcygeal region, and pineal gland, although many unusual sources have also been reported.

34. **b. Undescended testis is an important predisposing factor.** The etiology of Leydig cell tumors is unknown. In contrast to germ cell tumors, there appears to be no association with cryptorchidism. The experimental production of Leydig cell tumors in mice after chronic estrogen administration or after intrasplenic testicular autografting is consistent with a

hormonal basis. The lesions are generally small, yellow to brown, and well circumscribed and rarely exhibit hemorrhage or necrosis. Microscopically, the tumors consist of relatively uniform, polyhedral, closely packed cells with round, slightly eccentric nuclei and eosinophilic granular cytoplasm with lipid vacuoles, brownish pigmentation, and occasional characteristic inclusions known as Reinke crystals. Pleomorphism with large and bizarre cell forms may occur, and mitotic figures may or may not be identified. None of these features appears to be consistently related to malignant potential. Virilizing types of congenital adrenocortical hyperplasia may also produce the endocrine signs and symptoms of interstitial cell tumors, so differential tests must be carried out to clarify the diagnosis.

35. **b. Lymphatic drainage has not been shown to cross over from right to left.** Lymphatics of the epididymis drain into the external iliac chain, affording locally extensive testicular tumors access to pelvic lymph nodes. Inguinal node metastasis may result from scrotal involvement by the primary tumor, prior inguinal or scrotal surgery, or retrograde lymphatic spread secondary to massive retroperitoneal lymph node deposits.

36. **c. Postganglionic sympathetic nerve fibers.** Modified (template) RPLND has significant advantages. By use of this technique, a complete dissection can be performed in the area most likely to be involved with retroperitoneal nodal disease, yet modification in a less likely area can spare some of the ejaculatory consequences. Two studies reported excellent return of ejaculation with nerve-sparing RPLND. These techniques involve removal of nodal-bearing tissue from around the postganglionic fibers, are somewhat more time consuming, and may require a steeper learning curve as well. Nonetheless, ejaculation can be preserved in 100% of patients and fertility is noted in 75% of patients undergoing this procedure.

37. **d. Pretreatment pulmonary metastases are an integral part of this classification.** In 1997, an international consensus was convened to address the multiplicity of prognostic systems. As a result of this meeting, a new prognostic classification was published: the International Germ Cell Consensus Classification (see Table 29-16). This validated model facilitates collaboration of clinical trials as well as providing a means of comparison of clinical results across studies. This collaboration provided agreement on the use of pretreatment serum tumor marker levels (AFP, βHCG, and lactate dehydrogenase) and metastases to organs other than the lung as poor-risk prognostic factors. The classification contains three subclassifications of good-, intermediate-, and poor-prognosis disease, but for clinical purposes patients are classified as having either good-risk (good and intermediate prognosis) disease or poor-risk (poor prognosis) disease. Chemotherapy is tailored according to this classification. For those patients predicted to have a more favorable outcome (i.e., good risk), the goals have been to maintain high cure rates while reducing treatment-related toxicity. Patients with minimal or moderate disease do well with standard chemotherapy, with response rates in the 91% to 95% category. Patients with advanced disease, however, had only a 53% therapeutic response. Therefore, more aggressive chemotherapy should be used in patients with advanced extent disease according to this category.

30

Surgery of Testicular Tumors

JOEL SHEINFELD • GEORG BARTSCH • GEORGE J. BOSL

QUESTIONS

1. A 23-year old man presented after undergoing transscrotal orchiectomy after presumed hydrocele surgery. Pathology reveals embryonal carcinoma with vascular invasion. Serum tumor markers, physical exam, and CT of the chest, abdomen, and pelvis are normal. Which of the following approaches is appropriate?
   a. Observation
   b. RPLND
   c. RPLND plus excision of scrotal scar
   d. RPLND plus scrotectomy and inguinal lymph node dissection
   e. RPLND plus scrotal and inguinal radiation
2. A 23-year-old man undergoes right orchiectomy for seminoma and undergoes chemotherapy for a 10-cm retroperitoneal mass. His tumor markers are normal both before and after treatment. After treatment the mass is 5 cm. Which is TRUE?
   a. Residual retroperitoneal disease can usually be resected completely.
   b. Probability of viable disease in the retroperitoneum is approximately 25%.
   c. Post-chemotherapy RPLND is associated with low morbidity.
   d. Post-chemotherapy radiation is warranted.
   e. Percutaneous biopsy is accurate.
3. Which of the following is TRUE regarding testicular anatomy?
   a. The right testicular vein drains to the right renal vein.
   b. The left testicular artery arises from the left renal artery.
   c. The left testis lymphatic drainage is to the interaortocaval and paracaval nodes.
   d. The right testis lymphatic drainage is to the paracaval, interaortocaval, and pre-aortic nodes.
   e. The right testicular artery arises from the right renal artery.
4. A 19-year-old man presents after undergoing four cycles of etoposide and platinum chemotherapy for NSGCT diagnosed by needle biopsy of a 5-cm para-aortic mass. The left testis, which had a 2 cm mass before treatment, is now without any abnormality on sonogram or physical examination and the tumor markers have normalized. Which of the following is appropriate treatment of the testes?
   a. Observation.
   b. Radiation.
   c. Radical inguinal orchiectomy.
   d. Biopsy and orchiectomy if viable disease remains.
   e. Bilateral orchiectomy.
5. Which of the following is the most common site for late recurrence of NSGCT?
   a. Retroperitoneum
   b. Lung
   c. Liver
   d. Brain
   e. Mediastinum
6. Which of the following associations is correct when describing the events of ejaculation?
   a. Lumbar sympathetics and bulbourethral muscle contraction
   b. Bladder neck contraction and pudendal somatic nerves
   c. Sympathetic fibers and bladder neck contraction
   d. Pelvic parasympathetics and emission
   e. Lumbar sympathetics and erection
7. During post-chemotherapy RPLND each of the following structures can be ligated without attendant morbidity EXCEPT:
   a. Inferior mesenteric vein
   b. Inferior mesenteric artery
   c. Right and left testicular arteries
   d. Right renal vein
   e. Lumbar arteries
8. Which of the following is FALSE regarding laparoscopic RPLND?
   a. Feasible when performed by experienced laparoscopists
   b. Well-established therapeutic efficacy
   c. Associated with shorter recovery times than open RPLND
   d. Less postoperative analgesic requirements than open RPLND
   e. Low morbidity in post-chemotherapy RPLND
9. A 23-year-old man undergoes right orchiectomy for a mixed NSGCT without vascular invasion. Physical examination and CT of the chest, abdomen, and pelvis are normal, and the patient's preoperative βHCG is elevated and remains elevated after orchiectomy. Which of the following is the most appropriate?
   a. Surveillance
   b. Two cycles of platinum-based chemotherapy
   c. Four cycles of etoposide and platinum or three cycles of bleomycin, etoposide, and platinum
   d. RPLND
   e. Radiation to retroperitoneum

10. A 33-year-old man undergoes left orchiectomy for NSGCT, and serum tumor markers normalize. Imaging reveals a 2-cm mass in the para-aortic region, and he undergoes primary RPLND. During the operation excessive bleeding leads to an incomplete resection. Pathology reveals four positive lymph nodes, the largest of which measures 3.5 cm with extranodal extension. Which of the following is the most appropriate therapy?
    a. Observation
    b. Redo RPLND
    c. Two cycles of platinum-based chemotherapy
    d. Four cycles of etoposide and platinum or three cycles of bleomycin, etoposide, and platinum
    e. Salvage chemotherapy
11. Abnormal fertility in testicular cancer patients is associated with all of the following EXCEPT:
    a. chemotherapy.
    b. primary germ cell defect.
    c. nerve-sparing RPLND.
    d. circulating levels of βHCG.
    e. radiation to scrotum.
12. Which of the following is the strongest risk factor for postoperative pulmonary complications in bleomycin treated patients?
    a. Preoperative pulmonary function test results
    b. Concentration of inspired oxygen during operation
    c. Overall fluid administered in the perioperative period
    d. History of acute bleomycin toxicity
    e. Age
13. A 25-year-old man undergoes four cycles of etoposide and platinum for stage IIb NSGCT. Post-chemotherapy CT of the chest, abdomen, and pelvis is normal. There was no teratoma in the primary tumor. What is the probability of residual teratoma or viable cancer in the retroperitoneum?
    a. 0%
    b. 5%
    c. 20%
    d. 45%
    e. 100%
14. Which of the following is the most common adjunctive procedure performed during post-chemotherapy RPLND?
    a. Splenectomy
    b. Left nephrectomy
    c. Right nephrectomy
    d. Vena caval resection
    e. Bowel resection
15. Which of the following is TRUE regarding resection of residual thoracic disease after chemotherapy for NSGCT?
    a. Unsafe to perform in conjunction with RPLND
    b. Unnecessary if retroperitoneal specimens reveal fibrosis
    c. More likely to reveal fibrosis in the setting of a solitary pulmonary mass and fibrosis in the retroperitoneum
    d. Not necessary to remove right lung nodule if left lung nodule reveals fibrosis
    e. Safely performed via same incision as RPLND
16. A 21-year-old man undergoes four cycles of etoposide and platinum after right-sided orchiectomy for mixed NSGCT. During post-chemotherapy RPLND, the para-aortic lymph nodes above the inferior mesenteric artery reveal viable germ cell tumor on frozen section. The remainder of the dissection should include:
    a. paracaval and interaortocaval tissue.
    b. interaortocaval tissue.
    c. paracaval, interaortocaval, and para-aortic tissue below the inferior mesenteric artery.
    d. no further tissue.
    e. right suprahilar tissue.
17. Malignant transformation, that is, into non–germ cell elements, is a feature associated with:
    a. seminoma.
    b. yolk sac tumors.
    c. embryonal carcinoma.
    d. teratoma.
    e. choriocarcinoma.
18. A 32-year-old man with bulky retroperitoneal NSGCT has completed induction primary chemotherapy with partial regression of a 10-cm interaortocaval mass. His AFP remains elevated. Appropriate management in this setting is:
    a. radiation therapy to the retroperitoneum.
    b. bilateral RPLND.
    c. modified RPLND.
    d. second-line chemotherapy.
    e. nerve-sparing RPLND.
19. Late relapse is a feature most commonly associated with:
    a. seminoma.
    b. yolk sac.
    c. embryonal carcinoma.
    d. choriocarcinoma.
    e. teratoma.
20. A 24-year-old man with stage IIC NSGCT completes induction chemotherapy with complete resolution of a 6-cm para-aortic mass. AFP has normalized; HCG is markedly elevated. Appropriate therapy at this point is:
    a. radiation therapy to the retroperitoneum.
    b. salvage chemotherapy.
    c. full RPLND.
    d. exploratory laparotomy.
    e. modified RPLND.
21. A 25-year-old man with stage IIC NSGCT has completed primary platinum-based chemotherapy. Tumor markers have normalized according to appropriate half-life and he underwent bilateral post-chemotherapy RPLND. Final pathology revealed a focus of yolk sac tumor. Appropriate therapy at this point is:
    a. careful observation.
    b. radiation therapy.
    c. two additional cycles of platinum-based chemotherapy.
    d. four additional cycles of platinum-based chemotherapy.
    e. re-exploration in 6 weeks.
22. The most common site of relapse for patients with clinical stage I on surveillance is the:
    a. brain.
    b. liver.
    c. chest.
    d. retroperitoneum.
    e. supraclavicular nodes.

23. The most common site for retroperitoneal recurrence after RPLND is the:
    a. interaortocaval region
    b. paracaval region
    c. para-aortic region
    d. interiliac region
    e. precaval region

24. After meticulous bilateral primary RPLND with negative lymph nodes, the most likely pattern of relapse includes:
    a. brain metastasis.
    b. liver metastasis.
    c. lung metastasis.
    d. elevated serum tumor markers.
    e. both c and d.

25. Arguments against primary chemotherapy for clinical stage I NSGCT include all of the following EXCEPT:
    a. possible nephrotoxicity, ototoxicity, neurotoxicity, and cardiovascular toxicity.
    b. potential late relapse secondary to chemorefractory elements, particularly teratoma.
    c. myelosuppression.
    d. risk of acute leukemia.
    e. retrograde ejaculation.

26. Incidence of teratoma in the retroperitoneum in patients with pathologic stage II NSGCT following primary RPLND is:
    a. 0% to 5%.
    b. 6% to 10%.
    c. 11% to 20%.
    d. 21% to 30%.
    e. >50%.

27. Late relapse of GCT is characterized by:
    a. poor clinical outcome.
    b. retroperitoneum most common site.
    c. elevated AFP.
    d. chemoresistance.
    e. all of the above.

ANSWERS

1. **c. RPLND plus excision of scrotal scar.** In the setting of scrotal contamination and clinical stage I disease the patient is best managed with RPLND and wide excision of the scrotal scar. Observation is not optimal owing to the presence of vascular invasion and scrotal contamination.

2. **b. Probability of viable disease in the retroperitoneum is approximately 25%.** Post-chemotherapy residual masses in the setting of pure seminoma are difficult to manage. The morbidity of complete RPLND is great owing to the severe desmoplastic reaction surrounding the tumor. Complete RPLND is rare. Residual masses greater than 3 cm are associated with a 27% chance of harboring viable malignancy in a study from Memorial Sloan-Kettering Cancer Center.

3. **d. The right testis lymphatic drainage is to the paracaval, interaortocaval, and pre-aortic nodes.** Lymphatic drainage is critical to the understanding of metastatic spread. The left testis drains mainly to the para-aortic nodes. However, the right testis drains into the interaortocaval, precaval, and preaortic lymph nodes. The right testicular vein drains directly into the vena cava, and the left vein drains into the left renal vein. Both testicular arteries arise from the aorta between the renal and inferior mesenteric arteries.

4. **c. Radical inguinal orchiectomy.** Delayed orchiectomy after chemotherapy is indicated because the testes represent are privileged site and are often refractory to chemotherapy. Up to 50% of testes removed in this setting will contain either viable germ cell tumor or teratoma (Simmonds, 1995).

5. **a. Retroperitoneum.** The most common site of late recurrence for both teratoma and viable NSGCT is the retroperitoneum.

6. **c. Sympathetic fibers and bladder neck contraction.** Lumbar sympathetic fibers control the act of emission innervating the seminal vesicles, vas deferens, and prostate. Bladder neck contraction is also controlled via sympathetic nerves and is necessary for antegrade ejaculation. Pudendal somatic nerves control the rhythmic contractions of the perineal muscles and bulbourethral muscle.

7. **d. Right renal vein.** The inferior mesenteric artery can be ligated in younger patients without ischemic injury to the colon providing the marginal arterial supply is intact. Lumbar arteries are routinely divided to expose the tissue behind the great vessels. The right renal vein has limited anastomotic flow, and ligation will lead to renal vein hypertension and loss of kidney function.

8. **b. Well-established therapeutic efficacy.** Although no randomized trial has been conducted, multiple studies describing the feasibility of LRPLND have been reported. In general the postoperative pain and recovery times are shorter than open RPLND. Because of the short median follow-up and the frequent use of adjuvant chemotherapy, no statement can yet be made regarding therapeutic efficacy.

9. **c. Four cycles of etoposide and platinum or three cycles of bleomycin, etoposide, and platinum.** This patient has stage I-S disease and RPLND alone in this setting is associated with a high incidence of postoperative persistently elevated tumor markers. Full induction chemotherapy is warranted with four cycles of platinum and etoposide or three cycles of platinum, etoposide, and bleomycin.

10. **d. Four cycles of etoposide and platinum or three cycles of bleomycin, etoposide, and platinum.** Because of the findings of viable disease, extranodal extension, and nodes greater than 2 cm this patient is not a good candidate for observation. The operation described is incomplete and no interaortocaval dissection was performed; therefore, it cannot be assumed that this patient is without evidence of disease and adjuvant chemotherapy with two cycles is not possible. Reoperation in this setting is not warranted unless there is a persistent mass after full induction chemotherapy.

11. **c. nerve-sparing RPLND.** Patients undergoing primary prospective nerve-sparing RPLND have similar paternity rates to testicular cancer patients on surveillance. The other choices are all either reversible or permanent causes of subnormal fertility in testicular cancer patients.

12. **c. Overall fluid administered in the perioperative period.** The single most important risk factor for postoperative pulmonary complications in patients previously treated with bleomycin is the overall fluid and blood transfusion requirements.

13. **c. 20%.** The interpretation of post-chemotherapy CT scans as normal or abnormal is subject to variability. In the three large series of RPLND in the setting of a "normal" CT scan the findings of teratoma or viable germ cell tumor ranged from 20% to 30%.

14. **b. Left nephrectomy.** The left kidney is the most common organ removed in most series of post-chemotherapy RPLND. Twenty percent of patients in the series of Nash and colleagues required nephrectomy, and these patients usually presented with hilar or suprahilar left-sided residual masses.

15. **c. More likely to reveal fibrosis in the setting of a solitary pulmonary mass and fibrosis in the retroperitoneum.** The predictors of fibrosis in thoracic specimens include fibrosis in the retroperitoneum, solitary mass, and pretreatment tumor markers. In the setting of fibrosis in the retroperitoneum there is a 30% chance of finding discordant histologic findings in the chest. Even in the presence of benign pathology in one lung there can still be teratoma or viable germ cell tumor in the contralateral lung.

16. **c. paracaval, interaortocaval, and para-aortic tissue below the inferior mesenteric artery.** The presence of left-sided viable disease makes full bilateral dissection mandatory. Prospective nerve-sparing techniques can be employed in this setting in select candidates to preserve antegrade ejaculation.

17. **d. teratoma.** Despite the histologically benign nature of teratoma, there is a risk of malignant transformation, that is, the development of non–germ cell malignant elements such as sarcoma or carcinoma. The overall incidence is 6% to 8% in the postchemotherapy setting, and the most common histologic subtypes include rhabdomyosarcoma and carcinoma.

18. **d. second-line chemotherapy.** Increased serum concentrations of AFP and βHCG after primary cisplatin-based chemotherapy are often characterized by unresectable, viable germ cell tumor; and second-line salvage chemotherapy is usually recommended for these nonresponders.

19. **e. teratoma.** Late relapse of germ cell tumor after definitive therapy is defined as recurrence occurring more than 2 years after completion of therapy and being without evidence of disease. Teratoma is the most common histologic subtype involved in cases of late relapse. This is likely due to its combination of prolonged doubling time and chemotherapy resistance.

20. **b. salvage chemotherapy.** Increased serum concentrations of AFP and βHCG after primary cisplatin-based chemotherapy are often characterized by unresectable, viable germ cell tumor, and second-line salvage chemotherapy is usually recommended for these nonresponders. If the complete resolution of radiographic abnormalities after chemotherapy seen in this patient were accompanied by normalization of tumor markers, then therapeutic options include observation versus post-chemotherapy RPLND. In this setting, 20% to 30% of patients will have either viable germ cell tumor or teratoma at the time of RPLND.

21. **c. two additional cycles of platinum-based chemotherapy.** The patient's prognosis is related to serum tumor marker level at the time of RPLND, prior treatment burden, and the pathologic findings for the resected specimen. If viable germ cell tumor is present at any site but all disease is completely resected, two additional cycles provide survival benefit in this subset of patients. Einhorn reported only 2 long-term survivors of 22 patients (9%) with completely resected viable germ cell tumor after cisplatin, bleomycin, and vinblastine chemotherapy if additional postoperative chemotherapy was not given. Fox and colleagues reported that 70% of patients with completely resected viable germ cell tumor after primary chemotherapy followed by two cycles of postoperative chemotherapy remained disease-free compared with none of 7 patients without additional chemotherapy.

22. **d. retroperitoneum.** Sixty to 70 percent of patients with stage I NSGCT who experience relapse on surveillance will have retroperitoneal metastasis (± elevated serum tumor markers). Approximately 90% of relapses occur the first year and almost 98% within the first 2 years.

23. **c. para-aortic region.** The most common site for retroperitoneal relapse after RPLND for both right and left primary tumors is the para-aortic region. There are two reasons for this: (1) this region is excluded in some published modified right-sided templates and (2) obtaining adequate exposure in this area is more technically demanding.

24. **e. both c and d.** Retroperitoneal ("infield") recurrences are rare after a meticulous bilateral RPLND. Systemic failures most commonly present as either lung nodules or rising serum tumor markers.

25. **e. retrograde ejaculation.** Chemotherapy does not impact antegrade ejaculation.

26. **d. 21% to 30%.** The Memorial Sloan-Kettering series reported a 21% incidence of teratomatous elements in patients with pathologic stage II NSGCT while the Indiana series reported a 30% incidence in this setting.

27. **e. all of the above.** Late relapse of GCT is characterized by 5-year survival rates under 50%. This setting is further characterized by chemoresistance, an elevated AFP, and the fact that 50% to 80% of the patients will have retroperitoneal disease.

31

Tumors of the Penis

CURTIS A. PETTAWAY • DONALD F. LYNCH, Jr. • JOHN W. DAVIS

QUESTIONS

1. Which of the following penile lesions does NOT have malignant potential?
   a. Balanitis xerotica obliterans
   b. Condylomata acuminata
   c. Coronal papillae
   d. Bowen's disease
   e. Leukoplakia
2. Which of the following infections is associated with cervical dysplasia?
   a. HIV infection
   b. Herpesvirus infection
   c. Gonorrhea
   d. Human papillomavirus (HPV) infection
   e. Lymphogranuloma venereum
3. What is the major difference between Bowen's disease and erythroplasia of Queyrat?
   a. Loss of rete pegs
   b. Keratin staining
   c. Viral etiologic agents
   d. Location
   e. Potential for metastasis
4. Kaposi's sarcoma of the AIDS-related (epidemic) type is associated with which of the following etiologic agents?
   a. HPV type 16
   b. Human herpesvirus (HHV) type 8
   c. HPV type 32
   d. *Haemophilus ducreyi* (chancroid [soft chancre])
   e. Coxsackievirus type 23
5. Where do penile cancers most commonly arise?
   a. Glans
   b. Shaft
   c. Frenulum
   d. Coronal sulcus
   e. Scrotum
6. Which of the following is not considered a risk factor for the development of squamous penile cancer?
   a. Cigarette smoke
   b. HPV infection
   c. Phimosis
   d. Gonorrhea
   e. Chewing tobacco
7. All of the following are preventive strategies to decrease the incidence of penile cancer EXCEPT which one?
   a. Circumcision after 21 years of age
   b. Avoiding sexual promiscuity
   c. Daily genital hygiene
   d. Avoiding cigarette smoke
   e. Circumcision before puberty
8. Which of the following statements regarding penile cancer is FALSE?
   a. Cancer may develop anywhere on the penis.
   b. Because of the associated discomfort, patients usually present to physicians within the first month of noting the lesion.
   c. Phimosis may obscure the nature of the lesion.
   d. Penetration of Buck's fascia and the tunica albuginea by the tumor permits invasion of the vascular corpora.
   e. Cancer cells reach the contralateral inguinal region because of lymphatic cross-communications at the base of the penis.
9. Before a treatment plan for penile cancer is initiated, which of the following is TRUE?
   a. Adequate biopsies to determine stage are unimportant, because all patients should be treated with amputation.
   b. Radiologic studies play no role in decision making.
   c. DNA flow cytometry should be performed on virtually all specimens, because it provides crucial information.
   d. Tumor stage and grade and vascular invasion status all provide prognostically important information.
   e. No disfiguring therapy is indicated, because spontaneous remissions have been noted in approximately 10% of cases.
10. Which of the following statements is TRUE regarding the natural history of penile cancer?
   a. Metastasis from the primary tumor often involves lung, liver, or bone as initial sites.
   b. Lymphatic drainage from the primary tumor is ipsilateral alone in most cases.
   c. Metastasis often initially involves spread from the corpora cavernosa to the pelvic lymph nodes.
   d. Metastasis initially involves inguinal lymph nodes beneath the fascia lata.
   e. Metastasis initially involves inguinal lymph nodes above the fascia lata.

11. Which of the following statements concerning hypercalcemia in patients with penile cancer is TRUE?
    a. It is more commonly due to massive bone metastases than bulky soft tissue metastases.
    b. It is often related to uremia due to ureteral obstruction.
    c. It may be due to the action of parathyroid hormone–like substances released from the tumor.
    d. It is related to the action of osteoblasts on bone formation.
    e. It is managed with aggressive diuretic administration as first-line therapy.
12. The following statements are true regarding imaging tests in patients with penile cancer EXCEPT which one?
    a. Both ultrasonography and MRI lack sensitivity for the detection of corpus cavernosum involvement.
    b. CT is not an appropriate test for determining primary tumor stage.
    c. CT may be beneficial in detecting enlarged inguinal nodes in obese patients or those who have had prior inguinal therapy.
    d. Lymphangiography can detect abnormal architecture in normal-sized lymph nodes.
    e. Inguinal palpation is preferred to CT and lymphangiography for determining inguinal nodal status.
13. According to the current 1997 version of the International Union Against Cancer/TNM staging system for penile cancer, which of the following statements is TRUE?
    a. Primary tumor stage is based on the size of the primary lesion.
    b. Lymph node stage is based on the resectability of involved nodes.
    c. Stage T2 tumors are based on biopsy and involve corpora cavernosa only.
    d. Large verrucous carcinomas are considered stage Ta.
    e. Stage T1 tumors may involve the urethra at the meatus.
14. What is the strongest prognostic factor for survival in penile cancer?
    a. The presence of lymph node metastasis
    b. The grade of the primary tumor
    c. The stage of the primary tumor
    d. The vascular invasion present in the primary tumor
    e. The extent of lymph node metastasis
15. Criteria for curative surgical resection (>70% 5-year survival) in patients treated for lymph node metastasis include all of the following EXCEPT which one?
    a. No more than two positive inguinal lymph nodes
    b. No positive pelvic lymph nodes
    c. Absence of extranodal extension of cancer
    d. Unilateral metastasis
    e. A single metastasis of only 6 cm
16. Surgical staging of the inguinal region is strongly considered under all of the following conditions EXCEPT which one?
    a. Palpable adenopathy
    b. Stage T2 or greater primary tumor
    c. Presence of vascular invasion in primary tumor
    d. Presence of predominantly high-grade cancer in primary tumor
    e. Stage Ta tumors
17. A watchful waiting strategy toward the management of the inguinal region in patients with no palpable adenopathy is recommended for all of the following situations EXCEPT which one?
    a. Primary tumor stage Tis
    b. Primary tumor stage Ta
    c. Primary tumor stage T1, grade I
    d. Primary tumor stage T1, grade II
    e. Noncompliant patients
18. Strategies to minimize the morbidity of inguinal staging in patients with no palpable adenopathy include all the following EXCEPT which one?
    a. Superficial inguinal lymph node dissection
    b. Modified complete inguinal dissection
    c. Standard ilioinguinal dissection
    d. Sentinel lymph node biopsy
    e. Intraoperative lymphatic mapping
19. Which of the following inguinal staging procedures is considered the 'gold standard' for detecting microscopic metastases while limiting both morbidity and false negative findings?
    a. Inguinal node biopsy
    b. Superficial inguinal dissection
    c. Sentinel lymph node dissection
    d. Fine-needle aspiration cytology
    e. Sentinel lymph node biopsy
20. For patients with proven unilateral metastasis all of the following surgical considerations are true EXCEPT which one?
    a. Ipsilateral ilioinguinal lymphadenectomy should be performed.
    b. A contralateral staging procedure is not indicated.
    c. A contralateral staging procedure is indicated.
    d. Both a superficial dissection and deep ipsilateral dissection are performed.
    e. Ipsilateral pelvic dissection provides useful prognostic information.
21. Adjuvant or neoadjuvant chemotherapy should be considered in addition to surgery for all of the following EXCEPT which one?
    a. Single pelvic nodal metastasis
    b. Extranodal extension of cancer
    c. Fixed inguinal masses
    d. Two unilateral inguinal nodes with focal metastases
    e. Single 6-cm inguinal lymph node
22. The majority of penile cancers are of which of the following histologic types?
    a. Melanoma
    b. Bowenoid papulosis
    c. Squamous cell carcinoma
    d. Epidemic Kaposi's sarcoma
    e. Verrucous carcinoma
23. Which of the following chemotherapeutic agents have been used in combination therapy for penile cancer?
    a. Bleomycin
    b. Methotrexate
    c. Cisplatin
    d. 5-Fluorouracil (5-FU)
    e. All of the above
24. Indications for radiation therapy as primary treatment for penile cancer include which of the following?
    a. Young, sexually active patient with a small lesion
    b. Patient refuses surgery
    c. Patient with inoperable tumor who needs local treatment but desires to retain the penis
    d. None of the above
    e. a, b, and c
25. Primary penile melanoma is thought to be rare for what reason?
    a. Penile skin is protected from exposure to the sun.
    b. Keratin content in penile skin is decreased.
    c. Penile blood supply precludes such tumor development.
    d. Effective topical chemotherapy exists.
    e. None of the above

26. Lymphomatous infiltration of the penis is most likely secondary to which condition?
    a. Autoimmune disorder
    b. Diffuse disease
    c. Metastasis from a distant primary tumor
    d. Chronic infection
    e. Previous venereal infection
27. What is the most frequently encountered sign of metastatic involvement of the penis?
    a. Pain
    b. Urethral discharge
    c. Ecchymoses
    d. Priapism
    e. Preputial swelling
28. Which of the following features of Buschke-Löwenstein tumor characterizes it as different from condyloma acuminatum?
    a. Propensity for early distant metastasis
    b. Disruption of the rete pegs
    c. Loss of pigmentation
    d. Autoamputation
    e. Invasion and destruction of adjacent tissue by compression
29. Which of the following statements about how verrucous carcinoma of the penis differs from classic Buschke-Löwenstein tumor is TRUE?
    a. The terms describe the same disease.
    b. Verrucous carcinoma sometimes exhibits spontaneous regression.
    c. Proportion of melanin pigment in verrucous carcinoma is higher than in Buschke-Löwenstein tumor.
    d. Simultaneous bilateral inguinal metastases occur commonly with Buschke-Löwenstein tumor.
    e. Circumcision is not protective for verrucous carcinoma.
30. Small lesions of erythroplasia of Queyrat may be successfully treated by which of the following?
    a. Topical 5% 5-FU
    b. Neodymium: yttrium-aluminum-garnet (Nd:YAG) laser
    c. Local excision
    d. External-beam radiation therapy
    e. All of the above

ANSWERS

1. **c. Coronal papillae.** Coronal papillae present as linear, curved, or irregular rows of conical or globular excrescences, varying from white to yellow to red, arranged along the coronal sulcus. They are considered acral angiofibromas. These lesions have not been associated with malignancy.
2. **d. Human papillomavirus (HPV) infection.** HPV is recognized as the principal etiologic agent in cervical dysplasia and cervical cancer.
3. **d. Location.** Carcinoma in situ of the penis is referred to by urologists and dermatologists as erythroplasia of Queyrat if it involves the glans penis, prepuce, or penile shaft and as Bowen's disease if it involves the remainder of the genitalia or perineal region.
4. **b. Human herpesvirus (HHV) type 8.** HHV type 8—also known as KSHV (Kaposi sarcoma-associated herpesvirus)—is strongly suspected to be the etiologic agent of epidemic (AIDS-related) Kaposi sarcoma.
5. **a. Glans.** Penile tumors may present anywhere on the penis but occur most commonly on the glans (48%) and prepuce (21%).
6. **d. Gonorrhea.** No convincing evidence has been found linking penile cancer to other factors such as occupation, other venereal diseases (gonorrhea, syphilis, herpes), marijuana use, or alcohol intake.
7. **a. Circumcision after 21 years of age.** Adult circumcision appears to offer little or no protection from subsequent development of the disease. These data suggest that the crucial period of exposure to certain etiologic agents may have already occurred at puberty and certainly by adult age, rendering later circumcision relatively ineffective as a prophylactic tool for penile cancer.
8. **b. Because of the associated discomfort, patients usually present to physicians within the first month of noting the lesion.** Patients with cancer of the penis, more than patients with other types of cancer, seem to delay seeking medical attention. In large series, from 15% to 50% of patients have been noted to delay medical care for more than a year.
9. **d. Tumor stage and grade and vascular invasion status all provide prognostically important information.** Confirmation of the diagnosis of carcinoma of the penis and assessment of the depth of invasion, the presence of vascular invasion, and histologic grade of the lesion by microscopic examination of a biopsy specimen are mandatory before the initiation of any therapy.
10. **e. Metastasis initially involves inguinal lymph nodes above the fascia lata.** The lymphatics of the prepuce form a connecting network that joins with the lymphatics from the skin of the shaft. These tributaries drain into the superficial inguinal nodes (the nodes external to the fascia lata).
11. **c. It may be due to the action of parathyroid hormone–like substances released from the tumor.** Parathyroid hormone and related substances may be produced by both tumor and metastases that activate osteoclastic bone resorption.
12. **a. Both ultrasonography and MRI lack sensitivity for the detection of corpus cavernosum involvement.** The sensitivity of ultrasonography for detecting cavernosum invasion was 100% in one study. This study confirmed the value of ultrasonography in assessing the primary tumor also reported by other investigators. For lesions suspected of invading the corpus cavernosum, both ultrasonography and contrast medium–enhanced MRI may provide unique information, especially when organ-sparing surgery is considered.
13. **d. Large verrucous carcinomas are considered stage Ta.** According to this staging system, designations for primary tumors are as follows: Tx indicates that the primary tumor cannot be assessed; T0 indicates no evidence of tumor; Tis indicates carcinoma in situ; Ta indicates noninvasive verrucous carcinoma; T1 indicates tumor invading subepithelial connective tissue; T2 indicates tumor invading corpus spongiosum or cavernosum; T3 indicates tumor invading urethra or prostate; and T4 indicates tumor invading other adjacent structures.
14. **e. The extent of lymph node metastasis.** The presence and extent of metastasis to the inguinal region are the most important prognostic factors for survival in patients with squamous penile cancer.
15. **e. A single metastasis of only 6 cm.** Taken together, these data suggest that the pathologic criteria associated with long-term

survival after attempted curative surgical resection of inguinal metastases (i.e., 80% 5-year survival) include (1) minimal nodal disease (up to two involved nodes in most series), (2) unilateral involvement, (3) no evidence of extranodal extension of cancer, and (4) the absence of pelvic nodal metastases.

16. **e. Stage Ta tumors.** Tumor histologic type associated with little or no risk for metastasis includes those patients with primary tumors exhibiting (1) carcinoma in situ or (2) verrucous carcinoma.

17. **e. Noncompliant patients.** Noncompliant patients should be in the high-risk category.

18. **c. Standard ilioinguinal dissection.** In patients with no evidence of palpable adenopathy who are selected to undergo inguinal procedures by virtue of adverse prognostic factors within the primary tumor, the goal is to define whether metastases exist with minimal morbidity for the patient. A variety of treatment options for this purpose have been reported and include (1) fine-needle aspiration cytology, (2) node biopsy, (3) sentinel lymph node biopsy, (4) extended sentinel lymph node dissection, (5) intraoperative lymphatic mapping, (6) superficial dissection, and (7) modified complete dissection.

19. **b. Superficial inguinal dissection.** One series found that the sensitivity of fine-needle aspiration cytology was approximately 71% in 18 patients with clinically negative lymph nodes. This finding and the technical difficulty with lymphangiography make aspiration less practical as a staging technique for patients with no palpable lymph nodes. Biopsies directed to a specific anatomic area can be unreliable in identifying microscopic metastasis and are no longer recommended.

20. **b. A contralateral staging procedure is not indicated.** Clinical support for a bilateral procedure is based on the finding of contralateral metastases in more than 50% of patients so treated, even if the contralateral nodal region was negative to palpation.

21. **d. Two unilateral inguinal nodes with focal metastases.** For patients requiring ilioinguinal lymphadenectomy because of the presence of metastases, adjuvant chemotherapy should be considered for those exhibiting more than two positive lymph nodes, extranodal extension of cancer, or pelvic nodal metastasis. Reports from one center further confirmed the value of adjuvant chemotherapy. Of 25 node-positive patients treated with adjuvant combination vincristine, bleomycin, and methotrexate (VBM), 82% survived 5 years, compared with 37% of 31 patients treated with surgery alone.

22. **c. Squamous cell carcinoma.** The majority of tumors of the penis are squamous cell carcinomas demonstrating keratinization, epithelial pearl formation, and various degrees of mitotic activity.

23. **e. All of the above.** 5-FU has been used as a continuous intravenous infusion in combination with cisplatin in a limited number of patients. VBM was administered in 12 weekly treatments to 17 patients as either a neoadjuvant (5 patients) or a postoperative (12 patients) treatment program at the Milan National Tumor Institute.

24. **e. a, b, and c.** Radiation therapy may be considered in a select group of patients: (1) young individuals presenting with small (2 to 4 cm), superficial, exophytic, noninvasive lesions on the glans or coronal sulcus; (2) patients refusing surgery as an initial form of treatment; and (3) patients with inoperable tumor or distant metastases who require local therapy to the primary tumor but who express a desire to retain the penis.

25. **a. Penile skin is protected from exposure to the sun.** Melanoma and basal cell carcinoma rarely occur on the penis, presumably because the organ's skin is protected from exposure to the sun.

26. **b. Diffuse disease.** When lymphomatous infiltration of the penis is diagnosed, a thorough search for systemic disease is necessary.

27. **d. Priapism.** The most frequent sign of penile metastasis is priapism; penile swelling, nodularity, and ulceration have also been reported.

28. **e. Invasion and destruction of adjacent tissues by compression.** The Buschke-Löwenstein tumor differs from condyloma acuminatum in that condylomata, regardless of size, always remain superficial and never invade adjacent tissue. Buschke-Löwenstein tumor displaces, invades, and destroys adjacent structures by compression. Aside from this unrestrained local growth, it demonstrates no signs of malignant change on histologic examination and does not metastasize.

29. **a. The terms describe the same disease.** Buschke-Löwenstein tumor is synonymous with verrucous carcinoma and giant condyloma acuminatum.

30. **e. All of the above.** When lesions are small and noninvasive, local excision, which spares penile anatomy and function, is satisfactory. Circumcision will adequately treat preputial lesions. Fulguration may be successful but often results in recurrences. Radiation therapy has successfully eradicated these tumors, and well-planned, appropriately delivered radiation results in minimal morbidity. Topical 5-FU as the 5% base causes denudation of malignant and premalignant areas while preserving normal skin. There are also reports of successful treatment with Nd:YAG laser.

32

Surgery of Penile and Urethral Carcinoma

DAVID S. SHARP • KENNETH W. ANGERMEIER

QUESTIONS

1. Biopsy of a penile lesion provides all of the following information EXCEPT:
   a. confirmation of the histologic diagnosis.
   b. initial assessment of tumor grade.
   c. depth of invasion.
   d. prognosis.
2. Laser therapy may provide effective treatment for all but which one of the following lesions?
   a. Invasive stage T2 lesions
   b. Carcinoma in situ
   c. Bowenoid papulosis
   d. Superficial stage Ta penile cancers
3. Techniques that may allow improved delineation of the extent of superficial penile cancer during laser therapy include all of the following EXCEPT:
   a. photodynamic diagnosis and autofluorescence.
   b. preparation of the treatment area with 5% acetic acid.
   c. loupe magnification.
   d. frozen section biopsies.
4. Mohs' micrographic surgery provides which of the following?
   a. Compromise of long-term local control
   b. Effective therapy for invasive tumors (stage T2 or greater)
   c. Retention of function and anatomic integrity of the penis
   d. Effective therapy for large lesions
5. All of the following statements regarding conservative surgical excision for penile carcinoma are true EXCEPT which one?
   a. Careful long-term surveillance following surgery is necessary.
   b. Frozen section biopsies are usually not needed during these procedures.
   c. Glans defects after tumor excision that are not amenable to primary closure may be covered with a split thickness skin graft or a flap of outer preputial skin.
   d. Glansectomy and circumcision remove the entire contents of the preputial cavity.
6. Successful local control by partial penectomy depends on which of the following?
   a. Division of the penis at least 2 cm proximal to the gross tumor
   b. Cleanliness of the patient
   c. Use of adjuvant chemotherapy
   d. Status of inguinal nodes
7. Partial penectomy:
   a. requires creation of a perineal urethrostomy.
   b. provides for normal sexual function in greater than 70% of men.
   c. is required less often than total penectomy.
   d. results in local recurrence rates of less than 10%.
8. Efforts designed to improve the accuracy of dynamic sentinel lymph node biopsy include all of the following EXCEPT:
   a. using an ultrasensitive gamma ray detection probe.
   b. routine inguinal exploration in the absence of radiotracer visualization.
   c. extended pathologic analysis of excised lymph nodes.
   d. intraoperative palpation of the wound for abnormal nodes.
9. When compared with the standard groin dissection, the modified groin dissection has all of the following features EXCEPT which one?
   a. The node dissection excludes regions lateral to the femoral artery and caudad to the fossa ovalis.
   b. The saphenous vein is preserved.
   c. The transposition of the sartorius muscle is eliminated.
   d. The required incision is longer.
10. Which of the following statements regarding radical ilioinguinal lymphadenectomy is TRUE?
    a. The fascia lata remains intact.
    b. The saphenous vein may be preserved in the setting of low volume disease.
    c. The rotation of the gracilis muscle is performed to cover the exposed femoral vessels.
    d. The femoral nerve is visualized superior to the iliacus fascia.
11. A pelvic node dissection for male penile cancer should include all of the following areas EXCEPT which one?
    a. Distal common iliac nodes
    b. Para-aortic and paracaval node dissection
    c. External iliac nodes
    d. Obturator group of nodes
12. Which of the following measures may help prevent lymphedema after a radical ilioinguinal node dissection?
    a. Preservation of Colles' fascia in the flap dissection
    b. Low-dose heparin in the perioperative period
    c. A 6-week delay between treatment of the primary tumor and the node dissection
    d. Postoperative bed rest and elastic stockings

13. What is the most frequent site of both stricture disease and urethral cancer in the male?
    a. Pendulous urethra
    b. Fossa navicularis
    c. Bulbomembranous urethra
    d. Prostatic urethra
14. Which of the following is true concerning distal urethral carcinoma in the male?
    a. Prognosis depends on histologic cell type.
    b. Penectomy is usually indicated for tumors infiltrating the corpus spongiosum.
    c. Prognosis is worse than bulbomembranous urethral cancer.
    d. Conservative surgical therapy is not effective.
15. When a delayed urethrectomy is performed in a male patient after radical cystectomy, which of the following is necessary to ensure a complete dissection and decrease the risk of a local recurrence?
    a. Removal of the fossa navicularis and urethral meatus
    b. Bilateral groin dissections
    c. Total penectomy
    d. Intraoperative ultrasound imaging
16. Which of the following statements regarding urethral tumor recurrence after cystectomy and orthotopic urinary diversion is FALSE?
    a. It seems to occur more frequently than after cutaneous diversion.
    b. Some patients with carcinoma in situ may be successfully treated with urethral infusion of BCG.
    c. Urethrectomy and cutaneous diversion can often be done using bowel from the existing neobladder.
    d. Surveillance consists of urine cytology and symptom assessment.
17. Possible causes for female urethral carcinoma include all of the following EXCEPT:
    a. childhood urinary tract infections.
    b. leukoplakia.
    c. chronic irritation or urinary tract infections.
    d. proliferative lesions such as caruncles.
18. What is the most common histologic type of proximal urethral cancer in women?
    a. Adenocarcinoma
    b. Squamous cell carcinoma
    c. Melanoma
    d. Transitional cell carcinoma
19. What is the most significant prognostic factor for local control and survival in female urethral cancer?
    a. Anatomic location and extent of the tumor
    b. Age at presentation
    c. Histologic type of the tumor
    d. Hematuria
20. Radiation therapy for female urethral carcinoma is most successful:
    a. as a single modality for proximal invasive tumors.
    b. when used in conjunction with chemotherapy for low-stage distal urethral tumors.
    c. at controlling distant metastatic disease.
    d. at controlling small lesions in the distal urethra.

ANSWERS

1. **d. prognosis.** Before the administration of therapy, a biopsy is required to provide histologic confirmation of the diagnosis of penile cancer and staging information by assessing the depth of microscopic invasion. Adjacent normal tissue should be included to evaluate invasion, a crucial differential point with regard to planning definitive surgery.
2. **a. Invasive stage T2 lesions.** Laser therapy has gained popularity in recent years for the treatment of premalignant lesions and carcinoma in situ (Bowen's disease, erythroplasia of Queyrat, bowenoid papulosis) and some stage Ta and small T1 penile cancers.
3. **c. loupe magnification.** Photodynamic visualization and autofluorescence have been described as aids to guiding frozen section biopsies during laser therapy of superficial penile cancer, whereas coating the treatment area with 5% acetic acid often results in acetowhite staining of occult areas of squamous cell carcinoma.
4. **c. Retention of function and anatomic integrity of the penis.** Mohs' micrographic surgery allows retention of function and anatomic integrity of the penis without compromising local control rates in small (<1 to 2 cm) superficial noninvasive and small T1 tumors and is contraindicated for larger or more invasive lesions.
5. **b. Frozen section biopsies are usually not needed during these procedures.** Frozen section biopsies are an essential component of conservative excision for penile carcinoma to help ensure complete tumor eradication.
6. **a. Division of the penis at least 2 cm proximal to the gross tumor.** Successful local control by partial penectomy depends on division of the penis at least 2 cm proximal to the gross tumor extent.
7. **d. results in local recurrence rates of less than 10%.** Partial penectomy results in a local recurrence rate of 0% to 8%. It is performed more often than total penectomy, does not generally require creation of a perineal urethrostomy, and provides for adequate sexual function in a relatively small percentage of men.
8. **a. using an ultrasensitive gamma ray detection probe.** Techniques reported to increase the accuracy of dynamic sentinel lymph node biopsy include preoperative inguinal ultrasound with needle biopsy of any suspicious nodes, routine inguinal exploration even in the absence of radiotracer visualization, intraoperative palpation of the wound for abnormal nodes, and extended pathologic analysis of any excised lymph nodes.
9. **d. The required incision is longer.** The modified groin dissection differs from the standard dissection in that (1) the skin incision is shorter; (2) the node dissection is limited, excluding regions lateral to the femoral artery and caudad to the fossa ovalis; (3) the saphenous veins are preserved; and (4) the transposition of the sartorius muscles is eliminated.

10. **b. The saphenous vein may be preserved in the setting of low volume disease.** In a radical inguinal lymphadenectomy, the fascia lata is divided longitudinally and the sartorius muscle is rotated to cover the femoral vessels. The femoral nerve is usually not seen as it lies beneath the iliacus fascia lateral to the femoral artery. In the setting of low volume nodal disease, it is acceptable to spare the saphenous vein if feasible in order to attempt to decrease the risk of lower extremity complications.
11. **b. Para-aortic and paracaval node dissection.** The pelvic lymphadenectomy includes the distal common iliac, external iliac, and obturator groups of nodes. No further therapeutic benefit is gained from proximal iliac or para-aortic node dissection.
12. **d. Postoperative bed rest and elastic stockings.** Efforts to minimize lymphedema during the initial postoperative period include applying thigh-high elastic wraps or stockings and elevating the foot of the bed.
13. **c. Bulbomembranous urethra.** The incidence of urethral stricture in men later developing a carcinoma of the urethra ranges from 24% to 76% and most frequently involves the bulbomembranous urethra, which is also the portion of the urethra most commonly involved by tumor.
14. **b. Penectomy is usually indicated for tumors infiltrating the corpus spongiosum.** In general, anterior urethral carcinoma is more amenable to surgical control, and the patient's prognosis is better than that for posterior urethral carcinoma, which is often associated with extensive local invasion and distant metastasis.
15. **a. Removal of the fossa navicularis and urethral meatus.** It is important that the fossa navicularis and meatus are also taken in the dissection because of the high incidence of involvement of the squamous epithelium.
16. **a. It seems to occur more frequently than after cutaneous diversion.** Studies to date suggest that urethral tumor recurrence after orthotopic urinary diversion is less common than after cutaneous diversion. In the presence of an orthotopic neobladder, urethral surveillance consists of urine cytology and symptom assessment. Success has been reported in selected patients treated with urethral infusion of BCG for urethral carcinoma in situ after orthotopic diversion. After urethrectomy, cutaneous diversion can often be done using bowel from the existing neobladder, eliminating the need to take additional small bowel out of circuit.
17. **a. childhood urinary tract infections.** Causes associated with subsequent development of malignancy include chronic irritation or urinary tract infections; proliferative lesions such as caruncles, papillomas, adenomas, and polyps; and leukoplakia of the urethra.
18. **b. Squamous cell carcinoma.** Carcinomas of the proximal or entire urethra tend to be high grade and locally advanced, with squamous cell carcinoma accounting for 60%; transitional cell carcinoma, 20%; adenocarcinoma, 10%; undifferentiated tumor and sarcomas, 8%; and melanoma, 2%.
19. **a. Anatomic location and extent of the tumor.** The most significant prognostic factor for local control and survival is the anatomic location and extent of the tumor (see Tables 32-2 and 32-3), with low-stage distal urethral tumors having a better prognosis than high-stage proximal urethral tumors.
20. **d. at controlling small lesions in the distal urethra.** Radiation therapy alone, as with surgical excision, is often sufficient to control small lesions in the distal urethra.

33

Surgery of the Penis and Urethra

GERALD H. JORDAN • STEVEN M. SCHLOSSBERG

QUESTIONS

1. With regard to the physical characteristics of tissue, which of the following statements is TRUE?
   a. They are a function of the collagen-elastin architecture as it is suspended in a mucopolysaccharide matrix.
   b. Only select tissues have inherent tissue tension.
   c. Extensibility can be used synonymously with compliance.
   d. Physical properties of grafts are a function of the superficial dermal or laminar area.
2. In tissue transfer terms, which of the following statements concerning grafts is TRUE?
   a. The process of take is more than 48 hours.
   b. A graft is tissue that is excised from a donor site that reestablishes its blood supply by revascularization.
   c. During inosculation, the first phase of take, the graft exists at below core body temperature.
   d. Conditions of take are a reflection of only the graft host bed (e.g., scarring, infection).
3. With regard to the microanatomy of the grafts using skin as a model, which of the following statements is TRUE?
   a. The intradermal plexus is at the interface of the superficial dermis and the deep dermis.
   b. The subdermal plexus is carried at the juncture of the deep dermis and the underlying tissue.
   c. The lymphatics are most richly distributed in the adventitial dermis.
   d. The adventitial dermis, because of its collagen content, accounts for the majority of the physical characteristics.
4. Grafts of all kinds can be termed *split thickness* or *full thickness*. Choose the best answer below with regard to these.
   a. A split-thickness skin graft exposes the vessels of the subdermal plexus.
   b. Exposing the subdermal plexus conveys less fastidious vascular characteristics.
   c. Mesh grafts are created by cutting slits in the epidermis or epithelium.
   d. A full-thickness skin graft is fastidious because of the nature of the subdermal plexus, among other variables.
5. With regard to the grafts used most commonly in genitourinary reconstructive surgery, which of the following statements is TRUE?
   a. Thin full-thickness skin is an optimal replacement for the tunica albuginea of the corpora cavernosa.
   b. Bladder epithelial graft is fastidious because of the nature of the superficial lamina.
   c. Buccal mucosa graft is thought to have a panlaminar plexus.
   d. Tunica vaginalis graft has proved to be a very reliable one for single-stage urethral reconstruction.
6. If a flap is classified according to elevation technique, which of the following statements is TRUE?
   a. All peninsula flaps would by definition be a random flap.
   b. An island flap would by definition be an axial flap.
   c. A true island flap could also be called a paddle.
   d. The microvascular free transfer flap relies on the principle of flap delay.
7. With regard to the anatomy of the penile shaft, which of the following statements is TRUE?
   a. Throughout most of the length of the penis, the septum is a true competent septum.
   b. The erectile tissues of the normal corpora cavernosa are separated from the tunica by the space of Smith.
   c. The dorsal arteries of the penis are carried in envelope fashion in the dartos fascia.
   d. The Buck's fascia is loosely areolar and lies immediately beneath the skin.
8. According to consensus, the urethra should be divided into six entities. Which of the following statements is most accurate?
   a. The fossa navicularis is that portion of the urethra that is most dorsally displaced with regard to the surrounding spongy erectile tissue.
   b. The bulbous urethral portion is invested by the thickest portion of the corpus spongiosum.
   c. The bulbous urethra at its proximal extent is part of the posterior urethra.
   d. The membranous urethra is invested by the most proximal aspect of the corpus spongiosum.

9. With regard to the arterial vascularization of the deep structures of the penis, which of the following statements is TRUE?
   a. The circumflex cavernosal arteries are uniform in number and distribution.
   b. The arteries to the bulb arborize into the spongy erectile tissue of the glans.
   c. The common penile artery represents the end continuation of the deep internal pudendal artery.
   d. The common penile artery divides to become the cavernosal artery and the dorsal arteries, after giving off the circumflex cavernosal arteries.
10. With regard to the innervation to the penis, which of the following statements is TRUE?
    a. The cavernosal nerves are purely parasympathetic and are the extensions of the nervi erigentes.
    b. The pudendal nerves accompany the vessels as they run through the obturator foramen.
    c. The dorsal nerve arises in Alcock's canal as a branch of the pudendal nerve.
    d. The dorsal nerves throughout their course are prominent, large nerve bundles.
11. With regard to Colles' fascia, which of the following statements is TRUE?
    a. Colles' fascia is the perineal component of Camper's fascia.
    b. Colles' fascia attaches at its posterior margin to the midline fusion of the ischial cavernosus muscle.
    c. Colles' fascia joins with the dartos fascia (tunica dartos) of the scrotum.
    d. Colles' fascia becomes contiguous with Buck's fascia in the posterior triangle of the perineum.
12. With regard to the anterior triangle of the perineum, which of the following statements is TRUE?
    a. The ischiocavernosus muscles laterally attach to the inner surface of the ischium and insert in the midline into Buck's fascia.
    b. The bulbous spongiosum muscles (midline fusion of the ischial cavernosus muscles) insert posteriorly to the anal sphincter.
    c. The perineal body represents a confluence of fascial structures.
    d. The perineal body has a prominent neurovascular pedicle within it that provides autonomic innervation to the pelvic diagram.
13. Select the correct statement from below.
    a. When one encounters the endoscopic findings consistent with urethral hemangioma, one must be alert to exclude the diagnosis of urethral carcinoma.
    b. Laser therapy has been very successfully employed for the management of large urethral hemangiomas.
    c. Reiter's syndrome includes the triad of stomatitis, arthritis, and urethritis.
    d. In Reiter's syndrome, the urethritis is usually mild and self-limiting.
14. Select the correct statement from below.
    a. Lichen sclerosus (BXO) is the genital manifestation of psoriasis.
    b. Lichen sclerosus (BXO) is a disease of middle-aged adults and is virtually never seen in younger adults or adolescents.
    c. Amyloidosis is a rare disease involving the urethra. It presents as a urethral mass, and patients may experience hematuria, dysuria, or urethral obstruction.
    d. In most cases in patients presenting with amyloidosis aggressive excision is often required.
15. Which of the following statements concerning urethral fistula associated with hypospadias repair is TRUE?
    a. Fistula closure, in the majority of cases, requires tissue transfer.
    b. In acute fistulas, resuturing and reinstitution of diversion should be considered.
    c. Fistulas associated with inflammatory strictures usually resolve with aggressive antibiotic therapy.
    d. Fistulas often recur, not because of a problem at the fistula site but because of stenosis or obstruction distal to the fistula site.
16. With regard to urethral meatal stenosis in childhood, which of the following statements is TRUE?
    a. Meatal stenosis is a frequent complication of phimosis.
    b. Meatal stenosis is frequently associated with upper tract changes, and all patients should be evaluated with ultrasonography and voiding cystourethrography.
    c. When ammoniacal meatitis is noted, often a short course of meatal dilation and steroid cream application will resolve the problem.
    d. When meatal stenosis is present, usually a dorsally based Y-V advancement flap repair is preferred.
17. When one is treating a patient with penile amputation, which of the following statements is TRUE?
    a. Replantation is not a consideration in self-inflicted injury, because most of these patients are chronically psychotic and will eventually try to amputate the penis again.
    b. If the distal part of the penis is not available, even if the amputation involves mostly skin with much of the shaft preserved, it is recommended that the remaining shaft be buried in the scrotum.
    c. The classic technique for replantation involves coaptation of the dorsal nerve, the deep dorsal vein, and the cavernosal arteries.
    d. The McRoberts technique of macro-replantation is not the preferred method of management for these patients, but when the situation warrants it, it is very successful.
18. With regard to the management of external trauma, which of the following statements is TRUE?
    a. Because of the nature of the genital tissues, aggressive initial débridement must be undertaken.
    b. The eventual effect of a genital burn may be to unacceptably tether and/or incarcerate the penis.
    c. The gracilis flap is ideally suited for coverage of large perineal or groin wounds.
    d. Complications of direct irradiation to the penis can usually be resolved with split-thickness skin grafts.
19. Concerning genital lymphedema, which of the following statements is TRUE?
    a. Reconstruction for lymphedema that is the consequence of the indirect effects of radiation is best accomplished with excision of the tissues and coverage with split-thickness skin grafts (STSGs).
    b. In reconstruction for lymphedema, it is essential to maintain the parietal tunica vaginalis of the testes intact with grafting over that location.
    c. When considering reconstruction for lymphedema, full-thickness skin grafts (FTSGs) are preferable because of the distribution of the lymphatics in the superficial (adventitial) dermis.
    d. In the case of genital lymphedema, it is not unusual for the immune response of the tissues to be altered and for patients to have significant involvement with genital papillomas.

20. Which of the following statements is most accurate concerning urethral stricture disease?

   a. It causes limitation of the urethral lumen because of the bulk of the scar.
   b. It most often is limited to the urethral epithelium.
   c. It implies a scarring process, usually involving both the epithelium and the underlying spongy erectile tissue of the corpora cavernosa.
   d. It causes limitation of the urethral lumen because of contraction and noncompliance of the scar.

21. Which of the following statements concerning posterior "urethral stricture" is TRUE?

   a. It involves the tissues of the epithelium as well as the underlying erectile tissues of the corpora cavernosa.
   b. It involves the tissues of the epithelium as well as the underlying erectile tissue of the corpus spongiosum.
   c. It is not a true stricture but rather fibrosis that results from distraction of the urethra.
   d. The stricture process can often be occult because of the unpredictable involvement of the urethral tissues.

22. Which of the following statements regarding strictures resulting from LS/BXO is true?

   a. They are usually associated with the scarring extending deeply into the corpus spongiosum.
   b. They usually begin as meatal stenosis associated with ammoniacal balanitis.
   c. They often resolve with the use of antibiotics.
   d. The process has been definitively shown to be the result of infectious inflammation of the urethral tissues caused by *Borrelia burgdorferi.*

23. When the urologist is treating a patient in retention or a patient experiencing difficult catheter placement, which of the following statements is TRUE?

   a. Endoscopy defines the nature of the difficulty.
   b. The patient can usually be effectively treated with filiform follower dilation.
   c. Optimal management may mean placement of a suprapubic catheter.
   d. Imaging results are usually not informative.

24. In determining the anatomy of the stricture, all of the following provide useful information EXCEPT which one?

   a. MRI
   b. High-resolution ultrasonography
   c. Contrast studies
   d. Urethroscopy

25. With regard to the modalities for evaluation of the urethra, which of the following statements is TRUE?

   a. Extravasation of contrast material during retrograde urethrography inevitably implies poor technique.
   b. Distention of the urethra during ultrasonographic study often confuses findings.
   c. Contrast material suitable for intravenous injection should be used for all retrograde urethra studies.
   d. Contrast material thickened with lubricating gels better define the stricture length.

26. With regard to planning of reconstruction for urethral stricture, which of the following statements is TRUE?

   a. Even if a patient does not have retention, placement of a suprapubic tube may help define strictured areas.
   b. Tightly stenotic areas should be dilated to pass endoscopes proximally.
   c. The effects of hydrodilation are manifested most immediately distal to the area of narrowest stenosis.
   d. Calibration of strictured areas to 16 Fr or greater reliably predicts the potential for segments to contract.

27. With regard to direct visual internal urethrotomy, which of the following statements is TRUE?

   a. Strictures are best incised at the 12-o'clock position because of the efficiency of most urethrotomies when used in this orientation.
   b. It can be associated with erectile dysfunction.
   c. In optimally selected patients, long-term success of internal urethrotomy is approximately 90%.
   d. Internal urethrotomy should be the first procedure considered for any stricture of the anterior urethra.

28. Concerning permanently implanted urethral stents, which of the following statements is TRUE?

   a. Long-term follow-up (10- and 11-year data) shows that if a permanently implanted stent is patent at 4.0 to 4.5 years, then long-term patency can be expected.
   b. Permanently implantable stents are indicated for short strictures of the bulbous urethra and, when so employed, are associated with short-term success in the range of approximately 84%.
   c. They are rarely complicated by persistent perineal pain.
   d. They are useful for short strictures of the pendulous urethra.

29. All of the following are either absolute or strong relative contraindications to the use of the Urolume stent EXCEPT which one?

   a. Distraction injuries of the membranous urethra
   b. Patients who have failed prior substitution urethral reconstruction
   c. Patients with short strictures of the bulbous urethra not associated with significant straddle trauma as the etiology of the stricture
   d. Patients who are younger than 50 years old who are reasonable candidates for urethral reconstruction

30. Concerning anterior urethral reconstruction, which of the following statements is TRUE?

   a. Excision and primary anastomosis treatment is severely limited and useful only for very proximal strictures 1 to 2 cm in length.
   b. Performance of the excision and primary anastomosis technique is facilitated by dissection of the corpus spongiosum to the level of the glans penis.
   c. Success requires total excision of the fibrosis with a widely spatulated anastomosis.
   d. Reconstruction is facilitated by development of the intracrural space with infrapubectomy.

31. With regard to techniques of urethral reconstruction, which of the following statements is TRUE?
    a. The Monseur technique employed the use of mesh split-thickness skin.
    b. Excision with strip anastomosis and onlay (augmented anastomosis) is an excellent form of reconstruction for strictures too long to be dealt with by excision and primary anastomosis only.
    c. The Barbagli operation combines the use of excision with staged augmented anastomosis.
    d. The use of spongioplasty maneuver requires the total excision of all spongiofibrosis.
32. With regard to genital skin flap operations for anterior urethral reconstruction, which of the following statements is TRUE?
    a. Flap operations are best applied as individual techniques and require the surgeon to become intimately familiar with the individual steps of all techniques.
    b. The operation can conceptually become one operation with multidimensional application.
    c. The operations are all based on mobilization of the extended Buck's fascia.
    d. The operations require a comfortable understanding of the extended circumflex iliac superficial vascular pattern.
33. With regard to flap procedures for anterior urethral reconstruction, which of the following statements is TRUE?
    a. The scrotal skin island is a problematic flap and should be avoided at all cost.
    b. The circular skin islands, mechanically, are facilitated by dividing the dartos fascial flaps ventrally.
    c. The "tubed flaps" in general are optimal for cases of short to moderate length strictures.
    d. The length of tubed segments can be limited by the aggressive mobilization of the corpus spongiosum.
34. With regard to strictures associated with lichen sclerosus/BXO, which of the following statements is TRUE?
    a. Urolume has proved to be an excellent option.
    b. Staged skin graft procedures have yielded excellent durable results.
    c. Because lichen sclerosus/BXO is a generalized skin condition, buccal mucosa has been considered for reconstruction with initial encouraging results.
    d. Flap techniques have provided excellent long-term success rates.
35. Which of the following statements concerning urethral distraction injuries is TRUE?
    a. They are usually associated with full-thickness spongiofibrosis.
    b. Although they can involve any part of the membranous urethra, they most frequently occur at the juncture of the membranous urethra with the bulbous urethra.
    c. They can be partial, and this difference is easily defined by contrast studies.
    d. They are best managed with an aligning catheter placed to traction.
36. Membranous urethral distraction injuries are:
    a. optimally first evaluated with contrast studies.
    b. often evaluated with an endoscope in the anterior urethra and a cystogram with the patient straining to void.
    c. always defined with simultaneous cystogram and retrograde urethrogram.
    d. always complicated by postoperative incontinence when contrast material is seen in the posterior urethra.
37. With regard to continence after reconstruction for membranous urethral distraction, which of the following statements is TRUE?
    a. Location of the injury along the course of the membranous urethra is not associated with continence postoperatively.
    b. Continence can be accurately predicted by contrast studies.
    c. Continence is best predicted by the appearance of the bladder neck on endoscopy.
    d. Continence is best addressed after a procedure to reestablish urethral continuity is performed.
38. All of the following maneuvers facilitate reconstruction of pelvic fracture urethral distraction injuries without creating chordee or foreshortening of the penis EXCEPT:
    a. development of the intracavernosal (intracrural) space.
    b. infrapubectomy.
    c. mobilization of the proximal corpus spongiosum.
    d. division of the attachment of the bulbospongiosum to the perineal body.
39. With regard to failures of reconstruction of posterior urethral distraction primary anastomotic technique, which of the following statements is TRUE?
    a. Most failures are due to technical anastomotic procedures.
    b. Long-segment failures are readily amenable to direct-vision internal urethrotomy with Urolume placement.
    c. Patients with one intact pudendal artery are at risk for ischemic stenosis of the corpus spongiosum.
    d. Patients with reconstitution of an injured pudendal vessel, even if reconstitution was a unilateral phenomenon, are excellent candidates for posterior urethral reconstruction.
40. In dealing with the entity of chordee without hypospadias, which of the following statements is TRUE?
    a. Correction of curvature is often achieved with mobilization of the corpus spongiosum alone.
    b. It often can be corrected with maneuvers that lengthen the foreshortened ventral skin.
    c. There is a stepwise progression of ventral dissection of dysgenetic tissues, correction of skin tethering, elevation of mobilization of the corpus spongiosum, midline ventral septotomy, and often dorsal plication.
    d. Division of the urethral is virtually always indicated.
41. With regard to congenital curvature of the penis, which of the following statements is TRUE?
    a. If length is an issue, the patient probably is more correctly characterized as having chordee without hypospadias.
    b. It is optimally managed with incision and grafting to avoid foreshortening of the penis.
    c. In most cases, despite dissection and incision of tissues that appear inelastic, most patients require incision with grafting.
    d. Correction is facilitated by tourniquet occlusion during artificial erections.
42. With regard to acquired curvatures of the penis that are not Peyronie's disease, which of the following statements is TRUE?
    a. Most are characterized by prominent dorsal scars.
    b. In most cases, global cavernosal veno-occlusive dysfunction (CVOD) is not a complicating factor.
    c. They are virtually never associated with "minimal" buckling trauma.
    d. Patients often have significant penile foreshortening.

ANSWERS

1. **a. They are a function of the collagen-elastin architecture as it is suspended in a mucopolysaccharide matrix.** All tissue has inherent physical characteristics, and those are extensibility, inherent tissue tension, and the vesicoelastic properties of stress relaxation and creep. The physical characteristics of a transferred unit are primarily a function of the helical arrangement of collagen along with the elastin cross-linkages. The collagen-elastin architecture is suspended in a mucopolysaccharide matrix that influences the vesicoelastic properties. The physical properties of skin and the other grafts appropriate for urethral reconstruction are by and large a function of the deep laminar or dermal layer. It is that layer that has the most abundant number of collagen elastin architecture.
2. **b. A graft is tissue that is excised from a donor site that reestablishes its blood supply by revascularization.** Tissue can be transferred as a graft (see Fig. 33-1). The term *graft* implies that tissue has been excised and transferred to a graft host bed, where a new blood supply develops via a process that has been termed *take*. Take requires approximately 96 hours and occurs in two phases. The initial phase, termed *imbibition*, takes about 48 hours, and during that phase the graft survives by 'drinking' nutrients from the adjacent graft host bed. During that phase, the graft temperature is less than core body temperature. The second phase, termed *inosculation*, also requires about 48 hours and is the phase during which true microcirculation is reestablished in the graft. During that phase, the temperature of the graft rises to core body temperature. Processes that interfere with the vascularity of the graft host bed thus interfere with graft take. The process of take is also influenced by the nature of the grafted tissue. Thus a split-thickness unit in most cases is much less fastidious from a vascular standpoint and also much less fastidious from the standpoint of total mass of the grafted tissue. However the tradeoff with split-thickness tissue is that it does not generally carry "the physical characteristics" and is thus prone to contraction. All of these conditions must be recognized and included in the planning process when one elects a form of reconstruction (i.e. primary versus staged).
3. **b. The subdermal plexus is carried at the juncture of the deep dermis and the underlying tissue.** The superficial plexus or intradermal plexus is carried at approximately the interface of the epithelium and the superficial dermis. The subdermal plexus exists at the interface of the deep dermis and the subcutaneous tissues. That skin is termed the *reticular dermis*. The superficial dermis and skin is termed the *adventitial dermis* and is equivalent to the superficial lamina. The majority of the lymphatics are in the deep dermal layer or reticular dermal layer, and this can be compared with the deep laminar layer. The collagen content of that layer is much greater than in the superficial layer. Thus it is that layer that is believed to account for the physical characteristics of the tissue. The intradermal or superficial plexus in most tissues is generally composed of many small vessels. The subdermal layer or deep plexus consists of much more sparsely distributed vessels, which are larger.
In the case of the bladder epithelial graft, the perforators connecting the deep plexus to the superficial plexus are much more frequently distributed than in skin. In buccal mucosa, the layered arrangement is lost and the microvasculature consists of a panlaminar plexus.
4. **d. A full-thickness skin graft is fastidious because of the nature of the subdermal plexus, among other variables.** If a graft is carried as a full-thickness unit (FTG), it carries the covering. It carries the superficial dermis or lamina with all of the characteristics attributable to that layer. In most cases, the plexus (subdermal plexus) is composed of larger vessels that are more sparsely distributed. The graft is thus fastidious in its vascular characteristics.
5. **c. Buccal mucosa graft is thought to have a panlaminar plexus.** In the case of the buccal mucosal graft, there is a panlaminar plexus. In the case of the bladder epithelial graft, there is a superficial and a deep plexus; however, the plexuses are connected by many more perforators. The dermal graft for years has been used to augment the tunica albuginea. Mature vein grafts show evidence of take to the vas vasorum. Other grafts that have been utilized for single-stage urethral reconstruction include rectal mucosa grafts, dermal grafts, and tunica vaginalis graft. The results using dermal grafts and tunica vaginalis grafts are not acceptable, and these grafts are not considered to be good grafts for urethral reconstruction. There are only a small series that have reported the use of rectal mucosal grafts. The precise process of take, to our knowledge, has not been well defined. In recent years, acellular collagen matrix has been proposed as an alternative to the grafts mentioned earlier. The precise mechanism of action of these "grafts" is not well defined. It may well be that these grafts serve as a biologic dressing only and then become placed by lateral ingrowths from the adjacent epithelial layer. The future probably lies in the use of cultured tissues for grafts.
6. **b. An island flap would by definition be an axial flap.** A peninsula flap is a flap in which the vascular and cutaneous continuity of the flap base are left intact. Peninsula flaps can be elevated on either random vasculature or axial vasculature, depending on the location of the donor site (see Fig. 33-3A). An island flap is a flap in which the vascular continuity is maintained; however, the cuticular continuity is divided (see Fig. 33-3B). The microvascular free transfer flap (free flap) (see Fig. 33-3C) has both the vascular continuity and the cuticular continuity interrupted. The vascular continuity is then reestablished at the recipient site. A true island flap is elevated on dangling vessels. The terminology thus should not be confused with what is most commonly used for urethral reconstruction, fascial flaps carrying skin islands or skin paddles (see Fig. 33-4B).
7. **b. The erectile tissues of the normal corpora cavernosa are separated from the tunica by the space of Smith.** The corpora cavernosa are not separate structures but constitute a single space with free communication through an incompetent midline septum, composed of multiple strands of elastic tissue similar to that making up the tunica albuginea. The erectile tissue is separated from the tunica albuginea by a thin layer of areolar connective tissue that was described by Smith. Buck's fascia is directly abutted to the tunica albuginea of the corpora cavernosa. Buck's fascia surrounds the adventitia of the corpora spongiosum in envelope fashion, and the dorsal neurovascular structures are contained in envelope fashion between the superficial and deep laminar of Buck's fascia on the dorsum. Buck's fascia is thus "diverted" to the deep structures (see Figs. 33-5 and 33-8A and B). The dartos fascia is loosely areolar and lies immediately beneath the skin. It is in that fascial layer that the arborizations of the superficial external pudendal vessels and the posterior scrotal vessels are carried (see Fig. 33-8C).
8. **b. The bulbous urethral portion is invested by the thickest portion of the corpus spongiosum.** The fossa navicularis is contained within the spongy erectile tissue of the glans penis and terminates at the junction of the urethral epithelium with the skin of the glans. The bulbous urethra is covered by the midline fusion of the ischiocavernosus musculature and is

invested by the bulbospongiosum of the proximal corpus spongiosum. It becomes larger and lies closer to the dorsal aspect of the corpus spongiosum, exiting from its dorsal surface prior to the posterior attachment of the bulbospongiosum to the perineal body. The membranous urethra is the portion that traverses the perineal pouch and is surrounded by the external urethral sphincter. This segment of the urethra is unattached to fixed structures, has the distinction of being the only portion of the male urethra that is not invested by another structure, and is lined with a delicate transitional epithelium (see Fig. 33-6).

9. **c. The common penile artery represents the end continuation of the deep internal pudendal artery.** The blood supply to the deep structures of the penis is derived from the common penile artery, which is the continuation of the internal pudendal artery after it gives off its perineal branch. From that point on it is termed the *common penile artery*. As it nears the urethral bulb, the artery divides into its three terminal branches as follows: (1) the bulbourethral arteries, which enter the proximal corpus spongiosum; (2) the dorsal artery, which travels along the dorsum of the penis contained in envelope fashion between the superficial and deep lamina of Buck's fascia; and (3) the cavernosal arteries, usually a single artery, which arise and penetrate the corpora cavernosa at the hilum and run the length of the penile shaft. The circumflex cavernosal arteries are given off at varying locations along the dorsal artery, but their distribution is neither uniform nor dependable (see Fig. 33-11).

10. **c. The dorsal nerve arises in Alcock's canal as a branch of the pudendal nerve there.** The cavernosal nerves are a combination of the parasympathetic and visceral afferent fibers that constitute the autonomic nerves of the penis. These provide the nerve supply to the erectile apparatus. The pudendal nerves enter the perineum with the internal pudendal vessels through the lesser sciatic notch at the posterior border of the ischiorectal fossa. They run in the fibrofascial pudendal canal of Alcock to the edge of the urogenital diaphragm (see Fig. 33-5). Each dorsal nerve of the penis arises in Alcock's canal as the first branch of the pudendal nerve. On the shaft, their fascicles fan out to supply proprioceptive and sensory nerve terminals in the tunica of the corpora cavernosa and sensory terminals in the skin.

11. **c. Colles' fascia joins with the dartos fascia (tunica dartos) of the scrotum.** Colles' fascia joins with the dartos fascia (tunica dartos) of the scrotum, and a fold of this fascia projects backward beneath the fibers of the bulbospongiosus muscle. Anteriorly, Colles' fascia fuses and becomes continuous with the membranous layer of the subcutaneous connective tissue of the anterior abdominal wall (Scarpa's fascia) (see Figs. 33-8C and 33-12A).

12. **a. The ischiocavernosus muscles laterally attach to the inner surface of the ischium and insert in the midline into Buck's fascia.** The ischiocutaneous muscles cover the crura of the corpora cavernosa. They attach to the inner surfaces of the ischium and ischial tuberosities on each side and insert at the midline into Buck's fascia, surrounding the crura at their junction below the arcuate ligament of the penis. The bulbospongiosus muscles are located in the midline of the perineum. They are attached to the perineal body posteriorly and to each other in the midline, as they encompass the bulbospongiosum and crura of the corpora cavernosa at the base of the penis. These muscles are confluent with the ischiocavernosus muscles laterally, and at their insertion into Buck's fascia (see Figs. 33-12A to D).

13. **d. In Reiter's syndrome, the urethritis is usually mild and self-limiting.** Because all reported cases of urethral hemangioma have been benign, management is dependent on the size and location of the lesion. For smaller lesions, laser treatment has been successful and produces less scarring. The preferred treatment for larger lesions is open excision and urethral reconstruction. Reiter's syndrome is characterized by a classic triad of arthritis, conjunctivitis, and urethritis. Urethral involvement is usually mild, self-limiting, and a minor portion of the disease.

14. **c. Amyloidosis is a rare disease involving the urethra. It presents as a urethral mass, and patients may present with hematuria, dysuria, or urethral obstruction.** *BXO* has in the past been the term used to describe the genital presentation of lichen sclerosus. By recent consensus conference, the term *BXO* has become synonymous with lichen sclerosus, and lichen sclerosus is the favored terminology. It is the most common cause of meatal stenosis. Lichen sclerosus appears as a whitish plaque that may involve the prepuce, glans penis, urethral meatus, and fossa navicularis. Several reports have suggested the association with chronic infection by a infection with the spirochete *Borrelia burgdorferi*. Although previously thought to be rare, lichen sclerosus (BXO) is commonly found at the time of circumcisions performed beyond the neonatal period. Long-term antibiotic therapy may also be helpful to improve the inflammation because secondary infection of the inflamed tissue may occur. We have typically used tetracycline, but a trial of long-term penicillin (or advanced-generation erythromycin) may be warranted. Amyloidosis, a rare disease, should be considered in the evaluation of any patient with a urethral mass. The differential diagnosis includes urethral neoplasm. Cystoscopy and transurethral biopsy is indicated. Patients may present with hematuria, dysuria, or urethral obstruction. Most patients can be followed expectantly.

15. **d. Fistulas often recur, not because of a problem at the fistula site but because of stenosis or obstruction distal to the fistula site.** Treatment of a urethral fistula must be directed not only toward the defect but also toward the underlying process leading to its development. In cases of urethral reconstruction, especially reconstruction for hypospadias, fistula often occurs or recurs because of distal obstruction and high-pressure voiding. After urethral surgery, fistulas can develop immediately or as delayed complications. Repair of the fistula may be delayed at a minimum of 6 months to allow for complete resolution of the inflammation. Fistulas associated with inflammatory strictures occur as periurethral tracts and develop secondary to high-pressure voiding of infected urine. Repair requires suprapubic drainage, and treatment of the infection requires incision and drainage of any abscesses present. One must be very cautious in treating the patient with urethral fistulas but without a chronic history of obstructive voiding symptoms. In many cases, fistula or periurethral abscess may be the hallmark symptom of urethral carcinoma.

16. **c. When ammoniacal meatitis is noted, often a short course of meatal dilation and steroid cream application will resolve the problem.** Meatal stenosis in the male child appears to be a consequence of circumcision, which allows for ammoniacal meatitis. In children seen with ammoniacal meatitis, we usually start them with meatal dilation using steroid cream. Within a week, the process seems to settle down. Anecdotally, the fusion of the ventral meatus skin, which causes meatal stenosis, seems to be avoided. Because childhood meatal stenosis truly represents a fusion of the ventral urethral meatus, dividing the thin membrane of fusion is preferred (see Fig. 33-16). This leaves the child with a slit-shaped meatus; the use of a dorsal Y-V maneuver can be required in special circumstances, but for most cases it can be avoided and should be because of the cosmetic deformity of the glans that it leaves.

17. **d. The McRoberts technique of macro-replantation is not the preferred method of management for these patients, but when the situation warrants it, it is very successful.** Often the

amputation is self-inflicted, usually during an acute psychotic break. This should not preclude replantation unless the patient adamantly refuses such treatment. Even then, with a court order and the agreement of two or more surgeons, replantation may be undertaken. If possible, microreplantation should be carried out. This technique consists of an anatomic approximation of the tunica albuginea of the corporal bodies, a spatulated two-layer anastomosis of the urethra. The dorsal nerves are coapted using an epineural technique unless the injury is distal, at which point a vesicular coaptation may be required. The dorsal vein is anastomosed, and the dorsal arteries are anastomosed. Anastomosis of the cavernosal arteries is not possible and should not be attempted. If the situation is such that microreplantation cannot be undertaken, then the technique described by McRoberts can be carried out. His series and other series show that a high degree of success can be expected after replantation without microvascular reanastomosis. In most of the patients, however, they will have numbness distal to the replant site. With microreplantation, it is not at all unusual for patients to have excellent sensation distal to the area of injury and to have resumption of normal erectile function.

If the patient presents with the distal part having been disposed of or otherwise unavailable, then the wound should be closed. Often the penis will have been stretched during the amputation and an excess of skin will have been removed, leaving a good length intact with denuded penile shaft structures. In that case, the corporal bodies would be closed, the urethral meatus must be spatulated, and the penis can be immediately covered with a split-thickness skin graft. If the injury involves the testes and the testes are avulsed as part of the injury, replantation is not an option because of the stretch injury to the spermatic vessels (see Fig. 33-22).

18. **b. The eventual effect of a genital burn may be to unacceptably tether and/or incarcerate the penis.** The physiologic functions of genital tissues cannot be accurately duplicated. The unique vascularity of genital tissue allows for less aggressive rather than more aggressive débridement. In many patients, the penis will have become incarcerated in contracted scar tissue after healing of the acute injury. Successful transposition of a gracilis musculocutaneous flap introduces compliant vascular tissue and skin into the area, allowing release of the penile shaft. The gracilis musculocutaneous flap is not particularly well suited for the coverage of large perineal or groin defects; however, the posterior thigh flap offers excellent bulky sensate tissues. Therapeutic radiation can produce chronic suppurative gangrene. These lesions are not amenable to reconstruction.

19. **a. Reconstruction for lymphedema that is the consequence of the indirect effects of radiation is best accomplished with excision of the tissues and coverage with STSGs.** Patients with lymphedema can readily undergo reconstruction. When the lymphedematous tissue has been excised, the testes will be free and, as in a degloving injury, they must be fixed in the midline in an anatomically correct position. The shaft of the penis should be covered with an STSG. If the scrotum cannot be closed, a meshed STSG is utilized to cover the testes, as described. Not uncommonly, these patients have hydroceles, the parietal tunica vaginalis must be excised, and grafting can be done directly onto the visceral tunica vaginalis of the testicles. Unlike the FTSF, split-thickness skin carries little of the reticular dermis and hence few of the lymphatic channels. Reaccumulation of lymphedema will occur within an FTSG and can recur in a thick STSG. In many cases of lymphedema limited to the genitalia, the posterior scrotal skin and the lateral scrotal skin are spared from the lymphedematous process. Thus, in some cases, primary closure after excision can be accomplished using these tissues. If grafting is required, using these tissues to blend the grafts into the groin and perineum technically is much easier. The lymphedematous process involves recurrent cellulitis, lymphedema, and the development of lymphangiectasia. Lymphangiectasia can look like genital papilloma; however, it is a very different process. If there is any question, biopsy can clarify the issue.

20. **d. It causes limitation of the urethral lumen because of contraction and noncompliance of the scar.** The term *urethral stricture* refers to anterior urethral disease. By virtue of the Consensus Conference, obliterative processes of the membranous urethra, such as those associated with pelvic fracture, would be referred to as pelvic fracture urethral distraction defects and other narrowing processes of the posterior urethra are correctly referred to as either contractures or stenoses. Thus the term *urethral stricture* describes a process that involves the urethral epithelium along with the spongy erectile tissue of the corpus spongiosum and this is referred to as spongiofibrosis. In some cases, the scarring process can extend through the tissues of the corpus spongiosum and into the adjacent tissues. It is contraction of the scar that reduces the urethral lumen.

21. **c. It is not a true stricture but rather fibrosis that results from distraction of the urethra.** By virtue of the Consensus Conference, narrowings of the posterior urethra are not referred to as strictures. Those obliterative processes associated with pelvic fracture are termed *pelvic fracture urethral distraction defects* (PFUDD). PFUDD is an obliterative process of the posterior urethra that has resulted in fibrosis and is the defect of distraction of the urethra in that area. Although the distraction defect can be lengthy in some cases, the actual process involving the tissues of the urethra is usually confined.

22. **a. They are usually associated with the scarring extending deeply into the corpus spongiosum.** Some evidence suggests that the progression of the stricture to eventually involve the entire anterior urethra may be due to high-pressure voiding that causes intravasation of urine into the glands of Littre, inflammation of these glands, and, perhaps, microabscesses and deep spongiofibrosis. Whether the urethral changes and eventual fibrosis are also related to bacterial injury, to our knowledge, has not been well defined. Literature does not show resolution of the stricture process with the use of antibiotics. Whereas the spirochete *Borrelia burgdorferi* has been implicated as being involved in lichen sclerosus elsewhere, there is no literature that absolutely implicates it in the process that we see on the genitalia referred to as lichen sclerosus/BXO.

23. **c. Optimal management may mean placement of a suprapubic catheter.** When a patient cannot void, an attempt is made to pass a urethral catheter. If the catheter does not pass, the nature of the obstruction is determined via dynamic retrograde urethrography. Thus, most cases are managed with acute dilation, and clearly there are many instances in which this is not the best course of for the patient. When there is doubt, we determine the nature of the stricture when possible, and not uncommonly we place a suprapubic cystostomy catheter to treat the acute situation and allow time for a more appropriate treatment plan to be devised. Although detailed imaging is not always available, flexible endoscopy is very useful in allowing a glide wire to be passed through the area of stenosis; however, the anatomy of this stricture process is not able to be determined just by endoscopy.

24. **a. MRI.** To devise an appropriate treatment plan, it is important to determine the location, length, depth, and density of the stricture (spongiofibrosis). The length and location of the stricture can be determined using radiographs, urethroscopy, and ultrasonography. The depth and density of

the scar in the spongy tissue can be deduced from the physical examination, the appearance of the urethra in contrast studies, the amount of elasticity noted on urethroscopy, and the depth and density of fibrosis as evidenced by ultrasonographic evaluation of the urethra, although the absolute length of spongiofibrosis may not be evident on ultrasonographic evaluation. MRI has been suggested as useful in patients with pelvic fracture urethral distraction, particularly in cases in which the anatomy of the pelvis has become significantly distorted. With regard to anterior urethral stricture, however, MRI has not been useful, with the exception of those cases in which there is urethral carcinoma. In those cases, MRI can provide invaluable information concerning the spread of the tumor.

25. **c. Contrast material suitable for intravenous injection should be used for all retrograde urethral studies.** Extravasation during retrograde urethrography is possible in patients in whom the urethra is markedly inflamed. For this reason, contrast studies should be carried out with contrast material that is suitable for intravenous injection. Contrast materials that have been thickened with lubricating jelly can be a source of problems and offer little benefit. Real-time ultrasonographic evaluation of the urethra after it has been filled with a lubricating jelly or saline has been described by McAninch. If the patient is not in a steep lateral oblique position for the retrograde urethrogram, the length of the stricture will be underestimated.

26. **a. Even if a patient does not have retention, placement of a suprapubic tube may help define strictured areas.** In selected patients, we have found it useful to place a suprapubic tube to defunctionalize the urethra. After 6 to 8 weeks, if there is going to be constriction of an area that was hydrodilated with voiding, the tendency for that constriction to occur should become apparent. It is imperative, however, to completely evaluate the urethra proximal and distal to the stricture with endoscopy and bougienage during surgery, to ensure that all of the involved urethra is included in the reconstruction. Whereas hydraulic pressure generated by voiding may keep segments proximal to the stricture patent, unless these segments are included in the repair, they are at risk for contraction after obstruction of the narrow caliber segment is relieved with reconstruction. For this reason, any abnormal areas of the urethra that are proximal to a narrow caliber segment of the stricture must be treated with suspicion. If the lumen does not appear to demonstrate evidence of diminished compliance, then we presume that area to be uninvolved in active stricture disease. However, coning down of the urethra suggests its involvement in the scar.

27. **b. It can be associated with erectile dysfunction.** Many surgeons have learned to perform internal urethrotomy by making a single incision at the 12-o'clock position. This location might be questioned, however, based on the location of the urethra within the corpus spongiosum. Distally, although the anterior aspect of the corpus spongiosum is thicker, a deep incision in the more distal aspects of the anterior urethra will certainly enter the corpora cavernosa, and these incisions have been associated with the creation of erectile dysfunction. The most common complication of internal urethrotomy is recurrence of stricture. Less commonly noted complications of internal urethrotomy include bleeding and extravasation of irrigation fluid into the perispongiosal tissues. One report using actuarial technique showed the curative success rate of internal urethrotomy to be 29% to 30% for all comers. Other evaluations have confirmed this success rate. However, there are a number of studies that do show which strictures best respond to internal urethrotomy. These are strictures of the bulbous urethra that are less than 1.5 cm in length and are not associated with dense or deep spongiofibrosis (i.e., straddle injuries). In those particular cases, long-term success has been shown to be 75% to 78%. For strictures outside the bulbous urethra, most studies do not show internal urethrotomy to have long-term success.

28. **b. Permanently implantable stents are indicated for short strictures of the bulbous urethra and, when so employed, are associated with short-term success in the range of approximately 84%.** Removable urethral stents are designed to prevent the process of epithelialization from incorporating the stent into the urethral wall and are left in place for as long as 6 months to a year before being removed. The greatest experience with these removable stents comes from Israel, and centers there report good success in small numbers. Removable urethral stents are currently only available in the United States as part of clinical trials. Permanently implantable stents have been approved for use in the United States for a number of years. Milroy's study shows a success rate of approximately 84% at 4.5 years using the permanently implantable Urolume endourethral stent. That success rate is almost identical to the initial data from the North American study. However, 11-year follow-up from the North American study does not show durability, and overall the success rate is less than 30%. Likewise, long-term data from Germany would indicate that the initial enthusiasm for the use of these stents has waned because of lack of durability. Young patients in particular complain of perineal pain often associated with vigorous activity even when the stent is properly implanted in the bulbous urethra. Placement of the stents in the pendulous portion of the urethra is contraindicated.

29. **c. Patients with short strictures of the bulbous urethra not associated with significant straddle trauma as the etiology of the stricture.** Patients who have had pelvic fracture urethral distraction injuries are not candidates for the use of the Urolume endoprosthesis. The use of the Urolume in these patients is specifically contraindicated. Patients who have undergone prior substitution urethral reconstruction, particularly when skin has been incorporated into the urethra, have been shown to be very poor candidates for implantation with the Urolume endoprosthesis. These patients are a strong relative contraindication. Patients who have had significant urethral straddle trauma have strictures that are associated with deep spongiofibrosis, and these patients are likewise not good candidates for implantation. There are many centers in Europe and South America, where the Urolume has been employed for 15 to 16 years that are now advocating the use of the Urolume endoprosthesis only in patients who are older than 50 years of age and/or who have other significant medical problems that would make the option of open urethral reconstruction less appealing.

30. **c. Success requires total excision of the fibrosis with a widely spatulated anastomosis.** It has now been demonstrated with certainty that the most dependable technique of anterior urethral reconstruction is the complete excision of the area of fibrosis, with a primary reanastomosis of the normal ends of the anterior urethra. The best results are achieved when the following technical points are observed: (1) the area of the fibrosis is totally excised; (2) the urethral anastomosis is widely spatulated, creating a large ovoid anastomosis; and (3) the anastomosis is tension free. With vigorous mobilization, development of the intercrural space, and detachment of the bulbospongiosum from the perineal body, significant lengths of stricture can be excised and reanastomosed. For very proximal bulbous strictures, tension-free anastomosis can be facilitated by the dissection of the membranous urethra. As a rule, the closer the stricture is to the membranous urethra, the longer it can be and still be reconstructed via anastomotic techniques.

The tenet that excision and primary anastomosis should be the goal for all bulbous strictures is one that is being further reinforced by current series published. While guideline lengths of 1 to 2 cm are valuable for planning, most would agree that if excision and primary anastomosis is possible it should be done, and, with aggressive dissection and the maneuvers described earlier, oftentimes strictures much longer than the "guideline lengths" can be so reconstructed.

31. **b. Excision with strip anastomosis and onlay (augmented anastomosis) is an excellent form of reconstruction for strictures too long to be dealt with by excision and primary anastomosis only.** A number of grafts have been used for reconstruction as follows: (1) full-thickness skin graft; (2) split-thickness skin graft for staged techniques; (3) the bladder epithelial graft; (4) the buccal mucosal grafts; and (5) in small series the rectal mucosal graft. The place of the acellular matrixes as well as cultured tissues is being studied at a number of institutions. Early reports are quite favorable, but long-term follow-up is lacking, and series size at this point is small.

    Monseur described a technique in which the urethra was opened on the dorsum and was then sewn open. Barbagli modified that operation by adding a graft to the opened stricturotomy. The place for spongioplasty has been debated. Spongioplasty is really only appropriate in the bulbous urethra, and certainly spongioplasty cannot be utilized if there is extensive spongiofibrosis involving the bulbospongiosum.

32. **b. The operation can conceptually become one operation with multidimensional application.** A number of applications of genital skin islands, mobilized on either the dartos fascia of the penis or the tunica dartos of the scrotum, have been proposed for repair of urethral stricture disease. In the past, these flap operations were considered to be separate procedures. We suggest that all of these procedures are really different applications of a single concept, proposed by the microinjection studies of Quartey. Skin islands, as mentioned, can be viewed as passengers on fascial flaps, and the design of flaps for urethral reconstruction can be paralleled to the design of flaps for reconstruction in general. These procedures utilizing skin islands oriented on the penile dartos fascia have been also useful for reconstruction of the fossa navicularis. There are three important considerations for the use of flaps in urethral reconstruction: (1) the nature of the flap tissue; (2) the vasculature of the flap; and (3) the mechanics of flap transfer. The skin must be nonhirsute for urethral reconstruction. In addition, for donor site consideration, it is most convenient to use the areas of redundant nonhirsute genital skin.

33. **d. The length of tubed segments can be limited by the aggressive mobilization of the corpus spongiosum.** The literature has made it clear that onlay procedures (graft or flap) are attended with a higher success rate than are tubularized skin islands. Tubularized grafts and skin islands should therefore be avoided, if possible. When tubularized segments cannot be avoided, the length of these segments can be limited by combining aggressive mobilization and excision. Tubularized flaps, without question, provide better results than tubularized grafts. There are now few small series that seek to avoid tubed flap reconstruction by using the combination of a graft spread-fixed to "reestablish the urethral plate" combined with flap onlay. At this point, there is only short follow-up but that short follow-up does suggest better results than pure tubed flap reconstruction.

34. **c. Because lichen sclerosus/BXO is a generalized skin condition, buccal mucosa has been considered for reconstruction with initial encouraging results.** Special mention must be made regarding reconstruction for strictures associated with LS/BXO. With the advent of flap techniques, many centers embraced these techniques for these strictures. However, analysis of results of these patients from several large centers has shown a very high recurrence rate. Because of that, these centers adjusted by applying staged graft techniques. Interestingly, staged graft techniques using skin grafts again had a very high recurrence rate on a number of analyses. It is theorized that because LS/BXO is a skin condition, the use of skin as a flap, a single-stage graft, or a staged graft does not preclude involvement of the skin with the LS/BXO inflammatory process. At the time of this writing, this center has completed a cursory assessment of our series of patients with LS/BXO-associated strictures who underwent reconstruction with flap-skin island techniques and skin graft. Preliminary results at our center are not as dismal as from other centers, but the success rate is clearly less (approximately 60%) than for non–LS/BXO-associated strictures. At present, a number of centers now believe that, for reconstruction of stricture associated with LS/BXO, staged buccal graft techniques should be employed. Short follow-up suggests better success with this approach.

35. **b. Although they can involve any part of the membranous urethra, they most frequently occur at the juncture of the membranous urethra with the bulbous urethra.** Urethral distraction injuries are the result of blunt pelvic trauma and accompany about 10% of pelvic fracture injuries. Although it is possible to totally disrupt the urethra with a straddle injury, these injuries most commonly involve only the bulbous urethra. Distraction injuries of the membranous urethra have been compared to plucking an apple (prostate) off its stem (the membranous urethra). This analogy implies that the injury most frequently occurs at the apex of the prostate. Experience shows that this is not the case, however, and the most frequent point of distraction is at the departure of the membranous urethra from the bulbospongiosum. In the postpubescent male, the injury seldom involves the prostatic urethra. In the prepubescent male, in whom the prostatic urethra is more fragile, the injury can extend into that area. Many injuries appear not to totally distract the entire circumference of the urethra. Instead, a strip of epithelium is left intact. In these patients, the placement of an aligning catheter may allow the urethra to heal virtually unscarred or with an easily managed stricture. Because of flexible endoscopy equipment, placement of an aligning catheter is relatively straightforward. Because of the ready availability of flexible cystoscopes, some centers are now evaluating acutely these injuries only with endoscopy. Aligning catheters are just what the name implies, a guide, not a mechanism for placing traction on the bladder and prostate.

36. **a. optimally first evaluated with contrast studies.** Although location of the distraction injury has been demonstrated to be an important factor in continence after reconstruction, this information should be a factor only in patient counseling before the reconstruction and not in the treatment approach. The length of the defect is an important consideration and must be determined as precisely as possible. Lack of contrast material in the posterior urethra gives some information, albeit inconclusive, about the integrity of the bladder neck. When the patient is successfully relaxing to void and the cystogram outlines the posterior urethra, a simultaneous retrograde urethrogram nicely outlines the length of the distraction defect. However, this situation is the exception rather than the rule, and retrograde urethrograms are most useful for determining whether the anterior urethra is normal. If the anterior urethra is normal, it has been our experience as well as that of others that a successful anastomotic repair is ensured. In fact, a primary anastomosis has been shown to be possible even with some involvement of the anterior urethra. Thus, primary anastomosis is unquestionably the goal in all of these patients

until it is proved impossible to do. When the proximal urethra is not visualized on simultaneous cystogram with urethrogram, endoscopy through the suprapubic tract in combination with retrograde urethrogram can be used to outline the defect.

37. **d. Continence is best addressed after a procedure to reestablish urethral continuity is performed.** We have found, and others have reported, that the competence of the bladder neck is difficult to accurately assess before the reestablishment of urethral continuity. Even in cases in which an obvious scar is noted to involve the bladder neck, follow-up of these patients after the urethral reconstruction establishes continuity of the urethra has found many patients with more than adequate continence. Still other patients are believed to have incontinence due to scar incarceration of the bladder neck. In our experience, however, this is an infrequent occurrence and the appearance of the bladder neck by any modality available is not predictive of continence. It is currently our practice to reestablish the continuity of the urethra, and in cases in which there are concerns about continence, to forewarn the patient before the urethral reconstruction.

38. **d. division of the attachment of the bulbospongiosum to the perineal body.** Development of the intracrural space, mobilization of the corpus spongiosum, infrapubectomy, and if needed, rerouting of the corpus spongiosum all shorten the course that the corpus spongiosum must traverse and allow for reconstruction without attendant chordee. Division of the attachments of the bulbospongiosum to the perineal body is, in fact, the maneuver that facilitates anterior urethral reconstruction. Whereas some centers prefer to divide the corpus spongiosum very proximally during the mobilization of the corpus spongiosum, the most favored mechanism mobilizes the entire bulbospongiosum, divides the proximal blood supply if it has not been disrupted by the trauma itself, and divides then through the area of the distraction fibrosis (see Figs. 33-44 to 33-47).

39. **d. Patients with reconstitution of an injured pudendal vessel, even if reconstitution was a unilateral phenomenon, are excellent candidates for posterior urethral reconstruction.** With the techniques discussed, or similar techniques, curative rates for reconstruction of posterior urethral distraction injuries are in the high 90% range according to the work of the authors. Failures are not, in large centers, due to technical problems (i.e., anastomotic restenosis). In general, failures are indicative of ischemia of the proximal corpus spongiosum with ensuring stenosis of the mobilized corpus spongiosum. We found that many patients had evidence of either unilateral or bilateral pudendal artery lesions but that most had evidence of vascular reconstitution. We found that patients with an intact pudendal artery on one side often were potent and were reliably cured with reconstruction. We found that patients with only reconstituted vessels, either unilateral or bilateral, never were potent but were reliably reconstructed.

40. **c. There is a stepwise progression of ventral dissection of dysgenetic tissues, correction of skin tethering, elevation of mobilization of the corpus spongiosum, midline ventral septotomy, and often dorsal plication.** Patients with chordee without hypospadias usually present with either ventral curvature or ventral curvature associated with torsion. In many cases, there are abnormalities of the ventral penile skin. In patients who have chordee without hypospadias, the photograph will reveal an erect penis commensurate with the size of the detumesced penis, whereas in the congenital curvature patient the erect penis will be noticeably large. Many of our patients are also evaluated preoperatively by our sex therapy colleague. Because of their congenital anomaly, these patients often become relatively reclusive and have poor self and genital images. Even in patients with obvious abnormalities of the corpus spongiosum (i.e., poor ventral fusion or frank bifid corpus spongiosum), wide mobilization usually reveals that it is not the corpus spongiosum that remains as the ventral limiting factor. In most patients, the penis will remain curved due to the inelasticity of the ventral aspect of the corpora cavernosa. If the epithelial tube has served as an adequate urethra (i.e., it is not stenotic), the morbidity of the urethral division and subsequent need for urethral reconstruction must be considered before undertaking such a procedure. In children, after mobilization and excision of the dysgenetic tissues, the residual chordee can usually be corrected by making a longitudinal incision with a sharp blade. If this maneuver is not sufficient, the dorsal neurovascular structures can be mobilized in concert with Buck's fascia and a small ellipse or ellipses of dorsal tunica albuginea excised and closed with watertight plicating sutures.

41. **a. If length is an issue, the patient probably is more correctly characterized as having chordee without hypospadias.** Patients with congenital curvature of the penis can have ventral, lateral (which is most often to the left), and/or unusually dorsal curvature. Patients usually present as otherwise healthy young men between the ages of 18 and 30. Many of these patients will have noticed curvature before puberty but will have presumed it to be normal. With puberty, however, they discover that the curvature is not normal. We do not routinely recommend a tourniquet device because constricting devices can conceal the proximal limits of the curvature. This is of most significance in cases of ventral curvatures that frequently extend proximally. In patients with ventral curvature, there may be some illusion of thickening of the dartos fascia and Buck's fascia, and in those patients, the fibrous tissue is mobilized and completely excised. After these issues are excised, the artificial erection is repeated and an occasional patient will have a completely straightened curvature. Most patients, however, suffer from a differential elasticity between the dorsal and ventral aspects of the corporal bodies, and although the curvature may have been lessened, it will persist, unless further procedures are done to straighten the penis. Because the size of the erect penis is usually not a problem in these cases of congenital curvature, we have chosen the second option. If the patient falls into the category of chordee without hypospadias, if shortness of the penis is an issue, we do not hesitate to use incisions with grafts to correct the curvature.

42. **b. In most cases, global cavernosal veno-occlusive dysfunction (CVOD) is not a complicating factor.** When a young man presents with an acquired curvature of the penis, one must always allow the possibility of Peyronie's disease. Occasionally, however, a patient or his initial care physician will ignore the stigmata of the trauma (often described as "minimal" by patients), and the patient will present with a noticeable lateral scar that causes both indentation of the lateral aspect of the penis and, in some cases, curvature. Patients who had preexisting lateral curvature may actually notice that their penis has been straightened by the trauma, but they are disturbed by the concavity caused by the scar. The pathology of a subclinical fracture of the penis is believed to be due to either the disruption of the outer longitudinal layer of the tunica albuginea during the buckling trauma only or the disruption of both layers of the tunica albuginea during buckling trauma but with preservation of Buck's fascia. These patients usually have normal erectile function, and there is no association with concomitant global CVOD. However, the association of CVOD and trauma of the penis continues to be seen, and some patients after fracture-type injuries of the penis will have significant problems with erectile dysfunction. These injuries

are not associated with shortening of the penis. It is the lack of erectile dysfunction and penile shortening that help distinguish these patients from those with Peyronie's disease. Although foreshortening of the penis is not a characteristic of either the injury itself or the resulting scar in either of these injuries, these patients are not thought to be best treated by approaching the opposite aspect of the scar and excising an ellipse of the tunica. This would result in bilateral scars, which will cause bilateral indentation of the penis, and although the penis will have been straightened by the correction, most patients are upset by the cosmetic and functional result of a near-circumferential indentation of the penis.

34

Surgery of Scrotum and Seminal Vesicles

JAY I. SANDLOW • HOWARD N. WINFIELD • MARC GOLDSTEIN

QUESTIONS

1. Which of the following vessels has the least direct contribution to the arterial supply of the vas deferens?
   a. Deferential artery
   b. Internal spermatic artery
   c. Superior vesicle artery
   d. Inferior epigastric artery
   e. Inferior epididymal artery
2. All of the following are reasons to utilize bilateral incisions when performing a vasectomy EXCEPT when:
   a. there is very little chance of dividing the same side twice.
   b. the longer testicular vasal remnant may decrease the likelihood of post-vasectomy congestive epididymitis.
   c. the time to azoospermia is decreased as compared with single incision.
   d. the longer testicular vasal remnant may make subsequent reversal more successful.
   e. All of the above are reasons to utilize bilateral incisions.
3. The best reason for utilizing the no-scalpel vasectomy technique is:
   a. it has a higher success rate than standard vasectomy with incision.
   b. patients are rendered sterile in less time.
   c. it is easier to learn than the standard technique.
   d. it results in a lower rate of complications, including hematoma and infection.
   e. it results in a higher rate of reversibility.
4. What is the estimated percentage of men who develop antisperm antibodies after vasectomy?
   a. 0% to 20%
   b. 20% to 40%
   c. 40% to 60%
   d. 60% to 80%
   e. >80%
5. Which of the following is an indication for repeat vasectomy?
   a. Painless sperm granuloma
   b. Motile sperm found in semen analysis 3 months after vasectomy
   c. Nonmotile sperm found in semen analysis 3 months after vasectomy
   d. Persistent testicular pain 3 months after vasectomy
   e. None of the above
6. After vasectomy, where in the reproductive tract does most of the pressure-induced injury occur?
   a. Testis
   b. Ejaculatory duct
   c. Epididymis
   d. Vas deferens
   e. Seminal vesicles
7. In discussing the management options for an adult with bilateral cryptorchidism, which of the following is correct?
   a. The patient has no chance of fathering children.
   b. Bilateral orchiopexy should be considered.
   c. Bilateral orchiectomy should be the treatment of choice.
   d. The patient should be counseled that he is at no greater risk for testicular cancer than the general population.
   e. Nothing should be done.
8. In the management of chronic orchialgia, which of the following statements is TRUE?
   a. Imaging studies are not indicated.
   b. Varicocele is never causative.
   c. Orchiectomy almost always relieves the pain.
   d. Denervation of the cord may offer relief in selected cases.
   e. Diagnostic epididymal puncture should be performed to rule out chronic epididymitis.
9. Which of the following is TRUE regarding hydrocelectomy?
   a. Hematoma is the least frequent complication.
   b. Jaboulay's bottleneck operation is associated with a high recurrence rate.
   c. Lord's plication is an ideal operation for longstanding postinfectious hydroceles.
   d. Sclerotherapy is the treatment of choice for young men of reproductive age.
   e. Jaboulay's bottleneck operation is associated with a low recurrence rate.

10. A nontransilluminating, nontender mass is noted in the epididymis on physical examination and confirmed to be solid by sonography. What is the most likely diagnosis?
    a. Epididymal cyst
    b. Adenomatoid tumor
    c. Spermatocele
    d. Testicular tumor
    e. Hydrocele
11. Which of the following is TRUE regarding retractile testes in adults?
    a. As in children, surgical repair is never indicated.
    b. A dartos pouch operation is the treatment of choice.
    c. Simple three-stitch orchiopexy of the tunica albuginea to the dartos, as for torsion prophylaxis, is effective in preventing retraction.
    d. Bilateral orchiopexy is necessary for unilateral retractile testis.
    e. Coexisting varicocele is common.
12. All of the following conditions can lead to orchialgia EXCEPT which one?
    a. Sperm granuloma
    b. Vasectomy
    c. Varicocele
    d. Chronic epididymitis
    e. Congenital absence of the vas deferens
13. What is the embryologic origin of the seminal vesicles?
    a. Müllerian duct
    b. Ectodermal ridge
    c. Distal mesonephric duct
    d. Swelling of the distal paramesonephric duct
    e. Neural crest cells
14. What percentage of the ejaculate volume is made up of seminal vesicle secretions?
    a. 5% to 10%
    b. 20% to 30%
    c. 60% to 80%
    d. 90%
    e. The seminal vesicle does not contribute to the seminal plasma volume.
15. What artery is the major blood supply to the seminal vesicle?
    a. Hypogastric
    b. Vesiculodeferential artery
    c. Inferior vesicle
    d. Internal iliac
    e. Deep dorsal penile
16. Decreased T1 signal intensity on MRI along with increased T2 intensity of seminal vesicles is indicative of which process?
    a. Inflammation of the seminal vesicles
    b. Hemorrhage within the seminal vesicles
    c. Seminal vesicle tumors
    d. Seminal vesicle cysts
    e. Normal seminal vesicles
17. Agenesis of the seminal vesicle is associated with significant ipsilateral renal anomalies. What is the embryologic reason for this?
    a. A genetic defect links seminal vesicle agenesis to renal agenesis.
    b. Mutation occurs of the cystic fibrosis transmembrane regulator gene.
    c. There was an insult to the mesonephric duct at approximately 12 weeks' gestation.
    d. There was an embryologic insult to the mesonephric duct earlier than 7 weeks' gestation.
    e. There is no association between agenesis of the seminal vesicle and ipsilateral renal anomalies.
18. What disorder is frequently associated with bilateral agenesis of the seminal vesicles?
    a. Cystic fibrosis
    b. Kartagener's syndrome
    c. Young's syndrome
    d. Kallmann's syndrome
    e. Klinefelter's syndrome
19. What causes the majority of seminal vesicle cysts?
    a. Genetic abnormality
    b. Obstruction of the ejaculatory duct
    c. Inflammation
    d. Renal agenesis
    e. Genetic abnormalities
20. What is the most common type of malignant neoplasm found in seminal vesicles?
    a. Primary adenocarcinoma
    b. Sarcoma
    c. Cystosarcoma phyllodes
    d. Metastatic tumors
    e. Amyloidosis
21. What is the best first test for a suspected seminal vesicle abnormality?
    a. CT
    b. Transrectal ultrasound
    c. MRI
    d. Fine-needle biopsy
    e. Vasography
22. Vasography is useful for providing information regarding all of the following EXCEPT:
    a. presence of seminal vesicle.
    b. level of obstruction of the seminal vesicle and/or ejaculatory duct.
    c. pathology of the seminal vesicle.
    d. epididymal or vasal obstruction.
    e. none of the above.
23. What is the best method to differentiate a benign from malignant seminal vesicle mass?
    a. Biopsy of the lesion
    b. Contrast medium–enhanced CT
    c. Gadolinium-enhanced MRI
    d. Transrectal ultrasound
    e. Rectal examination
24. What is the best surgical approach to a congenital lesion of the seminal vesicle?
    a. The perineal route because this has the quickest recovery
    b. The transcoccygeal route because these are usually large lesions
    c. The laparoscopic route so that the ipsilateral kidney can be dealt with concomitantly and recovery may be shorter
    d. The paravesical route because this has a lower incidence of postoperative erectile dysfunction
    e. The transvesical route because rectal injury is much less likely
25. What is the best indication for the transcoccygeal approach to the seminal vesicle?
    a. Need for exploration of the ipsilateral kidney
    b. Patient with previous suprapubic and/or perineal surgery
    c. Patient wishing to maintain potency
    d. Patient with bilateral large seminal vesicle lesions
    e. None of the above

26. In a patient with a seminal vesicle abscess, the treatment of choice is:

    a. laparoscopic unroofing.
    b. transvesical excision of the seminal vesicle.
    c. aspiration and antibiotic instillation.
    d. endoscopic unroofing via deep transurethral resection.
    e. retropubic approach to unroof the abscess.

27. A strong indication for varix ligation would include:

    a. nonpalpable (subclinical) varices.
    b. varices and adolescent testicular growth retardation.
    c. inguinal/scrotal needle like pain.
    d. presence of varices and an epididymal cyst.
    e. complete absence of sperm in ejaculate.

ANSWERS

1. **c. Superior vesicle artery.** The superior vesicle artery does not supply the vas deferens, whereas all of the other arteries listed have a branch to the vas.
2. **c. the time to azoospermia is decreased as compared with single incision.** Reasons include no chance of dividing the same side twice as there is with a single midline incision; it is much easier to divide the vas far from the testis with bilateral incisions, thus possibly preventing post-vasectomy congestive pain; and the longer the testicular vasal remnant, the greater the likelihood of a successful vasectomy reversal (if desired).
3. **d. it results in a lower rate of complications, including hematoma and infection.** This method eliminates the incision, results in fewer hematomas and infections, and leaves a much smaller wound than conventional methods of accessing the vas deferens for vasectomy.
4. **d. 60% to 80%.** Vasectomy disrupts the blood-testis barrier, resulting in detectable levels of serum antisperm antibodies in 60% to 80% of men.
5. **b. Motile sperm found in semen analysis 3 months after vasectomy.** If any motile sperm are found in the ejaculate 3 months after vasectomy, consideration should be given to repeating the procedure.
6. **c. Epididymis.** The brunt of pressure-induced damage after vasectomy falls on the epididymis and efferent ductules.
7. **b. Bilateral orchiopexy should be considered.** Adults with undescended testes have a substantially increased risk of testis tumors. Although orchiopexy does not reduce that risk, it allows for surveillance. Furthermore, bilateral orchiopexy in adults can result in induction of spermatogenesis and pregnancy.
8. **d. Denervation of the cord may offer relief in selected cases.** Microsurgical total denervation of the spermatic cord is a measure with reported success in 80% of cases in several small series.
9. **e. Jaboulay's bottleneck operation is associated with a low recurrence rate.** The Jaboulay bottleneck operation, in which the sac edges are sewn together behind the cord, reduces the chance of recurrence caused by reapposition of the edges of the hydrocele sac.
10. **b. Adenomatoid tumor.** Most nontransilluminable solid epididymal masses are benign adenomatoid tumors.
11. **b. A dartos pouch operation is the treatment of choice.** Creation of a dartos pouch will keep the testis well down into the scrotum and permanently prevent retraction.
12. **e. Congenital absence of the vas deferens.** Chronic orchialgia can result from vasectomy and its associated effects, such as sperm granuloma. It can also be due to varicocele and chronic infection. However, vasal agenesis is not likely to lead to testicular pain.
13. **c. Distal mesonephric duct.** The seminal vesicle develops as a dorsolateral bulbous swelling of the distal mesonephric duct at approximately 12 fetal weeks.
14. **c. 60% to 80%.** The secretions from the seminal vesicle contribute 60% to 80% of the ejaculate volume.
15. **b. Vesiculodeferential artery.** The blood supply to the seminal vesicle is from the vesiculodeferential artery, a branch of the umbilical artery.
16. **a. Inflammation of the seminal vesicles.** Seminal vesiculitis shows decreased signal intensity on the T1-weighted image, whereas T2-weighted image intensity is higher than that of both fat and the normal seminal vesicle.
17. **d. There was an embryologic insult to the mesonephric duct earlier than at 7 weeks' gestation.** Unilateral agenesis of the seminal vesicles has an incidence of 0.6% to 1% and may be associated with unilateral absence of the vas deferens, as well as ipsilateral renal anomalies. The embryologic insult is believed to occur before 7 weeks' gestation.
18. **a. Cystic fibrosis.** Seventy to 80 percent of men with bilateral absence of the vas deferens or seminal vesicles are carriers of the genetic mutation associated with cystic fibrosis. Conversely, 80% to 95% of men with cystic fibrosis have bilateral absence of the vas deferens or seminal vesicles.
19. **b. Obstruction of the ejaculatory duct.** Cysts of the seminal vesicles may be either congenital or acquired and are thought to be due to obstruction of the ejaculatory duct.
20. **d. Metastatic tumors.** Very few primary tumors of the seminal vesicles have been reported. It is more common for carcinoma of the bladder, prostate, or rectum, or lymphoma, to secondarily involve the seminal vesicles.
21. **b. Transrectal ultrasound.** Transrectal ultrasonography is the preferred initial test for seminal vesicle abnormality, owing to its low invasiveness, ease of performance, and ability to perform concomitant transrectal biopsies.
22. **c. pathology of the seminal vesicle.** Vasography does not provide accurate information of the pathologic condition of the seminal vesicles in patients with vesiculitis, cysts, or tumors.
23. **a. Biopsy of the lesion.** Transrectal ultrasound and biopsy of the seminal vesicle mass is accurate and easily accomplished.
24. **c. The laparoscopic route so that the ipsilateral kidney can be dealt with concomitantly and recovery may be shorter.** Although data are limited for laparoscopic excision of benign seminal vesicle disease alone, this approach appears to afford superb visualization with minimal postoperative morbidity and shorter hospitalization, compared with the open surgical alternatives.
25. **b. Patient with previous suprapubic and/or perineal surgery.** In individuals for whom the perineal or supine position may be difficult to maintain, or for those who have had multiple suprapubic or perineal surgeries, the transcoccygeal approach may be useful.

26. **d. endoscopic unroofing via deep transurethral resection.** If the abscess is in the portion of the seminal vesicle adjacent to the prostate, a deep transurethral resection into the prostatic substance just distal to the bladder neck, at the 5 o'clock or 7 o'clock position, may be effective in relieving the problem.

27. **b. varices and adolescent testicular growth retardation.** Varix ligation is indicated only in patients with clinically apparent varicocele and male factor infertility, adolescent testicular growth retardation, or scrotal pain not attributable to another pathologic process. Treatment of patients with subclinical varices remains controversial.

SECTION VIII

RENAL PHYSIOLOGY AND PATHOPHYSIOLOGY

35

Renal Physiology and Pathophysiology

DANIEL A. SHOSKES • ALAN W. MCMAHON

QUESTIONS

1. Which of the following is true about the AT1 receptor?
   a. More pronounced vasoconstriction on the afferent rather than the efferent arteriole
   b. Receptor for angiotensin I
   c. Protects against ischemia-reperfusion injury by intrarenal dilation
   d. Mediates increased release of aldosterone
   e. Not expressed in the kidney
2. Which of the following statements about endothelin is FALSE?
   a. Stimulation of endothelin-1 (ET-1) decreases sodium excretion.
   b. Endothelin is the most potent vasoconstrictor yet identified.
   c. ET-1 release is inhibited by nitric oxide.
   d. ET-1 release stimulates aldosterone secretion.
   e. ET-1 release reduces renal blood flow.
3. Which of the following is a vasodilator of the renal artery?
   a. Endothelin
   b. Carbon monoxide
   c. Atrial natriuretic peptide
   d. Norepinephrine
   e. Angiotensin II
4. Which of the following is FALSE regarding carbon monoxide and the enzyme HO?
   a. Hemoxygenase-2 (HO-2) is a constitutive enzyme.
   b. HO-1 is an inducible enzyme.
   c. Increased carbon monoxide (CO) increases ischemia-reperfusion injury in the kidney.
   d. HO-1 expression helps to maintain renal medullary blood flow.
   e. HO-1 produces CO through the catabolism of heme.
5. Which of the following regarding erythropoiesis is FALSE?
   a. Reduced erythropoiesis and anemia are common in chronic renal disease.
   b. Erythropoiesis is inhibited by low circulating oxygen tension.
   c. During chronic inflammation, erythropoiesis is decreased.
   d. The kidney makes most of the erythropoietin in the body.
   e. There are erythropoietin receptors in many organs of the body.
6. Which of the following is TRUE about sodium and the kidney?
   a. By definition, hypernatremia is always associated with elevated total body sodium content.
   b. Normal compensation for hyponatremia is decreased ADH secretion and thirst suppression.
   c. Abnormal elevation of serum lipids can lead to a measured false elevation of serum sodium.
   d. If asymptomatic hyponatremia does not improve within 24 hours, intravenous hypertonic saline should be started.
   e. In therapy for symptomatic hyponatremia, the goal should be a normal serum sodium value of 135 mEq/L within 48 hours.
7. The syndrome of inappropriate antidiuretic hormone secretion (SIADH):
   a. is associated with decreased aquaporin expression in the kidney.
   b. is always seen in patients with hypervolemia.
   c. is associated with high total body sodium.
   d. is triggered by low circulating volume.
   e. may be treated with lithium or demeclocycline.

8. Which of the following regarding therapy for hyponatremia is FALSE?
   a. Fluid overload as a result of hypertonic saline infusion should be treated with a loop diuretic such as furosemide.
   b. Too rapid correction can lead to a cerebral demyelination syndrome.
   c. Aggressive therapy should be discontinued when the serum sodium concentration is raised 10% or symptoms subside.
   d. Intranasal desmopressin is a useful adjuvant therapy.
   e. For acute severe hyponatremia with symptoms, a typical infusion rate of hypertonic saline would be 1 mL/kg/hr.
9. Which of the following is TRUE about diabetes insipidus?
   a. May be classified as nephrogenic or urogenic
   b. Associated with inappropriately concentrated urine
   c. Associated with hypervolemia
   d. Associated with mutations of the genes producing aldosterone
   e. Maximum concentrating ability of the kidney is impaired due to loss of the medullary osmotic gradient
10. Which of the following regarding potassium is FALSE?
    a. ACE inhibitors may be a cause of hypokalemia.
    b. Potassium is primarily an intracellular ion.
    c. Acidosis drives potassium out of the cell into the circulation.
    d. High sodium load in the distal tubule promotes potassium excretion.
    e. Upper limit for safe intravenous potassium infusion is 40 mEq/hr.
11. Which of the following regarding hyperkalemia is FALSE?
    a. Hemolysis of the blood sample may falsely elevate the measured potassium.
    b. Hyperkalemia can cause peaked T waves on the ECG.
    c. All patients with a serum potassium value > 5.5 mEq/L require immediate therapy.
    d. Nebulized albuterol can reduce serum potassium by promoting intracellular shift of potassium.
    e. Intravenous calcium does not lower serum potassium but is given to protect the heart from the effects of hyperkalemia.
12. Which of the following is TRUE about acid handling?
    a. Normal pH in the blood is 7.56 to 7.60.
    b. Normal body metabolism produces less than 1000 mmol of acid per day.
    c. All acids produced by metabolism can be excreted by the lungs.
    d. Immediate response to an acid load is through buffers in the blood.
    e. NH_4 is the most important buffer in the blood.
13. Which of the following regarding renal handling of acid is FALSE?
    a. Most bicarbonate is reabsorbed in the distal collecting tubule.
    b. Lungs can excrete volatile acid, but the kidneys must excrete fixed acid.
    c. Carbonic anhydrase catalyzes the production of H^+ and HCO_3^- from H_2O and CO_2.
    d. Chronic respiratory acidosis should lead to increased H^+ in the kidney.
    e. Ammonium ion (NH_4^+) is produced from glutamine, primarily by proximal tubular cells.
14. A patient has a blood pH of 7.2. Which of the following must be TRUE?
    a. The patient has a pure metabolic acidosis.
    b. The patient has a pure respiratory acidosis.
    c. The patient has acidemia.
    d. The patient's blood buffer system is not working.
    e. The patient has a mixed acid-base disturbance.
15. Which of the following is TRUE about acidosis?
    a. Increasing the blood HCO_3^- level increases the anion gap.
    b. Direct bicarbonate loss from the kidney would lead to metabolic acidosis and a normal anion gap.
    c. Lactic acidosis usually presents as a non–anion gap metabolic acidosis.
    d. Appropriate respiratory compensation for a metabolic acidosis is decreased respiration with an increased P_{CO_2}.
    e. It is not possible to have both a respiratory and metabolic acidosis at the same time.
16. Which of the following regarding renal tubular acidosis (RTA) is FALSE?
    a. The hallmark of RTA Type I is a hyperchloremic metabolic acidosis with a high urinary pH (>5.5) in the presence of persistently low serum HCO_3^-.
    b. Type I RTA is also called distal RTA.
    c. Type II RTA is more common in children.
    d. The hallmark of type IV RTA is hypokalemia.
    e. The form of RTA most commonly associated with renal calculi is type I.
17. Which of the following regarding metabolic alkalosis is FALSE?
    a. Paradoxical aciduria may occur due to distal tubule injury.
    b. Excessive nasogastric fluid loss can lead to metabolic alkalosis that is chloride responsive.
    c. Appropriate respiratory compensation is decreased respiration and increased P_{CO_2}.
    d. Hyperaldosteronism can lead to chloride-resistant metabolic alkalosis.
    e. Therapy for chloride responsive metabolic alkalosis requires replacement of chloride AND fluid volume.
18. Which of the following is NOT a function of ADH?
    a. Increase aquaporin-2 insertion into the luminal membrane of the collecting duct
    b. Increase urea transporter insertion into the luminal membrane of the collecting duct
    c. Increase systemic vascular resistance
    d. Increase sodium reabsorption
    e. Increase free water excretion in response to hypernatremia
19. Which of the following is TRUE about vitamin D metabolism?
    a. Vitamin D deficiency is uncommon in chronic renal failure.
    b. Dermally synthesized cholecalciferol is the most potent form of vitamin D.
    c. Dermally synthesized cholecalciferol must be hydroxylated by both the liver and kidney for maximal potency.
    d. Vitamin D activity is mediated through membrane bound vitamin D receptors.
    e. Vitamin D increases renal excretion of calcium.
20. Which of the following regarding parathyroid hormone (PTH) is FALSE?
    a. PTH secretion is increased by hypocalcemia.
    b. PTH secretion is increased by hyperphosphatemia.
    c. PTH receptors are found mainly in bone and kidney.
    d. PTH increases calcium and phosphorus reabsorption in the distal tubule.
    e. PTH helps regulate 1,25(OH)-vitamin D levels by increasing 1α-hydroxylase activity.

21. Which of the following statements regarding renal blood flow (RBF) is TRUE?
    a. RBF is equal in all parts of the kidney.
    b. RBF accounts for 5% to 10% of cardiac output.
    c. Blood enters the glomerulus through the afferent arteriole and exits through the efferent venule.
    d. RBF is similar in men and women.
    e. RBF is one of the determinants of the glomerular filtration rate.

22. All of the following can increase total GFR EXCEPT increased:
    a. RBF.
    b. intraglomerular (hydraulic) pressure.
    c. glomerular permeability.
    d. efferent arteriolar resistance.
    e. functioning nephron number.

23. All of the following are important in GFR regulation EXCEPT:
    a. afferent arteriolar tone.
    b. distal tubule chloride concentrations.
    c. angiotensin II.
    d. nitric oxide.
    e. serum osmolarity.

24. All of the following statements regarding GFR assessment are true EXCEPT:
    a. plasma creatinine is an accurate marker of early reductions in GFR.
    b. inulin clearance is an accurate but impractical measurement of GFR.
    c. 24-hour creatinine clearance overestimates GFR by 10% to 20%.
    d. use of the four variable MDRD formula improves the accuracy of the plasma creatinine.
    e. plasma urea is an unreliable estimate of GFR.

25. Which of the following regarding glucose handling in the kidney is FALSE?
    a. Glucose is freely filtered across the glomerulus.
    b. Glucose reabsorption is facilitated by specific glucose transporters in the PCT.
    c. Glucose reabsorption is linked to bicarbonate reabsorption in the PCT.
    d. Glucose reabsorption is 100% up to plasma glucose levels of 400 mg/dL.
    e. Glucose reabsorption is a passive process.

26. Which of the following about the proximal convoluted tubule is FALSE?
    a. It functions as a bulk transporter, rather than a fine tuner, of ultrafiltrate.
    b. It is able to increase or decrease reabsorption rates in response to changes in GFR.
    c. It has a minor role in sodium reabsorption.
    d. It reabsorbs 80% of filtered water, mainly through aquaporin-1 water channels.
    e. It is the major site of bicarbonate reabsorption.

27. All of the following are true regarding the loop of Henle EXCEPT:
    a. it is responsible for the generation of a hypertonic medullary interstitium, which is necessary for urinary concentration.
    b. it is able to increase or decrease reabsorption rates in response to changes in GFR.
    c. the descending limb is highly water permeable.
    d. the thin ascending limb actively reabsorbs sodium, chloride, and urea.
    e. the thick ascending limb is impermeable to water.

28. Which of the following about the thick ascending limb of the loop of Henle is FALSE?
    a. Twenty-five percent of filtered sodium is actively reabsorbed via the furosemide sensitive NKCC2 co-transporter.
    b. Calcium and magnesium reabsorption is inhibited by furosemide.
    c. Potassium is reabsorbed and returned to the systemic circulation via ROMK channels.
    d. It is the site of uromodulin secretion.
    e. Ten to 20 percent of filtered bicarbonate is reabsorbed in the TALH.

29. Regarding the distal convoluted tubule, all the following are true EXCEPT:
    a. DCT reabsorbs 10% of filtered sodium via the thiazide-sensitive NCC co-transporter.
    b. sodium reabsorption is dependent solely on luminal sodium concentrations.
    c. calcium reabsorption is paracellular and influenced by sodium re-absorption.
    d. magnesium reabsorption is transcellular via luminal magnesium channels.
    e. loop diuretics increase sodium reabsorption in the DCT.

30. All of the following are TRUE about the collecting tubule EXCEPT:
    a. the collecting tubule is designed for fine tuning, rather than bulk transport, of ultrafiltrate.
    b. sodium reabsorption is regulated by aldosterone and occurs passively through luminal sodium channels.
    c. potassium reabsorption is dependent on both aldosterone and luminal flow rates.
    d. the collecting tubule is impermeable to water at all times.
    e. intercalated cells are largely responsible for acid-base regulation in the collecting tubule.

ANSWERS

1. **d. Mediates increased release of aldosterone.** AT1, the receptor for angiotensin II, mediates the release of aldosterone. Intrarenal dilatation is mediated through AT2.
2. **a. Stimulation of the endothelin-1 (ET-1) decreases sodium excretion.** Despite reduction in renal blood flow, stimulation of ET1 by endothelin increases net sodium excretion.
3. **b. Carbon monoxide.** The others are vasoconstrictors.
4. **c. Increased carbon monoxide (CO) increases ischemia-reperfusion injury in the kidney.** CO is protective against renal ischemia-reperfusion injury.
5. **b. Erythropoiesis is inhibited by low circulating oxygen tension.** Erythropoiesis is increased by low circulating oxygen tension.
6. **b. Normal compensation for hyponatremia is decreased ADH secretion and thirst suppression.**
7. **e. may be treated with lithium or demeclocycline.** Both lithium or demeclocycline may be used to treat SIADH.
8. **d. Intranasal desmopressin is a useful adjuvant therapy.** Desmopressin is useful to treat hypernatremia caused by diabetes insipidus.
9. **e. Maximum concentrating ability of the kidney is impaired due to loss of the medullary osmotic gradient.** In both nephrogenic and neurogenic diabetes insipidus, maximum concentrating ability of the kidney is impaired owing to loss of the medullary osmotic gradient.
10. **a. ACE inhibitors may be a cause of hypokalemia.**
11. **c. All patients with a serum potassium value > 5.5 mEq/L require immediate therapy.** Patients with mild elevation of potassium, especially when chronic and not associated with ECG changes, do not require emergent therapy.
12. **d. Immediate response to an acid load is through buffers in the blood.**
13. **a. Most bicarbonate is reabsorbed in the distal collecting tubule.** Most bicarbonate reabsorption in the kidney occurs in the proximal tubule.
14. **c. The patient has acidemia.** The only thing that is certain with a low pH is that there is an acidemia. This may be caused by metabolic, respiratory, or mixed disorders.
15. **b. Direct bicarbonate loss from the kidney would lead to metabolic acidosis and a normal anion gap.** Direct bicarbonate loss is "measured" in the anion gap and therefore leads to metabolic acidosis with a normal anion gap.
16. **d. The hallmark of type IV RTA is hypokalemia.** RTA type IV is most commonly associated with hyperkalemia. Aldosterone deficiency or resistance leads to decreased secretion of potassium in the distal tubule.
17. **a. Paradoxical aciduria may occur due to distal tubule injury.** Metabolic alkalosis is often associated with hypovolemia and elevated aldosterone. In an attempt to conserve sodium and water, H^+ may be exchanged with sodium, leading to aciduria, despite the presence of systemic alkalosis.
18. **e. Increase free water excretion in response to hypernatremia.** ADH decreases free water excretion in response to hypernatremia in an attempt to return plasma osmolality back to normal.
19. **c. Dermally synthesized cholecalciferol must be hydroxylated by both the liver and kidney for maximal potency.** Cholecalciferol is minimally active, but potency increases 100 times after it is hydroxylated at the 1- and 25-position to form calcitriol.
20. **d. PTH increases calcium and phosphorus reabsorption in the distal tubule.** PTH increases phosphorus excretion in the kidney.
21. **e. RBF is one of the determinants of the glomerular filtration rate.**
22. **c. glomerular permeability.** Glomerular permeability is already maximal under normal conditions for water and small solutes, so GFR will not increase significantly with increased glomerular permeability. Rather, one sees increased filtration of larger substances such as albumin.
23. **e. serum osmolarity.** GFR is not affected significantly by serum osmolality.
24. **a. plasma creatinine is an accurate marker of early reductions in GFR.** Plasma creatinine is a very insensitive marker of early reductions in GFR, because increases in tubular secretion of creatinine keep plasma levels from rising until there has been a significant reduction in GFR.
25. **d. Glucose reabsorption is 100% up to plasma glucose levels of 400 mg/dL.** The reabsorptive threshold for glucose is about 200 mg/dL. Plasma levels above this result in urinary glucose wasting.
26. **c. It has a minor role in sodium reabsorption.** The PCT accounts for 65% of sodium reabsorption, the most of any tubular segment.
27. **d. the thin ascending limb actively reabsorbs sodium, chloride, and urea.** Reabsorption of sodium, chloride, and urea occurs passively in the thin ascending limb.
28. **c. Potassium is reabsorbed and retuned to the systemic circulation via ROMK channels.** Potassium is recycled in the TALH rather than reclaimed, so that luminal potassium concentrations change very little.
29. **c. calcium reabsorption is paracellular and influenced by sodium reabsorption.** Calcium reabsorption is transcellular via $ECaC_1$ channels, and paracellular calcium movement is inhibited by claudin 8.
30. **d. the collecting tubule is impermeable to water at all times.** Water permeability is low in the basal state but increases markedly under the influence of ADH.

36

Renovascular Hypertension and Ischemic Nephropathy

ANDREW C. NOVICK • AMR FERGANY

QUESTIONS

1. The rate-limiting step in the renin-angiotensin-aldosterone cascade is:
   a. secretion of angiotensinogen by the liver.
   b. conversion of angiotensinogen to angiotensin I.
   c. conversion of angiotensin I to angiotensin II.
   d. secretion of aldosterone from the adrenal cortex.
   e. secretion of adrenocorticotropic hormone from the anterior pituitary.
2. The major site of synthesis of systemic renin is the:
   a. liver.
   b. lung.
   c. brain.
   d. kidney.
   e. adrenal gland.
3. Renin secretion is mediated by all of the following EXCEPT:
   a. diminished potassium delivery to the distal tubule.
   b. diminished chloride delivery to the distal tubule.
   c. diminished stretch of the afferent arteriole.
   d. β-adrenergic stimulation of the kidney.
   e. exogenous prostaglandins.
4. Angiotensin-converting enzyme (ACE):
   a. is a specific enzyme that converts angiotensin I to angiotensin II.
   b. is a nonspecific enzyme that has several functions in vivo.
   c. forms angiotensin I from angiotensinogen.
   d. is the only enzyme in the formation of angiotensin II that cannot be pharmacologically modulated.
   e. is the major enzyme for degradation of angiotensin II.
5. Angiotensin II stimulates all the following actions EXCEPT:
   a. cardiac muscle hypertrophy.
   b. thirst.
   c. vasoconstriction.
   d. secretion of aldosterone.
   e. secretion of epinephrine.
6. Under conditions of decreased renal perfusion, angiotensin II regulates glomerular filtration through:
   a. afferent arteriolar vasodilatation.
   b. afferent arteriolar vasoconstriction.
   c. efferent arteriolar vasodilatation.
   d. efferent arteriolar vasoconstriction.
   e. main renal artery vasoconstriction.
7. Experimental models of renovascular hypertension are characterized by:
   a. close resemblance to human clinical renovascular hypertension.
   b. early volume dependent phase of hypertension.
   c. late renin-dependent phase of hypertension.
   d. constant sensitivity to ACE inhibition.
   e. dynamic change through different pathophysiologic phases.
8. Atheroembolism (cholesterol embolism):
   a. frequently contributes to deterioration of renal function in patients with atherosclerotic renal artery stenosis.
   b. occurs mainly in young patients with fibrous renal artery disease.
   c. is usually managed by exploration and immediate surgical repair.
   d. is usually managed by percutaneous transluminal angioplasty.
   e. is a benign phenomenon, usually limited to the lower extremities, that rarely involves the kidney.
9. The presence of anatomic renal artery stenosis:
   a. indicates that surgical or endovascular repair is necessary.
   b. should be excluded in every patient with high blood pressure.
   c. is only significant if stenosis is more than 70%.
   d. is only significant if associated with other vascular (e.g., aortic) disease.
   e. is exclusively the result of renal artery atherosclerosis.

10. The diagnosis of renal artery stenosis:
    a. is usually confirmed through laboratory testing.
    b. is based on wide radiologic screening of asymptomatic patients.
    c. is based on radiologic confirmation of clinically suspicious cases.
    d. is generally not pursued in azotemic patients.
    e. can be confirmed by clinical examination alone.

11. Definitive diagnosis of renal artery stenosis is currently provided through:
    a. duplex ultrasonography.
    b. rapid sequence intravenous urography.
    c. intraoperative digital subtraction angiography.
    d. magnetic resonance angiography.
    e. intra-arterial angiography.

12. Duplex ultrasonography as a tool to diagnose renal artery stenosis:
    a. has the advantage of providing excellent anatomic detail.
    b. is limited by the need to transport patients to an imaging facility.
    c. can provide all the necessary information for treatment of patients with ischemic nephropathy.
    d. is not useful as a screening test for patients where renal artery stenosis is suspected.
    e. has the advantage of mobility, widespread availability, noninvasiveness, and no effect on renal function.

13. Carbon dioxide digital subtraction angiography:
    a. is an invasive diagnostic modality that is especially useful in patients with renal insufficiency.
    b. is a noninvasive diagnostic technique that minimizes the risk associated with iodinated contrast angiography.
    c. is associated with a higher incidence of arterial wall trauma than is standard angiography.
    d. cannot be used if angioplasty is contemplated.
    e. is associated with a high incidence of allergic complications and gas embolism.

14. Medical management for patients with renal artery stenosis:
    a. rarely succeeds in controlling hypertension.
    b. is the best chance for maintaining renal function.
    c. is appropriate therapy for young patients with ischemic nephropathy.
    d. is generally preferred for children.
    e. is appropriate therapy for older patients with mild hypertension.

15. Nephrectomy as a treatment option for renal artery stenosis:
    a. is indicated for hypertension caused by a unilateral, small, poorly functioning kidney.
    b. is indicated for bilateral renal artery stenosis provided that total renal function is normal.
    c. is usually indicated in cases of ischemic nephropathy rather than renovascular hypertension.
    d. should be performed exclusively using open surgical technique and not laparoscopically.
    e. rarely provides long-term therapeutic benefit even in properly selected cases.

16. Revascularization of ischemic kidneys:
    a. should be performed only in patients with ischemic nephropathy.
    b. should be performed only in patients with renovascular hypertension.
    c. provides inferior long-term benefit compared with medical management.
    d. leads to stabilization, but not improvement, of renal function.
    e. may be performed surgically or percutaneously.

17. Percutaneous transluminal angioplasty of the renal arteries:
    a. can be performed under ultrasonographic guidance.
    b. is currently performed using coaxial dilators placed through the femoral artery.
    c. currently employs a dilatation balloon passed through the femoral or axillary artery.
    d. is useful only for cases of atherosclerotic renal artery disease.
    e. is the preferred modality for treating branch renal artery disease.

18. The best therapeutic results after percutaneous angioplasty can be expected with the following arterial lesions:
    a. renal artery aneurysm.
    b. ostial renal artery atherosclerotic stenosis.
    c. branch renal artery atherosclerotic stenosis.
    d. main renal artery fibrous stenosis.
    e. branch renal artery fibrous stenosis.

19. Complications of percutaneous angioplasty:
    a. should never be managed surgically.
    b. include contrast allergy as well as femoral and renal artery trauma.
    c. occur in 30% to 50% of cases.
    d. are not related to operator experience.
    e. should always be managed by immediate surgery.

20. Technical success for percutaneous angioplasty in cases of fibrous dysplasia can be expected to be:
    a. less than 50%.
    b. 50% to 60%.
    c. 65% to 75%.
    d. 75% to 85%.
    e. 90% or more.

21. Results of percutaneous angioplasty in cases of atherosclerotic renal artery stenosis are worse than in cases of fibrous disease because:
    a. atherosclerotic plaque is more difficult to dilate using angiographic balloons.
    b. atherosclerotic lesions are tighter and do not allow passage of the guidewire.
    c. femoral artery atherosclerosis usually precludes arterial access.
    d. renal artery atherosclerotic lesions are usually ostial and part of aortic wall plaque.
    e. renal artery atherosclerosis usually involves arterial branches and responds poorly to dilatation.

22. The use of endovascular stents as treatment for renal artery stenosis:
    a. has increased the rate of emergency surgery because of complications of angioplasty.
    b. has increased the rate of immediate postangioplasty success.
    c. is reserved mainly for cases of fibrous renal artery stenosis.
    d. is the preferred technique for angioplasty in children.
    e. necessitates arterial access through the axillary artery.

23. Continued deterioration of renal function after renal artery stent placement may be due to all of the following EXCEPT:
    a. acute thrombosis of the renal artery.
    b. cholesterol embolism.
    c. a slightly larger stent than the renal artery diameter.
    d. restenosis of the renal artery.
    e. progressive glomerulosclerosis.
24. Which of the following statements regarding atherosclerotic renal artery disease is incorrect?
    a. It is the most common type of renal artery disease.
    b. It is more common in men than in women.
    c. It is usually not associated with manifestations of generalized atherosclerosis.
    d. It is more common in patients older than 50 years of age.
    e. It usually involves the proximal 2 cm of the main renal artery.
25. The most useful clinical marker or markers of progressive atherosclerotic renal artery obstruction are:
    a. poorly controlled hypertension.
    b. poorly controlled hypertension and a decrease in kidney size.
    c. poorly controlled hypertension and an increase in serum creatinine level.
    d. a decrease in kidney size and an increase in serum creatinine level.
    e. all of the above.
26. All of the following represent clinical clues to the presence of atherosclerotic renal artery disease EXCEPT:
    a. evidence of generalized atherosclerosis.
    b. patient age younger than 50 years.
    c. unilateral small kidney.
    d. mild azotemia.
    e. severe hypertension.
27. The most common cause of unilateral renal atrophy in patients older than 50 years of age is:
    a. congenital hypoplasia.
    b. chronic pyelonephritis.
    c. atherosclerotic renal artery disease.
    d. fibrous renal artery disease.
    e. chronic glomerulonephritis.
28. Clinical clues suggesting renal salvageability with complete arterial occlusion include all of the following EXCEPT:
    a. kidney size greater than 9 cm.
    b. angiographic evidence of collateral vascular supply.
    c. nondiseased glomeruli as seen on a renal biopsy specimen.
    d. function of the involved kidney as revealed by isotope renography.
    e. absence of contralateral compensatory renal hypertrophy.
29. The percentage of end-stage renal disease cases that are currently thought to be caused by ischemic nephropathy is:
    a. 0% to 5%.
    b. 6% to 10%.
    c. 15% to 20%.
    d. 50% to 60%.
    e. 80% to 90%.
30. The natural history of renal artery atherosclerosis is best characterized as being:
    a. unpredictable and varying in each case.
    b. gradually improving.
    c. progressive and unremitting.
    d. not a threat to renal function.
    e. associated with remissions and exacerbation.
31. Renal artery stenosis causing ischemic nephropathy is:
    a. most commonly due to atherosclerosis of the renal arteries.
    b. easy to diagnose because of characteristic symptoms.
    c. usually occurs in young, healthier patients.
    d. results in mild renal impairment of no clinical significance.
    e. usually diagnosed as focal disease affecting the renal arteries.
32. The class of antihypertensive drugs having a specific deleterious effect on renal function in cases of renal artery stenosis is:
    a. vasodilators.
    b. calcium channel blockers.
    c. ACE inhibitors.
    d. β-adrenergic blockers.
    e. ganglion blockers.
33. Which of the following investigations is best suited as an initial screening test for renal artery stenosis in a 65-year-old woman with generalized atherosclerosis, diabetes mellitus, and a serum creatinine value of 2.5 mg/dL?
    a. CT angiography
    b. Intra-arterial digital subtraction angiography
    c. Captopril test
    d. Duplex ultrasonography of the renal arteries
    e. Determination of differential renal vein renin
34. Which of the following best describes the outcome of patients with ischemic nephropathy who undergo dialysis?
    a. They have the poorest survival of all patients.
    b. They have the best survival of all patients.
    c. Infection is the major cause of mortality.
    d. Long-term survival is a realistic goal.
    e. Complications with vascular access make peritoneal dialysis a better choice.
35. Patients with end-stage renal failure from ischemic nephropathy:
    a. are always beyond the point of regaining renal function with revascularization.
    b. are the best candidates for revascularization.
    c. may be suitable candidates for revascularization if renal salvage criteria are met.
    d. tolerate permanent dialysis exceptionally well.
    e. should undergo only angioplasty for revascularization.
36. Which of the following is the most common type of renal arterial aneurysm?
    a. Fusiform
    b. Saccular
    c. Dissecting
    d. Post-traumatic
    e. Intrarenal
37. A 30-year-old healthy woman is evaluated for hypertension and noted to have a 4-cm noncalcified renal artery aneurysm. Factors that affect treatment include all the following EXCEPT:
    a. the absence of calcification.
    b. the patient's age.
    c. the absence of hematuria.
    d. the size of the aneurysm.
    e. hypertension.
38. Arteriovenous fistulas resulting from needle biopsy of the kidney:
    a. generally heal spontaneously within 2 weeks.
    b. are not amenable to transcatheter angiographic occlusion.
    c. usually require total or partial nephrectomy for treatment.
    d. generally heal spontaneously within 18 months.
    e. are an uncommon cause of acquired renal arteriovenous fistulas.

39. In which of the following clinical settings is surgical excision of a renal arterial aneurysm clearly NOT indicated?
    a. Dissecting aneurysm
    b. Calcified aneurysm 1.5 cm in diameter
    c. Aneurysm causing hypertension
    d. Noncalcified aneurysm 3.0 cm in diameter
    e. Aneurysm increasing in size on sequential angiograms

40. Renal arterial aneurysms may cause hypertension through all of the following mechanisms EXCEPT:
    a. extrinsic compression of renal arterial branches.
    b. turbulent blood flow within an aneurysm.
    c. associated arteriolar nephrosclerosis.
    d. associated renal artery stenosis.
    e. peripheral renal embolism.

41. The most common cause of an acquired renal arteriovenous fistula is:
    a. blunt renal trauma.
    b. renal carcinoma.
    c. renal surgery.
    d. penetrating renal trauma.
    e. closed renal biopsy.

42. The most common method of surgical treatment of symptomatic congenital arteriovenous fistulas has been:
    a. aortorenal bypass with saphenous vein.
    b. total or partial nephrectomy.
    c. bench surgery and autotransplantation.
    d. individual ligation of interconnecting arteriovenous channels.
    e. aortorenal bypass with hypogastric artery.

43. The most appropriate method of management for a patient with unilateral renal arterial embolism secondary to a myocardial ventricular aneurysm is:
    a. systemic anticoagulation.
    b. observation.
    c. aortorenal bypass.
    d. surgical renal artery embolectomy.
    e. segmental renal arterial resection and reanastomosis.

44. Which of the following statements regarding acute renal arterial thrombosis is FALSE?
    a. It commonly occurs in the proximal two thirds of the main renal artery.
    b. It may be due to trauma.
    c. It more commonly involves the right renal artery.
    d. It may be due to atherosclerosis.
    e. It may be managed with percutaneous intra-arterial infusion of streptokinase.

45. Combined repair of aortic and renal artery atherosclerosis:
    a. is recommended to decrease patient morbidity from multiple procedures.
    b. has a low morbidity in cases of bilateral renal artery repair.
    c. can be performed with a combination of open and endovascular repair.
    d. should not be performed using a combination of open and endovascular repair.
    e. cannot be performed as a staged procedure.

46. Regarding selection of patients for endovascular treatment (stenting) of atherosclerotic renal artery stenosis:
    a. any patient with renal artery stenosis should be offered this procedure.
    b. procedure-related morbidity is so low that most patients are good candidates.
    c. most unselected patients have good results with acceptable morbidity.
    d. selection criteria should be as strict as surgical selection to minimize patient morbidity.
    e. higher morbidity than open surgery results in fewer number of suitable patients.

47. Which of the following is correct regarding treatment of renal artery aneurysms?
    a. Conservative management by observation is the most appropriate strategy.
    b. If surgery is required, nephrectomy is the best option.
    c. Endovascular stents have no role in managing this condition.
    d. Ex-vivo repair with autotransplantation is sometimes required.
    e. Rupture of the aneurysm is the only indication for treatment.

48. In patients with significant renal artery stenosis to a solitary kidney:
    a. volume expansion with decreasing renin secretion occurs.
    b. the acute phase of renovascular hypertension is severe and prolonged.
    c. there is minimal risk of ischemic nephropathy.
    d. medical management with ACE inhibitors is optimal.
    e. medical management with antihypertensive medication is usually easy to achieve.

49. An 18-year-old man is found to be hypertensive (BP 190/110 mm Hg). Subsequent evaluation includes renal angiography, which reveals a unilateral tight (90%) renal artery stenosis that is smooth and associated with an intimal dissection and prominent collateral vessels. What should be done?
    a. Medical treatment is the long-term treatment of choice.
    b. Emergency open surgical repair should be undertaken.
    c. This lesion will not progress; observation is the best option.
    d. Percutaneous angioplasty should be undertaken after institution of medical treatment.
    e. A threat to renal function may necessitate dialysis.

50. An 82-year-old man is being evaluated angiographically for aortic atherosclerotic disease. An acute deterioration of renal function occurs over the following 2 days. All of the following statements are true EXCEPT which one?
    a. Repeat angiography to exclude renal artery thrombosis and possible emergency revascularization is needed.
    b. Atheroembolism may be the reason for deterioration of renal function.
    c. Nephrotoxicity from radiographic contrast agent may be responsible for renal function deterioration.
    d. Duplex ultrasound of the renal artery is a reasonable study to exclude renal artery thrombosis.
    e. Supportive care as needed is the best option in this situation.

ANSWERS

1. **b. conversion of angiotensinogen to angiotensin I.** The basic cascade of the renin-angiotensin-aldosterone system (RAAS) involves conversion of angiotensinogen to angiotensin I through the action of renin. This is the rate-limiting step for the entire system, and, accordingly, control of renin release regulates the activity of the whole system.
2. **d. kidney.** Renin is a single polypeptide chain aspartyl protease that is secreted from the juxtaglomerular cells of the afferent arteriole. The kidney is the major site of renin production, although renin mRNA is found in several other tissues where the local renin-angiotensin system functions.
3. **a. decreased potassium delivery to the distal tubule.** Reduction of distal tubule salt delivery stimulates renin secretion and vice versa. Although sodium was initially thought to be responsible for this action, it now appears that the signal for macula densa–controlled renin release is the alteration of tubular chloride concentration.
4. **b. is a nonspecific enzyme that has several functions in vivo.** ACE is expressed in several tissues where the local RAAS functions. Renal ACE is localized to the glomerular endothelial cells and the proximal tubule brush border, where it might play a role in cleaving filtered protein for reabsorption. Within the central nervous system (CNS), ACE is found in several locations, where it functions in the local RAAS. This local CNS RAAS is thought to have dipsogenic and hypertensive effects as well as to stimulate vasopressin secretion. Adrenal ACE is found predominantly in the medulla, where it is thought to stimulate catecholamine secretion. ACE is found abundantly in the testes and prostate, in the Leydig cells, and in cytoplasmic droplets in sperm. In the female reproductive tract, ACE is found in follicular and fallopian tube oocytes. The precise role of ACE in the reproductive system has not been elucidated.
5. **e. secretion of epinephrine.** Angiotensin II acts directly on the adrenal glomerulosa cells to stimulate aldosterone secretion, which is accomplished through increased desmolase activity and increased conversion of corticosterone to aldosterone. This serves to augment the salt reabsorptive actions of angiotensin II to conserve sodium. Vasoconstriction and release of aldosterone occur immediately and are of short duration, supporting the role of angiotensin II in maintaining tissue perfusion in hypovolemia. Other actions such as vascular growth, and ventricular hypertrophy are slower in onset and longer in duration, lasting for several days or weeks.
6. **d. efferent arteriolar vasoconstriction.** One of the most important actions of angiotensin II is the autoregulation of glomerular filtration rate (GFR) in response to changes in renal perfusion. This action is effected through changes in vascular resistance as well as mesangial cell tone. Angiotensin II causes a marked increase in efferent arteriolar resistance in cases of renal hypoperfusion but does not affect afferent arteriolar resistance unless there is an increase in renal perfusion pressure. The result of this disproportionate increase in efferent over afferent resistance is an increase in capillary hydraulic pressure, and subsequently in filtration pressure, maintaining GFR in the face of decreased renal perfusion.
7. **e. dynamic change through different pathophysiologic phases.** Renovascular hypertension has been demonstrated in two models of experimental Goldblatt hypertension: the two-kidney, one-clip model (2K,1C), in which one renal artery is clipped and the contralateral kidney is in place and normal; and the one-kidney, one-clip model (1K,1C), in which one renal artery is clipped and the contralateral kidney is removed. Both models do not remain static but rather pass through an acute phase, a transition phase, and then a final chronic phase. In cases of 2K,1C hypertension, a chronic phase is eventually reached after several days or weeks when unclipping of the stenotic kidney fails to normalize blood pressure. In this chronic phase, the elevated perfusion pressure as well as high levels of angiotensin II have resulted in widespread arteriolar damage to the contralateral kidney. Excretory function (natriuresis) of the contralateral kidney declines, resulting in extracellular volume expansion, decrease of circulating angiotensin II levels, and gradual development of a "volume-dependent" type of hypertension.
8. **a. frequently contributes to deterioration of renal function in patients with atherosclerotic renal artery stenosis.** The organs most commonly affected by atheroembolism are the kidney, spleen, pancreas, and gastrointestinal tract. Renal effects take the form of deteriorating renal function, usually after a precipitating event. The decline in renal function can vary in severity from slowly progressive to rapid acute renal failure. Gradual improvement of renal function occurs after the event, but recurrent episodes lead to progressive loss of renal function with time.
9. **c. is only significant if stenosis is more than 70%.** Renal artery stenosis becomes hemodynamically significant when the stenosis exceeds 70% of the lumen. Most patients with hypertension suffer from essential hypertension and, thus, are not indicated for investigations for renal arterial disease. Renal artery stenosis can be the result of atherosclerosis, fibromuscular dysplasia, as well as other less common diseases.
10. **c. is based on radiologic confirmation of clinically suspicious cases.** The clinical clues serve in the selection of patients who should be studied for the possible presence of renal artery stenosis. For patients with suspected renovascular hypertension, a number of tests are available for functional diagnosis of renovascular hypertension. These tests (plasma renin activity, captopril test, captopril renography, and renal vein renin assays) diagnose hyperactivity of the RAAS but provide no anatomic information regarding the offending arterial lesion. Anatomic delineation of the arterial lesion guides the treatment decisions and is obtained by intra-arterial angiography, which remains the most definitive study and the "gold standard" against which other diagnostic techniques are compared.
11. **e. intra-arterial angiography.** Intra-arterial angiography remains the gold standard for diagnosing renal artery disease, and it is the test against which other tests are compared. However, angiography is not suitable for use as a preliminary screening tool for all patients suspected of having renal artery stenosis.
12. **e. has the advantage of mobility, widespread availability, noninvasiveness, and no effect on renal function.** Duplex ultrasonography of the renal arteries is a noninvasive anatomic study that has shown excellent ability for screening and diagnosis of renal artery stenosis. The equipment is mobile and can be moved to critically ill patients. It is also widespread, relatively easy to use, and does not depend on kidney function nor affect kidney function. It does not provide anatomic detail because it depends on measuring blood flow velocity in the renal artery and comparing that to the blood flow velocity in the aorta.
13. **a. is an invasive diagnostic modality that is especially useful in patients with renal insufficiency.** Carbon dioxide has been introduced as a contrast agent for intra-arterial injection in an effort to reduce contrast nephrotoxicity from iodinated contrast material. Carbon dioxide has no effect on renal function, making it an ideal agent for use in patients with renal insufficiency.

14. **e. is appropriate therapy for older patients with mild hypertension.** In patients with atherosclerotic renal vascular hypertension, more vigorous attempts at medical management are warranted, because these patients are older and often have extrarenal vascular disease. Therefore, multiple-drug regimens that control blood pressure are often the preferred approach.

15. **a. is indicated for hypertension caused by a unilateral, small, poorly functioning kidney.** Advances in both surgical renal vascular reconstruction and medical antihypertensive therapy have limited the role of total or partial nephrectomy in the management of patients with renal artery disease. These operations are only occasionally indicated in patients with severe arteriolar nephrosclerosis, severe renal atrophy, noncorrectable renal vascular lesions, and renal infarction.

16. **e. may be performed surgically or percutaneously.** Intervention with surgery or endovascular therapy is best reserved for patients whose hypertension cannot be adequately controlled or when renal function is threatened by advanced vascular disease.

17. **c. currently employs a dilatation balloon passed through the femoral or axillary artery.** The original Gruntzig coaxial technique utilizes an 8 or 9 Fr renal guiding catheter through which a 4.3 or 4.5 Fr balloon catheter is passed over a guide wire traversing the stenotic segment through a femoral arterial puncture. Modification of the original technique and balloon catheters have allowed the use of a 5 Fr femoral artery puncture through which a 5 Fr diagnostic catheter is passed to the renal artery using the Seldinger technique. An axillary approach may be used to perform renal percutaneous transluminal angioplasty when the renal arteries originate at an acute angle from the abdominal aorta as well as in cases with severe pelvic atherosclerosis, occlusion, or the presence of bypass grafts in the pelvic or abdominal areas.

18. **d. main renal artery fibrous stenosis.** The results of angioplasty for fibrous dysplasia of the main renal artery have been excellent and equal to those obtained with surgical revascularization; therefore, angioplasty is the initial treatment of choice in such cases.

19. **b. include contrast allergy as well as femoral and renal artery trauma.** The complications of percutaneous transluminal angioplasty include those of standard angiography (complications related to arterial puncture and to the use of iodinated contrast material), as well as specific complications related to manipulation of the renal arteries. Transient deterioration of renal function is the most frequent complication and is related to the contrast load delivered during the procedure. Technical mishaps during percutaneous transluminal angioplasty may lead to an intimal dissection or even thrombosis of the renal artery.

20. **e. 90% or more.** Percutaneous transluminal angioplasty is usually performed in cases of fibrous dysplasia without stent placement and has become the primary modality of treatment for these lesions. With the use of modern equipment and increasing experience with the technique, technical success has been more than 90%. A beneficial blood pressure response—that is, cure of hypertension or improvement in blood pressure control—can be expected in more than 80% and up to 100% of cases.

21. **d. renal artery atherosclerotic lesions are usually ostial and part of aortic wall plaque.** Renal artery stenosis in cases of arteriosclerosis obliterans is usually bilateral and ostial or very proximal in the main renal artery. In most ostial cases, this represents encroachment of the atherosclerotic plaque in the abdominal aorta upon the origin of the renal artery rather than primary renal artery disease. The patients affected by atherosclerotic renal artery stenosis are also different from patients with fibrous dysplasia of the renal arteries in that they are generally older and have a number of comorbid medical conditions as well as generalized atherosclerosis affecting the coronary and carotid arteries or the peripheral vascular tree. Associated essential hypertension and nephrosclerosis are usually present. All of the previously mentioned factors, as well as the propensity for atheroembolism in patients with generalized arteriosclerosis obliterans, make percutaneous transluminal angioplasty in cases of arteriosclerosis obliterans renal artery stenosis less successful and associated with higher morbidity (and some mortality) than in cases of fibrous dysplasia.

22. **b. has increased the rate of immediate postangioplasty success.** In the only prospective study comparing percutaneous transluminal angioplasty alone versus the procedure with stenting in ostial atherosclerosis, 85 patients were randomized to receive either treatment. Technical success was higher in the group receiving stents (88% vs. 57%), and patency at 6 months was 75% for patients in the group receiving stents versus 29% for the patients undergoing the procedure alone. In patients with successful primary procedures, restenosis occurred in 14% of the patients with stents and in 48% of patients undergoing percutaneous transluminal angioplasty alone. Stenting for immediate or late failure of the procedure was required in 12 (of 42) patients in the group undergoing percutaneous transluminal angioplasty alone. This study reflects the overall higher success of percutaneous transluminal angioplasty with stenting in treating ostial atherosclerosis when compared with the procedure alone and probably also justifies the increasing trend to perform primary stenting in these cases to avoid exposing patients to a secondary procedure.

23. **c. a slightly larger stent than the renal artery diameter.** Complications of percutaneous transluminal angioplasty with stenting were not found to be significantly different from those of percutaneous transluminal angioplasty alone in a prospective study comparing both procedures. Specifically, rates in both groups for bleeding-related complications were 19% and for cholesterol embolism were 10%; the rate for access site pseudoaneurysm and renal artery injury was slightly higher with stent placement (7% vs. 5%). Transient deterioration of renal function secondary to contrast nephrotoxicity was noted in 24% of patients undergoing the procedure alone and in 21% of patients undergoing the procedure with stent placement.

24. **c. It is usually not associated with manifestations of generalized atherosclerosis.** Recent epidemiologic studies indicate that atherosclerotic renal artery disease is quite common in patients with generalized atherosclerosis obliterans, regardless of whether renovascular hypertension is present.

25. **d. a decrease in kidney size and an increase in the serum creatinine level.** Clinical follow-up of patients in our study also revealed that significantly more patients with progressive disease developed deterioration of overall renal function (a decrease in kidney size or an increase in the serum creatinine level) compared with patients with stable disease. Interestingly, serial blood pressure control was equivalent in these two groups, indicating that it is not a useful clinical marker for progressive atherosclerotic renal artery stenosis.

26. **b. patient age younger than 50 years.** Studies indicate that clinical screening for atherosclerotic renal artery disease is appropriate in older patients with most or all of the following features: (1) evidence of generalized atherosclerosis; (2) a decrease in the size of one or both kidneys; (3) renal insufficiency, even of a mild extent, particularly in patients with no obvious underlying cause; (4) the development of progressive azotemia after restoration of normotension with medical antihypertensive therapy; (5) coronary artery disease; (6) a history of congestive heart failure; and (7) peripheral vascular disease.

27. **c. atherosclerotic renal artery disease.** The screening of patients for atherosclerotic renal artery disease is based in part on an early (1965) study by Gifford and colleagues. These investigators found that in 53 of 75 older patients (71%) with unilateral renal atrophy, the renal atrophy was caused by stenosing atherosclerotic renal artery disease. Of equal importance was the finding that 22 of these 53 patients (42%) also had unsuspected atherosclerotic renal artery disease involving the opposite normal-sized kidney. Subsequently, Lawrie and colleagues reviewed 40 patients with renal atrophy caused by total arterial occlusion and noted contralateral atherosclerotic renal artery stenosis in 31 patients (78%). These observations underscore the high incidence of renal artery disease, often bilateral, in patients with generalized atherosclerosis and diminished renal size.

28. **e. absence of contralateral compensatory renal hypertrophy.** Complete occlusion of the renal artery most often ends in irreversible ischemic damage of the involved kidney. In some patients with gradual arterial occlusion, however, the viability of the kidney can be maintained through the development of collateral arterial supply. Helpful clinical clues suggesting renal salvageability in such cases include the following: (1) angiographic demonstration of retrograde filling of the distal renal arterial tree, by collateral vessels on the side of the total arterial occlusion; (2) a renal biopsy showing well-preserved glomeruli; (3) kidney size greater than 9 cm; and (4) function of the involved kidney as revealed by isotope renography or intravenous pyelography. When such criteria are present, restoration of normal renal arterial flow can lead to recovery of renal function.

29. **b. 6% to 10%.** The exact incidence of end-stage renal disease caused by atherosclerotic renal artery disease in the United States is not known. In a report from England, Scoble and colleagues prospectively performed renal arteriography in all new patients with end-stage renal disease during an 18-month period. Atherosclerotic renal artery disease was the cause of end-stage renal disease in 6% of all patients and in 14% of patients older than 50 years of age. Approximately 300,000 patients in the United States are currently being maintained by chronic dialysis. Their median age is greater than 60 years, and a majority of patients have evidence of generalized atherosclerosis obliterans. Although the exact number of patients with end-stage renal disease caused by atherosclerotic renal artery disease is not known, these data suggest that there are several thousand patients in this category.

30. **c. progressive and unremitting.** Natural history data clearly show that atherosclerotic renal artery disease progresses in many patients and that loss of functioning renal parenchyma is a common sequela of such progression.

31. **a. most commonly due to atherosclerosis of the renal arteries.** Atherosclerosis of the renal arteries, usually as part of generalized atherosclerosis, is the most common cause of ischemic nephropathy. This is a silent disease that required clinical suspicion for diagnosis. The condition usually occurs in older patients with generalized atherosclerosis and can progress to significant renal impairment and the need for renal replacement therapy.

32. **c. ACE inhibitors.** Another important clinical clue to the presence of significant atherosclerotic renal artery stenosis is the development of progressive azotemia after medical control of blood pressure in patients with significant hypertension. ACE inhibitor agents can lead to deterioration of renal function through loss of efferent arteriolar vasoconstrictor tone in the kidney.

33. **d. Duplex ultrasonography of the renal arteries.** Duplex ultrasonography offers significant advantages as a diagnostic tool for renal artery stenosis. It is noninvasive, uses portable equipment that is relatively inexpensive and widely available, does not utilize iodinated contrast material, and has no effect on renal function. Azotemia does not affect the results of the study, and no discontinuation of antihypertensive medications is required.

34. **a. They have the poorest survival of all patients.** Patients with renal vascular disease as the cause of end-stage renal disease had the poorest survival of all patients who have had dialysis, with a 27-month median survival time and a 12% 5-year survival rate.

35. **c. may be suitable candidates for revascularization if renal salvage criteria are met.** Occasional patients with end-stage renal disease from ischemic nephropathy have been encountered in whom renal function has been salvageable with revascularization. The basis for this has been the presence of chronic bilateral total renal arterial occlusion when, fortuitously, the viability of one or both kidneys has been maintained through collateral vascular supply. In such cases, revascularization can yield dramatic recovery of renal function.

36. **b. Saccular.** Saccular aneurysms are the most common type and account for about 75% of renal artery aneurysms. They generally occur at the bifurcation of the renal artery, perhaps because of an inherent weakness in the wall of the artery at this point.

37. **c. the absence of hematuria.** Factors that appear to predispose to aneurysmal rupture include absent or incomplete calcification, aneurysmal diameter greater than 2.0 cm, coexisting hypertension, and pregnancy (females of child-bearing age).

38. **d. generally heal spontaneously within 18 months.** Approximately 70% of fistulas occurring after needle biopsy of the kidney close spontaneously within 18 months.

39. **b. Calcified aneurysm 1.5 cm in diameter.** A small (<2.0 cm) well-calcified renal arterial aneurysm in an asymptomatic normotensive patient does not require operative intervention. These aneurysms can be followed with serial plain abdominal radiographs to detect any change in size.

40. **c. associated arteriolar nephrosclerosis.** The majority of renal arterial aneurysms are small and asymptomatic. Renovascular hypertension is reported to occur in 15% to 75% of patients and may be due to turbulent flow within an aneurysm, associated arterial stenosis, dissection, arteriovenous fistula formation, thromboembolism, or compression of adjacent arterial branches by a large aneurysm.

41. **e. closed renal biopsy.** Acquired fistulas are the most common type of fistula, accounting for 70% to 75% of all renal arteriovenous fistulas. On angiography, they appear as solitary communications between an artery and a vein. By far the most common cause is iatrogenic trauma resulting from needle biopsy of the kidney.

42. **b. total or partial nephrectomy.** Various operations have been used in the surgical treatment of renal arteriovenous fistulas. Most congenital or cirsoid fistulas have been managed with total or partial nephrectomy because of the difficulty of completely excising the many small communicating vessels.
43. **a. systemic anticoagulation.** Patients with unilateral renal arterial embolic occlusion generally have serious underlying extrarenal disease and are best managed nonoperatively with systemic anticoagulation.
44. **c. It more commonly involves the right renal artery.** Renal arterial thrombosis commonly involves the proximal or middle third of the main renal artery, whereas renal arterial embolization generally involves peripheral arterial branches. Acute arterial occlusion is more common on the left side because of the more acute angle between the left renal artery and the aorta.
45. **c. can be performed with a combination of open and endovascular repair.** The morbidity of a combined repair especially when both renal arteries are involved is especially high, and this justifies a staging technique, where the renal arteries are repaired separate from the aorta, or a combined open/endovascular approach.
46. **d. selection criteria should be as strict as surgical selection to minimize patient morbidity.** Procedure-related morbidity from renal artery stenting is substantial with possible mortality. This requires attention to patient comorbidities before recommending the procedure. At the same time, the chance of a beneficial outcome should be carefully evaluated with regard to the renal function, the size of the kidneys, as well as the anatomic distribution of disease.
47. **d. Ex-vivo repair with autotransplantation is sometimes required.** A variety of treatment methods are available for treatment of renal artery aneurysms. Surgical repair commonly requires ex-vivo reconstruction and autotransplantation due to involvement of the branches of the renal artery. Endovascular stents have recently been used to exclude the aneurysm from the main renal artery and effectively treat it. Nephrectomy should be the last resort in complicated cases. Such treatment modalities should be instituted before complications, especially rupture of the aneurysm, occur.
48. **a. volume expansion with decreasing renin secretion occurs.** In patients with stenosis to the artery of a solitary kidney, the situation is similar to a one-kidney, one-clip experimental model of renovascular hypertension. The acute renin-dependent phase of hypertension is short, rapidly passing into the chronic phase characterized by volume expansion and gradually decreasing renin secretion. In the clinical situation, medical management is usually difficult, and the patients face the risk of developing ischemic nephropathy and deterioration of renal function. Acute deterioration of renal function can be precipitated by the use of ACE inhibitors in this situation.
49. **d. Percutaneous angioplasty should be undertaken after institution of medical treatment.** This appearance is typical of an intimal fibroplasia. These lesions are usually progressive and can result in intimal dissection with occlusion of the main renal artery or its branches. Renal function is not usually threatened in unilateral lesions. Long-term medical treatment is not a good option in younger patients to avoid the complications of long-term treatment, which does not stop disease progression. Initial control of blood pressure should be undertaken medically followed by an attempt at endovascular repair, which is usually successful. Surgical revascularization should be reserved for failure of percutaneous angioplasty.
50. **a. Repeat angiography to exclude renal artery thrombosis and possible emergency revascularization is needed.** This scenario is most commonly explained by atheroembolism to the kidneys after manipulation of an atherosclerotic aorta. Less common causes may be contrast nephrotoxicity or thrombosis of the renal arteries. The best option is to provide supportive care to the patient as needed and avoid further manipulation of the aorta. Duplex ultrasound is a good noninvasive test to assess patency of the main renal artery if occlusion or thrombosis is suspected.

SECTION IX

PATHOPHYSIOLOGY OF URINARY TRACT OBSTRUCTION

37

Pathophysiology of Urinary Tract Obstruction

VERNON M. PAIS JR. • JACK W. STRANDHOY • DEAN G. ASSIMOS

QUESTIONS

1. What of the following is unique to obstructive nephropathy as compared with hydronephrosis?
   a. Renal function impairment
   b. Bilateral ureteral dilation
   c. Unilateral ureteral dilation
   d. Calyceal blunting
   e. None of the above
2. Which of these urinary changes occur after relief of bilateral ureteral obstruction?
   a. Increased sodium excretion
   b. Decreased phosphate excretion
   c. Decreased potassium excretion
   d. Decreased magnesium excretion
   e. None of the above
3. Which of the following is thought to play a role in postobstructive diuresis after release of bilateral ureteral obstruction?
   a. Increased renal aquaporin-2 water channels
   b. Increased renal aquaporin-3 water channels
   c. Decreased ADH
   d. Increased atrial natriuretic peptide
   e. Increased aldosterone
4. After 5 hours of unilateral ureteral obstruction, which of the following occurs in the obstructed kidney?
   a. Increased renal plasma flow
   b. Increased glomerular filtration
   c. Shift of blood flow from the outer to the inner cortex
   d. Increased sodium delivery to the macula densa
   e. Decrease in renal vein renin levels
5. Atrial natriuretic peptide induces which of the following?
   a. Decrease in urinary sodium excretion
   b. Increase in afferent arteriolar dilation
   c. Increase in efferent arteriolar dilation
   d. Decrease in glomerular tubular feedback
   e. Increase in renin production
6. Which of the following occurs after bilateral ureteral obstruction?
   a. Shift of blood flow to the outer renal cortex
   b. Decrease in atrial natriuretic peptide
   c. Decrease in collecting system pressure during the first day
   d. Increase in renal plasma flow at 8 hours
   e. None of the above
7. Which of the following may promote tubular interstitial fibrosis in the obstructed kidney?
   a. Increase in renal metalloproteinase levels
   b. Increase in expression of transforming growth factor-β
   c. Administration of enalapril
   d. Administration of losartan
   e. Decrease in phosphorylation of SMAD proteins
8. A difference between unilateral (UUO) and bilateral ureteral obstruction (BUO) is that:
   a. fractional excretion of sodium after relief of obstruction is greater in BUO.
   b. atrial natriuretic peptide levels are higher in UUO.
   c. risk of postobstructive diuresis is less with BUO.
   d. urinary pH is higher in UUO.
   e. new-onset hypertension is more common with UUO.

9. Which of the following is true of compensatory renal growth?
   a. Glomerular number increases.
   b. Insulin-like growth factor-1 is inhibitory.
   c. It increases with age.
   d. Hypertrophic and hyperplastic growth occur.
   e. It is more common with partial obstruction.
10. The chance for renal recovery after ureteral obstruction is most influenced by:
    a. early relief of obstruction.
    b. presence of extrarenal pelvis.
    c. presence of a solitary kidney.
    d. uninfected urine.
    e. normal blood pressure.
11. Which of the following is expected in a kidney that has been obstructed for 1 month?
    a. Increased renal pelvic pressure
    b. Reduced Na^+, K^+-ATPase activity
    c. Reduced urinary pH
    d. Reduced tubulointerstitial fibrosis
    e. Increased aquaporin-2 water channels
12. Reduced expression of sodium transporters in the obstructed kidney may be due to:
    a. reduced delivery of sodium to the nephron.
    b. renal ischemia.
    c. increased renal interstitial pressure.
    d. increased PGE_2.
    e. all of the above.
13. A reduction in concentrating ability of the obstructed kidney is due to:
    a. decreased ADH expression.
    b. maintenance of a medullary hypertonicity and reduced GFR.
    c. increased renal aquaproin-1 water channels.
    d. decreased renal aquaporin-2 water channels.
    e. urea backflux from the inner medullary collecting duct.
14. A persistent concentrating defect after relief of bilateral ureteral obstruction (BUO) is primarily due to:
    a. continued excessive secretion of atrial natriuretic peptide.
    b. decreased synthesis of aquaporins.
    c. decreased synthesis of cyclic AMP.
    d. persistent hypokalemia.
    e. decreased release of ADH from the posterior pituitary.
15. In studies of complete UUO for 24 hours, renal blood flow has been shown to:
    a. briefly cease with ureteral clamping and then gradually return toward control.
    b. gradually decline over the course of the constriction.
    c. increase by 25% and remain elevated during the obstruction.
    d. increase over an hour and then steadily decrease.
    e. remain unchanged during clamping and undergo reactive hyperemia upon release.
16. Ureteral, and tubular, pressure changes in experimental unilateral ureteral occlusion over 24 hours are characterized by:
    a. a continued increase due to urine secretion.
    b. an immediate decrease as flow ceases.
    c. an increase followed by a decrease.
    d. no change due to extravasation of tubule fluid.
    e. no change due to contralateral renal compensation.
17. Which of the following have been implicated in the initial rise in renal blood flow in UUO?
    a. Adenosine and bradykinin
    b. Atrial natriuretic peptide and platelet-activating factor
    c. Dopamine and acetylcholine
    d. Prostaglandin and nitric oxide
    e. Endothelin and angiotensin II
18. Experimental evidence has implicated which of the following vasoconstrictor lipids with the decreased renal blood flow in the third phase of UUO?
    a. Ergosterol
    b. Plasminogen activating inhibitor-1
    c. Prostaglandin E_2
    d. Leukotriene C_4
    e. Thromboxane A_2
19. Which of the following best explains the greater fractional excretion of sodium that follows the release of BUO compared with UUO?
    a. Better preserved glomerular filtration rate with UUO than with BUO
    b. Greater expansion of extracellular volume with BUO than with UUO
    c. More contralateral compensation with BUO than with UUO
    d. Less renal vasoconstriction with BUO than with UUO
    e. More secretion of aldosterone with BUO than with UUO
20. Obstruction causes which of the following disturbances in the renal regulation of acid-base balance?
    a. Decreased bicarbonate reclamation in the proximal tubule
    b. Decreased H^+-ATPase expression in the collecting duct
    c. Greater buffering of acid loads by glutamine breakdown into NH_3
    d. Decreased proportion of H^+ buffered as titratable acid rather than as NH_4^+
    e. Urine pH above 7.4
21. Ureteral obstruction causes which of the following metabolic increases in the kidney?
    a. ATP synthesis
    b. Glycolytic capacity in the cortex
    c. Medullary consumption of oxygen
    d. Ratio of lactate to pyruvate in renal tissue
    e. Utilization of glucose metabolism by the proximal tubule
22. Which of the following contribute(s) to obstruction-induced tubulointerstitial fibrosis?
    a. Angiotensin II
    b. Metalloproteinase inhibitors
    c. Transforming growth factor-β
    d. Nuclear factor-κB
    e. All of the above
23. Obstruction induces apoptosis, or programmed cell death, of nephrons. Tumor necrosis factor-α causes inflammation in the kidney and stimulates which key family of enzymes involved in apoptosis?
    a. Aminopeptidases
    b. Caspases
    c. Metalloproteinases
    d. Phosphatases
    e. Reverse transcriptases

24. A 36-year-old man has severe, acute right flank pain. Which imaging study should be performed?
    a. Excretory urogram
    b. Contrast enhanced CT
    c. Unenhanced CT
    d. Unenhanced MRI
    e. Renal ultrasonography

25. Which of the following studies best predicts whether renal functional recovery will occur after reconstruction of an obstructed kidney?
    a. Diuretic-MAG-3 scan
    b. Diuretic-DTPA scan
    c. Duplex ultrasound of the kidneys
    d. DMSA renogram
    e. Unenhanced magnetic resonance urogram

26. A 40-year-old man has anorexia, fatigue, and a serum creatinine value of 4.6 mg/dL. CT reveals severe bilateral hydronephrosis and a retroperitoneal soft tissue mass encasing the great vessels and ureters. The next step is:
    a. CT-guided biopsy of the mass.
    b. open surgical biopsy of the mass.
    c. placement of bilateral ureteral stents.
    d. corticosteroid therapy.
    e. ureterolysis.

27. Pelvic lipomatosis is associated with:
    a. cystitis glandularis.
    b. prostatic urethral elongation.
    c. bladder neck elevation.
    d. extrinsic compression of the rectum.
    e. all of the above.

28. Which of the following may cause either intrinsic or extrinsic obstruction of the ureter in women?
    a. Gravid uterus
    b. Endometriosis
    c. Tubo-ovarian abscess
    d. Ovarian remnant
    e. Fibroid uterus

29. A 69-year-old woman has bilateral ureteral obstruction secondary to locally invasive cervical cancer. What is the likelihood of stent failure within the first 3 months?
    a. 5%
    b. 15%
    c. 30%
    d. 50%
    e. 90%

30. Which of the following is not characteristic of hydronephrosis of pregnancy?
    a. Right side more commonly affected
    b. Most prevalent in the third trimester
    c. Ureteral dilation above the pelvic brim
    d. Ureteral dilation below the pelvic brim
    e. Usually resolves by 6 weeks post partum

31. A patient has asymptomatic unilateral, mild hydronephrosis 1 week after repair of an abdominal aortic aneurysm. Serum creatinine value is normal. The next step is:
    a. corticosteroid therapy.
    b. tamoxifen therapy.
    c. ureteral stent placement.
    d. exploratory laparotomy.
    e. observation with serial imaging.

32. In a patient with an obstructing ureteral stone, administration of nonsteroidal anti-inflammatory drugs will induce all of the following changes EXCEPT reduction in:
    a. collecting system pressure.
    b. renal blood flow.
    c. renal aquaporin-2 water channels.
    d. diuresis.
    e. pain score.

33. A 55-year-old, otherwise healthy woman has a chronically obstructed left kidney and normal right kidney. Which differential renal function for the left kidney would best serve as a cutoff point below which nephrectomy should be performed and above which salvage should be considered?
    a. 5%
    b. 10%
    c. 25%
    d. 35%
    e. 45%

ANSWERS

1. **a. Renal function impairment.** The term *obstructive nephropathy* should be reserved for the damage to the renal parenchyma that results from an obstruction to the flow of urine anywhere along the urinary tract. The term *hydronephrosis* implies dilatation of the renal pelvis and calyces and can occur without obstruction.

2. **a. Increased sodium excretion.** There is a profound increase in sodium excretion after relief of bilateral ureteral obstruction. This is due to ANP, and perhaps reduced sodium transporters. The massive natriuresis enhances excretion of phosphate, potassium, and magnesium.

3. **d. Increased atrial natriuretic peptide (ANP).** The accumulation of extracellular volume stimulates the synthesis and release of ANP, which promotes increased GFR and sodium excretion. Decreases in the aquaporin water channels in the kidney further promote the diuresis.

4. **c. Shift of blood flow from the outer to the inner cortex.** There is a shift of blood flow from the outer to inner cortex with UUO that is opposite to that which is seen with BUO. At the 5-hour interval of UUO there is a reduction in renal plasma flow and GFR that results in diminished sodium delivery to the macula densa.

5. **b. Increase in afferent arteriolar dilation.** By promoting dilation of the afferent arteriole and constriction of the efferent arteriole, ANP increases GFR. It also decreases the sensitivity of tubuloglomerular feedback, inhibits renin release, and increases the ultrafiltration coefficient.

6. **a. Shift of blood flow to the outer renal cortex.** There is a shift of blood flow to the outer renal cortex with BUO in contrast to the reversed pattern with UUO.

7. **b. Increase in expression of transforming growth factor-β (TGF-β).** There is increased expression of TGF-β with obstruction that contributes to an increase in the extracellular matrix of the kidney and promotes inflammation. TGF-β is activated by angiotensin II, and animal models have demonstrated that pharmacologic methods of inhibiting angiotensin II reduces the fibrosis occurring after obstruction.

8. **a. fractional excretion of sodium after relief of obstruction is greater in BUO.** The increase fractional excretion of sodium in BUO is due to volume expansion resulting in increased levels of ANP and the overall increased solute load.

9. **d. Hypertrophic and hyperplastic growth occur.** Compensatory renal growth of the unaffected kidney has been demonstrated, and animal models indicate that both hyperplastic and hypertrophic growth can occur. These growth patterns may depend on the age of the subject. Insulin-like growth factor-1 is thought to stimulate this event. It is more prominent in the immature kidney. Animal models have demonstrated that glomerular number does not increase during this process.

10. **a. early relief of obstruction.** Although the other distractors influence recovery of renal function after release of obstruction, prompt eradication of obstruction provides the best chance for salvage.

11. **b. Reduced Na^+, K^+-ATPase.** Obstruction results in a reduction in sodium transporters including Na^+, K^+-ATPase. It also promotes tubulointerstitial fibrosis, reduction in aquaporin channels, and acidification defects. The collecting system pressure should not be increased at this interval.

12. **e. all of the above.** All of the factors listed may contribute to a reduction in sodium transporters.

13. **d. decreased renal aquaporin-2 water channels.** The concentrating defect that occurs with obstruction is not due to inadequate levels of ADH. Choices b, c, and e result in enhanced concentrating ability whereas a reduction in aquaporin-2 water channels does the opposite.

14. **b. decreased synthesis of aquaporins.** Li and coworkers (2001) showed that the polyuria after release of BUO correlated with a decreased expression of aquaporins 1, 2, and 3. Over a 30-day period, the expressions of AQP-2 and -3 gradually normalized but the expression of AQP-1 remained decreased. The reduced rate of synthesis and mobilization of water channels into the nephron membranes accounts for a decreased response to exogenous vasopressin or cyclic AMP.

15. **d. increase over an hour and then steadily decrease.** Renal blood flow initially rises in the first phase because of afferent arteriolar vasodilatation. In phase 2, efferent arteriolar constriction keeps ureteral pressure elevated but in phase 3 both preglomerular and postglomerular vasoconstriction reduces renal blood flow and ureteral pressure.

16. **c. an increase followed by a decrease.** The first phase is characterized by a rise in both ureteral pressure and renal blood flow lasting 1 to 1.5 hours. This is followed by a decline in RBF and a continued increase in ureteral (tubular) pressure lasting until the fifth hour of occlusion. The final phase involves a further decline in RBF and a progressive decline in ureteral pressure.

17. **d. Prostaglandin and nitric oxide.** Studies during the early, vasodilatory phase of UUO have shown that the increase in RBF can be prevented by prostaglandin synthesis inhibitors such as indomethacin or other NSAIDs. Intravenous administration of indomethacin before ureteral ligation results in a decline in renal blood flow without the initial vasodilatation. In addition, administration of NO synthesis inhibitors such as L-NAME or L-NMMA attenuates the initial rise in RBF with occlusion in rats, and when L-NMMA was discontinued the rise in RBF was restored in 10 minutes. These findings provide evidence for a role of prostaglandins and nitric oxide in reducing preglomerular afferent arteriolar vascular resistance in the early phase of UUO.

18. **e. Thromboxane A_2.** In the vasoconstrictive, established phase of UUO inhibitors of thromboxane synthesis have shown reduced vasoconstriction, reduced renal TxB_2 production, the stable metabolite of TxA_2, and an increase in the ratio of prostacyclin to thromboxane production. Administration of a thromboxane receptor blocker also improved renal function in rats after 24 hours of UUO.

19. **b. Greater expansion of extracellular volume with BUO than with UUO.** With bilateral obstruction, the contralateral renal unit does not have the opportunity for compensation as with UUO. Extracellular volume may be greatly expanded so that postobstructive diuresis is most commonly seen in this type of obstruction. After relief of BUO, the increased extracellular volume with attendant salt and water buildup, urea and other osmolytes, and increased production of atrial natriuretic peptide and potentially other natriuretic substances all contribute to a profound natriuresis and a FE_{Na} that is greater than after relief of UUO.

20. **b. Decreased H^+-ATPase expression in the collecting duct.** The cumulative evidence shows a major acidification defect in the distal nephron. Release of obstruction does not result in bicarbonaturia, indicating that proximal reclamation remains intact. There is a defect in the proximal handling and breakdown of glutamine, which means that a higher proportion of protons are buffered as titratable acid. Best evidence indicates a defect in the expression of H^+-ATPase in the collecting duct. Even so, because there is a deficit in filtered and excreted phosphate, fewer protons can be buffered by phosphate so that the pH of the urine may be lower in spite of a total net decrease in H^+ secretion.

21. **d. Ratio of lactate to pyruvate in renal tissue.** Obstruction causes a shift from oxidative metabolism to anaerobic respiration. This results in a reduction of renal ATP levels and an increase in the renal lactate to pyruvate ratio. The proximal tubule has relatively little glycolytic capacity and uses ketone bodies, fatty acids, glutamine, and lactate for mitochondrial ATP synthesis. The proximal convoluted tubule cannot utilize glucose for oxidative metabolism.

22. **e. All of the above.** See Figure 37-3 for an overview of the processes leading up to inflammation and increased matrix synthesis and components of fibrosis. Tubule cells, macrophages, and fibroblasts all contribute to the fibrotic process. The mediators of angiotensin II, growth factors, and cytokines contribute to the process and offer opportunities for pharmacologic intervention.

23. **b. Caspases.** Cysteinyl aspartate-specific proteinases (caspases) are known to mediate apoptotic cell death in obstructed kidneys. This is a family of 12 enzymes, and caspase 3 and 8 are best correlated with renal cell apoptosis. Increases in TNF-α and binding of its two receptors initiate events along with stimulation of NF-κB. Growth factors modify the process and offer opportunities for therapeutic intervention.

24. **c. Unenhanced CT.** The reported overall accuracy of unenhanced CT for the detection of ureteral calculi is 97%. Smith and colleagues (1995) demonstrated its superiority over EXU. Contrast-enhanced CT is unnecessary, and the contrast may, in fact, obscure visualization of the calculus. Standard MRI does not reliably identify calculi. The sensitivity of Doppler

ultrasonography in the evaluation of acute colic with suspected obstruction has been reported to be 52% (Chen et al, 1993).

25. **d. DMSA renogram.** The DMSA renogram has been shown to be superior to DTPA or MAG3 for the prediction of renal recovery (Thompson and Gough, 2001). Although some have successfully used these other radiotracers to predict functional recovery, the cortical phase of the renogram is the critical factor. Doppler ultrasound and MRU have not been demonstrated to predict renal recovery.

26. **c. placement of bilateral ureteral stents.** In the acutely ill patient, initial therapy should be directed at draining the obstructed kidneys. Biopsy should be undertaken after metabolic stabilization. An underlying malignancy may be present in 8% to 10% of cases of suspected retroperitoneal fibrosis. This is most commonly obtained percutaneously, but open surgical biopsy may be necessary. Definitive therapy of retroperitoneal fibrosis, whether medical or surgical, should be delayed until after adequate drainage has been obtained and malignancy has been excluded.

27. **e. all of the above.** Cystitis glandularis is present in 40% of patients with pelvic lipomatosis. Elongation of the prostatic urethra and elevation of the bladder neck are commonly encountered mechanical effects of the pelvic lipomatosis and may preclude rigid cystoscopy. Hence the urologist should be aware of these and prepared to perform flexible cystoscopy if needed. Extrinsic compression of the rectum has also been identified in these patients.

28. **b. Endometriosis.** In the female patient, the gravid uterus, endometrial implants, a tubo-ovarian abscess, an ovarian remnant, and fibroids all may cause extrinsic compression and obstruction of the ureter. The ureter is involved in 15% to 20% of endometriosis of the urinary tract. In addition to extrinsic obstruction, ureteral implants may involve the ureteral lumen and cause intrinsic obstruction.

29. **d. 50%.** Ureteral stenting is recognized to be less effective in the management of extrinsic ureteral obstruction, particularly when it is due to malignancy. In a prospective study, a 56% failure rate was noted at 3 months. A similar study noted that over 40% of those stents that ultimately failed had failed within 6 days of initial placement. If ureteral stenting is performed in patients with extrinsic obstruction due to malignancy, close follow-up is warranted.

30. **d. Ureteral dilation below the pelvic brim.** Hydronephrosis of pregnancy is common, occurring in 43% to 100% of women. Although it occurs two to three times more commonly on the right, it may be bilateral. It becomes progressively more common throughout gestation and may persist through the first postpartum week in one third of patients. It should resolve in the majority of patients by 6 weeks post partum. Because a component of the obstruction is due to mechanical obstruction by the gravid uterus at the pelvic brim, hydroureter commonly extends down to this point. Hydroureter between the pelvic brim and the UVJ, however, can be suggestive of another cause of obstruction, such as a calculus in the distal ureter.

31. **e. observation with serial imaging.** Hydronephrosis in the early postoperative period is common and resolves spontaneously in a majority of these patients. Intervention may be required if symptoms arise or renal functional impairment is noted.

32. **c. renal aquaporin-2 water channels.** NSAIDs have been shown to significantly reduce pain in patients treated for acute ureteral obstruction. NSAIDs have also been demonstrated to reduce renal blood flow and collecting system pressure. This may contribute to the reduction in diuresis seen after relief of obstruction. An additional mechanism for the reduced collecting system pressure and reduced diuresis is an NSAID-mediated preservation of aquaporin-2 water channels, preventing the downregulation of aquaporin-2 channels otherwise seen in the obstructive setting.

33. **b. 10%.** The usual cutoff point for nephrectomy is 10% or less of total renal function being supplied by the affected kidney. This has not been prospectively studied but is based on common clinical practice, and as such this must be tempered by clinical insight into the overall status of the patient.

38

Management of Upper Urinary Tract Obstruction

THOMAS H. S. HSU • STEVAN B. STREEM • STEPHEN Y. NAKADA

QUESTIONS

1. Which of the following is considered a contraindication to transureteroureterostomy?
   a. History of retroperitoneal fibrosis
   b. History of urothelial malignancy
   c. History of nephrolithiasis
   d. All of the above
   e. b and c
2. Which of the following regarding the flap procedures for UPJO surgical repair is FALSE?
   a. The flap procedures generally rely on large, redundant extrarenal pelvis.
   b. The flap procedures can be useful in the presence of a relatively long segment of ureteral stricture or narrowing.
   c. A spiral flap can bridge a strictured or narrow area of shorter length.
   d. The flap procedures are not suitable in the setting of crossing vessels.
   e. A vertical flap can bridge a strictured or narrow area of longer length.
3. Foley Y-V plasty is appropriate for which of the following?
   a. Anterior crossing vessel
   b. Duplication of collecting system
   c. Redundant renal pelvis
   d. High ureteral insertion
   e. Small intrarenal pelvis
4. Which of the following is important to achieving successful outcome in surgical management of ureteropelvic junction obstruction?
   a. Funnel-shaped transition between the renal pelvis and ureter
   b. Dependent drainage
   c. Watertight anastomosis
   d. Tension-free anastomosis
   e. All of the above
5. Which of the following type of pyeloplasty (open or laparoscopic) is indicated in the case of an associated aberrant crossing vessel
   a. Foley Y-V plasty
   b. Culp-DeWeerd spiral flap
   c. Scardino-Prince vertical flap
   d. Ligation and transection of the crossing vessel
   e. Dismembered pyeloplasty
6. Which of the following regarding the transperitoneal approach to laparoscopic pyeloplasty is FALSE?
   a. It is used most widely among laparoscopic urologists performing pyeloplasty.
   b. Watertight, tension-free anastomosis is the surgical objective.
   c. It provides more familiar anatomy.
   d. It provides working space equivalent to that in retroperitoneal approach.
   e. External surgical drain is absolutely necessary.
7. A 25-year-old man presents with persistent and worsening right flank pain. He underwent a laparoscopic pyeloplasty 3 years ago that failed within 1 year after the surgery. Consequently, he underwent an attempt at cautery-wire balloon incision and percutaneous antegrade endopyelotomy for persistent right UPJ obstruction, both of which failed. CT shows moderate cortical loss in the right kidney with normal-appearing left kidney. A renogram reveals 35% differential function on the affected side, and a diuretic study demonstrates functional obstruction (half-life > 30 min). What is the next approach?
   a. Indwelling internal ureteral stent that is changed every 3 to 4 months
   b. Ureterocalicostomy
   c. Davis intubated ureterotomy
   d. Ileal ureter
   e. Renal autotransplantation
8. Additional bladder mobility can be achieved via transection of the:
   a. contralateral inferior vesical artery.
   b. ipsilateral inferior vesical artery.
   c. contralateral superior vesical artery.
   d. ipsilateral superior vesical artery.
   e. ipsilateral gonadal artery.
9. The general contraindications to ileal ureter creation include the following EXCEPT:
   a. renal insufficiency with serum creatinine greater than 2 mg/dL.
   b. inflammatory bowel disease.
   c. small intrarenal pelvis.
   d. bladder dysfunction.
   e. radiation enteritis.

10. Retrocaval ureter results from which of the following?
    a. Persistence of anterior cardinal veins
    b. Persistence of posterior cardinal veins
    c. Duplication of inferior vena cava
    d. Aberrance of lumbar veins
    e. Retroaortic renal veins

11. The most common cause of retroperitoneal fibrosis is:
    a. drug-induced etiology.
    b. infection.
    c. lymphoma.
    d. breast cancer.
    e. idiopathy.

12. In a psoas hitch, a structure particularly susceptible to injury is the:
    a. obturator nerve.
    b. genitofemoral nerve.
    c. iliohypogastric nerve.
    d. ilioinguinal nerve.
    e. sacral nerve.

13. Normal bladder capacity and function without outlet obstruction are critical to the success of all the following EXCEPT:
    a. ileal ureteral substitution.
    b. psoas hitch.
    c. endoscopic incision of transmural ureter.
    d. ureteroneocystostomy.
    e. Boari flap.

14. All of the following are true for retroperitoneal fibrosis EXCEPT which one?
    a. Retroperitoneal fibrotic mass generally centers on the distal aorta at L4-L5 and wraps around the ureters, leading to hydronephrosis via extrinsic compression on the ureters or interference with ureteral peristalsis.
    b. Laboratory evaluation may show an elevated erythrocyte sedimentation rate, moderate leukocytosis, anemia, and variable renal insufficiency associated with electrolyte abnormalities.
    c. Initial management of RPF in the presence of hydronephrosis and uremia includes emergent decompression by percutaneous nephrostomy or indwelling ureteral stents.
    d. Medical therapy has no role in the treatment of retroperitoneal fibrosis.
    e. Both open and laparoscopic ureterolysis may be applied successfully.

15. A 40-year-old woman with a history of hypertension and recurrent nephrolithiasis presents with a 5-cm proximal right ureteral stricture following an iatrogenic injury in a recent abdominal surgery. She has an indwelling right nephrostomy tube for over 6 months. Her baseline serum creatinine is 2.5 mg/dL. Renal scan shows split function of 65% in the right kidney. Her bladder capacity is found to be less than 300 mL. What would be the appropriate step of management for her right kidney?
    a. Ureteroureterostomy
    b. Boari flap
    c. Autotransplant
    d. Transureteroureterostomy
    e. Ileal ureter

16. Which of the following is FALSE regarding ileal ureter substitution?
    a. Ischemic necrosis of the ileal segment may occur and should be considered if signs of an acute abdomen are present.
    b. Patients with worsening metabolic abnormalities associated with a progressively dilating ileal ureter should be evaluated for vesicourethral dysfunction.
    c. Malignancy may arise from ileal ureter, warranting surveillance postoperatively.
    d. Significant electrolyte abnormalities and renal insufficiency are unusual if preoperative renal function is normal.
    e. None of the above.

17. Which of the following is not associated with retroperitoneal fibrosis?
    a. β-Adrenergic blocker
    b. Aspirin
    c. Ergot alkaloids
    d. Abdominal aortic aneurysm
    e. Abdominal radiotherapy

18. Ureteropelvic junction (UPJ) obstruction in the neonate is most frequently found as a result of:
    a. maternal-fetal ultrasonography.
    b. voiding cystourethrography.
    c. diuretic renography.
    d. abdominal radiography.
    e. physical examination.

19. Which of the following studies can be diagnostic for functional obstruction at the UPJ?
    a. Retrograde pyelography
    b. Three-dimensional helical CT
    c. Diuretic renography
    d. Renal ultrasound
    e. Renal angiography

20. A 62-year-old man presents with left flank pain. Intravenous pyelography reveals delayed excretion and hydronephrosis to the level of a 2.5-cm calculus at the UPJ. Percutaneous stone extraction is accomplished without difficulty, but a postextraction nephrostogram reveals hydronephrosis to the level of the UPJ without residual stone. A follow-up nephrostogram 1 week later is unchanged. What is the next step?
    a. Removal of the nephrostomy tube
    b. Diuretic renography
    c. CT scan abdomen/pelvis
    d. Antegrade nephrostogram
    e. Whitaker pressure-perfusion test

21. Which of the following clinical situations is most predictive of failure after percutaneous endopyelotomy?
    a. Renal ptosis
    b. Ipsilateral stones
    c. Ipsilateral renal function
    d. Moderate to severe hydronephrosis and crossing vessels
    e. Chronic flank pain

22. The major concern with crossing vessels and UPJ obstruction is:
    a. risk of bleeding.
    b. decreased endopyelotomy success.
    c. ureteral ischemia.
    d. risk of arteriovenous malformation.
    e. diminished visibility intraoperatively.

23. Which modality generally has the lowest success rate in treating UPJ obstruction?
    a. Antegrade endopyelotomy
    b. Retrograde ureteroscopic endopyelotomy
    c. Retrograde balloon dilation
    d. Laparoscopic pyeloplasty
    e. Hot-wire balloon cautery endopyelotomy
24. The most appropriate location for endoscopic incision of a proximal ureteral stricture is:
    a. lateral.
    b. anterior.
    c. medial.
    d. posterior.
    e. anterolateral.
25. The best treatment option for a patient with a functional left ureteroenteric anastomotic stricture is:
    a. balloon dilation.
    b. laser endoureterotomy.
    c. sequential rigid dilation.
    d. cautery balloon endoureterotomy.
    e. open repair.

ANSWERS

1. **d. All of the above.** Relative contraindications include history of nephrolithiasis, retroperitoneal fibrosis, urothelial malignancy, chronic pyelonephritis, and abdominopelvic radiation.
2. **e. A vertical flap can bridge a strictured or narrow area of longer length.** Flap procedures can be useful in situations involving relatively long segments of ureteral narrowing or stricture. Of the various flap procedures, a spiral flap can bridge a strictured or narrow area of longer length. The flap procedures are not appropriate in the setting of crossing vessels.
3. **d. High ureteral insertion.** The Foley Y-V plasty is designed for repair of a UPJ obstruction secondary to a high ureteral insertion. It is specifically contraindicated when transposition of lower pole vessels is necessary. In situations requiring concomitant reduction of redundant renal pelvis, this technique is also of little value.
4. **e. All of the above.** For any surgical repair of UPJ obstruction, the resultant anastomosis should be widely patent and completed in a watertight fashion without tension. In addition, the reconstructed UPJ should allow a funnel-shaped transition between the pelvis and the ureter that is in a position of dependent drainage.
5. **e. Dismembered pyeloplasty.** In the presence of crossing aberrant or accessory lower pole renal vessels associated with UPJ obstruction, a dismembered pyeloplasty is the only method to allow transposition of the UPJ in relation to these vessels.
6. **d. It provides working space equivalent to that in retroperitoneal approach**. Transperitoneal laparoscopic pyeloplasty provides larger working space relative to retroperitoneoscopic approach. Together with more familiar anatomy, transperitoneal approach is used most commonly in the laparoscopic urologic community to date.
7. **b. Ureterocalicostomy.** Direct anastomosis of the proximal ureter to the lower calyceal system is a well-accepted salvage technique for the failed pyeloplasty.
8. **c. contralateral superior vesical artery.** In psoas hitch, transection of contralateral superior vesical artery can be helpful to bridge the gap to the ipsilateral ureteral end, thereby achieving tension-free anastomosis.
9. **c. Small intrarenal pelvis.** In ileal segment usage, small intrarenal pelvis is not considered as a contraindication. In such a scenario, ileocalicostomy can be performed successfully.
10. **b. Persistence of posterior cardinal veins.** Retrocaval ureter results from the persistence of the posterior cardinal veins.
11. **e. idiopathy.** In the majority of cases of retroperitoneal fibrosis, no clear etiology can be identified.
12. **b. genitofemoral nerve.** Genitofemoral nerve injury is well known to occur in psoas hitch procedures.
13. **c. endoscopic incision of transmural ureter.** Normal bladder function without significant outlet obstruction is crucial to the success of ileal ureteral substitution, psoas hitch, Boari flap, and ureteroneocystostomy.
14. **d. Medical management has no role in treatment of retroperitoneal fibrosis.** Although corticosteroids do not reverse the established fibrosis, further inflammatory reaction and fibrosis with their associated symptomatology and sequelae may be minimized. Current data seem to suggest that patients who have the evidence of active inflammation—manifested by increased erythrocyte sedimentation rate, leukocytosis, or active inflammation on a biopsy—are more likely to respond to corticosteroid therapy.
15. **c. Autotransplant.** Ureteroureterostomy is inappropriate for a 5-cm upper ureteral defect. Boari flap is inappropriate for a small bladder capacity. Transureteroureterostomy is contraindicated in the patient with history of recurrent nephrolithiasis. Ileal ureter is contraindicated in the presence of elevated serum creatinine above 2 mg/dL. Autotransplant is appropriate for this particular patient.
16. **e. None of the above.** All of the statements regarding ileal ureter use are true.
17. **b. Aspirin.** Drugs such as ergot alkaloids and β-adrenergic blockers have been identified or implicated in patients with retroperitoneal fibrosis with identifiable etiology. Radiation therapy for retroperitoneal malignancy is also known to produce a residual fibrotic mass leading to secondary ureteral obstruction. Abdominal aortic aneurysm may cause significant retroperitoneal inflammatory reaction, leading to fibrosis and ureteral obstruction.
18. **a. maternal-fetal ultrasonography.** The current widespread use of maternal ultrasonography has led to a dramatic increase in the number of asymptomatic newborns being diagnosed with hydronephrosis, many of whom are subsequently found to have UPJ obstruction.
19. **c. Diuretic renography.** Provocative testing with a diuretic urogram may allow accurate diagnosis of UPJ obstruction. Renal ultrasound, CT, and retrograde pyelogram give anatomic assessments of the UPJ without quantitatively assessing urinary drainage and function.

20. **e. Whitaker pressure-perfusion test.** When there remains some doubt as to the clinical significance of a dilated collecting system, placement of percutaneous nephrostomy allows access for pressure perfusion studies. In the pressure perfusion test, as first described by Whitaker in 1973 and then modified in 1978, the renal pelvis is perfused with normal saline or dilute radiographic contrast solution and the pressure gradient across the presumed area of obstruction is determined. Renal pelvic pressures in excess of 15 to 22 cm are highly suggestive of a functional obstruction. While diuretic renography is useful for diagnosis as well, the Whitaker test is ideal for this situation because a nephrostomy tube is already in situ.

21. **d. Moderate to severe hydronephrosis and crossing vessels.** Consideration of any of the less invasive alternatives to open operative intervention must take into account individual anatomy, including, but not limited to, the degree of hydronephrosis, overall and ipsilateral renal function, and, in some cases, the presence of crossing vessels or concomitant calculi. One study found that endopyelotomy success rates were less than 50% when significant hydronephrosis and crossing vessels were identified preoperatively.

22. **b. decreased endopyelotomy success.** There is evidence that crossing vessels lower the success rate of endopyelotomy from several investigators; and when such patients were culled from the pool of candidates available for treatment of UPJ obstruction, endopyelotomy success rates improved in most studies. Although crossing vessels remain controversial, certainly reports indicate the risk of bleeding is not a reason to avoid endopyelotomy if the incision is directed properly.

23. **c. Retrograde balloon dilation.** McClinton reported long-term follow-up data on balloon dilation of the UPJ, finding a success rate of only 42%, which was significantly lower than the initial publications would indicate.

24. **a. lateral.** Proximal ureteral strictures are incised laterally, similar to UPJ strictures. Posterior incision is offered to UPJ obstruction patients who have failed open pyeloplasty. Distal strictures are incised anteriorly, as are strictures of the middle ureter.

25. **e. open repair.** There are several studies linking poor outcomes with endoscopic management of left ureteroenteric strictures. This may be a result of diminished blood flow to the ureter, because the left ureter requires more mobilization than the right side at the time of diversion. With open repair, reports demonstrate an 80% success rate, although these are often challenging cases.

39

Renal and Ureteral Trauma

JACK W. McANINCH • RICHARD A. SANTUCCI

QUESTIONS

1. What method is used to perform 'one-shot' intraoperative IVP in a 50-kg woman?
   a. Inject a 50-mL bolus of intravenous contrast agent followed by a full IVP series, including abdominal compression to evaluate the ureters.
   b. Inject a 100-mL bolus of intravenous contrast agent followed in exactly 10 minutes by a flat plate of the abdomen on the operating room table.
   c. Inject a 50-mL bolus of intravenous contrast agent followed in exactly 10 minutes by a flat plate of the abdomen on the operating room table.
   d. Determine the patient's serum creatinine level before administration of intravenous contrast agent to make sure that she will not experience renal failure as a result of reaction to the contrast agent.
   e. Inject 100 mL of intravenous contrast and obtain a kidney, ureter, bladder (KUB) scan once the patient is safely out of surgery.
2. What is the best option for repair of midureteral transection after a stab wound?
   a. Ureteroureterostomy
   b. Transureteroureterostomy
   c. Boari flap
   d. Nonabsorbable sutures
   e. Intraperitonealization of the ureteral anastomosis
3. When ureteroureterostomy is performed, which of the following is required?
   a. Postoperative retroperitoneal suction drain
   b. Postoperative nephrostomy drain
   c. Spatulated, watertight repair
   d. Nonabsorbable sutures
   e. Intraperitonealization of the ureteral anastomosis
4. Which maneuver is cited as a cause of ureteral injury during stone basketing?
   a. Ureteroscopy without dilating the ureteral orifice first
   b. Ureteroscopy in nondilated systems
   c. Use of the holmium laser
   d. Pulsatile saline irrigation to assist visualization
   e. Persistence in stone basketing attempts in the face of a ureteral tear
5. Which of the following is a contraindication to transureteroureterostomy for repair of significant lower ureter injury?
   a. History of urolithiasis
   b. History of ureteral trauma
   c. Obesity
   d. Neurogenic bladder
   e. Spinal fracture
6. What is the treatment of choice for a ureteral contusion by a high-velocity bullet?
   a. Observation
   b. Ureteral stent placement
   c. Transureteroureterostomy
   d. Ureteroureterostomy
   e. Oversewing the contusion with healthy ureteral tissue
7. Which imaging technique is most useful for detecting ureteral injuries after trauma?
   a. CT without use of contrast material
   b. CT with use of contrast agent, obtained immediately after injection of the contrast agent
   c. CT with the use of contrast material, obtained 20 minutes after injection of the contrast agent
   d. Intravenous pyelography
   e. Furosemide (Lasix) renography
8. Which of the following statements is TRUE about ureteral injuries during laparoscopy?
   a. Total number of injuries has stayed steady over the years.
   b. Surgery for endometriosis greatly increases the risk.
   c. Bipolar cautery use during tubal ligation eliminates risk.
   d. Most are recognized immediately.
   e. Indigo carmine dye eliminates the risk of injury.

ANSWERS

1. **b. Inject a 100-mL bolus of intravenous contrast agent followed in exactly 10 minutes by a flat plate of the abdomen on the operating room table.** Only a single film is taken 10 minutes after intravenous injection (IV push) of 2 mL/kg of contrast material.
2. **a. Ureteroureterostomy.** Ureteroureterostomy, so-called end-to-end repair in injuries to the upper two thirds of the ureter, is common (up to 32% of one large series) and has a reported success rate as high as 90%.
3. **c. Spatulated, watertight repair.** Repair ureters under magnification with spatulated, tension-free, stented, watertight anastomosis, placing retroperitoneal drains afterward.
4. **e. Persistence in stone basketing attempts in the face of a ureteral tear.** One factor cited as a cause of injury was the persistence in stone basket attempts after recognition of a ureteral tear, and current recommendations are to stop and place a ureteral stent.
5. **a. History of urolithiasis.** Some authors believe that this operation is contraindicated in patients with a history of urothelial calculi.
6. **d. Ureteroureterostomy.** Ureteral contusions, although the most "minor" of ureteral injuries, often heal with stricture or break down later if microvascular injury results in ureteral necrosis. Severe or large areas of contusion should be treated with excision and ureteroureterostomy.
7. **c. CT with the use of contrast material, obtained 20 minutes after injection of the contrast agent.** Because modern helical CT scanners can obtain images before intravenous contrast dye is excreted in the urine, delayed images must be obtained (5 to 20 minutes after contrast material injection) to allow contrast material to extravasate from the injured collecting system, renal pelvis, or ureter.
8. **b. Surgery for endometriosis greatly increases the risk.** A large percentage of ureteral injuries after gynecologic laparoscopy occur during electrosurgical or laser-assisted lysis of endometriosis.

SECTION X

RENAL FAILURE AND TRANSPLANTATION

Renal Transplantation

JOHN M. BARRY • MARK L. JORDAN

QUESTIONS

1. The incidence of patients starting renal replacement therapy for end-stage renal disease (ESRD) in the United States is between that of which two cancers?
   a. Breast and prostate
   b. Prostate and bladder
   c. Bladder and kidney
   d. Kidney and testis
   e. Bladder and testis
2. ESRD in adults is defined as an irreversible glomerular filtration rate (GFR) of less than how many milliliters per minute and a serum creatinine level of greater than how many milligrams per deciliter?
   a. 5 mL/min, 10 mg/dL
   b. 10 mL/min, 8 mg/dL
   c. 15 mL/min, 6 mg/dL
   d. 20 mL/min, 5 mg/dL
   e. 20 mL/min, 4 mg/dL
3. The most common form of treatment for adults with ESRD is:
   a. kidney transplantation.
   b. chronic ambulatory peritoneal dialysis.
   c. in-center hemodialysis
   d. home hemodialysis.
   e. in-center peritoneal dialysis.
4. When was the first human-to-human kidney transplantation performed?
   a. 1908
   b. 1926
   c. 1933
   d. 1951
   e. 1954
5. Which of the following renal diseases has a high probability of recurrence in patients with a kidney transplant, resulting in failure of the kidney graft?
   a. Chronic glomerulonephritis
   b. Focal segmental glomerulosclerosis
   c. IgA nephropathy
   d. Alport's syndrome
   e. Autosomal dominant polycystic kidney disease
6. Lymphoproliferative disorders are most commonly associated with which of the following viruses?
   a. Herpes simplex virus type 1
   b. Varicella-zoster virus
   c. Epstein-Barr virus (EBV)
   d. Cytomegalovirus virus (CMV)
   e. Coxsackievirus
7. To reduce the risk of cancer recurrence, a minimum waiting time of how many cancer-free years from the time of last cancer treatment is recommended for patients who have had invasive malignancies?
   a. 1
   b. 2
   c. 3
   d. 4
   e. 5
8. A disadvantage of intestinal augmentation cystoplasty in an anephric hemodialysis patient is:
   a. hyperkalemia.
   b. hypernatremia.
   c. metabolic acidosis.
   d. metabolic alkalosis.
   e. mucus.

9. Pretransplant nephrectomy is indicated for:
   a. hypertension controlled with medication.
   b. prior renal infection.
   c. renal calculi unsuitable for minimally invasive procedures.
   d. 200 mg/dL proteinuria.
   e. most polycystic kidneys.

10. The best renal imaging protocol for a living renal donor to define renal anatomy and renal vasculature and to rule out renal stones is:
    a. kidney, ureter, bladder (KUB) radiography and selective renal arteriography.
    b. magnetic resonance nephrotomography and angiography.
    c. helical CT without and with intravenous contrast.
    d. helical CT without and with intravenous contrast and a KUB radiograph.
    e. renal ultrasonography and selective renal arteriography.

11. After living donor nephrectomy, the renal donor is expected to have what level of total renal function?
    a. 50%
    b. 65%
    c. 75%
    d. 90%
    e. 95%

12. Kidney transplant survival rates are poorest for which of the following donor categories?
    a. sibling
    b. parent
    c. spouse
    d. standard criteria deceased
    e. expanded criteria deceased

13. The initial goals of resuscitation of the brain-dead cadaver donor are systolic blood pressure of what level and urinary output exceeding how many milliliters per kilogram per hour?
    a. 100 mm Hg, 0.25 mL/kg/hr
    b. 60 mm Hg, 0.5 mL/kg/hr
    c. 90 mm Hg, 0.5 mL/kg/hr
    d. 90 mm Hg, 0.3 mL/kg/hr
    e. 80 mm Hg, 0.4 mL/kg/hr

14. Which of the following is required for the cellular sodium-potassium pump to maintain a high intracellular concentration of potassium and a low intracellular concentration of sodium?
    a. ADP
    b. ATP
    c. CMP
    d. CTP
    e. Nitric oxide

15. The best solution for preservation of all abdominal organs is:
    a. EuroCollins.
    b. Collins 2.
    c. Sach's solution.
    d. University of Wisconsin (UW) solution.
    e. Lactated Ringer's solution with heparin.

16. A cadaver kidney transplant recipient receives points on the national waiting list for all of the following EXCEPT:
    a. time on the waiting list.
    b. age younger than 18 years.
    c. panel reactive antibody (PRA) level greater than 80%.
    d. histocompatibility.
    e. full-time employment.

17. In the absence of significant recipient arteriosclerosis, the renal artery is usually anastomosed to the:
    a. aorta.
    b. external iliac artery.
    c. common iliac artery.
    d. internal iliac artery.
    e. internal pudendal artery.

18. The renal vein is usually anastomosed to the recipient's:
    a. inferior vena cava.
    b. common iliac vein.
    c. external iliac vein.
    d. posterior gluteal vein.
    e. internal iliac vein.

19. The standard method of urinary tract reconstruction during renal transplantation is:
    a. ureteropyelostomy.
    b. ureteroureterostomy.
    c. ureteroneocystostomy.
    d. vesicopyelostomy.
    e. cutaneous ureterostomy.

20. The usual intravenous solution for urine volume replacement after renal transplantation is:
    a. 0.25% saline.
    b. 0.45% saline.
    c. 0.45% saline in D5W.
    d. 0.90% saline.
    e. D5W.

21. The risk of a hyperacute rejection after kidney transplantation is high when which of the following crossmatch is positive?
    a. B-cell flow
    b. T-cell flow
    c. B-cell microlymphocytotoxicity
    d. T-cell microlymphocytotoxicity
    e. DR-cell

22. Which of the following immunosuppressants inhibits cell cycle progression?
    a. Azathioprine
    b. Mycophenolate mofetil
    c. Cyclosporine
    d. Tacrolimus
    e. Sirolimus

23. Which of the following paired immunosuppressants have similar mechanisms of action and toxicity?
    a. Azathioprine and cyclosporine
    b. Azathioprine and tacrolimus
    c. Basiliximab and mycophenolate mofetil
    d. Cyclosporine and tacrolimus
    e. OKT3 and mycophenolate mofetil

24. Which of the following two drugs have been used to reduce calcineurin inhibitor dosing and cost while maintaining blood levels and immunosuppressive effect?
    a. Diltiazem and ketoconazole
    b. Prednisone and azathioprine
    c. Basiliximab and daclizumab
    d. Equine antilymphocyte globulin and azathioprine
    e. Mycophenolate mofetil and azathioprine

25. Steroid-resistant rejection is often treated with:
    a. thymoglobulin.
    b. glucocorticoids.
    c. sirolimus.
    d. daclizumab.
    e. mycophenolate mofetil.

26. Prophylaxis against *Pneumocystis* infection is best achieved with:
    a. trimethoprim-sulfamethoxazole.
    b. erythromycin.
    c. ciprofloxacin.
    d. cephalexin.
    e. minocycline.

27. Prophylaxis against cytomegalovirus infection is best done with:
    a. trimethoprim-sulfamethoxazole.
    b. erythromycin.
    c. ganciclovir.
    d. basiliximab.
    e. minocycline.

28. A cadaver kidney transplant recipient has a serum creatinine level of 1.9 mg/dL. A large, asymptomatic perigraft fluid collection is aspirated, and the creatinine level is 2.0 mg/dL. What is the most likely diagnosis?
    a. Hydrocele
    b. Lymphocele
    c. Perinephric abscess
    d. Hematoma
    e. Urinoma

29. Which of the following interferes with the tubular secretion of creatinine and can cause an increase in serum creatinine levels?
    a. Azathioprine
    b. Trimethoprim
    c. Mycophenolate mofetil
    d. Tacrolimus
    e. Basiliximab

30. Fluconazole is prescribed to treat cystitis caused by yeast. Which of the following medications will need to have the dose reduced?
    a. Muromonab CD3
    b. Prednisone
    c. Tacrolimus
    d. Azathioprine
    e. Mycophenolate mofetil

31. Hemorrhagic cystitis in an immunosuppressed patient has been associated with which of the following viruses?
    a. Cytomegalovirus
    b. Adenovirus
    c. Herpes simplex virus type 1
    d. Herpes simplex virus type 2
    e. Polyoma virus

32. Which of the following antihypertensive agents is least likely to cause erectile dysfunction?
    a. Propranolol
    b. Clonidine
    c. Methyldopa
    d. Labetalol
    e. Lisinopril

33. A successful kidney transplant recipient and his wife desire to have a child. What is the recommended length of time in months between transplantation and impregnation?
    a. 3
    b. 6
    c. 9
    d. 12
    e. 24

34. At what frequency would preterm delivery be expected in a pregnant kidney transplant recipient?
    a. 10%
    b. 20%
    c. 30%
    d. 40%
    e. 50%

35. The most common cancer after kidney transplantation is:
    a. skin.
    b. cervix.
    c. Kaposi sarcoma.
    d. thyroid.
    e. breast.

36. A kidney transplant recipient has recurrent superficial transitional cell carcinoma of the urinary bladder. Each of the following treatments is acceptable EXCEPT:
    a. fulguration.
    b. thiotepa instillation
    c. mitomycin instillation.
    d. BCG instillation.
    e. doxorubicin instillation

37. Hyperlipidemia is most often associated with which of the following three-drug combinations?
    a. Prednisone, cyclosporine, sirolimus
    b. Antithymocyte globulin, tacrolimus, mycophenolate mofetil
    c. Mycophenolate mofetil, tacrolimus, basiliximab
    d. Cyclosporine, tacrolimus, mycophenolate mofetil
    e. Daclizumab, mycophenolate mofetil, azathioprine

ANSWERS

1. **b. Prostate and bladder.** The estimated number of patients starting renal replacement therapy each year for ESRD in the United States is about 335 per million population. The two most common urologic cancers, in order, are prostate and bladder, and the incidence of ESRD is between them.

2. **b. 10 mL/min, 8 mg/dL.** Permanent renal failure in adults is commonly defined as an irreversible GFR of less than 10 mL/min or a serum creatinine level of greater than 8.0 mg/dL.

3. **c. in-center hemodialysis.** In-center hemodialysis is the predominant form of therapy for adults with ESRD. In the United States, it accounts for about 60% of all treated ESRD patients.

4. **c. 1933.** In 1933, the first human renal allograft was performed by Voronoy in the Ukraine. The recipient was a 26-year-old woman who had attempted suicide by ingesting mercuric chloride. The donor was a 66-year-old man whose kidney had been removed 6 hours after death.

5. **b. Focal segmental glomerulosclerosis.** Patients with focal segmental glomerulosclerosis, hemolytic-uremic syndrome, or primary oxalosis should be counseled about the significant probability of disease recurrence and the risk of secondary graft failure.

6. **c. Epstein-Barr virus (EBV).** EBV titers are determined in children, and, for the EBV-seronegative child, a kidney from an EBV-seronegative donor is preferred to reduce the risk of a post-transplant lymphoproliferative disorder, the most common de novo malignancy in pediatric organ transplant recipients.

7. **b. 2.** To reduce the risk of cancer recurrence, a waiting time of 2 to 5 cancer-free years from the time of last cancer treatment is recommended for patients who have had invasive malignancies.

8. **e. mucus.** A urothelial-lined augmentation is best because mucus does not have to be rinsed from the bladder on a regular basis.

9. **c. renal calculi unsuitable for minimally invasive procedures.** The generally accepted indications for pretransplant nephrectomy include the following: renal stones not cleared by minimally invasive techniques or lithotripsy; solid renal tumors with or without acquired renal cystic disease; polycystic kidneys that are symptomatic, extend below the iliac crest, have been infected, or have solid tumors; persistent antiglomerular basement membrane antibody levels; significant proteinuria not controlled with medical nephrectomy or angioablation; recurrent pyelonephritis; and grade 4 or 5 hydronephrosis.

10. **d. helical CT with and without intravenous contrast and a KUB radiograph.** Three-dimensional CT angiography without and with intravenous contrast followed by a radiograph of the abdomen has been widely accepted for use with living renal donors because it satisfactorily excludes stone disease, demonstrates renal and vascular anatomy, and defines the urinary collecting system, all with minimal donor morbidity and at reasonable expense.

11. **c. 75%.** Hyperfiltration injury has not been a problem for living renal donors. Endogenous creatinine clearance rapidly approaches 70% to 80% of the preoperative level, and this has been shown to be sustained for more than 10 years. The development of late hypertension is nearly the same as that for the general population, and the development of proteinuria is negligible.

12. **e. Expanded criteria deceased.** Kidney transplant survival rates are poorest when the quality of the kidney is the worst. Expended criteria deceased kidney donors are older than the age of 60 years or are older than the age of 50 years and have two of the following: death from cerebrovascular accident, hypertension, or serum creatinine > 1.5 mg/dL.

13. **c. 90 mm Hg, 0.5 mL/kg/hr.** The initial goals of resuscitation of the brain-dead cadaver donor are a systolic blood pressure of 90 mm Hg and a urinary output exceeding 0.5 ml/kg/hr.

14. **b. ATP.** ATP is required for the cellular sodium-potassium pump to maintain a high intracellular concentration of potassium and a low intracellular concentration of sodium.

15. **d. University of Wisconsin (UW) solution.** The UW solution minimizes cellular swelling with the impermeable solutes lactobionate, raffinose, and hydroxyethyl starch. Phosphate is used for its hydrogen ion buffering qualities, adenosine is for ATP synthesis during reperfusion, glutathione is a free radical scavenger, allopurinol inhibits xanthine oxidase and the generation of free radicals, and magnesium and dexamethasone are membrane-stabilizing agents. A major advantage of this preservation solution has been its utility as a universal preservation solution for all intra-abdominal organs.

16. **e. full-time employment.** A point system that has evolved in the United States for the selection of cadaver kidney transplant recipients that includes the following variables: waiting time; human leukocyte antigen panel reactive antibody greater than 80%; age < 17 years; donor of kidney, liver segment, lung segment, partial pancreas, or small bowel segment; and histocompatibility.

17. **d. internal iliac artery.** The renal artery is usually anastomosed to the end of the internal iliac artery or to the side of the external iliac artery.

18. **c. external iliac vein.** The renal vein, with or without an extension, is usually anastomosed end-to-side to the external iliac vein.

19. **c. ureteroneocystostomy.** Urinary tract reconstruction is usually by antireflux ureteroneocystostomy, of which there are several techniques.

20. **b. 0.45% saline.** Intravenous fluid that contains 5% dextrose is given to replace estimated insensible losses, and 0.45% saline in 0% dextrose is given at a rate equal to the previous hour's urinary output. This is to prevent hyperglycemia and an osmotic diuresis when the urinary output is very high.

21. **d. T-cell microlymphocytotoxicity crossmatch.** Hyperacute rejection is very rare when the T-cell microlymphocytotoxicity crossmatch between recipient serum and donor lymphocytes is negative.

22. **e. Sirolimus.** Sirolimus (formerly called rapamycin) inhibits cell cycle progression.

23. **d. Cyclosporine and tacrolimus.** Cyclosporine and tacrolimus have similar mechanisms of action, effectiveness, and cost, but slightly different side effect profiles, and they are not used together.

24. **a. Diltiazem and ketoconazole.** Diltiazem and ketoconazole have been used to reduce cyclosporine dosing and cost while maintaining blood levels and immunosuppressive effect.

25. **a. thymoglobulin.** Conventional treatment for acute renal allograft rejection is high-dose pulses of glucocorticoids. Treatment of steroid-resistant rejection is with antilymphocyte antibody preparations such as muromonab-CD3 and thymoglobulin.

26. **a. trimethoprim-sulfamethoxazole.** Commonly used regimens to prevent infections include trimethoprim-sulfamethoxazole for 3 months for prophylaxis against *Pneumocystis* pneumonia.

27. **c. ganciclovir.** Prophylaxis against cytomegalovirus disease is possible with ganciclovir, acyclovir, valacyclovir, or cytomegalovirus immune globulin.

28. **b. Lymphocele.** Lymph, urine, and blood can be differentiated from each other by creatinine and hematocrit determinations. Lymph has a creatinine concentration that is the same as serum, urine has a creatinine concentration higher than that of serum and approaching that of bladder urine, and blood has a high hematocrit level when compared with the other two fluids.

29. **b. Trimethoprim.** Trimethoprim interferes with the tubular secretion of creatinine, and this can cause an increase in serum creatinine levels.

30. **c. Tacrolimus.** Cyclosporine and tacrolimus doses usually have to be reduced when ketoconazole or fluconazole is given because these drugs interfere with the metabolism of both of those immunosuppressants.

31. **b. Adenovirus.** Hemorrhagic cystitis can be caused by adenovirus. The disease is usually self-limited and resolves within a week or two.

32. **e. Lisinopril.** Erectile dysfunction can be due to any one or a combination of factors. Included are the antihypertensives clonidine, methyldopa, propranolol, and labetalol. ACE inhibitors, calcium channel blockers, and α-adrenergic blockers are relatively "penis friendly." Lisinopril is an ACE inhibitor.

33. **d. 12 months.** Among male recipients who have fathered children, there has been no increase in congenital abnormalities in the offspring. However, it is recommended that impregnation be delayed for at least 1 year after transplantation.

34. **e. 50%.** Successful renal transplantation usually restores female fertility. In a report based on thousands of pregnancies in renal transplant recipients, Davison and Milne noted, among other findings, that 50% of the deliveries were preterm.

35. **a. skin.** Immunosuppressed patients are more likely to develop cancer than age-matched control subjects in the general population. Among several thousand tumors that occurred in renal transplant recipients, the common cancers, in order, were skin, lymphoma, Kaposi sarcoma, carcinomas of the cervix, renal tumors, and carcinomas of the vulva and perineum.

36. **d. BCG instillation.** BCG should be avoided for the treatment of superficial transitional cell carcinoma of the bladder in immunosuppressed kidney transplant recipients because of the risk of systemic infection and the likelihood of diminished therapeutic response.

37. **a. Prednisone, cyclosporine, sirolimus.** Prednisone, cyclosporine, and sirolimus all result in hyperlipidemia.

41

Etiology, Pathogenesis, and Management of Renal Failure

DAVID A. GOLDFARB • JOSEPH V. NALLY JR. • MARTIN J. SCHREIBER JR.

QUESTIONS

1. Creatinine clearance overestimates GFR in renal insufficiency because:
   a. tubular creatinine reabsorption is increased.
   b. creatinine production is decreased.
   c. proportion of tubular creatinine secretion is increased.
   d. total body creatinine is increased.
   e. glomerular creatinine selectivity is increased.
2. In patients with occult renal artery stenosis, ACE inhibitors cause acute renal failure due to:
   a. sodium retention.
   b. increased antidiuretic hormone.
   c. afferent arteriolar vasoconstriction.
   d. efferent arteriolar vasodilation.
   e. decreased sympathetic nervous system activity.
3. Six days after partial nephrectomy in a solitary kidney the patient is oliguric. Large amounts of fluid are coming from the flank drain. The serum creatinine value increases from 1.7 to 3.2 mg/dL. The next step in management is:
   a. renal angiography.
   b. CT scan with intravenous contrast.
   c. renal scan.
   d. immediate surgical exploration.
   e. MRI.
4. After a 7-hour complex urethral reconstruction performed in the extended lithotomy position, a patient has severe thigh and buttocks pain. The creatine phosphokinase (CPK) is dramatically elevated. The next step is:
   a. dopamine infusion.
   b. plasmapheresis.
   c. dobutamine infusion.
   d. forced alkaline diuresis.
   e. dialysis.
5. The sentinel cellular change in renal ischemic injury is:
   a. loss of cell polarity.
   b. depletion of ATP.
   c. alteration of Na^+ metabolism.
   d. increased intracellular Ca^{2+}.
   e. increased oxidant stress.
6. The renal structure at greatest risk for ischemic injury is the:
   a. afferent arteriole.
   b. cortical collecting duct.
   c. juxtaglomerular apparatus.
   d. straight segment (S3) proximal tubule.
   e. distal convoluted tubule.
7. A patient with acute renal failure has a urinary sodium value of 10 mEq/L, urinary osmolality of 650 mOsm/kg, and a renal failure index of < 1. Urinalysis shows 10 to 20 RBC/HPF, 3 to 5 WBC/HPF, 2+ proteinuria, and RBC casts. The most likely diagnosis is:
   a. acute tubular necrosis.
   b. prerenal azotemia.
   c. acute glomerulonephritis.
   d. acute interstitial nephritis.
   e. obstruction.
8. When renal impairment is demonstrated in a patient, the first therapeutic intervention should be to:
   a. begin low dose dopamine.
   b. administer a cardiac inotropic agent.
   c. restore adequate circulating blood volume.
   d. administer a loop diuretic.
   e. begin a mannitol infusion.
9. Loop diuretics are of benefit in the management of ATN owing to:
   a. improved patient survival.
   b. decreased metabolic demand.
   c. decreased hypoxic cell swelling.
   d. free radical scavenging.
   e. increased renal vascular resistance.
10. Regarding the pharmacologic management of acute renal failure:
    a. mannitol has a demonstrated beneficial effect.
    b. outcome results are improved in patients who respond to loop diuretics.
    c. atrial natriuretic peptide is associated with hypertension.
    d. calcium channel blockers adversely affect renal outcomes.
    e. growth factors prevent renal ischemic injury.

11. Dopamine therapy in acute renal failure:
    a. causes efferent arteriolar vasodilation.
    b. is recommended for routine use after renal transplantation.
    c. is effective due to improved cardiac function.
    d. is an unproven treatment.
    e. improves patient survival.

12. A patient with ATN after partial nephrectomy has a serum potassium value of 6.9 mEq/L and widening of the QRS complex on ECG. The initial step in management should be:
    a. intravenous calcium.
    b. intravenous insulin and glucose.
    c. sodium polystyrene sulfonate resin (Kayexalate).
    d. intravenous furosemide.
    e. dialysis.

13. A patient with a serum creatinine value of 2.7 mg/dL requires renal angiography. The best way to protect renal function is:
    a. saline diuresis.
    b. pre-study mannitol.
    c. furosemide before study.
    d. dopamine throughout the study.
    e. atrial natriuretic factor before study.

14. In response to a reduction in renal mass, a number of events occur within the kidney that include all of the following EXCEPT:
    a. activation of the sympathetic nervous system.
    b. hyperfiltration.
    c. glomerular hypertrophy.
    d. intrarenal vascular occlusion.
    e. interstitial fibrosis.

15. A 65-year-old man has a radical nephrectomy. The estimated GFR by MDRD equation is 56 mL/min. Follow-up should include:
    a. low protein diet.
    b. renal transplant evaluation.
    c. nephrology consult for stage 3 CKD.
    d. reassessment of kidney function every few months.
    e. loop diuretics.

16. A hypertensive patient with CKD should take an ACE inhibitor to:
    a. improve renal function.
    b. prevent progressive kidney disease.
    c. improve cardiac ejection fraction.
    d. enhance glycemic control.
    e. control blood lipids.

17. The most common cause for ESRD in the United States is:
    a. FSGS.
    b. MPGN (type 2).
    c. membranous glomerulonephritis.
    d. autosomal dominant polycystic kidney disease.
    e. diabetes mellitus.

18. The most accurate monitoring tool for assessment of progression of renal failure is:
    a. urinary creatinine clearance.
    b. Cockcroft-Gault formula.
    c. serum creatinine.
    d. MDRD study equation.
    e. iothalamate GFR measurement.

19. A hypertensive 38-year-old man has a serum creatinine value of 2.4 mg/dL. The urinalysis has 10 to 20 RBC/HPF, 3+ protein, and RBC casts. Ultrasound shows echogenic kidneys without hydronephrosis. The best way to achieve a diagnosis is with:
    a. renal angiography.
    b. renal biopsy.
    c. retrograde pyelography.
    d. MRI.
    e. spiral CT.

20. In addition to an ACE inhibitor, patients with CKD would benefit from which drug to help slow the progression of renal disease:
    a. α-adrenergic blocker.
    b. thiazide diuretic.
    c. HMG-CoA reductase inhibitor (statin).
    d. β-adrenergic blocker.
    e. nitrate.

21. Chronic renal failure patients treated with an ACE inhibitor may experience a decrease in residual renal function in the setting of:
    a. unilateral renal artery stenosis.
    b. concomitant treatment with an α-adrenergic blocker.
    c. acquired renal cystic disease.
    d. left ventricular hypertrophy.
    e. autosomal dominant PKD with cysts larger than 10 cm.

22. The best renal replacement therapy for an otherwise healthy 37-year-old woman with chronic interstitial nephritis is:
    a. preemptive transplantation.
    b. stabilization with hemodialysis for 1 year, then transplant.
    c. stabilization with peritoneal dialysis for 1 year, then transplant.
    d. home hemodialysis.
    e. peritoneal dialysis with an automated cycler.

23. Based on the National Kidney Foundation K/DOQI Clinical Guidelines, dialysis should be initiated in chronic renal failure patients except when:
    a. the weekly KrT/V urea is less than 2.
    b. the patient has more than 6% involuntary reduction of edema free water.
    c. the body weight is less than 90% of standardized body weight for NHANES II.
    d. the reduction of albumin is by more than 0.3 g/dL.
    e. the hematocrit is higher than 25%.

24. Late referral for dialysis is associated with:
    a. hematocrit < 20%.
    b. Kt/V > 2.
    c. increased mortality rate.
    d. vascular access problems.
    e. increased edema-free body weight.

25. The strongest predictor of hospitalization in chronic dialysis patients is:
    a. African-American race.
    b. hematocrit < 30%.
    c. glomerulonephritis.
    d. poor nutritional status.
    e. age < 30 years.

ANSWERS

1. **c. proportion of tubular creatinine secretion is increased.** Serum creatinine is produced at a constant rate by muscle and more accurately reflects the GFR. When renal function deteriorates, tubular secretion represents an increasing proportion of creatinine excretion. Therefore, creatinine clearance may overestimate the GFR as renal function slowly declines when measured in the steady state.
2. **d. efferent arteriolar vasodilatation.** Angiotensin II has selectively greater vasoconstrictor effects on the efferent than on the afferent arteriole, whereas vasodilatory prostaglandins cause afferent arteriolar vasodilatation. Drugs that block angiotensin II synthesis (ACE inhibitors), block angiotensin II receptor binding (angiotensin II receptor antagonists), or inhibit vasodilatory prostaglandin synthesis (nonsteroidal anti-inflammatory drugs) may cause ARF in selected clinical settings.
3. **c. renal scan.** Ways to confirm urinary extravasation include intravenous administration of a vital dye excreted by the kidneys (e.g., indigo carmine or methylene blue) and radiographic demonstration of a fistula (isotope renography, retrograde pyelography, cystography, CT). Renal scan can assess perfusion and also demonstrate extravasation.
4. **d. forced alkaline diuresis.** The combination of renal hypoperfusion and the nephrotoxic insult of myoglobin or hemoglobin within the proximal tubule may result in acute tubular necrosis (ATN). Early recognition of this disorder is crucial, because a forced alkaline diuresis is indicated to minimize nephrotoxicity.
5. **b. depletion of ATP.** The sentinel biochemical event in renal ischemia is the depletion of ATP, which is the major energy currency for cellular work.
6. **d. straight segment (S3) proximal tubule.** The S3 segment of the proximal tubule is associated with the greatest ischemic damage. Other structures that sustain injury in this region include the medullary thick ascending limb, which is metabolically active and rich in the energy-requiring Na^+, K+-ATPase.
7. **c. acute glomerulonephritis.** A low fractional excretion of sodium (or renal failure index) may be associated with either prerenal azotemia or acute glomerulonephritis. These entities could be separated clinically by examination of the urinalysis results. Conditions associated with prerenal azotemia would have a bland urinalysis, whereas proteinuria, RBCs, and RBC casts would be seen with acute glomerulonephritis.
8. **c. restore adequate circulating blood volume.** During the initial stages, a trial of parenteral hydration with isotonic fluids may correct ARF secondary to prerenal causes.
9. **b. decreasing metabolic demand.** They decrease active NaCl transport in the thick ascending limb of Henle and thereby limit energy requirements in the metabolically active segment, which often bears the greatest ischemic insult.
10. **a. mannitol has a demonstrated beneficial effect.** Mannitol has shown some benefit in the clinical setting of ARF, particularly when administered prophylactically or within a short time after an ischemic or nephrotoxic insult.
11. **d. is an unproven treatment.** Results of clinical studies have not conclusively proved that dopamine infusion improves ARF.
12. **a. intravenous calcium.** Priorities for treatment of acute hyperkalemia with electrocardiographic changes include stabilizing the electrical membrane of the cardiac conduction system, which may be accomplished with the use of intravenous calcium salts. These have an immediate effect and a rather short duration of action.
13. **a. saline diuresis.** A study by Solomon and coworkers confirmed that prestudy intravenous hydration with saline was crucial in limiting the nephrotoxic effect of radiocontrast agents in patients with preexisting azotemia. The addition of either a loop diuretic or mannitol did not improve outcome.
14. **d. intrarenal vascular occlusion.** In response to reduced nephron mass, a mosaic of events occurs linking sympathetic nervous system activation, renal structural remodeling, altered gene expression and regulation, and several regulatory mechanisms for progression.
15. **c. nephrology consult for stage 3 CKD.** According to the National Kidney Foundation (K/ DOQI) guidelines, this patient indeed has stage 3 CKD. A nephrologist should be observing this patient and appropriate preventive strategies instituted for preservation of kidney function and minimizing the impact of comorbidities.
16. **b. prevent progressive kidney disease.** ACE inhibitors work by hemodynamic and nonhemodynamic mechanisms to slow the progression of renal disease.
17. **e. diabetes mellitus.** Diabetes mellitus and hypertension account for the greatest percentage of cases, followed by glomerular diseases (e.g., FSGS, membranous glomerulonephritis) and then secondary glomerulonephritis associated with systemic diseases (e.g., systemic lupus erythematosus, Wegener's granulomatosis).
18. **e. iothalamate GFR measurement.** The iothalamate GFR assay is the "gold standard" for measuring renal function, but it requires a dedicated staff and laboratory to carry out the tests.
19. **b. renal biopsy.** For definitive diagnosis, a renal biopsy is required to aid prognosis and therapy decisions, especially in the setting of abnormal renal function.
20. **c. HMG Co-A reductase inhibitor (statin).** Evidence now supports the role of statin drugs in reducing fibrosis and mesangial proliferation. They should be incorporated into renal protective strategies.
21. **e. autosomal dominant PKD with cysts larger than 10 cm.** Individuals with bilateral renal artery stenosis and autosomal dominant PKD patients with cyst size greater than 10 cm may also experience a decrease in residual renal function while being given ACE inhibitor therapy.
22. **a. preemptive transplantation.** A comparison of outcomes suggests that renal transplantation is the best overall treatment for ESRD patients.
23. **e. the hematocrit is higher than 25%.** The K/DOQI guidelines recommend that dialysis be initiated when the weekly renal Krt/Vurea decreases to less than 2, unless all three of the following criteria are met: (1) stable or increased edema-free body weight, (2) randomized protein equivalent of total nitrogen appearance greater than 0.8, and (3) absence of clinical symptoms and signs attributable to uremia. The patient should begin some sort of renal replacement therapy if Krt/Vurea is < 2 and $> 6\%$ involuntary reduction of edema-free weight exists or the patient weighs $< 90\%$ of standard body weight from the National Health and Nutrition Examination Survey III standard, or there is a reduction in albumin by ≥ 0.3 g/dL.

24. **c. increased mortality rate.** Historically, mortality among late referrals for dialysis is consistently higher than among those with more timely initiated renal replacement therapy patterns.

25. **d. poor nutritional status.** The strongest predictors of the number of hospitalizations per year of patients at risk include low serum albumin, decreased activity level, diabetes mellitus as a primary cause of ESRD, peripheral vascular disease, white race, increasing age, and congestive heart failure. Both nutritional status (levels of serum albumin, creatinine, transferrin, and prealbumin, and lean body mass) and inflammatory response (e.g., C-reactive protein) are independent predictors of hospitalization in chronic hemodialysis patients.

SECTION XI

URINARY LITHIASIS AND ENDOUROLOGY

42

Urinary Lithiasis: Etiology, Epidemiology, and Pathogenesis

MARGARET S. PEARLE • YAIR LOTAN

QUESTIONS

1. Which ethnic/racial group has the highest prevalence of stone disease?

   a. African Americans
   b. Hispanics
   c. Caucasians
   d. Asians
   e. American Indians

2. The geographic area associated with the highest incidence of calcium oxalate stone disease is the:

   a. Northeast.
   b. Southeast.
   c. Southwest.
   d. West.
   e. Northwest.

3. Which of the following occurs when the concentration product of urine falls in the metastable range?

   a. Urine is supersaturated.
   b. Homogeneous nucleation occurs.
   c. Solubility product is reduced.
   d. Urinary inhibitors decrease the formation product.
   e. Nucleation never occurs.

4. What is the point at which nucleation occurs in pure solutions?

   a. Formation product
   b. Concentration product
   c. Solubility product
   d. Saturation ratio
   e. Concentration product ratio

5. What is the process by which nucleation occurs in pure solutions?

   a. Homogeneous nucleation
   b. Heterogeneous nucleation
   c. Epitaxy
   d. Aggregation
   e. Agglomeration

6. What is the proteinaceous component of stones called?

   a. Concentric lamination
   b. Protein-crystal complex
   c. Matrix
   d. Nephrocalcin
   e. Osteocalcin

7. Citrate inhibits calcium oxalate stone formation by:

   a. increasing urine pH.
   b. lowering urine magnesium levels.
   c. increasing urinary saturation of sodium urate.
   d. complexing calcium.
   e. lowering urine pH.

8. Approximately what percentage of dietary calcium is absorbed by the intestine?

   a. 10% to 25%
   b. 20% to 35%
   c. 30% to 45%
   d. 40% to 55%
   e. 50% to 65%

9. Calcium is maximally absorbed in which portion of the gastrointestinal tract?
   a. Stomach
   b. Jejunum
   c. Jejunum and proximal ileum
   d. Ileum
   e. Ascending colon
10. Which vitamin D metabolite stimulates intestinal calcium absorption?
   a. 1,25-Dihydroxyvitamin D
   b. 1,25-Dihydroxyvitamin D_1
   c. 1,25-Dihydroxyvitamin D_2
   d. 1,25-Dihydroxyvitamin D_3
   e. 1,25-Dihydroxyvitamin D_4
11. Which hormone is responsible for regulating renal phosphate reabsorption?
   a. Parathyroid hormone
   b. Thyroxine
   c. Cortisol
   d. Nephrocalcin
   e. Calcitriol
12. Metabolic acidosis can result from a defect in which of the following?
   a. Acid excretion
   b. Bicarbonate excretion
   c. Acid or bicarbonate excretion
   d. Acid reabsorption
   e. Acid or bicarbonate reabsorption
13. What effect does metabolic acidosis have on citrate metabolism?
   a. It reduces citrate excretion.
   b. It increases citrate excretion.
   c. It reduces citrate reabsorption.
   d. It increases citrate reabsorption.
   e. It has no effect.
14. Absorptive hypercalciuria is associated with:
   a. hypercalcemia.
   b. low to normal PTH levels.
   c. elevated PTH levels.
   d. fasting hypercalciuria.
   e. suppressed 1,25-dihyroxyvitamin D_3.
15. What is the underlying abnormality of renal hypercalciuria?
   a. Enhanced calcium filtration
   b. Enhanced calcium secretion
   c. Enhanced calcium reabsorption
   d. Primary renal wasting of calcium
   e. Primary renal storage of calcium
16. What is the prevalence of stone disease in patients with hyperparathyroidism?
   a. 1%
   b. 5%
   c. 10%
   d. 15%
   e. 20%
17. In the inpatient setting, what is the most common cause of hypercalcemia?
   a. Injection
   b. Immobilization
   c. Malignancy
   d. Endocrine disorder
   e. Medical induction
18. Sarcoidosis is associated with hypercalciuria for which of the following reasons?
   a. Absorptive hypercalciuria
   b. Renal hypercalciuria
   c. Resorptive hypercalciuria
   d. Acidosis
   e. Medical induction
19. What is the primary cause of enteric hyperoxaluria?
   a. Excessive intake of oxalate
   b. Reduced excretion of oxalate
   c. Increased fat in the diet
   d. Decreased fat in the diet
   e. Malabsorption
20. Renal handling of oxalate is best described by:
   a. complete glomerular filtration.
   b. complete glomerular filtration and proximal tubular secretion.
   c. complete glomerular filtration and proximal tubular reabsorption.
   d. proximal tubule secretion.
   e. proximal tubule secretion and nearly complete proximal tubule reabsorption.
21. The etiology of low urinary pH in uric acid stone formers with type II diabetes mellitus is:
   a. defective ammoniagenesis
   b. impaired urinary bicarbonate excretion
   c. lactic acidosis
   d. glucosuria
   e. ketoacidosis
22. In idiopathic calcium oxalate stone formers, Randall's plaques originate in the:
   a. basement membrane of the thin loops of Henle.
   b. terminal collecting ducts.
   c. medullary interstitium.
   d. vasa recta.
   e. papillary tip.
23. In calcium oxalate stone formers, Randall's plaques are composed of:
   a. calcium oxalate.
   b. brushite.
   c. calcium carbonate.
   d. calcium apatite.
   e. uric acid.
24. Urinary saturation of calcium oxalate is determined:
   a. primarily by urinary calcium concentration.
   b. primarily by urinary oxalate concentration.
   c. equally by urinary calcium and oxalate concentrations.
   d. primarily by urinary pH.
   e. primarily by urinary volume.

25. *Oxalobacter formigenes* reduces urinary oxalate by:
    a. reducing intestinal calcium absorption, leading to decreased luminal free oxalate and reduced oxalatc absorption.
    b. degrading urinary oxalate in infected urine.
    c. increasing urinary oxalate reabsorption.
    d. inhibiting the intestinal oxalate transporter.
    e. utilizing oxalate as a substrate in the intestine, thereby reducing intestinal oxalate absorption.
26. Which of the following organisms is most likely to produce urease?
    a. *Staphylococcus aureus*
    b. *Escherichia coli*
    c. *Streptococcus pneumoniae*
    d. *Serratia marcescens*
    e. *Chlamydia*
27. The mechanism responsible for type I (distal) renal tubular acidosis is:
    a. impaired bicarbonate reabsorption in the proximal tubule.
    b. defective H^+-ATPase in the distal tubule that is unable to excrete excess acid.
    c. impaired bicarbonate reabsorption in the distal tubule.
    d. impaired excretion of non-titratable acids.
    e. hypoaldosteronism.
28. Patients with Lesch-Nyhan syndrome treated with high doses of allopurinol are at risk for formation of stones of which of the following compositions?
    a. Hypoxanthine
    b. Uric acid
    c. Xanthine
    d. 2,8-Dihydroxyadenine
    e. Calcium apatite
29. The etiology of ammonium acid urate stone formation in patients abusing laxatives is:
    a. recurrent infections with urease-producing bacteria.
    b. chronic dehydration and excessive uric acid excretion.
    c. increased ammoniagenesis.
    d. urinary phosphate deficiency and intracellular acidosis.
    e. chronic dehydration, intracellular acidosis, and low urinary sodium.
30. What is the primary mechanism of action of citrate in preventing stones?
    a. Reducing the excretion of calcium
    b. Reducing the excretion of oxalate
    c. As a complexing agent of calcium
    d. As a complexing agent of oxalate
    e. As a complexing agent of phosphate
31. Typically, hypomagnesuria is associated with what other abnormality?
    a. Hypercalciuria
    b. Hyperoxaluria
    c. Hyperuricosuria
    d. Hypocitraturia
    e. Renal tubular acidosis
32. Type I (distal) renal tubular acidosis (RTA) is characterized by which abnormality?
    a. Hyperkalemia
    b. Hypochloremia
    c. Alkalosis
    d. Hypercitraturia
    e. None of the above
33. What is the primary defect of type II (proximal) RTA? Failure of bicarbonate reabsorption in the
    a. glomerulus.
    b. proximal tubule.
    c. loop of Henle.
    d. distal tubule.
    e. collecting duct.
34. The most common abnormality identified in patients with uric acid stones is:
    a. acidic urine.
    b. alkaline urine.
    c. low uric acid concentration.
    d. high uric acid concentration.
    e. RTA.
35. The factors influencing uric acid stone formation include which of the following?
    a. Urinary pH
    b. Urinary concentration of uric acid
    c. Uric acid excretion
    d. All of the above
    e. None of the above
36. Urease-producing bacteria hydrolyze urea to which of the following?
    a. Uric acid
    b. Carbon monoxide
    c. Carbon dioxide
    d. Ammonium
    e. Carbon dioxide and ammonium
37. What is the most common composition of vesical calculi in noninfected urine?
    a. Calcium oxalate
    b. Calcium phosphate
    c. Struvite
    d. Cystine
    e. Uric acid
38. What is the most common anatomic abnormality in children that is believed to be responsible for stone formation?
    a. Calyceal obstruction
    b. Infundibular obstruction
    c. Ureteropelvic obstruction
    d. Ureteral obstruction
    e. Ureterovesical obstruction

ANSWERS

1. **c. Caucasians.** The highest prevalence of stone disease in both men and women occurs in Caucasians. In men the lowest prevalence occurs in African Americans, whereas Asian women have been found to have the lowest prevalence in one series.

2. **b. Southeast.** According to hospital discharge rates among U.S. veterans, calcium oxalate stone disease is most prevalent in the Southeast.

3. **a. Urine is supersaturated.** The solubility product refers to the point of saturation where dissolved and crystalline components in solution are in equilibrium. Addition of any more crystals to the solution will result in precipitation of crystals. In this supersaturated urine (metastable state), crystallization can occur on preexisting crystals but spontaneous crystallization occurs only when the concentration product exceeds the formation product. In the metastable state, the presence of inhibitors prevents or delays crystallization.

4. **c. Solubility product.** The point at which saturation is reached and crystallization begins is referred to as the thermodynamic solubility product (Ksp).

5. **a. Homogeneous nucleation.** The process by which nuclei form in pure solutions is called homogeneous nucleation.

6. **c. Matrix.** Depending on their type, kidney stones contain between 10% and 65% of noncrystalline material or matrix. Extensive investigations have characterized matrix as a derivative of several of the mucoproteins of urine and serum.

7. **d. complexing calcium.** Citrate inhibits stone formation by complexing calcium, thereby lowering urinary saturation of calcium oxalate. In addition it inhibits spontaneous precipitation of calcium oxalate and agglomeration of calcium oxalate crystals. It also inhibits calcium oxalate and calcium phosphate crystal growth, with its effect of calcium phosphate crystal growth more pronounced than on calcium oxalate crystal growth. Lastly, it prevents heterogeneous nucleation of calcium oxalate by monosodium urate.

8. **c. 30% to 45%.** Of the calcium content of the average Western adult diet, 30% to 45% (300 to 400 mg) is absorbed.

9. **c. Jejunum and proximal ileum.** Calcium is probably maximally absorbed in the jejunum and the proximal portion of the ileum.

10. **d. 1,25-Dihydroxyvitamin D_3.** It is generally accepted that 1,25-dihydroxyvitamin D_3 is the vitamin D metabolite that is the most potent stimulator of intestinal calcium absorption.

11. **a. Parathyroid hormone.** Parathyroid hormone is the major hormonal regulator of renal phosphate reabsorption.

12. **a. Acid excretion.** A defect in either acid excretion or bicarbonate reabsorption can lead to metabolic acidosis.

13. **a. It reduces citrate excretion.** Metabolic acidosis reduces citrate excretion by augmenting citrate reabsorption and mitochondrial oxidation.

14. **b. low to normal PTH levels.** The underlying pathophysiologic abnormality in absorptive hypercalciuria is overabsorption of calcium from the intestine, resulting in a transient decrease in serum calcium, which suppresses PTH secretion. The increased filtered load of calcium and the suppressed PTH lead to increased urinary excretion of calcium. Serum calcium concentration remains normal because the increased intestinal absorption of calcium is matched by increased renal excretion. Fasting hypercalciuria may occur in severe cases of absorptive hypercalciuria type I but is more typical of renal calcium leak or resorptive hypercalciuria.

15. **d. Primary renal wasting of calcium.** In this condition, the underlying abnormality is a primary renal wasting of calcium.

16. **a. 1%.** The prevalence of stone disease in hyperparathyroidism is only about 1%.

17. **c. Malignancy.** In an inpatient setting, it is the most common cause of hypercalcemia.

18. **a. Absorptive hypercalciuria.** The sarcoid granuloma produces 1,25-dihydroxyvitamin D_3, causing increased intestinal calcium absorption, hypercalcemia, and hypercalciuria.

19. **e. Malabsorption.** Malabsorption from any cause, including small bowel resection, intrinsic disease, or jejunoileal bypass, increases the colonic permeability of oxalate as the result of exposure of the colonic epithelium to bile salts.

20. **b. complete glomerular filtration and proximal tubular secretion.** Oxalate excretion in the kidney occurs by both glomerular filtration and secretion. Nearly all plasma oxalate is ultrafiltrable and is filtered at the glomerulus. A secretary pathway also exists, but it is unlikely that reabsorption of oxalate occurs to any appreciable degree.

21. **a. defective ammoniagenesis.** Patients with type II diabetes mellitus typically exhibit characteristics of the metabolic syndrome, including insulin resistance. Although peripherally, insulin resistance leads to typical symptoms of diabetes, insulin resistance at the level of the kidney leads to impaired ammoniagenesis, by way of reduced production of ammonia from glutamine and reduced activity of the Na^+/H^+ exchanger in the proximal tubule that is responsible for either the direct transport or trapping of ammonium in the urine. The result is reduced urinary ammonium and low urine pH.

22. **a. basement membrane of the thin loops of Henle.** In idiopathic calcium oxalate stone formers, Randall's plaques have been found to originate in the basement membrane of the thin loops of Henle. From there, they extend through the medullary interstitium to a subepithelial location where they serve as an anchoring site for calcium oxalate stone formation.

23. **d. calcium apatite.** Randall's plaques are invariably composed of calcium apatite, which serve as an anchoring site onto which calcium oxalate crystals can adhere and grow.

24. **c. equally by urinary calcium and oxalate concentrations.** Urinary saturation of calcium oxalate is strongly, positively correlated with urinary calcium and oxalate concentrations. Both contribute equally to urinary saturation of calcium oxalate. Urinary volume and pH are inversely correlated with urinary saturation of calcium oxalate.

25. **e. utilizing oxalate as a substrate in the intestine, thereby reducing intestinal oxalate absorption.** *Oxalobacter formigenes* is an oxalate-degrading bacterium found in the intestinal lumen that utilizes oxalate as an energy source, thereby reducing luminal oxalate and intestinal oxalate absorption. *Oxalobacter* is not found in urine.

26. **a. *Staphylococcus aureus*.** Although *Proteus* species are most commonly associated with struvite stones, more than 90% of *Staphylococcus aureus* organisms produce urease and are therefore associated with struvite stone formation.

27. **b. defective H^+– ATPase in the distal tubule that is unable to excrete excess acid.** A defective H+-ATPase in the distal tubule has been implicated in the inability to excrete excess acid in

the presence of an oral acid load among patients with distal RTA. Type II, or proximal RTA, is characterized by impaired bicarbonate reabsorption in the proximal tubule, and type IV RTA is common in diabetics with chronic renal damage who demonstrate aldosterone resistance.

28. **c. Xanthine.** Patients with Lesch-Nyhan syndrome suffer from an inherited deficiency of the purine salvage enzyme hypoxanthine-guanine phosphoribosyltransferase, which leads to the accumulation of hypoxanthine that is ultimately converted to uric acid. Allopurinol inhibits xanthine oxidase, which is responsible for converting hypoxanthine to xanthine and xanthine to uric acid. High doses of allopurinol in these patients leads to the accumulation of hypoxanthine and xanthine, but because xanthine is less soluble in urine than hypoxanthine, xanthine stones form.

29. **e. chronic dehydration, intracellular acidosis, and low urinary sodium.** Subjects who abuse laxatives are chronically dehydrated, resulting in intracellular acidosis. In addition, urinary sodium is very low from sodium loss as a result of the laxatives. In this environment, urate preferentially complexes with the abundant ammonium rather than sodium and produces ammonium acid urate stones.

30. **c. As a complexing agent of calcium.** The primary mechanism of action of citrate is as a complexing agent for calcium.

31. **d. Hypocitraturia.** Most patients with hypomagnesuria also have hypocitraturia.

32. **e. None of the above.** Distal RTA is characterized by hypokalemic, hyperchloremic, non–anion gap metabolic acidosis and a urinary pH consistently above 6.0.

33. **b. proximal tubule.** The primary defect here is a failure of bicarbonate reabsorption in the proximal tubule, leading to urinary bicarbonate excretion.

34. **a. acidic urine.** Patients with uric acid stones often have prolonged periods of acidity in the urine.

35. **d. All of the above.** Three factors are involved in uric acid urolithiasis. First, patients tend to excrete excessively acid urine at a relatively fixed, low urinary pH. Second, they may absorb, produce, or excrete more uric acid than patients without gout or uric acid stones. Third, urinary volume is diminished in these patients.

36. **e. Carbon dioxide and ammonium.** Urease-producing bacteria hydrolyze urea to carbon dioxide and ammonium molecules.

37. **e. Uric acid.** In contrast to renal stones, bladder stones are usually composed of uric acid (in noninfected urine) or struvite (in infected urine).

38. **c. Ureteropelvic obstruction.** In those series that provide a breakdown of anatomic lesions responsible for stone formation, ureteropelvic junction obstruction is the most common lesion.

43

Medical Management of Nephrolithiasis

PAUL K. PIETROW • GLENN M. PREMINGER

QUESTIONS

1. Patients with enteric hyperoxaluria are most likely to form stones composed of:
   a. calcium phosphate.
   b. calcium oxalate.
   c. magnesium ammonium phosphate.
   d. uric acid.
   e. cystine.
2. The risk factor most associated with recurrent stone formation in patients with inflammatory bowel disease is:
   a. hyperabsorption of oxalate in the jejunum.
   b. hyperexcretion of calcium from the distal tubule.
   c. diminished citrate absorption in the terminal ileum.
   d. hyperabsorption of calcium in the small bowel.
   e. increased colonic absorption of free oxalate.
3. Hypocitraturia in patients with inflammatory bowel disease or chronic diarrhea syndrome is due to:
   a. persistent bicarbonate losses.
   b. hypokalemia.
   c. metabolic acidosis.
   d. intracellular acidosis.
   e. all of the above.
4. The optimum treatment for patients with enteric hyperoxaluria includes:
   a. calcium supplements, potassium citrate, and increased oral fluid intake.
   b. dietary restriction of oxalate.
   c. thiazides and potassium citrate.
   d. allopurinol.
   e. pyridoxine.
5. The most important factor predisposing patients to gouty diathesis is:
   a. hypercalciuria.
   b. low urinary pH.
   c. hypocitraturia.
   d. low urine volumes.
   e. hyperuricosuria.
6. The initial laboratory test that provides the most important diagnostic clue in patients with uric acid calculi is:
   a. urine pH.
   b. serum uric acid levels.
   c. urine sodium.
   d. urine calcium.
   e. urine uric acid levels.
7. The most appropriate medical treatment of a patient with gouty diathesis is:
   a. allopurinol.
   b. thiazides.
   c. increased fluids.
   d. dietary calcium restriction.
   e. potassium citrate.
8. A patient with recurrent uric acid calculi is placed on oral medical treatment and returns for follow up 3 months later. He is noted to have significantly elevated urinary uric acid levels as compared with his first 24-hour urine collection. This finding is due to:
   a. increased production of endogenous uric acid.
   b. failure to avoid high sodium foods.
   c. increased solubility of uric acid.
   d. increased consumption of red.
   e. inhibition of xanthine oxidase.
9. A patient with uric acid calculi is placed on alkali therapy but returns 1 year later having passed 2 calcium phosphate stones. A repeat 24-hour urine demonstrates a urine pH of 7.4, a urinary citrate of 450 mg/day, and a urinary uric acid of 875 mg/day. The most likely cause for recurrent stone formation is:
   a. cessation of potassium citrate.
   b. increase in oral purine intake.
   c. decrease in solubility of uric acid.
   d. excess alkalization.
   e. increase in saturation of oxalate.

10. A patient with gouty diathesis is started on sodium bicarbonate therapy and urinary pH is maintained between 6.3 and 6.7. Calcium oxalate stones may form due to:

   a. sodium inhibiting calcium reabsorption in the proximal tubule.
   b. homogeneous nucleation of calcium oxalate.
   c. undiagnosed hypercalciuria.
   d. lack of allopurinol in medical management regimen.
   e. reduction in monosodium urate.

11. A 58-year-old Hispanic female with a history of recurrent urinary tract infections treated three to four times in the past 18 months is seen by her family physician. At present she is asymptomatic. She has no history of nephrolithiasis. Renal ultrasound demonstrates moderate left hydronephrosis and a large density within the renal pelvis with posterior shadowing. KUB with tomography reveals a poorly opacified dendritic stone in the renal pelvis and lower pole calyces. Prior urine cultures have *Proteus* and *Klebsiella* species. The stone composition of this patient is most likely:

   a. calcium oxalate.
   b. uric acid.
   c. magnesium ammonium phosphate.
   d. cystine.
   e. hydroxyapatite.

12. The most significant factor contributing to stone formation in patients with struvite calculi is:

   a. gouty diathesis.
   b. recurrent urinary tract infections.
   c. family history.
   d. hyperoxaluria.
   e. hypercalciuria.

13. The most common cause of recurrent stone disease in a patient having undergone "sandwich" therapy for a staghorn calculus is:

   a. hypomagnesuria.
   b. hyperoxaluria.
   c. retained stone fragments.
   d. renal tubular acidosis.
   e. hypercalciuria.

14. Which of the following treatments is contraindicated for patients with recurrent struvite calculi?

   a. Orthophosphate
   b. Fluoroquinolones
   c. Thiazide diuretics
   d. Acetohydroxamic acid
   e. Calcium channel blockers

15. Acetohydroxamic acid contributes to reducing infection stone formation by:

   a. reversing associated metabolic defects.
   b. preventing recurrent urinary tract infections.
   c. alkalization of the urine.
   d. irreversibly inhibiting urease.
   e. all of the above.

16. A 12-year-old boy is seen for evaluation of recurrent nephrolithiasis. He has spontaneously passed three stones over the previous 4 years and has recently undergone shock wave lithotripsy twice without success. He has been treated in the past with an unknown medication, but this was discontinued because the parents believed it was of no benefit. Urinalysis demonstrates hexagonal crystals. The likely metabolic diagnosis contributing to this patient's recurrent stone formation is:

   a. hypocitraturia.
   b. hyperoxaluria.
   c. low urine volumes.
   d. gouty diathesis.
   e. cystinuria.

17. First-line medical treatment for the prevention of recurrent cystine stones would be aimed at:

   a. urinary acidification.
   b. increasing the solubility of cystine.
   c. decreasing urinary sodium.
   d. decreasing the solubility of cystine.
   e. binding of cystine within the intestines.

18. α-Mercaptopropionylglycine (α-MPG, Thiola) may be helpful in the management of cystinuria because it:

   a. acts as a diuretic, further decreasing urinary cystine concentration.
   b. is significantly more effective than D-penicillamine.
   c. can be used as both an oral and intrarenal chemolytic agent.
   d. has equivalent efficacy at increasing solubility with reduced toxicity as compared with D-penicillamine.
   e. adequately alkalizes the urine, obviating the need for potassium citrate.

19. Three years after initiating treatment for cystine stones with Thiola, 800 mg/day, a patient returns with a follow-up 24-hour urine collection demonstrating a significant reduction in cystine excretion from 740 to 250 mg/day. Urine volume is 775 mL/day. He has two additional stones. The reason for recurrent stone formation is:

   a. increased age, thereby exacerbating the disorder.
   b. decreased efficacy of Thiola.
   c. continued supersaturation of urinary cystine.
   d. continued hypocitraturia.
   e. increased urine acidity.

20. A 19-year-old white woman with a 6-year history of recurrent stone disease is found to have multiple bilateral renal calculi by renal ultrasound during an evaluation for recurrent flank pain. She reports having passed more than 10 stones in the previous 2 years. Review of the renal ultrasound indicates no evidence of hydronephrosis. KUB and tomograms demonstrate 5 stones on the left and 8 stones on the right, all less than 4 mm. She has a strong family history of stones with three first-degree relatives and two cousins with nephrolithiasis. Urine pH is consistently above 6.8. Stone compositions have been mixed calcium phosphate and calcium oxalate. The most definitive test to identify this disorder would demonstrate:

   a. decreased serum parathyroid hormone levels.
   b. persistently elevated urine calcium.
   c. inability to reduce the urine pH below 5.3.
   d. normalization of hypercalciuria.
   e. marked increase in urinary uric acid levels with initiation of treatment.

21. Which of the following is NOT a cause of hypocitraturic calcium nephrolithiasis?
    a. Thiazide-induced hypocitraturia
    b. Absorptive hypercalciuria type I
    c. Distal renal tubular acidosis
    d. Metabolic acidosis
    e. Chronic diarrheal syndrome
22. The most appropriate treatment for patients with renal tubular acidosis is:
    a. thiazides.
    b. allopurinol.
    c. sodium alkali.
    d. acetohydroxamic acid.
    e. potassium alkali.
23. Renal tubular acidosis may be associated with nephrolithiasis due to:
    a. hypercalciuria and hypocitraturia.
    b. hyperoxaluria and hypercalcemia.
    c. hyperuricosuria.
    d. hypocitraturia with normal urine magnesium.
    e. hypercitraturia and hypercalciuria.
24. Chronic metabolic acidosis may cause:
    a. increased parathyroid hormone levels.
    b. significantly reduced bone density.
    c. hypercalcemia.
    d. increased intestinal calcium absorption.
    e. all of the above.
25. To accurately diagnose a patient with renal leak hypercalciuria, one must identify both:
    a. increased intestinal calcium absorption and hyperthyroidism.
    b. renal leak of calcium and normal intestinal calcium absorption.
    c. hypoparathyroidism and increased intestinal calcium absorption.
    d. secondary hyperparathyroidism and renal calcium leak.
    e. primary hyperparathyroidism and increased intestinal calcium absorption.
26. Which of the following findings would support the diagnosis of renal leak hypercalciuria?
    a. Hypocitraturia
    b. Diminished urinary cyclic AMP excretion
    c. Normocalciuria on a calcium-restricted diet
    d. Decreased urinary sodium with thiazide challenge
    e. Low or low/normal radial bone density
27. The primary abnormality in patients with renal leak hypercalciuria is considered to be:
    a. impairment of renal tubular reabsorption of calcium.
    b. excessive mobilization of calcium from bone.
    c. increased 1,25-$(OH)_2$ vitamin D levels.
    d. elevation of serum parathyroid hormone levels.
    e. hyperabsorption of intestinal calcium.
28. Which of the following mechanisms explains the effectiveness of thiazides in treating patients with renal leak hypercalciuria? Thiazides:
    a. bind calcium in the intestinal tract.
    b. cause intracellular volume depletion.
    c. correct the renal leak of calcium by augmenting calcium reabsorption in the proximal tubule.
    d. directly inhibit calcium absorption.
    e. restore normal serum 1,25-$(OH)_2$ vitamin D levels.
29. Which of the following medications is contraindicated in this renal leak hypercalciuria disorder, because it will cause a negative calcium balance?
    a. Trichlormethiazide
    b. Sodium cellulose phosphate
    c. Orthophosphate
    d. Acetohydroxamic acid
    e. Allopurinol
30. The primary defect in patients with absorptive hypercalciuria is considered to be:
    a. primary hyperabsorption of intestinal calcium.
    b. hypersecretion of parathyroid hormone.
    c. renal leak of calcium.
    d. bone disease.
    e. excessive dietary intake of calcium-containing foods.
31. The most appropriate initial treatment for patients with absorptive hypercalciuria is:
    a. sodium cellulose phosphate.
    b. allopurinol.
    c. potassium citrate.
    d. limited dietary calcium.
    e. phosphate binders.
32. Which of the following is NOT a potential complication of sodium cellulose phosphate?
    a. Hyperoxaluria
    b. Hyperuricosuria
    c. Hypomagnesuria
    d. Negative calcium balance with secondary hyperparathyroidism
    e. Gastrointestinal upset
33. After 18 months of chlorthalidone treatment, a patient with hypercalciuria is doing well with no further stone formation. However, 8 months later, while still on thiazides, she passed a small stone. The most likely cause of her recurrent stone formation is:
    a. excessive intake of dietary calcium.
    b. inappropriate fluid management.
    c. excessive sodium intake.
    d. thiazide-induced hypocitraturia.
    e. cessation of medications.
34. A patient with absorptive hypercalciuria is continued on chlorthalidone and potassium citrate without problems for 18 months and then passes two stones spontaneously. She claimed that she was still on her medications. The most likely cause of her continued stone formation is:
    a. excessive calcium intake.
    b. heterogeneous nucleation of calcium oxalate.
    c. high dietary sodium intake.
    d. bone mobilization of calcium.
    e. exacerbation of intestinal calcium absorption.
35. The metabolic condition in a patient with absorptive hypercalciuria type II is:
    a. a less severe form of absorptive hypercalciuria type I.
    b. controlled by a calcium restricted diet.
    c. not characterized by a renal leak of calcium.
    d. characterized by an increased intestinal absorption of calcium.
    e. all of the above.
36. The most appropriate treatment in a patient with absorptive hypercalciuria type II may include all of the following EXCEPT:
    a. moderate intake of high calcium-containing foods.
    b. limit sodium intake.
    c. increase fluids to maintain urine volumes greater than 2 L/day.
    d. restrict dietary oxalate.
    e. intake of potassium citrate.

ANSWERS

1. **b. calcium oxalate.** Patients with enteric hyperoxaluria are more likely to form calcium oxalate stones, owing to increased urinary excretion of oxalate and decreased inhibitory activity from hypocitraturia, secondary to chronic metabolic acidosis and hypomagnesuria. In addition, fluid losses from persistent diarrhea from inflammatory bowel disease may cause an extremely concentrated environment suitable for stone formation.

2. **e. increased colonic absorption of free oxalate.** Intestinal hyperabsorption of oxalate in patients with enteric hyperoxaluria is the most significant risk factor leading to recurrent calculus formation. Intestinal transport of oxalate is primarily increased because of the effects of bile salts and fatty acids on the permeability of colonic intestinal mucosa to oxalate. The total amount of oxalate absorbed may also be increased because of an enlarged intraluminal pool of oxalate available for absorption. Intestinal fat malabsorption characteristic of ileal disease will exaggerate calcium soap formation, limit the amount of "free" calcium to complex to oxalate, and thereby raise the oxalate pool available for absorption.

3. **e. all of the above.** Acid-base status probably is the most important factor in the renal handling of citrate. Hypokalemia with its induced intracellular acidosis (caused by bicarbonate loss from chronic diarrhea) will reduce urinary citrate both by enhancing renal tubular resorption and reducing the synthesis of citrate. Therefore, in patients with enteric hyperoxaluria where bicarbonate loss and hypokalemia both contribute to metabolic acidosis, the hypocitraturia is often profound.

4. **a. calcium supplements, potassium citrate, and increased oral fluid intake.** The initial goals of medical management are to rehydrate and reverse metabolic acidosis. Hydration is at times difficult in some patients because an increase in oral fluids may exacerbate diarrhea. Hydration and potassium citrate will contribute to the reversal of the metabolic acidosis, as well as enhance the excretion of citrate to increase its inhibitory effects on stone formation. Calcium supplements will bind excess oxalate within the intestine, thereby reducing intestinal oxalate absorption. Calcium citrate may offer an ideal calcium supplement in this condition because it should reduce urinary oxalate and increase urinary citrate. Thiazides may worsen metabolic acidosis and hypokalemia through its diuretic effects and renal potassium losses. Colon resection may be of benefit in those patients refractory to medical management, because the primary site of intestinal absorption of oxalate is the large bowel.

5. **b. low urinary pH.** Although low urine volumes and hyperuricosuria contribute to the possibility of uric acid stone formation, the most critical determinant of the crystallization of uric acid remains urinary pH. In addition, uric acid stones may be formed in patients with primary gout with associated severe hyperuricosuria and other secondary causes of purine overproduction such as myeloproliferative states, glycogen storage disease, and malignancy.

6. **a. urine pH.** Patients with gouty diathesis and uric acid stones will characteristically have urinary pH lower than the dissociation constant for uric acid (5.5). In fact, many will have a urine pH consistently close to 5.0. Whereas serum and urine uric acid levels may be elevated in patients with uric acid calculi, the urine pH remains the most cost-effective means of screening for this condition as well as monitoring therapy.

7. **e. potassium citrate.** Allopurinol will decrease the production of uric acid by inhibiting xanthine oxidase in the purine metabolic pathway but is most effective in patients with extremely elevated levels of uric acid (urinary uric acid > 1500 mg/day). In addition, increasing total urine volume will decrease the concentration of uric acid to assist in preventing stone formation. However, raising the urinary pH above the dissociation constant of uric acid is the key to prevent recurrent uric acid stone formation and correcting gouty diathesis. The urine pH should be maintained between 6.0 and 6.5. Thiazides and calcium restriction have limited roles in the medical treatment of uric acid stone patients.

8. **c. increased solubility of uric acid.** With adequate alkali therapy, this patient has been able to raise the urine pH above the dissociation constant of uric acid. The solubility of uric acid is more than 10 times greater at a pH of 7 than at a pH of 5. Therefore, patients may initially present with low/normal 24-hour urinary uric acid levels because the uric acid will precipitate out of solution in the acid urinary environment. Once the urine has been alkalized, all of the uric acid will come back into solution, causing a significant increase in the urinary uric acid.

9. **d. excess alkalization.** Excessive alkalization with urinary pH values above 7.0 may result in calcium phosphate stone formation. Alkali therapy with potassium citrate should aim to keep the urinary pH between 6.5 and 7.0 when treating patients with gouty diathesis.

10. **a. sodium inhibiting calcium reabsorption in the proximal tubule.** Patients treated with sodium alkali will occasionally begin forming calcium oxalate stones due to an excess sodium load that will inhibit reabsorption of calcium in the proximal tubule, thereby causing hypercalciuria. In addition, heterogeneous nucleation of calcium oxalate induced by monosodium urate may occur in those individuals with hyperuricosuria. Thus, potassium-based alkali, usually in the form of potassium citrate, is the treatment of choice for patients with gouty diathesis.

11. **c. magnesium ammonium phosphate.** Ascending urinary tract infections with urea-splitting organisms, such as *Proteus* species, will metabolize urea to ammonia. Ammonuria, in conjunction with a matrix composed of organic compounds, carbonate apatite, inflammatory cells, and bacteria, results in the rapid formation of an "infection" calculus, eventually progressing into a mineralized, dense stone. Bacteria trapped within the stone perpetuate the recurrent urinary tract infections, and further stone formation eventually develops into the classic staghorn calculus.

12. **b. recurrent urinary tract infections.** Etiologic factors involved with infection calculi include a history of recurrent urinary tract infections and potential anatomic or physiologic abnormalities. It is important to remember that these patients may also have underlying metabolic disorders, such as hypercalciuria, which could contribute to the stone formation. These disorders are most commonly found in patients with mixed stone composition (i.e., struvite and calcium calculi). A comprehensive metabolic evaluation is warranted in these patients.

13. **c. retained stone fragments.** After removal of an infected struvite calculus, the most common cause of recurrent stone formation is failure to completely eradicate the calculus. Surgical therapy may leave retained fragments of infected stone within calyces, thus allowing infection to persist. Underlying metabolic disorders may also contribute to recurrent stone formation, but persistent calculus remains the most important risk factor.

14. **a. Orthophosphate.** "Struvite stones," "infection stones," or "triple-phosphate stones" all refer to calculi composed of magnesium ammonium phosphate or carbonate apatite. Because phosphate is a major component of these two salts, phosphate therapy would be contraindicated in cases of infection calculi because this medication may promote further stone formation.
15. **d. irreversibly inhibiting urease.** Acetohydroxamic acid (AHA), a competitive inhibitor of the bacterial enzyme urease, will reduce the urinary saturation of struvite and retard stone formation. When given at a dose of 250 mg orally three times a day, this medication can prevent the recurrence of new stones and inhibit the growth of existing stones in patients with chronic urea-splitting infections. AHA can also cause dissolution of small stones. However, up to 30% of patients will experience minor side effects, including headache, nausea, vomiting, anemia, rash, or alopecia. In addition, 15% of patients have developed deep venous thrombosis while on long-term treatment. Therefore, careful monitoring is required when using this medication.
16. **e. cystinuria.** Cystinuria is a complex autosomal recessive disorder of amino acid transport involving cystine, ornithine, lysine, and arginine. Supersaturation of the urine will occur in patients with the homozygous state. Therefore, it is unusual to see a family history with cystine stones and the age at onset is often in the first or second decade.
17. **b. increasing the solubility of cystine.** Increasing the solubility of cystine is the mainstay of treating this disorder. Therefore, medical therapy is aimed at dissociating cystine into cysteine, which is 200 times more soluble than cystine. Solubility increases dramatically when this disulfide exchange occurs, effectively preventing further stone formation.
18. **d. has equivalent efficacy at increasing solubility with reduced toxicity as compared with D-penicillamine.** D-Penicillamine and α-MPG are equally effective in their ability to decrease urinary cystine levels. However, studies have demonstrated that α-MPG is significantly less toxic than D-penicillamine. Moreover, the side effects that may occur with α-MPG are also less severe. However, if a patient has been doing well on D-penicillamine with no significant complications, there is no need to switch medications.
19. **c. continued supersaturation of urinary cystine.** The primary goal of medical therapy is to reduce the urinary cystine concentration below the solubility limit of 200 to 250 mg/L of urine. Because many of these patients present at a young age, compliance may be difficult. Even though this patient's cystine excretion has been reduced to 250 mg/day by the α-MPG therapy, his cystine concentration remains > 300 mg/L. Therefore, a combination of medication along with an increased urine output is essential to reduce the urinary cystine concentration. Long-term follow-up is necessary to ensure maintenance of cystine undersaturation.
20. **c. inability to reduce the urine pH below 5.3.** Renal tubular acidosis is a clinical syndrome of chronic metabolic acidosis resulting from renal tubular abnormalities while glomerular filtration is relatively well preserved. Although patients may present with many different symptoms and physical findings, renal stone formation is a well-recognized manifestation of distal renal tubular acidosis (dRTA). Patients with the incomplete form of dRTA are not persistently acidemic despite their inability to lower urinary pH with an acid load. These patients are able to compensate for their acidification defect and remain in acid-base balance by increasing ammonia synthesis and ammonium excretion as a buffering mechanism.

    The initial identification of incomplete dRTA is often a chance finding. Many of these patients will present with recurrent nephrolithiasis or may be referred for evaluation after the discovery of nephrocalcinosis after routine abdominal radiographs. Most patients will have normal serum electrolytes, yet they will have a high-normal urine pH along with significant hypocitraturia. The diagnosis of incomplete dRTA can be confirmed by inadequate urinary acidification after an ammonium chloride loading test.
21. **b. Absorptive hypercalciuria type I.** Urinary citrate is a potent inhibitor of stone formation particularly in excess of 600 mg/day on a 24-hour urine collection. Hypocitraturia can be a result of any acidotic state, because acidosis will cause both decreased endogenous renal citrate production as well as increased renal tubular absorption of citrate. Hypokalemia induced by thiazide wasting of potassium will cause intracellular metabolic acidosis, thus utilizing citrate and reducing excretion in a manner similar to metabolic acidosis. Chronic diarrheal syndromes promote intestinal loss of alkali as well as dehydration, resulting in metabolic acidosis and reduced urinary citrate levels.
22. **e. potassium alkali.** In the past, sodium alkali has been the treatment of choice for chronic therapy in patients with distal renal tubular acidosis. It was given either in the form of sodium bicarbonate or Shohl's solution (a combination of sodium citrate and citric acid). Although sodium alkali is beneficial in correcting the acidosis, excess sodium may be detrimental to calcium metabolism, especially with respect to nephrolithiasis. Sodium alkali therapy has been complicated by the development of calcium stones (calcium phosphate or calcium oxalate), especially when the urinary pH is above 7.0. Potassium citrate has been shown to reduce the excretion of urinary calcium, whereas sodium alkali has no effect on urinary calcium. Therefore, potassium alkali, usually in the form of potassium citrate (Poly Citra K or Urocit-K) is the recommended first-line therapy.
23. **a. hypercalciuria and hypocitraturia.** Hypocitraturia, commonly seen in patients with distal renal tubular acidosis, promotes the formation of nephrolithiasis due to reduced inhibitory action of urinary citrate. In addition, hypercalciuria will occur due to mobilization of calcium from bone and impaired renal tubular absorption of calcium, both as a result of chronic acidosis.
24. **b. significantly reduced bone density.** It is well established that metabolic acidosis may cause a negative calcium balance as a result of impaired renal tubular reabsorption of calcium in the proximal tubule, leading to excessive renal loss of calcium. In addition, intestinal calcium absorption is diminished in patients with persistent acidosis. Slow dissolution of bone mineral can also be identified as calcium and phosphate act as buffering mechanisms to correct the acidosis. Chronic acidosis has been cited as a major factor in the genesis of bone disease.
25. **d. secondary hyperparathyroidism and renal calcium leak.** To confirm the diagnosis of renal hypercalciuria, evidence for secondary hyperparathyroidism and renal leak of calcium must be present. Both of these values can be obtained during the fasting urinary calcium test. Before arrival at the physician's office, it is essential that patients have adhered to a calcium- and sodium-restricted diet for at least 12 hours before testing to eliminate the effects of absorbed calcium on fasting calcium excretion. Three hundred milliliters of distilled water is consumed 12 and 9 hours before the fasting urine collection to ensure adequate hydration. At 7 AM, patients empty their bladder completely, discard the urine, and drink another 600 mL of distilled water. Urine is then collected as a pooled sample for a 2-hour period (7 to 9 AM). A fasting serum blood

is obtained at the end of the 2-hour period. The serum sample is analyzed for parathyroid hormone levels. The fasting urine sample is assayed for calcium and creatinine. Fasting urinary calcium is expressed as milligrams per deciliter of glomerular filtrate because it is reflective of renal function. To obtain this value, urinary calcium in milligrams per milligrams of creatinine is multiplied by serum creatinine in milligrams per deciliter. Normal fasting urinary calcium is < 0.11 mg/dL glomerular filtrate.

26. **e. Low or low/normal radial bone density.** Patients with renal hypercalciuria may display a low or low/normal radial bone density. The diminished bone density is a result of the secondary hyperparathyroidism, which causes stimulation of parathyroid hormone and subsequent production of 1,25 $(OH)_2$ vitamin D. Both PTH and vitamin D will act on bone to mobilize calcium and cause a loss in bone density. Calcium restriction has no effect in managing renal hypercalciuria.

27. **a. impairment of renal tubular reabsorption of calcium.** The primary abnormality in renal hypercalciuria is an impairment in proximal renal tubular calcium reabsorption. This urinary calcium wasting and subsequent reduction in serum calcium concentration stimulates the production of parathyroid hormone. As a result, vitamin D synthesis in the kidney is stimulated. Both PTH and vitamin D will increase bone resorption and absorption of intestinal calcium increasing the circulating concentration and filtered load of calcium, often causing significant hypercalciuria. Unlike primary hyperparathyroidism, serum calcium is normal and the state of hyperparathyroidism is secondary.

28. **c. correct the renal leak of calcium by augmenting calcium reabsorption in the proximal tubule.** Thiazide is the primary medical treatment of renal hypercalciuria and has been shown to correct the renal leak of calcium by augmenting the calcium reabsorption in the distal tubule. In addition, thiazides cause extracellular volume depletion, thereby stimulating proximal tubular reabsorption of calcium. A positive calcium balance ensues, with correction of the secondary hyperparathyroidism.

29. **b. Sodium cellulose phosphate.** Sodium cellulose phosphate is a calcium-binding resin that inhibits the absorption of calcium in the intestine. This medication will further exaggerate secondary hyperparathyroidism in patients with renal hypercalciuria by binding the intestinal calcium being absorbed to compensate for the renal calcium loss. Therefore, sodium cellulose phosphate should only be used in cases of absorptive hypercalciuria, where the object of treatment is to reduce the primary defect of intestinal calcium hyperabsorption.

30. **a. primary hyperabsorption of intestinal calcium.** The basic abnormality in absorptive hypercalciuria type I is the intestinal hyperabsorption of calcium. The consequent increase in the circulating concentration of calcium enhances the renal filtered load and suppresses parathyroid function. Hypercalciuria results from the combination of increased filtered load and reduced renal tubular reabsorption of calcium, a function of parathyroid suppression. The excessive renal loss of calcium compensates for the high calcium absorption from the intestinal tract and helps to maintain serum calcium in the normal range.

31. **e. phosphate binders.** Sodium cellulose phosphate (SCP) does not correct the primary intestinal defect in this condition. However, SCP will bind calcium within the gut, making it less available for absorption. Complications of SCP treatment may include induction of hyperoxaluria as well as hypomagnesemia because sodium cellulose phosphate will bind cations other than calcium. In addition, sodium cellulose phosphate, if used in patients with other types of hypercalciuria, can perpetuate a negative calcium balance by parathyroid stimulation. SCP should be used only in patients with severe type I absorptive hypercalciuria. Although widely used to treat this condition, thiazides are not considered selective medical therapy for type I absorptive hypercalciuria. Thiazides do not correct the basic abnormality of increased calcium intestinal absorption but will augment calcium reabsorption in the distal tubule. In addition, extracellular volume depletion indirectly stimulates proximal tubular reabsorption of calcium.

32. **b. Hyperuricosuria.** Sodium cellulose phosphate will bind calcium in the intestinal tract to aid in correcting hypercalciuria of type I absorptive hypercalciuria. This may result in excess filtered load of oxalate, because calcium is no longer available to bind oxalate in the gut for excretion. Sodium cellulose phosphate will bind other cations, causing hypomagnesemia due to intestinal losses. In addition, sodium cellulose phosphate, if used in patients with other types of hypercalciuria, can perpetuate a negative calcium balance by parathyroid stimulation and further calcium wasting. A common adverse effect of sodium cellulose phosphate is gastrointestinal upset, occasionally causing cessation of therapy.

33. **d. thiazide-induced hypocitraturia.** Intracellular acidosis resulting from thiazide-induced hypokalemia will augment renal tubular reabsorption of citrate with resultant hypocitraturia. The reduction in the inhibitory effects of hypocitraturia may promote further stone formation. Therefore, potassium repletion is necessary if long-term thiazide treatment is anticipated. Our potassium supplement of choice is potassium citrate, either in pill or liquid preparations.

34. **c. high dietary sodium intake.** A high dietary sodium intake has two deleterious effects in this case. An excess sodium load will inhibit reabsorption of calcium in the proximal tubule, thereby causing hypercalciuria. Moreover, sodium will block the hypocalciuric action of thiazides. Therefore, patients placed on thiazide diuretics for management of hypercalciuria should also be placed on a dietary sodium restriction.

35. **e. all of the above.** Absorptive hypercalciuria type II is believed to be a less severe form of absorptive hypercalciuria type I. Placing a patient on a calcium-restricted diet will normalize their urinary calcium excretion. However, patients with hypercalciuria type I have a high urinary calcium excretion despite dietary modifications. Appropriate therapy for absorptive hypercalciuria type II would be to moderate calcium intake and maintain a high fluid intake to maintain urine output greater than 2 L/day. A severe dietary calcium restriction is not indicated, because significant dietary modifications may exacerbate stone disease.

36. **d. restrict dietary oxalate.** Initial treatment of patients diagnosed with absorptive hypercalciuria type II includes moderating dietary calcium intake to reduce the filtered calcium load, increasing fluid intake to maintain urine output greater than 2 L/day, limiting sodium intake to reduce the calciuric effects of sodium on proximal tubular reabsorption of calcium, and initiating potassium citrate to alkalize the urine and reduce calcium stone formation.

44

Surgical Management of Upper Urinary Tract Calculi

JAMES E. LINGEMAN • BRIAN R. MATLAGA • ANDREW P. EVAN

QUESTIONS

1. What percentage of renal calculi can be successfully managed with extracorporeal shockwave lithotripsy (ESWL)?
   a. 90% to 95%
   b. 80% to 85%
   c. 70% to 75%
   d. 60% to 65%
   e. 50% to 55%
2. The best predictor of post-PNL urosepsis is which of the following cultures?
   a. preoperative bladder urine
   b. intraoperative bladder urine
   c. stone
   d. preoperative blood
   e. intraoperative blood
3. What is the risk of mortality from an untreated struvite staghorn stone?
   a. Less than 10%
   b. 10% to 30%
   c. 30% to 50%
   d. 50% to 70%
   e. Greater than 70%
4. The increased risk of residual fragments after ESWL of large-volume calculi is of particular importance for patients with stones composed of:
   a. brushite.
   b. uric acid.
   c. struvite.
   d. calcium oxalate monohydrate.
   e. calcium oxalate dihydrate.
5. What is the single most important factor when choosing among ESWL, ureteroscopic stone removal (URS), and percutaneous nephrolithotomy (PNL) for renal calculi?
   a. Stone composition
   b. Stone location
   c. Anatomic abnormalities
   d. Stone burden
   e. Body habitus
6. What is the preferred treatment for a known brushite stone former harboring a lower pole renal calculus 25 mm in diameter?
   a. ESWL
   b. ESWL with ureteral stenting
   c. Flexible ureteroscopy with holmium laser lithotripsy
   d. PNL
   e. Laparoscopic pyelolithotomy
7. What is the preferred initial treatment for staghorn calculi?
   a. ESWL with ureteral stenting
   b. Flexible ureteroscopy with holmium laser lithotripsy
   c. PNL
   d. Extended pyelolithotomy with multiple radial nephrotomies
   e. Anatrophic nephrolithotomy
8. Which of these is the most difficult stone composition to fragment with ESWL?
   a. Calcium oxalate dihydrate
   b. Calcium oxalate monohydrate
   c. Struvite
   d. Hydroxyapatite
   e. Uric acid
9. What is the preferred treatment approach for a symptomatic patient with a 1.5-cm stone in a lower pole calyceal diverticulum?
   a. ESWL
   b. Flexible ureteroscopy
   c. PNL
   d. PNL with fulguration of the diverticulum
   e. Laparoscopic diverticulectomy
10. What is the preferred initial treatment for a 10-mm stone in the renal pelvis of a horseshoe kidney with minimal hydronephrosis?
    a. ESWL
    b. Flexible ureteroscopy
    c. PNL
    d. Laparoscopic pyelolithotomy
    e. Symphysiotomy with pyelolithotomy

11. What is the preferred treatment approach for a 10-mm renal calculus in a patient who weighs 375 pounds?
    a. ESWL
    b. Flexible ureteroscopy
    c. PNL
    d. ESWL using the "blast path" technique
    e. Open surgery
12. What is the preferred treatment option for a symptomatic patient with a 1.5-cm renal calculus and a coagulopathy?
    a. ESWL
    b. ESWL after administration of fresh frozen plasma
    c. Indwelling ureteral stent
    d. Flexible ureteroscopy
    e. PNL
13. Residual fragments after ESWL have been associated with which of the following?
    a. Hypertension
    b. Increased rate of recurrent stones
    c. Decreased rate of recurrent stones
    d. Perinephric hematomas
    e. Hematuria
14. What is the most sensitive test for identifying residual fragments after PNL?
    a. Nephrotomograms
    b. MRI
    c. Ultrasonography
    d. Noncontrast CT
    e. Contrast-enhanced CT
15. Factors affecting the probability of spontaneous passage of ureteral calculi include all of the following except which one?
    a. Stone size
    b. Stone location
    c. Stone composition
    d. Degree of hydronephrosis
    e. Duration of symptoms
16. Irreversible loss of renal function can occur within what time period when a completely obstructing ureteral stone is present?
    a. 1 week
    b. 2 to 4 weeks
    c. 4 to 6 weeks
    d. More than 6 weeks
    e. 3 months
17. A first-time stone former is diagnosed with a 4-mm proximal ureteral calculus. The best initial management is:
    a. ureteroscopic laser lithotripsy.
    b. ureteral stent placement.
    c. ESWL.
    d. expectant management.
    e. ESWL with ureteral stent placement.
18. What is the stone-free rate for patients with ureteral stones < 1 cm, located in the proximal ureter and treated primarily with ESWL? Between
    a. 90% and 100%
    b. 80% and 90%
    c. 70% and 80%
    d. 60% and 70%
    e. 50% and 60%
19. Ureteral stent placement when ESWL is performed for ureteral stones is appropriate for all of the following reasons except which one?
    a. Solitary kidney
    b. Relief of severe symptoms
    c. Enhancement of stone fragmentation
    d. Relief of obstruction
    e. Localization of difficult-to-visualize stones
20. What is the stone-free rate for patients with ureteral stones < 1 cm located in the proximal ureter and treated with flexible ureteroscopy? Between
    a. 90% and 100%
    b. 80% and 90%
    c. 70% and 80%
    d. 60% and 70%
    e. 50% and 60%
21. What is the stone-free rate for patients with ureteral stones < 1 cm located in the distal ureter and treated with rigid ureteroscopy? Between
    a. 90% and 100%
    b. 80% and 90%
    c. 70% and 80%
    d. 60% and 70%
    e. 50% and 60%
22. Metabolic changes associated with pregnancy that are relevant to urolithiasis include all of the following except which one?
    a. Absorptive hypercalciuria
    b. Hypercalcemia
    c. Hyperuricosuria
    d. Increased citrate excretion
    e. Increased magnesium excretion
23. What is the preferred initial diagnostic study for suspected urolithiasis in pregnant patients
    a. Kidney, ureter, and bladder (KUB)
    b. Tailored intravenous pyelography (i.e., two or three films)
    c. Renal ultrasonography
    d. Spiral CT
    e. MRI
24. The optimal management of a 28-week pregnant patient with a 6-mm proximal ureteral calculus that is refractory to conservative therapy is:
    a. ESWL
    b. PNL
    c. URS
    d. Placement of internalized double-J stent
    e. Placement of percutaneous nephrostomy drain
25. The risk of ureteral perforation is greatest with which of the following intracorporeal lithotripsy technologies?
    a. EHL
    b. Holmium laser
    c. Pulsed dye laser
    d. Ultrasonic lithotripsy
    e. Ballistic lithotripsy
26. The risk of retrograde stone propulsion is greatest with which of the following intracorporeal lithotripsy technologies?
    a. EHL
    b. Holmium laser
    c. Pulsed dye laser
    d. Ultrasonic lithotripsy
    e. Ballistic lithotripsy

27. The coumarin dye wave length (540 nm) of the pulsed dye laser is not absorbed by which of the following?
    a. Calcium oxalate dihydrate
    b. Calcium oxalate monohydrate
    c. Cystine
    d. Struvite
    e. Uric acid
28. What are the preferred initial power settings for holmium laser lithotripsy of ureteral stones?
    a. 0.6 J, 6 Hz
    b. 0.6 J, 10 Hz
    c. 1.0 J, 10 Hz
    d. 1.2 J, 10 Hz
    e. 1.0 J, 15 Hz
29. Which intracorporeal lithotripsy technology fragments the highest percentage of stones?
    a. Ultrasound
    b. Ballistic lithotripsy
    c. Coumarin dye laser
    d. Holmium laser
    e. Electrokinetic lithotripsy
30. Which intracorporeal lithotripsy technology has the least risk of ureteral perforation?
    a. Ultrasound
    b. Ballistic
    c. Holmium laser
    d. EHL
    e. Erbium laser
31. Energy sources for ESWL include all of the following except which one?
    a. Electrohydraulic
    b. Holmium laser
    c. Piezoelectric
    d. Electromagnetic
    e. Microexplosive
32. What is a major disadvantage of sonographic imaging for ESWL?
    a. Inability to visualize ureteropelvic junction (UPJ) stones
    b. Exposure to ionizing radiation
    c. Inability to visualize radiolucent stones
    d. Expense of ultrasonography systems
    e. Inability to visualize ureteral stones
33. Factors influencing the amount of pain during ESWL include all but which of the following?
    a. Power level applied
    b. Stone composition
    c. Type of shock wave generator
    d. Shock wave energy density at the point of skin penetration
    e. Stone location
34. Which lithotripter produces the highest stone-free rates?
    a. Wolf Piezolith 2300
    b. Siemens Lithostar
    c. Modified Dornier HM3
    d. Unmodified Dornier HM3
    e. HealthTronics LithoTron
35. Possible mechanisms producing stone fragmentation during ESWL include all of the following EXCEPT which one?
    a. Compression fracture
    b. Spallation
    c. Acoustic cavitation
    d. Dynamic fatigue
    e. Vaporization
36. What percentage of kidneys experience trauma during ESWL?
    a. 0% to 20%
    b. 20% to 40%
    c. 40% to 60%
    d. 60% to 80%
    e. 80% to 100%
37. Risk factors that will enhance the bioeffects of shock waves include all of the following EXCEPT which one?
    a. Older than 60 years
    b. Younger than 18 years (pediatric population)
    c. Stone burden
    d. Preexisting hypertension
    e. Reduced renal mass
38. The primary insult to the kidney exposed to shock waves occurs in which of the following tissues?
    a. Blood vessels
    b. Proximal tubules
    c. Renal papillae
    d. Glomeruli
    e. Renal capsules
39. Which of the following is an absolute contraindication to PNL?
    a. Morbid obesity
    b. Uncorrected coagulopathy
    c. Neurogenic bladder
    d. Pelvic kidney
    e. Horseshoe kidney
40. What is the most common secondarily infecting organism after percutaneous stone removal?
    a. *Proteus mirabilis*
    b. *Klebsiella oxytoca*
    c. *Pseudomonas aeruginosa*
    d. *Staphylococcus epidermidis*
    e. *Enterococcus (Streptococcus) faecalis*
41. What is the initial step in performing PNL?
    a. Percutaneous puncture of the renal collecting system
    b. Placement of a double-J ureteral stent
    c. Insertion of a ureteral catheter
    d. Administration of intravenous contrast material
    e. Antegrade placement of a guide wire into the ureter
42. What is the preferred site of puncture into the renal collecting system during access for PNL?
    a. Upper pole infundibulum
    b. Anterior lower pole calyx
    c. Posterior lower pole calyx
    d. Upper pole calyx
    e. Renal pelvis
43. Risk factors for colon injury during PNL include all of the following EXCEPT which one?
    a. Horseshoe kidney
    b. Kyphoscoliosis
    c. Access lateral to the posterior axillary line
    d. Previous jejunoileal bypass for obesity
    e. Upper pole puncture
44. To minimize the risk of lung and pleura injury during supracostal upper pole access for PNL:
    a. the puncture should be performed during full expiration.
    b. the puncture should be performed during full inspiration.
    c. CO_2 should be injected through the ureteral catheter to identify the upper pole calyx.
    d. the puncture should be done with local anesthesia.
    e. the puncture should be performed by a radiologist.

45. Indications for supracostal access during PNL include all of the following EXCEPT which one?
    a. Predominant stone distribution in the upper pole
    b. Access to the UPJ or proximal ureter required
    c. Cystine stones
    d. Multiple lower pole infundibula and calyces containing stone material
    e. Horseshoe kidneys

46. When performing PNL and endopyelotomy in the same setting, the optimal point of entry is:
    a. posterior upper pole calyx.
    b. posterior lower pole calyx.
    c. anterior upper pole calyx.
    d. anterior lower pole calyx.
    e. renal pelvis.

47. During access for PNL, what is the preferred initial wire?
    a. Amplatz super stiff
    b. Benson
    c. Hydrophilic glide
    d. Lunderquist
    e. J-tipped movable core

48. What is the most common serious error in PNL access?
    a. Not using an Amplatz sheath
    b. Overadvancement of the dilator/sheath
    c. Anterior calyceal puncture
    d. Ultrasonographically guided puncture
    e. Using telescoping metal dilators

49. What is the appropriate irrigating solution for PNL?
    a. 3% sorbitol
    b. Sterile water
    c. Glycine
    d. Dilute contrast material
    e. 0.9% saline

50. Middle or upper pole access for PNL in horseshoe kidneys is preferred for all of the following reasons EXCEPT which one?
    a. Higher incidence of retrorenal colon
    b. Malrotation of the renal collecting system
    c. Incomplete ascent of horseshoe kidneys
    d. Anterior medial location of lower pole calyces
    e. Facilitated access to the UPJ or upper ureter

51. What is the most significant complication of PNL?
    a. Hemorrhage
    b. Extravasation of irrigation fluid
    c. Incomplete stone removal
    d. Urinary tract infection
    e. Pleural effusion

52. What is the risk of arteriovenous fistula formation after PNL?
    a. 1 in 10
    b. 1 in 100
    c. 1 in 200
    d. 1 in 500
    e. 1 in 1000

53. If uncontrolled bleeding persists after nephrostomy tube placement after PNL, what would the preferred approach be?
    a. Insertion of a double-J stent
    b. Administration of furosemide (Lasix) to promote diuresis
    c. Surgical exploration
    d. Immediate angiography
    e. Insertion of a Kaye tamponade balloon

54. If a retroperitoneal injury to the colon is diagnosed after PNL, what is the usually preferred management?
    a. Surgical exploration and repair
    b. Diverting colostomy with later definitive repair
    c. Leaving the nephrostomy tube in for 2 weeks to allow the tract to mature
    d. Insertion of a double-J stent and withdrawal of the nephrostomy tube into the colon
    e. Immediate removal of the nephrostomy tube

55. The use of double-J stents to reduce the risk of steinstrasse after ESWL has been demonstrated to be beneficial for what size of stones? Greater than:
    a. 5 mm
    b. 10 mm
    c. 15 mm
    d. 20 mm
    e. 25 mm

56. Indications for flexible ureteroscopy for the management of renal calculi include all of the following EXCEPT which one?
    a. Failed ESWL
    b. Morbid obesity
    c. Cystine calculi
    d. Anticoagulant therapy
    e. Staghorn stones

ANSWERS

1. **b. 80% to 85%.** The majority of "simple" renal calculi (80% to 85%) can be treated satisfactorily with ESWL.

2. **c. stone culture.** The best predictor of post-PNL urosepsis is stone culture or renal pelvic urine culture results.

3. **b. 10% to 30%.** The 10-year mortality rate of untreated staghorn stones was 28%, versus 7.2% in patients treated with surgery.

4. **c. struvite.** Struvite stones must be removed completely to minimize the risk of continued urea-splitting bacteriuria.

5. **d. Stone burden.** Stone burden (size and number) is perhaps the single most important factor in deciding the appropriate treatment modality for a patient with kidney calculi.

6. **d. PNL.** The Lower Pole Stone Study Group compared URS and PNL for patients with 10- to 25-mm lower pole stones and found a significant difference in stone clearance, with only 40% of the URS cohort stone free at 3 months versus 76% of the PNL cohort.

7. **c. PNL.** The management of staghorn stones with a combined approach must be viewed as primarily percutaneous, with ESWL being used only as adjunct to minimize the number of accesses required.

8. **b. Calcium oxalate monohydrate.** Cystine and brushite are the stones most resistant to ESWL, followed by calcium oxalate monohydrate. Next, in descending order, are hydroxyapatite, struvite, calcium oxalate dihydrate, and uric acid stones.

9. **c. PNL.** The percutaneous approach for the management of patients with calyceal diverticular stones provides the patient with the best chance of becoming stone and symptom free.

10. **a. ESWL.** ESWL can achieve satisfactory results in properly selected patients, such as those with small stones (<1.5 cm) in the presence of normal urinary drainage. For larger stones or when there is evidence of poor urinary drainage, PNL should be used as the primary approach.

11. **b. Flexible ureteroscopy.** Retrograde ureteroscopic intrarenal surgery may be the preferred modality of treatment for morbidly obese patients when the stone burden is not excessively large.

12. **d. Flexible ureteroscopy.** When anticoagulation cannot be temporarily discontinued, the use of ureteroscopy in combination with holmium laser lithotripsy is preferred. One study reported that even when patients' coagulopathies were not fully corrected, stones could be successfully treated with no increase in hemorrhagic complications.

13. **b. Increased rate of recurrent stones.** At follow-up (1.6 to 85.4 months), 43% of the patients with residual fragments had a significant symptomatic episode or required intervention.

14. **d. Noncontrast CT.** Although flexible nephroscopy is often considered the "gold standard" for assessing residual stones after PNL, the routine use of flexible nephroscopy has been challenged by studies showing the high sensitivity of noncontrast CT in detecting residual stones. Noncontrast CT had 100% sensitivity for detecting residual stones after PNL in 36 patients evaluated by both CT and flexible nephroscopy.

15. **c. Stone composition.** One study analyzed 75 patients with ureteral calculi and found that the interval to stone passage was highly variable and dependent on stone size, location, and side. Stones that were smaller, more distal, and on the right side were more likely to pass spontaneously. In another study, duration of symptoms before presentation was the most influential factor, followed by the degree of hydronephrosis.

16. **b. 2 to 4 weeks.** Even with complete ureteral obstruction, irreversible loss of renal function does not occur for more than 2 weeks but can progress to total renal unit loss at up to 6 weeks.

17. **d. expectant management.** The majority of ureteral stones less than 5 mm will pass spontaneously and therefore can be treated with expectant management.

18. **b. Between 80% and 90%.** For stones smaller than 1 cm, the stone-free rate for ESWL was 84%.

19. **c. Enhancement of stone fragmentation.** Although early reports supported the routine use of a ureteral stent to bypass ureteral stones before ESWL, data analyzed by the American Urological Association ureteral calculi guidelines panel showed no improvement in fragmentation with stenting, and therefore routine stent placement before ESWL was discouraged. However, ureteral stent placement is appropriate for other indications, such as management of pain, relief of obstruction, and stones that are difficult to visualize, and is mandatory in a patient who has a solitary obstructed kidney.

20. **a. Between 90% and 100%.** A review of the current literature shows excellent results for flexible ureteroscopic lithotripsy utilizing the holmium laser for proximal ureteral calculi, with a mean stone-free rate of 95% and a low associated rate of ureteral perforation and stricture.

21. **a. Between 90% and 100%.** A review of the current literature shows excellent results for rigid ureteroscopic lithotripsy utilizing the holmium laser for distal ureteral calculi, with a mean stone-free rate of 95% associated with a low perforation and stricture rate of about 1%.

22. **b. Hypercalcemia.** Pregnancy induces a state of absorptive hypercalciuria and mild hyperuricosuria that is offset by increased excretion of urinary inhibitors such as citrate and magnesium, as well as increased urinary output. The metabolic changes in pregnancy do not influence the rate of new stone occurrence. However, paradoxically, it has been suggested that metabolic alterations in urine may contribute to accelerated encrustation of stents during pregnancy.

23. **c. Renal ultrasonography.** To avoid the small risk of radiation, ultrasonography has become the first-line diagnostic study for urolithiasis in pregnancy.

24. **c. URS.** Improvements in ureteroscopic technology and intracorporeal lithotripters have made it possible to successfully access and treat any stone in the upper urinary tract, even in the pregnant patient. Pregnancy is a contraindication to ESWL, PNL requires prolonged anesthesia and radiation exposure, and ureteral stents and nephrostomy tubes have been reported to encrust at an accelerated rate in the pregnant patient.

25. **a. EHL.** The major disadvantage of EHL is its propensity to damage the ureteral mucosa and its association with ureteral perforation.

26. **e. Ballistic lithotripsy.** Ballistic lithotripsy is accompanied by a relatively high rate of stone propulsion of between 2% and 17% when ureteral stones are treated. The holmium laser has been associated with a reduced potential for causing retropulsion owing to the weak shock wave that is typically induced during holmium laser lithotripsy.

27. **c. Cystine.** The coumarin wavelength was chosen because it is absorbed by all stone materials other than cystine but not by surrounding tissues. Cystine calculi do not absorb the 504 nm laser light and, thus, are not fragmented with the coumarin-pulsed dye laser.

28. **a. 0.6 J, 6 Hz.** It is recommended to commence treatment using low-pulse energy (i.e., 0.6 J) with a pulse rate of 6 Hz and increase the pulse frequency (in preference to increasing the pulse energy) as needed to speed fragmentation.

29. **d. Holmium laser.** The ability of the holmium laser to fragment all stones regardless of composition is a clear advantage over the coumarin-pulsed dye laser. Successful fragmentation of ureteral stones of all compositions is reported in 91% to 100% of the cases with a mean stone-free rate of 95%. Currently, the holmium laser is the most effective and versatile intracorporeal lithotripter with a good margin of safety.

30. **b. Ballistic.** When compared with EHL or ultrasonic or laser lithotripsy, ballistic devices have a significantly lower risk of ureteral perforation.

31. **b. Holmium laser.** There are three primary types of shock wave generators: electrohydraulic (Spark Gap), electromagnetic, and piezoelectric. Microexplosive generators have also been produced but have not gained mainstream acceptance.

32. **e. Inability to visualize ureteral stones.** Sonographic localization of a kidney stone requires a highly trained operator. Furthermore, localization of stones in the ureter is difficult or impossible.

33. **b. Stone composition.** The discomfort experienced during ESWL is related directly to the energy density of the shock wave as it passes through the skin as well as the size of the focal point, parameters that are affected by all of the choices listed except for stone composition.

34. **d. Unmodified Dornier HM3.** To date, despite the proliferation of lithotripters and the variety of solutions devised for stone targeting and shock wave delivery, no other lithotripter system has convincingly equaled or surpassed the results produced by the unmodified Dornier HM3 device.

35. **e. Vaporization.** Several potential mechanisms for ESWL stone breakage have been described: (1) spall fracture, (2) squeezing, (3) shear stress, (4) superfocusing, (5) acoustic cavitation, and (6) dynamic fatigue.

36. **e. 80% to 100%.** ESWL is now known to induce acute structural changes in the treated kidney in a majority, if not all, patients. Morphologic studies using both MRI and quantitative radionuclide renography have suggested that 63% to 85% of all ESWL patients treated with an unmodified HM3 lithotripter exhibit one or more forms of renal injury within 24 hours of treatment.

37. **c. Stone burden.** Patients with existing hypertension are at increased risk for the development of perinephric hematomas as a consequence of ESWL. Age is a factor on both ends of the scale in that children and the elderly both appear to be at a greater risk for structural and functional changes after exposure to shock waves. These responses are probably related to a reduction in the large renal reserve present in most healthy adult patients.

38. **a. Blood vessels.** Macroscopically, the acute changes noted in dog and pig kidneys treated with a clinical dose of shock waves are strikingly similar to those described for patients. This lesion is predictable in size, is focal in location, and is unique in the types of injuries (primarily vascular insult) induced. Regions of damage reveal rupture of nearby thin-walled veins, walls of small arteries, and glomerular and peritubular capillaries, which correlates with the vasoconstriction measured in both treated and untreated kidneys. These observations show that both the microvasculature and the nephron are susceptible to shock wave damage; however, the primary injury appears to be a vascular insult.

39. **b. Uncorrected coagulopathy.** Uncorrected coagulopathy and an active, untreated urinary tract infection are two absolute contraindications to PNL.

40. **d. *Staphylococcus epidermidis.*** Cephalosporins are the most appropriately used antibiotics for prophylaxis of surgical procedures in noninfected stone cases, because the most common secondarily infecting organism is *S. epidermidis.*

41. **c. Insertion of a ureteral catheter.** When performed as a single-stage procedure, PNL is initiated by the cystoscopic placement of a ureteral catheter.

42. **c. Posterior lower pole calyx.** Because the posterior calyces are generally oriented so that the long axis points to the avascular area of the renal cortex, a posterolateral puncture directed at a posterior calyx would be expected to traverse through the avascular zone.

43. **e. Upper pole puncture.** A puncture placed too laterally may injure the colon. The position of the retroperitoneal colon is usually anterior or anterolateral to the lateral renal border. Therefore, risk of colon injury is usually only with a very lateral (lateral to the posterior axillary line) puncture. Posterior colonic displacement is more likely in thin female patients, with very little retroperitoneal fat, and/or elderly patients, as well as in patients with jejunoileal bypass resulting in an enlarged colon. Other factors increasing the risk of colon injury include anterior calyceal puncture, previous extensive renal operation, horseshoe kidney, and kyphoscoliosis. A retrorenal colon is more frequently noted on the left side.

44. **a. the puncture should be performed during full expiration.** A supracostal puncture should be performed only during full expiration.

45. **c. Cystine stones.** A supracostal puncture is indicated when the predominant distribution of stone material is in the upper calyces; when there is an associated UPJ stricture requiring endopyelotomy; in cases of multiple lower pole infundibula and calyces containing stone material or an associated ureteral stone; in staghorn calculi with substantial upper pole stone burden; and in horseshoe kidneys.

46. **a. posterior upper pole calyx.** A posterior upper pole calyx puncture, typically through a supracostal approach, aligns the axis of puncture with the UPJ. This allows the treating urologist to perform endopyelotomy with a rigid nephroscope, while exerting minimal torque on the instrument.

47. **c. Hydrophilic glide.** The hydrophilic glide wire is preferred for entering the collecting system, because it is the most flexible and maneuverable wire available.

48. **b. Overadvancement of the dilator/sheath.** Overadvancement of the dilator/sheath is the most common serious error in access for PNL and may result in significant trauma to the renal collecting system and/or excessive hemorrhage.

49. **e. 0.9% saline.** Physiologic solutions should be used for irrigation during PNL to minimize the risk of dilutional hyponatremia in the event of large volume extravasation.

50. **a. Higher incidence of retrorenal colon.** The optimal point of entry for a horseshoe kidney is through a posterior calyx, which is typically more medial than in the normal kidney because of the altered renal axis and rotation associated with the midline fusion. An upper pole collecting system puncture is often appealing, because the entire kidney is usually subcostal. In most cases, the lower pole calyces are anterior and inaccessible percutaneously.

51. **a. Hemorrhage.** Bleeding is the most significant complication of PNL, with transfusion rates varying from less than 1% to 10%.

52. **c. 1 in 200.** Bleeding from an arteriovenous fistula or pseudoaneurysm requiring emergency embolization is seen in less than 0.5% of patients.

53. **e. Insertion of a Kaye tamponade balloon.** If bleeding is not controlled by nephrostomy tube placement and clamping, a Kaye nephrostomy tamponade balloon catheter should be placed (Cook Urological, Spencer, IN). The Kaye nephrostomy tube incorporates a low-pressure, 12-mm balloon that may be left inflated for prolonged periods to tamponade bleeding from the nephrostomy tract.

54. **d. Insertion of a double-J stent and withdrawal of the nephrostomy tube into the colon.** Colonic injury is an unusual complication often diagnosed on a postoperative nephrostogram. Typically, the injury is retroperitoneal; thus, signs and symptoms of peritonitis are infrequent. If the perforation is extraperitoneal, management may be expectant with placement of a ureteral catheter or double-J stent to decompress the collecting system and by withdrawing the nephrostomy tube from an intrarenal position to an intracolonic position, thus serving as a colostomy tube. The colostomy tube is left in place for a minimum of 7 days and is removed after a nephrostogram or a retrograde pyelogram shows no communication between the colon and the kidney.

55. **d. Greater than 20 mm.** Stents may be particularly advantageous with stones larger than 20 mm.

56. **e. Staghorn stones.** One study reported the first large series (208 patients) of renal calculi treated by retrograde intrarenal surgery using a flexible deflectable ureteroscope after 1 to 2 weeks of ureteral stenting. The indications for the procedure included patients in whom ESWL had failed (single stone of <1 cm or up to 5 particles of <5 mm), radiolucent stones (<1.5 cm), concomitant ureteral and renal stones, renal stones associated with intrarenal stenosis, nephrocalcinosis or urinary diversion, patients with a need for complete stone removal (e.g., pilots), and patients with bleeding disorders. A ureteroscopic approach to the treatment of staghorn stones has been described, although not widely accepted.

45

Ureteroscopy and Retrograde Access

BEN H. CHEW • JOHN D. DENSTEDT

QUESTIONS

1. When inserting the flexible ureteroscope over a guidewire, difficulty is encountered advancing the endoscope past the ureteral orifice. What is the next step?
   a. Dilate the ureter with a balloon.
   b. Rotate the scope 90 to 180 degrees.
   c. Dilate the ureter with a 8/10 Fr coaxial dilator.
   d. Switch to the semi-rigid ureteroscope.
   e. Remove the second (safety) wire.
2. Which method of intracorporeal lithotripsy when combined with flexible ureteroscopy is effective against all types of stone compositions?
   a. Electrohydraulic lithotripsy
   b. Pulsed-dye laser
   c. Holmium:YAG laser
   d. Pneumatic lithotripsy
   e. Ultrasonic lithotripsy
3. Ureteral dilation to facilitate ureteroscopy:
   a. is necessary in every case.
   b. is necessary when performing endoscopy above the iliac vessels.
   c. is necessary for rigid ureteroscopy.
   d. is necessary for flexible ureteroscopy.
   e. is not necessary in every case.
4. Placement of a ureteral stent after ureteroscopy and stone manipulation is recommended if:
   a. the stone was removed by a basket with no remaining fragments.
   b. ureteral trauma occurred intraoperatively.
   c. the rigid ureteroscope was used.
   d. the stone was located in the kidney.
   e. pneumatic lithotripsy was used.
5. The incidence of ureteral stricture post ureteroscopy increases with:
   a. flexible ureteroscopy.
   b. use of the holmium:YAG laser for intracorporeal lithotripsy.
   c. an indwelling stent.
   d. ureteral perforation.
   e. hydronephrosis and an obstructing stone.
6. The holmium:YAG laser emits at which of the following wavelengths?
   a. 1064 nm
   b. 2100 nm
   c. 504 nm
   d. 755 nm
   e. 10,200 nm
7. The holmium:YAG laser energy transmits which of the following distances when used in a fluid environment?
   a. 10 mm
   b. 0.1 mm
   c. 2 cm
   d. 0.5 mm
   e. 0.01 mm

ANSWERS

1. **b. Rotate the scope 90 to 180 degrees.** Rotating the scope 90 to 180 degrees usually allows the flexible scope to be advanced. This maneuver takes into account the offset working channel of the ureteroscope and will allow the body of the scope to enter into the ureteral orifice.
2. **c. Holmium:YAG laser.** This method of intracorporeal lithotripsy is effective against all stone composition including cystine, calcium phosphate, and calcium oxalate monohydrate stones. The holmium:YAG laser delivers photothermal energy that results in stone vaporization. The pulsed-dye laser requires coumarin and operates at a wavelength of 504 nm, which is not absorbed by cystine or calcium oxalate monohydrate, thus making these stones resistant to the pulsed-dye laser. EHL lithotripsy is less effective in fragmenting hard stones such as calcium oxalate monohydrate or cystine. Rigid probes used with ultrasound or pneumatic lithotripsy cannot be used with flexible ureteroscopy.
3. **e. is not necessary in every case.** The advent of smaller ureteroscopes and intracorporeal lithotriptors has resulted in techniques that do not routinely require ureteral dilation in order to advance ureteroscopes beyond the ureteral orifice or proximally up the ureter.

4. **b. ureteral trauma occurred intraoperatively.** Randomized controlled clinical trials demonstrate that the rate of complications is equal whether patients have stents placed or not after ureteroscopy and lithotripsy. Indications to stent after ureteroscopy include ureteral trauma, ureteral perforation, impacted stone with significant edema, large stone burden, or ureteral dilation > 10 Fr. Ureteral stents are also left indwelling for passive ureteral dilation over 7 to 10 days if attempts at ureteroscopic access are unsuccessful.

5. **d. ureteral perforation.** The ureteral stricture rate in uncomplicated ureteroscopic cases ranges from 1% to 2%. If the ureter is perforated intraoperatively, the rate increases to about 6%. A ureteral stent is left indwelling to provide drainage and reduce the incidence of subsequent ureteral stricture formation.

6. **b. 2100 nm.** The neodymium:YAG laser operates at 1064 nm, the pulsed-dye laser at 504 nm, the alexandrite laser at 755 nm, and the CO_2 laser at 10,200 nm.

7. **d. 0.5 mm.** The depth of penetration of the holmium:YAG laser is 0.5 mm when used in liquid because the energy is rapidly absorbed in water, thus making this modality very safe.

46

Percutaneous Management of the Upper Urinary Tract

MANTU GUPTA • MICHAEL C. OST • JAY B. SHAH • ELSPETH M. MCDOUGALL • ARTHUR D. SMITH

QUESTIONS

1. Which of the following is the best indication for percutaneous nephrostomy over ureteral stenting for drainage of a renal unit?
   a. UPJ obstruction
   b. Distal ureteral calculus
   c. Forniceal rupture
   d. Pyonephrosis
   e. Ureteral stricture
2. What is the main source of radiation exposure to the urologist?
   a. Rays reflected off the image intensifier
   b. Scatter from the collimator
   c. Directly from the x-ray emission tube
   d. Rays that have penetrated through the patient's body
   e. Scatter from the table and patient
3. Which of the following technical features is most important for a fluoroscopic C-arm unit to minimize exposure?
   a. Rotation to change angle of x-ray delivery
   b. Collimation to minimize area radiated
   c. Boost mechanism to obtain high quality images
   d. Image hold function
   e. Continuous fluoroscopy
4. In which of the following situations is the scattered radiation to the operator greatest?
   a. Multiple short pulses for fluoroscopy
   b. Emission tube above the table
   c. Emission tube under the table
   d. Image intensifier over the table
   e. Image intensifier as close to the patient's body as possible
5. In which of the following situations of puncture is arterial bleeding most likely?
   a. Direct posterolateral
   b. Inferior pole
   c. Superior pole
   d. Medial puncture
   e. Mid pole
6. When bleeding occurs during the initial dilation of the tract with Amplatz dilators, what approach should be undertaken?
   a. Take out the dilator and observe
   b. Perform angiography and embolization
   c. Insert the next larger size dilator
   d. Abandon site and do access in different location
   e. Take out dilator and endoscopically fulgurate site of bleeding
7. The bull's-eye sign is observed on the fluoroscopic screen when the needle hub:
   a. is superimposed on the needle shaft, and the plane of the needle is in line with the x-ray beam.
   b. is near the needle shaft, giving the appearance of an arrow.
   c. is superimposed on the needle shaft and the plane of the needle is vertical to the x-ray beam.
   d. is off the fluoroscopic image, and the plane of the needle is horizontal to the x-ray beam.
   e. and needle tip are apart from each other as much as possible, giving the appearance of an arrow.
8. How is the depth of needle penetration monitored?
   a. By feeling the resistance of tissues being penetrated
   b. By injection of contrast medium through the needle
   c. By rotation of the C-arm back to the vertical position
   d. By aspiration of urine from the collecting system
   e. By fluoroscopy in the same plane as the puncture
9. Triangulation is the preferred technique for gaining access to which structure?
   a. Renal pelvis
   b. Calyx above the 12th rib
   c. Posterior, lower pole calyx
   d. Transplant kidney
   e. Posterior upper pole calyx
10. At the end of the percutaneous procedure, before placement of a tube, there is oozing from the nephrostomy tract. What would be the best initial management?
    a. Nephrostomy catheter, clamping it to allow tamponade
    b. Tamponade balloon catheter
    c. Large-bore nephrostomy tube
    d. Angiography for embolization
    e. Exploration in the operating room

11. Dilation of the nephrostomy tract should always be performed:
    a. after placement of a second guide wire.
    b. over a hydrophilic-coated guide wire.
    c. using a balloon dilating catheter.
    d. using the stiff metallic Alken dilators.
    e. using the Amplatz system of progressive dilators.
12. The insertion of the second safety guide wire must be performed:
    a. through a double-lumen catheter.
    b. to prevent excessive bleeding.
    c. to prevent loss of access.
    d. by inexperienced surgeons.
    e. when the stone is larger than 1 cm.
13. Which event is least likely to happen if excessive force is exerted during dilation with fascial dilators?
    a. Displacement of the guide wire
    b. Perforation of the collecting system
    c. Kinking of the guide wire
    d. Injury to the ureter
    e. Loss of renal access
14. A pregnant woman needs to undergo percutaneous drainage of the upper urinary system because of an obstructing stone. Which approach is *least* acceptable?
    a. Percutaneous nephrostomy under ultrasound guidance
    b. Ureteroscopy and stone removal
    c. Cystoscopic placement of a ureteral stent
    d. Ureteroscopy and laser lithotripsy
    e. Retrograde ureteropyelogram with fluoroscopic guidance
15. Tract dilation with the Amplatz dilators should always be performed:
    a. in a stepwise fashion at 2-Fr intervals.
    b. up to 34 Fr.
    c. at 6-Fr intervals.
    d. in two steps to 34 Fr.
    e. not at all—too dangerous.
16. The 8-Fr catheter that is included in the Amplatz set:
    a. prevents kinking of the wire.
    b. helps establish a tract to the bladder.
    c. allows placement of a safety wire.
    d. is hydrophilic so it slides easily.
    e. is completely radiolucent.
17. The optimal tract reaches the:
    a. renal hilum.
    b. ureteropelvic junction.
    c. renal pelvis.
    d. calyx.
    e. infundibulum.
18. Ideally, the final inner diameter of the working sheath should exceed the tube or instrument that is finally going to be inserted by how much?
    a. 1 to 2 Fr
    b. 2 to 4 Fr
    c. 8 to 10 Fr
    d. 10 to 12 Fr
    e. 14 to 16 Fr
19. A characteristic "waist" is evident fluoroscopically when which of the following devices is used for tract dilation?
    a. Amplatz dilators
    b. Alken dilators
    c. Balloon dilating catheters
    d. Teflon-coated catheters
    e. Single step devices
20. What is the main disadvantage of the Cope catheter?
    a. It needs to be removed under fluoroscopic control.
    b. It has tight loop formation and encrustation at the end hole that may make removal difficult.
    c. It is more likely to get infected than other catheters due to the coating material used on the loop mechanism.
    d. It has a high risk of eroding through the renal pelvis.
    e. It is uncomfortable because of large size.
21. Which nephrostomy tube would be advisable for an obese patient?
    a. Foley catheter
    b. Malecot catheter
    c. Single pigtail stent
    d. Nephroureteral stent
22. The main advantage of subcostal access to the upper pole by triangulation is that it:
    a. places less torque on the renal parenchyma.
    b. allows the shortest access tract to be created.
    c. minimizes the risk of pleural injury.
    d. affords easier access to the renal pelvis.
    e. is easier to perform than other methods of access.
23. What percentage of patients requires angiography and embolization after percutaneous procedures?
    a. 0.8% to 1.5%
    b. 2% to 3%
    c. 9% to 10%
    d. 12% to 15%
    e. 19% to 20%
24. Injury to the colon is most likely during percutaneous procedures:
    a. in thin females.
    b. in obese males.
    c. in patients who have had prior gallbladder surgery.
    d. on the left side.
25. Which approach has the best success rate for treatment of a stone-bearing lower pole calyceal diverticulum?
    a. Indirect percutaneous
    b. Retrograde ureteroscopic
    c. Direct percutaneous
    d. Open partial nephrectomy
    e. Laparoscopic
26. At which pressure is the Whitaker test unequivocally positive?
    a. 5 cm H_2O
    b. 10 cm H_2O
    c. 15 cm H_2O
    d. 25 cm H_2O
27. For percutaneous management of a renal cyst, which of the following is the most effective form of therapy?
    a. Percutaneous drainage alone
    b. Intrarenal drainage of the cyst
    c. Sclerosis of the cyst
    d. Endoscopic fulguration of the cyst wall
28. All of the following are risk factors for the development of fungal bezoars except:
    a. immunocompromised status.
    b. interstitial cystitis.
    c. neurogenic bladder.
    d. chronic antibiotic use.
    e. diabetes mellitus.

ANSWERS

1. **d. Pyonephrosis.** Pus in the kidney often drains poorly through small tubes and thus requires a larger drainage catheter than a ureteral stent. In patients presenting with acute pyonephrosis, percutaneous nephrostomy drainage is associated with minimal morbidity, facilitates definitive treatment, and provides therapeutic benefit. In all of the other choices, adequate drainage is usually provided by a ureteral stent.
2. **e. Scatter from the table and the patient.** The major source of the radiation dose received by the urologist is scattered radiation from the patient, hence the recommendation that the image intensifier be placed as close to the patient as possible.
3. **d. Image hold function.** Use of a last-image-hold feature is of great importance in reducing the overall irradiation time. It allows for inspection of anatomic detail without "thinking with a foot on the pedal." Collimation also helps minimize radiation exposure for the patient and surgeon.
4. **b. Emission tube above the table.** When the tube is above the operating table, there is a combination of leakage and scattered radiation. However, when the image intensifier is placed superiorly, radiation leakage is minimized, as the emission tube is shielded by an additional layer of material. The scattered radiation to the operator is also reduced.
5. **d. Medial puncture.** In more than 50% of kidneys, the posterior segmental artery is located in the middle or upper half of the posterior renal surface, and it may be damaged with an excessively medial needle puncture of an upper calyx. A direct posterior puncture that is too medial risks injury to the posterior segmental artery, which is the artery most commonly injured in endourologic procedures.
6. **c. Insert the next larger size dilator.** Bleeding during tract dilation is expected and is usually secondary to small parenchymal vessels. Effective tamponade can be used by progressively dilating until the working sheath is placed. The working sheath can be used to limit bleeding from the percutaneous tract.
7. **a. the needle hub is superimposed on the needle shaft, and the plane of the needle is in line with the x-ray beam.** An 18-gauge translumbar angiography needle is advanced in the plane of the fluoroscopic beam with the C-arm in the 30-degree position (see Fig. 46-16). The appropriate direction for needle advancement is determined by obtaining a bull's-eye sign on the fluoroscopic screen. This effect can be observed only when the needle hub is superimposed on the needle shaft and is evident when the plane of the needle is the same as that of the x-ray beam.
8. **c. By rotation of the C-arm back to the vertical position.** The depth of needle penetration is monitored by rotating the C-arm back to the vertical position.
9. **b. Calyx above the 12th rib.** One of the more frequently used techniques to access any calyx above the 12th rib without risking pleural injury is triangulation (see Fig. 46-18).
10. **c. Large-bore nephrostomy tube.** Most bleeding after percutaneous renal surgery is parenchymal and is recognized after removal of the working sheath. In these situations the simplest and most effective initial management is to place a large tube that closely mimics the size of the working sheath. Should this measure fail, the other measures mentioned can be utilized.
11. **a. after placement of a second guide wire.** A safety wire is of paramount importance and should be introduced before dilating the tract to its final working diameter.
12. **c. to prevent loss of access.** The safety guide wire allows re-access to the collecting system should the primary guide wire become dislodged or kinked.
13. **d. Injury to the ureter.** All of the others can be a direct result of excessive force, but ureteral injury is rare.
14. **e. Retrograde ureteropyelogram with fluoroscopic guidance.** Ultrasonographically guided nephrostomy puncture is preferred for pregnant women in whom there is a need for decompression of an obstructed kidney. Cystoscopic stent insertion and ureteroscopic stone extraction/lithotripsy may also be undertaken but all attempts should be made to avoid or minimize the use of radiation.
15. **a. in a stepwise fashion at 2-Fr intervals.** The tract is initially dilated until the curved 8-Fr Teflon catheter can be inserted over the wire. The larger dilators are tapered to fit over this catheter and should be done sequentially at 2-Fr intervals.
16. **a. prevents kinking of the wire.** Because of its flexibility, the 8-Fr catheter can pass easily into the ureter, sliding over the guide wire and protecting and stabilizing the guide wire to prevent kinking during progressive dilation. In addition, this catheter allows larger dilators to slide easily over it but is not hydrophilic coated.
17. **d. calyx.** The most stable tract that does not risk vascular injury enters a renal calyx. Dilators must be advanced over the working guide wire until they enter the calyceal lumen. However, further insertion may damage the integrity of the pelvicalyceal system and should be avoided.
18. **b. 2 to 4 Fr.** The final inner diameter of the working sheath should exceed the tube or instrument size by 2 to 4 Fr to allow adequate flow of fluid. This maintains low pressure within the collecting system to prevent sepsis and renal injury and allows adequate inflow of irrigant for clarity of vision. If the inner diameter of the working sheath is 30 Fr, a 26-Fr nephroscope can be easily inserted.
19. **c. Balloon dilating catheters.** As the balloon is inflated, a characteristic "waist" appears in areas of high resistance, such as the renal capsule or a previous operative scar (see Fig. 46-24).
20. **b. It has tight loop formation and encrustation at the end hole that may make removal difficult.** The main problem is that if a tight loop forms and the end hole becomes encrusted, the catheter becomes very difficult to remove.
21. **a. Foley catheter.** In obese and hypermobile patients, nephrostomy tubes can easily be pulled out. The Foley catheter balloon helps prevent dislodgement compared with the other types of tubes listed.
22. **c. minimizes risk of pleural injury.** Subcostal access prevents pleural injury but does not do any of the other things listed.
23. **a. 0.8% to 1.5%.** Of patients undergoing percutaneous renal procedures, 0.8% to 1.5% required angiography and embolization for uncontrolled bleeding.
24. **a. in thin females.** Colonic perforation is a rare complication of the percutaneous procedures, being reported in less than 1% of cases. It has been reported in thin females with right retrorenal colons.
25. **c. Direct percutaneous approach.** A ureteroscopic approach is difficult for lower pole diverticula, an indirect approach is usually doomed to failure, and open and laparoscopic approaches are more invasive.

26. **d. 25 cm H_2O.** Normal pelvic pressures range from 5% to 15%. If the difference in pressure between the renal pelvis and the bladder is less than 13 to 15 cm H_2O, the system is unobstructed. In contrast, a renal pelvis/bladder pressure differential greater than 22 cm H_2O indicates obstruction. A pressure difference of 15 to 22 cm H_2O is considered equivocal.
27. **d. Endoscopic fulguration of the cyst wall.** Drainage alone usually results in reaccumulation of fluid, and sclerosis of the cyst is potentially dangerous because of the medial location (resultant UPJ obstruction has been reported).
28. **b. interstitial cystitis.** Interstitial cystitis is not a risk factor for the development of fungal bezoars. Neurogenic bladder, chronic antibiotic use, diabetes mellitus, and immunocompromised conditions (elderly age, HIV, transplant patients, premature infants) are known risk factors for fungal bezoars.

SECTION XII

NEOPLASMS OF THE UPPER URINARY TRACT

47

Renal Tumors

STEVEN C. CAMPBELL • ANDREW C. NOVICK • RONALD M. BUKOWSKI

QUESTIONS

1. What is the most accurate imaging study for characterizing a renal mass?
   a. Intravenous pyelography
   b. Ultrasonography
   c. CT with and without contrast enhancement
   d. MRI
   e. Renal arteriography
2. A hyperdense renal cyst may also be termed a:
   a. Probable malignancy.
   b. Bosniak II cyst.
   c. Bosniak III cyst.
   d. Bosniak IV cyst.
   e. Probable angiomyolipoma.
3. The primary indication for fine-needle aspiration of a renal mass is which suspected clinical diagnosis?
   a. Renal cell carcinoma
   b. Renal oncocytoma
   c. Renal adenoma
   d. Renal metastasis
   e. Renal angiomyolipoma
4. Postoperative surveillance after radical nephrectomy for T1N0M0 renal cell carcinoma should include:
   a. No imaging studies
   b. Chest radiograph yearly
   c. Chest radiograph and abdominal CT yearly
   d. Chest radiograph yearly and abdominal CT every 2 years
   e. Chest radiograph and abdominal CT every 2 years
5. The major disadvantage of partial nephrectomy compared with radical nephrectomy for localized low-stage renal cell carcinoma is the increased risk of:
   a. perioperative renal failure.
   b. perioperative hemorrhage.
   c. postoperative distant metastasis.
   d. postoperative tumor recurrence in remnant kidney.
   e. postoperative tumor recurrence in perirenal lymph nodes.
6. After partial nephrectomy for T2N0M0 renal cell carcinoma, it is necessary to perform surveillance abdominal CT with what frequency?
   a. Never
   b. Every 6 months
   c. Every year
   d. Every 2 years
   e. Every 4 years
7. After partial nephrectomy of a solitary kidney, what is the most effective method of screening for hyperfiltration nephropathy?
   a. Urinary dipstick test for protein
   b. 24-hour urinary protein measurement
   c. Iothalamate glomerular filtration measurement
   d. Serum creatinine measurement
   e. Renal biopsy
8. What is an important prerequisite for successful laparoscopic cryoablation of a renal tumor?
   a. Slow freezing
   b. Rapid thawing
   c. A single freeze-thaw cycle
   d. A double freeze-thaw cycle
   e. Freezing of tumor to a temperature of −10°C

9. What is the most accurate and preferred imaging modality for demonstrating the presence and extent of an inferior vena caval tumor thrombus?
   a. Abdominal ultrasonography
   b. Transesophageal ultrasonography
   c. CT
   d. MRI
   e. Contrast venacavography
10. In patients undergoing complete surgical excision of renal cell carcinomas, the lowest 5-year survival rate is associated with which factor?
    a. Perinephric fat involvement
    b. Microvascular renal invasion
    c. Subdiaphragmatic inferior vena caval involvement
    d. Intra-atrial tumor thrombus
    e. Lymph node involvement
11. A 45-year-old man has a 5-cm renal cell carcinoma in the upper pole of a solitary left kidney and a single 2-cm left lower lung metastasis. What is the best treatment?
    a. Initial immunotherapy, then partial nephrectomy
    b. Partial nephrectomy, then immunotherapy
    c. Staged partial nephrectomy and pulmonary lobectomy
    d. Simultaneous partial nephrectomy and pulmonary lobectomy
    e. Simultaneous radical nephrectomy and pulmonary lobectomy
12. What is the approximate overall objective response rate to IL-2 monotherapy in patients with metastatic renal cell carcinoma?
    a. 5%
    b. 10%
    c. 15%
    d. 20%
    e. 25%
13. Which treatment will yield the highest response rate in patients with metastatic renal cell carcinoma?
    a. IL-2
    b. IFN-α
    c. IL-2 and 5-fluorouracil
    d. IFN-α and dendritic cell
    e. IL-2 and IFN-α
14. Which of the following statements is true of a diagnosis of renal adenoma?
    a. It can be made primarily on the basis of histologic criteria.
    b. It can be rendered only if tumor size is less than 1.0 cm.
    c. It is commonly made at autopsy.
    d. It requires specific immunohistochemical staining.
    e. It can be confirmed by electron microscopy.
15. A healthy 62-year-old man is referred after renal biopsy of a 3.0-cm centrally located renal mass. The biopsy is interpreted as renal oncocytoma. The other kidney is normal, the serum creatinine level is 1.0 mg/dL, and there is no evidence of metastatic disease. What is the best next step?
    a. Observation with follow-up abdominal CT in 3 months
    b. Radical nephrectomy
    c. Laparoscopic exposure and renal cryoablative therapy
    d. Partial nephrectomy
    e. Observation with follow-up renal ultrasonography in 6 to 12 months
16. Tuberous sclerosis is similar to von Hippel-Lindau disorder in which of the following respects?
    a. Propensity toward development of seizure disorders
    b. Similarity of cutaneous lesions
    c. Common development of adrenal tumors
    d. Frequent involvement of cerebral cortex with vascular lesions
    e. Mode of genetic transmission
17. A 48-year-old woman with a history of seizure disorder presents with recurrent gross hematuria and left flank pain. Abdominal CT shows a large left perinephric hematoma associated with a 3.0-cm left renal angiomyolipoma. There are also multiple right renal angiomyolipomas ranging in size from 1.5 to 6.5 cm. What is the best management of the left renal lesion?
    a. Selective embolization
    b. Radical nephrectomy
    c. Observation
    d. Partial nephrectomy
    e. Laparoscopic exposure and renal cryoablative therapy
18. Which of the following statements is TRUE regarding multiloculated cystic nephromas?
    a. They are complex cystic lesions that are typically classified as Bosniak II.
    b. They are malignant 2% to 5% of the time.
    c. They are more common in men than in women.
    d. They are characterized by bimodal age distribution.
    e. They are readily differentiated from renal cell carcinoma on the basis of appropriate imaging studies.
19. Which environmental factor is most generally accepted as a risk factor for renal cell carcinoma?
    a. Radiation therapy
    b. Antihypertensive medications
    c. Tobacco use
    d. Diuretics
    e. High-fat diet
20. Which of the following manifestations is restricted to certain families with the von Hippel-Lindau disorder?
    a. Renal cell carcinoma
    b. Pancreatic cysts or tumors
    c. Epididymal tumors
    d. Pheochromocytoma
    e. Inner ear tumors
21. Renal cell carcinoma develops in what percentage of patients with the von Hippel-Lindau disorder?
    a. 0% to 20%
    b. 21% to 40%
    c. 41% to 60%
    d. 61% to 80%
    e. 81% to 100%
22. What is the most common cause of death in patients with the von Hippel-Lindau syndrome?
    a. Renal failure
    b. Cerebellar hemangioblastoma
    c. Unrelated medical disease
    d. Pheochromocytoma
    e. Renal cell carcinoma
23. The von Hippel-Lindau syndrome tumor suppressor protein regulates the expression of which of the following mediators of biologic aggressiveness for renal cell carcinoma?
    a. Basic fibroblast growth factor
    b. Vascular endothelial cell growth factor
    c. Epidermal growth factor receptor
    d. Hepatocyte growth factor (scatter factor)
    e. P-glycoprotein (multiple drug resistance efflux protein)
24. What do the hereditary papillary renal cell carcinoma syndrome and von Hippel-Lindau syndrome have in common?
    a. Mode of genetic transmission
    b. Chromosome 3 abnormalities
    c. Propensity toward tumor formation in multiple organ systems
    d. Inactivation of a tumor suppressor gene
    e. Nearly complete penetrance

25. Mutation of the *MET* proto-oncogene in hereditary papillary renal cell carcinoma leads to:
    a. increased expression of hepatocyte growth factor.
    b. increased sensitivity to vascular endothelial growth factor.
    c. inactivation of a tumor suppressor gene that regulates cellular proliferation.
    d. constitutive activation of the receptor for hepatocyte growth factor.
    e. increased expression of vascular endothelial growth factor.
26. P-glycoprotein is a transmembrane protein that is involved in:
    a. immunotolerance.
    b. resistance to high-dose IL-2 therapy.
    c. resistance to cisplatin therapy.
    d. resistance to radiation therapy.
    e. efflux of large hydrophobic compounds, including many cytotoxic drugs.
27. What is the primary proangiogenic molecule in conventional renal cell carcinoma?
    a. Basic fibroblast growth factor
    b. Hepatocyte growth factor
    c. Vascular endothelial cell growth factor
    d. Epidermal growth factor
    e. Transforming growth factor-β
28. Which of the following is most likely to demonstrate an infiltrative growth pattern?
    a. Sarcomatoid variants of conventional renal cell carcinoma
    b. High-grade granular variants of conventional renal cell carcinoma
    c. High-grade papillary renal cell carcinoma
    d. Moderate-grade transitional cell carcinoma of the renal pelvis
    e. Classic variant of chromophobe cell carcinoma
29. What is the most common mutation identified in sporadic conventional renal cell carcinoma?
    a. Activation of the *MET* proto-oncogene
    b. Activation of the von Hippel-Lindau tumor suppressor gene
    c. Inactivation of the von Hippel-Lindau tumor suppressor gene
    d. Inactivation of *TP53*
    e. Inactivation of genes on chromosome 9
30. Which of the following cytogenetic abnormalities is among those commonly associated with papillary renal cell carcinoma?
    a. Trisomy of chromosome 7
    b. Trisomy of the Y chromosome
    c. Loss of chromosome 17
    d. Loss of all or parts of chromosome 3
    e. Loss of chromosome 7
31. What percentage of renal cell carcinomas are chromophobe cell carcinomas?
    a. 0% to 2%
    b. 4% to 5%
    c. 8% to 10%
    d. 12% to 15%
    e. 18% to 25%
32. Most renal medullary cell carcinomas are:
    a. found in patients with sickle cell disease.
    b. diagnosed in the fifth decade of life.
    c. responsive to high-dose chemotherapy.
    d. genetically and histologically similar to papillary renal cell carcinoma.
    e. metastatic at the time of diagnosis.
33. Which paraneoplastic syndrome associated with renal cell carcinoma can often be managed or palliated medically?
    a. Polycythemia
    b. Stauffer's syndrome
    c. Neuropathy
    d. Hypercalcemia
    e. Cachexia
34. A healthy 64-year-old man is found to have a 6.0-cm solid, heterogeneous mass in the hilum of the right kidney. CT of the abdomen and pelvis shows interaortocaval lymph nodes enlarged to 2.5 cm. A chest radiograph and a bone scan have negative results, and the contralateral kidney is normal. The serum creatinine level is 1.0 mg/dL. What is the next best step?
    a. Right radical nephrectomy and regional or extended lymph node dissection
    b. Abdominal exploration, sampling of the enlarged lymph nodes, and possible radical nephrectomy pending frozen section analysis
    c. CT-guided percutaneous biopsy of the lymph nodes
    d. CT-guided percutaneous biopsy of the tumor mass
    e. Systemic immunotherapy followed by radical nephrectomy
35. Which of the following patients would be a good candidate for percutaneous biopsy of a renal mass?
    a. A 42-year-old man with a 2.5-cm Bosniak III complex renal cyst
    b. An 88-year-old man with angina and a 1.7-cm solid, enhancing renal mass
    c. A 32-year-old woman with bilateral solid, enhancing renal masses ranging in size from 1.5 to 4.0 cm
    d. A 48-year-old woman with a 3.5-cm solid, enhancing renal mass with fat density present
    e. A 38-year-old woman with a fever, urinary tract infection, and 3.5-cm solid, enhancing renal mass
36. A 67-year-old man undergoes radical nephrectomy and inferior vena caval thrombectomy (level 2 thrombus). The primary tumor is otherwise confined to the kidney, and the lymph nodes are not involved. What is the approximate 5-year cancer-free survival rate?
    a. 15% to 25%
    b. 26% to 35%
    c. 36% to 45%
    d. 46% to 60%
    e. 61% to 75%
37. Important prognostic factors for patients with metastatic renal cell carcinoma include which of the following?
    a. Age
    b. Performance status
    c. Degree of renal function
    d. Primary tumor size
    e. Tumor grade
38. What is the most common form of renal sarcoma?
    a. Liposarcoma
    b. Rhabdosarcoma
    c. Fibrosarcoma
    d. Leiomyosarcoma
    e. Angiosarcoma

39. Which of the following statements about renal lymphoma is TRUE?
    a. Five to 10 percent of all lymphomas involving the kidney are primary tumors.
    b. Radiographic patterns manifested by renal lymphoma are diverse and can be difficult to differentiate from renal cell carcinoma.
    c. Percutaneous biopsy is rarely indicated if renal lymphoma is suspected.
    d. Renal failure associated with renal lymphoma is most often due to extensive parenchymal replacement by the malignancy.
    e. Most common pattern of renal involvement is from direct extension from adjacent retroperitoneal lymph nodes.
40. Which of the following would be considered diagnostic for renal angiomyolipoma?
    a. Hyperechoic pattern on ultrasonography
    b. Enhancement of > 30 Hounsfield units (HU) on CT
    c. Small area with HU of < −20 units on nonenhanced CT
    d. Aneurismal changes on renal arteriogram
    e. Positive signal on T2-weighted images of MRI
41. The main limitation of renal mass biopsy is:
    a. risk of needle tract seeding.
    b. difficulty differentiating the eosinophilic variants of RCC from renal oncocytoma.
    c. risk of pneumothorax.
    d. risk of hemorrhage.
    e. high incidence of inadequate tissue sampling.
42. Which of the following features is typically required for the diagnosis of renal adenoma in a clinical setting?
    a. Tumor size < 3 cm
    b. Low to moderate grade
    c. Papillary architecture
    d. Nonconventional histology
    e. Noncentral location
43. Which of the following tumors is most likely to be a malignant RCC?
    a. 2.5-cm hyperechoic complex cyst, with no enhancement with IV contrast
    b. 6.0-cm complex cyst with 4 thin septa
    c. 5.0-cm cyst with thin, curvilinear calcification
    d. 11-cm cyst with water density and homogeneous nature
    e. 3.0-cm tumor with fat associated with calcification
44. A reliable finding for the diagnosis of renal oncocytoma is:
    a. trisomy of chromosomes 7 and 17.
    b. central, stellate scar on CT.
    c. spokewheel pattern on renal angiography.
    d. multiple mitochondria on electron microscopy.
    e. hypervascular pattern.
45. A distinctive finding for renal angiomyolipoma is:
    a. positive staining for vimentin.
    b. unique cytokeratin expression pattern.
    c. positive staining for HMB-45.
    d. multiple microsomes on electron microscopy.
    e. occasional aneuploidy.
46. A distinctive finding for mixed epithelial cell tumor of the kidney is:
    a. positive staining for estrogen or progesterone receptors.
    b. bimodal age distribution.
    c. peak incidence in 6th decade of life.
    d. presentation as a poorly enhancing solid renal mass, often herniating into the collecting system.
    e. male predominance.
47. A common and pathogenic cytogenetic finding in children with RCC is:
    a. VHL mutation
    b. *MET* oncogene mutation
    c. *TP53* mutation
    d. *TFE3* mutations
    e. *PTEN* mutations
48. The central mediator for loss of VHL protein function is:
    a. HIF-1α.
    b. PEGF.
    c. Erythropoietin.
    d. VEGF.
    e. TP53.
49. Most tumors at various sites in the VHL syndrome share which of the following characteristics?
    a. Malignant behavior
    b. Hypervascularity
    c. Rapid growth rate
    d. High nuclear grade
    e. Symptomatic presentation
50. One major difference between hereditary papillary RCC syndrome and VHL is:
    a. Pattern of genetic inheritance
    b. Age at onset
    c. Sex distribution
    d. Incidence of metastasis
    e. Incidence of associated tumors in nonrenal organ systems
51. Which syndrome is most likely to exhibit aggressive behavior of RCC?
    a. VHL
    b. Hereditary papillary RCC syndrome
    c. Hereditary leiomyomatosis and RCC syndrome
    d. Birt-Hogg-Dubé syndrome
    e. Familial oncocytosis
52. Spontaneous pneumothorax is occasionally observed in which of the following?
    a. VHL
    b. Hereditary papillary RCC syndrome
    c. Hereditary leiomyomatosis and RCC syndrome
    d. Birt-Hogg-Dubé syndrome
    e. Familial oncocytosis
53. Chromophobe RCC is thought to be partly related to:
    a. oncocytoma.
    b. type 2 papillary RCC.
    c. granular RCC.
    d. mesoblastic nephroma.
    e. mixed epithelial stromal tumor of the kidney.
54. A diagnostic finding for collecting duct carcinoma is:
    a. central location and infiltrative growth pattern
    b. aggressive clinical course
    c. *TP53* mutation
    d. positive staining for *Ulex europeus* lectin
    e. sensitivity to chemotherapy
55. Sarcomatoid differentiation is most commonly observed with which histologic subtypes of RCC:
    a. conventional and chromophilic.
    b. chromophilic and chromophobe.
    c. conventional and collecting duct.
    d. conventional and chromophobe.
    e. chromophobe and collecting duct.

56. Which of the following factors has greatest utility for predicting bone metastasis from RCC?

   a. Tumor size
   b. Tumor grade
   c. Performance status
   d. Elevated alkaline phosphatase
   e. Invasion of the perinephric fat

57. The main utility of PET scan for the evaluation of patients with RCC is?

   a. Correlation with response to therapy
   b. Correlation with histologic subtype to help guide therapy
   c. High sensitivity
   d. High specificity
   e. High negative predictive power

58. Which of the following has correlated with better survival for conventional RCC?

   a. Increased expression of CA-9
   b. Increased TP53 staining
   c. Bone metastasis compared with other sites
   d. Thrombocytopenia
   e. Male sex

59. The prognosis for a 3-cm tumor infiltrating the renal sinus fat is:

   a. similar to a pT1bN0 tumor.
   b. similar to a pT2N0 tumor.
   c. similar to a pT3a tumor with invasion of the perinephric fat laterally.
   d. worse than a pT3a tumor with invasion of the perinephric fat laterally.
   e. similar to a pT3a tumor with ipsilateral adrenal involvement.

60. The most powerful prognosticator for RCC is:

   a. tumor stage.
   b. tumor grade.
   c. performance status.
   d. histologic subtype.
   e. integrated analysis.

61. Risk of local recurrence is highest in which of the following situations?

   a. pT3b tumor after radical nephrectomy and IVC thrombectomy
   b. VHL patient after partial nephrectomy with wedge resection of a single tumor
   c. Multifocal papillary RCC after partial nephrectomy with 3 wedge resections
   d. A 3.5-cm tumor after cryoablation
   e. A 2.5-cm centrally located tumor after radiofrequency ablation

62. The most useful prognostic factors for renal sarcoma are:

   a. tumor size and grade.
   b. tumor stage and grade.
   c. histologic subtype and stage.
   d. tumor stage and ploidy status.
   e. margin status and grade.

63. Which of the following renal tumors has the best prognosis?

   a. Sarcoma
   b. Carcinoid
   c. Adult Wilms' tumor
   d. PNET
   e. Small cell carcinoma

64. Which cytokine produces the highest durable complete regression rate in patients with metastatic RCC?

   a. IFN-α
   b. IFN-α + IL-2
   c. IL-2
   d. IL-12
   e. IFN-γ

65. Which of the following metastatic RCC tumors is most likely to benefit from cytokine therapy?

   a. Papillary carcinoma
   b. Clear cell carcinoma
   c. Medullary carcinoma
   d. Collecting duct carcinoma
   e. Chromophobe carcinoma

66. A 46-year-old man presents to your office with several recent episodes of gross hematuria. He has an unremarkable medical history and is otherwise well. Physical examination reveals a 3-cm right supraclavicular lymph node. A contrast-enhanced CT scan reveals an 8-cm right renal mass and multiple pulmonary nodules in both lung bases. A lymph node biopsy demonstrates metastatic clear cell carcinoma. Which of the following should be considered?

   a. Therapy with IL-2 + IFN-α
   b. Symptomatic care
   c. Right renal artery embolization
   d. Cytoreductive nephrectomy
   e. Medroxyprogesterone therapy

67. Randomized trials have demonstrated increased time to progression in patients with refractory metastatic clear cell carcinoma after treatment with which of the following agents?

   a. IL-2
   b. Sorafenib
   c. IFN-α
   d. SU011248
   e. IFN-α + vinblastine

68. Standard postoperative adjuvant therapy for patients at high risk of recurrence after nephrectomy includes which of the following?

   a. IL-2
   b. Sorafenib
   c. Autologous tumor vaccine
   d. Observation
   e. IFN-α

69. A 58-year-old woman had a nephrectomy 6 years previously for a grade 2 clear-cell carcinoma. She was incidentally found to have three left-sided pulmonary nodules (two < 1.0 cm, other 2.5 cm). A physical examination is normal, as are all blood chemistries. CT of the brain, lungs, abdomen, and pelvis show three pulmonary nodules with no associated hilar or mediastinal adenopathy, and a bone scan is normal. Which of the following should be considered?

   a. Therapy with high dose IL-2
   b. Biopsy of a pulmonary nodule
   c. Mediastinoscopy followed by resection of the pulmonary nodules
   d. Observation
   e. IFN-α therapy

70. Agents targeting which of the following signaling pathways in clear cell cancers have significant antitumor effects in patients with metastatic disease?

    a. EGF/EGFR
    b. TP53
    c. VEGF/PDGF
    d. TGF-α
    e. All of the above

71. The rationale for cytoreductive nephrectomy followed by immunotherapy with cytokines in patients with synchronous metastatic RCC includes all of the following EXCEPT:

    a. removal of tumor burden.
    b. removal of source of tumor-associated immunosuppressive factors.
    c. reversal of acquired immune dysfunction.
    d. improved tolerance to cytokine therapy.
    e. improved T-lymphocyte function.

ANSWERS

1. **c. CT with and without contrast enhancement.** A dedicated (thin-slice) renal CT scan remains the single most important radiographic image for delineating the nature of a renal mass. In general, any renal mass that enhances with administration of intravenous contrast material on CT should be considered a renal cell carcinoma until proved otherwise.

2. **b. Bosniak II cyst.** Category II lesions are minimally complicated cysts that are benign but have some radiologic findings that cause concern. Classic hyperdense renal cysts are small (<3 cm), round, and sharply marginated and do not enhance after administration of contrast material.

3. **d. Renal metastasis.** Fine-needle aspiration or biopsy is of limited value in the evaluation of renal masses. The major problem with this technique is the high incidence of falsely negative biopsies in patients with renal malignancy. The primary indication for needle aspiration or biopsy of a renal mass occurs when a renal abscess or infected cyst is suspected or when differentiating renal cell carcinoma from metastatic malignancy or renal lymphoma.

4. **a. No imaging studies.** Surveillance for recurrent malignancy after radical nephrectomy for renal cell carcinoma can be tailored according to the initial pathologic tumor stage. All patients should be evaluated with a medical history, physical examination, and selected blood studies on a yearly or twice-yearly basis. For patients with T1N0M0 tumors, routine postoperative radiographic imaging is not necessary because of the low risk of recurrent malignancy.

5. **d. postoperative tumor recurrence in remnant kidney.** The major disadvantage of nephron-sparing surgery is the risk of postoperative local tumor recurrence in the operated kidney, which has occurred in up to 10% of patients.

6. **d. Every 2 years.** Surveillance for recurrent malignancy after nephron-sparing surgery for renal cell carcinoma can be tailored according to the initial pathologic tumor stage. A yearly chest radiograph is recommended after nephron-sparing surgery for T2N0M0 tumors because the lung is the most common site of postoperative metastasis. Abdominal or retroperitoneal tumor recurrence is uncommon in the latter group, particularly early after nephron-sparing surgery, and these patients require only occasional follow-up abdominal CT; the authors recommend that this be done every 2 years.

7. **b. 24-hour urinary protein measurement.** Patients who undergo nephron-sparing surgery for renal cell carcinoma may be left with a relatively small amount of renal tissue. The patients are at risk for developing long-term renal functional impairment from hyperfiltration renal injury. Because proteinuria is the initial manifestation of the phenomenon, a 24-hour urinary protein measurement should be obtained yearly in patients with a solitary remnant kidney to screen for hyperfiltration nephropathy.

8. **d. A double freeze-thaw cycle.** Renal cryosurgery is an emerging nephron-sparing treatment option for renal cell carcinoma. The aim of cryosurgery is to ablate the same predetermined volume of tissue that would have been removed had a conventional surgical excision been performed. Established critical prerequisites for successful cryosurgery include rapid freezing, gradual thawing, and a repetition of the freeze-thaw cycle.

9. **d. MRI.** MRI is a noninvasive and accurate modality for demonstrating both the presence and the distal extent of vena caval involvement, and this has become the preferred diagnostic study at most centers.

10. **e. Lymph node involvement.** In most studies, the presence of lymph node or distant metastases has carried a dismal prognosis that is not appreciably altered by radical surgical extirpation.

11. **d. Simultaneous partial nephrectomy and pulmonary lobectomy.** The subset of patients with metastatic renal cell carcinoma and a solitary metastasis, estimated at between 1.6% and 3.2% of patients, may derive benefit from nephrectomy with resection of the metastatic lesion.

12. **c. 15%.** A recent review of clinical results in 1714 patients treated with IL-2 monotherapy indicated an overall objective response rate of 15.4%.

13. **e. IL-2 and IFN-α.** The single-agent activity of IFN-α and IL-2 in patients with metastatic renal cell carcinoma and preclinical observations indicating that these cytokines may have synergistic antitumor activity led to studies examining their combined use in the treatment of this disease. A recent review of 1411 patients receiving IFN-α and IL-2 in phase I or II trials indicated an overall objective response rate of 20.6%, with a 4.4% complete response rate.

14. **c. It is commonly made at autopsy.** Small, evidently benign, solid renal cortical lesions have been found at autopsy with an incidence of 7% to 23% and have been designated renal adenomas.

15. **b. Radical nephrectomy.** Most renal oncocytomas cannot be differentiated from malignant renal cell carcinomas on the basis of clinical or radiographic means. Given these uncertainties about a preoperative diagnosis, most authors have emphasized the need to treat these tumors aggressively with exploration and nephron-sparing surgery or radical nephrectomy dependent on the clinical circumstances.

16. **e. Mode of genetic transmission.** Approximately 20% of angiomyolipomas are found in patients with the tuberous sclerosis (TS) syndrome, an autosomal dominant disorder characterized by mental retardation, epilepsy, and adenoma sebaceum, a distinctive skin lesion.

17. **a. Selective embolization.** Most patients with acute or potentially life-threatening hemorrhage will require total nephrectomy if exploration is done, and if the patient has TS,

bilateral disease, preexisting renal insufficiency, or other medical or urologic disease that could affect renal function in the future, selective embolization should be considered. In such circumstances, selective embolization can temporize and in many cases will prove to be definitive treatment.

18. **d. They are characterized by bimodal age distribution.** Multiloculated cystic nephroma is a characteristic renal lesion with a bimodal age distribution and a benign clinical course.

19. **c. Tobacco use.** The only generally accepted environmental risk factor for renal cell carcinoma is tobacco use, although the relative associated risks have been modest, ranging from 1.4 to 2.3 when compared with controls. All forms of tobacco use have been implicated, with risk increasing with cumulative dose or pack-years.

20. **d. Pheochromocytoma.** The familial form of the common clear-cell variant of renal cell carcinoma is the von Hippel-Lindau syndrome. Major manifestations include the development of renal cell carcinoma, pheochromocytoma, retinal angiomas, and hemangioblastomas of the brain stem, cerebellum, or spinal cord. Penetrance for all of these traits is far from complete, and some, such as pheochromocytomas, tend to be clustered in certain families but not in others.

21. **c. 41% to 60%.** Renal cell carcinoma develops in about 50% of patients with von Hippel-Lindau syndrome and is distinctive for early age at onset, often developing in the third, fourth, or fifth decades of life, and for bilateral and multifocal involvement.

22. **e. Renal cell carcinoma.** With improved management of the central nervous system manifestations of the disease, renal cell carcinoma has now become the most common cause of mortality in patients with von Hippel-Lindau syndrome.

23. **b. Vascular endothelial cell growth factor.** Data suggest that inactivation or mutation of the von Hippel-Lindau gene leads to dysregulated expression of hypoxia inducible factor-1, an intracellular protein that plays an important role in regulating cellular responses to hypoxia, starvation, and other stresses. This, in turn, leads to a severalfold upregulation of the expression of vascular endothelial growth factor (VEGF), the primary proangiogenic growth factor in renal cell carcinoma, contributing to the pronounced neovascularity associated with this carcinoma.

24. **a. Mode of genetic transmission.** Studies of families with hereditary papillary renal cell carcinoma have demonstrated an autosomal dominant mode of transmission.

25. **d. constitutive activation of the receptor for hepatocyte growth factor.** Missense mutations of the *MET* proto-oncogene at 7q31 were found to segregate with the disease, implicating it as the relevant genetic locus. The protein product of this gene is the receptor tyrosine kinase for the hepatocyte growth factor (also known as scatter factor), which plays an important role in the regulation of the proliferation and differentiation of epithelial and endothelial cells in a wide variety of organs, including the kidney. Most of the mutations in hereditary papillary renal cell carcinoma have been found in the tyrosine kinase domain of *MET* and apparently lead to constitutive activation.

26. **e. efflux of large hydrophobic compounds, including many cytotoxic drugs.** P-glycoprotein is a 170-kDa transmembrane protein expressed by 80% to 90% of renal cell carcinomas that acts as an energy-dependent efflux pump for a wide variety of large hydrophobic compounds, including several cytotoxic drugs.

27. **c. Vascular endothelial cell growth factor.** The primary angiogenesis inducer in clear cell renal cell carcinoma appears to be VEGF, which is suppressed by the wild-type von Hippel-Lindau protein under normal conditions and is dramatically upregulated during tumor development.

28. **a. Sarcomatoid variants of conventional renal cell carcinoma.** Most renal cell carcinomas are round to ovoid and circumscribed by a pseudocapsule of compressed parenchyma and fibrous tissue rather than a true histologic capsule. Unlike upper tract transitional cell carcinomas, most renal cell carcinomas are not grossly infiltrative, with the notable exception of some sarcomatoid variants.

29. **c. Inactivation of the von Hippel-Lindau tumor suppressor gene.** Chromosome 3 alterations and von Hippel-Lindau mutations are common in conventional renal cell carcinoma, and mutation or inactivation of this gene has been found in 75% of sporadic cases.

30. **a. Trisomy of chromosome 7.** The cytogenetic abnormalities associated with papillary renal cell carcinoma are characteristic and include trisomy of chromosomes 7 and 17 and loss of the Y chromosome.

31. **b. 4% to 5%.** Chromophobe cell carcinoma is a distinctive histologic subtype of renal cell carcinoma that appears to be derived from the cortical portion of the collecting duct. It represents 4% to 5% of all renal cell carcinomas.

32. **e. metastatic at the time of diagnosis.** Renal medullary carcinoma is a relatively new histologic subtype of renal cell carcinoma that occurs almost exclusively in association with sickle cell trait. It is typically diagnosed in young African Americans, often in the third decade of life. Many cases are both locally advanced and metastatic at the time of diagnosis. Most patients have not responded to therapy and have succumbed to their disease in a few to several months.

33. **d. Hypercalcemia.** Hypercalcemia has been reported in up to 13% of patients with renal cell carcinoma and can be due to either paraneoplastic phenomena or osteolytic metastatic involvement of the bone. The production of parathyroid hormone-like peptides is the most common paraneoplastic etiology, although tumor-derived 1,25-dihydroxyvitamin D_3 and prostaglandins may contribute in a minority of cases. Medical management includes vigorous hydration followed by diuresis with furosemide and the selective use of bisphosphonates, corticosteroids, and/or calcitonin.

34. **a. Right radical nephrectomy and regional or extended lymph node dissection.** This approach will help to stage the nodes and remove the primary tumor. Nodes this size may still be inflammatory. Data also suggest that removal of the nodess may have a benefical effect in this setting. RCC is still primarily a disease treated with surgery.

35. **e. A 38-year-old woman with a fever, urinary tract infection, and a 3.5-cm solid, enhancing renal mass.** Patients with flank pain, a febrile urinary tract infection, and a renal mass may be considered for percutaneous biopsy or aspiration to establish a diagnosis of renal abscess rather than malignancy.

36. **d. 46% to 60%.** Venous involvement was once thought to be a poor prognostic finding for renal cell carcinoma, but more recent studies suggest that most patients with tumor thrombi can be salvaged with an aggressive surgical approach. These studies document 45% to 69% 5-year survival rates for patients with venous tumor thrombi as long as the tumor is otherwise confined to the kidney.

37. **b. Performance status.** Systemic metastases portend a particularly poor prognosis for renal cell carcinoma, with 1-year survival of less than 50%, 5-year survival of 5% to 30%, and 10-year survival of 0% to 5%. For patients with asynchronous metastases, the metastasis-free interval has proved to be a useful

prognosticator, as it reflects the tempo of disease progression. Other important prognostic factors for patients with systemic metastases include performance status, the number and sites of metastases, anemia, and hypercalcemia.

38. **d. Leiomyosarcoma.** Leiomyosarcoma is the most common histologic subtype of renal sarcoma, accounting for 50% to 60% of such tumors.

39. **b. Radiographic patterns manifested by renal lymphoma are diverse and can be difficult to differentiate from renal cell carcinoma.** CT is the radiographic modality of choice for the diagnosis of renal lymphoma and for monitoring the response to therapy. Renal lymphoma can present as multiple distinct renal masses; a solitary renal mass, which can be difficult to differentiate from renal cell carcinoma; diffuse renal infiltration; or direct invasion of the kidney from enlarged retroperitoneal nodes.

40. **c. Small area with HU of < −20 on nonenhanced CT.** The presence of even a small focus of fat, as evidenced by HU of < −20 on a nonenhanced CT scan, is diagnostic for AML. The findings described in a, b, and d are all suggestive but not diagnostic for renal AML.

41. **b. difficulty differentiating the eosinophilic variants of RCC from renal oncocytoma.** The main limitation of renal mass biopsy is difficulty differentiating renal oncocytoma, the most common benign renal mass, from eosinophilic variants of conventional, chromophilic, and chromophobic RCC on biopsy material. The risk of complications is low in the modern era with the use of smaller gauge needles, and needle tract seeding with RCC appears to be a rare event.

42. **c. Papillary architecture.** Most pathologists will not make the diagnosis of renal adenoma in a nonautopsy setting unless the lesion is low grade, small (<1.0 cm), and of papillary architecture.

43. **e. 3.0-cm tumor with fat associated with calcification.** Tumors with calcification associated with fat are uncommon but are almost always malignant RCC. In this setting the fat is thought to be a reactive process related to tumor necrosis. Calcification is virtually never seen in association with AML. The lesions described in a to c are Bosniak II renal cysts, with risk of malignancy of <10%. The lesion described in d is simple cyst and highly likely to be benign despite large size.

44. **d. multiple mitochondria on electron microscopy.** A distinctive and diagnostic feature of renal oncocytoma is the presence of multiple mitochondria on electron microscopy. Suggestive radiographic findings including central stellate scar on CT or spokewheel pattern on renal angiography have been described but can be seen with RCC and are absent in many oncocytomas. Trisomy of 7 and 17 is found in papillary RCC, not renal oncocytoma.

45. **c. positive staining for HMB-45.** AML will stain positive for HMB-45 in most cases, and this can be used to confirm the diagnosis in challenging cases. This antigen, which was originally found in association with melanoma, is expressed by most AMLs.

46. **a. positive staining for estrogen or progesterone receptors.** MESTK most commonly presents in perimenopausal woman, often with a history of hormonal therapy or hormonal manipulation. Most stain positive for estrogen or progesterone receptors. Most present as a complex renal cyst, typically Bosniak III.

47. **d. *TFE3* mutation.** Mutations or translocations involving the *TFE3* site are common in children with RCC.

48. **a. HIF-1α.** Inactivation of the VHL protein or loss of its function allows HIF-1α to accumulate, leading to a variety of downstream events, including upregulation of VEGF, erythropoietin, and PEGF. HIF-1α is the primary mediator of these events.

49. **b. Hypervascularity.** Tumors in the VHL syndrome include adrenal pheochromocytoma, retinal angiomas, cerebellar and brain stem hemangioblastoma, RCC, and others. Most are relatively slow growing and asymptomatic if patients are evaluated and screened in a proactive manner. The common feature is that almost all are hypervascular.

50. **e. Incidence of associated tumors in nonrenal organ systems.** The incidence of nonrenal tumors is low in the familial papillary RCC syndrome in contrast to patients with VHL, who commonly develop tumors in the eyes, spinal cord, cerebellum, adrenal, inner ear, epididymis, and pancreas.

51. **c. Hereditary leiomyomatosis and RCC syndrome.** Malignant behavior is particularly common in the hereditary leiomyomatosis and RCC syndrome, and proactive and aggressive management is recommended.

52. **d. Birt-Hogg-Dubé syndrome.** Lung cysts and spontaneous pneumothoraces are well described and relatively common findings in the Birt-Hogg-Dubé syndrome.

53. **a. oncocytoma.** Both chromophobe RCC and renal oncocytoma are derived from the distal tubules, and both are commonly observed in the Birt-Hogg-Dubé syndrome. There are also some overlapping cytogenetic changes, all suggesting a potential relationship for these renal tumors.

54. **d. positive staining for *Ulex europeus* lectin.** *Ulex europeus* lectin is expressed by the normal collecting duct, and tumor staining suggests origin from this structure. Most collecting duct tumors are centrally located and exhibit infiltrative growth pattern and aggressive clinical course, but this is also true for poorly differentiated TCCs of the renal pelvis or centrally located sarcomatoid RCC.

55. **d. conventional and chromophobe.** Sarcomatoid differentiation is most commonly found in association with conventional and chromophobe RCC.

56. **c. Performance status.** Poor performance status (PS) can be used to segregate patients when deciding whether to obtain a bone scan for metastatic RCC. Shvarts and colleagues (2004) have shown that patients with good performance status (ECOG performance status = 0), no evidence of extraosseous metastases, and no bone pain were extremely low risk for bone metastasis and did not benefit from bone scanning. They recommended a bone scan for all other patients, and the incidence of bone metastasis in this group was > 15%.

57. **d. High specificity.** PET scan for RCC has been shown to have high specificity but suboptimal sensitivity for the evaluation of metastatic sites for RCC. Its main role at present is for troubleshooting in the evaluation of equivocal situations.

58. **a. Increased expression of CA-9.** Increased CA-9 expression, which is associated with loss of function of the VHL protein, is associated with better survival, suggesting that VHL-independent tumors may have increased pathogenesis. Increased *TP53* staining correlates with mutation of the gene, because the mutated protein has a prolonged half life in the cell. Bone metastasis has been controversial, with some studies suggesting a worse prognosis but others refuting this.

59. **d. worse than a pT3a tumor with invasion of the perinephric fat laterally.** Invasion of the peri-sinus fat medially has been shown to be a poor prognostic sign. Medial invasion places the tumor in proximity to the venous system and likely increases the risk of metastatic dissemination. Ipsilateral adrenal involvement is even worse, and some have proposed

reclassifying these tumors as pT4 if due to direct local extension or M+ otherwise, consistent with a hematogenous route of dissemination.

60. **e. integrated analysis.** Integrated analysis of a variety of factors including tumor stage and grade, performance status, tumor necrosis, and histologic subtype has yielded the most powerful prognostication for RCC.

61. **b. VHL patient after partial nephrectomy with wedge resection of a single tumor.** Local recurrence after partial nephrectomy for VHL disease is common if patients are observed long term owing to multifocal tumor diathesis. These kidneys have been shown to harbor several hundred incipient tumors, and the risk of local recurrence is thus high during longitudinal follow-up.

62. **e. margin status and grade.** Margin status and tumor grade are the primary prognostic factors for sarcoma. Patients with high-grade disease are at risk for systemic metastasis, and those with low-grade disease are at risk for local recurrence.

63. **b. Carcinoid.** All of these tumor types have a relatively poor prognosis except for renal carcinoid, which tends to be associated with good outcomes in most patients.

64. **c. IL-2.** Recent randomized clinical trials utilizing high dose IL-2 and previous single-arm trials have demonstrated a 5% to 8% rate of durable complete regression in carefully selected patients.

65. **b. Clear cell carcinoma.** Recent retrospective analyses have demonstrated that patients with metastatic clear cell cancers are the most likely group to benefit from therapy with cytokines such as IL-2 or IFN-α.

66. **d. Cytoreductive nephrectomy.** Cytoreductive nephrectomy followed by cytokine treatment in patients with synchronous metastatic RCC is associated with modest improvement in overall patient survival.

67. **b. Sorafenib.** A recent blinded placebo-controlled, randomized trial in patients with cytokine-refractory metastatic clear cell cancer has demonstrated that oral administration of sorafenib (BAY 43-9006), a tyrosine kinase inhibitor of VEGFR and PDGFR, produces a doubling of TTP with very acceptable side effects.

68. **d. Observation.** All randomized postoperative adjuvant trials in patients with resected RCC have failed to demonstrate improvement in survival or TTP. The standard approach continues to be periodic observation.

69. **c. Mediastinoscopy followed by resection of the pulmonary nodules.** Patients with pulmonary nodules related to remote renal tumors may have prolonged survival following resection of the nodule(s). No evidence has demonstrated a routine role for use of preoperative or postoperative cytokine therapy.

70. **c. VEGF/PDGF.** Recent clinical trials with SU011248 and sorafenib demonstrate tumor response rates > 30% or significant decreases in the rate of tumor progression. Both of these drugs are orally administered tyrosine kinase inhibitors that are multifunctional and inhibit VEGFR and PDGFR.

71. **d. improved tolerance to cytokine therapy.** Studies suggest patients with synchronous metastatic RCC have a high frequency of acquired immune dysfunction involving T-lymphocytes. The abnormalities described include increased T-cell apoptosis, impaired proliferative responses, and tumor-associated immunosuppressive factors. Cytoreductive nephrectomy may improve these abnormalities. No data demonstrate better patient tolerance to cytokine therapy.

48

Urothelial Tumors of the Upper Urinary Tract

ROBERT C. FLANIGAN

QUESTIONS

1. The most consistent predictor of invasiveness in upper tract cancers is:
   a. deep tumor biopsy.
   b. tumor ploidy.
   c. CT estimation of depth of invasion.
   d. tumor grade.
   e. nuclear matrix protein level.
2. Nodal status in the TNM staging of upper tract tumors mandates a stage of N3 if:
   a. multiple lymph node metastases are found.
   b. lymphatic disease is unresectable.
   c. any lymph node is > 5 cm in dimension.
   d. lymph nodes show extranodal extension.
   e. more than 4 lymph nodes are involved.
3. Percutaneous resection of upper tract cancer is typically indicated for:
   a. tumors of the upper pole calyx.
   b. large-volume disease.
   c. squamous cell carcinoma.
   d. bilateral cancers.
   e. low grade cancers.
4. A risk factor associated with the diagnosis of upper tract urothelial cancer is:
   a. chronic inflammation.
   b. young age.
   c. alcohol consumption.
   d. chronic aspirin use.
   e. male sex.
5. The most important prognostic factor in predicting survival after treatment of an upper tract cancer is tumor:
   a. ploidy.
   b. grade.
   c. chromosome 9 deletion.
   d. TP53 status.
   e. stage.
6. The most typical radiologic presentation of upper tract tumors is:
   a. hydronephrosis.
   b. extravasation of contrast.
   c. renal contour abnormality.
   d. radiolucent filling defect.
   e. a single dilated calyx.
7. The risk of upper tract cancer developing after a diagnosis of bladder cancer is higher in patients with:
   a. ureteral reflux.
   b. low-stage cancer.
   c. a single bladder lesion.
   d. absence of CIS.
   e. squamous cell carcinoma.

ANSWERS

1. **d. tumor grade.** Given the significant difficulty with getting biopsies of the upper tract that are deep and representative enough to determine invasiveness of urinary tract tumors, grade has been shown in multiple studies to be the best predictor of invasion.
2. **c. any lymph node is > 5 cm in dimension.** In the current TNM staging system the number of lymph nodes involved with tumor is important in stages N1 and N2, but in N3 the only factor of importance is a metastatic node of more than 5 cm.
3. **b. large-volume disease.** Percutaneous, in contrast to ureteroscopic, resection is more efficient and reliable in patients in whom the lesion to be resected is large volume. This is purely a technical consideration.
4. **a. chronic inflammation.** Of the factors listed here, only a history of chronic infection has been associated with upper tract urothelial cancer. Other important factors include smoking, Balkan nephropathy, analgesic usage, and occupational factors.

5. **e. stage.** Despite the fact that grade, ploidy, and TP53 status are probably prognostic factors in upper tract cancers, tumor stage remains to date the most significant predictor.

6. **d. radiolucent filling defect.** Although upper tract tumors can present with the listed findings, a filling defect remains the most common presentation and illustrates the need for contrast usage in a radiologic test that identifies the entire urothelium, including the ureters.

7. **a. ureteral reflux.** High-stage cancer, multiple lesions, and CIS presence are risk factors predicting recurrence. Reflux after resection of a tumor overlying a ureteral orifice has been associated with a higher incidence of urinary tract recurrence in many studies.

49

Management of Urothelial Tumors of the Renal Pelvis and Ureter

ARTHUR I. SAGALOWSKY • THOMAS W. JARRETT

QUESTIONS

1. Which factor is the major determinant of the type of treatment for upper tract urothelial tumors?
   a. Size
   b. Number
   c. Stage and grade
   d. Contralateral renal function
   e. Level of lesion
2. What is (are) the most common symptom(s) of localized upper tract tumors?
   a. None, inasmuch as such tumors are incidental findings
   b. Flank pain
   c. Frequency
   d. Dysuria and hematuria
   e. Weight loss and fatigue
3. Which of the following statements is TRUE regarding flank pain in patients with upper tract tumors?
   a. It is rare.
   b. It signifies invasive disease.
   c. It indicates invasion into adjacent structures.
   d. It correlates with stage.
   e. None of the above.
4. In patients with upper tract tumors, what is the most common finding on imaging studies of the urinary tract?
   a. A mass
   b. A filling defect
   c. Hydronephrosis
   d. Nonfunction
   e. Delayed function
5. The majority of renal pelvis tumors are of which type?
   a. Papillary and invasive
   b. Papillary and noninvasive
   c. Sessile and invasive
   d. Sessile and noninvasive
   e. Mixed papillary and sessile
6. Most ureteral tumors are:
   a. sessile.
   b. high grade and noninvasive.
   c. low grade and noninvasive.
   d. medium grade and low stage.
   e. low grade and invasive.
7. What is the most common location of ureteral tumors?
   a. Ureteropelvic junction
   b. Proximal
   c. Middle
   d. Distal
   e. Intramural
8. After complete conservative treatment of a ureteral tumor (i.e., segmental excision or endoscopic ablation), which of the following is true?
   a. Ipsilateral recurrence is common.
   b. Recurrence is rare.
   c. Recurrence most likely is contralateral.
   d. Recurrence signifies incomplete initial therapy.
   e. Recurrence in the renal pelvis is common.
9. What is the major factor predisposing to recurrence of upper tract tumors?
   a. Incomplete therapy
   b. Multifocal field change
   c. Implantation during instrumentation
   d. Normal ureteral peristalsis
   e. Periureteral spread
10. What is the main factor for outcome in patients with multifocal upper tract tumors?
    a. Determined mainly by stage
    b. Poor without early radical surgery
    c. Poor independent of stage
    d. Determined by the rate of recurrence
    e. Poor regardless of the extent of surgery
11. What is the single most important determinant of outcome in the treatment of upper tract tumors?
    a. Grade
    b. Stage
    c. Early diagnosis
    d. Extent of surgery
    e. Size and focality of lesion
12. What is the earliest site of spread of proximal ureteral tumors?
    a. Lung and bone
    b. Liver and bone
    c. Lung and liver
    d. Pelvic nodes
    e. Para-aortic nodes

13. Reasons to consider nephron-sparing surgery for patients with upper tract tumors include all of the following EXCEPT which one?
    a. Bilateral tumors
    b. Unreliable follow-up
    c. Balkan nephropathy
    d. Diabetic nephropathy
    e. Solitary kidney
14. A 60-year-old diabetic man is diagnosed with a 4-cm, grade 2 to 3/3 transitional cell tumor of the renal pelvis. Serum creatinine value is 2.2 mg/dL. What is the recommended treatment?
    a. Ureteroscopic ablation
    b. Antegrade percutaneous resection
    c. Pyelotomy and tumor excision
    d. Radical nephroureterectomy
    e. Ileal ureteral substitution
15. A 57-year-old man with a grade 3, stage T2 tumor of the proximal ureter is undergoing radical nephroureterectomy. Correct management of the ureter requires which of the following?
    a. Ligation and division as far as exposure allows
    b. Ureterectomy in continuity with the kidney
    c. Ligation and division at the juxtavesical portion
    d. Complete distal ureterectomy with a bladder cuff
    e. Ligation and division 4 cm distal to the tumor and a negative margin on frozen section
16. Which statement is most correct regarding the role of lymphadenectomy in conjunction with radical nephroureterectomy?
    a. It should not be performed.
    b. It is helpful for determining prognosis.
    c. It is associated with a high morbidity rate.
    d. It decreases the occurrence of distant relapse.
    e. It is therapeutic.
17. A 46-year-old woman has a 2.5-cm stage Ta, grade 2 transitional cell tumor of the mid ureter. Initial treatment consists of "complete" ureteroscopic laser ablation of the tumor. Six months later there is a recurrent 2-cm tumor of the same stage and grade at the same location in the ureter. What should the next step in management be?
    a. Segmental ureterectomy
    b. Nephroureterectomy
    c. Ureteroscopic ablation
    d. Antegrade resection
    e. Antegrade resection followed by instillation of mitomycin
18. A 38-year-old man has a brief episode of gross hematuria. His initial evaluation included the following, all of which results were normal: bladder wash cytology, intravenous urography, cystoscopy, bladder biopsy, urethral biopsy, and bilateral retrograde pyelography. The upper tract cytologic result is positive for the right and negative for the left. What is the next step in management?
    a. Repeat upper tract cytology in 6 months
    b. Ureteropyeloscopy
    c. Right nephroureterectomy
    d. Intravesical bacille Calmette-Guérin (BCG)
    e. Right nephrostomy and infusion of BCG
19. After radical nephroureterectomy for a stage T3 transitional cell carcinoma (TCC) of the renal pelvis, which of the following is TRUE?
    a. Local relapse is the main limitation to survival.
    b. Adjuvant radiation decreases local relapse.
    c. Adjuvant chemotherapy increases survival.
    d. Adjuvant radiation does not improve survival.
    e. Adjuvant radiation plus chemotherapy increases survival.
20. Which of the following statements is TRUE regarding metastatic TCC of the upper urinary tract?
    a. It is not chemosensitive.
    b. It responds to the same chemotherapy as that used for bladder cancer.
    c. It is uniquely sensitive to taxanes.
    d. It is uniquely sensitive to interleukin-2.
    e. It responds best to debulking surgery plus chemotherapy.
21. A 46-year-old man is diagnosed with a 2-cm grade 3 tumor of the left renal pelvis. He is otherwise healthy. Acceptable treatment options include which of the following?
    a. Ureteroscopic ablation of the tumor.
    b. Percutaneous resection of the tumor followed by BCG therapy.
    c. Laparoscopic nephroureterectomy.
    d. Open nephroureterectomy.
    e. Both c and d.
22. After a total laparoscopic nephroureterectomy, surveillance of the ipsilateral ureteral orifice is done by which modality?
    a. Interval cystoscopy and ureteroscopy of the stump
    b. Cystoscopy with retrograde pyelography
    c. Cystoscopy and urine cytology
    d. Radiographic imaging with CT
    e. No specific surveillance of the distal ureter required
23. When endoscopic treatment of TCC of the upper urinary tract is used, ureteroscopy is generally preferred for which type of tumors?
    a. Small papillary tumors of the renal pelvis or ureter
    b. Large-volume tumors of the renal pelvis
    c. Small papillary tumors in the upper tracts of patients with previous urinary diversion
    d. Large bulky tumors of the lower pole of the kidney
    e. Large parenchymal invasive tumors of the renal pelvis
24. Which of the following is NOT a distinct advantage of the ureteroscopic approach?
    a. Decreased morbidity rate when compared with percutaneous renal surgery
    b. Maintenance of a closed system without exposure of nonurothelial surfaces to tumor cells
    c. Higher risk of tumor implantation outside the urinary tract
    d. Ease of access to the entire urinary tract without extensive dilatation of the ureteral orifice
    e. Usually can be done on an outpatient basis
25. A 60-year-old man who had undergone prior urinary diversion and a right nephroureterectomy is diagnosed with a grade 1 tumor of the lower pole collecting system of his solitary kidney. What is the optimal approach for this patient?
    a. Ureteroscopy with laser therapy of the lower pole tumor
    b. Nephroureterectomy
    c. Open lower pole partial nephrectomy
    d. Placement of a nephrostomy tube and BCG therapy
    e. Percutaneous access and resection of the lower pole tumor

26. Which of the following statements regarding adjuvant therapy for upper tract TCC is the most accurate?
    a. Adjuvant therapy with BCG has shown a definite advantage with regard to survival and tumor recurrence rates.
    b. Adjuvant therapy with mitomycin has shown a definite improvement with regard to survival and tumor recurrence rates.
    c. Although many studies have shown responses to instillation therapy, no significant improvement in survival or recurrence rate has been demonstrated.
    d. The most common complication of instillation therapy is systemic absorption of the agent.
    e. Granulomatous disease of the kidney is rare after upper tract BCG therapy.
27. An otherwise healthy 50-year-old man presents with a grade 1 tumor of the intramural ureter. The endoscopic approach or approaches that are acceptable options are which of the following?
    a. Ureteroscopic treatment.
    b. Transurethral resection of the ureteral orifice and distal ureter.
    c. Percutaneous antegrade ureteroscopy.
    d. Placement of a ureteral stent and BCG therapy.
    e. Both a and b.
28. Which of the following statements is NOT true regarding follow-up after treatment of upper urinary tract TCC?
    a. Patients undergoing conservative (organ-sparing) therapy need interval endoscopy of the ipsilateral urinary tract for tumor recurrence.
    b. Follow-up should be identical for all patients regardless of tumor stage or grade.
    c. Efficient and cost-effective follow-up should be based on tumor grade and stage.
    d. Cross-sectional imaging with CT or MRI is necessary with high-grade and high-stage tumors to assess for local recurrence and metastatic spread.
    e. All patients need interval evaluation of the contralateral urinary tract to assess for bilateral disease.
29. A 67-year-old patient with a solitary kidney has a large tumor of the renal pelvis. His urinary cytologic result is negative, and CT shows no evidence of invasive disease. What is the best course of action?
    a. Radical nephroureterectomy and hemodialysis
    b. Single-stage percutaneous access and resection of the entire tumor
    c. Single-stage ureteroscopic treatment of the entire tumor
    d. Endoscopic evaluation and biopsy with continued endoscopic therapy only if the pathologic evaluation shows a low potential for tumor progression
    e. Laparoscopic nephroureterectomy and hemodialysis
30. All of the following statements regarding the percutaneous approach to upper tract TCCs are true EXCEPT which one?
    a. The nephrostomy tract can be maintained for immediate postoperative surveillance nephroscopy.
    b. Tumor seeding of the nephrostomy tract is a common complication.
    c. Adjuvant therapy with BCG can be given through the established nephrostomy.
    d. The larger endoscopes used for percutaneous removal of TCC allow for tumor staging as well as grading.
    e. Percutaneous tumor resection has a higher morbidity rate when compared with a ureteroscopic approach.

ANSWERS

1. **c. Stage and grade.** Treatment may be based primarily on the risk the tumor poses and the efficacy of specific treatment rather than on other considerations.
2. **d. Dysuria and hematuria.** The common symptoms of localized disease (hematuria and dysuria) and advanced upper tract tumors (weight loss, fatigue, anemia, and bone pain) are similar in type and frequency to those of bladder cancer.
3. **e. None of the above.** Flank pain caused by obstruction by tumor or clot is more prevalent in upper tract tumors, being reported in 10% to 40% of cases. Flank pain in patients with upper tract tumors does not correlate with either locally advanced tumor stage or worse prognosis, as is the case with bladder cancer.
4. **b. A filling defect.** A filling defect is the most common finding on imaging studies.
5. **a. Papillary and invasive.** Approximately 85% of renal pelvis tumors are papillary; the remainder are sessile. In contrast to the majority of bladder tumors' being noninvasive, 50% to 60% of renal pelvis tumors are invasive.
6. **c. low grade and noninvasive.** Although invasion is still more common among ureteral tumors than among bladder tumors, 55% to 75% of ureteral tumors are low grade and low stage.
7. **d. Distal.** Ureteral tumors occur in the distal, middle, or proximal segment in 70%, 25%, and 5% of cases, respectively.
8. **a. Ipsilateral recurrence is common.** After conservative treatment, ipsilateral upper tract tumor recurrence is common in a proximal to distal direction and is seen in 33% to 55% of cases.
9. **b. Multifocal field change.** The high rate of ipsilateral recurrence is due in part to a multifocal field change.
10. **a. Determined mainly by stage.** Tumor multifocality per se does not lessen patient survival independent of stage.
11. **b. Stage.** The single most important determinant of outcome is tumor stage.
12. **e. Para-aortic nodes.** Renal pelvis and upper ureteral tumors spread initially to para-aortic and paracaval nodes, whereas distal ureteral tumors spread to pelvic nodes.
13. **b. Unreliable follow-up.** Reasons to consider nephron sparing include the presence of a tumor in a solitary kidney, synchronous bilateral tumors, or a predisposition to form multiple recurrences, as in endemic Balkan nephropathy.
14. **d. Radical nephroureterectomy.** Radical nephroureterectomy with excision of a bladder cuff is recommended for large, high-grade, invasive tumors of the renal pelvis and proximal ureter.

15. **d. Complete distal ureterectomy with a bladder cuff.** The role of complete distal ureterectomy with excision of a bladder cuff in radical nephroureterectomy for upper tract tumors is well established. The risk of tumor recurrence in a remaining ureteral stump is 30% to 75%.
16. **b. It is helpful for determining prognosis.** The rationale for continuing regional lymphadenectomy is that it adds little time or morbidity to the surgery, is important for prognosis, and may occasionally have therapeutic value.
17. **a. Segmental ureterectomy.** Segmental ureterectomy and ureteroureterostomy are indicated for noninvasive grade 1 and 2 tumors of the proximal ureter or midureter that are too large for complete endoscopic ablation and for grade 3 or invasive tumors when nephron sparing for preservation of renal function is a factor. Repeated endoscopic ablation of the tumor is not categorically incorrect. However, the rapid and large tumor recurrence is a matter of concern and favors segmental ureterectomy.
18. **b. Ureteropyeloscopy.** Occasionally, one is faced with a patient who has an isolated positive cytologic result from the upper urinary tract. By definition, the patient should have negative results from intravenous urography and retrograde pyelography, cystoscopy, and biopsy from the bladder and urethra. Ureteropyeloscopy is indicated in such cases, because the yield for direct visualization of small lesions is superior to that of retrograde pyelography.
19. **d. Adjuvant radiation does not improve survival.** In one series of patients with tumor stages of T2, T3, or N+, all patients with local relapse also had distant relapse, leading the authors of the report to conclude that adjuvant radiation is not beneficial. Another retrospective review of patients with stage T3 disease with or without adjuvant radiation found that radical nephroureterectomy alone provides a high rate of local control. Adjuvant radiation for high-stage disease does not decrease local relapse or protect against a high rate of distant failure.
20. **b. It responds to the same chemotherapy as that used for bladder cancer.** The systemic chemotherapy regimens offered for treatment of patients with metastatic urothelial tumors of the upper urinary tract are the same as those used for transitional cell carcinoma of the bladder.
21. **e. Both c and d.** Percutaneous management is acceptable in patients with low-grade (grade 1) disease regardless of the status of the contralateral kidney. Patients with grade 3 disease do poorly regardless of the modality chosen but should probably undergo nephroureterectomy to maximize cancer therapy (provided that they are medically fit). Radical nephroureterectomy with excision of a bladder cuff is recommended for large, high-grade invasive tumors of the renal pelvis and proximal ureter. Nephroureterectomy can be performed either completely laparoscopically or assisted with an open incision in the lower abdomen. The indications for laparoscopic nephroureterectomy are the same as those for open nephroureterectomy.
22. **e. No specific surveillance of the distal ureter required.** No surveillance is needed because the ureter has been removed in identical manner to the open surgical counterpart.
23. **a. Small papillary tumors of the renal pelvis or ureter.** The ureteroscopic approach to tumors is generally favored for ureteral and smaller renal tumors. Tumors of the upper urinary tract can be approached in a retrograde or antegrade manner. The approach chosen depends largely on the tumor location and size. In general, a retrograde ureteroscopic approach is used for low-volume ureteral and renal tumors. An antegrade percutaneous approach is preferred for larger tumors of the upper ureter or kidney, or those that cannot be adequately manipulated in a retrograde approach because of location (i.e., lower pole calyx) or previous urinary diversion.
24. **c. Higher risk of tumor implantation outside the urinary tract.** The advantages of a ureteroscopic approach are lower morbidity than the percutaneous and open surgical counterparts and the maintenance of a closed system. With a closed system, nonurothelial surfaces are not exposed to the possibility of tumor seeding.
25. **e. Percutaneous access and resection of the lower pole tumor.** A percutaneous approach may avoid the limitations of flexible ureteroscopy, especially when working in complicated calyceal systems or areas that are difficult to access such as the lower pole calyx or the upper urinary tract of patients with urinary diversion.
26. **c. Although many studies have shown responses to instillation therapy, no significant improvement in survival or recurrence rate has been demonstrated.** Many studies have described small retrospective uncontrolled series of patients undergoing therapy with thiotepa, mitomycin, and BCG. Although the cumulative experience appears encouraging, no individual study has shown statistical improvement with relation to survival and recurrence rates.
27. **e. Both a and b.** When a tumor protrudes from the ureteral orifice, complete ureteroscopic ablation of the tumor or aggressive transurethral resection of the entire most distal ureter can be performed with acceptable results.
28. **b. Follow-up should be identical for all patients regardless of tumor stage or grade.** All patients should be assessed at 3-month intervals the first year after they are rendered tumor-free by endoscopic or open surgical approaches. If an organ-sparing approach is chosen, the ipsilateral urinary tract must be assessed as well as the remainder of the urinary tract. The frequency and duration of the follow-up depend largely on the grade and stage of the lesion but are usually every 6 months for several years and then annually. Metastatic restaging is required in all patients at significant risk for disease progression to local or distant sites. This group includes those with high-grade and/or high-stage disease, who should be assessed by use of cross-sectional imaging, chest radiography, liver function tests, and selective use of bone scanning.
29. **d. Endoscopic evaluation and biopsy with continued endoscopic therapy only if the pathologic evaluation shows a low potential for tumor progression.** Endoscopic management is completed only after the pathologic evaluation shows that the patient is an acceptable candidate for continued minimally invasive endoscopic management. If the tumor is high grade or invasive, the patient should proceed to nephroureterectomy and dialysis, provided that he or she is medically fit.
30. **b. Tumor seeding of the nephrostomy tract is a common complication.** A major concern of the percutaneous approach is potential seeding of nonurothelial surfaces with tumor cells. Although there have been several reported cases of nephrostomy tract infiltration with high-grade tumors, there were no reported occurrences in the three largest series. Tract seeding is a possibility but appears to be an uncommon event.

50

Open Surgery of the Kidney

ANDREW C. NOVICK

QUESTIONS

1. What is the maximum period of unprotected warm ischemia that can be tolerated with no permanent loss of renal function?
   a. 10 minutes
   b. 20 minutes
   c. 30 minutes
   d. 45 minutes
   e. 60 minutes
2. What is the single most effective and commonly employed method of protecting the kidney from warm ischemic damage?
   a. Mannitol
   b. Inosine
   c. Calcium channel blockers
   d. Surface hypothermia
   e. Perfusion hypothermia
3. Renal ischemia is most damaging to which of the following parts of the nephron?
   a. Proximal tubule
   b. Descending limb of Henle's loop
   c. Ascending limb of Henle's loop
   d. Distal tubule
   e. Renal medulla
4. Renal ischemic damage from temporary renal vascular occlusion during surgery can be minimized by which of the following?
   a. Leaving the kidney covered with ice slush for 10 minutes before beginning the renal operation
   b. Occlusion of both the renal artery and the renal vein
   c. Intermittent unclamping and reclamping of the renal artery
   d. Intermittent unclamping and reclamping of the renal artery and vein
   e. Adjunctive intra-arterial injection of mannitol
5. The thoracoabdominal approach for radical nephrectomy is most advantageous in which of the following settings?
   a. Large upper pole left renal tumor
   b. Large upper pole right renal tumor
   c. Large central (hilar) renal tumor
   d. Renal tumor with extensive lymphadenopathy
   e. Renal tumor with level I vena caval thrombus
6. What is the most important surgical aspect of radical nephrectomy with respect to prevention of recurrent malignancy postoperatively?
   a. Removal of the ipsilateral adrenal gland
   b. Preliminary ligation of the renal artery
   c. Preliminary ligation of the renal artery and vein
   d. Removal of the kidney outside Gerota's fascia
   e. Performance of complete regional lymphadenectomy
7. The least common location of vena caval hemorrhage during retroperitoneal surgery is at the level of the:
   a. lumbar veins.
   b. right gonadal vein.
   c. left gonadal vein.
   d. renal veins.
   e. right adrenal vein.
8. What is the most effective adjunctive technique for radical nephrectomy and vena caval thrombectomy with an intra-atrial thrombus?
   a. Cardiopulmonary bypass
   b. Cardiopulmonary bypass with hypothermic circulatory arrest
   c. Caval-atrial shunt
   d. Pringle maneuver
   e. Thoracic aortic arch occlusion
9. What is the maximum period of deep hypothermic circulatory arrest that can safely be maintained for most patients?
   a. 20 minutes
   b. 30 minutes
   c. 40 minutes
   d. 60 minutes
   e. 80 minutes
10. Adjunctive venovenous bypass (caval-atrial shunt) is most helpful for removal of a vena caval thrombus in which setting?
    a. Tumor invasion of vena caval wall
    b. Intra-atrial vena caval thrombus
    c. Previous open heart surgery
    d. Subhepatic vena caval thrombus
    e. Intrahepatic vena caval thrombus

11. Acceptable criteria for performing partial nephrectomy with localized unilateral renal cell carcinoma and a normal opposite kidney include which of the following?
    a. Single tumor ≤ 6 cm, located in the upper or lower renal pole
    b. Single tumor ≤ 6 cm, any renal location
    c. Single tumor ≤ 4 cm, any renal location
    d. Up to two tumors ≤ 4 cm, any renal location
    e. Single tumor ≤ 4 cm, located in the upper or lower renal pole
12. The major disadvantage of partial nephrectomy compared with radical nephrectomy for localized low-stage renal cell carcinoma is the increased risk of which of the following?
    a. Perioperative renal failure
    b. Perioperative hemorrhage
    c. Postoperative distant metastasis
    d. Postoperative tumor recurrence in the remnant kidney
    e. Postoperative tumor recurrence in perirenal lymph nodes
13. What is the preferred surgical approach for performing partial nephrectomy for malignancy?
    a. Anterior subcostal transperitoneal
    b. Anterior subcostal extraperitoneal
    c. Flank extraperitoneal
    d. Posterior extraperitoneal
    e. Thoracoabdominal
14. What is the single most useful imaging study for surgical planning when performing partial nephrectomy for malignancy?
    a. Renal MRI with coronal and sagittal views
    b. Selective renal arteriography with oblique views
    c. Selective renal venography
    d. Intraoperative ultrasonography
    e. Three-dimensional renal CT
15. When a transverse partial resection of the upper half of the kidney is performed, particular care must be taken to avoid injury to which of the following renal arterial branches?
    a. Apical
    b. Anterior superior
    c. Posterior
    d. Anterior inferior
    e. Basilar
16. When partial nephrectomy for renal cell carcinoma is performed, what is the primary indication for surgical enucleation?
    a. Centrally located tumors
    b. von Hippel-Lindau disease
    c. Tuberous sclerosis
    d. Multiple sporadic tumors
    e. Papillary tumors
17. Which surgical technique is seldom necessary for performing partial nephrectomy for malignancy?
    a. Wedge resection of lateral tumor
    b. Transverse renal resection
    c. Segmental polar resection
    d. Wedge resection of central tumor
    e. Extracorporeal renal resection
18. What are the two most common complications after partial nephrectomy for renal malignancy?
    a. Hemorrhage and acute renal failure
    b. Hemorrhage and urinary fistula
    c. Urinary fistula and ureteral obstruction
    d. Urinary fistula and acute renal failure
    e. Ureteral obstruction and acute renal failure
19. After partial nephrectomy for pT2N0M0 renal cell carcinoma, it is necessary to perform surveillance abdominal CT how frequently?
    a. Never
    b. Every 6 months
    c. Every year
    d. Every 2 years
    e. Every 4 years
20. After partial nephrectomy in a solitary kidney, what is the most effective method of screening for hyperfiltration nephropathy?
    a. Urinary dipstick test for protein
    b. 24-hour urinary protein measurement
    c. Iothalamate glomerular filtration measurement
    d. Serum creatinine measurement
    e. Renal biopsy
21. Progressive renal artery obstruction with ischemic atrophy of the kidney is least likely to occur in which of the following?
    a. Atherosclerosis
    b. Medial fibroplasia
    c. Perimedial fibroplasia
    d. Intimal fibroplasia
    e. Intramural dissection
22. Surgical treatment of a renal artery aneurysm is indicated when it is:
    a. calcified and larger than 2 cm.
    b. noncalcified and larger than 2 cm.
    c. associated with medial fibroplasia.
    d. noncalcified, of any size.
    e. associated with atherosclerosis.
23. What is the primary indication for endovascular stenting of the renal artery?
    a. Intimal fibroplasia
    b. Ostial atherosclerosis
    c. Medial fibroplasia
    d. Nonostial atherosclerosis
    e. Renal artery aneurysm
24. Revascularization to preserve renal function for atherosclerotic renal artery disease is primarily indicated in which situation?
    a. 80% Right renal artery stenosis, normal left renal artery, serum creatinine level 4.0 mg/dL
    b. Bilateral 80% renal artery stenosis, serum creatinine level 2.1 mg/dL
    c. 50% Right renal artery stenosis, 80% left renal artery stenosis, serum creatinine level 1.6 mg/dL
    d. Bilateral 50% renal artery stenosis, serum creatinine level 4.5 mg/dl
    e. 80% Stenosis of the renal artery to a solitary kidney, serum creatinine level 4.5 mg/dL
25. What is the preferred technique for surgical revascularization of the right kidney in patients with severe atherosclerotic disease of both the abdominal aorta and the renal artery?
    a. Abdominal aortorenal bypass
    b. Thoracic aortorenal bypass
    c. Aortic endarterectomy
    d. Hepatorenal bypass
    e. Iliorenal bypass
26. What is the most common complication after direct end-to-end anastomosis of the right hepatic and renal arteries?
    a. Hepatic dysfunction
    b. Common bile duct obstruction
    c. Ischemic cholecystitis
    d. Renal artery thrombosis
    e. Portal vein injury

27. What is the preferred incision for performing thoracic aortorenal revascularization of the left kidney?
    a. Bilateral anterior subcostal transperitoneal
    b. Anterior midline transperitoneal
    c. Supracostal flank extraperitoneal
    d. Thoracoabdominal
    e. Anterior midline transperitoneal with median sternotomy
28. When aortorenal bypass is performed, what is the optimal bypass graft source for renal artery replacement?
    a. Polytetrafluoroethylene
    b. Gonadal vein
    c. Cephalic vein
    d. Saphenous vein
    e. Hypogastric artery
29. Operative mortality after surgical revascularization for atherosclerotic renal artery disease can be reduced by all of the following EXCEPT which one?
    a. Preoperative screening for coronary disease
    b. Preoperative screening for cerebrovascular disease
    c. Avoidance of an operation on a diseased abdominal aorta
    d. Bilateral simultaneous renal revascularization
    e. Perioperative pulmonary wedge pressure monitoring
30. Surgical unroofing of renal cysts in autosomal dominant polycystic kidney disease is most likely to result in which of the following?
    a. Improvement of hypertension
    b. Improvement of renal function
    c. Extended stabilization of renal function
    d. Relief of associated pain
    e. Reduced frequency of urinary infections
31. What is the preferred surgical approach for performing surgery on a horseshoe kidney?
    a. Dorsal lumbotomy
    b. Flank extraperitoneal
    c. Anterior midline transperitoneal
    d. Anterior subcostal extraperitoneal
    e. Thoracoabdominal
32. When performing a partial nephrectomy for renal cell carcinoma, the minimum necessary margin of normal parenchyma around the tumor is:
    a. 2 mm.
    b. 4 mm.
    c. 6 mm.
    d. 8 mm.
    e. 10 mm.
33. Compared with open partial nephrectomy, laparoscopic partial nephrectomy is associated with an increased risk of postoperative:
    a. infection.
    b. hemorrhage.
    c. ileus.
    d. ureteral obstruction.
    e. urinary fistula.
34. A 52-year-old man previously underwent a left partial nephrectomy through a flank incision. He is now undergoing a right partial nephrectomy through a flank incision. Flexion with elevation of the kidney rest during this second operation may result in:
    a. hypotension.
    b. respiratory distress.
    c. hemorrhage.
    d. ischemic left renal damage.
    e. ischemic right renal damage.

ANSWERS

1. **c. 30 minutes.** The extent of renal damage after normothermic arterial occlusion depends on the duration of the ischemic insult. Canine studies have shown that warm ischemic intervals of up to 30 minutes can be sustained with eventual full recovery of renal function. For periods of warm ischemia beyond 30 minutes, there is generally significant immediate functional loss and late recovery of renal function is either incomplete or absent.
2. **d. Surface hypothermia.** Local hypothermia is the most efficacious and commonly employed method for protecting the kidney from ischemic damage. Lowering renal temperature reduces energy-dependent metabolic activity of the cortical cells, with a resultant decrease in both the consumption of oxygen and the breakdown of ATP. In-situ renal hypothermia can be achieved with external surface cooling or perfusion of the kidney with a cold solution instilled into the renal artery. These two methods are equally effective; however, the latter is an invasive technique that requires direct entry into the renal artery. Surface cooling of the kidney is a simpler and more widely used method that has been accomplished by a variety of techniques, such as surrounding the kidney in a cold solution.
3. **a. Proximal tubule.** Histologically, renal ischemia is most damaging to the proximal tubular cells, which may show varying degrees of necrosis and regeneration, whereas the glomeruli and blood vessels are generally spared.
4. **a. Leaving the kidney covered with ice slush for 10 minutes before beginning the renal operation.** Most urologists currently prefer ice slush cooling for surface renal hypothermia because of its relative ease and simplicity. The mobilized kidney is surrounded with a rubber sheet on which sterile ice slush is placed to completely immerse the kidney. An important caveat with this method is to keep the entire kidney covered with ice for 10 to 15 minutes immediately after occluding the renal artery and before commencing the renal operation. This amount of time is needed to obtain core renal cooling to a temperature (approximately 20°C) that optimizes in situ renal preservation.
5. **b. Large upper pole right renal tumor.** The thoracoabdominal approach is desirable for performing radical nephrectomy in patients with large tumors involving the upper portion of the kidney. It is particularly advantageous on the right side, where the liver and its venous drainage into the upper vena cava can

limit exposure and impair vascular control as the tumor mass is being removed.

6. **d. Removal of the kidney outside Gerota's fascia.** Perhaps the most important aspect of radical nephrectomy is removal of the kidney outside Gerota's fascia because capsular invasion with perinephric fat involvement occurs in 25% of patients.

7. **c. left gonadal vein.** During performance of radical nephrectomy, intraoperative hemorrhage can occur from the inferior vena cava or its tributaries. Lumbar veins enter the posterolateral aspect of the vena cava at each vertebral level, and undue traction on the cava can result in their avulsion with troublesome bleeding. A second predictable bleeding site is the entry of the right gonadal vein into the anterolateral surface of the vena cava. A third predictable site of bleeding lies at the level of the renal veins, where large lumbar veins will often course posteriorly from the left renal vein just lateral to the aorta, or from the posterior aspect of the vena cava close to the entry of the right renal vein. A fourth predictable site of bleeding is at the level of the right adrenal vein, which enters the inferior vena cava.

8. **b. Cardiopulmonary bypass with hypothermic circulatory arrest.** In patients with renal cell carcinoma and an intrahepatic or suprahepatic inferior vena cava thrombus, the difficulty of surgical excision is significantly increased. Several different surgical maneuvers have been used to provide adequate exposure, prevent severe bleeding, and achieve complete tumor removal in this setting. At the Cleveland Clinic, we have preferred to employ cardiopulmonary bypass with deep hypothermic circulatory arrest for most patients with complex supradiaphragmatic tumor thrombi and for all patients with right atrial tumor thrombi. We initially reported a favorable experience with this approach in 43 patients, and a subsequent study has shown excellent long-term cancer-free survival after its use in patients with right atrial thrombi.

9. **c. 40 minutes.** When the patient is under deep hypothermic circulatory arrest, the entire interior lumen of the vena cava can be directly inspected to ensure that all fragments of thrombus are completely removed. Hypothermic circulatory arrest can be safely maintained for at least 40 minutes without incurring a cerebral ischemic event.

10. **e. Intrahepatic vena caval thrombus.** In patients with nonadherent supradiaphragmatic vena caval tumor thrombi that do not extend into the right atrium, venovenous bypass in the form of a caval-atrial shunt is a useful technique.

11. **c. Single tumor ≤ 4 cm, any renal location.** Studies have clarified the role of partial nephrectomy in patients with localized unilateral renal cell carcinoma and a normal contralateral kidney. These data indicate that radical nephrectomy and partial nephrectomy provide equally effective curative treatment for such patients who present with a single small (<4 cm), and clearly localized renal cell carcinoma.

12. **d. Postoperative tumor recurrence in the remnant kidney.** The major disadvantage of partial nephrectomy for renal cell carcinoma is the risk of postoperative local tumor recurrence in the operated kidney, which has been observed in 4% to 6% of patients. These local recurrences are most likely a manifestation of undetected microscopic multifocal renal cell carcinoma in the renal remnant.

13. **c. Flank extraperitoneal.** It is usually possible to perform partial nephrectomy for malignancy in situ by using an operative approach that optimizes exposure of the kidney and by combining meticulous surgical technique with an understanding of the renal vascular anatomy in relation to the tumor. We employ an extraperitoneal flank incision through the bed of the 11th or 12th rib for almost all of these operations; we occasionally use a thoracoabdominal incision for very large tumors involving the upper portion of the kidney. These incisions allow the surgeon to operate on the mobilized kidney almost at skin level and provide excellent exposure of the peripheral renal vessels.

14. **e. Three-dimensional renal CT.** Three-dimensional volume-rendered CT is a new noninvasive imaging modality that can accurately depict the renal parenchymal and vascular anatomy in a format familiar to urologic surgeons. The data integrate essential information from arteriography, venography, excretory urography, and conventional two-dimensional CT into a single imaging modality, and this method obviates the need for more invasive imaging.

15. **c. Posterior.** When a transverse resection of the upper part of the kidney is performed, care must be taken to avoid injury to the posterior segmental renal arterial branch, which may also occasionally supply the basilar renal segment. Preoperative selective renal arteriography with oblique views is integral to identifying and preserving the posterior segmental artery at surgery and to thereby avoid devascularizing a major portion of the healthy remnant kidney.

16. **b. von Hippel-Lindau disease.** The technique of enucleation is currently employed only in occasional patients with von Hippel-Lindau disease and multiple low-stage encapsulated tumors involving both kidneys.

17. **e. Extracorporeal renal resection.** Although some urologic surgeons have found that almost all patients undergoing partial nephrectomy for renal cell carcinoma can be managed satisfactorily in situ, others have continued to recommend an extracorporeal approach for selected patients.

18. **d. Urinary fistula and acute renal failure.** A study has detailed the incidence and clinical outcome of technical or renal-related complications occurring after 259 partial nephrectomies for renal tumors at the Cleveland Clinic. The most common complications were urinary fistula formation and acute renal failure.

19. **d. Every 2 years.** Surveillance for recurrent malignancy after nephron-sparing surgery for renal cell carcinoma can be tailored according to the initial pathologic tumor stage. Abdominal or retroperitoneal tumor recurrence is uncommon in pT2 patients, particularly early after nephron-sparing surgery, and these patients require only occasional follow-up abdominal CT; the author recommends that this be done every 2 years in this category.

20. **b. 24-hour urinary protein measurement.** Patients with more than 50% reduction in overall renal mass are at greater risk for proteinuria, glomerulopathy, and progressive renal failure. Structural or functional renal damage in such cases is usually antedated by the appearance of proteinuria. Therefore, the follow-up of patients after partial nephrectomy in a solitary kidney should include a 24-hour urinary protein determination in addition to the usual renal function and tumor surveillance studies.

21. **b. Medial fibroplasia.** For patients with renovascular hypertension caused by fibrous dysplasia, candidacy for surgical intervention is guided by the specific pathologic process, as determined by angiographic findings, and its associated natural history. Medical management of medial fibroplasia is the initial approach because loss of renal function from progressive obstruction is uncommon, and intervention is reserved for those patients with difficult-to-control hypertension. Renal artery disease caused by intimal or perimedial fibroplasia is often associated with progressive obstruction, which can result in ischemic renal atrophy.

22. **b. noncalcified and larger than 2 cm.** Renal artery aneurysms may require repair when they result in significant hypertension or for prevention of rupture when they are larger than 2 cm and noncalcified.

23. **b. Ostial atherosclerosis.** Whereas percutaneous transluminal angioplasty is associated with a successful blood pressure result for nonostial atherosclerosis, the long-term success rate with ostial lesions is poor owing to a higher incidence of restenosis. The results with endovascular stenting for ostial lesions are better than those with percutaneous transluminal angioplasty.

24. **b. Bilateral 80% renal artery stenosis, serum creatinine level 2.1 mg/dL.** Knowledge of the natural history of atherosclerotic renal artery disease permits identification of patients at risk for ischemic nephropathy. Those at highest risk are patients with high-grade stenosis (>75%) involving the entire renal mass (bilateral disease or disease in a solitary kidney). Intervention in these patients is for the purpose of preservation of renal function.

25. **d. Hepatorenal bypass.** Hepatorenal bypass is the preferred vascular reconstructive technique for patients with a troublesome aorta who require right renal revascularization.

26. **c. Ischemic cholecystitis.** Despite the resulting total or segmental hepatic dearterialization in patients with direct end-to-end anastomosis of the right hepatic and renal arteries, postoperative liver function study results have remained normal. However, the gallbladder is more susceptible to ischemic damage and may undergo necrosis when its blood supply from the right hepatic artery is interrupted.

27. **d. Thoracoabdominal.** For left renal revascularization, a left thoracoabdominal incision is made below the 8th rib and extended medially across the midline. This incision provides excellent simultaneous exposure of the thoracic aorta and renal artery with no need for extensive abdominal visceral mobilization.

28. **e. Hypogastric artery.** Although a variety of surgical revascularization techniques are available for treating patients with renal artery disease, aortorenal bypass with a free graft of autogenous saphenous vein or hypogastric artery remains the preferred method in patients with a nondiseased abdominal aorta. An arterial autograft is theoretically advantageous.

29. **d. Bilateral simultaneous renal revascularization.** In recent years, several policies have been adopted to reduce operative mortality after surgical revascularization in patients with atherosclerotic renal artery disease. These include preliminary screening and correction of existing coronary or cerebrovascular occlusive disease, avoidance of bilateral simultaneous renal operations, and reliance on methods of revascularization that avoid operation on a badly diseased aorta.

30. **d. Relief of associated pain.** Multiple cyst punctures and unroofing of cysts (Rovsing's operation) do not appear to improve renal function or prevent further deterioration. However, this approach can provide long-term pain relief in symptomatic patients.

31. **d. Anterior subcostal extraperitoneal.** When surgery on a horseshoe kidney is performed, an anterior subcostal extraperitoneal approach is preferred. This provides good access to the isthmus as well as to the pelvis and ureter, which are rotated anteriorly.

32. **a. 2 mm.** Recent data have shown that, as long as a histologic tumor-free margin of resection is present, the width of the resection margin is of no biologic or prognostic significance.

33. **b. hemorrhage.** Recent data have shown that there is an increased risk of intraoperative and postoperative renal hemorrhage with laparoscopic partial nephrectomy, compared with open partial nephrectomy. There is no significant difference in the incidence of other general or urologic complications.

34. **e. ischemic right renal damage.** Renal dysfunction may be associated with staged bilateral renal operations through the flank. Specifically, when performing the second renal operation, flexion with elevation of the kidney rest may cause ischemic damage to the previously operated contralateral kidney, which has become fixed in place due to postoperative scarring. In such cases, the second flank operation should be performed without elevating the kidney rest. Alternatively, an anterior surgical approach may be elected for the second operation.

51

Laparoscopic Surgery of the Kidney

JAY T. BISHOFF • LOUIS R. KAVOUSSI

QUESTIONS

1. Contraindications to laparoscopic kidney surgery include all of the following EXCEPT which one?
   a. Severe cardiopulmonary disease
   b. Uncorrected coagulopathy
   c. Prior extensive abdominal surgery
   d. Peritonitis
   e. Untreated infection
2. Laparoscopic radical nephrectomy through a transperitoneal approach compared with the retroperitoneal approach results in all of the following EXCEPT which one?
   a. Similar operative times
   b. Comparable hospital stay
   c. Equivalent postoperative narcotic requirements
   d. A slower return to oral intake
   e. Quicker ligation of artery
3. Simple nephrectomy is indicated in the treatment of all of the following renal diseases EXCEPT which one?
   a. Renovascular hypertension
   b. Symptomatic acquired renal cystic disease
   c. Nephrosclerosis
   d. Symptomatic autosomal dominant polycystic disease (ADPKD)
   e. Indeterminate enhancing renal mass
4. During a laparoscopic simple nephrectomy, dissection of the ureter:
   a. is performed after dissection of the upper pole and the renal hilum.
   b. is avoided since the ureter is fragile and may tear.
   c. is performed early in the procedure and the ureter divided soon after recognition.
   d. assists in the identification and dissection of renal artery and vein.
   e. is avoided in order to prevent bleeding from the gonadal vessels.
5. Safe dissection of the renal hilum is accomplished by all of the following maneuvers EXCEPT which one?
   a. Elevation of the lower pole of the kidney
   b. Identification of the psoas muscle and tendon
   c. Medial retraction of large and small bowel
   d. Layer by layer dissection of renal hilum
   e. Traction on the gonadal vein
6. Acceptable means of extracting the kidney specimen, after laparoscopic radical nephrectomy, includes use of all of the following EXCEPT which one?
   a. Entrapment device
   b. Extraction through hand assist device with wound protector
   c. Direct removal through extended incision
   d. Entrapment in LapSac
   e. Morcellation in LapSac
7. Laparoscopic renal biopsy is not indicated in which of the following cases?
   a. Uncontrolled hypertension
   b. Failed percutaneous biopsy
   c. Anticoagulation
   d. Morbid obesity
   e. Solitary kidney
8. What is the most common complication after laparoscopic renal biopsy?
   a. Inadequate tissue sample
   b. Infection
   c. Pneumonia
   d. Hemorrhage
   e. Flank pain
9. Which of the following statements concerning the laparoscopic treatment and evaluation of symptomatic and indeterminate renal cysts is accurate?
   a. It is contraindicated, because aspiration is effective and has a low complication rate.
   b. It allows rapid localization of intraparenchymal cysts.
   c. It is contraindicated in patients with autosomal dominant polycystic kidney disease.
   d. It allows biopsy and conversion to nephrectomy in case of malignancy.
   e. It is contraindicated because the collecting system may be entered during the procedure.
10. All of the following statements about laparoscopic cyst decortication for the treatment of symptomatic ADPKD are accurate EXCEPT which one?
    a. It is often necessary to unroof 100 cysts to relieve pain.
    b. The collecting system is prone to injury.
    c. The renal cysts are not close to the renal hilum.
    d. Nephrectomy may be necessary in renal failure.
    e. Laparoscopic ultrasound may be needed to identify cysts.

11. Symptomatic nephroptosis is a rare condition that:
    a. is most common in middle-aged, obese females.
    b. can be diagnosed by renal ultrasound.
    c. may be present when the kidney descends more than one vertebral body.
    d. is usually associated with irritable bowel and fibromyalgia.
    e. should be shown to cause obstruction of the kidney before repair.

12. Laparoscopic pyelolithotomy is indicated in all of the following cases EXCEPT which one?
    a. Failed extracorporeal shockwave lithotripsy (ESWL)
    b. Pelvic or otherwise ectopic kidney
    c. Failed attempt to fragment cystine stone
    d. Pregnancy with symptomatic ureteropelvic junction (UPJ) stone
    e. Failed ureteroscopic stone extraction

13. Which of the following statements is FALSE concerning the laparoscopic treatment of a symptomatic calyceal diverticulum with stones?
    a. Stones can be evacuated.
    b. Lining can be fulgurated.
    c. Fat can be inserted to prevent recurrence.
    d. Location can be readily identified by surface changes.
    e. Retroperitoneal or transperitoneal approach can be used.

14. In the treatment of urologic malignancy, port site seeding has been most frequently described in which condition?
    a. Renal cell carcinoma
    b. Prostate cancer
    c. Testicular cancer
    d. Transitional cell carcinoma
    e. Penile cancer

15. Steps to prevent port site seeding include all of the following EXCEPT which one?
    a. Minimizing direct handling of specimen
    b. Avoiding morcellation in LapSac
    c. Performing wide en bloc resection
    d. Removing all tissue in protective sac
    e. Draping surgical field before extraction

16. Which of the following statements concerning the preoperative clinical staging of renal cell carcinoma with CT is TRUE?
    a. It is more likely to lead to overstaging than understaging of a renal mass.
    b. It allows accurate staging in 35% to 55% of patients.
    c. It is an inadequate study to allow morcellation of renal specimens.
    d. It should be correlated with renal angiography.
    e. It is inadequate to predict lymph node involvement.

17. Laparoscopic radical nephrectomy is contraindicated in which of the following cases?
    a. History of ipsilateral renal surgery including ESWL
    b. Perinephric inflammation in CT
    c. Prior transabdominal surgery
    d. Tumors invading into adrenal gland or perinephric tissues (T3a)
    e. Tumors grossly extending into the vena cava to the level of the liver

18. Which of the following statements concerning morcellation of a radical nephrectomy specimen is TRUE?
    a. It should not be performed, because pathologic staging information is lost.
    b. It should be performed after placement of the kidney in an Endocatch retrieval device.
    c. It is associated with a high incidence of trocar site seeding.
    d. It should be monitored intra-abdominally with the laparoscope.
    e. It should not be performed after placement of the kidney in a LapSac.

19. What is the approximate actuarial 5-year disease-free survival rate and overall survival rate for clinically localized renal cell carcinoma patients treated with laparoscopic radical nephrectomy?
    a. 95% to 100%
    b. 85% to 94%
    c. 75% to 84%
    d. 65% to 74%
    e. 55% to 64%

20. What is the reported approximate overall complication rate from laparoscopic radical nephrectomy?
    a. 40% to 45%
    b. 30% to 35%
    c. 20% to 25%
    d. 10% to 15%
    e. 0% to 5%

21. All of the following are true about hand-assisted laparoscopic nephrectomy EXCEPT which one?
    a. It is used for large T2 radical nephrectomy specimens.
    b. It allows compression with the hand for partial nephrectomy.
    c. It is contraindicated in ADPKD.
    d. It allows dissection of the distal ureter.
    e. It allows complex reconstruction if required.

22. Which of the following is an advantage of hand-assisted nephrectomy over laparoscopic nephrectomy? Ability to
    a. elevate the lower pole of the kidney
    b. remove the specimen intact
    c. separate the adrenal from the upper pole of the kidney
    d. perform bilateral procedures
    e. rapidly control bleeding with direct pressure

23. The approximate incidence of hernia formation at the hand-assisted site has been reported to be:
    a. <1%.
    b. 2%.
    c. 4%.
    d. 6%.
    e. >6%.

24. After laparoscopic partial nephrectomy with ureteral irrigation cooling, renal hilar vessel control, wide excision of a 3-cm mid-pole tumor, closure of the collecting system, placement of oxidized cellulose bolster, closure of renal parenchyma, and ischemic time of 41 minutes, a patient is asymptomatic. A CT obtained on postoperative day 21 shows gas in the area of the nephron-sparing surgery site. The most common cause of the air in this particular case is:
    a. postoperative hematoma.
    b. postoperative urinoma from collecting system injury.
    c. abscess in the area of resection.
    d. oxidized cellulose used in reconstruction.
    e. necrotic renal parenchyma.

25. Laparoscopic partial nephrectomy mimics open partial nephrectomy in all of the following ways EXCEPT which one?
    a. Tissue is removed under direct vision.
    b. Margin status is determined at the time of surgery.
    c. Inspection of the surface allows identification and treatment of multifocal disease.
    d. Collecting system cannot be reconstructed to prevent urinoma formation.
    e. Arterial occlusion with hypothermia can be performed.
26. Laparoscopic partial nephrectomy is a recent advancement in the treatment of small T1 renal tumors. What is the reported approximate 3-year cancer specific survival rate?
    a. 95%
    b. 90%
    c. 85%
    d. 80%
    e. 75%
27. Laparoscopic cryosurgical ablation of renal tumors requires which of the following?
    a. Tumor tissue temperatures less than −20°C
    b. CT monitoring of the ice ball
    c. MRI monitoring of the ice ball
    d. Intraoperative ultrasound monitoring of the ice ball
    e. A double freeze cycle
28. Reported complications of laparoscopic cryosurgical ablation of renal tumors include all of the following EXCEPT which one?
    a. Tumor recurrence
    b. Urinary fistula formation
    c. Hemorrhage
    d. Small bowel obstruction
    e. Skin necrosis
29. Which of the following statements concerning radiofrequency ablation of renal tumors is TRUE?
    a. It can be reliably monitored using ultrasound and MRI.
    b. It requires tissue temperatures of > 45°C to induce tissue necrosis.
    c. It causes increased tissue temperatures indirectly through local ion vibration.
    d. It must be delivered with a temperature-based feedback system.
    e. It results in little temperature drop from the center of the probe to the periphery.
30. Approximately what percent of patients having traditional flank incisions report concern over body image alteration after open renal surgery?
    a. 5%
    b. 10%
    c. 20%
    d. 40%
    e. 60%
31. Common areas of postoperative bleeding after laparoscopic kidney surgery include all of the following EXCEPT which one?
    a. Adrenal gland
    b. Large bowel mesentery
    c. Gonadal vessels
    d. Psoas muscle
    e. Ureteral stump
32. Which of the following statements concerning bowel injuries during laparoscopic surgery is TRUE?
    a. They occur in 1/100 cases.
    b. They are usually the result of Veress needle placement.
    c. They most commonly involve the large bowel.
    d. They are the result of electrocautery in half of the cases.
    e. They are usually recognized at the time of surgery.
33. The presentation of unrecognized bowel injury most commonly involves all of the following signs or symptoms EXCEPT which one?
    a. Pain out of proportion at one trocar site
    b. Nausea
    c. Diarrhea
    d. Low-grade fever
    e. Elevated white blood cell count
34. Seventy percent of complications in laparoscopic nephrectomy have been reported to occur during the first how many cases?
    a. 5
    b. 10
    c. 20
    d. 30
    e. 40
35. Conversion from laparoscopic to open kidney surgery occurs most often during procedures performed for which indication?
    a. Malignancy
    b. Stones
    c. Obstruction
    d. Infection
    e. Renovascular hypertension
36. What is the most common cause for conversion from laparoscopic to open surgery?
    a. Failure to progress
    b. Inability to visualize the renal hilum
    c. Perinephric adhesions
    d. Difficulty finding the ureter
    e. Bleeding

ANSWERS

1. **c. Prior extensive abdominal surgery.** Prior abdominal surgery may alter the choice between transperitoneal or retroperitoneal approaches, patient positioning, and placement site of trocars, but it is not a contraindication to laparoscopic surgery.
2. **d. A slower return to oral intake.** In a randomized clinical trial between the transperitoneal and retroperitoneal laparoscopic approach to the kidney the two approaches were found to be similar in outcomes. However, the transperitoneal approach had a faster return to oral intake compared with the retroperitoneal group.
3. **e. Indeterminate enhancing renal mass.** Indications include renovascular hypertension, symptomatic acquired renal cystic disease in dialysis patients, nephrosclerosis, symptomatic patients with autosomal dominant polycystic disease, chronic pyelonephritis, reflux/obstructive nephropathy, multicystic dysplastic kidney, and post-kidney transplant hypertension.

4. **d. assists in the identification and dissection of the renal artery and vein.** Once identified, the ureter is elevated and followed proximally to the lower pole and hilum of the kidney. The ureter is not divided at this time, because it can be used to help elevate the kidney.
5. **e. Traction on the gonadal vein.** Traction on the gonadal vein will not always help with dissection of the renal hilum and on the right side excessive traction can tear the gonadal at the insertion on the vena cava. Elevation of the kidney at the lower pole places the hilar vessels on stretch which will help with dissection especially when the bowel has been retracted medially, allowing visualization of the hilum and vessels.
6. **c. Direct removal through extended incision.** Unsuspected carcinoma has been reported and can cause extraction site seeding. Tissue should not be extracted directly through a wound or trocar site.
7. **a. Uncontrolled hypertension.** Renal biopsy under direct vision is indicated in three primary categories: failed percutaneous needle biopsy, anatomic variations, and high risk of bleeding complication. Factors that may make a patient unsuitable for percutaneous biopsy include morbid obesity, multiple bilateral cysts, body habitus that makes localization impossible, and a solitary functioning kidney.
8. **d. Hemorrhage.** Hemorrhage is the most common major complication associated with laparoscopic renal biopsy.
9. **d. It allows biopsy and conversion to nephrectomy in case of malignancy.** The edge of the cyst and base if suspicious should be carefully inspected and biopsies performed using 5-mm laparoscopic biopsy forceps. If there is no evidence of malignancy, the parenchymal surface of the cyst wall can be fulgurated with electrocautery or the argon beam coagulator. Surgical cellulose (Surgicel, Johnson & Johnson, Arlington, TX) can be packed into the cyst base. If malignancy is noted, the patient should have a partial or radical nephrectomy, as indicated. Once the decortication is complete, careful inspection for hemostasis should be performed.
10. **c. The renal cysts are not close to the renal hilum.** Perihilar cysts can be difficult to visualize and can usually be identified with laparoscopic ultrasound because they can be in close proximity to the renal hilum, which is often distorted by renal cysts. Furthermore, ultrasound will help locate deeper cysts that may be causing pain and are not always readily seen on the surface of the kidney.
11. **e. should be shown to cause obstruction of the kidney before repair.** Either erect and supine intravenous urograms or renal scans documenting obstruction are the best diagnostic studies for nephroptosis. Descent of the symptomatic kidney by two vertebral bodies and obstruction or diminished flow to the symptomatic side should be documented before surgical repair.
12. **d. Pregnancy with a symptomatic UPJ stone.** Laparoscopy has been performed during pregnancy to treat malignancy, but in the pregnant patient other less invasive treatments would be recommended before laparoscopy. Individuals to be considered for this approach include those in whom extracorporeal shock wave lithotripsy, percutaneous, or ureteroscopic procedures have failed; patients with unusual anatomy such as a pelvic kidney; and patients with stones resistant to fragmentation such as those of cystine composition.
13. **d. Location is readily identified by surface changes.** Once the surface of the kidney is uncovered the exact location of the stone and diverticulum can be very difficult to find. The surgeon should plan ahead and have fluoroscopy available and have the patient on a table that allows fluoroscopy to locate the stone.
14. **d. Transitional cell carcinoma.** In the laparoscopic staging and treatment of transitional cell carcinoma there have been seven reports of port-site seeding and four reports of renal cell carcinoma.
15. **b. Avoiding morcellation in LapSac.** Morcellation of radical nephrectomy specimens in a LapSac has not been associated with an increased incidence of port-site seeding or metastatic recurrence of renal cell carcinoma.
16. **a. It is more likely to lead to overstaging than understaging of a renal mass.** One study concluded that clinical CT staging of low-stage renal tumors is reliable and tends to overstage rather than understage renal tumors.
17. **e. Tumors invading into adrenal gland to the level of the liver. (T3a).** Contraindications to laparoscopic radical nephrectomy include tumors with vena cava extension to the level of the liver.
18. **d. It should be monitored intra-abdominally with the laparoscope.** If the specimen is to be morcellated, a LapSac (Cook Urological, Spencer, IN) fabricated from a double layer of plastic and nondistensible nylon is used. This sac has been shown to be impermeable to bacteria and tumor cells even after use for morcellation.
19. **b. 85% to 94%.** The 5-year disease-free survival is 91%, and the overall 15-year survival is 94%.
20. **d. 10% to 15%.** Complications occurred in 15% of the laparoscopic patients and 24% of the open surgery patients.
21. **c. It is contraindicated in ADPKD.** ADPKD is not a contraindication to laparoscopy or hand-assisted nephrectomy. The large size and weight of the specimen in ADPKD patients can make laparoscopic surgery difficult and the hand can be useful for dissection and manipulation of the kidney.
22. **e. Rapidly control bleeding with direct pressure.** One of the greatest benefits of hand-assisted kidney surgery is the ability to rapidly control bleeding that would otherwise require conversion to open surgery or to permit conversion in a more controlled fashion.
23. **c. 4%.** Several series have shown the incidence of hernia formation to be approximately 4% and most appearing 3 months or greater from the time of surgery.
24. **d. oxidized cellulose used in reconstruction.** Oxidized cellulose (Surgicel, Johnson & Johnson) is often placed in the defect created after removal of the renal mass. In the early postoperative period this may appear as a gas-containing abscess, due to air in the gauze spaces, when no real infection is present. This appearance on CT has been reported as long as 30 days after surgery.
25. **d. Collecting system cannot be reconstructed to prevent urinoma formation.** An extension of laparoscopy in the treatment of small renal lesions has been the partial nephrectomy, which mimics the fundamentals of open surgery. Tissue is removed under direct vision with margin status being assessed intraoperatively. Direct vision and laparoscopic ultrasonography permit the laparoscopist to identify multifocal tumors, determine an adequate surgical margin, and maintain orientation with respect to the collecting system and renal hilum. If necessary, the collecting system can be resected with the surgical specimen to obtain adequate margins and then repaired and different techniques are now available to create cold ischemic conditions.
26. **a. 95%.** Allaf and associates have reported on their series of 48 patients treated with LNSS for T1 renal tumors less than 4 cm. The mean tumor size was 2.4 cm (range: 1.0 to 4 cm). This study has one of the longest follow-up periods to date at a mean follow-up of 38 months (range: 22 to 84 months) with

two recurrences. In a patient with VHL a new tumor was seen at the edge of the initial LNSS site 18 months after surgery and the second was in a patient who demonstrated a new tumor remote for the original surgical site 46 months after his first procedure.

27. **a. Tumor tissue temperatures less than −20°C.** Chosy and colleagues (1996) demonstrated that a renal tissue temperature less than −20°C was necessary to create tissue necrosis. Uchida and coworkers evaluated renal cancer cell lines in culture by phase microscopy 24 hours after subjecting them to 60 minutes of −5, −10, −20 and −30°C. About 95% of renal cancer cells survived after cooling for 60 minutes at temperature about −10°C but only 15% survived at a temperature of −20°C. Schmidlin and colleagues also found the threshold temperature for complete tissue ablation to be −16.1°C.

28. **e. Skin necrosis.** Potential complications of cryosurgery include urinary fistula formation, post-treatment hemorrhage, and injury to adjacent structures to include the collecting system, bowel, and liver. Given that even momentary contact of the active cryoprobe can lead to necrosis and fibrosis, disastrous results could soon follow. One study in a porcine model noted severe adhesions between cryoablated kidney and overlying bowel in nonretroperitonealized kidneys. There was no evidence of bowel injury or fistulas. Another study reported the complication of small bowel obstruction when the cryoprobe inadvertently contacted a loop of small bowel during porcine laparoscopic renal cryoablation. Certain reports of short-term local tumor recurrences mandate further investigation to predict cryotherapy's ultimate role in the treatment of renal tumors.

29. **c. It causes increased tissue temperatures indirectly through local ion vibration.** The probe carries an alternating current of high-frequency radio waves that causes the local ions to vibrate, and the resistance in the tissue creates heat to the point of desiccation (thermal coagulation).

30. **e. 60%.** Recently reports of patient concern over body image alteration after renal surgery have appeared in the literature. These studies show that flank incisions, as traditionally made for open surgery and some hand-assisted cases, result in significantly larger, postoperative, surface area and volume changes on the operated side compared with the noninvolved flank. Patients reported dissatisfaction with the body changes occurring in up to 60% of flank incisions.

31. **d. Psoas muscle.** Common areas of postoperative intra-abdominal bleeding include the adrenal gland, mesentery, gonadal vessels, and ureteral stump.

32. **d. They are the result of electrocautery in half of the cases.** One of the most devastating complications occurring as a result of laparoscopic surgery is that of unrecognized bowel injury. Because only 10% of the laparoscopic instrument is in the visual field, these injuries can occur out of the surgeon's field of view. The combined incidence of bowel injury in the literature is 1.3 per 1000 cases. Most injuries (69%) are not recognized at the time of surgery. Small bowel segments account for 58% of injuries, followed by colon (32%) and stomach (7%). Fifty percent of bowel injuries are caused by electrocautery, and 32% occur during Veress needle or trocar insertion.

33. **e. Elevated white blood cell count.** Patients with unrecognized bowel injury after laparoscopy typically present with persistent and increased trocar site pain at the site closest to the bowel injury. Later signs and symptoms include nausea, diarrhea, anorexia, low-grade fever, persistent bowel sounds, and a low or normal white blood cell count.

34. **c. 20 cases.** In fact, 70% of the complications occurred during the first 20 cases at each institution. A learning curve of approximately 20 laparoscopic nephrectomy cases is also supported by other reports.

35. **d. Infection.** The majority of patients who had conversion to open surgery had infectious causes of renal pathology as the leading indication for kidney removal.

36. **e. Bleeding.** Bleeding was the most common cause of open conversion, followed by inability to visualize the renal hilum for dissection.

52

Ablative Therapy of Renal Tumors

MICHAEL MARBERGER • JULIAN MAUERMANN

QUESTIONS

1. Renal tumors best suited for energy based ablation techniques are:
   a. multifocal benign tumors.
   b. perihilar tumors less than 3 cm in diameter.
   c. recurrent tumors after previous nephron-sparing nephrectomy for renal cell carcinoma.
   d. spherical tumors restricted to the lower pole of the kidney.
   e. unifocal exophytic peripheral tumors less than 3 cm in diameter.
2. Complete ablation of a renal tumor is most reliably documented by:
   a. negative follow-up biopsy.
   b. complete loss of enhancement on serial follow-up CT or MRI.
   c. loss of enhancement and progressive size reduction on serial follow-up CT or MRI.
   d. homogeneous hyperechogenicity and progressive shrinkage of the lesion at serial follow-up ultrasonography.
   e. absence of clinical signs of tumor progression.
3. Based on clinical data an adequate temperature for cell death of tumor cells during renal cryosurgery is:
   a. –4°C.
   b. 0°C maintained over 15 minutes.
   c. –40°C.
   d. –15°C.
   e. –180°C.
4. Intraoperative monitoring of an effective cryolesion can be achieved by:
   a. real-time ultrasound monitoring of the advancing ice ball, targeting extension 1 cm beyond the tumor margins.
   b. thermometry with thermocouples at the tumor margin targeting a temperature of –40°C.
   c. real-time MRI monitoring of the advancing ice ball, targeting an extension 1 cm beyond the tumor margins.
   d. real-time MRI thermometry, targeting tumor margin temperatures –40°C.
   e. all of the above.
5. The most common complication of renal cryoablation is:
   a. renal vein thrombosis.
   b. renal failure.
   c. urinary fistula.
   d. pancreatic injury.
   e. hemorrhage from the cryolesion after thawing and probe removal.
6. With radiofrequency ablation the developing lesion is reliably monitored by:
   a. intraoperative Doppler ultrasonography.
   b. intraoperative MRI.
   c. real-time tissue thermometry with thermosensors on the electrode.
   d. impedance tomography.
   e. none of the above.
7. The most important issue to increase the size of radiofrequency (RF) lesions is:
   a. using higher RF currents.
   b. applying RF currents faster to achieve better heating.
   c. clamping the hilar vessels.
   d. reducing impedance by improving current conductivity.
   e. using bipolar electrodes.
8. High-intensity focused ultrasound achieves targeted tissue ablation by:
   a. localized thermal and cavitation processes.
   b. mitotic toxicity.
   c. disrupting microperfusion.
   d. cavitation.
   e. initiating shock waves.
9. Which of the listed ablative technologies has been proven equally effective to partial nephrectomy in the treatment of a 4-cm renal tumor?
   a. Cryoablation
   b. Radiofrequency ablation
   c. High-intensity focused ultrasound ablation
   d. Microwave coagulation
   e. None of the above
10. The main theoretical advantage of "radiosurgical" ablation over thermal ablation techniques is:
    a. faster cell kill.
    b. technical simplicity.
    c. real-time imaging of the evolving lesion.
    d. not influenced by renal perfusion.
    e. less damage to surrounding tissues.

ANSWERS

1. **e. unifocal exophytic peripheral tumors less than 3 cm in diameter.** With small exophytic, peripheral tumors, radiographic complete remission was achieved in 50 of 51 (98%) masses treated in one series whereas this was only accomplished in 16 of 22 (72%) masses located centrally, although of comparable size.

2. **c. loss of enhancement and progressive size reduction on serial follow-up CT or MRI.** Complete loss of contrast enhancement on follow-up CT or MRI has been considered a sign of complete tissue destruction. Of note, viable residual tumor has been demonstrated in nonenhancing lesions after radiofrequency (RF) ablation. The lesion should also show progressive shrinking after therapy as proof of remission, although this may take months and is less pronounced after radiofrequency ablation.

3. **c. –40°C.** Using intraoperative ultrasound monitoring and targeting thermosensor-controlled margin temperatures of –40°C, double-freeze sequences were performed with one to three cryoprobes. With a median follow-up of 16 months only one patient had a biopsy-confirmed recurrent tumor. Postoperative morbidity was moderate, with 5 patients needing some intervention after cryoablation to control bleeding from the ablation site.

4. **e. all of the above.** In clinical practice real-time monitoring of the advancing ice ball with an extension 10 mm beyond the tumor margin has proven a reliable clinical endpoint. Thermometry with thermocouples at the tumor margin targeting a margin temperature of –40°C and on-line MRI monitoring have been reported comparable.

5. **e. hemorrhage from the cryolesion after thawing and probe removal.** Morbidity is low and mainly consists of probe site pain and paresthesia, and minor hemorrhage, with a higher incidence after percutaneous cryoablation.

6. **e. none of the above.** Because of the low intrinsic contrast between normal and ablated tissues and artifacts from gas bubble formation, real-time imaging of the developing thermal lesion with intraoperative ultrasonography, MRI, or CT has proven unreliable. In general, imaging techniques are only used to place the electrodes (see Fig. 52-2), and RF per se is monitored by measuring temperature and/or impedance changes, usually with feedback from thermosensors integrated at the end of the RF tines.

7. **d. reducing impedance by improving current conductivity.** The electrically conductive agent facilitates the delivery of energy from the electrode to surrounding tissue, rendering it a much larger, "virtual" electrode. Impedance remains lower, and larger volumes are ablated.

8. **a. localized thermal and cavitation processes.** As an ultrasound wave propagates through biologic tumors, it is progressively absorbed and energy is converted to heat. If the ultrasound beam is brought to a tight focus at a selected depth within the body, the high energy density produced in this region results in temperatures exceeding the threshold of protein denaturation. With higher site intensities, cavitation phenomena occur, which are more difficult to control.

9. **e. None of the above.** At present only renal masses smaller than 3 cm in diameter and located peripherally on the convexity of the kidney, in an easily accessible position, can be considered curable. Standard nephron-sparing procedures achieve excellent results in tumor of this size, so that energy ablative techniques only appear justified if a less-invasive approach is mandated because the patient has significant comorbidity.

10. **d. not influenced by renal perfusion.** In contrast to thermal ablation techniques, radiation destroys dividing tumor cells by mitosis-linked death. Being temperature independent, a loss of efficacy near larger vessels is avoided.

SECTION XIII

THE ADRENALS

53

The Adrenals

E. DARRACOTT VAUGHAN, JR. • JON D. BLUMENFELD

QUESTIONS

1. Why are the adrenals quite large at birth?
   a. A large fetal adrenal cortex
   b. A large fetal adrenal medulla
   c. An ectopic gonadal tissue
   d. A fusion to the kidney
   e. An adrenal hemorrhage
2. What is the best imaging study to help diagnose adrenal hemorrhage in the newborn?
   a. CT
   b. Ultrasonography
   c. MRI
   d. Intravenous pyelography (IVP)
   e. Adrenal venography
3. Uncommonly, the right adrenal vein is joined by what vein?
   a. The right renal vein
   b. The portal vein
   c. A hepatic vein
   d. The gastroepiploic
   e. A pancreatic vein
4. Ectopic adrenocortical tissue was found how often in female children?
   a. 0%
   b. 2%
   c. 3%
   d. 5%
   e. 10%
5. Why is it important to identify the left inferior phrenic vein during left adrenalectomy?
   a. To avoid renal vein injury
   b. To avoid diaphragmatic injury
   c. Because it is the main adrenal venous drainage
   d. As a guide to the aorta
   e. Because troublesome bleeding results if it is damaged
6. What are the principal androgens from the adrenal?
   a. Dehydroepiandrosterone (DHEA) and androstenedione
   b. DHEA and cortisol
   c. Androstenedione and cortisol
   d. DHEA and aldosterone
   e. Aldosterone and androstenedione
7. What stimulates the cascade leading to cortisol secretion?
   a. Enkephalins
   b. Melanocyte-stimulating hormone
   c. Antidiuretic hormone
   d. Corticotropin (ACTH)
   e. Angiotensin II
8. What is the major control mechanism for aldosterone secretion?
   a. ACTH
   b. Angiotensin II
   c. High potassium level
   d. High sodium level
   e. Low potassium level
9. What is the hallmark of the presence of adrenal tumors in women who present with hirsutism?
   a. Testosterone and DHEA
   b. DHEA and cortisol
   c. Testosterone and cortisol
   d. DHEA and aldosterone
   e. Testosterone and aldosterone
10. What is the primary metabolite of adrenal medullary catecholamines?
    a. Metanephrine
    b. Dopamine
    c. Norepinephrine
    d. Epinephrine
    e. Vanillylmandelic acid

11. What is the most common cause of Cushing's syndrome?
    a. Adrenal carcinoma
    b. Adrenal adenoma
    c. Cushing's disease
    d. Ectopic ACTH
    e. Ectopic corticotropin-releasing factor
12. What is one cause of Cushing's syndrome that is often forgotten?
    a. Exogenous steroid use
    b. Adrenal carcinoma
    c. Adrenal adenoma
    d. Ectopic ACTH
    e. Pituitary adenoma
13. What is a cause of pseudo-Cushing's syndrome?
    a. Obesity
    b. Hypertension
    c. Diabetes
    d. Depression
    e. Congestive heart failure
14. What is the most direct way to determine the presence of Cushing's syndrome?
    a. Plasma ACTH assay
    b. Three 24-hour urinary cortisol determinations
    c. Measurement of diurnal variations of cortisol
    d. Plasma cortisol assay
    e. High-dose dexamethasone administration
15. The common "metabolic syndrome" has been found in association with which adrenal disorder?
    a. Pheochromocytoma
    b. Primary hyperaldosteronism
    c. Adrenal cysts
    d. Adrenogenital syndrome
    e. Cushing's syndrome
16. What is a new test to identify increased cortisol secretion?
    a. Plasma cortisol
    b. Urinary 17-OH steroids
    c. Urinary 17-ketosteroids
    d. Late night salivary cortisol measurement
    e. The dexamethasone suppression test
17. What is the most common reason that dexamethasone suppression tests are now utilized?
    a. To identify adrenal carcinoma
    b. To identify pseudo-Cushing's syndrome
    c. To identify adrenal adenoma
    d. To identify pituitary adenoma
    e. To identify ectopic ACTH
18. Currently, what is the ideal way to determine whether a patient has ACTH-dependent or ACTH-independent hypercortisolism?
    a. 24-hour cortisone excretion assay
    b. Concurrent measurement of ACTH and cortisone
    c. Measurement of diurnal variation of plasma cortisone
    d. Low-dose dexamethasone test
    e. High-dose dexamethasone test
19. What is the most direct way to demonstrate pituitary hypersecretion of ACTH?
    a. Plasma ACTH assay
    b. Brain MRI
    c. Brain CT
    d. Plasma cortisol assay
    e. Petrosal venous sinus sampling of ACTH
20. What characterizes Nelson's syndrome?
    a. Ectopic ACTH secretion
    b. Ectopic corticotropin-releasing hormone secretion
    c. Multiple endocrine tumors
    d. Pituitary tumor after bilateral adrenalectomy
    e. Recurrent cortical tissue after bilateral adrenalectomy
21. What is the best test to identify an adrenal cause of Cushing's syndrome during pregnancy?
    a. IVP
    b. Sonography
    c. MRI
    d. CT
    e. Adrenal venography
22. What is the size that best delineates adrenal benign tumors from adrenal malignancies?
    a. 5 cm
    b. 6 cm
    c. 3 cm
    d. 7 cm
    e. 4 cm
23. Which adrenal pathologic diagnoses are characterized by signal intensity ratio on a T2-weighted MR image?
    a. Neural tumors, carcinoma, metastatic lesions
    b. Neural tumors, adenoma, myelolipoma
    c. Carcinoma, adenoma, incidentaloma
    d. Metastatic lesions, adenoma, carcinoma
    e. Neural tumors, adenoma, carcinoma
24. How many adrenalectomies would have to be performed to find one case of adrenal carcinoma if all adrenals greater than 1.5 cm were removed?
    a. 1,000
    b. 2,000
    c. 3,000
    d. 4,000
    e. 5,000
25. What is a useful pathologic method for delineating large benign adrenal adenomas from adrenal carcinoma?
    a. Electron microscopy
    b. Transforming growth factor-β assay
    c. Masson's trichrome stain
    d. Hematoxylin-eosin stain
    e. Flow cytometry
26. What is the 5-year survival rate for patients with adrenocortical carcinoma?
    a. 15%
    b. 25%
    c. 35%
    d. 45%
    e. 55%
27. What is the usual management of a simple adrenal cyst that is asymptomatic?
    a. Drainage
    b. Observation
    c. Open surgical removal
    d. Laparoscopic removal
    e. Drainage and sclerosis

28. What unrecognized adrenal disorder should be considered in a cancer patient who is critically ill?
    a. Addison's disease
    b. Conn's syndrome
    c. Cushing's disease
    d. Nelson's syndrome
    e. Carney's syndrome

29. What are the primary biochemical characteristics of primary hyperaldosteronism?
    a. Hypokalemia, high plasma renin activity (PRA), high aldosterone level
    b. Hypokalemia, low PRA, high aldosterone level
    c. Hyperkalemia, low PRA, high aldosterone level
    d. Hyperkalemia, high PRA, high aldosterone level
    e. Normokalemia, high PRA, high aldosterone level

30. What is the important control that must be utilized before ruling out hypokalemia in a patient with hyperaldosteronism?
    a. Low sodium diet
    b. Low potassium diet
    c. High potassium diet
    d. Normal sodium intake
    e. Low calcium diet

31. What is the response to a postural stimulation test in a patient with hyperaldosteronism caused by an adenoma?
    a. Rise in PRA, rise in aldosterone
    b. Rise in PRA, fall in aldosterone
    c. Fall in PRA, fall in aldosterone
    d. Fall in PRA, rise in aldosterone
    e. Stable PRA, rise in aldosterone

32. What is the best method for lateralizing aldosterone secretion in a patient with primary hyperaldosteronism?
    a. 19-Iodocholesterol scan
    b. Adrenal venography
    c. MRI
    d. Ultrasonography
    e. Adrenal vein sampling

33. In a patient with primary hyperaldosteronism resulting from a solitary adenoma, what preparation should be used to determine that the patient is ready for unilateral adrenalectomy?
    a. Blood pressure control and sodium repletion
    b. Sodium and potassium repletion
    c. Blood pressure control and potassium repletion
    d. Thiazide diuretic for blood pressure control
    e. Blood volume repletion

34. What is the appropriate treatment of the patient with primary hyperaldosteronism resulting from bilateral hyperplasia when there is no lateralization of aldosterone secretion?
    a. Spironolactone
    b. A β-adrenergic blocker
    c. An angiotensin-converting enzyme inhibitor
    d. Hydrochlorothiazide
    e. Phenoxybenzamine

35. What is the cure and improvement rate in patients with primary hyperaldosteronism resulting from an adrenal adenoma after adrenalectomy?
    a. 60%
    b. 70%
    c. 80%
    d. 90%
    e. 100%

36. What percentage of patients with pheochromocytoma presents without hypertension?
    a. 5%
    b. 10%
    c. 15%
    d. 20%
    e. 25%

37. What characterizes catechol-induced myocardiopathy?
    a. Low cardiac ejection fraction
    b. Hepatic dysfunction
    c. Irreversible cardiac disease
    d. Malignant hypertension
    e. Encephalopathy

38. In what groups are multiple pheochromocytomas or ectopic catecholamine-secreting paragangliomas found?
    a. Children, those with multiple endocrine adenoma (MEA), familial groups
    b. Children, those with MEA, women
    c. Children, those with MEA, elderly
    d. Those with MEA, women, elderly
    e. Familial groups, children, women

39. What radiologic test is of most value in localizing a pheochromocytoma in a patient with the biochemical characteristics of the disease?
    a. Angiography
    b. CT
    c. MRI
    d. Sonography
    e. IVP

40. What is the appropriate preoperative preparation for a patient with a pheochromocytoma
    a. β-Adrenergic blockade alone
    b. Hydrochlorothiazide
    c. Angiotensin-converting enzyme inhibitor
    d. α-Adrenergic blockade with phenoxybenzamine
    e. Spironolactone

41. What is the primary use of partial adrenalectomy?
    a. pheochromocytoma
    b. bilateral tumors
    c. adrenal adenoma
    d. adrenal carcinoma
    e. myelolipoma

42. What is the approach of choice for most adrenal tumors?
    a. Posterior
    b. Modified posterior
    c. Laparoscopic
    d. Transabdominal
    e. Thoracoabdominal

ANSWERS

1. **a. A large fetal adrenal cortex.** The adrenal weight at birth is quite large (5 to 10 g) because of the fetal adrenal cortex, which may play a major role in fetal embryogenesis and homeostasis.
2. **c. MRI.** Adrenal hemorrhage at the time of birth is a condition now readily diagnosed by MRI.
3. **c. A hepatic vein.** First observed with laparoscopic adrenal surgery, an unnamed branch from the liver may join the adrenal vein before entering the inferior vena cava.
4. **a. 0%.** While ectopic adrenocortical tissue was found in 2.7% of males at the time of groin dissection, none was found in females.
5. **e. Because troublesome bleeding results if it is damaged.** Not well recognized is the left inferior phrenic vein, which typically communicates with the adrenal vein but then courses medially and can be injured during dissection of the medial edge of the gland.
6. **a. Dehydroepiandrosterone (DHEA) and androstenedione.** The principal androgens are DHEA, dehydroepiandrosterone sulfate (DHEAS), and androstenedione.
7. **d. Corticotropin (ACTH).** ACTH is produced from a large protein (290 amino acids) termed pro-opiomelanocortin (POMC). Other POMC-derived peptides include β-lipotropin, α- and β-melanocyte-stimulating hormone, β-endorphin, and methionine-enkephalin (see Fig. 53-9). ACTH secretion is characterized by an inherent diurnal rhythm leading to parallel changes in cortisol and ACTH. ACTH secretion is reciprocally related to the circulating cortisol level.
8. **b. Angiotensin II.** In contrast to glucocorticoids and adrenal androgens, the primary physiologic control of aldosterone secretion is angiotensin II.
9. **a. Testosterone and DHEA.** Elevated serum concentrations of testosterone and DHEA are the hallmark of the presence of adrenal tumors in women who present with hirsutism.
10. **e. Vanillylmandelic acid.** The primary metabolite in the urine is vanillylmandelic acid, with metanephrine, normetanephrine, and their derivatives contributing to total metabolic products.
11. **c. Cushing's disease.** Cushing's disease accounts for 75% to 85% of patients with endogenous Cushing's syndrome.
12. **a. Exogenous steroid use.** An exogenous source of Cushing's syndrome should always first be excluded because therapeutic steroids are the most common cause. Often the patient does not even realize that he or she is using a steroid-containing preparation, especially creams or lotions.
13. **d. Depression.** Patients with nonendocrine disorders that mimic the clinical and sometimes biochemical manifestations of Cushing's syndrome must be separated from those patients with true Cushing's syndrome; these patients have been said to have pseudo-Cushing's syndrome. Abnormally regulated cortical secretion, albeit mild, may exist in as many as 80% of patients with major depression.
14. **b. Three 24-hour urinary cortisol determinations.** At the present time, the determination of 24-hour excretion of cortisol in the urine is the most direct and reliable index of cortisol secretion. One study recommended that urinary cortisol should be measured in two and preferably three consecutive 24-hour urine specimens collected on an outpatient basis.
15. **e. Cushing's syndrome.** Early case studies of patients with the "metabolic syndrome" have found subclinical Cushing's syndrome in 3% of patients.
16. **d. Late night salivary cortisol measurement.** Salivary late night collection with a new device to measure salivary cortisol concentration is being used by endocrinologists.
17. **b. To identify pseudo-Cushing's syndrome.** These low-dose suppression tests are now reserved primarily for patients with equivocal 24-hour urinary cortisol excretion and are especially useful for identifying patients with pseudo-Cushing's syndrome.
18. **b. Concurrent measurement of ACTH and cortisone.** The ideal way to determine whether a patient has ACTH-dependent or ACTH-independent hypercortisolism is the concurrent measurement of both plasma ACTH (corticotropin) and cortisol.
19. **e. Petrosal venous sinus sampling of ACTH.** The most direct way to demonstrate pituitary hypersecretion of ACTH is to measure its level in the petrosal venous sinus and compare that level to the peripheral level.
20. **d. Pituitary tumor after bilateral adrenalectomy.** Generally, patients with severe Cushing's disease did well after bilateral adrenalectomy through a bilateral posterior approach with resolution of the disease. Ten to 20 percent of patients, however, subsequently developed pituitary tumors, usually chromophobe adenomas, perhaps caused by the lack of hypothalamic/pituitary feedback and high ACTH and related compounds. This entity, *termed Nelson's syndrome*, may arise many years after bilateral adrenalectomy.
21. **c. MRI.** The authors have used MRI to identify an adenoma in a pregnant patient with Cushing's syndrome.
22. **a. 5 cm.** CT may underestimate the size of an adrenal lesion, and one study suggested that exploration be performed when the lesion is more than 5 cm on CT scans or MR images.
23. **a. Neural tumors, carcinoma, metastatic lesions.** There are a number of entities other than adrenal carcinoma, however, that can cause high intensity, including neural tumors, metastatic tumors to the adrenal, and hemorrhage into a variety of adrenal lesions.
24. **d. 4,000.** Most adrenal carcinomas are greater than 5 cm and are rarely less than 2 cm, whereas small benign adenomas are found on autopsy in 7% of patients over 70.
25. **e. Flow cytometry.** One study reported that flow cytometry accurately demonstrated aneuploid stem lines in four cases classified histologically as carcinoma.
26. **c. 35%.** Except for testosterone-secreting tumors, adrenocortical carcinomas are highly malignant, with both local and hematogenous spread and a 5-year survival rate of about 35%.
27. **b. Observation.** Most asymptomatic adrenal cysts are observed. Symptomatic cysts can be drained with or without sclerosis, or resected with a laparoscopic technique.
28. **a. Addison's disease.** Adrenal insufficiency may be an important aspect of the care of a patient with cancer and may be due to replacement of the adrenals with metastases, infiltration with lymphoma, hemorrhagic necrosis in association with anticoagulation, or sepsis as well as impaired adrenal steroidogenesis in patients receiving aminoglutethimide, ketoconazole, mitotane, or suramin. Addison's disease is rare, the death rate being approximately 0.3 per 100,000, with the most common cause being either tuberculosis or adrenal atrophy. Other causes include malignant infiltration.
29. **b. Hypokalemia, low PRA, high aldosterone level.** The syndrome of primary hyperaldosteronism is now identified by

the combined findings of hypokalemia, suppressed PRA, and high urinary and plasma aldosterone levels in hypertensive patients.

30. **d. Normal sodium intake.** Because severe hypokalemia occurs less frequently in patients with restricted dietary sodium intake, certain authors do not recommend screening patients for this syndrome unless they are adequately salt loaded.

31. **b. Rise in PRA, fall in aldosterone.** In patients with primary aldosteronism with highly autonomous aldosterone production, plasma aldosterone levels decrease during this test, reflecting the influence of the diurnal fall in ACTH, which is normally a relatively minor stimulus for aldosterone production. The PRA level rises.

32. **e. Adrenal vein sampling.** Adrenal vein sampling of aldosterone remains the cornerstone for localization of aldosterone production.

33. **c. Blood pressure control and potassium repletion.** Adrenalectomy should be preceded by several weeks of adequate control of hypertension and correction of hypokalemia and other metabolic abnormalities.

34. **a. Spironolactone.** The cornerstone of medical therapy in primary aldosteronism caused by bilateral hyperplasia is spironolactone (Aldactone), a competitive antagonist of the aldosterone receptor.

35. **d. 90%.** Hypertension was either cured or improved to an acceptable target in more than 90% of the patients with an adenoma.

36. **b. 10%.** About 10% of pheochromocytomas are found in normotensive patients.

37. **a. Low cardiac ejection fraction.** One specific entity that has gained more recognition is catecholamine-induced cardiomyopathy. Experimentally injected catecholamines can cause foci of myocardial necrosis, with inflammation and fibrosis. These patients may have a reduction in blood pressure because of a global reduction in myocardial pump functions, considered to be due to both a downregulation of β-receptors and a decrease of viable myofibrils.

38. **a. Children, those with multiple endocrine adenoma (MEA), familial groups.** Familial pheochromocytomas may be divided into different types of genetic abnormalities. Pheochromocytomas occur in MEA type 2, a triad including pheochromocytoma, medullary carcinoma of the thyroid, and parathyroid adenomas. Pheochromocytoma may also be a part of multiple endocrine neoplasia type 3. In contrast to adults, children manifest a higher incidence of familial pheochromocytomas (10%) and bilaterality (24%).

39. **c. MRI.** There are multiple uses of MRI in patients with pheochromocytoma. The test appears to be as accurate as CT in identifying lesions, while having a characteristically bright, "light bulb" image on T2-weighted study (see Figs. 53-41 and 53-42). In addition, sagittal and coronal imaging can give excellent anatomic information about the relationship between the tumor and the surrounding vasculature as well as the draining venous channels (see Figs. 53-42 and 53-43). We believe that MRI should be the initial scanning procedure in patients with biochemical findings of a pheochromocytoma.

40. **d. α-Adrenergic blockade with phenoxybenzamine.** Phenoxybenzamine hydrochloride (Dibenzyline), a long-acting α-adrenergic blocker, controls blood pressure in patients with pheochromocytoma.

41. **b. bilateral tumor.** A major use of partial adrenalectomy is in patients at risk for multiple adrenal tumors such as von Hippel-Lindau type 2 patients.

42. **c. Laparoscopic.** Laparoscopy offers a shorter length of hospital stay, a decrease in postoperative pain, a shorter time to return to preoperative activity level, improved cosmesis, and reduced morbidity in the fragile patient afflicted with Cushing's disease.

54

Surgery of the Adrenal Glands

GEORGE K. CHOW • MICHAEL L. BLUTE

QUESTIONS

1. Which statement is FALSE?
   a. The right adrenal gland rests higher than the left adrenal gland.
   b. The right adrenal gland tends to lie in a retrocaval position.
   c. The right adrenal vein usually drains into the vena cava directly.
   d. The left adrenal gland receives arterial branches from the left inferior phrenic artery, aorta, and left renal artery.
   e. None of the above.
2. Absolute contraindications for laparoscopic adrenalectomy include:
   a. bleeding diathesis.
   b. adrenal mass size greater than 12 cm.
   c. adrenocortical carcinoma with adrenal vein thrombus.
   d. a and c are correct.
   e. a, b, and c are correct.
3. All of the following statements are true regarding adrenal cortical carcinoma EXCEPT which one?
   a. Adrenal masses larger than 6 cm are always carcinoma.
   b. CT can distinguish infiltrative from well-encapsulated tumors.
   c. Adrenal cortical carcinoma is a relative contraindication for laparoscopic surgery.
   d. Removal should not be attempted via the posterior lumbodorsal open approach.
   e. All of the above are true.
4. Intraoperative ultrasound helps laparoscopic adrenalectomy by:
   a. locating the adrenal gland.
   b. identifying the adrenal vein.
   c. locating an adrenal mass.
   d. a and c.
   e. a, b, and c.
5. During a right adrenalectomy, severe bleeding starts. The possible causes include all the following EXCEPT:
   a. right adrenal vein avulsion at origin on vena cava.
   b. avulsion of the right hepatic vein branch.
   c. disruption of adrenal capsule.
   d. inadvertent ligation of upper pole renal artery.
   e. all of the above.
6. Which of the following statements is TRUE regarding laparoscopic partial nephrectomy?
   a. The adrenal vein can be taken without compromising the adrenal glands venous drainage.
   b. Enucleation of mass can be performed with ultrasonic scalpel.
   c. Laparoscopic partial nephrectomy is facilitated by intraoperative ultrasound.
   d. a and c are true.
   e. a, b, and c are true.
7. Which of the following statements about postoperative addisonian crisis is TRUE?
   a. It is the result of contralateral adrenal activation.
   b. It can occur with fever and hypotension.
   c. It is managed by administration of spironolactone.
   d. It occurs only after laparoscopic adrenalectomy.
   e. All of the statements are true.
8. A pregnant woman with hypertension presents to the clinic. In her case, to distinguish pheochromocytoma from PIH (pregnancy-induced hypertension or "pre-eclampsia") which of the following is TRUE?
   a. PIH is never paroxysmal whereas pheochromocytoma-related hypertension can be.
   b. Proteinuria occurs with PIH not pheochromocytoma.
   c. The hypertension of PIH typically occurs in the first trimester, whereas pheochromocytoma hypertension can occur at any stage of pregnancy.
   d. a and b are true.
   e. a, b, and c are true.
9. Clinical indications for partial adrenalectomy include all of the following EXCEPT:
   a. solitary adrenal gland.
   b. bilateral adrenal tumors.
   c. Von Hippel-Lindau disease.
   d. multiple endocrine neoplasia type I.
   e. multiple endocrine neoplasia type IIA.

ANSWERS

1. **e. None of the above.** The right adrenal gland sits in a retrocaval position and lies in a more cephalad position than its left confrere. The venous drainage of the right adrenal gland can be variable but typically drains directly into the vena cava. In contrast, the left renal vein receives tributaries from the left adrenal vein and left gonadal vein. In some instances, a lumbar vein can drain directly into the left renal vein. Arterial supply is often more numerous and variable than the venous drainage. The adrenal glands receive arterial branches from the aorta, renal artery, and phrenic arteries.
2. **d. a and c are correct.** With improvements in technical skill and equipment, larger adrenal masses are being approached laparoscopically. There is no clear limit to the size of an adrenal that can be removed laparoscopically. Various size limits have been suggested in the past. However, case reports continue to be published describing ever larger masses that have been removed laparoscopically. Therefore, size should be a relative contraindication for laparoscopic surgery, and a surgeon's experience and skill must be factored into the decision making process. Larger masses are more likely to be adrenocortical carcinoma that can directly invade into surrounding organs, rendering them very difficult to resect laparoscopically. However, adrenocortical carcinomas can be resected laparoscopically as long as there is no suspicion of tumor extension into surrounding structures. The presence of adrenal vein tumor thrombus should be considered an absolute contraindication to the laparoscopic approach. Finally, severe coagulopathy should be considered an absolute contraindication for laparoscopic surgery.
3. **a. Adrenal masses larger than 6 cm are always carcinoma.** As was noted in the answer to question 3, there is no definite size that correlates absolutely with adrenocortical carcinoma. Many forms of adrenal pathology can exceed 6 cm, including adrenal cysts, pheochromocytomas, adrenal hemorrhage, and so on. Adrenocortical carcinoma is not a contraindication for laparoscopic surgery. However, certain conditions that can exist with adrenocortical carcinoma (organ invasion, tumor thrombus) are. Cross-sectional imaging (CT and MRI) are critical for making such distinctions.
4. **e. a, b, and c.** Intraoperative ultrasound can assist with the identification of important structures during laparoscopy. This is especially true when operating on morbidly obese patients with lots of retroperitoneal fat. The direct localization of an adrenal mass can assist with ablative therapy or partial adrenalectomy.
5. **d. inadvertent ligation of upper pole renal artery.** All of the vascular injuries noted cause bleeding except ligation of an upper pole renal artery. Ligation of this artery would result in upper pole devascularization not hemorrhage.
6. **e. a, b, and c are true.** Although the adrenal vein is the principal route of venous drainage, in most instances there are smaller vessels that can be relied on to drain the adrenal should the adrenal vein be ligated. Laparoscopic partial adrenalectomy has been described using a laparoscopic stapler and enucleation with ultrasonic scalpel. Intraoperative ultrasound is an invaluable tool for localizing the tumor during partial adrenalectomy.
7. **b. It can present with fever and hypotension.** Addisonian crisis or acute adrenal insufficiency can occur after adrenalectomy or be due to other nonsurgical causes (e.g., adrenal hemorrhage and tuberculosis). Patients can present with back/abdominal pain, nausea, vomiting, diarrhea, hypotension, fever, hypoglycemia, and hyperkalemia. Removal of an adrenal gland can trigger addisonian crisis if there has been endocrine suppression (not activation) of the contralateral adrenal gland. Addisonian crisis is usually managed by steroid replacement, both glucocorticoid and mineralocorticoid (fludrocortisone).
8. **d. a and b are true.** PIH typically occurs in the third trimester and is distinguished from pheochromocytoma by the presence of proteinuria and the absence of paroxysmal symptoms.
9. **d. multiple endocrine neoplasia type I.** All of the answers correspond to strong clinical reasons to consider partial nephrectomy, namely, conditions that result in solitary adrenal gland or multifocal/bilateral adrenal disease. Multiple endocrine neoplasia type I is not associated with adrenal tumors and therefore is not a reason for considering partial adrenalectomy.

SECTION XIV

URINE TRANSPORT, STORAGE, AND EMPTYING

55

Physiology and Pharmacology of the Renal Pelvis and Ureter

ROBERT M. WEISS

QUESTIONS

1. During development, the ureteral lumen is obliterated and then recanalizes. Which of the following substances appears to be involved in this recanalization process?
   a. Prostaglandin E_2
   b. c-Kit
   c. Angiotensin
   d. Calcitonin gene–related peptide (CGRP)
   e. Acetylcholine
2. Caspases are involved in:
   a. smooth muscle relaxation.
   b. smooth muscle contraction.
   c. hysteresis.
   d. apoptosis.
   e. calcium sequestration.
3. The resting membrane potential is primarily determined by the distribution of which of the following ions across the cell membrane and the preferential permeability of the cell membrane to that ion?
   a. Potassium
   b. Sodium
   c. Calcium
   d. Chloride
   e. Barium
4. With excitation of the ureteral cell, an action potential is formed. Which of the following pairs of ions is responsible for the upstroke of the action potential?
   a. Potassium and calcium
   b. Sodium and chloride
   c. Calcium and sodium
   d. Potassium and sodium
   e. Calcium and chloride
5. Which of the following must be phosphorylated for smooth muscle contraction to occur?
   a. Actin
   b. Myosin
   c. Calmodulin
   d. Calcium
   e. Troponin
6. The primary site for intracellular storage of calcium is:
   a. mitochondria.
   b. caveolae.
   c. nucleolus.
   d. actin.
   e. endoplasmic reticulum.
7. The second messenger involved in β-adrenergic agonist–induced ureteral relaxation is:
   a. cyclic AMP.
   b. cyclic GMP.
   c. nitric oxide.
   d. inositol 1,4,5-triphosphate (IP_3).
   e. diacylglycerol (DG).
8. The enzyme that degrades cyclic GMP is:
   a. guanylyl cyclase.
   b. myosin light chain kinase.
   c. phosphodiesterase.
   d. phospholipase C.
   e. nitric oxide synthase (NOS).
9. The enzyme that degrades cyclic AMP is:
   a. adenylyl cyclase.
   b. myosin light chain kinase.
   c. phosphodiesterase.
   d. phospholipase C.
   e. NOS.

10. Nitric oxide causes smooth muscle relaxation. In doing so, it activates which of the following enzymes?
    a. Guanylyl cyclase
    b. Myosin light chain kinase
    c. Phosphodiesterase
    d. Phospholipase C
    e. NOS

11. The substrate for NOS is:
    a. cyclic AMP.
    b. cyclic GMP.
    c. GTP.
    d. L-arginine.
    e. L-citrulline.

12. Inducible NOS (iNOS) is:
    a. nicotinamide adenine dinucleotide phosphate (NADPH) independent and calcium independent.
    b. NADPH independent and calcium dependent.
    c. NADPH dependent and calcium independent.
    d. NADPH dependent and calcium dependent.
    e. nitric oxide dependent and calcium dependent.

13. The enzyme involved in the formation of DG is:
    a. adenylyl cyclase.
    b. guanylyl cyclase.
    c. phosphodiesterase.
    d. protein kinase C.
    e. phospholipase C.

14. DG increases the activity of which enzyme?
    a. Adenylyl cyclase
    b. Guanylyl cyclase
    c. Phosphodiesterase
    d. Protein kinase C
    e. Phospholipase C

15. An agent that prevents reuptake of norepinephrine in nerve terminals and thus potentiates and prolongs the activity of norepinephrine is:
    a. tyrosine.
    b. monoamine oxidase.
    c. imipramine.
    d. tetramethylammonium.
    e. tetraethylammonium.

16. Norepinephrine is synthesized from:
    a. tyrosine.
    b. arginine.
    c. choline.
    d. cocaine.
    e. imipramine.

17. Which of the following inhibits ureteral and renal pelvic contractile activity?
    a. Substance P
    b. Neurokinin A
    c. Neuropeptide K
    d. Neuropeptide Y
    e. CGRP

18. Which of the following collagen types is associated with ureteral obstruction?
    a. Type I collagen
    b. Type II collagen
    c. Type III collagen
    d. Type IV collagen
    e. Type V collagen

19. The enzyme involved in prostaglandin synthesis is:
    a. phospholipase C.
    b. cyclooxygenase.
    c. protein kinase C.
    d. phosphodiesterase.
    e. ATPase.

20. With ureteral obstruction, prostaglandins are involved in a process that aids in the preservation of renal function. What is this process?
    a. Afferent arteriole vasoconstriction
    b. Afferent arteriole vasodilatation
    c. Efferent arteriole vasoconstriction
    d. Efferent arteriole vasodilatation
    e. Glomerular vasoconstriction

21. Which of the following agents could theoretically cause urinary retention?
    a. Bethanechol
    b. BAY K 8644
    c. Prostaglandin $F_{2\alpha}$
    d. Verapamil
    e. Substance P

22. Which of the following is a β-adrenergic agonist?
    a. Cromakalim
    b. Physostigmine
    c. Propranolol
    d. Phenoxybenzamine
    e. Isoproterenol

23. Which of the following conditions must be present for urine to pass efficiently from the ureter into the bladder?
    a. Intraluminal ureteral contractile pressure must be above 40 cm H_2O.
    b. The ureterovesical junction must relax.
    c. Intraluminal ureteral contractile pressures must be greater than intravesical baseline pressures.
    d. Intravesical contractile pressures must be less than 40 cm H_2O.
    e. The bladder must relax just before contraction of the ureter.

24. What is normal baseline or resting ureteral pressure?
    a. 0 to 5 cm H_2O
    b. 5 to 10 cm H_2O
    c. 10 to 15 cm H_2O
    d. 15 to 20 cm H_2O
    e. 20 to 25 cm H_2O

25. The Laplace equation expresses the relationship between the variables that affect intraluminal pressure. Which of the following conforms to the Laplace relationship
    a. Tension = (radius × wall thickness)/pressure
    b. Tension = (radius × pressure)/wall thickness
    c. Tension = (wall thickness × pressure)/radius
    d. Pressure = (radius × wall thickness)/tension
    e. Pressure = (radius × tension)/wall thickness

26. Factors that facilitate ureteral stone passage include:
    a. increased hydrostatic pressures proximal to the calculus and relaxation of the ureter in the region of the stone.
    b. increased hydrostatic pressures proximal to the calculus and contraction of the ureter in the region of the stone.
    c. decreased hydrostatic pressures proximal to the calculus and relaxation of the ureter in the region of the stone.
    d. decreased hydrostatic pressures proximal to the calculus and contraction of the ureter in the region of the stone.
    e. decreased contractile pressures proximal to the calculus and contraction of the ureter in the region of the stone.

27. Which of the following hormones inhibits ureteral contractility?
   a. Bombesin
   b. Thyroxine
   c. Estrogen
   d. Aldosterone
   e. Progesterone

28. A drug that has efficacy in managing ureteral colic is:
   a. bethanechol.
   b. prostaglandin $F_{2\alpha}$.
   c. physostigmine.
   d. indomethacin.
   e. ephedrine.

29. Which of the following is a calcium-binding protein that plays a role in smooth muscle contraction?
   a. Connexin43
   b. Calmodulin
   c. Cromakalim
   d. Survivin
   e. Myosin

30. The resting or the contractile force developed at any given length, in the ureter, depends on the direction in which the change in length is occurring. This is referred to as:
   a. viscoelasticity.
   b. creep.
   c. hysteresis.
   d. stress relaxation.
   e. compensatory relaxation.

31. Which of the following is noted to be expressed before initiation of ureteral peristaltic activity?
   a. Prostanoids
   b. Nitric oxide
   c. c-Kit
   d. Myosin light chain
   e. Phosphodiesterase

32. Apoptosis plays an important role in:
   a. ureteral contraction.
   b. ureteral relaxation.
   c. ureteral pacemaker activity.
   d. branching of the ureteral bud.
   e. maintenance of the ureteral resting membrane potential.

33. Ureteral pacemaker activity is amplified by:
   a. prostanoids.
   b. norepinephrine.
   c. CGRP.
   d. cyclic GMP.
   e. potassium channel openers.

ANSWERS

1. **c. Angiotensin.** At a point during development, the ureteral lumen is obliterated and then recanalizes. It appears that angiotensin acting through the AT2 receptor is involved in the recanalization process. Knockout mice for the *ATR2* gene have congenital anomalies of the kidney and urinary tract, which include multicystic dysplastic kidneys, megaureters, and ureteropelvic junction obstructions.

2. **d. apoptosis.** Programmed cell death, or apoptosis, is involved in branching of the ureteric bud and subsequent nephrogenesis, and inhibitors of caspases, which are factors in the signaling pathway of apoptosis, inhibit ureteral bud branching.

3. **a. Potassium.** When a ureteral muscle cell is in a nonexcited or resting state, the electrical potential difference across the cell membrane, the transmembrane potential, is referred to as the resting membrane potential (RMP). The RMP is determined primarily by the distribution of potassium ions (K^+) across the cell membrane and by the permeability of the membrane to potassium ions.

4. **c. Calcium and sodium.** When the ureteral cell is excited, its membrane loses its preferential permeability to K^+ and becomes more permeable to calcium ions (Ca^{2+}) that move inward across the cell membrane, primarily through L-type Ca^{2+} channels, and give rise to the upstroke of the action potential.

5. **b. Myosin.** The most widely accepted theory suggests that phosphorylation of myosin is involved in the contractile process.

6. **e. endoplasmic reticulum.** Calcium release from tightly bound storage sites (i.e., the endoplasmic or sarcoplasmic reticulum) increases the Ca^{2+} concentration in the sarcoplasm.

7. **a. cyclic AMP.** Cyclic AMP is believed to mediate the relaxing effects of β-adrenergic agonists in a variety of smooth muscles.

8. **c. phosphodiesterase.** Another cyclic nucleotide, cyclic GMP, also can cause smooth muscle relaxation. Cyclic GMP is synthesized from GTP via the enzyme guanylyl cyclase and is degraded to 5′-GMP by a phosphodiesterase.

9. **c. phosphodiesterase.** Phosphodiesterase activity that can degrade both cyclic AMP and cyclic GMP has been demonstrated in the canine ureter, and various inhibitors can preferentially inhibit the breakdown of one or the other cyclic nucleotide.

10. **a. Guanylyl cyclase.** Nitric oxide released from the nerve activates the enzyme guanylyl cyclase in the smooth muscle cell, with the resultant conversion of guanosine triphosphate to cyclic GMP with resultant smooth muscle relaxation (see Fig. 55-12).

11. **d. L-arginine.** NOS converts L-arginine to nitric oxide and L-citrulline in a reaction that requires nicotinamide adenine dinucleotide phosphate (NADPH).

12. **c. NADPH dependent and calcium independent.** An inducible NOS isoform, iNOS, is NADPH dependent but Ca^{2+} independent and has been identified in ureteral smooth muscle.

13. **e. phospholipase C.** Some actions of α_1-adrenergic and muscarinic cholinergic agonists and a number of other hormones, neurotransmitters, and biologic substances are associated with an increase in intracellular Ca^{2+} and are related to changes in inositol lipid metabolism. These agonists combine with a receptor on the cell membrane, and the agonist-receptor complex, in turn, activates an enzyme, phospholipase C, that leads to the hydrolysis of polyphosphatidylinositol 4,5-bisphosphate, with the formation of two second messengers, IP_3 and DG (see Fig. 55-13).

14. **d. Protein kinase C.** DG binds to an enzyme, protein kinase C, causes its translocation to the cell membrane, and, by reducing the concentration of Ca^{2+} required for protein kinase C activation, results in an increase in this enzyme's activity.

15. **c. imipramine.** The greatest percentage of the norepinephrine is actively taken up (reuptake or neuronal uptake) into the neuron. Neuronal reuptake regulates the duration that norepinephrine is in contact with the innervated tissue and thus regulates the magnitude and duration of the catecholamine-induced response. Agents such as cocaine and imipramine (Tofranil), which inhibit neuronal uptake, potentiate the physiologic response to norepinephrine.

16. **a. tyrosine.** Norepinephrine, the chemical mediator responsible for adrenergic transmission, is synthesized in the neuron from tyrosine.

17. **e. CGRP.** Tachykinins and CGRP are neurotransmitters released from peripheral endings of sensory nerves. Tachykinins stimulate contractile activity and CGRP inhibits contractile activity.

18. **c. Type III collagen.** Increased amounts of collagen type III are seen in a variety of obstructed ureteral states.

19. **b. cyclooxygenase.** The "primary" prostaglandins, PGE_1, PGE_2, and $PGF_{2\alpha}$, are synthesized from the fatty acid arachidonic acid by enzymatic reactions involving two cyclooxygenase (COX) isoforms, COX-1 and COX-2.

20. **b. Afferent arteriole vasodilatation.** Indomethacin has been employed in the management of ureteral colic. The beneficial effects are probably due to indomethacin's inhibition of the prostaglandin-mediated vasodilatation that occurs subsequent to obstruction. The vasodilatation theoretically would result in an increase in glomerular capillary pressure and subsequent increase in pelviureteral pressure.

21. **d. Verapamil.** The calcium channel blockers verapamil, D-600 (a methoxy derivative of verapamil), diltiazem, and nifedipine have been shown to inhibit ureteral activity. These inhibitory effects are accompanied by decreases in action potential duration, number of oscillations on the plateau of the guinea pig action potential, excitability, and rate of rise and amplitude of the action potential. High concentrations of verapamil and D-600 cause a complete cessation of electrical and mechanical activity. Similar inhibition of bladder activity can occur.

22. **e. Isoproterenol.** Isoproterenol, a β-adrenergic agonist, depresses contractility.

23. **c. Intraluminal ureteral contractile pressures must be greater than intravesical baseline pressures.** The theoretical aspects of the mechanics of urine transport within the ureter were described in detail by Griffiths and Notschaele in 1983; these are depicted in Figure 55-19. At normal flow rates, as the renal pelvis fills, a rise in renal pelvic pressure occurs, and urine is extruded into the upper ureter, which is initially in a collapsed state. The contraction wave originates in the most proximal portion of the ureter and moves the urine in front of it in a distal direction. The urine that had previously entered the ureter is formed into a bolus. To propel the bolus of urine efficiently, the contraction wave must completely coapt the ureteral walls, and the pressure generated by this contraction wave provides the primary component of what is recorded by intraluminal pressure measurements. The bolus that is pushed in front of the contraction wave lies almost entirely in a passive, noncontracting part of the ureter.

24. **a. 0 to 5 cm H_2O.** Baseline or resting ureteral pressure is approximately 0 to 5 cm H_2O.

25. **b. Tension = (radius × pressure)/wall thickness.** The Laplace equation expresses the relationship between the variables that affect intraluminal pressure: pressure = (tension × wall thickness)/radius.

26. **a. increased hydrostatic pressures proximal to the calculus and relaxation of the ureter in the region of the stone.** Two factors that appear to be most useful in facilitating stone passage are an increase in hydrostatic pressure proximal to a calculus and relaxation of the ureter in the region of the stone.

27. **e. Progesterone.** Several studies have shown an inhibitory effect of progesterone on ureteral function. Progesterone has been noted to increase the degree of ureteral dilatation during pregnancy and to retard the rate of disappearance of hydroureter in postpartum women.

28. **d. indomethacin.** Indomethacin, by reducing pelviureteral pressure and thus pelviureteral wall tension, might eliminate some of the pain of renal colic that is dependent on distention of the upper urinary tract.

29. **b. Calmodulin.** With excitation, there is a transient increase in the sarcoplasmic Ca^{2+} concentration from its steady-state concentration of 10^{-8} to 10^{-7} M to a concentration of 10^{-6} M or higher. At this higher concentration, Ca^{2+} forms an active complex with the calcium-binding protein calmodulin. Calmodulin without Ca^{2+} is inactive (see Fig. 55-8). The calcium-calmodulin complex activates a calmodulin-dependent enzyme, myosin light-chain kinase (see Fig. 55-8). The activated myosin light-chain kinase, in turn, catalyzes the phosphorylation of the 20,000-dalton light chain of myosin (see Fig. 55-9). Phosphorylation of the myosin light chain allows activation by actin of myosin Mg^{2+}-ATPase activity, leading to hydrolysis of ATP and the development of smooth muscle tension or shortening (see Fig. 55-10).

30. **c. hysteresis.** Because the ureter is a viscoelastic structure, the resting or contractile force developed at any given length depends on the direction in which change in length is occurring and on the rate of length change. This is referred to as hysteresis; for the ureter, at any given length, the resting force is less and contractile force is greater when the ureter is allowed to shorten than when the ureter is being stretched (see Fig. 55-14).

31. **c. c-Kit.** This tyrosine kinase receptor is important in the development of pacemaker activity and peristalsis of the gut (Der-Silaphet et al, 1998). Pezzone and colleagues (2003) identified c-kit positive cells in the mouse ureter. The expression of c-kit was noted to be upregulated in the embryonic murine ureter before its development of unidirectional peristaltic contractions (David et al, 2005). Incubation of isolated cultured embryonic murine ureters with antibodies that neutralize c-Kit activity alters ureteral morphology and inhibits unidirectional peristalsis. c-Kit positive cells have been identified in the human ureter (Metzger et al, 2004).

32. **d. branching of the ureteral bud.** Programmed cell death, or apoptosis, is involved in branching of the ureteric bud and subsequent nephrogenesis. Inhibitors of caspases, which are involved in the apoptotic signaling pathway, inhibit ureteral bud branching (Araki et al, 1999).

33. **a. prostanoids.** The ionic conduction underlying pacemaker activity in the upper urinary tract is due to the opening and slow closure of voltage-activated L-type Ca^{2+} channels, which are amplified by prostanoids (Santicioli et al, 1995a). This is opposed by the opening and closure of voltage and Ca^{2+}-dependent K^+ channels. It has been suggested that prostaglandins and excitatory tachykinins, released from sensory nerves, help maintain autorhythmicity in the upper urinary tract through maintenance of Ca^{2+} mobilization. Tetrodotoxin and blockers of the autonomic nervous system, both parasympathetic and sympathetic, have little effect on peristalsis, suggesting that autonomic neurotransmitters have little role in maintaining pyeloureteral motility.

56

Physiology and Pharmacology of the Bladder and Urethra

NAOKI YOSHIMURA • MICHAEL B. CHANCELLOR

QUESTIONS

1. Sacral-evoked response testing measures nerve conduction time via which pathways?
   a. Somatic afferent, sympathetic efferent
   b. Somatic afferent, somatic efferent
   c. Sympathetic afferent, somatic efferent
   d. Sympathetic afferent, parasympathetic efferent
   e. Parasympathetic afferent, sympathetic efferent
2. During the resting state, bladder smooth muscle electrical activity is characterized by which of the following statements?
   a. Concentration of K^+ ions is higher on the outside of the cell membrane.
   b. Concentration of Na^+ ions is higher on the inside of the cell membrane.
   c. Cell membrane is preferentially permeable to K^+.
   d. Cell membrane is preferentially permeable to Na^+.
   e. Inside of the cell membrane is positive with respect to the outside.
3. A 31-year-old woman, 2 weeks after complete C6 spinal cord injury, has a urodynamic study that demonstrates detrusor areflexia. The most likely urodynamic finding 2 years later is:
   a. detrusor overactivity.
   b. detrusor areflexia.
   c. detrusor overactivity with detrusor-sphincter dyssynergia.
   d. detrusor areflexia with decreased bladder compliance.
   e. detrusor areflexia with detrusor-sphincter dyssynergia.
4. Urinary tract smooth muscle contractility is inhibited by:
   a. propranolol.
   b. nifedipine.
   c. phenylephrine.
   d. acetylcholine.
   e. substance P.
5. Phosphodiesterase inhibitors cause smooth muscle relaxation by inhibiting:
   a. calmodulin binding.
   b. production of cyclic GMP.
   c. production of cyclic AMP.
   d. degradation of phospholipase C.
   e. degradation of cyclic GMP.
6. The most common urodynamic finding in sacral level spinal cord injury is:
   a. detrusor hyperreflexia.
   b. detrusor hyperreflexia with detrusor-external sphincter dyssynergia.
   c. detrusor areflexia.
   d. poor detrusor compliance.
   e. normal urodynamics.
7. During physiologic filling bladder compliance is most affected by:
   a. perivesical ganglia activity.
   b. peripheral nerve activity.
   c. sacral spinal cord activity.
   d. suprasacral spinal cord activity.
   e. bladder wall viscoelasticity.
8. Increased bladder wall tension is directly related to:
   a. decreased bladder size.
   b. decreased intravesical pressure.
   c. increased intravesical pressure.
   d. thin bladder wall.
9. When the hypogastric nerve is stimulated, what is the primary neurotransmitter released at the ganglionic level?
   a. Acetylcholine
   b. Adenosine triphosphate
   c. Dopamine
   d. Norepinephrine
   e. Prostaglandin $F_{2\alpha}$
10. Pudendal nerve block may be useful in the treatment of neuropathic bladder dysfunction in patients with:
    a. lower motor lesions with spastic bladder.
    b. lower motor lesions with spastic sphincter.
    c. upper motor lesions with atonic bladder.
    d. upper motor lesions with spastic sphincter.
    e. upper motor lesions with vesicoureteral reflux.
11. Postganglionic sympathetic nerve fibers to the bladder release:
    a. acetylcholine.
    b. epinephrine.
    c. nitric oxide.
    d. norepinephrine.
    e. vasoactive intestinal polypeptide.

12. The bladder contraction and simultaneous urethral relaxation during voiding are coordinated by a reflex center located in the:
    a. hypothalamus.
    b. basal ganglia.
    c. medulla.
    d. pons.
    e. thoracic cord.
13. The sudden rise in detrusor pressure seen at the onset of carbon dioxide cystometry is due to:
    a. tonic contraction of the bladder.
    b. phasic contraction of the bladder.
    c. viscoelastic properties of the bladder.
    d. sacral reflex arc.
    e. bladder-urethral reflex arc.
14. The first event to occur with normal micturition is:
    a. relaxation of the bladder neck.
    b. relaxation of the prostate and prostatic capsule.
    c. relaxation of the external striated sphincter.
    d. contraction of the bladder body.
    e. contraction of the bladder trigone.
15. In patients with hypersensitive bladder dysfunction, intravesical capsaicin instillation may potentially benefit the patient by blockade of:
    a. glycosaminoglycan receptor.
    b. serotonin reuptake.
    c. Aδ fiber afferents.
    d. C-fiber afferents.
    e. tachykinin receptor.
16. Painful bladder sensations are conveyed by which nerve(s)?
    a. Hypogastric
    b. Pelvic
    c. Pudendal
    d. Pelvic and hypogastric
    e. Pelvic and pudendal
17. Smooth muscle contraction results from phosphorylation of which protein?
    a. Actin
    b. Caldesmon
    c. Desmin
    d. G-protein
    e. Myosin
18. Which of the following is NOT a characteristic of detrusor interstitial cells?
    a. Participates in spontaneous activity of the bladder
    b. Linked by gap junctions
    c. Located in the suburothelial space between urothelium and nerve endings
    d. Similar to myofibroblasts (urothelial interstitial cells)
    e. Triggers bladder pain
19. Neurally mediated relaxation of the urethra during voiding occurs by release of:
    a. Nitric oxide from sympathetics
    b. Nitric oxide from parasympathetics
    c. VIP from sympathetics
    d. VIP from parasympathetics
    e. Neuropeptide-Y from sympathetics
20. Influx of which ion/chemical is responsible for generation of action potential by bladder smooth muscle cells?
    a. Calcium
    b. Potassium
    c. Sodium
    d. Chloride
    e. Nitric oxide
21. The decrease in bladder compliance is due to what change in connective tissue component?
    a. Decreased elastin
    b. Decreased type I collagen
    c. Decreased type II collagen
    d. Increased type III collagen
    e. Increased type V collagen
22. Acetylcholine binds predominately to which of the five muscarinic receptor(s) to induce bladder contraction?
    a. M1
    b. M2
    c. M1 and M2
    d. M2 and M3
    e. M2 and M4
23. Which adrenergic receptor participates in human detrusor muscle relaxation during the storage phase?
    a. β_1
    b. β_2
    c. β_3
    d. α_1
    e. α_2
24. Substance P is located in which types of nerves?
    a. Afferent
    b. Efferent
    c. Afferent and efferent
    d. Aδ fibers
    e. Spinal cord interneurons
25. Which hormone increases α-adrenergic receptors density in the urethra?
    a. LHRH
    b. Dihydrotestosterone
    c. Testosterone
    d. Estrogen
    e. Testosterone and estrogen
26. Which is the most important excitatory neurotransmitter in the central nervous system to facilitate micturition?
    a. Acetylcholine
    b. GABA
    c. Norepinephrine
    d. Glutamate
    e. Serotonin
27. Which central nervous system neurotransmitter inhibits micturition?
    a. Acetylcholine
    b. Substance P
    c. Norepinephrine
    d. Glutamate
    e. Serotonin
28. What is the function of delta and mu opioid receptors in the spinal cord?
    a. Opioid receptors do not participate in the micturition reflex.
    b. They enhance bladder sensation.
    c. They inhibit descending pontine-spinal signaling.
    d. They stimulate bladder contraction.
    e. They inhibit bladder contraction.

29. Which nerves trigger normal micturition?
    a. Sympathetic nerves
    b. Myelinated Aδ afferent nerves
    c. Unmyelinated C-fiber afferent nerves
    d. Both Aδ and C-fiber afferent nerves
    e. None of the above

30. Which nerve triggers uninhibited bladder contractions induced by a spinal micturition reflex in the cat model of chronic spinal cord transection?
    a. Sympathetic
    b. Aδ
    c. C-fiber
    d. Both Aδ and C-fiber
    e. None of the above

31. Botulinum toxin relaxes detrusor muscle tone by:
    a. antagonizing vanilloid receptors.
    b. blocking SNARE proteins.
    c. enhancing nitric oxide release.
    d. presynaptic neurovesical reuptake inhibition.
    e. postsynaptic neurovesical antagonist.

ANSWERS

1. **b. Somatic afferent, somatic efferent.** Sacral-evoked response testing or measurement of sacral latency is accomplished by electrical stimulation of the skin of the penis while recording activity of the bulbocavernosus muscle. Both the afferent and efferent limbs of this reflex arc are somatic nerves. At present, no clinically useful neurophysiologic study exists that directly measures nerve conduction over autonomic nerves that supply the lower urinary tract or penis.

2. **c. Cell membrane is preferentially permeable to K^+.** During the resting state the cell membrane is preferentially permeable to K^+. The tendency of K^+ is to move from the inside of the cell where it is more concentrated to the outside of the cell membrane. This outward migration of potassium creates an electrical gradient across the cell membrane with the inside of the cell membrane being negative with respect to the outside.

3. **c. detrusor overactivity with detrusor-sphincter dyssynergia.** After spinal cord injury (SCI), patients generally develop a spinal shock phase that lasts approximately 4 weeks. During spinal shock, the detrusor is areflexic. In patients with complete high SCI, the long-term urodynamic manifestation is most commonly detrusor overactivity with detrusor-sphincter dyssynergia. Incomplete SCI generally demonstrates detrusor overactivity with or without detrusor sphincter-dyssynergia. In 10% to 15% of patients with cervical SCI, detrusor areflexia may be a permanent finding. The variability of urodynamic findings in SCI emphasizes the need for careful urodynamic evaluation and follow-up in all patients with SCI.

4. **b. nifedipine.** Phenylephrine is an α-adrenergic agonist, acetylcholine is a muscarinic cholinergic agonist, and substance P is a tachykinin. All three agents stimulate smooth muscle contractility. Propranolol is a β-adrenergic antagonist and blocks the inhibitory effects of β-adrenergic agonists such as isoproterenol. Nifedipine is a calcium channel blocker and inhibits the inward movement of calcium across the cell membrane that is needed for the upstroke of the smooth muscle action potential and for supplying the calcium that is required for contractility.

5. **e. degradation of cyclic GMP.** Cyclic GMP is a second messenger for nitric oxide that activates protein kinases promoting smooth muscle relaxation. Cyclic GMP is degraded to GMP by phosphodiesterase. A phosphodiesterase inhibitor potentiates the effect of cyclic GMP. Ca^{2+} binding to calmodulin is the first step in the initiation of smooth muscle contraction that activates myosin-light chain kinase.

6. **c. detrusor areflexia.** Sacral level spinal injury most commonly results in cauda equina injury. This lower motor neuron injury presents as paralysis of bladder. Only a small number of patients with detrusor areflexia have poor detrusor compliance.

7. **e. bladder wall viscoelasticity.** The elastic and viscoelastic properties of the bladder are the main determinate of compliance during filling. Although neurogenic influences may be operative in late stages of filling, it is clearly these passive properties that are the main determinant of the pressure/volume curve. When these properties are destroyed, as in fibrosis of the bladder wall, markedly decreased compliance is produced.

8. **c. increased intravesical pressure.** Laplace's law states that there is a direct relationship between wall tension (T) and intravesical pressure (P) and bladder size (R = radius). $T = P \times R/2$. Large increases in intravesical pressure, especially a hypertrophic, small-capacity bladder, can dramatically elevate bladder wall tension.

9. **a. Acetylcholine.** All preganglionic efferent autonomic fibers release acetylcholine whether or not they are anatomically parasympathetic or sympathetic. The term *cholinergic* refers to all those receptor sites where acetylcholine is a primary neurotransmitter, including the autonomic ganglion cells, neuromuscular junctions of somatic nerve fibers, and the junction of all postganglionic parasympathetic fibers. Cholinergic receptor sites are divided into two major classes: muscarinic and nicotinic. Muscarinic sites include all autonomic effector cells. Nicotinic sites are on autonomic ganglia, such as those referred to in this question, and the motor endplates of skeletal muscle.

10. **d. upper motor lesions with spastic sphincter.** The pudendal nerve innervate the striated muscle sphincter. Temporary (lidocaine) or permanent block (alcohol) of the pudendal nerve may inhibit detrusor-sphincter dyssynergia. This form of treatment has not been popular however, because complete bilateral blockade of the pudendal nerves is not easy and has the side effect of impotency.

11. **d. norepinephrine.** Postganglionic sympathetic nerves are traditionally noradrenergic and release norepinephrine. Other substances released include neuropeptide Y (NPY) and adenosine triphosphate (ATP). Vasoactive intestinal polypeptide (VIP) often coexists with acetylcholine in parasympathetic postganglionic nerves. However, "sympathetic" does not ALWAYS mean "noradrenergic" because in some tissues (e.g., sweat glands) sympathetics release acetylcholine.

12. **d. pons.** The center for integration and coordination of bladder and urethral activity during voiding is located in the pons (the pontine micturition center) based on animal electrophysiology studies and lesioning or PET scans in human. The basal ganglia and medulla seem to be involved in modulation of detrusor activity and perhaps in facilitation of detrusor contractility but not integration of bladder and urethral response.

13. **c. viscoelastic properties of the bladder.** Sudden stretch off detrusor muscle strips, in vivo preparations, or human bladder during cystometry causes a sudden rise in pressure that is due entirely to passive viscoelastic properties of the bladder. Clinically, this rise in pressure may stimulate a detrusor contraction. Because the phenomenon is a passive one, it does not require intact innervation.

14. **c. relaxation of the external striated sphincter.** Synchronous pressure/flow/EMG studies have demonstrated that the initiation of micturition reflex is characterized by a sudden and complete relaxation of the striated external sphincter followed by detrusor contraction, opening of the bladder neck, and uroflow.

15. **d. C-fiber afferents.** Capsaicin inhibits C-fiber afferent activity because TRPVI vanilloid receptors that bind to capsaicin are predominantly located in C-fibers. Although there are solid animal studies of capsaicin blockade of bladder inflammation, clinical data are scant. Only uncontrolled trials suggest that bladder hypersensitivity and pain are mediated by C-fiber afferents and that the symptoms are improved with intravesical capsaicin therapy.

16. **d. Pelvic and hypogastric.** Bladder pain due to overdistention is mediated by the hypogastric nerve. Bladder pain from inflammatory stimuli is mediated by pelvic nerves.

17. **e. Myosin.** Phosphorylation of myosin by myosin light chain kinase results in smooth muscle contraction. This process is critical for contraction of the ureter, vas deferens, bladder, and corporeal smooth muscle.

18. **e. Triggers bladder pain.** Interstitial cells or myofibroblasts have been identified in the suburethral space and are unique cells linked by gap junctions. Interstitial cells may play a pacemaker role in initiating or participating in the generation or propagation of spontaneous bladder activity. Interstitial cells have not been linked with triggering bladder pain.

19. **b. Nitric oxide from parasympathetics.** During voiding, active contraction of the bladder occurs through parasympathetically mediated cholinergic contraction. In addition, parasympathetically mediated urethral smooth muscle relaxation occurs. An abundance of experimental data indicates that nitric oxide is responsible for this relaxation.

20. **a. Calcium.** Influx of calcium results in action potential generation in smooth muscle cells.

21. **d. Increased type III collagen.** An increase in type III collagen results in decreased bladder compliance.

22. **d. M2 and M3.** Binding of acetylcholine to predominately M2 and M3 muscarinic receptors results in bladder contraction.

23. **c. β3.** Stimulation of β3 adrenergic receptors in the human detrusor results in the direct relaxation of the detrusor smooth muscle. β-Adrenoceptor–mediated relaxation of the human detrusor was not blocked by selective β_1 and/or β_2-adrenoceptor antagonists but is blocked by selective β_3-adrenoceptor antagonists. β_3 agonists are under evaluation for treatment of the overactive bladder.

24. **a. Afferent.** Substance P is located exclusively in afferent nerves.

25. **d. Estrogen.** Only estrogen has been shown to increases the number of α-adrenergic receptors.

26. **d. Glutamate.** Glutamate plays an essential role as an excitatory neurotransmitter in the central nervous system to facilitate voiding. It is facilitatory at the levels of bladder afferents, spinal neurons, descending projection from the pons, within the pons, and in the brain.

27. **e. Serotonin.** Serotonin acts as a neurotransmitter in the spinal cord to inhibit micturition.

28. **e. They inhibit bladder contraction.** Delta and mu opioid receptors in the spinal cord and the brain regulate micturition threshold volume and inhibit bladder contraction.

29. **b. Myelinated Aδ afferent nerves.** Aδ myelinated pelvic nerve afferents are responsible for triggering normal micturition. C-fibers are unmyelinated afferent nerves.

30. **c. C-fiber.** After spinal cord transection, unmyelinated C-fiber afferents in the pelvic nerve trigger a spinal micturition reflex in the cat. In the rat, C-fiber afferents are responsible for nonvoiding uninhibited bladder contractions, although voiding bladder contractions are still dependent on Aδ fiber afferent nerves.

31. **b. blocking SNARE proteins.** Botulinum toxin inhibits neurotransmitter release at the neuromuscular junction by cleaving the neuron terminal cytosolic translocation SNARE proteins, thus preventing neurovesical fusion with the plasma membrane.

57

Pathophysiology and Classification of Voiding Dysfunction

ALAN J. WEIN

QUESTIONS

1. Which of the following best describes normal bladder behavior during the filling-storage phase of the micturition cycle?
   a. Low compliance due to elastic properties
   b. High compliance due to elastic properties
   c. Low compliance due to elastic and viscoelastic properties
   d. High compliance due to elastic and viscoelastic properties
   e. High compliance due to a low relaxation coefficient of the lamina propria
2. A patient who has significantly and urodynamically dangerous decreased compliance because of a replacement by collagen of other components of the stroma is generally best managed by:
   a. pharmacologic regimen.
   b. hydraulic distention.
   c. nerve section.
   d. augmentation cystoplasty.
   e. neuromodulation.
3. The "guarding reflex" refers to the:
   a. abrupt increase in striated sphincter activity seen with a cough during normal bladder filling/storage.
   b. spinal sympathetic inhibition of parasympathetic ganglion activity.
   c. gradual increase in striated sphincter activity seen during normal bladder filling/storage.
   d. gradual inhibition of the pontine-mesencephalic micturition center by the cerebral cortex during normal bladder filling/storage.
   e. gradual inhibition of the sacral spinal cord ventral nuclei by the pontine-mesencephalic brainstem during normal bladder filling/storage.
4. The primary effect of the spinal sympathetic reflexes that are evoked in animals during bladder filling and that facilitate bladder filling/storage is:
   a. neurally mediated stimulation of the α-adrenergic receptors in the area of the smooth sphincter.
   b. neurally mediated stimulation of the β-adrenergic receptors in the bladder body smooth musculature.
   c. direct inhibition of detrusor motor neurons in the sacral spinal cord.
   d. neurally mediated inhibition of cholinergic receptors in the area of the bladder body.
   e. neurally mediated sympathetic modulation of cholinergic ganglionic transmission.
5. The organizational center for the micturition reflex in an intact neural axis is the:
   a. pontine mesencephalic formation in the brain stem.
   b. frontal area of the cerebral cortex.
   c. parietal area of the cerebral cortex.
   d. cerebellum.
   e. sacral spinal cord.
6. Involuntary bladder contractions are most commonly seen in association with:
   a. sacral spinal cord neurologic disease or injury.
   b. infrasacral neurologic disease or injury.
   c. suprasacral neurologic disease or injury.
   d. peripheral nerve neurologic disease or injury.
   e. interstitial cystitis.
7. Using the functional classification system, the usual lower urinary tract dysfunction seen after a stroke would be categorized as:
   a. failure to store because of the bladder (overactivity).
   b. combined deficit (failure to store because of the bladder, failure to empty because of striated sphincter dyssynergy).
   c. combined deficit (failure to store because of the bladder, failure to empty because of a nonrelaxing outlet).
   d. failure to store because of the bladder (hypersensitivity).
   e. failure to store because of the outlet.

8. In the International Continence Society (ICS) classification system the disorder described in question 7 would be characterized as during storage:
   a. overactive neurogenic detrusor activity increased sensation, low bladder capacity, incompetent urethral closure mechanism; during voiding, normal detrusor activity, abnormal urethral function (dysfunctional voiding).
   b. normal detrusor function, increased sensation, low bladder capacity, normal urethral closure mechanism; during voiding, normal detrusor activity, abnormal urethral function (dysfunctional voiding).
   c. overactive neurogenic detrusor activity, normal sensation, normal bladder capacity, incompetent urethral closure mechanism; during voiding, normal detrusor activity, normal urethral function.
   d. stable detrusor activity, reduced sensation, low bladder capacity, normal urethral closure mechanism; during emptying, normal detrusor activity, abnormal urethral function (dysfunctional voiding).
   e. overactive neurogenic detrusor activity, normal sensation, low capacity, normal compliance, normal urethral closure function; during emptying, normal detrusor activity, normal urethral function.
9. In the ICS current terminology, "detrusor hyperreflexia" has been replaced by:
   a. detrusor instability.
   b. idiopathic detrusor overactivity.
   c. hyperactive bladder.
   d. neurogenic detrusor overactivity.
   e. neurogenic detrusor instability.
10. In the Krane-Siroky urodynamic classification system, a patient with post–cerebrovascular accident voiding dysfunction characterized by urgency, frequency, and urge incontinence would most commonly be characterized as having:
    a. detrusor areflexia, striated sphincter dyssynergia, smooth sphincter dyssynergia.
    b. detrusor hyperreflexia, striated sphincter synergia, smooth sphincter dyssynergia.
    c. detrusor hyperreflexia, striated sphincter dyssynergia, smooth sphincter synergia.
    d. detrusor areflexia, striated sphincter synergia, smooth sphincter dyssynergia.
    e. detrusor hyperreflexia, striated sphincter synergia, smooth sphincter dyssynergia.
11. In the Lapides classification system, a patient with post–cerebrovascular accident voiding dysfunction characterized by urgency, frequency, and urge incontinence would most commonly be characterized as having:
    a. sensory neurogenic bladder.
    b. motor paralytic bladder.
    c. uninhibited neurogenic bladder.
    d. reflex neurogenic bladder.
    e. autonomous neurogenic bladder.
12. A reflex neurogenic bladder, as described in the Lapides system classification, is characteristically seen in which of the following? In a patient with:
    a. traumatic spinal cord injury between the sacral spinal cord and the brain stem.
    b. traumatic spinal cord injury between the sacral spinal cord and conus medullaris.
    c. cerebrovascular accident and insulin-dependent diabetes mellitus.
    d. non–insulin-dependent diabetes mellitus.
    e. multiple sclerosis.
13. In the Bors-Comarr system of classification, the term *unbalanced*, when applied to a patient with an upper motor neuron (UMN) lesion, implies:
    a. cerebellar lesion.
    b. involuntary bladder contractions during filling.
    c. areflexic bladder.
    d. decreased bladder compliance during filling.
    e. sphincter dyssynergia.
14. In the Bors-Comarr system, a patient with post–cerebrovascular accident voiding dysfunction characterized by urgency, frequency, and urge incontinence would most commonly be characterized as having:
    a. a UMN lesion, complete, balanced.
    b. a UMN lesion, complete, imbalanced.
    c. an lower motor neuron (LMN) lesion, complete, imbalanced.
    d. an LMN lesion, incomplete, balanced.
    e. a UMN lesion/LMN lesion, complete, balanced.

ANSWERS

1. **d. High compliance due to elastic and viscoelastic properties.** The normal adult bladder response to filling at a physiologic rate is an almost imperceptible change in intravesical pressure. During at least the initial stages of bladder filling, after unfolding of the bladder wall from its collapsed state, this very high compliance ($\Delta V/\Delta P$) of the bladder is due primarily to its elastic and viscoelastic properties. Elasticity allows the constituents of the bladder wall to stretch to a certain degree without any increase in tension. Viscoelasticity allows stretch to induce a rise in tension followed by a decay (stress relaxation) when the filling (stretch stimulus) slows or stops.
2. **d. augmentation cystoplasty.** The viscoelastic properties of the stroma (bladder wall less smooth muscle and epithelium) and the urodynamically relaxed detrusor muscle account for the passive mechanical properties and normal bladder compliance seen during filling. The main components of stroma are collagen and elastin. When the collagen component increases, compliance decreases. This can occur with various types of injury, chronic inflammation, bladder outlet obstruction, and neurologic decentralization. Once decreased compliance occurs because of a replacement by collagen of other components of the stroma, it is generally unresponsive to pharmacologic manipulation, hydraulic distention, or nerve section. Most often, under those circumstances, augmentation cystoplasty is required to achieve satisfactory reservoir function.
3. **c. gradual increase in striated sphincter activity seen during normal bladder filling/storage.** There is a gradual increase in urethral pressure during bladder filling, contributed to by at least the striated sphincter element and perhaps by the smooth sphincteric element as well. The rise in urethral pressure seen during the filling/storage phase of micturition can be correlated with an increase in efferent pudendal nerve impulse frequency and in electromyographic activity of the periurethral striated musculature. This constitutes the efferent limb of a spinal

somatic reflex, the so-called guarding reflex, which results in a gradual increase in striated sphincter activity during normal bladder filling and storage.

4. **e. neurally mediated sympathetic modulation of cholinergic ganglionic transmission.** Does the nervous system affect the normal bladder response to filling? At a certain level of bladder filling, spinal sympathetic reflexes facilitatory to bladder filling/storage are clearly evoked in animals, a concept developed over the years by deGroat and associates, who have also cited indirect evidence to support such a role in humans. This inhibitory effect is thought to be mediated primarily by sympathetic modulation of cholinergic ganglionic transmission. Through this reflex mechanism, two other possibilities exist for promoting filling/storage. One is neurally mediated stimulation of the predominantly α-adrenergic receptors in the area of the smooth sphincter, the net result of which would be to cause an increase in resistance in that area. The second is neurally mediated stimulation of the predominantly β-adrenergic receptors (inhibitory) in the bladder body smooth musculature, which would cause a decrease in bladder wall tension. McGuire has also cited evidence for direct inhibition of detrusor motor neurons in the sacral spinal cord during bladder filling that is due to increased afferent pudendal nerve activity generated by receptors in the striated sphincter. Good evidence also seems to exist to support a tonic inhibitory effect of other neurotransmitters on the micturition reflex at various levels of the neural axis. Bladder filling and consequent wall distention may also release autocrine-like factors that influence contractility (e.g., nitric oxide, prostaglandins, and peptides).

5. **a. pontine mesencephalic formation in the brain stem.** Although the origin of the parasympathetic neural outflow to the bladder, the pelvic nerve, is in the sacral spinal cord, the actual organizational center for the micturition reflex in an intact neural axis is in the brain stem, and the complete neural circuit for normal micturition includes the ascending and descending spinal cord pathways to and from this area and the facilitatory and inhibitory influences from other parts of the brain.

6. **c. suprasacral neurologic disease or injury.** Involuntary contractions (IVCs) are most commonly seen associated with suprasacral neurologic disease or after suprasacral neurologic injury; however, they may also be associated with aging, inflammation or irritation of the bladder wall, bladder outlet obstruction, or stress urinary incontinence, or they may be idiopathic.

7. **a. failure to store because of the bladder (overactivity).** The classic symptoms of post-stroke lower urinary tract dysfunction are urgency, frequency, and possible urgency incontinence. The urodynamic findings are generally detrusor overactivity during filling/storage with normal sensation and synergic sphincter activity during voluntary or involuntary emptying, unless the patient attempts to inhibit the involuntary contractions with striated sphincter contraction. This translates very simply in the functional system to a failure to store because of the bladder. See Tables 57-1 and 57-5.

8. **e. overactive neurogenic detrusor activity, normal sensation, low capacity, normal compliance, normal urethral closure function; during emptying, normal detrusor activity, normal urethral function.** The micturition dysfunction of a stroke patient with urgency incontinence would most likely be classified during storage as overactive neurogenic detrusor function, normal sensation, low capacity, normal compliance, and normal urethral closure function. During voiding, the dysfunction would be classified as normal detrusor activity and normal urethral function, assuming that no anatomic obstruction existed. See Table 57-6.

9. **d. neurogenic detrusor overactivity.** The Standardization Subcommittee of the ICS made some changes in definitions of terms (published as a committee report in 2002). One change was to eliminate the terms *detrusor hyperreflexia* and *instability* and replace them with *neurogenic detrusor overactivity* and *idiopathic detrusor activity* (Urology 61:37, 2003).

10. **b. detrusor hyperreflexia, striated sphincter synergia, smooth sphincter dyssynergia.** When exact urodynamic classification is possible, this system provides a truly precise description of the voiding dysfunction that occurs. If a normal or hyperreflexic detrusor exists with coordinated smooth and striated sphincter function and without anatomic obstruction, normal bladder emptying should occur.

    Detrusor hyperreflexia is most commonly associated with neurologic lesions above the sacral spinal cord. Striated sphincter dyssynergia is most common after complete suprasacral spinal cord injury, following the period of spinal shock. Smooth sphincter dyssynergia is seen most classically in autonomic hyperreflexia, when it is characteristically associated with detrusor hyperreflexia and striated sphincter dyssynergia.

    Detrusor areflexia may be secondary to bladder muscle decompensation or to various other conditions that produce inhibition at the level of the brain stem micturition center, sacral spinal cord, bladder ganglia, or bladder smooth muscle. Patients with a voiding dysfunction secondary to detrusor areflexia generally attempt bladder emptying by abdominal straining, and their continence status and the efficiency of their emptying efforts are determined by the status of their smooth and striated sphincter mechanisms.

11. **c. uninhibited neurogenic bladder.** Lapides contributed significantly to the classification and care of the patient with neuropathic voiding dysfunction by slightly modifying and popularizing a system originally proposed by McLellan in 1939. Lapides' classification differs from that of McLellan in only one respect, and that is the division of the group "atonic neurogenic bladder" into sensory neurogenic bladder and motor neurogenic bladder. This remains one of the most familiar systems to urologists and nonurologists because it describes in recognizable shorthand the clinical and cystometric conditions of many types of neurogenic voiding dysfunction. An uninhibited neurogenic bladder was described originally as resulting from injury or disease to the "corticoregulatory tract." The sacral spinal cord was presumed to be the micturition reflex center, and this corticoregulatory tract was believed to normally exert an inhibitory influence on the sacral micturition reflex center. A destructive lesion in this tract would then result in overfacilitation of the micturition reflex. Cerebrovascular accident, brain or spinal cord tumor, Parkinson's disease, and demyelinating disease were listed as the most common causes in this category. The voiding dysfunction is most often characterized symptomatically by frequency, urgency, and urge incontinence, and urodynamically by normal sensation with IVC at low filling volumes. Residual urine is characteristically low unless anatomic outlet obstruction or true smooth or striated sphincter dyssynergia occurs. The patient can generally initiate a bladder contraction voluntarily but is often unable to do so during cystometry because sufficient urine storage cannot occur before the IVC is stimulated.

12. **a. traumatic spinal cord injury between the sacral spinal cord and the brain stem.** Reflex neurogenic bladder describes the post–spinal shock condition that exists after complete interruption of the sensory and motor pathways between the sacral spinal cord and the brain stem. Most commonly, this occurs in traumatic spinal cord injury and transverse myelitis, but it may occur with extensive demyelinating disease or any

process that produces significant spinal cord destruction as well. Typically, there is no bladder sensation and there is inability to initiate voluntary micturition. Incontinence without sensation generally results because of low-volume IVC. Striated sphincter dyssynergia is the rule. This type of lesion is essentially equivalent to a complete UMN lesion in the Bors-Comarr system.

13. **e. sphincter dyssynergia.** This system applies only to patients with neurologic dysfunction and considers three factors: (1) the anatomic localization of the lesion; (2) the neurologic completeness or incompleteness of the lesion; and (3) a designation as to whether lower urinary tract function is balanced or unbalanced. The latter terms are based solely on the percentage of residual urine relative to bladder capacity. *Unbalanced* signifies the presence of greater than 20% residual urine in a patient with a UMN lesion or 10% in a patient with an LMN lesion. This relative residual urine volume was ideally meant to imply coordination (synergy) or dyssynergia between the smooth and striated sphincters of the outlet and the bladder, during bladder contraction or during attempted micturition by abdominal straining or the Credé method.

14. **a. a UMN lesion, complete, balanced.** In this system, *UMN bladder* refers to the pattern of micturition that results from an injury to the suprasacral spinal cord after the period of spinal shock has passed, assuming that the sacral spinal cord and the sacral nerve roots are intact and that the pelvic and pudendal nerve reflexes are intact. *LMN bladder* refers to the pattern resulting if the sacral spinal cord or sacral roots are damaged and the reflex pattern through the autonomic and somatic nerves that emanate from these segments is absent. This system implies that if skeletal muscle spasticity exists below the level of the lesion, the lesion is above the sacral spinal cord and is by definition a UMN lesion. This type of lesion is characterized by IVCs during filling. If flaccidity of the skeletal musculature below the level of a lesion exists, an LMN lesion is assumed to exist, implying detrusor areflexia. Exceptions occur and are classified in a mixed lesion group characterized either by IVCs with a flaccid paralysis below the level of the lesion or by detrusor areflexia with spasticity or normal skeletal muscle tone neurologically below the lesion level. *UMN lesion, complete, imbalanced* implies a neurologically complete lesion above the level of the sacral spinal cord that results in skeletal muscle spasticity below the level of the injury. IVC occurs during filling, but a residual urine volume of greater than 20% of the bladder capacity is left after bladder contraction, implying obstruction in the area of the bladder outlet during the involuntary detrusor contraction. This obstruction is generally due to striated sphincter dyssynergia, typically occurring in patients who are paraplegic and quadriplegic with lesions between the cervical and the sacral spinal cord. Smooth sphincter dyssynergia may be seen as well in patients with lesions above the level of T6, usually in association with autonomic hyperreflexia. *LMN lesion, complete, imbalanced* implies a neurologically complete lesion at the level of the sacral spinal cord or of the sacral roots, resulting in skeletal muscle flaccidity below that level. Detrusor areflexia results, and whatever measures the patient may use to increase intravesical pressure during attempted voiding are not sufficient to decrease residual urine to less than 10% of bladder capacity.

58

Urodynamic and Video-urodynamic Evaluation of Voiding Dysfunction

ANDREW C. PETERSON • GEORGE D. WEBSTER

QUESTIONS

1. A patient complains of urinary frequency, urgency, and nocturia. He is best described as having:
   a. obstructive symptoms.
   b. irritative symptoms.
   c. prostatism.
   d. storage symptoms.
   e. voiding symptoms.
2. Urinary continence in a neurologically intact male with an involuntary bladder contraction is maintained by:
   a. volitional contraction of the distal sphincter mechanism.
   b. reflex contraction of the distal sphincter.
   c. volitional contraction of the proximal sphincter mechanism.
   d. reflex contraction of the proximal sphincter mechanism.
   e. none of the above.
3. A woman who complains of unconscious leakage may have all of the following EXCEPT:
   a. bladder instability.
   b. intrinsic sphincter deficiency.
   c. vesicovaginal fistula.
   d. urge incontinence.
   e. overflow incontinence.
4. All of the following statements about symptom scores such as the International Prostate Symptom Score (IPSS) and International Continence Society (ICS) male questionnaire are true EXCEPT which one?
   a. They have been validated psychometrically.
   b. They help assess the severity and degree of bother of the lower urinary tract symptoms.
   c. They do not correlate well with urodynamic indices.
   d. They help differentiate between patients who have obstruction and those who do not.
   e. They are not sex specific.
5. Which of the following statements regarding bladder diaries is FALSE? They
   a. allow for quantitation of urinary output.
   b. help determine whether excessive frequency is due to low capacity or polyuria.
   c. correlate well with the patient's subjective estimate of urinary frequency.
   d. assist in the planning of behavioral therapy.
   e. help document triggers for urinary incontinence.
6. Which of the following statements about the bulbocavernosus reflex (BCR) is TRUE?
   a. It tests the integrity of L5-S1 cord segments.
   b. Its absence confirms the presence of a neurologic lesion.
   c. It is the contraction of the gluteus muscles in response to the squeezing of the glans.
   d. It may be maintained in patients with incomplete sacral lesions.
   e. None of the above.
7. All of the following are necessary in the routine workup of a patient with neurogenic bladder EXCEPT:
   a. an upper urinary tract study such as an ultrasonogram or renal scan.
   b. an assessment of reflexes.
   c. a cystoscopy.
   d. a urinalysis.
   e. a serum creatinine assay.
8. Which of the following statements is TRUE about urodynamics?
   a. If the study does not demonstrate unstable contractions, the patient does not have detrusor instability.
   b. A study showing detrusor instability proves that it is the cause of the patient's symptoms.
   c. If a study does not reproduce the patient's symptoms, it is not diagnostic.
   d. It is best to initially use the most sophisticated urodynamics test to make a diagnosis.
   e. None of the above.
9. Clear indications for urodynamic study include all of the following EXCEPT:
   a. patients with persistent LUTS despite presumably adequate therapy.
   b. patients in whom therapy may be hazardous.
   c. women with mixed incontinence after prior anti-continence procedures.
   d. patients with spinal cord injury.
   e. children with isolated nocturnal enuresis.

10. All of the following statements about patient preparation and precautions are true EXCEPT which one?
    a. Urodynamics should be deferred in patients with a urinary tract infection.
    b. Ideally, patients should not have an indwelling Foley catheter before the study.
    c. Ideally, drugs that affect bladder function should be stopped before the study.
    d. Routine antibiotic prophylaxis is needed for all patients.
    e. Patient cooperation is crucial for a successful test.
11. Which of the following statements about autonomic dysreflexia is FALSE?
    a. It is an exaggerated sympathetic response to visceral stimulation.
    b. If a patient experiences it during a urodynamic study, the bladder should be emptied immediately.
    c. It occurs in patients with spinal cord lesions above T6.
    d. Pretreatment with an α-adrenergic blocker or calcium channel blocker may be helpful.
    e. It manifests with sweating, headache, hypertension, and flushing below the level of the lesion.
12. Which of the following statements is TRUE regarding cystometrography (CMG)?
    a. The reference point for external transducers is the umbilicus.
    b. Pressures should be zeroed to atmospheric pressure.
    c. It is the measurement of intravesical pressure during voiding.
    d. Air bubbles in the pressure lines cause increases in pressure measurement.
    e. None of the above.
13. Which of the following statements about fluid factors that affect CMG is FALSE?
    a. Rapid fill rates can produce instability.
    b. Alkaline fluids may result in increased bladder capacity.
    c. Acidic fluids may inhibit unstable contractions.
    d. Rapid fill rates are those that are faster than 100 mL/min.
    e. Fluid temperature should be as close to body temperature as possible.
14. Which of the following statements about detrusor pressure (Pdet) is TRUE?
    a. It is determined with single-channel urodynamics.
    b. It is the component of bladder pressure created by extravesical forces.
    c. It is calculated by adding intravesical pressure (Pves) and abdominal pressure (Pabd).
    d. True changes in Pdet are independent of changes in Pves.
    e. None of the above.
15. The following variables are routinely measured by CMG EXCEPT:
    a. capacity.
    b. compliance.
    c. sensation.
    d. stability.
    e. obstruction.
16. Which of the following statements is TRUE of compliance?
    a. It is the change in volume for given change in pressure.
    b. It is a measure of outlet resistance.
    c. Measured compliance is affected by fill rate.
    d. The normal pressure rise during the course of a cystogram test is 50 cm H_2O.
    e. None of the above.
17. Detrusor overactivity, or an unstable bladder contraction is:
    a. defined as an involuntary pressure rise of greater than 20 cm H_2O.
    b. always demonstrated in patients with urge incontinence.
    c. called neurogenic detrusor overactivity in neurologically intact patients.
    d. inhibited in a patient with sensory urgency.
    e. is always symptomatic.
18. Which of the following statements about provocative testing and pitfalls in CMG is FALSE?
    a. Bethanechol testing is unreliable in diagnosing neurogenic bladder.
    b. The ice water test is used to differentiate upper motor neuron lesions from lower motor neuron lesions.
    c. Vesicoureteral reflux may improve measured bladder compliance.
    d. If the bladder outlet is incompetent, it may be necessary to be occluded with a Foley catheter for accurate measurement.
    e. None of the above.
19. Which of the following statements about detrusor leak-point pressure (DLPP) is TRUE? It is:
    a. the lowest pressure causing urine leakage with abdominal straining.
    b. a reflection of resistance of the urethra to the bladder.
    c. associated with a higher risk of upper tract damage when less than 20.
    d. not affected by catheter size.
    e. determined by bladder outlet resistance.
20. Which of the following statements about Valsalva leak-point pressure (VLPP) is TRUE?
    a. A normally positioned and functioning urethra can be caused to leak by straining.
    b. A low Valsalva leak-point means that stress incontinence is the sole cause of incontinence.
    c. There is good correlation between Valsalva leak-point pressure and maximum urethral closing pressure.
    d. The Valsalva leak-point pressure is the highest abdominal pressure that causes incontinence.
    e. None of the above.
21. A high VLPP may be caused by each of the following EXCEPT:
    a. prolapse.
    b. anxiety.
    c. poor bladder compliance.
    d. large catheter size.
    e. All of the above cause a high VLPP.
22. Which of the following statements about uroflow is TRUE?
    a. The uroflow pattern of a plateau with a prolonged flow time is diagnostic of bladder outlet obstruction.
    b. Qmax is affected by age in patients of both sexes.
    c. A difference in Qmax on repeated testing may be spurious.
    d. All voids of less than 150 mL should be disregarded.
    e. A flow rate of greater than 15 mL/s rules out bladder outlet obstruction.
23. Which of the following statements about pressure-flow studies is TRUE?
    a. Size of the urethral filling catheter does not seem to be important.
    b. If a patient is unable to void, he has abnormal detrusor activity (acontractile detrusor).
    c. Postmicturition contractions are more common in patients with detrusor overactivity than in those without.
    d. Normal postvoid residual rules out bladder outlet obstruction.
    e. Bladder outlet obstruction can be diagnosed only if Pdet is greater than 100 cm H_2O.

24. Which of the following is true of the Abrams-Griffith (AG) nomogram?
    a. It uses the maximum detrusor pressure during voiding as the most important variable.
    b. It clearly divides patients into obstructed versus unobstructed groups.
    c. It can help grade the degree of obstruction by calculating the AG number.
    d. It has been validated for use in both men and women with obstruction.
    e. It is based on the detrusor contractility being the only important variable in diagnosing bladder outlet obstruction.

25. Which of the following is true of the ICS nomogram?
    a. It is based on the fact that the various models of urethral resistance are different.
    b. It allows for continuous grading of obstruction by calculating the bladder outlet obstruction index (BOOI).
    c. It is essentially identical to the Schaffer nomogram in appearance.
    d. It is intended for use in females with possible bladder outlet obstruction.
    e. It relies solely on flow rate, obviating the need for invasive testing.

26. Ambulatory urodynamics is thought to be advantageous over conventional urodynamics because it:
    a. predominantly uses natural filling and allows the subject to reproduce normal activities.
    b. does not require much patient compliance.
    c. is less likely to document insignificant detrusor overactivity.
    d. can better classify patients as obstructed versus unobstructed.
    e. tends to exaggerate the magnitude of low bladder compliance.

27. Advantages of video-urodynamics include the ability to:
    a. determine the presence and location of obstruction.
    b. determine the significance of an open bladder neck.
    c. diagnose detrusor sphincter dyssynergy.
    d. determine the significance of vesicoureteral reflux.
    e. all of the above.

28. Which statement about kinesiologic sphincter electromyography (EMG) is TRUE? It:
    a. determines whether the bladder and external sphincter are coordinated.
    b. helps to diagnose neuropathy.
    c. measures latency responses.
    d. tests the integrity of peripheral nervous pathways.
    e. requires the use of an oscilloscope.

29. Detrusor sphincter dyssynergy (DSD):
    a. is the technical term for dysfunctional voiding in neurologically impaired patients.
    b. is the term for delayed sphincter relaxation in patients with Parkinson's disease.
    c. typically occurs in patients with suprasacral cord injuries.
    d. is the relaxation of the bladder neck that occurs during a detrusor contraction.
    e. is the normal response of the external sphincter during unstable bladder contraction.

30. On neurophysiologic testing, neuropathy is implied by:
    a. polyphasic potentials that constitute greater than 15% of all activity.
    b. complex repetitive discharges.
    c. positive sharp waves.
    d. fibrillation potentials.
    e. all of the above.

31. Signal processing includes all of the following factors EXCEPT:
    a. amplification.
    b. filtration.
    c. integration.
    d. differentiation.
    e. display.

32. A 70-year-old man with a history of dementia is being evaluated for urinary incontinence. The initial workup before urodynamics should include all of the following EXCEPT:
    a. urinalysis with culture
    b. mental status exam
    c. medication and review
    d. uroflow and postvoid residual
    e. baseline upper tract imaging study (renal ultrasound, nuclear scan)

33. Normal function of the lower urinary tract is characterized by:
    a. storage of urine at low pressure.
    b. storage of urine at high pressure.
    c. voiding of urine at high pressure.
    d. high activity of the urinary sphincter on electromyelogram during voiding.
    e. closed bladder neck during voiding.

34. Which of the following factors will influence results of a video-urodynamic study?
    a. Rate of infusion
    b. Temperature of the fluid
    c. pH of the fluid
    d. Presence of vesicoureteral reflux
    e. All of the above

35. Which of the following may be recorded during a video-urodynamic study?
    a. Electromyelogram
    b. Voiding cystourethrogram
    c. Uroflow data
    d. Valsalva leak-point pressure
    e. All of the above

36. Possible technical reasons for problems with signal trends action from the intravesical catheter include all of the following EXCEPT:
    a. poor position of the catheter within the bladder.
    b. air bubbles within the line.
    c. obstruction or kinking of the tubing.
    d. fast, rather than physiologic, fill rate.
    e. equipment malfunction (poor connection of transducer to sensor).

37. All of the following about transducers are true EXCEPT which one?
    a. Fluid-filled transducers are zeroed at that level of the symphysis pubis.
    b. The measurement of bladder pressures using the microtip transducer is independent of its position within the bladder.
    c. Bladder pressure is measured in cm H_2O.
    d. To decrease the amount of error, external transducers connected to fluid-filled tubing are used for abdominal and vesical measurements.
    e. All of the above.

38. All of the following are true about catheters EXCEPT which one?
    a. The smallest possible diameter of catheter is used to prevent artifact during the study.
    b. Simultaneous filling and pressure transduction are performed with a dual-lumen 7-Fr catheter.
    c. When using single-lumen infusion catheters, 5 Fr or smaller sizes are desirable to prevent artifact during the urination phase of the study.
    d. When using a rectal balloon catheter, the balloon is filled to only 10% to 20% capacity.
    e. The suprapubic placement of catheters is reserved only in specific circumstances such as stricture disease.

39. All of the following about uroflow are true EXCEPT which one?
    a. The documented flow curve is always smoothed by hand to exclude computer analysis error.
    b. The maximum flow rate (Qmax) is not dependent on the total volume voided.
    c. Different machines are calibrated to density of the fluid used to obtain accurate measurements.
    d. Flow rates decline with age in men but remain stable in women.
    e. Uroflow curve shape gives evidence without the aid of pressure-flow studies or video-urodynamics as to the etiology of the urination symptoms.

ANSWERS

1. **d. storage symptoms.** *Voiding symptoms* is the term used to replace *obstructive symptoms* and includes the symptoms of hesitancy, slow stream, intermittency, straining to void, terminal dribbling, and a feeling of incomplete emptying. *Storage symptoms* replaces the term *irritative symptoms* for the symptoms of frequency, nocturia, urgency, and urge incontinence.

2. **a. volitional contraction of the distal sphincter mechanism.** With an involuntary bladder contraction, the bladder neck automatically opens and continence must be maintained by the volitional contraction of the distal sphincter mechanism.

3. **d. urge incontinence. In some patients, incontinence occurs in the absence of any obvious increase in intra-abdominal pressure, without an urge to void or any conscious recognition that leakage is occurring.** This is called unconscious incontinence and may be secondary to unstable bladder contractions, intrinsic sphincter deficiency, overflow incontinence, or extraurethral incontinence, such as that caused by a fistula.

4. **d. They help differentiate between patients who have obstruction and those who do not.** Although the IPSS has been formally validated with both clinimetric and psychometric principles, the symptoms it grades are not specific to benign prostatic hyperplasia and are also common in women. Furthermore, although the system tests the degree to which symptoms are present and bothersome, they do not correlate with urodynamic indices such as the presence of detrusor instability or bladder outlet obstruction. In fact, symptomatic patients with bladder outlet obstruction do not have significantly different scores from those who are not obstructed (who have detrusor dysfunction).

5. **c. correlate well with the patient's subjective estimate of urinary frequency. A 3- to 5-day voiding diary is one of the most helpful tools in the assessment of voiding dysfunction.** From this record, the total 24-hour urinary output, number of voids, voiding interval, diurnal distribution, timing and triggers for incontinence, and functional bladder capacity may be determined. In fact, it may be more reliable than the patient's own history, because there is often no correlation between the number of voids per patient history compared with the number documented on a voiding diary.

6. **d. It may be maintained in patients with incomplete sacral lesions.** The normal BCR is the contraction of the anal sphincter and bulbocavernosus muscles in response to such maneuvers as placing an examining finger in the patient's rectum and then either squeezing the glans penis or clitoris or pulling on an indwelling Foley catheter. This is primarily a test of the integrity of spinal cord segments S2-S4. Thirty percent of neurologically intact females have an absent BCR, and patients with incomplete sacral lesions may maintain the reflex, and thus the presence or absence of the reflex does not establish the diagnosis of a neurologic lesion.

7. **c. cystoscopy.** In the routine evaluation of a patient with a neurogenic bladder, an assessment of reflexes, a urinalysis, a serum creatinine assay, and a baseline upper tract imaging study (intravenous pyelogram, ultrasonogram, or renal scan) are indicated. Endoscopic evaluation of the lower urinary tract is not indicated in the routine screening of patients with neurogenic bladder.

8. **c. If a study does not reproduce the patient's symptoms, it is not diagnostic.** The goal in performing a urodynamic study is to answer specific questions related to the patient's storage and voiding functions. Nitti noted three important principles: (1) a study that does not duplicate the patient's symptoms is not diagnostic; (2) failure to record an abnormality does not rule out its existence; and (3) not all abnormalities detected are clinically significant.

9. **e. children with isolated nocturnal enuresis.** Clear indications for some type of urodynamic investigation, however, include patients with persistent LUTS despite presumed appropriate therapy and patients in whom potential therapy may be hazardous (one would want to be sure of the correct diagnosis before instituting such therapy). Other indications for some type of urodynamic investigation include women with recurrent incontinence in whom surgery is planned, those with a confusing mix of stress and urge symptoms, and those with associated voiding problems. All neurologically impaired patients who have neurogenic bladder dysfunction should undergo urodynamic study to characterize the nature of the detrusor and sphincter problem and to determine prognosis and management. Children with isolated nocturnal enuresis rarely have abnormalities that are identified by routine laboratory-based urodynamic investigations.

10. **d. Routine antibiotic prophylaxis is needed for all patients.** Urodynamic studies are invasive and have been associated with morbidity, including urinary retention, hematuria, urinary tract infection, and pain. Studies should be deferred in the presence of urinary tract infection and ideally should not be performed after recent instrumentation (e.g., cystoscopy). Urinary tract infection and indwelling catheters may result in altered bladder dynamics (e.g., loss of compliance, reduced capacity) that may not otherwise exist. Patients who are catheter dependent ideally should have the catheter removed and have clean intermittent catheterization for a period of time before the urodynamic study is undertaken. Many pharmacologic agents can significantly affect detrusor or

sphincteric function, and either patients should stop these medications or their impact on the urodynamic study should be taken into account. Routine oral prophylactic antibacterial drugs are not necessary.

11. **e. It manifests with sweating, headache, hypertension, and flushing below the level of the lesion.** Autonomic dysreflexia is an exaggerated sympathetic nervous system response to afferent visceral stimulation that occurs in patients with high neurologic lesions above the sympathetic outflow tract (at or above T6). It manifests with symptoms such as sweating, headache, flushing above the level of the lesion, severe (possibly life-threatening) hypertension, and reflex bradycardia. If the patient begins to experience these symptoms during a urodynamic study, the bladder should be emptied immediately and the patient given an antihypertensive, such as sublingual nifedipine (10 mg) or intravenous hydralazine if the condition does not resolve rapidly. In patients with a known diagnosis of autonomic dysreflexia, blood pressure should be monitored throughout the test and pretreatment with sublingual nifedipine or an α-adrenergic blocking agent may be used.
12. **b. Pressures should be zeroed to atmospheric pressure.** Cystometry is the measurement of intravesical pressure during the course of bladder filling. When external transducers are used, the reference point is the superior edge of the pubic symphysis. All systems should be zeroed to atmospheric pressure, and it is crucial that there are no air bubbles in any of the transducers or tubing that could otherwise cause pressure dampening or dissipation.
13. **c. Acidic fluids may inhibit unstable contractions.** An alkaline pH (>8.5) has been noted to increase bladder capacity in patients with instability, whereas an acidic solution (pH < 3.5) can provoke instability in otherwise stable bladders.
14. **e. None of the above.** A shortcoming of single-channel cystometry is that the measured Pves represents a summation of the pressure caused by bladder wall events (e.g., detrusor contraction, Pdet), and the pressure caused by extravesical sources (e.g., abdominal straining, Pabd). Thus, when there is a rise in bladder pressure recorded using single-channel cystometry (Pves), one cannot be sure whether this is due to a bladder contraction or to increases in intra-abdominal pressure that are transmitted to the bladder, or both. The use of multichannel cystometry, whereby a catheter that records abdominal pressure is used in addition to an intravesical catheter, allows for the determination of the contributions of the individual components of Pves, Pdet, and Pabd. Because Pdet is the component of Pves that is created by the contractile forces within the bladder wall, it is the critical pressure to measure. However, it cannot be measured directly; it is rather obtained by subtracting the abdominal pressure from the total vesical pressure (Pdet = Pves – Pabd), which is done electronically. Pabd is generally recorded by a catheter placed in the rectum. The rectum is close to the bladder and thus theoretically the intra-abdominal pressure experienced by both should be similar. A change in either Pabd or Pdet should be accompanied by a change in Pves. If Pabd changes independently of Pves, then the subtracted Pdet will also change, but this will be an artifact (poor pressure transmission, rectal contraction); true detrusor pressure cannot change in the absence of a change in Pves.
15. **e. obstruction.** During the course of cystometry, information is sought regarding four bladder characteristics: (1) capacity, (2) sensation, (3) compliance, and (4) the occurrence of involuntary contractions.
16. **c. Measured compliance is affected by fill rate.** Bladder compliance is defined as the change in bladder pressure for a given change in volume. It is a measure of bladder elasticity and reflects the sum of two forces: a mechanical force proportional to the amount of collagen present in the bladder wall and a neuromuscular force called tonus. The measured compliance is also variably dependent on the fill rate. Customarily, the pressure rise during the course of CMG in the normal bladder will be only 6 to 10 cm H_2O (see Fig. 58-6).
17. **d. is inhibited in a patient with sensory urgency.** The unstable bladder is one that can be demonstrated to contract either spontaneously or with provocative maneuvers during filling cystometry while the patient is trying to inhibit micturition. When it occurs in a patient with neurologic disease (e.g., spinal cord injury, cerebrovascular accident, demyelinating disease), it is called neurogenic detrusor overactivity; in the absence of neurologic disease, it is called idiopathic detrusor overactivity. The absence of documented instability on CMG does not rule out its existence. As many as 40% of people with motor urge incontinence will not demonstrate detrusor overactivity on CMG.
18. **c. Vesicoureteral reflux may improve measured bladder compliance.** The bethanechol supersensitivity test was originally described by Lapides and colleagues to try to distinguish between a neurogenic and a myogenic cause in a patient with an acontractile bladder. It is based on the observation that after an organ is deprived of its nerve supply, it develops hypersensitivity to the normal excitatory neurotransmitters for that organ. The test has been shown to be unreliable, however. A positive test by itself does not indicate a neurogenic bladder and a negative test does not rule it out. The ice water test was first described by Bors and Blinn in 1957 as a way to differentiate upper from lower motor neuron lesions. It is based on the principle that mucosal temperature receptors can elicit a spinal reflex contraction of the detrusor, a reflex that is normally inhibited by supraspinal centers. On cystometry, if the bladder outlet is incompetent, urine may leak around the filling catheter and a low bladder compliance may be not be diagnosed because the bladder is never adequately filled (e.g., spinal dysraphism, severe intrinsic sphincter deficiency in an older woman). In this scenario, the CMG test should be repeated using a Foley catheter for bladder filling, with the distended catheter balloon pulled down to occlude the bladder neck. In patients with massive reflux, large volumes of the filling solution reflux into the dilated upper tracts and a low capacity/low compliance detrusor may be missed because of this "pop off" mechanism.
19. **b. a reflection of resistance of the urethra to the bladder.** DLPP is defined as the lowest bladder pressure (in the absence of a detrusor contraction) at which leakage occurs across the urethra. As such, it is a reflection of the resistance of the urethra to the bladder and a measure of the storage pressures in the bladder (i.e., compliance). An important concept in urodynamics is the fact that bladder outlet resistance is the main determinant of detrusor pressure. If the outlet resistance is high, a higher bladder pressure will be needed to overcome this resistance and cause leakage. McGuire's group found that in myelodysplastic patients (who have elevated outlet resistance due to fixed external sphincters), those with DLPP values greater than 40 cm H_2O were at significantly higher risk for upper tract deterioration (hydronephrosis, reflux) than those with DLPP values less than 40 cm H_2O. Catheter size has not been standardized for the test, but it appears that catheter size can affect the results.
20. **e. None of the above.** VLPP or abdominal leak-point pressure is the lowest abdominal pressure that causes leakage of urine across the urethra in the absence of a bladder contraction. Whereas the detrusor pressure tends to force the urethral sphincter open, the abdominal pressure will not open a

urethral sphincter if the urethra is normally positioned and closed. If leakage is caused by an increase in abdominal pressure, then the urethra must be abnormal. If there is no leakage at high pressures (>150 cm H_2O), then the urethra is unlikely to be the cause of the patient's incontinence and rather the bladder is the more likely culprit. However, the converse is not true (i.e., a low VLPP does not rule out a significant detrusor-related component to the incontinence). A poor correlation between VLPP and MUCP has been noted by several authors, which is not surprising because the MUCP is a reflection of the urethral resistance to detrusor pressure and as such is more related to the DLPP than to the VLPP.

21. **c. poor bladder compliance.** There is evidence that VLPP is affected by catheter size and that anterior vaginal wall prolapse (i.e., cystocele) may artificially elevate the VLPP. Other potential artifacts are related to patient anxiety and cooperation.

22. **c. A difference in Qmax on repeated testing may be spurious.** The flow pattern, that is, the shape of the flow tracing, can sometimes be used to make a presumptive diagnosis, although it cannot be used to make a definitive diagnosis. The typical obstructed flow pattern has a plateau-shaped curve with a prolonged flow time, sustained low flow rate, and increased time to Qmax. This is not diagnostic of outlet obstruction because detrusor hypocontractility can give a similar tracing. Furthermore, a high flow rate (>15 mL/s) does not rule out bladder outlet obstruction. In men Qmax decreases with age, whereas in women it is not influenced by age. It has been documented that 40% of men have a difference in Qmax of at least 2 mL/s between voids and 20% of men may have a difference of at least 4 mL/s. Thus, it has been recommended by some that multiple flow rates be recorded to increase the likelihood that a representative flow is achieved. The volume voided probably has the greatest effect on peak flow rate, and it is generally accepted that voided volumes of less than 150 mL generate inaccurate flow patterns and parameters. However, voids of less than 150 mL can provide useful information (particularly in truly obstructed patients) and thus should not be discarded.

23. **c. Postmicturition contractions are more common in patients with detrusor overactivity than in those without.** Catheter size may influence the results of pressure-flow studies, and the larger the catheter, the greater the chance that the catheter will cause some degree of outlet obstruction. Failure to void during a pressure-flow study does not in and of itself indicate a functional abnormality, because many patients find it difficult to void in the setting of the urodynamic laboratory. Postvoid residual urine is the volume of urine remaining in the bladder immediately after voiding. Although the testing situation often leads to inefficient voiding and a falsely elevated residual urine volume, the absence of residual urine does not exclude infravesical obstruction or bladder dysfunction. Postmicturition contraction (after-contraction) is a reiteration of the detrusor contraction after flow has ceased, and its magnitude is typically greater than that of the micturition pressure at maximum flow. These are not well understood, but they seem to be more common in patients with unstable or hypersensitive bladders. There is no consensus regarding a critical value for pressure and flow that is diagnostic for obstruction. Outlet obstruction is suggested by a pressure-flow study in which low flow occurs despite a detrusor contraction of adequate force, duration, and speed, regardless of the actual numerical values.

24. **c. It can help grade the degree of obstruction by calculating the AG number.** The degree of obstruction can be graded by using the AG number, which is derived from the equation for the slope of the line that divides the obstructed group from the equivocal group on the AG nomogram and is calculated by the formula AG number = PdetQmax – 2Qmax.

25. **b. It allows for continuous grading of obstruction by calculating the bladder outlet obstruction index (BOOI).** A continuous grading of obstruction is possible by calculating the BOOI, which is essentially the AG number, given by the formula: BOOI = PdetQmax – 2Qmax.

26. **a. predominantly uses natural filling and allows the subject to reproduce normal activities.** Ambulatory urodynamic monitoring (AUM) is defined as any functional test of the lower urinary tract predominantly utilizing natural filling of the urinary tract and reproducing the subject's normal activity. As such, the unphysiologic nature of conventional urodynamics (filling by rapid infusion through a catheter, monitoring in a laboratory setting) is avoided and the patient may move about and continue with the activities of daily living that may trigger the presenting symptoms (e.g., urgency, incontinence). However, the patient must play an active role in the performance of AUM because the test is not confined to a laboratory with staff monitoring. This reliance on patient compliance may be a source of significant error. Studies have shown that AUM is more sensitive than conventional CMG in the detection of detrusor overactivity, in both symptomatic and asymptomatic subjects, and furthermore that AUM can detect detrusor overactivity in patients in whom CMG is nondiagnostic. However, the significance of this increased detection of DI is unclear, given the high incidence found in asymptomatic patients. Studies have shown that in neurogenic patients, filling pressures with AUM tend to be significantly lower than those with conventional CMG, and patients with hydronephrosis and high end filling pressures (and low compliance) on CMG were found to have normal filling pressures on AUM. Instead, these patients were found to have increased phasic detrusor activity on AUM that correlated with the presence of upper tract changes. It has therefore been hypothesized that the high end filling pressure (and thus low compliance) seen on conventional CMG may, in fact, be an artifact related to the high phasic activity on AUM being converted to low compliance by the more rapid (and unphysiologic) filling of conventional CMG. AUM has not been clearly demonstrated to better classify patients as having obstructed versus unobstructed conditions.

27. **e. all of the above.** Simultaneous fluoroscopic screening of the bladder outlet during voiding and while pressure-flow data are being recorded helps to identify the site of the obstruction as being at the bladder neck, prostatic urethra, or distal sphincter mechanism (see Fig. 58-12). It is particularly useful in the identification of bladder neck dysfunction and in the identification of dyssynergia of the proximal and distal sphincter mechanisms in neurogenic patients; in determining whether an open bladder neck in the absence of a detrusor contraction in a woman with stress incontinence may be a sign of intrinsic sphincter deficiency; and in identifying and characterizing pathology that can be associated with complex voiding dysfunction including reflux, diverticula, fistulas, and stones.

28. **a. It determines whether the bladder and external sphincter are coordinated.** Clinically, the most important information obtained from sphincter EMG is whether there is coordination or discoordination between the external sphincter and the bladder.

29. **c. typically occurs in patients with suprasacral cord injuries.** DSD typically occurs in patients with suprasacral spinal cord injury in which there is an interruption of the

spinobulbar-spinal pathways that normally coordinate the detrusor and sphincter muscles.

30. **e. all of the above.** Normal muscle may have up to 15% of its activity in the form of such polyphasic potentials; however, when the amount of polyphasic activity is significantly greater than this, neuropathy is implied. Spontaneous firing of groups of muscle fibers may be seen in denervated muscles and causes complex repetitive discharges. Positive sharp waves are seen in denervated muscle and are closely associated with fibrillation potentials. The fibrillation potential is characterized as a low amplitude and very short signal seen with muscle denervation.

31. **e. display.** Signal processing is the process by which the raw data are amplified, filtered, and converted to a recorded signal that may be interpreted as one urodynamic datum. Transducers sense the signal, which is then processed by amplification. Filtration, integration, differentiation, and conversion from analog to digital are all parts of this process. The urodynamic datum is then displayed either on chart, magnetic tape, oscilloscope, or computer (Rowan, 1987).

32. **e. Baseline upper tract imaging study (renal ultrasound, nuclear scan).** In patients with dementia and new-onset urination symptoms, a screening history, physical examination with complete review of medications, and neurologic evaluation are imperative. We believe the noninvasive uroflow and bladder scan should be performed before any invasive urodynamic testing because these can often answer many of the questions the patient presents with. Upper tract imaging studies are required in those with lower urinary tract findings that may cause damage over time.

33. **a. storage of urine at low pressure.** The optimum function of the lower urinary tract includes low-pressure storage, stable detrusor muscle, and coordinated urination phase. The voiding or micturition phase should include coordinated relaxation of the sphincter, contraction of the detrusor muscle, with near-complete evacuation of urine with high flow and low pressure.

34. **e. All of the above.** The infusion rate can affect outcomes of urodynamics with faster than normal rates promoting detrusor instability. The acidity of the infusing can cause unstable contractions artificially, as can temperature, as seen with the ice water test. Vesicoureteral reflux may change compliance readings as well as volume data.

35. **e. All of the above.** Video-urodynamics gives information with both pressure readings as well as fluoroscopic images for all phases of bladder activity, including filling, storage, and emptying. This is the most complex form of bladder testing utilizing intravesical pressure catheters and real-time fluoroscopic imaging while using contrast media as a filling agent.

36. **d. fast, rather than physiologic fill rate.** During urodynamics the clinician must have an understanding of the clinical question to be answered, basic physiology, basic biophysics, and a practical working knowledge of the equipment being used. Sources of artifact in pressure monitoring include poor placement of catheters, kinking of the catheter tubing or the catheter itself, air within the system that inhibits conductance of the signal, poor connection of the transducer with sensor equipment, and malfunction of computer equipment or sensor. One must be familiar with the basic mechanical parameters of the urodynamic equipment being used. The rate of fill may result in detrusor overactivity however, it should not produce artifact during pressure measurements directly.

37. **b. The measurement of bladder pressures using the microtip transducer is independent of its position within the bladder.** Pressure measurements performed with fluid-filled transducers are independent of the location of the tip of the transducer within the bladder. Microtip transducers, however, are dependent on their location within the bladder, thus possibly giving artifact. Fluid-filled transducers should be zeroed at the level of the symphysis pubis (Rowan, 1987).

38. **c. When using single-lumen catheters, 5-Fr or smaller sizes are desirable to prevent artifact during the urination phase of the study.** Catheters smaller then 6 Fr may limit the infusion rate and pressure provided by the pump during the filling phase of urodynamics to 20 to 30 mL/min. This may result in an offset of the amount of fluid actually pumped into the bladder versus what is recorded by the pump. Therefore, all volumes and pressure readings will be suspect. The current recommendation is for use of a two-lumen catheter 6 Fr or larger.

39. **b. The maximum flow rate (Qmax) is not dependent on the total volume voided.** Qmax is physiologically dependent on the bladder volume. As the bladder volume increases, detrusor muscle fibers become more stretched. At volumes greater than 400 to 500 mL, contractility may decrease because of this stretch. This may vary between individuals and with the type and degree of pathology (Schafer et al, 2002). It is important that the patient fully understand how the measurements are being recorded during uroflow. Disk-type flowmeters are susceptible to flow direction and thus, depending on where the stream hits the disk, different flow rate measurements may be possible. Therefore, the flow curves must be inspected visually to rule out artifacts and the patient must be appropriately instructed as to how to conduct the study. (Grino et al, 1993).

59

Lower Urinary Tract Dysfunction in Neurologic Injury and Disease

ALAN J. WEIN

QUESTIONS

1. What is the general pattern of voiding dysfunction secondary to neurologic lesions above the level of the brain stem?
   a. Involuntary bladder contractions, smooth sphincter dyssynergia, striated sphincter synergy.
   b. Involuntary bladder contractions, smooth sphincter synergy, striated sphincter synergy.
   c. Involuntary bladder contractions, smooth sphincter synergy, striated sphincter dyssynergia.
   d. Detrusor hypocontractility, smooth sphincter synergy, striated sphincter synergy.
   e. Detrusor areflexia, smooth sphincter synergy, striated sphincter synergy.
2. What is the general pattern of voiding dysfunction that results from complete lesions of the spinal cord above the level of S2 after recovery from spinal shock?
   a. Involuntary bladder contractions, smooth sphincter dyssynergia, striated sphincter synergy.
   b. Involuntary bladder contractions, smooth sphincter synergy, striated sphincter synergy.
   c. Involuntary bladder contractions, smooth sphincter synergy, striated sphincter dyssynergia.
   d. Detrusor hypocontractility, smooth sphincter synergy, striated sphincter synergy.
   e. Detrusor areflexia, smooth sphincter synergy, striated sphincter synergy.
3. Which of the following is the most common long-term expression of lower urinary tract dysfunction after a cerebrovascular accident (CVA)?
   a. Detrusor areflexia
   b. Lack of sensation of filling
   c. Impaired bladder contractility
   d. Striated sphincter dyssynergia
   e. Detrusor overactivity
4. Urinary incontinence is most likely to occur in a patient after a CVA if which of the following areas is affected?
   a. Internal capsule
   b. Basal ganglia
   c. Thalamus
   d. Cerebellum
   e. Hypothalamus
5. In a post-CVA patient who exhibits urgency and frequency but no incontinence, the state of striated sphincter activity can most commonly be best described as:
   a. uninhibited relaxation.
   b. dyssynergia.
   c. fixed voluntary tone.
   d. pseudodyssynergia.
   e. myotonus.
6. You are asked to evaluate and treat a 65-year-old man who has sustained a stroke but who is otherwise in good health. He has symptoms of hesitancy, straining to void, urgency, and frequency. The optimal next step in management is:
   a. anticholinergic therapy
   b. transurethral resection of the prostate
   c. transurethral incision of the bladder neck and prostate
   d. clean intermittent catheterization
   e. full urodynamic evaluation.
7. When considering the subject of voiding dysfunction associated with brain tumors, which of the following areas is more likely to be associated with urinary retention than with urinary incontinence?
   a. Pituitary gland
   b. Cerebellum
   c. Posterior fossa
   d. Hypothalamus
   e. Frontal cortex
8. The most common pattern of micturition in children and adults who have cerebral palsy (CP) and no other complicating neurologic condition is:
   a. abnormal filling/storage because of detrusor overactivity; normal emptying.
   b. normal filling/storage; normal emptying.
   c. normal filling/storage; abnormal emptying because of smooth sphincter dyssynergia.
   d. normal filling/storage; abnormal emptying because of striated sphincter dyssynergia.
   e. abnormal filling/storage because of detrusor overactivity; abnormal emptying because of striated sphincter dyssynergia.

9. The most common urodynamic findings in those individuals with cerebral palsy who do exhibit lower urinary tract dysfunction are:
   a. detrusor areflexia, coordinated sphincters.
   b. detrusor overactivity, smooth sphincter dyssynergia, striated sphincter dyssynergia.
   c. detrusor overactivity, smooth sphincter synergy, striated sphincter dyssynergia.
   d. decreased detrusor compliance, coordinated sphincters.
   e. detrusor overactivity, coordinated sphincters.

10. Deficiency of which of the following compounds in the nigrostriatal pathway accounts for most of the classic clinical motor features of Parkinson's disease (PD)?
    a. Dopamine
    b. Norepinephrine
    c. Acetylcholine
    d. Serotonin
    e. L-Dopa

11. The most common urodynamic abnormality found in patients with voiding dysfunction secondary to PD is:
    a. impaired sensation during filling.
    b. striated sphincter dyssynergia.
    c. striated sphincter bradykinesia.
    d. detrusor overactivity.
    e. impaired detrusor contractility.

12. Which of the following is more common in patients with PD than in patients with multiple system atrophy (MSA)?
    a. Intrinsic sphincter deficiency
    b. Evidence of striated sphincter denervation on an electromyogram
    c. Decreased compliance
    d. Incontinence after transurethral resection of the prostate
    e. Disease diagnosis preceding voiding and erectile symptoms

13. The lesions seen in multiple sclerosis most commonly affect which of the following locations in the nervous system?
    a. Thoracic spinal cord
    b. Sacral spinal cord
    c. Cervical spinal cord
    d. Lumbar spinal cord
    e. Midbrain

14. Which of the following urodynamic findings is least common in patients with multiple sclerosis and voiding dysfunction?
    a. Detrusor overactivity
    b. Detrusor areflexia
    c. Impaired detrusor contractility
    d. Striated sphincter dyssynergia
    e. Smooth sphincter dyssynergia

15. The incidence of upper urinary tract deterioration is greatest in which of the following?
    a. Multiple sclerosis
    b. Multiple system atrophy
    c. Parkinson's disease
    d. Spinal cord injury
    e. Diabetes

16. Which of the following most accurately reflects the number of patients with HIV/AIDS, overall, with moderate or severe voiding problems?
    a. 15% or less
    b. 15% to 25%
    c. 25% to 40%
    d. 40% to 60%
    e. 60% to 80%

17. The sacral spinal cord terminates in the cauda equina at approximately the spinal column level of:
    a. T10.
    b. L1.
    c. L2.
    d. L3.
    e. S1.

18. In spinal shock, findings generally include all of the following EXCEPT:
    a. acontractile bladder.
    b. areflexic bladder.
    c. open bladder neck.
    d. absent guarding reflex.
    e. maximal urethral closure pressure above normal.

19. All of the following are risk factors for upper urinary tract deterioration in a patient with a suprasacral spinal cord injury EXCEPT:
    a. high-pressure storage.
    b. high detrusor leak-point pressure.
    c. chronic bladder overdistention.
    d. high abdominal leak-point pressure.
    e. vesicourethral reflux with infection.

20. The presence of true detrusor striated sphincter dyssynergia implies a neurologic lesion between the:
    a. a neurologic lesion between the pons and the sacral spinal cord.
    b. a neurologic lesion between the cerebral cortex and the pons.
    c. a neurologic lesion between the cervical and the sacral spinal cord.
    d. a neurologic lesion between the sacral spinal cord and the striated sphincter.
    e. normal sensation in the presence of involuntary bladder contractions.

21. A spinal cord injury at which of the following cord levels would be most likely to be associated with autonomic hyperreflexia?
    a. Cervical
    b. Thoracic
    c. Lumbar
    d. Sacral
    e. Cauda equina

22. Which of the following is least characteristic as a finding in autonomic hyperreflexia?
    a. Headache before bladder contraction
    b. Hypertension
    c. Flushing above the level of the lesion
    d. Tachycardia
    e. Sweating above the level of the lesion

23. The most common urodynamic findings in a male with autonomic hyperreflexia include all but:
    a. detrusor overactivity.
    b. decreased compliance.
    c. striated sphincter dyssynergia.
    d. smooth sphincter dyssynergia.
    e. decreased bladder capacity.

24. Which of the following is not among the treatments for, or prophylaxis of, autonomic hyperreflexia?
    a. α-Adrenergic blockade
    b. β-Adrenergic blockade
    c. Ganglionic blockade
    d. Spinal anesthesia
    e. General anesthesia

25. In a male patient with detrusor striated sphincter dyssynergia, a high detrusor leak-point pressure, high-pressure vesicoureteral reflux, and beginning upper urinary tract deterioration, which of the following is least likely, as an isolated procedure, to halt or reverse the upper tract changes?
    a. Ureteral reimplantation
    b. Augmentation cystoplasty
    c. Dorsal root ganglionectomy
    d. Anticholinergic therapy and intermittent catheterization
    e. Sphincterotomy
26. The American Paraplegic Society guidelines for urologic care of spinal cord injury include all but:
    a. annual follow-up after injury for 5 to 10 years, then every other year if doing well.
    b. upper and lower urinary tract evaluation initially and yearly for 5 to 10 years, then every other year.
    c. cystoscopy annually for those with an indwelling catheter.
    d. urodynamic evaluation initially, yearly for 5 to 10 years, then every other year.
    e. neurologic evaluation initially and yearly for an indefinite period.
27. In a patient with voiding dysfunction secondary to myelomeningocele who has slightly decreased compliance, detrusor areflexia, and low-pressure moderate to severe vesicoureteral reflux, which of the following urodynamic changes would be most likely after ureteral reimplantation alone?
    a. Compliance increased
    b. Voiding pressure decreased
    c. Valsalva leak-point pressure decreased
    d. Maximum urethral closure pressure decreased
    e. Maximum bladder capacity decreased
28. The symptoms of voiding dysfunction in a child with tethered cord syndrome present most commonly after which of the following precipitating factors?
    a. Urinary tract infection
    b. Meningitis
    c. Puberty
    d. Cystoscopy
    e. Growth spurt
29. A classic "sensory neurogenic bladder" (Lapides classification system) is most commonly produced by:
    a. herpes zoster.
    b. herpes simplex.
    c. transverse myelitis.
    d. pernicious anemia.
    e. sacral spinal cord injury.
30. Patients who have voiding dysfunction secondary to lumbar disk disease most commonly present with which of the following symptoms and urodynamic findings?
    a. Retention; involuntary bladder contractions
    b. Incontinence; involuntary bladder contractions
    c. Retention; decreased bladder compliance
    d. Difficulty voiding; normal bladder compliance
    e. Incontinence; normal bladder compliance
31. The combination that best describes the type of permanent voiding dysfunction that can occur after radical pelvic surgery is:
    a. exertional (or stress) incontinence; detrusor areflexia.
    b. urgency incontinence; detrusor overactivity.
    c. reflex incontinence; detrusor areflexia.
    d. urgency incontinence; detrusor overactivity.
    e. exertional (or stress) incontinence; detrusor overactivity.
32. What is optimal management for a 65-year-old man who has had a first occurrence of urinary retention after radical pelvic surgery?
    a. Anticholinergic therapy
    b. Clean intermittent catheterization
    c. Transurethral resection of the prostate
    d. External sphincterotomy
    e. Bethanechol chloride
33. The urodynamic parameter most likely to distinguish urinary retention due to prostatic obstruction from urinary retention due to "classic diabetic cystopathy" is:
    a. uroflow.
    b. residual urine volume.
    c. bladder compliance.
    d. vesical pressure.
    e. detrusor pressure.
34. Detrusor striated sphincter dyssynergia is least expected to occur with which of the following conditions?
    a. Multiple sclerosis
    b. Spinal cord injury
    c. Stroke
    d. Autonomic hyperreflexia
    e. Transverse myelitis
35. Differentiation of bladder neck obstruction from dysfunctional voiding is most easily and accurately made by:
    a. filling cystometry.
    b. voiding cystometry.
    c. cystourethroscopy.
    d. flowmetry and residual urine determination.
    e. video-urodynamic study.
36. Which of the following is not a typical finding in a patient with Fowler's syndrome?
    a. Female younger than 30 years of age
    b. Unable to void for a day or more with no urgency
    c. Bladder capacity of less than 1 liter
    d. Increasing lower abdominal discomfort
    e. EMG abnormalities
37. Which of the following with the typical history is the most specific study to make the diagnosis of Fowler's syndrome?
    a. Striated sphincter needle EMG recording
    b. Striated sphincter patch EMG recording
    c. Neurologic examination
    d. Spinal MRI examination
    e. Detrusor pressure/urinary flow recording
38. Which of the following has proved to be successful in treating the urologic manifestations of Fowler's syndrome?
    a. Estrogen therapy
    b. Progesterone therapy
    c. Baclofen therapy
    d. Botulinum toxin injection therapy
    e. Neuromodulation
39. There is an increased incidence of urinary incontinence after prostatectomy in men with:
    a. hyperthyroidism.
    b. myasthenia gravis.
    c. schizophrenia.
    d. gastroparesis.
    e. Isaacs' syndrome.

ANSWERS

1. **b. Involuntary bladder contractions, smooth sphincter synergy, striated sphincter synergy.** Neurologic lesions above the level of the brain stem that affect micturition generally result in involuntary bladder contractions with smooth and striated sphincter synergy. Sensation and voluntary striated sphincter function are generally preserved. Areflexia may occur, however, either initially or as a permanent dysfunction.
2. **c. Involuntary bladder contractions, smooth sphincter synergy, striated sphincter dyssynergia.** Patients with complete lesions of the spinal cord between spinal cord levels T6 and S2, after they recover from spinal shock, generally exhibit involuntary bladder contractions without sensation, smooth sphincter synergy, but striated sphincter dyssynergia. Those with lesions above T6 may experience, in addition, smooth sphincter dyssynergia and autonomic hyperreflexia.
3. **e. Detrusor overactivity.** The most common long-term expression of lower urinary tract dysfunction after a CVA is detrusor hyperreflexia. Sensation is variable but is classically described as generally intact, and thus the patient has urgency and frequency with hyperreflexia.
4. **a. Internal capsule.** Previous descriptions of the voiding dysfunction after a CVA have all cited the preponderance of detrusor hyperreflexia with coordinated sphincter activity. It is difficult to reconcile this with the relatively high incontinence rate that occurs, even considering the probability that a percentage of these patients had an incontinence problem before the CVA. Tsuchida and coworkers (1983) and Khan and associates (1990) made early significant contributions in this area by correlating the urodynamic and CT pictures after CVA. They reported that patients with lesions in only the basal ganglia or thalamus have normal sphincter function. This means that when an impending involuntary contraction or its onset was sensed, these patients could voluntarily contract the striated sphincter and abort or considerably lessen the effect of an abnormal micturition reflex. The majority of patients with involvement of the cerebral cortex and/or internal capsule were unable to forcefully contract the striated sphincter under these circumstances.
5. **d. pseudodyssynergia.** Some authors have described striated sphincter dyssynergia in 5% to 21% of patients with brain disease and voiding dysfunction. This is incompatible with accepted neural circuitry. I agree with those who believe that true detrusor-striated sphincter dyssynergia does not occur in this situation. Pseudodyssynergia may indeed occur during urodynamic testing of these patients. This refers to an electromyographic (EMG) sphincter "flare" during filling cystometry, which is secondary to attempted inhibition of an involuntary bladder contraction by voluntary contraction of the striated sphincter.
6. **e. full urodynamic evaluation.** Poor flow rates and high residual urine volumes in a male with pre-CVA symptoms of prostatism generally indicate prostatic obstruction, but a full urodynamic evaluation is advisable before committing a patient to mechanical outlet reduction primarily to exclude detrusor hyperactivity with impaired contractility as a cause of symptoms.
7. **c. Posterior fossa.** The areas that are most frequently involved with associated micturition dysfunction are the superior aspects of the frontal lobe. When voiding dysfunction occurs, it generally consists of detrusor hyperreflexia and urinary incontinence. These individuals may have a markedly diminished awareness of all lower urinary tract events and, if so, are totally unable to even attempt suppression of the micturition reflex. Smooth and striated sphincter activity is generally synergic. Pseudodyssynergia may occur during urodynamic testing. Fowler (1999) reviewed the literature on frontal lobe lesions and bladder control. She cited instances of resection of a tumor relieving the micturition symptoms for a period of time, raising the question of whether the phenomenon of tumor-associated bladder hyperreflexia was a positive one (activating some system) rather than a negative one (releasing a system from control). Urinary retention has also been described in patients with space-occupying lesions of the frontal cortex, in the absence of other associated remarkable neurologic deficits. Posterior fossa tumors may be associated with voiding dysfunction (32% to 70%, based on references cited by Fowler). Retention or difficulty voiding is the rule, with incontinence being rarely reported.
8. **b. normal filling/storage; normal emptying.** Most children and adults with only CP have urinary control and what seems to be normal filling/storage and normal emptying. The actual incidence of voiding dysfunction is somewhat vague, because the few available series report findings predominantly in those who present with voiding symptoms. One study estimated that a third or more of children with CP are so affected. When an adult with CP presents with an acute or subacute change in voiding status, however, it is most likely unrelated to CP.
9. **e. detrusor overactivity, coordinated sphincters.** In those individuals with CP who exhibit significant dysfunction, the type of damage that one would suspect from the most common urodynamic abnormalities seems to be localized above the brain stem. This is commonly reflected by detrusor overactivity and coordinated sphincters. Spinal cord damage can occur, however, and probably accounts for those individuals with CP who seem to have evidence of striated sphincter dyssynergia.
10. **a. Dopamine.** PD is a neurodegenerative disorder of unknown cause that affects primarily the dopaminergic neurons of the substantia nigra but also heterogeneous populations of neurons elsewhere. The most important site of pathology is the substantia nigra pars compacta, the origin of the dopaminergic nigrostriatal tract to the caudate nucleus and putamen. Dopamine deficiency in the nigrostriatal pathway accounts for most of the classic clinical motor features of PD.
11. **d. detrusor overactivity.** The most common urodynamic finding is detrusor overactivity. The pathophysiology of detrusor overactivity most widely proposed is that the basal ganglia normally have an inhibitory effect on the micturition reflex, which is abolished by the cell loss in the substantia nigra.
12. **e. Disease diagnosis preceding voiding and erectile symptoms.** One study compared the clinical features of 52 patients with probable MSA and 41 patients with PD. Of patients with MSA, 60% had their urinary symptoms precede or present with their symptoms of parkinsonism. Of patients with PD, 94% had been diagnosed for several years before the onset of urinary symptoms. In patients with MSA, urinary incontinence was a significant complaint in 73%, whereas 19% had only frequency and urgency without incontinence. Sixty-six percent of the patients with MSA had a significant postvoid residual volume (100 to 450 mL). In patients with PD, frequency and urgency were the predominant symptoms in 85%, and incontinence was the primary complaint in 15%. In only 5 of 32 patients with PD in whom residual urine volume was measured was it significant. Ninety-three percent of the men with MSA questioned about erectile function reported erectile failure, and in 13 of 27 of these the erectile dysfunction preceded the diagnosis of MSA. Seven of the 21 men with PD had erectile failure, but in all these men the diagnosis of erectile dysfunction followed the diagnosis of PD by 1 to 4 years.

The initial urinary symptoms of MSA are urgency, frequency, and urge incontinence, occurring up to 4 years before the diagnosis is made, as does erectile failure. Cystourethrography or video-urodynamic studies generally reveal an open bladder neck (intrinsic sphincter deficiency), and many patients exhibit evidence of striated sphincter denervation on motor unit electromyography. The smooth and striated sphincter abnormalities predispose women to sphincteric incontinence and make prostatectomy hazardous in men.

13. **c. Cervical spinal cord.** The demyelinating process most commonly involves the lateral corticospinal (pyramidal) and reticulospinal columns of the cervical spinal cord.
14. **e. Smooth sphincter dyssynergia.** Detrusor overactivity is the most common urodynamic abnormality detected, occurring in 34% to 99% of cases in reported series. Of the patients with overactivity, 30% to 65% have coexistent striated sphincter dyssynergia. Up to 60% of those with overactivity may have impaired detrusor contractility, a phenomenon that can considerably complicate treatment efforts. Bladder areflexia may also occur; reports of its frequency vary but generally average from 5% to 20%. Generally, the smooth sphincter is synergic.
15. **d. Spinal cord injury.** Progressive neurologic diseases cause upper tract damage much less commonly than spinal cord injury, even when associated with severe disability and spasticity (Wyndaele et al, 2005).
16. **a. 15% or less.** How common are voiding problems overall in patients with HIV infection and AIDS? One study prospectively investigated voiding function in 77 men and 4 women with HIV infection or AIDS consecutively attending an outpatient clinic. Eight of these (10%) had moderate subjective voiding problems, whereas 2 (2%) had severe problems. The authors thought that in only 4% of patients did the nature of the disturbance warrant urodynamic examination and concluded that urinary voiding symptoms are only a modest problem; overall in an HIV/AIDS population, neuropathic bladder dysfunction is rare and mostly occurs in the late stages of the disease (Gyrtrup et al, 1995).
17. **c.** Spinal column (bone) segments are numbered by the vertebral level, and these have a different relationship to the spinal cord segmental level at different locations. The sacral spinal cord begins at about spinal column level T12-L1. The spinal cord terminates in the cauda equina at approximately the spinal column level of L2.
18. **c. open bladder neck.** Spinal shock includes a suppression of autonomic activity as well as somatic activity, and the bladder is acontractile and areflexic. Radiologically, the bladder has a smooth contour with no evidence of trabeculation. The bladder neck is generally closed and competent unless there has been prior surgery or, in some cases, thoracolumbar and presumably sympathetic injury. The smooth sphincter mechanism seems to be functional. Some EMG activity may be recorded from the striated sphincter, and the maximum urethral closure pressure is lower than normal but still maintained at the level of the external sphincter zone; however, the normal guarding reflex is absent and there is no voluntary control.
19. **d. high abdominal leak-point pressure**. As with all patients with neurologic impairment, a careful initial evaluation and periodic follow-up evaluation must be performed to identify and correct the following risk factors and potential complications: bladder overdistention, high pressure storage, high detrusor leak-point pressure, vesicoureteral reflux, stone formation (lower and upper tracts), and complicating infection especially in association with reflux.
20. **a. a neurologic lesion between the pons and sacral spinal cord.** A diagnosis of striated sphincter dyssynergia implies a neurologic lesion that interrupts the neural axis between the pontine-mesencephalic reticular formation and the sacral spinal cord.
21. **a. Cervical.** Autonomic hyperreflexia represents an acute massive disordered autonomic (primarily sympathetic) response to specific stimuli in patients with SCI above the level of T6 to T8 (the upper level of the sympathetic outflow). It is more common with cervical (60%) than thoracic (20%) injuries.
22. **d. Tachycardia.** Symptomatically, autonomic hyperreflexia is a syndrome of exaggerated sympathetic activity in response to stimuli below the level of the lesion. The symptoms are pounding headache, hypertension, and flushing of the face and body above the level of the lesion with sweating. Bradycardia is a usual accompaniment, and tachycardia or arrhythmia may be present.
23. **b. decreased compliance.** In autonomic hyperreflexia, the urodynamic picture is that of a suprasacral SCI. Smooth sphincter dyssynergia is generally found as well, at least in men.
24. **b. β-Adrenergic blockade.** Acutely the hemodynamic effects may be managed with parenteral ganglionic or α-adrenergic blockade. Any endoscopic procedure in susceptible patients ideally should be done with the patient under spinal or carefully monitored general anesthesia.
25. **a. Ureteral reimplantation.** The best initial treatment for reflux in a patient with voiding dysfunction secondary to neurologic disease or injury is to normalize lower urinary tract urodynamics as much as possible. Depending on the clinical circumstances, this may be by pharmacotherapy, urethral dilatation (in the myelomeningocele patient), neuromodulation, deafferentation, augmentation cystoplasty, or sphincterotomy. If this fails, the question of whether to operate on such patients for correction of the reflux or to correct the reflux while performing another procedure (e.g., augmentation cystoplasty) is not an easy one, because correction of reflux in an often very thickened bladder may not be an easy task.
26. **e. neurologic evaluation initially and yearly for an indefinite period.** All but e were specific recommendations (Linsenmeyer and Culkin, 1999).
27. **e. Maximum bladder capacity decreased.** One must remember the potential artifact that significant reflux can introduce into urodynamic studies. Measured bladder capacity may be more and measured pressures at given inflow volumes may be less than those after reflux correction. The apparent significance of detrusor overactivity may thus be underestimated.
28. **e. Growth spurt.** One study pointed out that, whereas children often develop symptoms of tethered cord after growth spurts, in adults the presenting symptoms often follow activities that stretch the spine, such as sports or motor vehicle accidents.
29. **d. pernicious anemia.** Although syphilitic myelopathy is disappearing as a major neurologic problem, involvement of the spinal cord dorsal columns and posterior sacral roots can result in a loss of bladder sensation and large residual urine volumes and therefore can be a cause of sensory neurogenic bladder. Another spinal cord cause of the classic sensory bladder is the now uncommon pernicious anemia. The most common cause is diabetes.
30. **d. Difficulty voiding; normal bladder compliance.** A study reported on findings in 114 patients with lumbar disk protrusion who were prospectively studied. The authors found

detrusor areflexia in 31 (27.2%) and normal detrusor activity in the remaining 83. All 31 patients with detrusor areflexia reported difficulty voiding with straining. Patients with voiding dysfunction generally present with these symptoms or in urinary retention. The most consistent urodynamic finding is that of a normally compliant areflexic bladder associated with normal innervation or findings of incomplete denervation of the perineal floor musculature.

31. **a. exertional (or stress) incontinence; detrusor areflexia.** When permanent voiding dysfunction occurs after radical pelvic surgery, the pattern is generally one of a failure of voluntary bladder contraction, or impaired bladder contractility, with obstruction by what seems urodynamically to be residual fixed striated sphincter tone, which is not subject to voluntarily induced relaxation. Often, the smooth sphincter area is open and nonfunctional. Decreased compliance is common in these patients, and this, with the "obstruction" caused by fixed residual striated sphincter tone, results in both storage and emptying failure. These patients often experience leaking across the distal sphincter area and, in addition, are unable to empty the bladder, because although intravesical pressure may be increased, there is nothing that approximates a true bladder contraction. The patient often presents with urinary incontinence that is characteristically most manifest with increases in intra-abdominal pressure. This is usually most obvious in females, because the prostatic bulk in males often masks an equivalent deficit in urethral closure function. Alternatively, patients may present with variable degrees of urinary retention.

32. **b. Clean intermittent catheterization.** The temptation to perform a prostatectomy should be avoided unless a clear demonstration of outlet obstruction at this level is possible. Otherwise, prostatectomy simply decreases urethral sphincter function and thereby may result in the occurrence or worsening of sphincteric urinary incontinence. Most of these dysfunctions will be transient, and the temptation to "do something" other than perform clean intermittent catheterization initially after surgery in these patients, especially in those with little or no preexisting history of voiding dysfunction, cannot be too strongly discouraged.

33. **e. detrusor pressure.** Detrusor contractility is classically described as being decreased in the end-stage diabetic bladder. Current evidence points to both sensory and motor neuropathy as being involved in the pathogenesis, the motor aspect per se contributing to the impaired detrusor contractility. The typically described classic urodynamic findings include impaired bladder sensation, increased cystometric capacity, decreased bladder contractility, impaired uroflow, and, later, increased residual urine volume. The main differential diagnosis, at least in men, is generally bladder outlet obstruction, because both conditions commonly produce a low flow rate. Pressure/flow urodynamic studies easily differentiate the two.

34. **c. Stroke.** True detrusor sphincter dyssynergia should exist only in patients who have an abnormality in pathways between the sacral spinal cord and the brain stem pontine micturition center, generally due to neurologic injury or disease.

35. **e. video-urodynamic study.** Objective evidence of outlet obstruction in these patients is easily obtainable by urodynamic study. Once obstruction is diagnosed, it can be localized at the level of the bladder neck by video-urodynamic study, cystourethrography during a bladder contraction, or micturitional urethral profilometry.

36. **c. Bladder capacity of less than 1 liter.** The criteria (Swinn and Fowler, 2001; Fowler, 2003) include a bladder capacity of over 1 liter with no sensation of urgency.

37. **a. Striated sphincter needle EMG recording.** Fowler's syndrome refers particularly to a syndrome of urinary retention in young women in the absence of overt neurologic disease. The typical history is that of a young woman younger than the age of 30 years who has found herself unable to void over the preceding day but with no sensation of urgency. MRI studies of the brain and the entire spinal cord are normal. On concentric needle electrode examination of the striated muscle of the urethral sphincter, however, Fowler and associates described a unique EMG abnormality. This abnormal activity, localized to the urethral sphincter, consists of a type of activity that would be expected to cause inappropriate contraction of the muscle. Sphincter activity consists of two components: complex repetitive discharges and decelerating bursts. This abnormal activity impairs sphincter relaxation.

38. **e. Neuromodulation.** Fowler reports that efforts to treat this condition by hormonal manipulation, pharmacologic therapy, or injections of botulinum toxin have been unsuccessful. This condition is highly responsive to neuromodulation, even in women who have had retention for many months or years.

39. **b. myasthenia gravis.** Any neuromuscular disease that affects the tone of the smooth or striated muscle of the distal sphincter mechanism can predispose an individual patient to a greater chance of urinary incontinence after even a well-performed transurethral or open prostatectomy. Myasthenia gravis is an autoimmune disease caused by autoantibodies to acetylcholine nicotinic receptors. This leads to neuromuscular blockade and hence weakness in a variety of striated muscle groups. The incidence of incontinence after prostatectomy is indeed greatly increased in patients with this disease.

60

Urinary Incontinence: Epidemiology, Pathophysiology, Evaluation, and Management Overview

VICTOR W. NITTI • JERRY G. BLAIVAS

QUESTIONS

1. Which of the following is not a symptom of incontinence?
   a. Stress incontinence
   b. Urge incontinence
   c. Mixed incontinence
   d. Overflow incontinence
   e. Nocturnal enuresis
2. Which of the following is the least relevant with respect to the impact of incontinence on society?
   a. Its prevalence
   b. Its incidence
   c. Its effect on quality of life
   d. The number of office visits it generates
   e. The number of operations it generates
3. Which of the following is not a risk factor for developing stress incontinence in women?
   a. Increasing age
   b. Recurrent urinary tract infection
   c. Pregnancy
   d. Vaginal delivery
   e. Obesity
4. Which of the following is FALSE with respect to the association between pregnancy and incontinence?
   a. The prevalence of incontinence during pregnancy is more than 30%.
   b. Compared with nulliparous women, those who had vaginal delivery one to four times had over twice the incidence of incontinence.
   c. Emergency cesarean section for obstructed labor significantly reduced the chances of subsequent incontinence.
   d. Elective cesarean section for obstructed labor significantly reduced the chances of subsequent incontinence.
   e. Incontinence that begins during pregnancy usually subsides within 1 year.
5. Incontinence in men:
   a. has an overall prevalence rate of about 2%.
   b. is associated with prostatic obstruction.
   c. is most commonly mixed incontinence.
   d. has half the prevalence of that in women.
   e. b and d.
6. Which of the following does not promote continence?
   a. Accommodation
   b. High bladder compliance
   c. Spinal reflex inhibition of sympathetic pathways to bladder
   d. Spinal reflex inhibition of somatic pathways
   e. Spinal reflex stimulation of bladder outlet
7. All of the following are thought to be important mechanisms for achieving continence in women EXCEPT:
   a. preventing urethral hypermobility.
   b. maintaining the integrity of the musculofascial connections between vaginal wall/urethra/levator complex and arcus tendineus fascial pelvis.
   c. preventing unequal movement of the anterior and posterior walls of the urethra during stress.
   d. maintaining the integrity of the pubourethral ligament and pubourethralis muscle.
   e. preventing laxity of the anterior vaginal wall.
8. Which of the following describes the urethral sphincter in men?
   a. The proximal urethral sphincter is composed of bladder neck, prostate, and prostatic urethra to the level of the verumontanum.
   b. The proximal urethral sphincter is innervated predominately by parasympathetic fibers from the pudendal nerve.
   c. The distal urethral sphincter is composed of the prostate-membranous urethra, rhabdosphincter, extrinsic paraurethral striated muscle, and connective tissue.
   d. a and c.
   e. a, b, and c.

9. Which of the following statements about post-prostatectomy incontinence is FALSE? It is caused by damage to the:
   a. proximal sphincter.
   b. distal sphincter.
   c. voluntary muscles of the distal sphincter.
   d. slow twitch fibers.
   e. c and d.

10. The detrusor leak-point pressure is useful in all of the following EXCEPT:
   a. female stress incontinence.
   b. myelodysplasia.
   c. radiation cystitis.
   d. L5 spinal cord tumor.
   e. radical hysterectomy.

11. Which of the following conditions is NOT associated with detrusor overactivity?
   a. Diabetes mellitus
   b. Cauda equina syndrome
   c. Pernicious anemia
   d. Prostatic obstruction
   e. Parkinson's disease

12. Which of the following statements about low bladder compliance is correct?
   a. It is calculated by $\Delta V/\Delta P$ where V is bladder volume and p is detrusor pressure.
   b. It is calculated by $\Delta P/\Delta V$ where V is bladder volume and p is detrusor pressure.
   c. It may result in upper tract damage when end detrusor pressure exceeds 40 cm H_2O.
   d. It is always associated with detrusor overactivity.
   e. a and c.

13. Which of the following is NOT a mechanism by which vaginal delivery might cause sphincteric incontinence?
   a. Mechanical injury to connective tissue support
   b. Vascular damage due to compression by the fetus
   c. Damage to pelvic nerves and/or muscles
   d. Direct injury to the lower urinary tract
   e. Injury to the spinal cord or nerves from spinal or epidural anesthesia

14. Intrinsic sphincter deficiency is caused by all of the following EXCEPT:
   a. urethral diverticulectomy.
   b. prolapse repair.
   c. radical hysterectomy.
   d. abdominal hysterectomy.
   e. a and c.

15. Transient causes of urinary incontinence include all of the following EXCEPT:
   a. impaction of stool.
   b. cystitis.
   c. diabetes mellitus.
   d. diabetes insipidus.
   e. c and d.

16. Which medication does not cause or exacerbate sphincteric incontinence?
   a. Imipramine
   b. Phentolamine
   c. Doxazosin
   d. Terazosin
   e. Tamsulosin

17. The single most important diagnostic criteria for urinary incontinence is:
   a. cystometry.
   b. direct visualization by the examiner.
   c. pad test.
   d. leak-point pressure.
   e. Q-tip test.

18. Which of the following is not considered to be an essential component of the initial evaluation of incontinence?
   a. Uroflow
   b. Determination of postvoid residual urine
   c. Urinalysis
   d. Assessment of its impact on quality of life
   e. Focal neurologic examination

19. Measurement of abdominal pressure during multichannel urodynamics is important because:
   a. abdominal pressure is a significant component of vesical pressure.
   b. it allows external sphincter function to be evaluated.
   c. total vesical pressure cannot be measured without it.
   d. detrusor pressure can be estimated from the subtraction of abdominal pressure from vesical pressure.
   e. a and d.

20. A cystometrogram (CMG):
   a. is the most accurate way to assess voiding function.
   b. normally shows a slow steady increase in bladder pressure as the bladder fills.
   c. is used to determine the pressure-volume relationship during bladder filling and storage.
   d. a and c.
   e. a, b, and c.

21. Urodynamic manifestations of bladder dysfunction include:
   a. detrusor overactivity.
   b. low bladder compliance.
   c. low abdominal leak-point pressure (ALPP).
   d. a and b.
   e. a, b, and c.

22. Abdominal leak-point pressure (ALPP) is:
   a. rarely below 60 cm H_2O in continent women.
   b. a measure of intrinsic bladder function.
   c. a measure of external sphincter function.
   d. the lowest vesical pressure at which urine passing through the urethra is associated with a rise in abdominal pressure.
   e. c and d.

23. Detrusor leak point pressure is:
   a. not valuable in patients with neurologic disease and associated incontinence.
   b. higher when outlet resistance is higher.
   c. a good predictor of outcomes for stress incontinence surgery.
   d. a predictor of upper tract damage when it exceeds 10 cm H_2O.
   e. the detrusor pressure at which urine passing through the urethra is associated with a rise in abdominal pressure.

24. Video-urodynamics:
    a. is the most precise diagnostic tool available for the evaluation of voiding function/dysfunction.
    b. according to the International Continence Society should be used routinely to evaluate incontinence.
    c. is most useful to confirm findings found on routine multichannel urodynamics.
    d. is not useful in cases of neurogenic voiding dysfunction and incontinence.
    e. is prone to more artifacts than non-video multichannel urodynamics.
25. The approach to treating the patient with incontinence is:
    a. predicated on a clear understanding of the underlying pathophysiology causing the symptom.
    b. usually the same, at least initially, regardless of the underlying condition.
    c. usually determined by the degree of bother to the patient.
    d. usually by protocol and rarely individualized.
    e. a and c.
26. Which of the following are barriers to curing incontinence?
    a. Frailty
    b. Economics
    c. Patient preference
    d. Access to health care professional
    e. All of the above
27. All of the following are accepted treatments for non-neurogenic incontinence caused by detrusor overactivity EXCEPT:
    a. behavioral modification.
    b. anticholinergic medications.
    c. treatment of coexisting bladder outlet obstruction.
    d. α-adrenergic agonists.
    e. sacral nerve neuromodulation.
28. Which of the following agents used to treat incontinence caused by detrusor overactivity does not have level 1 evidence (randomized controlled trials) to support its effectiveness?
    a. Oxybutynin
    b. Tolterodine
    c. Imipramine
    d. Trospium
    e. Solifenacin
29. Augmentation enterocystoplasty is:
    a. usually effective to treat detrusor overactivity but has little effect on decreased compliance.
    b. best in elderly patients with detrusor overactivity.
    c. contraindicated in patients with non-neurogenic detrusor overactivity.
    d. supported by level 1 evidence.
    e. associated with metabolic disturbances and stone formation.
30. Pelvic floor muscle training for stress incontinence:
    a. is best suited for elderly patients with severe incontinence who are not surgical candidates.
    b. has well-established exercise protocols that should be strictly adhered to for optimal results.
    c. has been shown to be superior to no treatment in randomized controlled trials.
    d. has been shown to work best when combined with biofeedback.
    e. b and d.
31. In postmenopausal women, estrogen replacement:
    a. should be used as first-line treatment for stress incontinence, either topically or systemically.
    b. has been shown to work best in treating stress incontinence with a significant component of ISD.
    c. improves symptoms of stress incontinence by increasing the volume of the submucosal layer of the urethra.
    d. is useful after failed surgical treatment for stress incontinence.
    e. should no longer be considered part of the routine treatment armamentarium for women with stress incontinence.
32. Which of the following concepts correctly explains contemporary thinking on the mechanism of action of surgery to treat stress incontinence secondary to urethral hypermobility? The urethra is:
    a. repositioned to a high retropubic (normal anatomic) position.
    b. passively compressed at all times.
    c. supported re-creating a proper backboard to resist increases in abdominal pressure.
    d. partially obstructed during increases in abdominal pressure and voiding.
    e. All of the above
33. According to the AUA Stress Incontinence Surgery Guidelines Panel, which of the following is TRUE?
    a. Slings are the procedures of choice for stress incontinence.
    b. All operations for stress incontinence have approximately equal efficacy.
    c. Patients should be informed of all available surgical procedures and the estimated risks and benefits, including complications and how they would be treated.
    d. Retropubic suspensions and sling procedures have better outcomes than transvaginal procedures.
    e. c and d.
34. Patients with mixed incontinence with a predominate stress component:
    a. usually respond well to anticholinergic medication.
    b. should never be treated surgically for stress incontinence because urge incontinence usually worsens.
    c. may have improvement in both stress and urge incontinence if treated with surgery for stress incontinence.
    d. should always be treated with a urethral bulking agent before surgery.
    e. are not effectively treated by any means.
35. For post-prostatectomy incontinence secondary to sphincter dysfunction:
    a. artificial urinary sphincter (AUS) is the 'gold standard' for all patients.
    b. AUS is never placed after radiation therapy.
    c. AUS and male perineal sling have comparable long-term results in men with moderate incontinence.
    d. urethral bulking agents are very effective for men with mild incontinence.
    e. c and d.

ANSWERS

1. **d. Overflow incontinence.** Overflow incontinence is not a symptom. It is a term used to describe incontinence associated with urinary retention.
2. **d. The number of office visits it generates.** Prevalence is the probability of having a disease or condition, in this case incontinence, within a defined population at a defined point in time. Incidence, on the other hand, is the probability of developing a disease or condition during a defined period of time. When determining social impact and allocation of health care resources, prevalence is the core important parameter.
3. **b. Recurrent urinary tract infection.** There is no reported causal relationship between recurrent urinary tract infection and stress incontinence.
4. **c. Emergency cesarean section for obstructed labor significantly reduced the chances of subsequent incontinence.** Groutz and associates (2004) found that the prevalence of stress incontinence 1 year after first delivery was similar among women who had a spontaneous vaginal delivery (10.3%) and those who had a cesarean section for obstructed labor (12%) ($P = 0.7$) but was significantly lower for those who had an elective cesarean section (3.4%, $P = 0.02$).
5. **e. b and d.** In men, urge incontinence dominates (40% to 80%). Its overall prevalence has been reported to range from 3% to 19%.
6. **d. Spinal reflex inhibition of somatic pathways.** During bladder storage, reflex activation of somatic (pudendal) pathways promotes continence by enhancing urethral striated muscle tone.
7. **a. preventing urethral hypermobility.** According to prevailing theories, all of these are important mechanisms for maintaining continence except for urethral hypermobility. Several studies have shown that there is no correlation between leak-point pressure and urethral mobility as measured by Q-tip angle and no correlation between urethral hypermobility and continence.
8. **d. a and c.** The proximal urethral sphincter is innervated by parasympathetic fibers that transverse the pelvic nerve.
9. **c. voluntary muscles of the distal sphincter.** Paralysis of the striated voluntary muscles does not cause incontinence and most men with post-prostatectomy incontinence do have preservation of voluntary control of these muscles, that is, they can contract their sphincter muscles and interrupt the stream.
10. **a. female stress incontinence.** The detrusor leak-point pressure is defined as the lowest detrusor pressure at which urinary leakage occurs in the absence of abdominal straining or a detrusor contraction. This is most useful in patients with low bladder compliance. Stress incontinence is assessed with the abdominal leak-point pressure.
11. **b. Cauda equina syndrome.** Cauda equina syndrome usually causes an areflexic or low compliance bladder.
12. **e. a and c.**
13. **e. Injury to the spinal cord or nerves from spinal or epidural anesthesia.** All of these injuries have been suggested as causes of incontinence after vaginal delivery except for injury to the spinal cord or nerves.
14. **e. a and c.** After urethral diverticulectomy, periurethral fibrosis may cause ISD. Radical hysterectomy may damage the sympathetic nerves.
15. **e. c and d.** Impaction of stool and cystitis are well-known causes of urinary incontinence. Incontinence usually subsides when the condition remits. Diabetes mellitus is associated with detrusor overactivity, likely on a neurologic basis, and can also cause polyuria. Polyuria is a reversible condition that can exacerbate incontinence and can be caused by both diabetes mellitus and diabetes insipidus.
16. **a. Imipramine.** Imipramine is a tricyclic antidepressant that is sometimes used to treat stress and urge incontinence because of its two mechanisms of action: norepinephrine uptake inhibition and anticholinergic effect. All of the others are α-adrenergic blocking agents that may cause relaxation of the proximal urethra, exacerbating stress incontinence.
17. **b. direct visualization by the examiner.** All of these are important aspect of characterizing incontinence, but none is as definitive as the examiner actually witnessing it.
18. **a. Uroflow.** Although useful in evaluating the possibility of urethral obstruction and impaired detrusor contractility, uroflow is not necessary in the initial evaluation.
19. **d. Detrusor pressure can be estimated from the subtraction of abdominal pressure from vesical pressure.** Vesical pressure is the sum of detrusor pressure and abdominal pressure. Detrusor pressure cannot be measured directly; it can only be estimated by subtracting abdominal pressure from vesical pressure.
20. **c. is used to determine the pressure-volume relationship during bladder filling and storage.** Voiding function is best attained by measuring detrusor pressure and uroflow. Normally, during bladder filling, at physiologic rates, there is little rise in pressure. This is due to a property of the bladder wall known as accommodation.
21. **a and b.** Abdominal leak-point pressure is a measure of sphincter strength, not a sign of bladder dysfunction.
22. **d. the lowest vesical pressure at which urine passing through the urethra is associated with a rise in abdominal pressure.** In continent women there is no leakage, so it is not possible to record a leak-point pressure.
23. **b. is higher when outlet resistance is higher.** A detrusor leak-point pressure > 40 cm H_2O is associated with a high likelihood of upper urinary damage.
24. **a. is the most precise diagnostic tool available for the evaluation of voiding function/dysfunction.** Because video-urodynamics measures and displays urodynamic findings with the radiographic appearance of the lower urinary tract, each parameter serves as a check against the other and, thus, provides the most accurate information.
25. **e. a and c.** Incontinence is a quality of life condition and, unless there are risk factors such as low bladder compliance, treatment is entirely elective and dependent on patient preferences. On the other hand, the most successful treatment is that which is based on a clear understanding of the underlying pathophysiology.
26. **e. All of the above.**
27. **d. α-adrenergic agonists.** α-Adrenergic agonists cause contraction of the smooth muscle of the urethra and bladder neck. They are sometimes used to treat sphincteric incontinence, but the results are marginal.
28. **c. Imipramine.** See Table 60-7.

29. **e. associated with metabolic disturbances and stone formation.** Augmentation cystoplasty is an effective treatment for patients of all ages with refractory detrusor overactivity. It is effective in abolishing detrusor overactivity and increasing bladder compliance but has not been subjected to randomized trials. It occasionally causes hyperchloremic metabolic acidosis and may be associated with stone formation.

30. **c. has been shown to be superior to no treatment in randomized controlled trials.** Pelvic floor muscle training is most effective in patients of any age with mild incontinence.

31. **e. should no longer be considered part of the routine treatment armamentarium for women with stress incontinence.** Recent large-scale studies have shown that estrogen therapy offers little or no benefit from estrogen replacement, either systemically or locally, for patients with stress incontinence. Furthermore, it may have harmful effects on cardiovascular disease and, unless given with progesterone, it can cause uterine cancer. It is no longer recommended for the treatment of stress incontinence.

32. **c. supported re-creating a proper backboard to resist increases in abdominal pressure.** Delancey's theory states that the endopelvic fascia connects the anterior vaginal wall to the arcus tendineus forming a hammock-like support structure upon which the bladder and urethra rest. During increases in abdominal pressure, the urethra is compressed against this hammock and it is the goal of stress incontinence surgery to re-create the hammock.

33. **e. c and d.** Retropubic suspensions and slings have a median cure/improvement rate of 83% at 4 years, considerably better than anterior repairs and needle suspensions.

34. **c. may have improvement in both stress and urge incontinence if treated with surgery for stress incontinence.** Recent data have shown that patients with mixed incontinence fare almost as well as those with pure stress incontinence after surgery for stress incontinence.

35. **a. artificial urinary sphincter (AUS) is the 'gold standard' for all patients.** The sphincter prosthesis has been subject to many well done studies since its inception in the early 1970s.

61

Overactive Bladder

PAUL ABRAMS • MARCUS DRAKE

QUESTIONS

1. Which definition or definitions appear in the current ICS terminology (2002)?
   a. Detrusor hyperreflexia
   b. Overactive bladder
   c. Idiopathic detrusor overactivity
   d. Hypertonic bladder
   e. Detrusor instability
2. Which symptoms are included in overactive bladder syndrome?
   a. Dysuria
   b. Straining
   c. Urge incontinence
   d. Bladder pain
   e. Frequency
3. In the community, what percentage of adults have overactive bladder symptoms?
   a. Less than 5%
   b. 5% to 12%
   c. 13% to 18%
   d. 18% to 25%
   e. More than 25%
4. Mixed incontinence includes:
   a. stress urinary incontinence.
   b. continuous incontinence.
   c. post-micturition leakage.
   d. incontinence during sexual intercourse.
   e. urge incontinence.
5. Which features are characteristics of urgency?
   a. Always leads to incontinence
   b. Builds up slowly
   c. Is usually felt suprapubically
   d. Develops quickly
   e. May lead to incontinence
6. Which statements are TRUE for detrusor overactivity (DO)?
   a. Phasic involuntary detrusor contractions
   b. Always accompanied by symptoms
   c. Is a urodynamic diagnosis
   d. Is a feature of the voiding phase of micturition
   e. Is often seen in neurologic disease
7. Detrusor overactivity can be diagnosed if:
   a. contractions are greater than 15 cm H_2O
   b. contraction is seen irrespective of size.
   c. there is urge incontinence but no contraction.
   d. leakage occurs during exercise.
   e. there is overactive bladder syndrome.
8. Which statements apply in hypotheses of detrusor pathophysiology?
   a. Afferent sensitization signifies an increased afferent firing rate in response to a standardized stimulus.
   b. The myogenic and peripheral autonomous hypotheses require abnormal propagation of excitation in the bladder wall.
   c. Synaptic reorganization in the spinal cord may contribute to neurogenic detrusor overactivity.
   d. Detrusor overactivity requires volitional control.
   e. The myovesical plexus comprises the ganglia and interstitial cells within the bladder wall.

ANSWERS

1. **b and c. Overactive bladder and Idiopathic detrusor overactivity.** *Overactive bladder* is a new term from the 2002 ICS report. *Idiopathic detrusor overactivity* replaces the term *detrusor instability*. *Detrusor hyperreflexia* is now replaced by *neurogenic detrusor overactivity*. Because the concept of tone is poorly understood the term *hypertonic bladder* is not recommended. *Detrusor instability* has been replaced by *idiopathic detrusor overactivity*.
2. **c and e. Urge incontinence and Frequency.** Urge incontinence is experienced by 50% of patients with OAB. Frequency is a nonspecific accompaniment to OAB in most patients. Stinging in the urethra is characteristic of urinary tract inflammation not OAB. In general, OAB patients do not strain unless they have coexisting detrusor underactivity.
3. **c. 13% to 18%.** Two large prevalence surveys in North America and Europe have shown the prevalence at 16%.
4. **a and e. Stress urinary incontinence and Urge incontinence.** Stress urinary incontinence and urge incontinence are parts of mixed incontinence. Continuous incontinence is rare and characterizes a fistula. Post-micturition leakage occurs after voiding rather than before voiding and is not part of the mixed incontinence picture. Incontinence during sexual intercourse has a number of causes but would not normally be included in mixed incontinence.
5. **d and e. Develops quickly and may lead to incontinence.** Urgency develops quickly, disturbing a patient's way of life,

and may lead to incontinence in the susceptible patient. Many patients, particularly those with good sphincteric function, do not have incontinence. Urgency is thought to be a symptom of rapid onset. Urgency is normally felt in the perineum.

6. **a, c, and e. Phasic involuntary detrusor contractions, is a urodynamic diagnosis, and is often seen in neurological disease.** Phasic involuntary detrusor contractions are characteristic of DO. Detrusor overactivity is a urodynamic diagnosis. Detrusor overactivity is often seen in neurologic disease and is known as neurogenic DO. In the elderly and in neurologic patients DO may be asymptomatic. Detrusor overactivity is a filling phase diagnosis.

7. **b. Contraction is seen irrespective of size.** This is correct, although the quality of the urodynamic trace requires a minimum contraction height. "Contractions are greater than 15 cm H_2O" is a pre-1988 ICS definition; subsequently it was realized that small contractions can cause significant symptoms. Urge incontinence but no contraction may be due to involuntary urethral relaxation. Leakage occurring during exercise is not a classic criterion for DO, although exercise can precipitate DO. Although the urodynamic demonstration of DO is often associated with OAB symptoms, either may occur independently of the other.

8. **a, b, c, and e. Afferent sensitization signifies an increased afferent firing rate in response to a standardized stimulus.** In theory, this could result in premature activation of the micturition reflex. **The myogenic and peripheral autonomous hypotheses require abnormal propagation of excitation in the bladder wall.** The myogenic hypothesis suggests direct propagation between muscle cells, the peripheral autonomous module hypothesis suggests propagation is through the myovesical plexus. **Synaptic reorganization in the spinal cord may contribute to neurogenic detrusor overactivity.** It could underlie reemergence of primitive reflexes. **The myovesical plexus comprises the ganglia and interstitial cells within the bladder wall** and is proposed as a structure analogous to the myenteric plexuses of the gut. Patients are unable to inhibit overactive contractions voluntarily.

62

Pharmacologic Management of Storage and Emptying Failure

KARL-ERIK ANDERSSON • ALAN J. WEIN

QUESTIONS

1. The effects of administration of antimuscarinic agent to an individual with an overactive bladder include all EXCEPT:
   a. increased total bladder capacity.
   b. depressed amplitude of involuntary bladder contractions.
   c. increased outlet resistance.
   d. increased volume to the first involuntary bladder contraction.
   e. increased mean volume voided.
2. Which of the following muscarinic receptor subtypes is the most common in human detrusor smooth muscle?
   a. M_1
   b. M_2
   c. M_3
   d. M_4
   e. M_5
3. Which of the following muscarinic receptor subtypes is predominantly responsible for the mediation of bladder contraction in human detrusor smooth muscle?
   a. M_1
   b. M_2
   c. M_3
   d. M_4
   e. M_5
4. The use of antimuscarinic agents to treat overactive bladder is limited by their lack of uroselectivity. Which of the following is not a recognized side effect of antimuscarinic agents?
   a. Dry mouth
   b. Constipation
   c. Cognitive dysfunction
   d. Bradycardia
   e. Blurred vision
5. Which of the following characteristics increases the possibilities for an antimuscarinic to pass the blood-brain barrier?
   a. High lipophilicity
   b. Large molecular size
   c. Low electrical charge
   d. Quaternary ammonium structure
   e. Small molecular size
6. As a therapeutic antimuscarinic agent, propantheline bromide is:
   a. receptor specific.
   b. tissue specific.
   c. poorly absorbed from the gastrointestinal tract.
   d. a tertiary ammonium compound.
   e. more effective than oxybutynin.
7. Oxybutynin exerts its clinical effects on the urinary bladder primarily by:
   a. calcium channel blockade.
   b. local anesthetic activity.
   c. inhibition of norepinephrine uptake.
   d. M_3 receptor blockade.
   e. M_1 receptor blockade.
8. The Committee on Pharmacologic Treatment of the Third International Consultation on Incontinence assessed agents according to the Oxford Guidelines, according to level of evidence and grade of recommendation with respect to treatment of detrusor overactivity. Which of the following did not receive a level of evidence rating of "1" and a grade of recommendation of "A"?
   a. Dicyclomine
   b. Flavoxate
   c. Trospium
   d. Tolterodine
   e. Oxybutynin
9. The pharmacologic characteristics of which class of drugs would suggest that they may be active during the filling/storage phase of micturition and effective in abolishing detrusor overactivity, yet with no effect on normal bladder contraction?
   a. Calcium antagonists
   b. Antimuscarinics
   c. Cyclooxygenase inhibitors
   d. Potassium channel openers
   e. β-Adrenoceptor antagonists
10. Which of the following pharmacologic actions is most probably responsible for the effects of oxybutynin when given systemically?
    a. Antimuscarinic, direct muscle relaxant, and local anesthetic actions
    b. Direct muscle relaxant effect alone
    c. Direct muscle relaxant effect and local anesthetic action
    d. Antimuscarinic and direct muscle relaxant effects
    e. Antimuscarinic effect

11. Which two of the following muscarinic receptor subtypes are not known to be involved in the potential antimuscarinic side effects of dry mouth, constipation, tachycardia, drowsiness, and blurred vision?
    a. M_1
    b. M_2
    c. M_3
    d. M_4
    e. M_5
12. The primary adverse event reported with the usage of oxybutynin-transdermal has been:
    a. tachycardia.
    b. dry mouth.
    c. constipation.
    d. application site reactions.
    e. blurred vision.
13. Which of the following agents is relatively selective for M_3 receptor blockade?
    a. Darifenacin
    b. Oxybutynin
    c. Solifenacin
    d. Tolterodine
    e. Trospium
14. Which of the following drugs have a theoretical advantage for causing less cognitive dysfunction and why?
    a. Darifenacin
    b. Oxybutynin
    c. Solifenacin
    d. Tolterodine
    e. Trospium
15. Of the following agents, which is actively excreted by the kidney in the proximal convoluted tubules?
    a. Darifenacin
    b. Oxybutynin
    c. Solifenacin
    d. Tolterodine
    e. Trospium
16. Which of the following pharmacologic actions of imipramine is least prominent?
    a. Sedative, on a central basis
    b. Block reuptake of norepinephrine in presynaptic nerve endings
    c. Block reuptake of serotonin in presynaptic nerve endings
    d. Antihistaminic, by blocking H1 receptors
    e. Direct antimuscarinic on bladder smooth muscle
17. Which of the following is NOT listed as a common side effect of imipramine?
    a. Peripheral antimuscarinic effects
    b. Weakness, fatigue
    c. Priapism
    d. Cardiac arrhythmia
    e. Hepatic dysfunction
18. Resiniferatoxin, as compared with capsaicin, exhibits which of the following properties?
    a. Greater desensitization at lower concentrations
    b. More early noxious side effects when administered intravesically
    c. More late side effects when administered intravesically
    d. Blockade of only Aδ fiber-mediated contraction
    e. Acts on non-vanilloid receptors
19. When used as an intradetrusor injection for detrusor overactivity, botulinum toxin A appears to exert its effects within what time frame and last for what time frame before reinjection is necessary?
    a. 3 weeks and 4 to 6 months
    b. 3 days and 6 to 9 months
    c. 2 hours and 6 to 9 months
    d. 1 week and 6 to 9 months
    e. 2 weeks and 4 to 6 months
20. α-Adrenergic agonists, in general, produce all but which of the following?
    a. An increase in maximum urethral pressure
    b. An increase in maximum urethral closure pressure
    c. A contraction of urethral smooth muscle
    d. A decrease in maximal bladder capacity
    e. An increase in bladder outlet resistance
21. The side effects of the α-adrenergic agonists include all of the following EXCEPT:
    a. tremor.
    b. palpitations.
    c. hypertension.
    d. somnolence.
    e. respiratory difficulties.
22. Which of the following agents has been reported to increase stroke risk in young women within 3 days of taking their first dose?
    a. Phenylpropanolamine
    b. Ephedrine
    c. Pseudoephedrine
    d. Midodrine
    e. Clenbuterol
23. In theory, which of the following agents, from the standpoint of potential efficacy and safety, would be preferred for the treatment of stress incontinence in a hypertensive individual?
    a. Ephedrine
    b. Propranolol
    c. Phenylpropanolamine
    d. Pseudoephedrine
    e. Clenbuterol
24. Which of the following statements is NOT true with respect to duloxetine hydrochloride?
    a. Significantly increases sphincteric muscle activity during filling/storage in an animal model
    b. A combined norepinephrine and serotonin reuptake inhibitor
    c. Lipophilic and well absorbed
    d. Effective in decreasing stress urinary incontinence episodes in women
    e. Not metabolized by the liver
25. Which of the following statements is FALSE with respect to desmopressin?
    a. It is classically used to test nocturnal enuresis.
    b. It is classically used to treat diabetes insipidus.
    c. It can be given orally or intranasally at the same doses.
    d. It suppresses urine production for 7 to 12 hours.
    e. It can be used in both children and adults.

26. A 75-year-old man placed on intranasal desmopressin therapy 3 days previously presents with a change of mental status and mental confusion. The most likely cause is:
   a. cognitive dysfunction due to antimuscarinic effect.
   b. hyponatremia.
   c. hypernatremia.
   d. hypokalemia.
   e. hyperkalemia.

27. With regard to bethanechol chloride, the least objective evidence exists to support which of the following statements?
   a. It has relatively selective in vitro action on urinary bladder and bowel.
   b. It has little or no nicotinic action.
   c. It is cholinesterase resistant.
   d. It causes in vitro contraction of bladder smooth muscle.
   e. It facilitates bladder emptying.

28. What oral dose of bethanechol chloride is required to produce the same urodynamic effects, at least in a denervated bladder, at the subcutaneous dose of 5 mg?
   a. 200 mg
   b. 100 mg
   c. 50 mg
   d. 25 mg
   e. 10 mg

29. Prostaglandins have been hypothesized to affect bladder activity through all but which of the following actions?
   a. Neuromodulation of efferent and afferent neurotransmission
   b. Sensitization to sensory stimuli (activation occurs with a lower degree of filling)
   c. Activation of certain sensory nerves
   d. Potentiation of acetylcholine release from cholinergic nerve terminals
   e. Potentiation of ATP release from urothelial mucosa

30. With respect to α-adrenergic receptors versus β-adrenergic receptors in the lower urinary tract, all but which of the following statements are TRUE?
   a. The α-adrenergic receptors are more prominent in the bladder base than are β-adrenergic receptors.
   b. The α_1-adrenergic receptors are more common than α_2-adrenergic receptors.
   c. The α-adrenergic receptors are less prominent in the bladder body than are β-adrenergic receptors.
   d. Bladder smooth muscle contraction is mediated predominantly by α_1-adrenergic receptors.
   e. Urethral smooth muscle contraction is mediated predominantly by α_1-adrenergic receptors.

31. Which of the following α-adrenergic blocking agents has significant antagonistic properties at both α_1 and α_2 receptor sites?
   a. Prazosin
   b. Terazosin
   c. Phenoxybenzamine
   d. Doxazosin
   e. Tamsulosin

32. Available data suggest that which of the following side effects is more common with tamsulosin than with either terazosin or doxazosin?
   a. Dizziness
   b. Asthenia
   c. Postural hypotension
   d. Palpitations
   e. Retrograde ejaculation

33. Which of the following agents or classes of agents, when administered systemically, will selectively relax the striated musculature of the pelvic floor?
   a. Benzodiazepines
   b. Dantrolene
   c. Baclofen
   d. Botulinum toxin
   e. None of the above

34. Which of the following is the most widely distributed inhibitory neurotransmitter in the mammalian central nervous system?
   a. γ-Aminobutyric acid (GABA)
   b. Glycine
   c. Glutamate
   d. Dopamine
   e. Norepinephrine

35. Baclofen (Lioresal) acts to decrease striated sphincter activity by which of the following mechanisms?
   a. Facilitating neuronal hyperpolarization through the $GABA_A$ receptor.
   b. Activating the $GABA_B$ receptor and depressing monosynaptic and polysynaptic excitation of motor neurons and interneurons in the spinal cord.
   c. Inhibiting excitation-contraction coupling in skeletal muscle by decreasing calcium release from the sarcoplasmic reticulum.
   d. Inhibiting excitation-contraction coupling by preventing calcium entry into the cell.
   e. Inhibiting acetylcholine release at the neuromuscular junction.

36. All but the following are true with regard to botulinum toxin EXCEPT which one?
   a. It has been reported to be useful in the treatment of striated sphincter dyssynergia via direct sphincteric injection.
   b. It has been reported to be useful in the treatment of detrusor overactivity by direct intradetrusor injection.
   c. It inhibits the release of acetylcholine and other transmitters at the neuromuscular junction of somatic nerve and striated muscle and the autonomic nerves in smooth muscle.
   d. It has been reported to be of use, via periurethral striated muscle injections, in the treatment of stress urinary incontinence.
   e. The immunologic subtype utilized for urologic use has primarily been Botox A.

ANSWERS

1. **c. increased outlet resistance.** Atropine and atropine-like agents will depress normal bladder contractions and involuntary bladder contractions of any cause. In such patients, the volume to the first involuntary bladder contraction will generally be increased, the amplitude of the involuntary bladder contraction decreased, and the total bladder capacity increased. Outlet resistance, at least as reflected by urethral pressure measurements, does not seem to be clinically affected.

2. **b. M_2.** On the basis of existing knowledge, it is now recommended that the designations M_{1-5} be used to describe both the

pharmacologic subtypes and the molecular subtypes of muscarinic acetylcholine receptors. The human urinary bladder smooth muscle contains a mixed population of M_2 and M_3 subtypes, with M_2 receptors being predominant (M_2 receptors predominate at least 3:1 over M_3 receptors not only on detrusor cells but also on other bladder structures, which may be of importance for detrusor activation).

3. **c. M_3.** The minor population of M_3 receptors is generally accepted at this time as being primarily responsible for the mediation of bladder contraction.
4. **d. Bradycardia.** In general, drug therapy for lower urinary tract dysfunction is hindered by a concept that can be expressed in one word: uroselectivity. The clinical utility of available antimuscarinic agents is limited by their lack of selectivity, responsible for the classic peripheral antimuscarinic side effects of dry mouth, constipation, blurred vision, tachycardia, and effects on cognitive function.
5. **a. High lipophilicity, c. Low electrical charge, and e. Small molecular size.** High lipophilicity, small molecular size, and low electrical charge increase the possibilities for an antimuscarinic to pass the blood brain barrier. Quaternary ammonium compounds pass into the central nervous system to a limited extent.
6. **c. poorly absorbed from the gastrointestinal tract.** Propantheline bromide (Pro-Banthine, others) was the classically described oral agent for producing an antimuscarinic effect in the lower urinary tract. It is a nonselective muscarinic antagonist. Propantheline is a quaternary ammonium compound, all of which are poorly absorbed after oral administration. There seems to be little difference between the antimuscarinic effects of propantheline on bladder smooth muscle and the effects of other classic antimuscarinic agents.
7. **d. M_3 receptor blockade.** Although the agents with mixed actions do relax smooth muscle in vitro by musculotropic activity and do have some local anesthetic properties, it is generally accepted that the clinical effects, at least of oxybutynin, occur solely through muscarinic blockade, as the other effects occur at much higher concentrations than its antimuscarinic actions. Oxybutynin chloride (Ditropan) is a potent muscarinic receptor antagonist with some degree of selectivity for M_3 and M_1 receptors.
8. **a. Dicyclomine and b. Flavoxate.** A level of evidence of "1" implies the presence of systematic reviews, meta-analyses, and good quality randomized controlled clinical trials. A grade of recommendation of "A" means that the agent is highly recommended, based on level "1" evidence. Dicyclomine received a level of evidence of "3," meaning that only case-controlled studies and case series existed as evidence for efficacy, and a grade of recommendation of "C," meaning that only level "4" studies (based on only expert opinion) or "majority evidence" existed. Flavoxate received a level of evidence of "2," meaning that either randomized control trials and/or good quality prospective cohort studies existed regarding its usage, but a grade of recommendation of "D," meaning that no recommendation for usage is possible because of inconsistent/inconclusive evidence. The complete listing of the Oxford Guidelines and the committee recommendations can be found in Tables 62-1 and 62-2.
9. **d. Potassium channel openers.** Opening of potassium channels and subsequent efflux of potassium will produce hyperpolarization of various smooth muscles, including the detrusor. This leads to a decrease in calcium influx with subsequent relaxation or inhibition of contraction. Theoretically, such drugs may be active during the filling/storage phase of micturition, abolishing detrusor overactivity with no effect on normal bladder contraction. Unfortunately, the first generation of potassium channel openers were found to be more potent as inhibitors of vascular than of detrusor muscle; and in clinical trials performed with these drugs, no bladder effects were found at doses that lowered blood pressure. However, new drugs with potassium-ATP channel opening properties have been described that may prove to be useful for the treatment of DO.
10. **e. Antimuscarinic effect.** Oxybutynin has several pharmacologic effects, some of which seem difficult to relate to its effectiveness in the treatment of detrusor overactivity. It has antimuscarinic, direct muscle relaxant, and local anesthetic actions. The local anesthetic action and direct muscle relaxant effect may be of importance when the drug is administered intravesically but probably play no role when it is given orally. In vitro, oxybutynin was shown to be 500 times weaker as a smooth muscle relaxant than as an antimuscarinic agent. Most probably, when given systemically, oxybutynin acts mainly as an antimuscarinic drug.
11. **d. M_4 and e. M_5.** The M_3 receptor has a primary role in salivation, bowel motility, and visual accommodation. The M_1 receptor is thought to be involved in cognition. The M_2 receptor is the primary cholinergic receptor in the heart, causing bradycardia when activated and, potentially, tachycardia, when blocked. The M_4 and M_5 receptors do not at this time seem to have a primary role in any of these organ systems.
12. **d. application site reactions.** The transdermal delivery of oxybutynin alters oxybutynin metabolism, reducing production of the primary metabolite, responsible for most of the side effects, to an even greater extent than extended release oxybutynin. The primary adverse event for this preparation has been application site reaction pruritus in 14% and erythema in 8.3%.
13. **a. Darifenacin.** Darifenacin is relatively selective for M_3 receptor blockade, meaning that, in vitro, the affinity for M_3 receptors is greater than for the other muscarinic receptors. This is only a relative selectivity, however, and whether this translates into either greater efficacy or greater tolerability has yet to be established.
14. **a. Darifenacin, d. Tolterodine, and e. Trospium.** The currently accepted theory as to why some antimuscarinic agents may cause cognitive dysfunction is antagonism of M_1 receptor activity in the brain. Theoretically, to have this side effect, an agent must be able to cross rather freely the blood-brain barrier and affect M_1 receptors to a significant extent. Darifenacin is relatively selective for M_3 receptor blockade, although it does cross the blood-brain barrier freely. Tolterodine, because of its low lipophilicity, relatively large molecular size, and charge status, is thought to have limited passage across the blood-brain barrier in a normal individual. Trospium, by virtue of its quaternary mean status, has limited passage across the blood-brain barrier in a normal individual.
15. **e. Trospium.** Darifenacin, oxybutynin, solifenacin, and tolterodine are all actively metabolized in the liver by the cytochrome P450 enzyme system. Trospium chloride is not metabolized to any significant degree in the liver. It is actively excreted by the proximal convoluted tubules in the kidney.
16. **e. Direct antimuscarinic on bladder smooth muscle.** All of these agents possess various degrees of at least three major pharmacologic actions: (1) they have central and peripheral antimuscarinic effects at some, but not all, sites; (2) they block the active transport system in the presynaptic nerve ending, which is responsible for the reuptake of the released amine neurotransmitters norepinephrine and serotonin; and (3) they are sedatives, an action that occurs presumably on a central basis but is perhaps related to antihistaminic properties. Imipramine has prominent systemic antimuscarinic effects but has only a weak antimuscarinic effect on bladder smooth muscle. A strong direct inhibitory effect on bladder smooth muscle does exist, however, that is neither antimuscarinic nor adrenergic.

17. **c. Priapism**. The most frequent side effects of the tricyclic antidepressants are those attributable to their systemic antimuscarinic activity. Allergic phenomena (including rash), hepatic dysfunction, obstructive jaundice, and agranulocytosis may also occur, but rarely. Central nervous system side effects may include weakness, fatigue, parkinsonian effect, fine tremor noted most in the upper extremities, manic or schizophrenic picture, and sedation, probably from an antihistaminic effect. Postural hypotension may also be seen, presumably on the basis of selective blockade (a paradoxical effect) of α_1-adrenergic receptors in some vascular smooth muscle. Tricyclic antidepressants can also cause excess sweating of obscure cause and a delay of orgasm or orgasmic impotence, whose cause is likewise unclear. They can also produce arrhythmias and interact in deleterious ways with other drugs, and so caution must be observed in their use in patients with cardiac disease.
18. **a. Greater desensitization at lower concentrations.** Resiniferatoxin (RTX) is an analog of capsaicin, approximately 1000 times more potent for desensitization but only a few hundred times more potent for excitation. Although both may have effects on Aδ fibers, this is speculative, and their primary action is to render sensitive primary afferents (C fibers) resistant to activation by natural stimuli.
19. **e. 2 weeks and 4 to 6 months.**
20. **d. A decrease in maximal bladder capacity**. The bladder neck and proximal urethra contain a preponderance of α_1-receptor sites, which, when stimulated, produce smooth muscle contraction. The static infusion urethral pressure profile is altered by such stimulation, which produces an increase in maximal urethral pressure and maximal urethral closure pressure. Various orally administered pharmacologic agents are available that produce α-adrenergic stimulation. Generally, outlet resistance is increased to a variable degree by such an action.
21. **d. somnolence.** Potential side effects of all of these agents include blood pressure elevation, anxiety, and insomnia due to stimulation of the central nervous system; headache; tremor; weakness; palpations; cardiac arrhythmias; and respiratory difficulties. They should be used with caution in patients with hypertension, cardiovascular disease, or hyperthyroidism.
22. **a. Phenylpropanolamine**. The Food and Drug Administration (FDA) originally asked manufacturers to stop selling PPA-containing drugs and to replace the ingredient with a safe alternative. Subsequently, it was taken off the market in the United States. The original request was based on a study reported by Kernan and colleagues in 2000 in the *New England Journal of Medicine*. In commenting on this article, the *Medical Letter* (Abramowicz and Zuccotti, 2000) noted that no case-control studies were available on the safety of phenylephrine, ephedrine, or pseudoephedrine but did note that case reports have associated ephedra alkaloids with hypertension, stroke, seizures, and death. The *Medical Letter* concluded: "Phenylpropanolamine may not be the only alpha-adrenergic agonist that can cause serious adverse effects when taken systemically in over-the-counter products marketed for nasal congestion or weight loss."
23. **b. Propranolol**. Theoretically, β-adrenergic blocking agents might be expected to "unmask" or potentiate an α-adrenergic effect, thereby increasing urethral resistance. Such treatment has been suggested as an alternative treatment to α-adrenergic agonists in patients with sphincteric incontinence and hypertension.
24. **e. Not metabolized by the liver.** Duloxetine hydrochloride is a combined norepinephrine and serotonin reuptake inhibitor that has been shown, in an animal model, to significantly increase urethral sphincteric muscle activity during the filling/storage phase of micturition. It is lipophilic, well absorbed, and extensively metabolized by the liver. Its effectiveness in the treatment of stress urinary incontinence in the female has been documented. At the time of this writing it was withdrawn from the FDA approval process and has not been resubmitted, but it has been approved for use in Europe.
25. **c. It can be given orally or intranasally at the same doses.** The synthetic antidiuretic hormone peptide analog DDAVP (1-deamino-8-D-arginine vasopressin), now more commonly known as desmopressin, has been utilized for the symptomatic relief of refractory nocturnal enuresis in both children and adults. The drug can conveniently be administered by intranasal spray at bedtime (10 to 40 μg) or as an oral preparation (100 to 400 μg) and effectively suppresses urine production for 7 to 12 hours.
26. **b. hyponatremia.** Side effects are relatively uncommon during desmopressin treatment, but there is a risk of water retention and hyponatremia, such that it is recommended that serum sodium concentration should be measured before and after a few days of treatment in elderly patients.
27. **e. It facilitates bladder emptying**. Many acetylcholine-like drugs exist, but only bethanechol chloride (Urecholine, Duvoid, others) exhibits a relatively selective in vitro action on the urinary bladder and gut with little or no nicotinic action. Bethanechol chloride is cholinesterase resistant and causes an in vitro contraction of smooth muscle from all areas of the bladder. Although it has been reported to increase gastrointestinal motility and has been used in the treatment of gastroesophageal reflux, and although anecdotal success in specific patients with voiding dysfunction seems to occur, there is no evidence to support its success in facilitating bladder emptying in series of patients when the drug was the only variable.
28. **a. 200 mg.** It is generally agreed that, at least in a "denervated" bladder, an oral dose of 200 mg is required to produce the same urodynamic effects as a subcutaneous dose of 5 mg.
29. **e. Potentiation of ATP release from urothelial mucosa.** Prostanoids are synthesized both locally in bladder muscle and mucosa, with synthesis being initiated by various physiologic stimuli such as detrusor muscle stretch, mucosal injury, neural stimulation, directly by ATP and by mediators of inflammation. Prostanoids have been reported to be useful in facilitating bladder emptying, with intravesical administration. Possible roles include (1) neuromodulators of efferent and afferent transmission; (2) sensitization; (3) activation of certain sensory nerves; and (4) potentiation of acetylcholine release from cholinergic nerve terminals through prejunctional prostanoid receptors.
30. **b. The α_1-adrenergic receptors are more common than α_2-adrenergic receptors.** The smooth muscle of the bladder base and proximal urethra contains predominantly α-adrenergic receptors, although β-adrenergic receptors are present. The bladder body contains both varieties of adrenergic receptors, with the β-adrenergic variety being more common. The human lower urinary tract contains more α_2- than α_1-adrenergic receptors, but prostatic smooth muscle contraction and human lower urinary tract smooth muscle contraction are mediated largely, if not exclusively, by α_1-adrenergic receptors.
31. **c. Phenoxybenzamine.** Phenoxybenzamine (Dibenzyline) was the α-adrenolytic agent originally used for the treatment of voiding dysfunction. It and phentolamine have blocking properties at both α_1-adrenergic and α_2-adrenergic receptor sites. Prazosin hydrochloride (Minipress) was the first potent selective α_1-adrenergic antagonist used to lower outlet resistance.

Terazosin (Hytrin) and doxazosin (Cardura) are two highly selective postsynaptic α_1-adrenergic blockers. Most recently, alfuzosin and tamsulosin (Flomax), both highly selective α_1-adrenergic blockers, have appeared and are marketed solely for the treatment of benign prostatic hyperplasia because of some reports suggesting preferential action on prostatic rather than vascular smooth muscle.

32. **e. Retrograde ejaculation.** Available data suggest that retrograde ejaculation and rhinitis are more common with tamsulosin, whereas dizziness and asthenia are more common with terazosin and doxazosin.

33. **e. None of the above.** There is no class of pharmacologic agents that will selectively relax the striated musculature of the pelvic floor.

34. **a. γ-Aminobutyric acid (GABA).** GABA and glycine have been identified as major inhibitory transmitters in the central nervous system. GABA is the most widely distributed inhibitory neurotransmitter in the mammalian central nervous system. GABA appears to mediate the inhibitory actions of local interneurons in the brain and presynaptic inhibition within the spinal cord.

35. **b. Activating the $GABA_B$ receptor and depressing monosynaptic and polysynaptic excitation of motor neurons and interneurons in the spinal cord.** Benzodiazepines potentiate the action of GABA by facilitating neuronal hyperpolarization through the $GABA_A$ receptor. Baclofen (Lioresal) depresses monosynaptic and polysynaptic excitation of motor neurons and interneurons in the spinal cord by activating $GABA_B$ receptors. Dantrolene (Dantrium) exerts its effects by a direct peripheral action on skeletal muscle. It is thought to inhibit the excitation-induced release of calcium ions from the sarcoplasmic reticulum of striated muscle fibers, thereby inhibiting excitation-contraction coupling and diminishing the mechanical force of contraction. Botulinum A toxin (Botox) is an inhibitor of acetylcholine release at the neuromuscular junction of somatic nerves on striated muscle.

36. **d. It has been reported to be of use, via periurethral striated muscle injections, in the treatment of stress urinary incontinence.** Intersphincteric injections of Botox A were first reported useful in the treatment of striated sphincter dyssynergia in 1990. The toxin blocks the release of acetylcholine and other transmitters from presynaptic nerve endings by interacting with the protein complex necessary for docking vesicles. This results in decreased muscle contractility and muscle atrophy at the injection site. The drug has been reported to be of use as well in the treatment of neurogenic detrusor overactivity and cases of non-neurogenic detrusor overactivity. There are seven immunologically distinct antigenic subtypes. Types A and B are in clinical use in urology, but most studies and treatments have been carried out with botulinum toxin A type. Intrasphincteric injections of botulinum toxin are not useful for stress incontinence. In fact, they can cause stress incontinence in a female.

63

Conservative Management of Urinary Incontinence: Behavioral and Pelvic Floor Therapy and Urethral and Pelvic Devices

CHRISTOPHER K. PAYNE

QUESTIONS

1. The consequences of urinary incontinence (UI) include an increased risk of all of the following EXCEPT:
   a. pressure ulcers.
   b. renal failure.
   c. urinary tract infections.
   d. admission to nursing homes.
   e. falls and fractures.
2. The annual medical expenditures for an average man with UI compared with one without incontinence are:
   a. 25% less.
   b. about the same.
   c. 25% more.
   d. 50% more.
   e. more than double.
3. Compared with Alzheimer's disease and asthma, NIH funding for incontinence research is:
   a. less than 1/10th.
   b. about half.
   c. about the same.
   d. 50% greater.
   e. more than double.
4. Nonsurgical treatments for UI are usually the preferred first-line interventions because of all of the following EXCEPT:
   a. pelvic floor rehabilitation is superior to surgery for stress incontinence.
   b. UI is not a uniformly progressive disease.
   c. nonsurgical treatments are safe and reversible.
   d. patients often request nonsurgical treatments.
   e. medical therapies are very effective for patients with OAB and urge incontinence.
5. Which of the following is an example of behavioral therapy?
   a. Use of a pessary to correct a cystocele
   b. Incontinence pads
   c. Vaginal EMG biofeedback training
   d. Discussion of normal bladder and sphincter function.
   e. Use of oxybutynin on an "as needed" basis
6. The behavioral technique most appropriate for an institutionalized, cognitively impaired individual is:
   a. timed voiding.
   b. bladder training.
   c. prompted voiding.
   d. fluid restriction.
   e. urge inhibition.
7. Which of the following statements is NOT an accurate description of the results of behavioral therapy?
   a. When behavioral therapy is combined with pharmacologic treatment of urge incontinence approximately 50% of patients will maintain good results after the drug is discontinued.
   b. Fantyl and colleagues demonstrated that behavioral approaches are equally effective for stress and urge incontinence.
   c. Behavioral therapy is equally successful with CMG negative, CMG positive, and neurogenic patients with OAB symptoms.
   d. Burgio demonstrated that behavioral therapy is as effective as medication for patients with urge and mixed incontinence.
   e. Outpatient behavioral therapy can be as successful as intensive inpatient regimens.
8. The accurate statement about cigarette smoking and UI is which one?
   a. Even low-level smoking increases the risk for UI.
   b. Smoking is strongly associated with SUI but not with OAB.
   c. Smoking cessation normalizes the risk of UI within 5 years.
   d. There are no clinical studies to determine the effectiveness of smoking cessation in the treatment of UI.
   e. Smoking cessation is only effective in the treatment of female SUI.

9. Evidence-based medicine supports which of the following recommendations?
   a. A 20% fluid restriction can be recommended as initial treatment for all OAB patients.
   b. Increasing alcohol use is linearly correlated with UI severity.
   c. Neither carbonated beverages nor tea appear to relate to UI symptoms.
   d. Decreasing caffeine intake improves continence.
   e. Acidic juices should be eliminated in patients with UI.
10. The correct statement(s) regarding obesity and UI is(are) which of the following?
    a. Obesity is strongly correlated with SUI only.
    b. Obesity is strongly correlated with OAB only.
    c. Obesity is strongly correlated with both SUI and OAB.
    d. Weight reduction can reduce UI in obese women.
    e. Weight reduction has not been shown to affect UI in obese women.
11. Accurate statements about pelvic floor muscle training (PFMT) include which of the following?
    a. Kegel initially described pelvic muscle exercises with use of biofeedback training.
    b. Approximately 50% of incontinent women cannot properly contract the pelvic muscles on command.
    c. "Training" emphasizes the need for a long-term treatment regimen.
    d. All of the above.
    e. None of the above.
12. All of the following statements about PFMT are true EXCEPT which one?
    a. Improved muscle strength correlates strongly with improvement in continence.
    b. They must be taught by a health care professional.
    c. With repeated exercise a muscle will develop improved responsiveness that may lead to a faster and/or stronger contraction.
    d. No single PFMT regimen has been proven most effective.
    e. Every-other-day exercise is recommended based on the exercise literature.
13. In preventing UI, the evidence supports routine use of PFMT in which of the following groups?
    a. All primiparous women, before delivery
    b. Primiparous women, after instrumented delivery
    c. All pregnant women, before delivery
    d. a and b
    e. All of the above
14. In treating established UI, the evidence supports routine use of PFMT in which of the following patient groups?
    a. All women with UI
    b. Women with SUI only
    c. Women with urgency incontinence only
    d. Men with post-prostatectomy incontinence
    e. None of the above
15. In treating established SUI in women, PFMT is proved to be more effective than:
    a. electrical stimulation.
    b. bladder training.
    c. vaginal cones.
    d. surgery.
    e. more effective than adrenergic agonist medications.
16. Which of the following is not a tool used in pelvic floor biofeedback therapy?
    a. Verbal coaching
    b. Vaginal cones
    c. Pressure perineometer
    d. Perineal EMG patches
    e. Neotonus device
17. Limitations/disadvantages of using biofeedback therapy for pelvic floor rehabilitation include:
    a. applicable only to SUI patients.
    b. inferior outcomes compared with PFMT alone.
    c. requires expensive equipment.
    d. requires motivated patient.
    e. requires long-term treatment.
18. Which of the following most accurately describes passive pelvic floor therapies (electrical and magnetic stimulation)?
    a. Patient motivation is the key to successful outcome.
    b. They are attractive options for patients unable to perform PFMT.
    c. Restoration of continence results from conversion of urethral skeletal muscle to predominantly fast-twitch fibers.
    d. Electrical stimulation is more effective than magnetic stimulation for SUI.
    e. Mixed incontinence patients are not candidates for these therapies.
19. Which of the following is NOT true of vaginal electrical stimulation therapy?
    a. E-stim appears to be superior to sham therapy for women with detrusor overactivity.
    b. E-stim decreased SUI episodes by 42% in a prospective, controlled trial.
    c. Optimal regimen for stimulation is twice per day in the induction phase.
    d. There has been no comparison between vaginal and peripheral surface E-stim with patch electrodes in the treatment of OAB symptoms.
    e. Long-term durability of stimulation results have not been established.
20. Electromagnetic stimulation therapy is:
    a. a simple, one-time office procedure performed using local anesthesia and sedation.
    b. the most effective nonsurgical treatment for female stress incontinence.
    c. much better tolerated than vaginal E-stim.
    d. a reasonable choice for the incontinent patient who is unable to identify the pelvic floor muscles.
    e. ineffective if a patient has detrusor instability.
21. In comparing biofeedback, electrical stimulation, and magnetic stimulation therapy for UI, which of the following statements is TRUE?
    a. Only biofeedback training is applicable to home therapy.
    b. Magnetic stimulation is an option for patients who will not accept vaginal instrumentation.
    c. If initially successful, biofeedback therapy has superior long-term results.
    d. All of the treatments require a skilled therapist to administer.
    e. All of the treatments depend on patient motivation.

22. When evaluating a patient with mixed incontinence for possible surgical therapy, which of the following devices will predict the response of the patient to an operation?

    a. A urethral meatal adhesive device
    b. A urethral stent
    c. A bladder neck support device
    d. None of the above
    e. All of the above

23. Vaginal support devices (pessaries):

    a. can be used on an "as needed" basis.
    b. cannot be used over the long term due to problematic local side effects.
    c. are likely to increase voiding difficulties and residual urine.
    d. are only indicated for those too ill to consider surgical correction.
    e. are more effective in treating stress incontinence due to intrinsic sphincter dysfunction.

24. Vaginal support devices (pessaries):

    a. may unmask occult stress incontinence in 50% of cystocele patients.
    b. can be used to determine if lower grade prolapse is symptomatic
    c. can be used to identify reversible urinary retention related to prolapse.
    d. All of the above
    e. None of the above

25. Patient satisfaction is directly related to:

    a. expectations.
    b. goal setting.
    c. goal achievement.
    d. surgical cure of stress incontinence.
    e. surgical cure of prolapse.

26. Treatment planning for the incontinent female requires all of the following EXCEPT:

    a. knowledge of the patient's goals and preferences.
    b. assessment of urethral support and pelvic anatomy.
    c. assessment of pelvic muscle strength.
    d. voiding diary.
    e. filling cystometry.

27. The maximum voided volume on a bladder diary correlates with what urodynamic parameter?

    a. Compliance
    b. Valsalva leak-point pressure
    c. Detrusor leak pressure
    d. Cystometric capacity
    e. Residual urine

28. When considering pelvic floor function in a female with UI those with:

    a. absent voluntary contraction have ISD and should be treated with a pubovaginal sling or periurethral injections.
    b. absent contraction are probably best served by biofeedback training.
    c. a weak contraction cannot benefit from PFMT alone.
    d. strong baseline contraction will benefit most from passive stimulation.
    e. strong baseline contraction cannot benefit from surgery since urethral closure is already high.

29. Almost all women with SUI can be offered effective nonsurgical therapy. Relative indications for surgical treatment of female SUI include all of the following EXCEPT:

    a. patient motivated to be completely dry.
    b. symptomatic prolapse.
    c. strong pelvic muscle contractions.
    d. severe leakage with minimal activity.
    e. associated OAB.

30. In planning treatment for a woman with urgency incontinence:

    a. if the bladder diary shows normal capacity early use of anticholinergic medications is appropriate.
    b. start with combination PFMT and anticholinergic medications.
    c. strong pelvic muscle contractions suggest more severe detrusor overactivity and a need for medical therapy.
    d. if the voiding interval is long more fluid intake is needed.
    e. timed voiding should begin with an interval 1 1/2 times the baseline interval.

31. Approved therapy for patients who fail conservative treatment of OAB includes:

    a. endoscopic injection of alcohol.
    b. endoscopic injection of collagen.
    c. endoscopic injection of botulinum toxin.
    d. sacral nerve stimulation.
    e. all of the above.

32. In comparing botulinum toxin injection therapy with sacral neuromodulation therapy for refractory OAB and urgency incontinence:

    a. botulinum toxin therapy is proved effective in the elderly patient with non-neurogenic detrusor overactivity.
    b. botulinum toxin must be repeated every 3 to 4 months to maintain effectiveness.
    c. neither is proved effective in the neurogenic population.
    d. patients implanted with a neurostimulator cannot undergo MRI.
    e. the initial cost is about equal.

33. In considering treatment options for the patient with mixed incontinence:

    a. surgical therapy may be more effective when the bladder diary demonstrates a good functional capacity.
    b. urodynamic studies are critical for treatment planning.
    c. electrical stimulation is ineffective.
    d. support of the bladder neck with a pessary will exacerbate the stress incontinence component.
    e. SUI surgery is indicated when medical therapy is ineffective.

ANSWERS

1. **b. renal failure.** In contrast to the other responses, UI does not commonly affect the upper urinary tracts. Lower urinary tract dysfunction can lead to renal failure when there are high storage pressures in the bladder. Incontinence can rarely coexist with high storage pressures in certain disorders such as neurogenic bladder with external sphincter dyssynergia and retention due to bladder outlet obstruction but these cases represent a small fraction of the incontinent population.
2. **e. more than double.** Recent data from the Urologic Diseases of America project sponsored by the National Institutes of Health have shown that treatment of incontinence is a major burden for the United States health care system.
3. **a. less than 1/10th.** Despite the high prevalence and significant costs associated with incontinence there has been very little federally funded research into the condition.
4. **a. pelvic floor rehabilitation is superior to surgery for stress incontinence.** Surgical therapy is clearly more effective than nonsurgical treatments for stress incontinence but delaying surgery does not prejudice the outcome and therefore it is appropriate and often desirable to use nonsurgical therapy initially.
5. **d. discussion of normal bladder and sphincter function.** Education is the cornerstone of behavioral therapy. Incontinent patients may have little understanding of normal lower urinary tract function. Instruction about normal function allows the patient to model his or her own behavior. Devices, biofeedback, and drug therapy are all nonsurgical approaches to treat incontinence but are best considered as supplements that are outside of standard behavioral therapy.
6. **c. Prompted voiding.** Cognitively impaired individuals need assistance and/or a reminder to void before incontinence occurs; this is referred to as "prompted voiding." Timed voiding, bladder training, and urge inhibition are used in the cognitively intact population. Fluid restriction is most appropriate when fluid intake is high, which is rarely the case in the cognitively impaired patients.
7. **c. Behavioral therapy is equally successful with CMG negative, CMG positive, and neurogenic patients with OAB symptoms.** There are little data examining the use of behavioral therapy in the neurogenic population. The 1983 study by Holmes showed poorer results with such patients. The other statements all accurately represent the results of clinical research cited in the chapter.
8. **d. There are no clinical studies to determine the effectiveness of smoking cessation in the treatment of UI.** Although there are many health reasons to promote smoking cessation, including reduced risk of bladder cancer, there are no data at this time to show that smoking cessation is helpful in restoring urinary continence.
9. **d. Decreasing caffeine intake improves continence.** The bulk of the evidence from both epidemiologic studies and prospective clinical trials support caffeine restriction in the treatment of UI.
10. **c. Obesity is strongly correlated with both SUI and OAB; and d. Weight reduction can reduce UI in obese women.** Obesity has been shown to correlate with both stress and urge incontinence in several epidemiologic studies. A prospective, randomized controlled trial enrolling women with BMI > 25 demonstrated 60% reduction in incontinence episodes in a treatment group that lost an average of 16 kg. Controls had no weight loss and decreased incontinence episodes by only 15%.
11. **d. All of the above.** Arnold Kegel, a California gynecologist, used biofeedback with a perineometer to teach pelvic muscle exercises. Bump demonstrated that half of women could not increase urethral closure pressure when asked to contract their pelvic muscles. Biofeedback whether from a therapist or a device is of little value unless the patient is committed to a program of regular home exercise to rehabilitate the muscles.
12. **a. Improved muscle strength correlates strongly with improvement in continence.** More research is needed to determine how PFMT improves continence and particularly if improvement in muscle bulk, contraction strength, contraction response, etc., are correlated with improved continence.
13. **d. a and b.** PFMT is recommended as first-line therapy for established incontinence and for prevention of incontinence selected cases. PFMT has proven efficacy for prevention in primiparous women and women after high risk deliveries such as instrumental delivery or delivery of a large infant. There are no data yet to prove effectiveness in preventing incontinence for all pregnant women.
14. **a. All women with UI.** PFMT is recommended as first-line therapy for all types of established incontinence in women.
15. **a. electrical stimulation.** More pragmatic research is needed to determine the comparative efficacy of various conservative therapies in the treatment of UI. At this time the evidence establishes that PFMT is more effective than electrical stimulation in treating female stress incontinence and less effective than surgery.
16. **e. Neotonus device.** The Neotonus device delivers passive magnetic stimulation as a means of pelvic floor rehabilitation; all of the other choices are means of delivering biofeedback.
17. **d. requires motivated patient.** Biofeedback is only a tool used to teach patients to control a bodily function such as urinary continence. It requires that the patient be motivated to practice the technique to establish mastery.
18. **b. They are attractive options for patients unable to perform PFMT.** Patients totally unable to perform a pelvic muscle contraction may become frustrated with biofeedback training; passive stimulation techniques can be used to stimulate the pelvic muscles and may be used to initiate rehabilitation in this population. Although the stimulation therapies depend on patient compliance they do not require effort.
19. **c. Optimal regimen for stimulation is twice per day in the induction phase.** A prospective, randomized trial demonstrated equal efficacy of every-other-day therapy when compared with daily treatments with vaginal electrical stimulation.
20. **d. a reasonable choice for the incontinent patient who is unable to identify the pelvic floor muscles.** Stimulation techniques can be effective for both stress and urge incontinence and depend only on patient compliance, not effort. They do require commitment to a course of therapy. There are both advantages and disadvantages of magnetic stimulation when compared with electrical stimulation that individual patients may find compelling.
21. **b. Magnetic stimulation is an option for patients who will not accept vaginal instrumentation.** Magnetic stimulation is an attractive option for the subset of patients who will not accept vaginal/rectal instrumentation because it can be delivered with the patient seated and fully clothed.
22. **c. A bladder neck support device.** If a bladder neck support device restores urinary continence then it is likely that

supportive surgical therapy (sling or suspension) will also be effective.

23. **a. can be used on an "as needed" basis.** Whereas pessaries were developed to be used chronically in the treatment of prolapse, some patients with incontinence find "as needed" use attractive when performing physically stressful activities that might stimulate incontinence.

24. **d. All of the above.** Pelvic relaxation can cause local discomfort, voiding dysfunction/urinary retention, and stress incontinence. Use of a pessary to restore normal anatomy can help predict when surgical correction will successfully relieve symptoms and identify cases where prolapse actually hides stress incontinence.

25. **c. goal achievement.** Patient satisfaction is not correlated with objective cure of stress incontinence or pelvic prolapse but is related to achieving specific goals.

26. **e. filling cystometry.** The patient's perspective drives decisions about treatment in quality of life disorders; the clinician can usually counsel patients accurately about treatment options after knowing the type of incontinence, the baseline voiding diary, and an assessment of anatomy. This mandates a history, physical examination, and bladder diary. Urodynamic testing is not required for treatment planning in most routine cases of female incontinence but can be useful in complicated cases and before surgical therapy when a higher degree of certainty is desired.

27. **d. Cystometric capacity.** The functional capacity on the voiding diary correlates with cystometric capacity at urodynamic testing.

28. **b. those with absent contraction are probably best served by biofeedback training.** While there is inadequate evidence, it seems logical to assume that patients who are unable to perform a pelvic muscle contraction will not be likely to succeed with PFMT unless some form of teaching or stimulation is added.

29. **e. associated OAB.** OAB sometimes resolves with correction of stress incontinence and is not a contraindication to surgical therapy; nevertheless patients with mixed incontinence are less likely to be cured of incontinence than those with pure stress leakage.

30. **c. strong pelvic muscle contractions suggest more severe detrusor overactivity and a need for medical therapy.** Patients who leak with urge despite good pelvic muscle contraction strength must have more powerful unstable contractions and thus more severe detrusor overactivity.

31. **d. sacral nerve stimulation.** Collagen is indicated for treatment of stress incontinence due to intrinsic sphincter dysfunction. Botox and alcohol injections have been used for OAB but are not FDA-approved therapies. Sacral nerve stimulation is an FDA-approved treatment for refractory OAB.

32. **d. patients implanted with a neurostimulator cannot undergo MRI.** Botulinum toxin injections have primarily been used in the neurogenic population and are not FDA approved for use in the urinary tract at this time. When effective, re-treatment in 6 to 12 months is expected. Disadvantages of sacral nerve stimulation include a high initial cost and a prohibition against MRI after stimulator implantation.

33. **a. surgical therapy may be more effective when the bladder diary demonstrates a good functional capacity.** Use of a bladder neck support device can be used to predict response to surgery in the patient with mixed incontinence. Electrical stimulation has been advocated by some as an ideal modality as high frequency E-stim can be used for the stress component and low frequency for the urge component. Urodynamic studies may be useful in treatment planning but are not necessary before use of noninvasive therapy. Surgical therapy is indicated when there is significant stress incontinence and reasonable bladder function. A good functional capacity on bladder diary indicates potential for good bladder storage whereas failure of medical therapy could be due simply to refractory detrusor overactivity.

64

Electrical Stimulation for Storage and Emptying Disorders

SANDIP P. VASAVADA • RAYMOND R. RACKLEY

QUESTIONS

1. The current approved indications for sacral neuromodulation are for the following EXCEPT:
   a. urinary urgency.
   b. urinary frequency.
   c. urge incontinence.
   d. interstitial cystitis.
   e. idiopathic nonobstructive urinary retention.
2. Which patient is probably not well suited for current neuromodulation therapies?
   a. A 65-year-old insulin-dependent diabetic man with bladder areflexia and nonobstructive urinary retention
   b. A 67-year-old woman status post CVA and now with urinary urgency and frequency
   c. A 41-year-old woman with urinary urge incontinence
   d. A 55-year-old woman status post vaginal sling surgery and urge incontinence
   e. A 36-year-old woman with a history of interstitial cystitis with minimal pain who voids between 20-25 times per day
3. What reflex or reflexes are responsible for modulation of bladder function?
   a. Guarding
   b. Bladder afferent loop
   c. Bladder bladder
   d. Bladder urethral
   e. a and b
4. Which of the following is (are) considered the major clinical concern(s) associated with performing a sacral rhizotomy?
   a. Pelvic pain
   b. Creation of bladder areflexia
   c. Abnormal sexual function
   d. Pelvic and lower extremity sensory or motor abnormalities
   e. c and d
5. The S3 sensory and motor response pattern to electrical stimulation is best described as having which one of the following?
   a. Plantarflexion of the entire foot with sensation in the leg and buttock
   b. Levator reflex (Bellow's reflex) and sensations in the leg and buttock
   c. Dorsiflexion of the great toe and Bellow's reflex and pulling sensation in the rectum, scrotum, or vagina
   d. Plantarflexion of the first three toes of the foot and sensation of pulling in the rectum or vagina
   e. Bellow's reflex (levator contraction) and sensation of pulling of the rectum
6. What is the main concern of performing MRI in the setting of neuromodulation and pacemaker type devices?
   a. Potential of dislodgement of the pacemaker
   b. Heating of the electrical leads
   c. Heating of the pacemaker itself
   d. Potentially fatal arrhythmias
   e. Significant neuromuscular injury risk
7. Which of the following represents the best clinical scenario in using neuromodulation therapy in a patient with multiple sclerosis (MS)?
   a. Detrusor sphincter dyssynergy
   b. Bedridden with significant functional incontinence
   c. Mild symptoms with no potential need for future MRI
   d. A poorly compliant bladder
   e. Areflexic bladder
8. What skeletal landmarks are associated with the S3 nerve foramen?
   a. 9 cm from the tip of the coccyx
   b. 11 cm from the tip of the coccyx
   c. 13 cm from the tip of the coccyx
   d. The inferior aspect of the sacral iliac joints
   e. a and d

9. Perhaps the main reason why neuromodulation devices are not currently approved for use in the U.S. by the FDA in pediatric patients is due to:
   a. lack of efficacy.
   b. potential worsening of neuromuscular function due to bony abnormalities (spina bifida and myelomeningocele).
   c. lack of data on growth of the spinal cord and nerve roots in the setting of neuromodulation devices.
   d. worsening of bowel function (Hinman bladder syndrome).
   e. excellent results with noninvasive therapies (transcutaneous electrical nerve stimulation) and therefore no reason to perform more invasive sacral neuromodulation in the long term.
10. The best option for a patient who has undergone a failed stage I sacral neuromodulation for severe refractory urge incontinence (Medtronic Interstim Stage I) is:
    a. anticholinergics.
    b. bilateral stimulation.
    c. radical cystectomy and ileal conduit.
    d. vaginal sling.
    e. bladder augmentation.
11. Which of the following statements is false about the dorsal genital nerve?
    a. Specific branches include the dorsal nerve of the penis in males and clitoral nerve in females.
    b. It is an afferent nerve that carries sensory information.
    c. Proximally, it carries sensory information from the hypogastric nerve.
    d. It is a pure sensory afferent nerve branch of the pudendal nerve.
    e. It has been proposed as a contributor to the pudendal pelvic nerve reflex.
12. An implantable pulse generator (IPG) infection would be best treated by:
    a. intravenous antibiotic
    b. oral antibiotics
    c. irrigation of the pocket
    d. removal of the entire device
    e. a and b
13. Which of the following statements about impedances is false?
    a. Impedance is best described as the resistance of flow of electrons through a circuit.
    b. If there is too much resistance, no current will flow (open).
    c. If there is too little resistance, excessive current will flow.
    d. If there is a broken circuit, electrons cannot flow and this will result in low impedance measurements.
    e. Unipolar measurements are most useful for identifying open circuits during impedance testing.
14. Which of the following are false about the Brindley device?
    a. It requires intact neuron pathways between the sacral cord and nuclei, pelvic nerve, and bladder to function.
    b. It works best in a state of long-term areflexic bladder function.
    c. It is most often used in patients with insufficient or nonreflex micturition after spinal cord injury.
    d. It is usually coupled with sacral posterior rhizotomy.
    e. Electrodes are applied extradurally to S2, S3, and S4 nerve roots.
15. Direct electrical stimulation of the bladder often results in all of the following EXCEPT:
    a. pelvic musculature contraction.
    b. erection.
    c. defecation.
    d. bladder neck opening.
    e. ejaculation.
16. All of the following statements regarding the use of the Brindley device are true EXCEPT:
    a. It requires intact neural pathways between the sacral cord and the bladder.
    b. Sacral posterior rhizotomy is generally performed.
    c. Myogenic decompensation is a contraindication.
    d. Electrodes are applied extradurally to sacral roots S2 to S4.
    e. It utilizes the principle of post-stimulation voiding.
17. All of the following statements regarding neurostimulation or neuromodulation are true EXCEPT:
    a. The desired effect of neurostimulation is through direct stimulation of nerves and muscles.
    b. Neurostimulation is mainly reserved for neurogenic conditions.
    c. Neurostimulation produces a delayed clinical response.
    d. The effect of neuromodulation is achieved through alteration of neurotransmission processes.
    e. Neuromodulation may be useful for neurogenic as well as non-neurogenic conditions.
18. Which of the following studies is (are) the most useful in predicting which patients will or will not respond to sacral neuromodulation?
    a. Uroflow/postvoid residual monitoring
    b. Voiding diary
    c. Urodynamics/EMG
    d. Percutaneous lead placement and trial stimulation
    e. c and d
19. Which of the following are relative clinical contraindications for excluding potential candidates for neuromodulation and neurostimulation therapies?
    a. Patients with significant anatomic abnormalities in the spine or sacrum may present challenges to gaining access.
    b. Patients who cannot manage their device or judge the clinical outcome due to mental incapacitation.
    c. Patients with physical limitations that prevent them from achieving normal pelvic organ function such as functional urinary incontinence.
    d. Patients who are noncompliant.
    e. All of the above.
20. Which of the following statements best characterizes bilateral S3 nerve root stimulation for sacral neuromodulation therapy?
    a. It is a rational consideration for salvage therapy or added benefit as the bladder receives bilateral innervation.
    b. It is an approach alternative to failed unilateral stimulation in patients with urinary retention.
    c. Initial basis for this approach produced in spinal cord-injured animal animal models suggests this may be a potential approach in humans.
    d. All of the above.
    e. a and c only.

21. Potential sites of selective nerve stimulation other than the S3 sacral root for neuromodulation therapies for pelvic health conditions include which of the following:
    a. S4 sacral root.
    b. Pudendal nerve.
    c. Dorsal genital nerve.
    d. Posterior tibial nerve.
    e. All of the above.

22. When troubleshooting the complication of IPG site discomfort or pain, which of the following statements best describes the necessary action(s) needed?
    a. Rule out IPG site infection by physical examination.
    b. Turn off the device and ask the patient if the discomfort is still present to differentiate IPG pocket site issues from IPG electrical output-related causes.
    c. If the IPG discomfort is output related, check whether bipolar stimulation is better than unipolar.
    d. If IPG site discomfort is output related, check impedances because a current leak may be present from the neuroelectrode to extension lead connection.
    e. All of the above.

23. When patients report recurrent symptoms after having achieved reduction or improvement of symptoms with sacral neuromodulation therapy, which of the following should be undertaken to evaluate the reason for the loss of clinical efficacy.
    a. Check the device settings for inadvertent on/off changes and battery performance.
    b. Evaluate the stimulation perception and anatomic localization for changes.
    c. Check for intermittent stimulation perception via positional changes of the patient because this may suggest lead migration or a loose lead connection.
    d. Obtain a radiograph to detect macro changes in the neuroelectrode position if findings in b and c are evident.
    e. All of the above.

ANSWERS

1. **d. interstitial cystitis.** Although used commonly for interstitial cystitis (IC) symptoms, urgency/frequency IC is not truly an indication for the sacral neuromodulation devices currently. Several groups have seen benefits of sacral neuromodulation in IC patients and there may be an expanding indication for this in the future.

2. **a. A 65-year-old insulin-dependent diabetic man with bladder areflexia and nonobstructive urinary retention.** It is implied that the end-organ response (bladder in this case) should have good function for sacral neuromodulation and, for that matter, any form of neuromodulation to work. Neurostimulation may be different but even if neurostimulation was used, simultaneous relaxation of the outlet would be required for a coordinated contraction and emptying phase to ensue.

3. **e. a and b.** Two important reflexes may play an important role in modulation of bladder function, the guarding reflex and the bladder afferent loop reflex. Both reflexes promote urine storage under sympathetic tone. The guarding reflex guards or prevents urine loss from times of cough or other physical stress that would normally trigger a micturition episode. Suprapontine input from the brain turns off the guarding reflex during micturition to allow efficient and complete emptying. The bladder afferent reflex works through sacral interneurons that then activate storage through pudendal nerve efferent pathways directed toward the urethral sphincter. Similar to the guarding reflex, the bladder afferent reflex promotes continence during periods of bladder filling and is quiet during micturition.

4. **e. c and d.** Bilateral anterior and posterior sacral rhizotomy or conusectomy converts a hyperreflexic bladder to an areflexic one. This alone may be inappropriate therapy because it also adversely affects the rectum, anal and urethral sphincters, sexual function, and the lower extremities. In an attempt to leave sphincter and sexual function intact, selective motor nerve section was originally introduced as a treatment to increase bladder capacity by abolishing only the motor supply responsible for involuntary contractions.

5. **c. Dorsiflexion of the great toe and Bellow's reflex and pulling sensation in the rectum, scrotum, or vagina.** The characteristic response of the S3 nerve distribution based on its lower innervation is to the levator musculature (Bellow's contraction) of the anus and ipsilateral great toe contraction. The other answers suggest either S2 stimulation (leg rotation) or S4 levator contraction.

6. **b. Heating of the electrical leads.** Although many concerns exist for MRI and pacemaker devices, it has been shown that the main concern is heating of the electrical leads. This may, in turn, traumatize blood vessels, nerve roots, or other structures that the leads, themselves, are next to. Currently, it is contraindicated to have an MRI in the presence of a pacemaker.

7. **c. Mild symptoms with no potential need for future MRI.** It is unknown whether subcategories of MS patients (DESD, areflexia, poor compliance) would be very good candidates for sacral neuromodulation, although it is doubtful based on disease severity alone. A mildly symptomatic patient without functional issues (e.g., can make it to the bathroom in time and no major mobility issues) probably makes sense as to the best patient.

8. **e. a and d.** The measurements for the rough vicinity of the S3 nerve foramen have been tested using the cross hair technique (Chai et al.) and simple measurements. The answers b and c are incorrect because they represent measurements from the anal verge (11 cm) and 13 cm is too far in general from the coccyx and would likely place one near S2 or S1.

9. **c. lack of data on growth of the spinal cord and nerve roots in the setting of neuromodulation devices.** Pediatric patients have undergone sacral neuromodulation in off label trials, but large scale use has been limited by lack of data on the growth of the pediatric patient and the relation of the sacral lead with regard to the sacral nerve roots, and so on. Whereas noninvasive therapies have worked, they are limited by the need for continued repeat therapy to maintain durability of result.

10. **e. bladder augmentation.** The patient should have tried and failed anticholinergic therapy before having the sacral neuromodulation therapy. Scheepens and coworkers have shown that bilateral stimulation, although logical, has not shown in

urge-incontinent patients to make much improvement. One could argue that contralateral lead placement should be attempted, but no prospective trials have shown that this makes a difference in outcomes. Vaginal sling and radical cystectomy is not indicated per se in this condition (sling is for stress incontinence, and cystectomy is too radical).

11. **c. Proximally, it carries sensory information from the hypogastric nerve.** The dorsal genital nerve is a terminal branch of the pudendal nerve and is being investigated for functional neuromodulation outcomes via a percutaneous approach. It does not carry information directly from the hypogastric nerve.
12. **d. removal of the entire device.** Because an IPG is a foreign body, it could harbor bacteria within a biofilm created by the infection. Accordingly, it is best to have it removed in its entirety. Antibiotics and irrigation for the most part are temporizing measures. Furthermore, there is a risk of an infection tracking along the sacral lead, which may create a sacral infection.
13. **d. If there is a broken circuit, electrons cannot flow and this will result in low impedance measurements.** Impedance describes the resistance to the flow of electrons through a circuit. Impedance or resistance is an integral part of any functioning circuit; however, if there is too much resistance, no current will flow (open). If there is too little resistance, you get excessive current flow resulting in diminished battery longevity (short). If the circuit is broken somehow, electrons cannot flow. *This is called an "open" circuit and impedance measurements are high.* Open circuits can be caused by a fractured lead or extension wires, loose connections, and so on.
14. **b. It works best in a state of long-term areflexic bladder function.** The chief applications of the Brindley device are in patients with inefficient or nonreflex micturition after SCI. Prerequisites for use are described by Madersbacher and Fisher (1993) as the following: (1) intact neural pathways between the sacral cord nuclei of the pelvic nerve and the bladder and (2) a bladder that is capable of contracting.
15. **d. bladder neck opening.** The spread of current to other pelvic structures whose stimulus thresholds are lower than that of the bladder has often resulted in (1) abdominal, pelvic, and perineal pain; (2) a desire to defecate or defecation; (3) contraction of the pelvic and leg muscles; and (4) erection and ejaculation in males. It has also been noted that the increase in intravesical pressure was generally not coordinated with bladder neck opening or with pelvic floor relaxation and that other measures to accomplish voiding may be necessary.
16. **d. Electrodes are applied extradurally to sacral roots S2 to S4.** Prerequisites for such usage were described in one study as (1) intact neural pathways between the sacral cord nuclei of the pelvic nerve and the bladder and (2) a bladder that is capable of contracting. The chief application is in patients with inefficient or no reflex micturition after spinal cord injury. Simultaneous bladder and striated sphincter stimulation is obviated by sacral posterior rhizotomy, usually complete, which also (1) eliminates reflex incontinence and (2) improves low bladder compliance, if present. Electrodes are applied intradurally to sacral roots 2, 3, and 4, but the pairs can be activated independently. The current Brindley stimulator utilizes the principle of poststimulus voiding, a term first introduced by Jonas and Tanagho. Relaxation time of the striated sphincter after a stimulus train is shorter than the relaxation time of the detrusor smooth muscle. Therefore, when interrupted pulse trains instead of continuous stimulus trains are used, poststimulus voiding is achieved between the pulse trains due to the higher sustained intravesical pressure when compared with the striated sphincter.
17. **c. Neurostimulation produces a delayed clinical response.** In neurostimulation, the use of electrical stimuli on nerves and muscles has mainly been developed for achieving immediate clinical responses in neurogenic conditions of pelvic organ dysfunction; whereas, in neuromodulation, the use of electrical stimuli to nerves has been developed for altering neurotransmission processes in cases of nonneurogenic as well as neurogenic conditions.
18. **d. Percutaneous lead placement and trial stimulation.** Despite all the studies done to date, there are no defined preclinical factors such as urodynamic findings that can predict which patients will or will not have a response to sacral neuromodulation. Thus, a trial of stimulation via a temporary or percutaneous lead placement is the best predictor of long-term clinical responsiveness.
19. **e. All of the above.** Whereas most patients are considered candidates for neurostimulation and neuromodulation therapies who have failed more conservative therapies, all of the above clinical considerations for excluding patients from this therapy should be considered. Furthermore, relative contraindications for patients who may be considering or who have an implantable electrical stimulation device are the issues of MRI and pregnancy, as outlined in the text.
20. **d. All of the above.** Bilateral stimulation has been suggested as an alternative, particularly in failed unilateral lead placements, for potential salvage or added benefit as the bladder receives bilateral innervation. The initial basis to consider bilateral stimulation was based on animal studies that demonstrated bilateral stimulation yielded a more profound effect on bladder inhibition than did unilateral stimulation. Only one clinical study has been performed to demonstrate the potential differences in unilateral versus bilateral stimulation (Scheepens, 2002). This study showed no significant difference in outcomes for unilateral versus bilateral stimulation with regard to urge incontinence, frequency, or severity of leakage in the OAB group, although, overall, results were impressive in both categories. The retention group patients had better parameters of emptying (volume per void) in bilateral as compared with unilateral stimulation.
21. **e. All of the above.** The introduction of new stimulation methods as well as application of these methods to all the different nerve locations listed will continue to provide improved treatment alternatives as shown in animal models and human applications. In addition, these innovations will provide the ability to further develop testable hypotheses of more basic questions on electrical neurostimulation, neuromodulation, and neurophysiology of the autonomic, somatic, and central pathways that regulate pelvic organ function.
22. **e. All of the above.** The probable causes of IPG site discomfort or pain are IPG pocket related or IPG output related. Pocket-related causes of discomfort include infection, pocket location (waistline), pocket dimension (too tight, too loose), seroma, and erosion. Turn off the IPG and determine if the discomfort is still present to differentiate pocket-related from output-related cause. If the discomfort is persistent, the cause is not related to the IPG electrical output. In the absence of clinical signs of infection, IPG pocket-related causes such as pocket size, seroma, and erosion should be considered. If the discomfort disappears, IPG electrical output is likely causing discomfort or pain. Output-related causes include sensitivity

to unipolar stimulation if this mode is used or a current leak as demonstrated by abnormal impedances.

23. **e. All of the above**. When the patient presents with recurrent symptoms, one should evaluate the stimulation perception. The possibilities are that the patient perceives the stimulation in a wrong location as compared with baseline, has no stimulation, or has intermittent stimulation based on lead migration or mechanical issues related to a loose connection or elevated impedances.

65

Retropubic Suspension Surgery for Female Incontinence

C. R. CHAPPLE

QUESTIONS

1. Urodynamic stress urinary incontinence (SUI) refers to incontinence occurring:
   a. during a cough on clinical examination.
   b. in the absence of urgency.
   c. in combination with detrusor overactivity.
   d. on coughing in association with urgency and demonstrable detrusor overactivity.
   e. on coughing in the absence of urgency and urge incontinence and with no demonstrable detrusor overactivity.
2. Anti-incontinence surgery via the retropubic route:
   a. does not address intrinsic sphincter deficiency.
   b. restores the same mechanism of continence that was present before the onset of incontinence.
   c. aims to improve the support to the urethrovesical junction and correct deficient urethral closure.
   d. is the most effective form of anti-incontinence surgery.
   e. is as effectively carried out laparoscopically as via an open approach.
3. Which of the following is most clearly established to be important in affecting the outcome of retropubic surgery?
   a. Increasing age
   b. Postoperative activity
   c. Coexisting medical morbidity
   d. Previous surgery
   e. Obesity
4. Intrinsic sphincter deficiency:
   a. is present in only 30% of patients with stress incontinence.
   b. is most probably present in the majority of women with stress incontinence.
   c. can be accurately identified on the basis of a Valsalva leak-point pressure.
   d. is an absolute contraindication to a retropubic suspension procedure.
   e. is clearly defined in the contemporaneous literature.
5. Retropubic colposuspension procedures may act via the following mechanisms:
   a. re-creating the normal continence mechanism.
   b. elevating the anterior vaginal wall and paravesical tissues toward the iliopectineal line.
   c. anchoring the obturator internus fascia to the iliopectineal line.
   d. suspending the bladder onto the periosteum of the symphysis pubis.
   e. strengthening the pubourethral ligaments.
6. In assessing the outcome of retropubic suspension surgery, which of the following is most important?
   a. Using objective urodynamic-based outcome criteria
   b. Improving symptoms from the patient's perspective
   c. Achieving complete continence
   d. Identifying the degree of improvement in the urethral closure pressure
   e. Having follow-up data of at least 6 months' duration
7. Which of the following is not an indication for retropubic repair of stress incontinence? A patient:
   a. who needs a concomitant hysterectomy that cannot be performed vaginally
   b. with urethral descent with straining and stress incontinence
   c. with limited vaginal access
   d. who frequently generates high intra-abdominal pressure due to a chronic cough
   e. with inadequate vaginal length or mobility of the vaginal tissues
8. Which of the following statements is TRUE regarding retropubic procedures for incontinence?
   a. It is important to avoid dissecting the old retropubic adhesions from prior incontinence procedures because these may contribute to continence.
   b. Nonabsorbable sutures are better than absorbable sutures for retropubic suspension procedures.
   c. It may be necessary to open the bladder to facilitate identification of the bladder margins and bladder neck.
   d. A urethral Foley catheter is preferred for bladder drainage because it is more comfortable and associated with fewer urinary tract infections and earlier resumption of voiding.
   e. The retropubic space must be drained after the procedure to prevent bleeding.

9. Which of the following statements is TRUE regarding the Marshall-Marchetti-Krantz (MMK) procedure?
   a. It is important to elevate the mid urethra and external sphincter in particular.
   b. It carries little risk of causing urethral obstruction.
   c. It is associated with osteitis pubis.
   d. A better than 90% cure rate can be expected in the long term.
   e. The sutures should incorporate a full thickness of the vaginal wall and lateral urethral wall.
10. Which of the following is TRUE of the Burch procedure?
   a. It is appropriate only for patients with adequate vaginal mobility and capacity.
   b. It is performed between the vagina and the arcus tendineus fasciae pelvis bilaterally.
   c. It is less effective than a transvaginal tape (TVT) procedure.
   d. It is less effective than a paravaginal repair.
   e. It is more effectively performed via a vaginal approach.
11. Laparoscopic retropubic colposuspension is advantageous over open colposuspension because it:
   a. is technically simple to perform.
   b. provides access for repair of an associated central defect cystocele.
   c. is more effective than an open colposuspension.
   d. is associated with shorter hospitalization and recovery times.
   e. is associated with shorter operating times.
12. Common complications specific to retropubic suspension procedures include:
   a. bladder denervation.
   b. detrusor sphincter dyssynergia.
   c. postoperative voiding difficulty.
   d. detrusor underactivity.
   e. genitourinary tract fistulas.
13. Postoperative voiding difficulty after a retropubic suspension procedure:
   a. is more likely if there is preexisting detrusor dysfunction.
   b. may be due to detrusor sphincter dyssynergia.
   c. is most likely to occur with undercorrection of the urethral axis.
   d. should be managed by urethrolysis within 1 month.
   e. occurs in less than 1% of patients.
14. Which of the following statements is TRUE regarding detrusor overactivity (DO) and retropubic suspension procedures?
   a. Preoperative DO is a contraindication to a retropubic suspension because it increases the risk of postoperative DO.
   b. New-onset DO after a suspension procedure performed for SUI invariably resolves within 3 months.
   c. DO occurs de novo, on average in less than 2% of the patients reported in the literature.
   d. A history of voiding symptoms and new-onset storage symptoms as well as a retropubically angulated urethra usually suggests obstruction.
   e. They are not causally related.
15. Prolapse is a reported complication of retropubic repairs, and?
   a. it is rarely associated with a central defect cystocele.
   b. genitourinary prolapse has been reported as a sequel to Burch colposuspension to occur in less than 10% of women.
   c. it may aggravate posterior vaginal wall weakness, predisposing to enterocele.
   d. it will be prevented by a synchronous hysterectomy.
   e. it occurs only rarely after a paravaginal repair.
16. From comparative studies in the literature, which is correct about open retropubic colposuspension? It is not
   a. as effective as a pubovaginal sling.
   b. effective in patients with a low leak-point pressure.
   c. more effective than an anterior colporrhaphy.
   d. more effective than a TVT procedure.
   e. more effective than a paravaginal repair.

ANSWERS

1. **e. on coughing in the absence of urgency and urge incontinence and with no demonstrable detrusor overactivity.** Stress incontinence is the symptom of involuntary loss of urine during situations of increased intra-abdominal pressure such as coughing or sneezing. The International Continence Society defines *urodynamic stress incontinence* as the involuntary loss of urine during increased intra-abdominal pressure during filling cystometry, in the absence of detrusor (bladder wall muscle) contraction (Abrams, 2002). Thus, urodynamic evaluation is a prerequisite for the diagnosis of urodynamic stress incontinence. It is not clear, however, especially from the clinical management standpoint, whether a urodynamic diagnosis is imperative for successful treatment of stress incontinence.
2. **c. aims to improve the support to the urethrovesical junction and correct deficient urethral closure.** Surgical procedures to treat SUI generally aim to improve the support to the urethrovesical junction and correct deficient urethral closure. There is disagreement, however, not only regarding the precise mechanism by which continence is achieved in the "normal asymptomatic female" and therefore not surprisingly how restoration of "normality" is reestablished via surgical manipulation. Anti-incontinence surgery is generally used to address the failure of normal anatomic support of the bladder neck and proximal urethra and intrinsic sphincter deficiency (ISD). It must be appreciated that anti-incontinence surgery does not necessarily work by restoring the same mechanism of continence that was present before the onset of incontinence. Rather, it works by a compensatory approach, creating a new mechanism of continence (Jarvis, 1994). The surgeon's preference, coexisting problems, and the anatomic features of the patient and her general health condition often influence the choice of procedure.
3. **d. Previous surgery.** Surgery for recurrent stress incontinence has a lower success rate. One study has reported that Burch colposuspension has an 81% success rate after one previous surgical procedure has failed, but this drops to 25% after two previous repairs and 0% after 3 previous operations (Petrou et al, 2001). Other series report excellent results for colposuspension carried out after prior failed surgery. Maher and coworkers (1999) and Cardozo and colleagues (1999) have both shown good objective (72% and 79%) and subjective (89% and 80%) success rates with repeat colposuspension at a mean follow-up of 9 months. Nitihara and colleagues (1999) reported a 69% subjective success at a mean follow-up of 6.9 years.

   The evidence on the duration of symptoms as a predictor of outcome is conflicting. Age may not be a contraindication to colposuspension with equivalent success rates in the elderly at long-term follow-up, although others reported less success with increasing age. Advice on the influence of levels of postoperative activity have been inadequately studied so that no recommendations can be made. There is limited evidence that medical comorbidity may impact on surgical outcomes depending on the outcomes selected. Obesity as a confounding variable is the subject of conflicting evidence in the literature and has not been studied in a prospective fashion. Approximately a fourth of women undergoing urodynamics have mixed urodynamic stress incontinence and detrusor overactivity. It is likely that the presence of concomitant detrusor overactivity lessens the success rate of surgery. There is no consensus in the literature as to whether the presence of intrinsic sphincter deficiency as assessed by urethral pressure profilometry has any influence on outcome of colposuspension.

4. **b. is most probably present in the majority of women with stress incontinence.** Hypermobility of the bladder neck and proximal urethra results from a weakening or loss of their supporting elements (ligaments, fasciae, and muscles), which in turn may be consequent on aging, hormonal changes, childbirth, and prior surgery. It seems likely that the majority of women with SUI will also have an element of intrinsic sphincteric weakness with a variable degree of loss of the normal anatomic support of the bladder neck and proximal urethra, resulting in hypermobility.

   A standardized test is not, however, available to differentiate the relative contributions of intrinsic sphincter deficiency and hypermobility; therefore, few studies have been able to accurately differentiate their individual contributions to the incontinence. Retropubic procedures act to restore the bladder neck and proximal urethra to a fixed, retropubic position and are used when hypermobility is thought to be an important factor in the development of that woman's stress incontinence. This may facilitate the function of a marginally compromised intrinsic urethral sphincter mechanism, but if significant ISD is present, SUI will persist despite efficient surgical repositioning of the bladder neck and proximal urethra.

5. **b. elevating the anterior vaginal wall and paravesical tissues toward the iliopectineal line.** Retropubic colposuspension urethral repositioning can be achieved by three distinctly different procedure principles (these are all based on a similar underlying principle, but in a spectrum in relation to the degree of the support and on elevations they achieve), and their outcomes differ somewhat in the longer term.

   The Burch colposuspension is the elevation of the anterior vaginal wall and paravesical tissues toward the iliopectineal line of the pelvic side wall using two to four sutures on either side (Burch, 1961). The vagino-obturator shelf repair aims to anchor the vagina to the obturator internus fascia and is a modification of a combination of the Burch and paravaginal defect repair with placement of the sutures laterally anchored to the obturator internus fascia rather than hitching the vagina up to the iliopectineal line (Turner-Warwick, 1986). The paravaginal defect repair aims to close a presumed fascial weakness laterally at the site of attachment of the pelvic fascia to obturator internus fascia (Richardson, 1976). The Marshall-Marchetti-Krantz procedure is the suspension of the vesicourethral junction (bladder neck) onto the periosteum of the symphysis pubis (Everard-Williams, 1947; Marshall et al, 1949). It aims to close the fascial defect rather than elevate the tissues in the paravesical area.

6. **b. Improving symptoms from the patient's perspective.** One or more high-quality validated symptom and quality of life instruments should be chosen at the outset of a clinical trial representing the patient's viewpoint, accurately defining baseline symptoms as well as any other areas where treatment may be beneficial, and assessing the objective severity and subjective impact of bother. Although many including the author believe that urodynamic studies are helpful in helping define the underlying pathophysiology in cases with incontinence, these studies have not been proven to have adequate sensitivity, specificity, or predictive value (Chapple et al, 2005). The recent International Consensus Meeting on Incontinence concluded that although urodynamic studies such as frequency volume charts and pad tests were useful there was inadequate evidence to justify pressure-flow studies for routine testing as either entry criteria or outcome measures in clinical trials, and it was recommended that most large-scale clinical trials should enroll subjects by carefully defined symptom-driven criteria when the treatment will be given on an empirical basis (Abrams et al, 2005).

7. **e. with inadequate vaginal length or mobility of the vaginal tissues.** Although it has been suggested that a retropubic colposuspension should be considered in patients who frequently generate high intra-abdominal pressure (e.g., those with chronic cough from obstructive pulmonary disease and women in strenuous occupations), it has also been argued that these patients may be better served by a pubovaginal sling as well.

   There may be specific indications for a retropubic approach for the correction of anatomic SUI, namely:

   1. A patient undergoing a laparotomy for concomitant abdominal surgery that cannot be performed vaginally.
   2. Where there is limited vaginal access.

   Conversely, contraindications include:

   1. If there is a history of prior failed incontinence procedures, the existence of significant sphincteric deficiency must be suspected, even if hypermobility exists, and consideration given to performing a pubovaginal sling.
   2. In cases with a pan–pelvic floor weakness, then a colposuspension should not be used in isolation but should be used as part of a comprehensive approach to the pelvic floor and be combined as appropriate with other alternative pelvic floor repair procedures. Although lateral defect cystocele and enterocele lend themselves to retropubic repair, a central defect cystocele, rectocele, and introital deficiency do not.
   3. In cases where there is an inadequate vaginal length or mobility of the vaginal tissues as for example after prior vaginal surgery or radiation therapy or such as that after a prior vaginal incontinence procedure.
   4. A retropubic colposuspension does not always adequately correct the associated vaginal prolapse that frequently coexists with bladder neck hypermobility.

8. **c. It may be necessary to open the bladder to facilitate identification of the bladder margins and bladder neck.** In open retropubic suspension procedures, good access to the retropubic space is crucial. This is best performed with the patient in the supine position with the legs abducted, in either a low or a modified dorsal lithotomy position using stirrups, allowing access to the vagina during the procedure and a perineoabdominal progression. A urethral Foley catheter is inserted; the catheter balloon is used for subsequent identification of the urethra and bladder neck and indeed is invaluable in allowing palpation of the edges of the bladder by appropriate manipulation. A Pfannenstiel or lower midline abdominal incision is made, separating the rectus muscles in the midline and sweeping the anterior peritoneal reflection off the bladder. It is essential to optimize the access to the retropubic space and if a Pfannenstiel skin incision is made it is advisable to utilize the suprapubic V modification described by Turner-Warwick and associates (1974). Likewise, whatever incision is made, extra valuable access to the retropubic space

is obtained by extending the division of the rectus muscles right down to the pubic bone and elevating the aponeurotic insertion of the rectus muscle right off the upper border of the pubic bone.

The retropubic space is then developed by teasing away the retropubic fat and underlying retropubic veins, from the back of the pubic bone. The bladder neck, anterior vaginal wall, and urethra are then easy to identify—often facilitated by the presence of the Foley balloon. In patients who have had previous retropubic surgery, the dissection is performed sharply and it is important to take down all old retropubic adhesions, particularly in the presence of a prior failed repair. If difficulty is encountered in the identification of the bladder neck, the bladder may be partially filled or even opened to identify its limits, and an examining finger in the vagina is invaluable in aiding the dissection (Symmonds, 1972; Gleason et al, 1976).

It is important to identify the lateral limits of the bladder as it reflects off the vaginal wall, because only in this manner can one avoid inadvertent suturing of the bladder itself. Dissection over the bladder neck and urethra in the midline is to be avoided so as to not damage the intrinsic musculature. The lateral bladder wall may be "rolled off" medially and cephalad from the vaginal wall using a mounted swab and by using countertraction with a finger in the vagina. In my experience it is not necessary to incise the endopelvic fascia. Occasional venous bleeding from the large vaginal veins can be controlled by suture ligature, although it often resolves with tying of elevating sutures. To aid in the identification of the lateral margin of the bladder, it is helpful to displace the balloon of the Foley catheter into the lateral recess, where it can be easily palpated through the bladder wall.

Suture Material

Absorbable sutures were used in the original descriptions of the MMK procedure (chromic catgut), Burch procedure (chromic catgut), and VOS procedure (PGA or PDS), whereas the original paravaginal repair used nonabsorbable sutures (silicon-coated Dacron). Fibrosis during subsequent healing is likely to be the most important factor in providing continued fixation of the perivaginal fascia to the suspension sites (Tanagho, 1996); nevertheless, some surgeons believe that a nonabsorbable suture material is better because of the risk of suture dissolution before the development of adequate fibrosis (Penson and Raz, 1996). Clearly, the choice of suspension suture material is a personal choice, but it must be remembered that nonabsorbent sutures eroding into the lumen of the bladder are a not uncommon complication and a not uncommon source of medical litigation (Woo et al, 1995).

Bladder Drainage

Some degree of immediate postoperative voiding difficulty can be expected after retropubic suspensions (Lose et al, 1987; Colombo et al, 1996). Immediately postoperative, bladder drainage may take the form of a urethral or a suprapubic catheter, generally based on surgeon preference. A voiding trial is usually performed around the 5th day postoperatively. However, there is some evidence that a suprapubic catheter may be advantageous with respect to a lower incidence of asymptomatic and febrile urinary tract infection and earlier resumption of normal bladder function (Andersen et al, 1985; Bergman et al, 1987). In addition, the use of a suprapubic tube is generally more comfortable, allows the patient to participate in catheter management, and avoids the need for self-clean intermittent catheterization. Catheterization can be discontinued when efficient voiding has resumed, which is usually indicated by a postvoid residual either less than 100 mL or less than 30% of the functional bladder volume.

Drains

A tube drain may be placed in the retropubic space when there is concern about ongoing bleeding from perivaginal veins that may prove difficult to control with suture and electrocautery. Often, tying the suspension sutures is sufficient to stop this bleeding, but, when it persists, drainage of the retropubic space is indicated. The drain is generally removed on the first to third day, when minimal output is noted.

9. **c. It is associated with osteitis pubis.** Complications occur in up to 21% of cases (Mainprize, 1988), and the placement of sutures through the pubic symphysis incurs the risk of osteitis pubis, a potentially devastating complication of the MMK procedure that has been reported in 0.9% to 3.2% of patients (Lee at al, 1979; Mainprize, 1988; Zorzos and Paterson, 1996). Patients usually present 1 to 8 weeks postoperatively with acute pubic pain radiating to the inner thighs, aggravated by moving. Physical examination reveals tenderness over the pubic symphysis, and radiography demonstrates haziness to the borders of the pubic symphysis and possibly lytic changes. Treatment is with bed rest, analgesics, and possibly corticosteroids (Lee at al, 1979).
10. **a. It is appropriate only for patients with adequate vaginal mobility and capacity.** The Burch retropubic colposuspension, which has undergone few modifications since its original description, is appropriate only if the patient has adequate vaginal mobility and capacity to allow the lateral vaginal fornices to be elevated toward and approximated to Cooper's ligament on either side.
11. **d. is associated with shorter hospitalization and recovery times.** Proposed advantages to the laparoscopic approach include improved intraoperative visualization, less postoperative pain, shorter hospitalization, and quicker recovery times (Liu, 1993). Disadvantages include greater technical difficulty with resultant longer operating times and higher operating costs (Paraiso et al, 1999).
12. **c. postoperative voiding difficulty.** As with any major abdominal or pelvic surgical procedure, intraoperative and perioperative complications that may occur after a retropubic suspension include bleeding, injury to genitourinary organs (bladder, urethra, ureter), pulmonary atelectasis and infection, wound infection or dehiscence, abscess formation, and venous thrombosis/embolism. Other common complications more specific to retropubic suspension procedures include postoperative voiding difficulty, detrusor overactivity, and vaginal prolapse.

    Nevertheless the reported incidence of these problems is relatively low. In their meta-analysis, Leach and associates (1997) noted a 3% to 8% transfusion rate for retropubic suspensions and no significant difference in the overall medical and surgical complication rates between retropubic suspensions, needle suspensions, anterior colporrhaphy, and pubovaginal slings.

    Ureteral obstruction has been reported rarely after Burch colposuspension, and it usually results from ureteral kinking after elevation of the vagina and bladder base, although direct suture ligation of the ureter can occur (Applegate et al, 1987). If identified intraoperatively, it is best remedied by removal of the offending ligature and temporary placement of a ureteral stent. The so-called post-colposuspension syndrome, which has been described as pain in one or both groins at the site of suspension, has been noted in up to 12% of patients after a Burch procedure (Galloway et al, 1987). More recently, Demirci and coworkers (2001) reported the occurrence of groin or suprapubic pain in 15 of 220 women (6.8%) after Burch colposuspension with a follow-up of 4.5 years.

13. **a. is more likely if there is preexisting detrusor dysfunction.** Postoperative voiding difficulty after any type of retropubic suspension is not uncommon, and undoubtedly its occurrence is more likely if there is preexisting detrusor dysfunction or denervation resulting from extensive perivesical dissection. In most cases, however, it is the result of overcorrection of the urethral axis, owing to sutures being inappropriately placed or excessively tightened. If they are placed too medially, sutures may also transfix the urethra or distort it.

    Preoperatively, at-risk patients may be identified by their history of prior voiding dysfunction or episodes of urinary retention. These women should be counseled carefully about the potential for postoperative voiding difficulty and the possible need for self-intermittent catheterization. Their incontinence should be of sufficient magnitude that its correction offsets the risk of the need for self-catheterization.

    Women with post-cystourethropexy voiding problems who have obstruction often do not exhibit the classic urodynamic features of obstruction. However, the history of postoperative voiding symptoms and associated new-onset bladder storage symptoms and a finding of a retropubically angulated and fixed urethra generally indicate that obstruction does exist (Carr and Webster, 1997). In such cases, revision of the retropubic suspension by releasing the urethra into a more anatomic position resolves voiding symptoms in up to 90% of cases (Webster and Kreder, 1990; Nitti and Raz, 1994; Carr and Webster, 1997).

    The meta-analysis by Leach and coworkers (1997) noted that the risk of temporary urinary retention lasting more than 4 weeks postoperatively was 5% for all retropubic suspensions, the risk for permanent retention was estimated to be less than 5%, and these risks were not significantly different from those for needle suspensions or pubovaginal slings.

14. **d. A history of voiding symptoms and new-onset storage symptoms as well as a retropubically angulated urethra usually suggests obstruction.** Bladder overactivity commonly accompanies anatomic SUI, and its incidence preoperatively has been reported to be as high as 30% in patients undergoing either first correction or repeated operations (McGuire, 1981). Provided that it is considered as a diagnosis, urodynamics is performed to show whether detrusor overactivity is present, an attempt at treatment of the related overactive bladder symptoms has been made (with or without success), and the patient has been advised that the presence of detrusor overactivity will increase the risk of continuing storage symptoms postoperatively. Then preoperative bladder overactivity does not contraindicate a retropubic suspension procedure, provided that anatomic SUI has also been demonstrated. In the majority of cases, the bladder overactivity symptoms resolve after surgical repair (McGuire, 1988). Leach and coworkers' meta-analysis (1997) found the risk of urgency after a retropubic suspension was 66% if urgency and detrusor overactivity were present preoperatively, 36% if there was urgency but no documented overactivity preoperatively, and only 11% if there was neither urgency nor overactivity preoperatively. There was no significant difference in the incidence of postoperative urgency between retropubic suspensions, needle suspensions, and pubovaginal slings. Postoperative urgency was noted in only 0.9% of Marshall-Marchetti-Krantz (MMK) cystourethropexy procedures in Mainprize and Drutz's meta-analysis of 15 series (1988), although Parnell and associates (1982) reported that 28.5% of their patients developed postoperative storage symptoms. Jarvis' meta-analysis (1994) of Burch procedures found the incidence of de novo bladder overactivity to be 3.4% to 18%. More recently, Smith and associates quote a figure for postoperative detrusor overactivity of 6.6% for colposuspension (range: 1.0% to 16.6%) whereas the incidence of postoperative urgency or urge incontinence after the paravaginal/VOS repair has been reported to be 0% to 6% (Shull and Baden, 1989; German et al, 1994; Colombo et al, 1996).

    For those patients in whom postoperative storage symptoms persist, are proven to be associated with detrusor overactivity, and are intractable to management with anticholinergic therapy and behavioral modification, surgical techniques including intravesical botulinum toxin therapy, neuromodulation, augmentation cystoplasty, or detrusor myectomy may be indicated.

    Bladder storage symptoms arising de novo after retropubic suspension may be associated with bladder outlet obstruction. This premise is supported by the frequent coexistence of these symptoms with impaired voiding after suspension procedures and confirmed by the finding that urethrolysis, by freeing the urethra from an obstructed position, often resolves both storage and voiding symptoms (Raz, 1981; Webster and Kreder, 1990).

15. **c. It may aggravate posterior vaginal wall weakness, predisposing to enterocele.** Retropubic suspensions alter vaginal and bladder base anatomy, and, thus, postoperative vaginal prolapse is a potential complication. Genitourinary prolapse has been reported as a sequel to Burch colposuspension in 22.1% of women (range: 9.5% to 38.2%) by Smith and associates (2005) in their review of the literature. The Burch procedure, because of lateral vaginal elevation, may aggravate posterior vaginal wall weakness, predisposing to enterocele. The incidence varies between 3% and 17% (Burch, 1961, 1968; Galloway et al, 1987; Wiskind et al, 1992); and because of this, prophylactic obliteration of the cul-de-sac of Douglas is sometimes considered when performing retropubic suspensions (Shull and Baden, 1989; Turner-Warwick and Kirby, 1993). However, simultaneous hysterectomy is not recommended prophylactically because it does not enhance the outcome of a retropubic suspension and should be performed only if there is concomitant uterine pathology (Milani et al, 1985; Langer et al, 1988). Although the Burch procedure and paravaginal/VOS repair both correct lateral defect cystourethroceles, recurrent cystourethroceles were noted in 11% and 39% of Burch procedures and paravaginal repairs, respectively (Colombo et al, 1996). In Mainprize and Drutz's review (1988), postoperative cystocele was noted in only 0.4% of patients after an MMK procedure.

    Wiskind and coworkers (1992) noted that 27% of patients who had undergone a Burch colposuspension developed prolapse requiring surgery: rectocele in 22%, enterocele in 11%, uterine prolapse in 13%, and cystocele in 2%. More recently it has been suggested that most women are asymptomatic and less than 5% have been reported to request further surgery (Smith et al, 2005). Ward and associates (2004) report 4.8% of women needing a posterior repair, whereas Kwon and colleagues (2003) report 4.7% requiring subsequent pelvic reconstruction.

    Because retropubic suspensions are unable to correct central defect cystoceles, patients must be carefully examined preoperatively to exclude their presence.

16. **d. more effective than a TVT procedure**. Comparisons between the MMK and the Burch procedures have generally yielded similar results. Three articles that reviewed the literature on incontinence procedures all found retropubic suspensions to be more effective than either needle suspensions or anterior colporrhaphies

(Jarvis, 1994; Black and Downs, 1996; Leach et al, 1997). Most studies in the literature have not demonstrated a significant difference in cure rates between retropubic suspensions (generally a Burch procedure) and pubovaginal slings (Jarvis, 1994; Black and Downs, 1996; Leach et al, 1997). The literature on the paravaginal repair is sparse. The only randomized study that compared the Burch procedure with a paravaginal repair found significantly greater subjective and objective cure with the Burch procedure (Colombo et al, 1996). At this point, TVT appears to be at least equivalent to the Burch colposuspension.

66

Vaginal Reconstructive Surgery for Sphincteric Incontinence and Prolapse

SENDER HERSCHORN

QUESTIONS

1. Which of the following statements about aging and urinary incontinence is TRUE?
   a. Urinary incontinence peaks in the younger age groups and remains stable throughout life.
   b. Urinary incontinence is more related to socioeconomic status than age.
   c. Stress incontinence predominates in young and middle-aged women, whereas mixed and urge incontinence predominate in surveys of older women.
   d. Urgency incontinence and stress incontinence tend to increase into the elderly age groups in various populations studied.
   e. Because methodologic factors interfere with interpretation, no conclusion regarding prevalence of incontinence and aging is possible.
2. Incidence rates of urinary incontinence are more difficult to ascertain than prevalence because they require:
   a. test-retest reliability.
   b. increased awareness of the problem.
   c. knowledge of the natural history of incontinence.
   d. repeated surveys of the same population.
   e. differing definitions of incontinence.
3. In the study from Oregon (Olsen et al, 1997), the lifetime risk of a woman undergoing a single operation for prolapse or incontinence by the age of 80 was:
   a. 2%.
   b. 11%.
   c. 33%.
   d. 56%.
   e. 74%.
4. Which of the following factors shows the strongest epidemiologic link to urinary incontinence?
   a. Menopause
   b. Obesity
   c. Episiotomy
   d. Chronic respiratory problems
   e. Pregnancy and childbirth
5. Which of the following muscles is not part of the levator ani?
   a. Pubococcygeus
   b. Puboanalis
   c. Puborectalis
   d. Iliococcygeus
   e. Coccygeus
6. Which of the following pelvic floor muscles can be palpated most easily on vaginal examination?
   a. Pyriformis
   b. Ischiococcygeus
   c. Pubococcygeus
   d. Obturator externus
   e. Iliococcygeus
7. Which of the following supportive structures is formed by fusion of the iliococcygeus and pubococcygeus muscles behind the rectum?
   a. Cardinal ligaments
   b. Arcus tendineus fasciae pelvis
   c. Levator plate
   d. Perineal membrane
   e. Puborectalis fascia
8. Which of the following statements about the urogenital diaphragm (perineal membrane) is NOT true? It
   a. closes the urogenital hiatus below the pelvic diaphragm.
   b. is contiguous with a parallel perianal diaphragm.
   c. has a sphincter-like effect at the distal vaginal wall.
   d. contributes to continence with connections to periurethral striated muscles.
   e. provides structural support for the distal urethra.
9. Central cystoceles result from:
   a. detachment of the paravaginal support from the arcus tendineus fasciae pelvis.
   b. breakage of the pubourethral ligaments.
   c. separation of the pubocervical fascia from the pubis.
   d. rupture of the posterior aspect of the arcus tendineus levator ani.
   e. weakness of the anterior vaginal wall or fascia.

10. The cardinal and uterosacral ligaments:
    a. support the uterine fundus to the lateral pelvic sidewalls.
    b. are the major source of support for the pubourethral ligamentous complex.
    c. hold the uterus and upper vagina in place on the levator plate.
    d. provide urethral support and closure.
    e. support the rectum via attachment to lateral prerectal fascia.
11. Which of the following defect is usually seen with level I defects?
    a. Urethrocele
    b. Cystocele
    c. Rectocele
    d. Vault prolapse
    e. Descending perineal syndrome
12. Which of the following is an example of a middle compartment defect?
    a. Central cystocele
    b. Rectocele
    c. Rectal prolapse
    d. Descending perineal syndrome
    e. Enterocele
13. Which of the following regarding symptoms of pelvic organ prolapse is TRUE?
    a. All women with pelvic organ prolapse have symptoms.
    b. Stress incontinence is inevitably an accompanying symptom even without a cystocele.
    c. They are usually specific to the prolapsing organ.
    d. Low back pain is always present.
    e. They may or may not be specific to the prolapsing compartment.
14. A 65 year-old woman presents with stage III anterior compartment prolapse. Stress incontinence had improved in the previous year. Which of the following statements about her evaluation is TRUE?
    a. No further lower urinary tract symptoms are necessary to ascertain.
    b. Occult or potential stress incontinence should be elicited.
    c. Cystoscopy and urodynamic studies are necessary to perform.
    d. MRI studies will provide a definitive diagnosis.
    e. Transvaginal ultrasound has been shown to be helpful in this situation.
15. The voiding diary, or frequency-volume chart, has been shown to:
    a. predict the outcome of stress incontinence surgery.
    b. confirm the result of the pad test.
    c. reflect symptoms most accurately.
    d. be independent of the patient's willingness to complete.
    e. check the validity of incontinence questionnaires.
16. The prevalence of severe hydronephrosis in patients with pelvic organ prolapse is reported to be:
    a. <1%.
    b. 5% to 10%.
    c. 12% to 18%.
    d. 20% to 25%.
    e. >30%.
17. Which of the following statements about clinical examination of anterior defects is TRUE?
    a. Physical examination has been shown to correlate well with MRI findings.
    b. The accuracy of clinical examination in assessing anterior defects has not yet been proven.
    c. It is a good predictor of the outcome of surgical therapy.
    d. It has been shown to have excellent test-retest reliability.
    e. It confirms symptoms in the vast majority of cases.
18. On speculum examination of the vaginal vault of a woman after hysterectomy, dimples seen at the 3 and 9 o'clock positions are the location of:
    a. Level 3 supports
    b. Pubocervical fascia
    c. Cardinal uterosacral ligaments
    d. Arcus tendineus fasciae pelvis
    e. Lateral rectal fascia
19. In the POPQ system for pelvic organ prolapse, which fixed structure is the reference point for prolapse?
    a. Hymenal ring
    b. Introitus
    c. Perineal body
    d. Ischial spine
    e. Genital hiatus
20. In the Pelvic Organ Prolapse Quantification (POPQ) system the perineal body is measured from the:
    a. middle of the urethral meatus to the posterior hymenal ring.
    b. anterior hymenal ring to anterior pouch of Douglas.
    c. midplane of the vagina to the introitus.
    d. anterior fornix to urethral meatus.
    e. posterior aspect of the genital hiatus to the midanal opening.
21. In the POPQ system for prolapse stage II is seen when:
    a. there is essentially complete vaginal eversion.
    b. no prolapse is demonstrated.
    c. the most distal portion of the prolapse is more than 1 cm above the level of the hymen.
    d. the most distal portion of the prolapse is 1 cm or less proximal or distal to the hymenal plane.
    e. the most distal portion of the prolapse protrudes more than 1 cm below the hymen but no farther than 2 cm less than the total vaginal length.
22. Which of the following statements about MRI of pelvic organ prolapse is TRUE?
    a. T1-weighted images give clearer soft tissue discrimination.
    b. It is more sensitive than cystocolpoproctography.
    c. Fast spin-echo T2-weighted sequences yield the clearest images.
    d. It is contraindicated in some patients because of the risk of ionizing radiation.
    e. It is the procedure of choice for assessing the degree of pelvic organ prolapse.
23. In the original Raz (1981) modification of the Pereyra needle suspension, all but which one of the following steps was new?
    a. Cystoscopic verification
    b. Entry into the retropubic space
    c. Digital guidance of the ligature carrier
    d. Placement of helical sutures into the periurethral connective tissue
    e. Urethrolysis if required
24. Bleeding from vaginal veins during the performance of a vaginal suspension for stress incontinence is usually treated by:
    a. Blood transfusion
    b. Laparotomy
    c. Angiographic embolization
    d. Vaginal sutures and packing
    e. Cystoscopy and suture removal

25. Which of the following statements about the results of transvaginal needle suspensions is TRUE?
    a. The long-term outcomes are still to be determined.
    b. Needle suspensions were more likely to fail after 1 year than open retropubic suspensions.
    c. The low morbidity permitted multiple repeated procedures in the same patient.
    d. The least invasive procedures had the highest patient acceptability rates.
    e. Permanent retention was an inevitable outcome.
26. Culdoplasty refers to which of the following?
    a. Obliteration of the vaginal lumen
    b. Resection of the vagina
    c. Attaching the vagina to the sacrotuberous ligament
    d. Plastic repair of the posterior vaginal wall
    e. Surgical obliteration of the cul-de-sac (pouch of Douglas)
27. Regarding the natural history of untreated pelvic organ prolapse, which of the following statements is TRUE?
    a. Occult weaknesses surface eventually.
    b. There is good correlation of symptoms and physical findings.
    c. There are little data on the natural history.
    d. Broad consensus exists on an adequate workup.
    e. Physical findings rather than symptoms determine the morbidity.
28. Which of the following statements about pessary use is TRUE?
    a. Pessaries are contraindicated in premenopausal women.
    b. Most women will discontinue pessary use within 2 months.
    c. Vaginal ulceration is an inevitable consequence.
    d. Pessaries are the mainstay of nonsurgical treatment.
    e. Masked stress incontinence is also effectively treated by the pessary.
29. Which of the following routes of delivery of low dose estrogen is most effective for urogenital atrophy?
    a. Oral
    b. Subcutaneous
    c. Intramuscular
    d. Intravenous
    e. Topical
30. Which of the following synthetic grafts has been shown to have the lowest rate of erosion?
    a. Expanded polytetrafluoroethylene (PTFE)
    b. Polyethylene
    c. Nylon
    d. Polypropylene
    e. Polyglactin
31. The maneuver to support the posterior aspect of a large cystocele during anterior colporrhaphy involves:
    a. imbricating the pubocervical fascia.
    b. supporting the repair with mesh.
    c. extending the repair to or through the arcus tendineus fasciae pelvis.
    d. incorporating the precervical or cardinal uterosacral complex.
    e. repairing the concomitant rectocele.
32. A paravaginal approach can be used to repair which of the following anterior wall defects?
    a. Lateral
    b. Central
    c. Anterior
    d. Posterior
    e. Distal
33. The addition of which of the following techniques to anterior colporrhaphy has been shown to be effective in addressing a lateral defect?
    a. Posterior colporrhaphy
    b. Enterocele repair
    c. Uterosacral suspension
    d. Grafting
    e. Injection of agents
34. What has been proposed as a cause of enterocele formation after a Burch procedure for stress urinary incontinence?
    a. Denervation of the vaginal wall
    b. Pelvic hematoma
    c. Urinary obstruction
    d. Alteration of the vaginal axis
    e. Effacement of the perineum
35. The standard treatment for symptomatic uterine prolapse is:
    a. hysterectomy only.
    b. hysterectomy plus prolapse repair.
    c. prolapse repair only.
    d. subtotal hysterectomy.
    e. complete pelvic floor mesh replacement.
36. Vaginal evisceration after vaginal hysterectomy is treated by:
    a. vaginal packing.
    b. endoscopic manipulation.
    c. bed rest and IV fluids.
    d. immediate surgery.
    e. sterile pessary.
37. Which structures travel just beneath the sacrospinous ligament and should be avoided during a sacrospinous ligament vault suspension?
    a. Pudendal vessels
    b. Hypogastric vessels
    c. Genitofemoral nerves
    d. Sciatic nerves
    e. Inferior gluteal arteries
38. The main vaginal site of recurrent pelvic relaxation after sacrospinous ligament vault suspension has been reported to be in the:
    a. vault.
    b. posterior wall.
    c. perineum.
    d. anterior wall.
    e. enterocele.
39. Which of the following vaginal vault suspension procedures has the greatest likelihood of ureteral injury?
    a. Sacrospinous ligament fixation
    b. Iliococcygeus suspension
    c. Uterosacral suspension
    d. Abdominal sacral colpopexy
    e. Laparoscopic sacral colpopexy
40. Abdominal sacral colpopexy has been compared with vaginal sacrospinous fixation. The results show that it:
    a. is more effective but takes longer.
    b. is equally effective.
    c. has largely been replace by laparoscopic procedures.
    d. narrows the vaginal canal and results in higher rates of dyspareunia.
    e. is associated with a higher rate of pudendal nerve damage.

41. A successful rectocele repair may accomplish all but which one of the following?
    a. Narrowing of the posterior aspect of the vaginal canal
    b. Plicating prerectal and pararectal fascia
    c. Narrowing of the vaginal caliber
    d. Narrowing of the posterior aspect of the levator (urogenital) hiatus with levator plication
    e. Preventing incontinence after anterior suspension

42. Which of the following is thought to cause dyspareunia after traditional rectocele repair?
    a. Persistence of enterocele
    b. Constipation
    c. Levator plication during the procedure
    d. Unrecognized rectal injury
    e. Persistence of the descending perineum syndrome

ANSWERS

1. **c. Stress incontinence predominates in young and middle-aged women, whereas mixed and urge incontinence predominate in older women.** When incontinence was classified by symptoms or urodynamics, in 21 of the 48 studies reviewed by Hampel and colleagues (1997), median prevalence of stress incontinence was 49%, followed by mixed and urge incontinence at 29% and 22%, respectively. In the EPINCONT study, over 50% of incontinence was stress, 36% was mixed, and 11% was urge (Hannestad et al, 2000). However, proportions of types differ by age. Stress incontinence predominates in young and middle-aged women whereas mixed and urge incontinence predominate in surveys of older women (Hunskaar et al, 2004, 2005).
2. **d. repeated surveys of the same population.** Incidence rates have been more difficult to ascertain because they require repeated surveys of the same population.
3. **b. 11%.** Olsen and coworkers, on the basis of chart reviews from a large managed care population in Oregon, reported that the lifetime risk of undergoing a single operation for prolapse or incontinence by age 80 was 11.1%.
4. **e. Pregnancy and childbirth.** Vaginal delivery is a major factor for the development of pelvic floor dysfunction in the majority of women (Bump and Norton, 1998). Most studies demonstrate a link between urinary incontinence and parity (Thomas et al, 1980; Yarnell et al, 1982; Hording et al, 1986; Sommer et al, 1990; Foldspang et al, 1992; Rortveit et al, 2001), although the level of risk is variable and lessens with age (Burgio et al, 1991; Rortveit et al, 2001). Parity and vaginal delivery are strong risk factors in pelvic organ prolapse (Mant et al, 1997; Hendrix et al, 2002). The labor and delivery process may cause the pelvic floor dysfunction as a result of nerve damage (e.g., afferents, pudendal, pelvic), muscular damage, and direct tissue stretching and disruption.
5. **e. Coccygeus.** The levator ani and coccygeus muscles that are attached to the inner surface of the minor pelvis form the muscular floor of the pelvis. With their corresponding muscles from the opposite side, they form the pelvic diaphragm (see Fig. 66-3). The levator ani is composed of two major muscles from medial to lateral: pubococcygeus and iliococcygeus (Kearney et al, 2004). The arcus tendineus of the levator ani is a dense connective tissue structure that runs from the pubic ramus to the ischial spine and courses along the surface of the obturator internus muscle.
6. **c. Pubococcygeus.** The pubococcygeus can be palpated during physical examination of the pelvis as a bulky muscular ridge on both right and left lateral side walls of the vagina, superior to the hymen. With contraction, it elevates the rectum, vagina, and urethra anteriorly and aids in compression of their lumens.
7. **c. Levator plate.** This median raphe between the anus and the coccyx is called the levator plate, the shelf on which the pelvic organs rest. It is formed by the fusion of the iliococcygeus and the posterior fibers of the pubococcygeus muscles. In the standing position, the levator plate is horizontal and supports the rectum and upper two thirds of vagina above it.
8. **b. It is contiguous with a parallel perianal diaphragm.** It bridges the gap between the inferior pubic rami bilaterally and the perineal body. It closes the urogenital (levator) hiatus, supports and has a sphincter-like effect at the distal vagina, and contributes to continence because it is attached to periurethral striated muscles. It also provides structural support for the distal urethra. The posterior triangle around the anus does not have a corresponding diaphragm or membrane.
9. **e. weakness of the anterior vaginal wall or fascia.** Weaknesses in the central part of the anterior vaginal wall or fascia give rise to cystocele from a central defect. Weakness in the lateral attachments to the arcus tendineus results in cystocele from a lateral or paravaginal defect. Combined defects with both central and lateral deficiency are also common (see Fig. 66-10).
10. **c. hold the uterus and upper vagina in place on the levator plate.** The cardinal and uterosacral ligaments hold the uterus and upper vagina in their proper place over the levator plate (Thompson, 1997).
11. **d. Vault prolapse.** Level I, or apical, defects are thought to be caused by loss of normal support of the upper paracolpium and parametrium and are associated with uterine prolapse, vaginal vault prolapse, and possibly enterocele.
12. **e. Enterocele.** Middle compartment defects involve the apical vaginal wall. Enteroceles are herniations of peritoneum-lined sacs containing abdominal contents such as small bowel or omentum (see Fig. 66-14).
13. **e. They may or may not be specific to the prolapsing compartment.** Symptoms caused by pelvic organ prolapse may or may not be specific to the prolapsing compartment(s), and the correlation of many pelvic symptoms with the extent of prolapse is weak (Mouritsen and Larsen, 2003; Burrows et al, 2004). Many women with pelvic organ prolapse have no symptoms, especially if the prolapse remains inside the vagina (Swift et al, 2003).
14. **b. Occult or potential stress incontinence should be elicited.** Many women with severe prolapse recall that as the prolapse worsened, their stress incontinence symptoms improved. Reducing the vaginal prolapse with a pessary or a speculum during the examination by the clinician can produce stress incontinence in up to 80% of clinically continent patients with severe prolapse (Fianu et al, 1985; Bump et al, 1988; Rosenzweig et al, 1992; Romanzi, 2002). This phenomenon has been termed *latent, masked, occult, or potential stress incontinence* and should be elicited when considering therapy.
15. **e. check the validity of incontinence questionnaires.** Voiding diaries, also known as micturition or bladder diaries and incontinence or frequency-volume charts, are widely used to assess frequency, nocturia, and incontinent episodes. The intake and voided volumes can also be recorded. They have been shown to exhibit test-retest reliability for incontinent episodes (Wyman et al, 1988) and have been used to check the validity of questionnaires (Donovan et al, 1996). They are helpful because they can portray the patient's daily picture of lower

urinary tract dysfunction. However, for accuracy they rely heavily on the patient's willingness and diligence to complete them. A 3-day diary has been suggested as optimal (Palnaes Hansen and Klarskov, 1998).

16. **a. <1%.** The prevalence of hydronephrosis in patients with pelvic organ prolapse is also low. Beverly and coworkers (1997) reported mild to moderate hydronephrosis in 6.8% and severe hydronephrosis in 0.9% of 323 patients with pelvic organ prolapse. The severe cases were seen only with uterine procidentia.
17. **b. The accuracy of clinical examination in assessing anterior defects has not yet been proven.**
18. **c. Cardinal uterosacral ligaments.** After hysterectomy, the vaginal cuff will have dimples at the 3 and 9 o'clock areas, at the locations of the cardinal uterosacral ligament attachments (Shull, 1993).
19. **a. Hymenal ring.** The POPQ system assigns negative numbers (in centimeters) to structures that have not prolapsed beyond the hymen and positive numbers to structures that protrude, with the plane of the hymen defined as zero (see Fig. 66-18). The hymen was selected as the reference point rather than introitus because it is more precisely identified (Bump et al, 1996a).
20. **e. posterior aspect of the genital hiatus to the midanal opening.**
21. **d. the most distal portion of the prolapse is 1 cm or less proximal or distal to the hymenal plane.**
22. **c. Fast spin-echo T2-weighted sequences yield the clearest images.** T1-weighted sequences can be obtained in a shorter time, resulting in less motion artifact, and are used as the initial imaging sequence. T2-weighted images have clearer soft tissue contrast discrimination. Very fast single-shot MR sequences have been developed for the evaluation of pelvic prolapse, allowing excellent visualization of the pelvic floor.
23. **a. Cystoscopic verification.** In 1981, Raz and coworkers reported a modification of the Pereyra procedure (see Fig. 66-22). The technique required an inverted U-shaped vaginal incision to improve access. It also was the first to enter the retropubic space sharply via the vaginal route by detaching the periurethral connective tissue and endopelvic fascia from the arcus tendineus and pelvic sidewall. Opening the retropubic space facilitates blind passage of the ligature carrier from the abdomen to the vaginal incision by allowing finger guidance, permitting urethrolysis if required, and allowing placement of helical sutures into the vaginal side of the periurethral connective tissue, which results in a more secure purchase of tissue. Another subsequent modification was the double-pronged ligature carrier that is passed twice via a midline suprapubic incision to retrieve the 1-0 nonabsorbable suture from each side.
24. **d. Vaginal sutures and packing.** Bleeding from retropubic dissection may be more problematic and is often a result of dissection too far laterally into the obturator fossa. Temporary vaginal packing along with digital compression can slow bleeding. Suture ligatures may be required. Vaginal closure with packing may tamponade bleeding that is not too brisk or flowing freely into the retropubic space. Rarely, abdominal exploration may be required to control bleeding. Transfusion requirement for endoscopic suspensions is estimated at 1%.
25. **b. Needle suspensions were more likely to fail after 1 year than open retropubic suspensions.** Nine trials with 347 women with needle suspensions were compared with 437 women who received comparison interventions. The results showed that needle suspensions were more likely to fail after 1 year than open retropubic suspensions (29% vs. 16%), and the difference in perioperative complications was not significant (23% vs. 16%).
26. **e. Surgical obliteration of the cul-de-sac (pouch of Douglas).** See Table 66-9.
27. **c. There are little data on the natural history.** There is still no consensus or guidelines regarding which tests constitute an adequate workup for patients before surgery, nor are the functional deficits and symptoms caused by pelvic organ prolapse and pelvic floor dysfunction totally specific or absolutely established (Mouritsen and Larsen, 2003; Burrows et al, 2004). It is therefore important for the surgeon to fully evaluate the patient clinically and record all of the symptoms and physical findings in a standardized manner, as discussed earlier. Because the various forms of organ prolapse are interrelated, owing to shared support mechanisms, it is generally recommended that all defects be repaired at the same time (Thompson, 1997; Raz et al, 1998; Kobashi and Leach, 2000) because occult weaknesses in other sites or new support defects may be acquired (Shull et al, 2002). Although this approach is supported by clinical experience and the reported occurrence of prolapse after retropubic urethropexy (Wiskind et al, 1992; Kjolhede et al, 1996) and vaginal vault suspension (Shull et al, 1992; Smilen et al, 1998), there are little data on the natural history of untreated pelvic organ prolapse and whether correction matters (Whiteside et al, 2004).
28. **d. Pessaries are the mainstay of nonsurgical treatment.** Pessaries are the mainstay of nonsurgical treatment and are of primarily two types: ring and support. Pessary use is widespread and may be successful in alleviating symptoms in the majority of women (Clemons et al, 2004) and occasionally improves the prolapse (Handa and Jones, 2002). Complications such as vaginal wall ulceration can be minimized by proper sizing, care, cleansing, and estrogen replacement therapy (Cundiff et al, 1998a). Stress incontinence may also be unmasked in about 20% of patients (Clemons et al, 2004). Sulak and coworkers (1993) reported that, despite effective management in women who refused surgery, there was a 20% discontinuation rate.
29. **e. Topical.** In postmenopausal women, estrogen therapy has been widely proposed for the preparation of the vagina before surgery. Because the estrogen dose required to improve urogenital atrophy is lower than that required for endometrial proliferation, administration of unopposed low dose estrogen is safe and effective (Robinson and Cardozo, 2003). The vaginal route of administration has also been found to correlate with better urogenital atrophy symptom relief, greater improvement in vaginal cytological findings, and higher serum estradiol levels than the oral, transcutaneous, or subcutaneous routes (Cardozo et al, 1998). A practical regimen is a 6-week preoperative course of vaginal estrogen cream (Kobashi and Leach, 2000). Long-term safety of various vaginal estrogen delivery systems has also been confirmed (Robinson and Cardozo, 2003).
30. **d. Polypropylene.** Type I polypropylene synthetic graft has the lowest rate of erosion (<3%) and is therefore the most commonly used (Cosson et al, 2003; Brubaker et al, 2005). However, there are great variations in the types of polypropylene and the surgeon must be aware of the different characteristics of thickness, flexibility, and stiffness.
31. **d. incorporating the precervical or cardinal uterosacral complex.** In the posterior aspect, approximating stitches can be placed in the pericervical fascia or cardinal uterosacral ligament complex for additional support.
32. **a. Lateral.** Lateral defects, causing mild to moderate cystoceles, can be repaired abdominally with a paravaginal repair.
33. **d. Grafting.** To improve the failure rate of cystocele repair, various graft materials have been used not only to buttress the

colporrhaphy but also to suspend the anterior wall to various parts of the lateral pelvic sidewall.

34. **d. Alteration of the vaginal axis.** Ventral fixation of the vagina, such as a Burch procedure, may also cause widening of the cul-de-sac with resultant enterocele formation (Wiskind et al, 1992; Jolhede et al, 1996).

35. **b. hysterectomy plus prolapse repair**. The standard treatment for symptomatic uterine prolapse is hysterectomy with procedure(s) to support the vaginal apex, address enterocele when indicated, repair coexisting anterior and posterior prolapse, and perform anti-incontinence procedures as needed.

36. **d. immediate surgery**. Vaginal evisceration is a rare but life-threatening surgical emergency that can arise after vaginal or abdominal hysterectomy, enterocele repair, dilatation and curettage, brachytherapy, vault suspension, or colpocleisis (Virtanen et al, 1996; Ginsberg et al, 1998; Verity and Bombieri, 2005). The evisceration repair operation can be done vaginally, abdominally, laparoscopically, or combined.

37. **a. Pudendal vessels.** Many important structures are in close proximity and must be avoided during the procedure. The hypogastric vessels lie superior and medial. The sciatic nerve and inferior gluteal artery exit the pelvis through the lower part of the greater sciatic foramen (Soames, 1995). The pudendal vessels and nerve and the nerve to the obturator internus travel around the ischial spine and reenter the pelvis through the lesser sciatic foramen, below the pelvic diaphragm. The sutures are placed 1.5 to 3 cm medial to the ischial spine, to avoid injury to the pudendal nerves and vessels, and through the substance of the ligament.

38. **d. anterior wall.** Recurrent pelvic relaxation developed in 109 (18%) patients, including 81 anterior vaginal wall defects, 32 vaginal vault eversions, 24 posterior vaginal wall prolapses, and 56 defects at unspecified or multiple sites. Reoperations were performed in 7 of 81 patients with anterior defects, 20 of 32 with vault eversion, and 4 of 24 with posterior wall prolapse. The relatively high recurrence or new onset of anterior vaginal prolapse has been mentioned earlier and ranges from 22% to 92% (Morley and DeLancey, 1988; Shull et al, 1992; Holley et al, 1995; Maher et al, 2001). It may be caused by exaggerated retroversion of the vagina with exposure of the anterior wall to greater abdominal pressure or possibly a neuropathy caused by the vaginal dissection (Benson et al, 1996). However, the overall results appeared better in a recent review of 2390 patients from Beer and Kuhn (2005). They reported a subjective cure rate of 70% to 98% and an objective cure rate based on physical examination of 67% to 96.8%. Recurrent prolapse in 2256 patients was reported at the vault in 3.6%, enterocele in 0.7%, cystocele in 4.6%, and rectocele in 1.5% of patients.

39. **c. Uterosacral ligament suspension**. Intraoperative ureteral injury has been reported as high as 11% (Barber et al, 2000a), underscoring the importance of performing intraoperative cystoscopy. If ureteral obstruction is suspected, the ipsilateral uterosacral stitches should be replaced or additional maneuvers, such as retrograde and stent, may be required.

40. **a. is more effective but takes longer**. Maher and colleagues (2004) concluded in their meta-analysis that abdominal sacral colpopexy is associated with a lower rate of recurrent vault prolapse and dyspareunia than the vaginal sacrospinous fixation. However, these benefits must be balanced against a longer operating time, longer time to return to activities of daily living, and increased cost of the abdominal approach.

41. **e. Preventing incontinence after anterior suspension.** The aims of traditional posterior colporrhaphy for the repair of rectocele are to (1) plicate the prerectal and pararectal fascia in the midline, (2) narrow the posterior aspect of the levator hiatus with levator plication, and (3) repair the perineal body (perineorrhaphy) (Raz et al, 1998). The repair effectively narrows the vaginal caliber.

42. **c. Levator plication during the procedure**. Dyspareunia or apareunia has been reported in 21% to 50% of patients (Francis and Jeffcoate, 1961; Haase and Skibsted, 1988; Kahn and Stanton, 1997) and is thought to be secondary to levator plication (Kahn and Stanton, 1997) or excessive tightness of the introitus or vagina.

67

Pubovaginal Sling

SEUNG-JUNE OH • JOHN T. STOFFEL • EDWARD J. MCGUIRE

QUESTIONS

1. The risk of an iatrogenic HIV infection from allogenic sling material is:
   a. 1:8,000.
   b. 1:80,000.
   c. 1:800,000.
   d. 1:8 million.
   e. 1:80 million.
2. An autologous fascial sling is indicated in the following conditions EXCEPT:
   a. proximal urethral incompetence in a myelodysplasic patient.
   b. urethral incompetence in a T12 spinal cord injury.
   c. urethral dysfunction after Miles operation.
   d. low urethral resistance combined with poor bladder compliance.
   e. loss of urethral closure function after treatment for a large urethral diverticulum.
3. An autologous sling procedure should be used rather than a synthetic suburethral sling procedure in the following patients with urinary incontinence EXCEPT:
   a. a 45-year-old woman with stress incontinence after removal of eroded synthetic sling.
   b. an 11-year-old girl with stress incontinence after severe pelvic trauma.
   c. a 36-year-old woman with urinary incontinence secondary to urethral erosion by chronic urethral catheter indwelling.
   d. a 51-year-old woman with persistent stress incontinence after multiple previous failed operations for urinary incontinence.
   e. a 48-year-old woman with stress incontinence associated with urethral hypermobility.
4. The risk of an iatrogenic Creutzfeldt-Jakob prion infection from allogenic sling material is:
   a. 1:3,500.
   b. 1:35,000.
   c. 1:350,000.
   d. 1:3.5 million.
   e. 1:35 million.
5. Which of the following statements regarding the sling materials is TRUE?
   a. HIV transmission is not a major concern in the use of allograft.
   b. Genetic materials can usually be removed during the processing of xenograft materials.
   c. Rectus fascia and fascia lata are seldom used for autologous materials.
   d. Porcine or bovine material is the least frequently used for the xenograft slings.
   e. There is almost no variation in the tensile strength according to the types of materials.
6. Which of the following statements regarding stress urinary incontinence is correct?
   a. It is important to identify poor bladder compliance before the surgical treatment for stress urinary incontinence.
   b. The timing for actually observed incontinence coincides exactly with peak abdominal pressure.
   c. The severity of stress urinary incontinence symptoms is correlated with the degree of urethral mobility.
   d. It is essential to detect overactive detrusor incontinence before the surgical treatment for stress urinary incontinence.
   e. Urethral pressure profile is an excellent parameter to determine the degree of intrinsic sphincteric deficiency.
7. Which description of the overactive bladder in stress urinary incontinence is correct?
   a. Overactive bladder symptoms are found in an average of 30% of the patients with stress urinary incontinence.
   b. OAB symptoms seem to affect the clinical outcome of surgical treatment of stress urinary incontinence.
   c. Most of the de-novo OAB symptoms after stress urinary incontinence usually do not disappear.
   d. In contrast to the OAB symptoms, urodynamically demonstrated detrusor overactivity is not a significant risk factor for the surgical outcome of stress urinary incontinence.
   e. Overall operative success for stress incontinence with respect of the resolution of OAB symptoms is different with various sling materials.
8. The following conditions are commonly associated with the low bladder compliance EXCEPT:
   a. pelvic trauma.
   b. post radical hysterectomy.
   c. chronic indwelling urethral catheter.
   d. post radiation therapy.
   e. meningomyelocele.

9. Which parameter is more closely correlated with leakage in the condition of stress urinary incontinence during a video-urodynamic study?
   a. Detrusor leak-point pressure
   b. Maximal urethral closing pressure
   c. Maximal flow rate
   d. Maximal detrusor contractile pressure
   e. Valsalva leak-point pressure
10. Which of the following descriptions of the maximal urethral closing pressure is correct? It
    a. measures the static tone of the urethra.
    b. correlates with the severity of stress incontinence.
    c. predicts surgical outcome.
    d. correlates with Valsalva leak-point pressure.
    e. distinguishes the presence or absence of stress incontinence.
11. Which is correct with regard to the practical measurement of Valsalva leak-point pressure?
    a. The measured pressure is detrusor pressure.
    b. The patient is positioned upright.
    c. The bladder is filled with 450 mL.
    d. Leakage at less than 100 cm H_2O indicates severe dysfunction.
    e. A normal urethra can show small amounts of leakage.
12. Cautions should be used in the interpretation of VLPP in the condition stress incontinence associated with:
    a. large cystocele.
    b. diabetes.
    c. prior pelvic trauma.
    d. prior bladder surgery.
    e. prior radical prostatectomy.
13. Which factor least affects the Valsalva leak-point pressure?
    a. Patient position
    b. Catheter diameter
    c. Bladder volume
    d. Detrusor pressure change
    e. Type of bladder filling media
14. Which is NOT correct regarding the typical determination of sling tension?
    a. Sling tension is usually applied with the vaginal retractor removed.
    b. Degree of sling tension applied is different in different types of patients.
    c. Application of tension can be minimal in patients with high VLPP.
    d. Compressive sling is required in patients with periurethral scarring.
    e. "No-tension" technique should be applied universally to avoid postoperative urinary retention.
15. Which of the following conditions is NOT commonly suitable for the crossover sling technique (compressive sling)?
    a. VLPP < 60 cm H_2O
    b. Urethral hypermobility
    c. Patients with myelodysplasia
    d. Many failed prior attempts at surgical treatment of incontinence
    e. Urethral closure and continent urinary diversion
16. What is the optimal site of urethra for the pubovaginal sling placement?
    a. Bladder neck and proximal urethra
    b. Mid urethra
    c. Around the external sphincter
    d. Distal third of the urethra
    e. Between the proximal urethra and mid urethra
17. Which of the following is the most important advantage from the autologous sling operation, different from the synthetic sling procedures?
    a. Urinary retention
    b. Urethral erosion
    c. Suprapubic pain
    d. Suprapubic tissue sarcoma
    e. Hematoma
18. Which figure is the closest to the contemporary overall success rate of the autologous pubovaginal sling for uncomplicated female stress urinary incontinence?
    a. 55% to 65%
    b. 60% to 80%
    c. 80% to 95%
    d. 90% to 95%
    e. >96%
19. Which is the best option for urinary incontinence if the correction of vaginal prolapse is necessary when the prolapse developed after a successful sling procedure?
    a. Observation
    b. Concomitant sling
    c. Biofeedback
    d. Medication
    e. Strict timed voiding

ANSWERS

1. **d. 1:8 million.**
2. **d. low urethral resistance combined with poor bladder compliance.** Poor bladder compliance can cause significant damage to the upper tract. This condition should be initially treated before any urethral procedure is undertaken.
3. **e. A 48-year-old woman with stress incontinence associated with urethral hypermobility.** Autologous sling procedure can be successfully indicated in complicated patients with stress incontinence or in cases where tissue erosion is anticipated with additional procedure.
4. **d. 1:3.5 million.**
5. **b. Genetic materials can usually be removed during the processing of xenograft materials.** Xenograft materials are also processed to remove cellular components.
6. **a. It is important to identify poor bladder compliance before the surgical treatment for stress urinary incontinence.** There is some time delay in actually observed incontinence after the peak

of the Pabd. The severity of stress urinary incontinence symptom is not well correlated with the degree of urethral mobility. It is not essential to detect detrusor overactivity in the treatment of stress urinary incontinence. Urethral pressure profile does accurately reflect the degree of intrinsic sphincteric deficiency.

7. **d. In contrast to the OAB symptoms, urodynamically demonstrated detrusor overactivity is not a significant risk factor for the surgical outcome of the stress urinary incontinence.** Based on the literature, neither OAB symptoms nor objectively determined overactive detrusor dysfunction can be regarded as risk factors for failure of operative therapy.
8. **a. pelvic trauma.** All of the others are well known to be closely related with poor bladder compliance.
9. **e. Valsalva leak-point pressure.**
10. **a. It measures the static tone of the urethra.** There is large overlap between the presence and absence of stress incontinence when the maximal urethral closing pressure (MUCP) is employed. MUCP does not correlate with the severity of stress incontinence, nor does it correlate with Valsalva leak-point pressure.
11. **b. The patient is positioned upright.** The patient is erect to measure the Valsalva leak point pressure. The measured pressure is the sum of Pdet and Pabd. The bladder is filled with 250 ml. Leakage at less than 40 cm H_2O indicates severe urethral dysfunction, whereas a normal urethra does not leak.
12. **a. large cystocele.** Vaginal prolapse interferes with leak-point pressure testing, apparently because the abdominal pressure is dissipated in the prolapse; and this makes the urethra appear better than it really is.
13. **e. Type of bladder filling media.** The patient position, catheter size, bladder volume, detrusor pressure change, and type of patient's efforts affect Valsalva leak-point pressure.
14. **e. "No-tension" technique should be applied universally to avoid postoperative urinary retention.** Universal application of the "no-tension" technique may result in suboptimal outcomes.
15. **b. Urethral hypermobility.** Crossover sling technique is a compressive sling, meaning an application of more tension. The other situations listed are indicated.
16. **a. Bladder neck and proximal urethra.**
17. **b. Urethral erosion.** Urethral erosion is very rare in the autologous sling procedure.
18. **c. 80% to 95%.**
19. **b. Concomitant sling.** If a vaginal prolapse does develop after a sling procedure, especially a cystocele, correction of the latter problem where it involves the arcus tendineus fasciae pelvis is likely to detach the sling from its fixation points with the development of recurrent stress incontinence. In these cases a well-supported urethra and good sling at the beginning of the procedure mean nothing. If the cystocele repair seems to loosen the sling, and produces new urethral mobility, it is best to redo the sling.

68

Tension-Free Vaginal Tape Procedures

ROGER DMOCHOWSKI • HARRIETTE SCARPERO • JONATHAN STARKMAN

QUESTIONS

1. Regarding the pathophysiology of incontinence:
   a. Hypermobility is the main underlying cause of stress urinary incontinence (SUI).
   b. Intrinsic urethral dysfunction (ISD) is rarely the primary etiology of SUI.
   c. ISD is the primary underlying cause of SUI for women with hypermobility being a secondary finding.
   d. The levator floor provides active compression to the proximal urethra.
   e. The extrinsic urethral skeletal sphincter is the primary mechanism for urinary continence.
2. The Integral Theory maintains that:
   a. the midurethral continence mechanism is active both passively and during stress events.
   b. the pubourethral ligaments are a secondary component of the complex.
   c. the pubourethral ligaments and pubococcygeal muscles provide a central support point that, during stress events, function to kink or functionally hinge the urethra, rendering continence.
   d. aging and childbirth have no effect on the midurethral support structures.
   e. the midurethral mechanism is intrinsically involved with bladder neck support.
3. The transvaginal tape(TVT or any midurethral sling) procedure incorporates all of the following EXCEPT:
   a. insertion trochars are used to transpose the implanted material into position.
   b. the synthetic material used is a wide porosity mesh.
   c. loose tension is placed on the sling material.
   d. the sling is sutured to the underlying tissues for fixation purposes.
   e. cystoscopy is a crucial component of the procedure.
4. In review of the efficacy outcomes obtained with mid-urethral procedures, which of the following is TRUE?
   a. Mid-urethral slings are less effective than open colposuspension procedures.
   b. Mid-urethral slings produce inferior results compared with laparoscopic colposuspensions.
   c. Postoperative voiding dysfunction is more common with mid-urethra procedures than with other types of suspension procedures.
   d. Mixed incontinence results are superior to those of pure stress incontinence.
   e. Five-year results demonstrate durability similar to one-year results.
5. In elderly patients, midurethral slings:
   a. are less effective than in younger patients.
   b. have rates of postoperative urgency higher than those in young patients.
   c. have satisfaction rates lower than those in young patients.
   d. have mixed incontinence resolution rates higher than those in young patients.
   e. result in postoperative urinary retention occurring more frequently.
6. When midurethral slings are performed at the time of prolapse surgery:
   a. risks of erosion and infection are higher than in cases in which only a sling is performed.
   b. concomitant hysterectomy has an adverse effect on incontinence outcome.
   c. rates of urethrolysis for postoperative retention are higher.
   d. occult incontinence is not adequately addressed.
   e. rates of retention are slightly higher than in those undergoing sling only.
7. When using midurethral slings as salvage procedures:
   a. complication rates are higher than when midurethral slings are done primarily.
   b. technique needs to be altered when done as a primary procedure.
   c. failure rates are unaffected by urethral hypermobility.
   d. bladder perforation is less than in primary cases.
   e. overall efficacy is similar to primary implantation.
8. Complications associated with midurethral slings include:
   a. bladder perforation injury rates range from 2% to 5%.
   b. voiding dysfunction ranges from 4% to 20%.
   c. de novo urgency occurs in 1% to 12%.
   d. wound healing is delayed in approximately 1%.
   e. all of the above.
9. Material-related erosions associated with midurethral slings are:
   a. decreased by the macroporous nature of the sling material.
   b. unaffected by tension placed on the slings.
   c. associated with vaginal erosions approximating 20%.
   d. associated with bladder erosion rates of 20%.
   e. do not affect outcomes or satisfaction.

10. In regard to erosions associated with midurethral slings:
    a. bladder erosions cannot be managed endoscopically in well-selected cases.
    b. vaginal erosions cannot be managed conservatively.
    c. erosions are not related to errant sling placement.
    d. symptoms are not usually associated with erosion.
    e. complete excision of exposed material is done.
11. Voiding dysfunction associated with midurethral slings is:
    a. not associated with changes in urodynamic parameters.
    b. predictable based on unique preoperative voiding parameters such as flow rate.
    c. managed by immediate sling release.
    d. managed initially conservatively, but sling release should be contemplated when persistent voiding trials are not successful.
    e. resolved by complete excision of the sling.
12. Complications associated with midurethral slings include:
    a. superficial vaginal material exposure.
    b. vascular perforation.
    c. intestinal perforation.
    d. significant hemorrhage requiring transfusion.
    e. all of the above.
13. Regarding the transobturator technique (TOT) the:
    a. surgical placement of the tape requires insertion through the adductor longus tendon.
    b. tape never traverses the gracilis or adductor magnus brevis muscles.
    c. anterior branch of the obturator artery is located at the medial aspect of the obturator foramen.
    d. tape remains above the perineal membrane and outside the true pelvis and does not penetrate the levator ani group.
    e. dorsal nerve of the clitoris is in close juxtaposition to the tape.
14. The TOT technique involves:
    a. either outside-in or inside-out approaches.
    b. no absolute requirement for cystoscopy.
    c. no risk of lower urinary tract injury.
    d. no risk of leg pain or dyspareunia.
    e. similar meshes in all different available kits.
15. Reported outcomes with the TOT:
    a. appear to be relatively similar regardless of whether intrinsic sphincter deficiency is present preoperatively.
    b. include bladder, but not urethral, injury being reported.
    c. indicate that vaginal erosion is similar regardless of the type of tape used.
    d. show that voiding dysfunction is significantly less with this technique as compared with the retropubic approach.
    e. are not affected by the presence of urethral hypermobility.

ANSWERS

1. **c. ISD is the primary underlying cause of SUI for women with hypermobility being a secondary finding.** Although urethral hypermobility is present in many women, most do not manifest incontinence and, therefore, intrinsic sphincteric deficiency (ISD) is considered to be the most important factor in women who experience urinary loss. The extrinsic urethral sphincter is not considered to be the primary mechanism for urinary continence in women. The ongoing debate regarding hypermobility and ISD is further compounded by the advent of midurethral slings, which clearly address hypermobility during stress events. Given the efficacy of midurethral slings, there has been some confusion regarding the role of hypermobility in promoting continence. However, most believe that the intrinsic urethral mechanism is of primary importance for urinary control.
2. **c. the pubourethral ligaments and pubococcygeal muscles provide a central support point that, during stress events, function to kink or functionally hinge the urethra rendering continence.** The integral theory places significant emphasis on the role of the pubourethral ligaments and the pubococcygeal muscles as central to urethral support during stress events. These structures actively function to provide a fulcrum around which the urethra rotates and subsequently is compressed during the stress event. Aging and childbirth clearly have a detrimental effect on the midurethral support mechanism. The midurethral mechanism is believed to be separate from the proximal urethral and bladder neck component of continence, although the latter component is considered to still have some importance in the overall passive control of urine. The midurethral continence mechanism only functions during active events and not during passive events and therefore has no function at rest.
3. **d. the sling is sutured to the underlying tissues for fixation purposes.** The TVT procedure incorporates several specific technical components. Insertion trocars are used either in a suprapubic or vaginal approach to assist in implantation of the material in the retropubic area. It is now well known that type 1 synthetic meshes are best because of their wide porosity. In addition, this mesh should be monofilamentous. Most authorities recommend loose tension only being placed on the TVT, although some authorities now are placing greater tension on the TVT, with success being established in patients with lesser degrees of hypermobility. No suture fixation is necessary to underlying periurethral fascia to anchor the sling. Cystoscopy is a vital component of this procedure to exclude urinary tract injury.
4. **e. Five-year results demonstrate durability similar to one-year results.** Five year (and now seven) longitudinal results have shown that mid-urethral slings have procedural durability in terms of efficacy. This efficacy is not substantially less than results obtained at one year. Randomized trials have demonstrated similar efficacy in patients undergoing either open colposuspensions or laparoscopic colposuspension procedures. Mid-urethral slings provide superior results compared with laparoscopic procedures. Although voiding dysfunction may be observed after any type of sling procedure, results suggest that mid-urethral slings are associated with less voiding dysfunction than either colposuspensions or bladder neck slings. Results with mixed incontinence are acceptable compared with other types of interventions for urinary incontinence but are less than those obtained in pure stress incontinence.
5. **b. have rates of postoperative urgency that are higher than those in young patients.** Elderly patients experience higher rates of postoperative urgency associated with any sling material, and this is true for the midurethral sling as well. However, elderly patients have results similar to their younger peers and therefore satisfaction rates are also similar to their younger peers. Mixed incontinence resolution rates are similar to the younger population, and actual postoperative retention occurs to a similar degree as in younger patients, but postoperative voiding function may be slightly higher in the older population.

6. **d. occult incontinence is not adequately addressed.** Midurethral slings performed at the time of prolapse surgery have now been shown to be safe and efficacious. Risks of erosion and infection are no greater than when the midurethral sling is performed as a primary isolated procedure. Concomitant hysterectomy has been shown not to have an adverse effect on continence status associated with these procedures. Additionally, rates of postoperative urethrolysis are no greater when the midurethral sling technology is combined with a prolapse correction. Rates of retention are also not appreciably higher in this population as compared with those women undergoing isolated slings only.
7. **e. overall efficacy is similar to primary implantation.** As salvage procedures, midurethral slings have overall efficacy similar to their use in primary implantation procedures. Complications should be no higher than when done as primary procedures. The technique remains the same, and no alteration is required. Success does appear to be reliant on hypermobility, and patients with less hypermobility would appear to have less overall functional success than those patients with greater hypermobility. Bladder perforation may be somewhat higher in this population than in primary cases.
8. **e. all of the above.** Complications with midurethral slings are an important part of informed consent. Bladder perforation ranges up to 5% and in some studies somewhat higher. Voiding function rates vary from 4% to 20%, and this variance is largely related to definitional reasons based on literature evidence. De novo urgency occurs with postoperative voiding dysfunction in up to 12% of patients, and wound healing can be affected in approximately 1% of patients; results represent dramatic improvement as compared with historic dense weave meshes.
9. **a. decreased by the macroporous nature of the sling material.** Erosion associated with midurethral slings is clearly decreased by the use of macroporous monofilament sling material (type 1). Tension may have a role in increasing erosion even in macroporous slings. Vaginal erosion rates and bladder erosion rates are very low and do not exceed 5% to 10% with these newer sling materials. When material erosions do occur, however, they have an adverse impact on overall patient satisfaction.
10. **e. complete excision of exposed material is done.** Management of erosions is complex and must be individualized. Primarily, all exposed material, whether it be vaginal or within the urinary tract, must be removed or in some manner covered. There have been successful reports of bladder management endoscopically, although this is contingent on absolute excision of all exposed material. Some authors have reported successful management of vaginal erosions with conservative use of topical estrogens and delayed primary closure as well as simple secondary tension healing. Erosions are clearly linked to technique, and errant sling placement has a high significance in creating erosions. Symptoms are usually associated with erosions especially in the urinary tract, but even vaginal erosions are associated with voiding symptomatology as well as persistent vaginal discharge and dyspareunia.
11. **d. managed initially conservatively, but sling release should be contemplated when persistent voiding trials are not successful.** Voiding dysfunction associated with midurethral slings is substantially less than with bladder neck slings but still occurs. Timing of intervention is dependent on surgeon experience but is trending toward earlier intervention. Most experts recommend a period of conservative management of a few days to 1 month. Persistent obstruction will require intervention. Urodynamic parameters are often affected in cases of persistent obstruction. Unfortunately, no preoperative factors are predictive of postoperative voiding dysfunction. Immediate release is not recommended because a short period of observation usually results in resolution of the voiding dysfunction. When sling release occurs, midline incision of the sling is all that is required; the entire sling does not need to be excised.
12. **e. all of the above.** Complications of technique include injury to surrounding structures and significant hemorrhage due to laceration of perivesical vessels. Intestinal and vascular complications lead to substantial morbidity including mortality.
13. **d. the tape remains above the perineal membrane and outside the true pelvis and does not penetrate the levator ani group.** The TOT technique is unique because it avoids (when done correctly) entry into the true pelvis and the levator group. Errant sling placement through the adductor longus tendon can result in substantial pain. Smaller muscle groups such as the magnus brevis and gracilis are often traversed by this technique, without substantive complication. The obturator vessels are lateral and superior to the area of insertion of the device. The dorsal nerve of the clitoris is separated from the trajectory of the device by at least 1 to 2 cm.
14. **a. either outside-in or inside-out approaches.** The TOT technique can be performed by insertion of the passing needles from either vaginal or obturator approaches. Associated risks of device use include leg pain, dyspareunia, and injury to surrounding structures. Cystoscopy is a useful safety adjunct and should be performed as an integral and necessary part of the TOT. Different kits use different meshes, and not all meshes are similar. The kit to be used should be evaluated critically for this parameter.
15. **a. appear to be relatively similar regardless of whether intrinsic sphincter deficiency is present preoperatively.** TOT outcomes are relatively similar to those seen with the retropubic slings, regardless of urethral function. Any urinary tract structure can be injured by the TOT, including the urethra and bladder. Vaginal erosion is clearly related to mesh type. Voiding dysfunction is similar to retropubic techniques. Less urethral hypermobility probably militates against success rates with TOT, such as those reported in women with higher degrees of urethral hypermobility.

69

Injection Therapy for Urinary Incontinence

RODNEY A. APPELL • J. CHRISTIAN WINTERS

QUESTIONS

1. What urodynamics parameter is affected in the treatment by injectable materials?
   a. Qmax—Maximal flow rate
   b. Pabd—Abdominal leak point pressure
   c. Pdet—Voiding detrusor pressure
   d. Pur—Maximal urethral closure pressure
   e. All of the above
2. When are injectables most successful?
   a. When patient has intrinsic sphincteric dysfunction (ISD)
   b. When patient has detrusor instability
   c. When patient has hypersensitivity
   d. All of the above
   e. None of the above
3. What factor most influences the positive results of treatment with injectables?
   a. Bladder capacity
   b. Viability of tissue at the injection site
   c. Cause of the incontinence
   d. Volume of injectable agent used
   e. Leak-point pressure
4. What is the correct site for injections for incontinence in men?
   a. Bulbous urethra
   b. Site is irrelevant
   c. Anastomotic line in post–radical prostatectomy
   d. Verumontanum in post-resection
   e. Proximal to the external sphincter.
5. How is postoperative urinary retention best handled?
   a. Self-catheterization with a small catheter
   b. Foley catheter for 24 hours
   c. Trochar cystotomy
   d. Acute urethral dilation with sounds
   e. α-Adrenergic blockers
6. What is the primary disadvantage to the use of injectables?
   a. Cost
   b. Allergic responses
   c. Need for reinjections
   d. Need for special equipment
   e. Pain and bleeding immediately post procedure
7. What is the most common complication from injection therapy?
   a. Transient urinary retention
   b. Irritative voiding symptoms
   c. Urinary tract infection
   d. Extravasation of injectable material
   e. Sepsis
8. What is the purpose of cross-linking bovine collagen with glutaraldehyde?
   a. To reduce infection rate
   b. To prevent urethral inflammation
   c. To prevent extravasation of collagen
   d. To reduce volume needed to gain urethrothelial coaptation
   e. To minimize immunoreactivity and increase resistance to collagenase
9. Suprapubic transvesical injections are routinely used in what circumstances?
   a. In females who cannot tolerate local anesthesia for intraurethral injections
   b. In any male patient
   c. In males or females with bladder neck contracture
   d. In males with failed transurethral attempts or with scarred urethras
   e. In patients with mixed incontinence problems (ISD and detrusor overactivity)
10. The optimal bulking agent has to meet all of the following standards EXCEPT:
    a. simple (easy) administration.
    b. no special equipment.
    c. must not migrate to other areas.
    d. easy quantification of material per patient per injection session.
    e. must not degrade (be inert).
11. The concept of implantable balloons for incontinence is less appealing than an injectable bulking agent for the following reasons EXCEPT:
    a. they require more difficult placement.
    b. they do not allow adjustments over time.
    c. they require special equipment.
    d. their manipulation requires regional or general anesthesia.
    e. they require surgery for removal or replacement.

12. Results with bulking agents have been similar thus far EXCEPT with:
    a. silicone
    b. PTFE (Teflon)
    c. autologous fat
    d. GAX-collagen
    e. zirconium-carbon beads
13. In reviewing data on males who have been treated with injectables, a major difficulty in interpreting data has been:
    a. differentiating neurogenic patients from post-prostatectomy patients.
    b. determining the number of injections required to reach dryness.
    c. assessing duration of dryness once it has been attained.
    d. differentiating post-radical prostatectomy patients from benign prostatic hyperplasia patients.
    e. conversion of patients from ISD as the cause of incontinence to overactive bladder problems.
14. One of the causes of failure to attain a good result initially in women is:
    a. instrumentation of the injected portion of the urethra.
    b. overinjection (too much injectable material).
    c. underinjection (too little injectable material).
    d. inexact placement of injectable material.
    e. urinary tract infection.
15. Which of the following materials have now been proved unsafe as an injectable agent?
    a. PTFE (Teflon)
    b. Silicone
    c. Zirconium-carbon beads
    d. All of the above
    e. None of the above
16. The disadvantage of periurethral injection over transurethral injection is:
    a. more bleeding.
    b. infection.
    c. longer learning curve.
    d. more extrusion of bulking material.
    e. sexual dysfunction.
17. The following is TRUE regarding the transurethral approach to injection therapy.
    a. It requires general anesthesia or intravenous sedation as a result of the instrumentation required.
    b. It can be done using a cystoscope, or an implanting device without the need for cystoscopy.
    c. Results are typically poorer than results after a periurethral approach.
    d. All currently available materials can be injected via a transurethral approach.
    e. Combination of b and d.
18. Which of the following is NOT true regarding the injectable agent Tegress?
    a. It is recommended to be injected using only the transurethral approach.
    b. It is a permanently implanted nonpyrogenic, injectable bulking agent composed of ethylene vinyl alcohol copolymer dissolved in dimethyl sulfoxide (DMSO).
    c. It requires a pressurized injection system.
    d. Exposed material is one of the more common adverse events after using Tegress.
    e. When injecting Tegress, volume injected is the most important parameter, not urethral coaptation.
19. Which of the following technology has been described to facilitate intraurethral injections?
    a. "Bent tip" needle for periurethral injections
    b. "Implacer" device for transurethral injections
    c. Ultrasonography to assess volume of material and configuration of material injected
    d. Antegrade (suprapubic) injections into the bladder neck
    e. All of the above
20. Which of the following regarding Durasphere is correct?
    a. Can be accomplished using local anesthesia with a pressurized injection system
    b. Can migrate
    c. Long-term results are superior to Contigen in randomized trials
    d. Consistently achieves durable, long-term correction of incontinence in many clinical trials
    e. Made of hydroxyapatite spheres in an aqueous gel
21. Which of the following statements is TRUE regarding urethral injection therapy in women:
    a. Periurethral injections are easier to perform and yield better results.
    b. Those with stress urinary incontinence can be offered urethral injection therapy as a method of treatment.
    c. Results of injections in those with mixed incontinence are similar to those with isolated stress urinary incontinence.
    d. The ideal patient for injection therapy is one with genuine stress incontinence and urethral hypermobility.
    e. None of the above.
22. Which agent is not currently approved by the U.S. Food and Drug Administration for the treatment of stress urinary incontinence in women?
    a. Polytetrafluoroethylene (PTFE)
    b. Glutaraldehyde cross-linked bovine collagen (GAX-collagen)
    c. Nonresorbable pyrolitic carbon-coated zirconium beads (Durasphere)
    d. Ethylene vinyl alcohol copolymer dissolved in dimethyl sulfoxide (Tegress)
    e. None of the above

ANSWERS

1. **b. Pabd—Abdominal leak point pressure.** One does not wish to increase resistance to Pdet just to obviate stress incontinence produced by increases in Pabd. Injectable materials can be used successfully in patients because they dramatically improve the ability of the urethra to resist increases in Pabd without changing voiding pressure or the Pdet at the time of leakage.
2. **a. When the patient has intrinsic sphincteric deficiency (ISD).** The ideal patient for the use of injectables is one with poor urethral function (ISD), normal bladder capacity and compliance, and good anatomic support. Contraindications to injectable agents include active urinary tract infection, untreated detrusor overactivity, and known hypersensitivity to the proposed injectable agent.
3. **b. Viability of tissue at the injection site.** The ability to do the procedure depends on tissue viability. For example, if a patient has a bladder neck contracture it must be recognized and

addressed before injectable therapy, and previous radiation therapy may limit the ability to do bulking without rupture of the urothelium, thus reducing the ability to coapt the walls of the urethra. Bladder capacity, the etiology of the incontinence, volume of agent used, and degree of ISD determined by leak-point pressure do not affect the ability to actually do the implant as viability of the tissue does.

4. **e. Proximal to the external sphincter.** The needle must be positioned proximal to the external sphincter, because injection into the sphincter has been associated with sphincter spasm and failure. To be effective, any injectable material must be injected into the urethra superior to the external sphincter.

5. **a. Self-catheterization with a small catheter**. If urinary retention should occur, clean intermittent catheterization should be utilized with a small 10-Fr to 14-Fr catheter.

6. **c. Need for reinjections**. Long-term results (>5 years) for all of these injectable procedures are scarce in the literature, and patients having been so treated have been observed for only short periods. The data available also do not take into consideration the reinjection rates, which run as high as 22% with collagen at 2 years after dryness is attained. This factor ultimately affects the cost of this therapy.

7. **b. Irritative voiding symptoms**. Irritative voiding symptoms develop in 20% of patients after injection of PTFE. More recent reports describe surprisingly high rates of irritative voiding symptoms. Corcos and Fournier (1999) demonstrated a 10% rate of de novo urgency and frequency, whereas Steele and colleagues (2000) stated that 50% of patients developed some degree of de novo detrusor overactivity.

8. **e. To minimize immunoreactivity and increase resistance to collagenase**. Cross linking with GAX results in a fibrillar collagen with resistance to collagenase digestion and significantly enhances persistence with stabilization preventing syneresis. GAX-collagen is a highly purified 35% suspension of bovine collagen in a phosphate buffer containing at least 95% of type I collagen and 1% to 5% of type III collagen prepared by selective hydrolysis of the nonhelicoidal amino-terminal and carboxyl-terminal segments (telopeptides) of the collagen molecules, which has the effect of decreasing the antigenicity and increasing the duration of the implant within the human body by increasing its resistance to collagenase.

9. **d. In males with failed transurethral attempts or with scarred urethras**. A newer method of injecting collagen in men by using a suprapubic antegrade approach is being employed. This approach has been described as using a flexible cystoscope placed through a suprapubic cystotomy. The antegrade approach has the advantage of direct visualization of the bladder neck and the injection of material into more supple, less scarred urethra. However, this has not won universal appeal with the newer agents and has only been used with collagen.

10. **b. no special equipment.** The optimal substance has to be inert and nondegradable. It must encapsulate and remain where injected, and it must neither lose bulk nor gain it (syneresis). It must not be too viscous, so that it can be injected with standard cystoscopic equipment used for other purposes under local anesthesia in an outpatient setting to help keep the procedure safe and cost effective. In addition, more accurate techniques for determining the quantity of material to inject in an individual must be developed to get the optimal result in a single treatment session.

11. **b. they do not allow adjustments over time**. Early experience with implantable microballoons (called Urovive) placed intraurethrally via a periurethral approach is encouraging; however, continued changes in the delivery device have delayed clinical trials in the United States. Another implantable balloon designed to have its volume adjusted once implanted via a completely periurethral approach (called ACT) is presently undergoing trials outside the United States. This balloon is placed completely outside the urethra at the level of the bladder neck and then filled through a port that remains accessible in the patient's labium, much like a pump mechanism from an artificial urinary sphincter. A disadvantage thus far has been the requirement for general or regional anesthesia for implantation.

12. **c. autologous fat**. Reports of studies with autologous fat have had less than impressive results. It appears that autologous fat undergoes a rapid rate of reabsorption because of its high water content.

13. **d. differentiating data on post-radicl prostatectomy patients from post-TURP patients.** On the male side, those patients with incontinence after prostatic resection for benign prostatic hyperplasia have often not been distinguished from those who have had a radical prostatectomy. For those with post-radical prostatectomy incontinence, it is often unclear which approach (retropubic or perineal) was employed. There has been very little in the way of objective reporting, with mostly subjective patient statements of cure, improvement, or failure. In addition, mixed techniques of injection and instrumentation are often intertwined.

14. **a. instrumentation of the injected portion of the urethra.** An effort should be made to avoid using instrumentation of the urethra and the risk of compressing the freshly placed implant by the endoscope.

15. **e. None of the above**. After injection of PTFE, the particles are noted to be found within lymphatics and blood vessels. Particles have also been found 1 year after injection in the pelvic lymph nodes, lungs, brain, kidneys, and spleen of animal models, and, although granuloma may form around the particles, no clinical reports of dysfunction of the organ involved have been noted.

16. **c. longer learning curve.** There is a tradeoff: the periurethral approach decreases bleeding complications, which hamper visualization and extrusion of the injected material but is associated with a much longer learning curve than the transurethral approach.

17. **e. Combination of b and d**. All of the currently available agents can be injected via a transurethral approach, and this can be done using a cystoscope or a urethral implanting device.

18. **c. It requires a pressurized injection system.** Tegress does not need a pressurized injection system to achieve implantation. It can be injected via a transurethral approach and 25-gauge needle without the need for a pressurized system.

19. **e. All of the above.** All of the mentioned technologies have been described to facilitate urethral injection therapy.

20. **b. Can migrate**. In a randomized multicenter trial, the results of Durasphere injections were not superior to that of collagen material, and Durasphere has been reported to migrate.

21. **b. Those with stress urinary incontinence can be offered urethral injection therapy as a method of treatment.** Although the ideal patient for urethral injection therapy has been described as one with genuine stress urinary incontinence and good anatomic support (no urethral hypermobility), the literature has demonstrated that all women with SUI regardless of anatomic urethral support can be offered injection therapy.

22. **a. Polytetrafluoroethylene** (**PTFE**). Although clinical data have been favorable, concerns regarding migration and safety of this material prevent its approval by the U.S. Food and Drug Administration.

70

Additional Therapies for Storage and Emptying Failure

M. LOUIS MOY • ALAN J. WEIN

QUESTIONS

1. The quoted rate of bladder rupture secondary to therapeutic overdistention of the bladder is:
   a. 20% to 25%.
   b. 10% to 20%.
   c. 5% to 10%.
   d. 1% to 4%.
   e. <1%.
2. Subarachnoid block generally accomplishes all but which of the following?
   a. Conversion of somatic spasticity to flaccidity
   b. Conversion of bladder hyperreflexia to areflexia
   c. Abolishment of autonomic hyperreflexia
   d. Completion of peripheral sensory loss where incomplete
   e. Improvement of reflexogenic erections
3. Which of the following represents the most devastating complication of subtrigonal infiltration of the pelvic plexus with phenol to treat urgency incontinence?
   a. Rectal fistula
   b. Urinary retention
   c. Vaginal fistula
   d. Decreased bladder compliance
   e. Stress incontinence
4. In a 70-year-old woman with urinary incontinence, which of the following is the most favorable characteristic for the use of an external urethral occlusion device?
   a. Moderate sphincteric incontinence
   b. Overactive bladder
   c. Cognitive impairment
   d. Moderate mixed incontinence
   e. Morbid obesity
5. The problems described as being associated with unstimulated graciloplasty include all but which of the following?
   a. Unsatisfactory sustained muscle contraction
   b. Passive obstruction
   c. Fibrosis of the muscle
   d. Active obstruction by tonic muscle contraction
   e. Necessity for prolonged leg adduction
6. Of the following, which is the main advantage of continuous suprapubic drainage over the urethral drainage?
   a. It is more comfortable.
   b. There is less risk of carcinoma.
   c. It is easier to replace.
   d. There is less bacteriuria.
   e. It obviates detrusor-related leakage.
7. The most significant complication that has been associated with the use of an external collecting device in the paraplegic male is:
   a. urine leakage.
   b. penile pressure necrosis.
   c. upper tract decompensation.
   d. its visibility.
   e. urinary infection.
8. All of the following accurately describe the factors associated with the Credé maneuver except which one?
   a. Funneling of the bladder outlet generally occurs.
   b. Increases in outlet resistance may occur.
   c. Vesicoureteral reflux is a relative contraindication.
   d. It is easier to perform in a thin than in an obese individual.
   e. It is most effective when outlet resistance is decreased.
9. In a young female paraplegic, the most effective way of initiating a bladder reflex contraction by "trigger voiding" is:
   a. squeezing the clitoris.
   b. digital rectal stimulation.
   c. pulling the skin of the pubis.
   d. pinching the skin of the thigh.
   e. rhythmic suprapubic manual pressure.
10. The preferred site of surgical sphincterotomy, when carried out transurethrally, is which of the following?
    a. 11 and 1 o'clock
    b. 3 and 9 o'clock
    c. 12 o'clock
    d. 5 and 7 o'clock
    e. 6 o'clock

11. Which of the following are necessary for successful clean intermittent catheterization?
    a. Patient motivation
    b. Hand dexterity
    c. Adequate urethral exposure
    d. Good training
    e. All of the above

12. All the following statements regarding acupuncture are true EXCEPT:
    a. it is a form of somatic sensory stimulation.
    b. it may facilitate bladder storage/filling.
    c. it is a standardized therapy.
    d. its mechanism of action is not clearly understood.
    e. it may involve the use of electrical stimulation.

ANSWERS

1. **c. 5% to 10%.** Therapeutic overdistention involves prolonged stretching of the bladder wall using hydrostatic pressure equal to systolic blood pressure. Improvement, when it occurs, is generally attributable to ischemic changes in the nerve endings or terminals in the bladder wall. Potential complications include bladder rupture (5% to 10%), hematuria, and retention.

2. **e. Improvement of reflexogenic erections**. Historically, a very central (subarachnoid block) type of interruption was not used solely for urologic indications but, rather, to convert a state of severe somatic spasticity to flaccidity and to abolish autonomic hyperreflexia. As a by-product, bladder hyperreflexia was converted acutely to areflexia. The flaccid bladder that resulted generally required additional therapy to empty or required clean intermittent catheterization. The obvious disadvantage of this type of procedure is a lack of selectivity, with unintended motor or sensory loss other than related to the bladder. Impotence was very common in males; and in those patients with some residual motor or sensory function, these functions were often significantly altered or lost.

3. **c. Vaginal fistula**. Transvesical infiltration of the pelvic plexus with phenol aims to produce a chemical neurolysis whose results parallel the surgical approaches outlined in the text. The potential risks of this procedure include urinary retention and vaginal fistula.

4. **a. Moderate sphincteric incontinence.** The ideal patient for such a device would be one with pure sphincteric incontinence that is mild to moderate, without significant bladder overactivity or decreased compliance, who desires active involvement in her treatment program, who desires immediate result, and who has the body habitus, manual dexterity, and cognitive ability to apply or insert the device and remove it.

5. **d. Active obstruction by titanic muscle contraction**. One 1998 study described unstimulated graciloplasty as an innovative idea but one that was associated with a number of problems: (1) the need for uncomfortable prolonged adduction of the leg to maintain sphincteric contraction; (2) unsatisfactory sustained muscle contraction due to the high content of fast-twitch, non–fatigue-resistant fibers; (3) loss of resting tension after dissection of the muscle, resulting in reduced contractility; (4) passive obstruction; (5) and the risk of fibrosis because the minor pedicles supplying the caudal segment of the gracilis as severed.

6. **a. It is more comfortable**. Occasionally, more often in females than in males, an indwelling catheter is a last resort type of therapy for long-term bladder drainage. Virtually all such patients have bacteriuria after a certain period. A contracted fibrotic bladder may be the ultimate result. Bladder calculi may form on the catheter or on the retention balloon. Urethral complications are relatively uncommon in females when proper care is exercised, but bladder spasm may occur, producing urinary incontinence around the catheter. The temptation to use a larger-bore catheter with a larger capacity balloon should be resisted, because the continuous use of such a drainage system combined with some pressure on the catheter may cause erosion of the bladder neck. A suprapubic catheter may be initially more comfortable and obviates urethral complications in the male, the main advantage of this type of continuous drainage over longer periods of time. Use of a suprapubic catheter does not, however, obviate urethral leakage with detrusor contraction, nor does it provide better drainage or less leakage in patients with sphincteric incontinence. When blockage or dislodgement occurs, nursing personnel may be reluctant to change this type of catheter without physician's assistance.

7. **b. penile pressure necrosis**. External collecting devices for the male (a condom or Texas catheter) are generally successful, insofar as urine collection is concerned, but are unacceptable to many patients because of the visible equipment required and the leaks of often foul-smelling urine that can result. Because many patients with neurogenic lower urinary tract dysfunction have impairment of sensation, it is easy for these devices to cause severe pressure necrosis of the penis. Maintaining an external urinary collection device is a major problem in some spinal cord injured patients. They are unable to maintain a device during vigorous voiding contraction, which is often associated with inadequate penile length. Because of recurrent laceration of the penile skin, temporary use of a Foley catheter is often dictated.

8. **a. Funneling of the bladder outlet generally occurs**. The Credé maneuver (manual compression of the bladder) is most effective in patients with decreased bladder tone who can generate an intravesical pressure greater than 50 cm H_2O with this maneuver and in whom outlet resistance is borderline or decreased. The Credé maneuver obviously requires adequate hand control. Straining at the time the Credé maneuver is applied is generally counterproductive because this increases intra-abdominal pressure and causes bulging of the abdominal wall, which then tends to lift the compressing hands off the fundus of the bladder. If the proper reflex arcs are intact, this also causes striated sphincter contraction. The Credé maneuver is obviously much easier in a patient with a lax, lean abdominal wall than in a person with a taut or obese one, and it is more readily performed in a child than an adult. Such "voiding" is unphysiologic and is resisted by the same forces that normally resist stress incontinence. Adaptive changes (funneling) of the bladder outlet generally do not occur with external compression maneuvers of any kind. As referred to previously, increases in outlet resistance (via a reflex mechanism) may actually occur. If adequate emptying does not occur, other types of therapy to decrease outlet resistance may be considered; however, these may adversely affect urinary continence. Vesicoureteral reflux is a relative contraindication to external compression or the Valsalva maneuver, especially in patients capable of generating a high intravesical pressure by doing so.

9. **e. rhythmic suprapubic manual pressure**. In most types of spinal cord injury or disease characterized by detrusor hyperreflexia, manual pressure sometimes provokes a reflex bladder contraction. Such "trigger voiding" is sometimes induced by

pulling of the skin or hair of the pubis, scrotum, or thigh; squeezing of the clitoris; or digital rectal stimulation. According to the classic reference, the most effective method of initiating a reflex contraction is rhythmic suprapubic manual pressure (seven or eight pushes every 3 seconds). Such activity is thought to produce a summation effect on the tension receptors in the bladder wall, resulting in an afferent neural discharge that activates that bladder reflex arc. Ideally, the contractions thus produced will be sustained and of adequate magnitude.

10. **c. 12 o'clock**. The 12 o'clock sphincterotomy, originally proposed by Maderbacher and Scott in 1975, remains the procedure of the choice for a number of reasons. The anatomy of the striated sphincter is such that its main bulk is anteromedial. The blood supply is primarily lateral, and thus there is little chance of significant hemorrhage with a 12 o'clock incision. There is some disagreement about the rate of postoperative erectile dysfunction in those individuals who preoperatively have erections. Estimates utilizing the 3 o'clock and 9 o'clock techniques vary from 5% to 30%, but, whatever the true figure is, it is clear that most would agree that this complication is far less common (approximately 5% with incision in the anteromedial position).

11. **e. All of the above**. Clean intermittent catheterization provides a safe and effective method for emptying the bladder in those who have emptying problems. Although it is the preferred method of bladder emptying due to a bladder cause, it is not suitable for all patients. The patients, especially if the bladder dysfunction is secondary to a neurologic lesion, must show adequate hand dexterity. Patients must also be motivated, because failure to perform CIC may be detrimental. They should also have good training in how to properly perform CIC and be able to obtain adequate exposure to the urethra.

12. **c. it is a standardized therapy**. Acupuncture is far from standardized and there exists a variety of techniques. Most studies have examined the use of acupuncture in the facilitation of bladder storage and filling and have shown some promising results. It usually involves the penetration of skin using a thin needle and the needles may be manipulated or electrically stimulated. The exact mechanism of action of acupuncture is not known but is a form of somatic sensory stimulation.

71

Geriatric Incontinence and Voiding Dysfunction

NEIL M. RESNICK • SUBBARAO V. YALLA

QUESTIONS

1. In people older than age 65, the prevalence of urinary incontinence is:
   a. 1% to 10%.
   b. 15% to 30%.
   c. 35% to 50%.
   d. 55% to 75%.
   e. 75% to 100%.
2. In demented elderly patients, incontinence:
   a. is inevitable.
   b. is virtually always due to detrusor hyperreflexia.
   c. is unlikely to respond to therapy.
   d. is multifactorial and often reversible.
   e. is treatable with a focus primarily on preventing skin breakdown.
3. Urinary incontinence in older people is usually:
   a. brought to a physician's attention by the patient.
   b. detected by the patient's primary physician.
   c. obvious to the urologist.
   d. detected by the physician but ignored.
   e. unknown to the patient's physician.
4. In older patients, uninhibited bladder contractions:
   a. are rare in asymptomatic patients.
   b. are primarily due to CNS pathology.
   c. are almost always the cause of incontinence.
   d. are inevitable with dementia.
   e. may not be the cause of incontinence.
5. After the history and physical examination, evaluation of the incontinent older patient should include:
   a. cystoscopy.
   b. video-urodynamics.
   c. postvoid residual assessment.
   d. urinary cytology.
   e. assessment of prostate size.
6. One of the following occurs as part of normal aging:
   a. urinary incontinence.
   b. small increase in serum creatinine concentration.
   c. uninhibited detrusor contractions.
   d. increase in bladder capacity.
   e. no change in urinary flow rate.
7. The cornerstone of treatment for persistent urge incontinence is:
   a. behavioral.
   b. flavoxate.
   c. oxybutynin.
   d. tolterodine.
   e. imipramine.
8. Acute urinary retention in an older man:
   a. indicates the need for surgical decompression.
   b. is treated effectively with α-adrenergic blockers.
   c. can occur with detrusor hyperactivity with impaired contractility.
   d. is treated effectively with bethanechol.
   e. requires treatment of the underlying urinary tract abnormality.
9. Incontinence management products (e.g., undergarments, pads):
   a. are reimbursed by insurance companies.
   b. should include menstrual pads.
   c. generally cost less than a dollar/day.
   d. should be chosen according to the type of incontinence rather than its severity.
   e. should be tailored to the individual.
10. The 5-year probability of an untreated older man with prostatism developing acute urinary retention is:
    a. 5% to 10%.
    b. 15% to 25%.
    c. 30% to 50%.
    d. 55% to 75%.
    e. 75% to 100%.
11. The voiding diary completed by an 83-year-old woman bothered by daytime incontinence discloses 800 mL output between 8 AM and 11 PM, and 1500 mL from 11 PM to 8 AM. Are the next steps TRUE or FALSE?
    a. Have her repeat it with a record of fluid intake.
    b. Give furosemide at 7 PM to reduce nocturnal excretion.
    c. Apply pressure gradient stockings to minimize peripheral edema.

12. Cystometry in a 78-year-old incontinent man reveals detrusor overactivity. If behavioral methods fail, the next step is to prescribe a bladder relaxant, TRUE or FALSE?

13. Anticholinergic agents should always be discontinued or substituted in an older patient who presents with incontinence. TRUE or FALSE?

14. A bladder relaxant medication with anticholinergic properties is contraindicated in older patients with cognitive impairment. TRUE or FALSE?

15. A bladder relaxant medication with anticholinergic properties is contraindicated in an older person with cognitive impairment who is currently taking an acetylcholinesterase inhibitor (AChEI, e.g., donepezil [Aricept]). TRUE or FALSE?

16. Anticholinergic bladder relaxants may, ironically, actually exacerbate incontinence through all but which one of the following mechanisms? Causing/exacerbating
    a. confusion
    b. impaired mobility
    c. dry mouth
    d. subacute urinary retention
    e. acute urinary retention

17. Desmopressin is an excellent agent for an older person with nocturia, especially if it is associated with incontinence that occurs predominantly at night. TRUE or FALSE?

ANSWERS

1. **b. 15% to 30%**. Although its prevalence increases with age, incontinence is abnormal at any age. Even in nursing home residents, where the average age is 85 and dementia and immobility affect more than half of residents, incontinence prevalence is 40% to 60%. More impressive is the fact that incontinence affects only slightly more than 50% of the most severely demented nursing home residents, provided they can transfer themselves from a bed to a chair and do not have other contributing factors; and even if they do, many of the factors fall into the category of transient incontinence and are reversible. Thus, incontinence is never the norm, no matter how old or frail the individual.
2. **d. is multifactorial and often reversible**. As just noted, incontinence is never normal, even with dementia. Detrusor overactivity (DO) is the most common type of lower urinary tract dysfunction among demented incontinent nursing home residents, but it is also the most common dysfunction among their dry peers. Moreover, incontinence in 40% of these individuals is not associated with DO but with obstruction (in men), stress incontinence (in women), or a combination of an outlet and a detrusor problem, and the cause does not correlate with either the presence or severity of dementia. Thus, it is no longer tenable to attribute incontinence a priori to DO. Because incontinence in the elderly is usually multifactorial, involving urinary tract as well as non–urinary tract contributions, it is often treatable. Even among nursing home patients, studies have documented more than a 50% reduction in incontinent episodes overall and full daytime continence in nearly 40% of residents. Particularly among demented individuals, nonurinary factors are prevalent and commonly include medication use, depression, fecal impaction, UTI, atrophic vaginitis, and disorders of fluid excretion. It is important to prevent skin breakdown, but this should not be the primary approach to the incontinent nursing home resident.
3. **e. unknown to any physician**. Despite the fact that incontinence is so common and amenable to therapy, most patients do not mention it to a physician. Reasons include embarrassment, misperception that it is a normal part of aging, belief that it is untreatable, fear of complications associated with its evaluation and treatment, or misconception that only major surgery can cure it. Moreover, when patients do mention it, most physicians either dismiss it as a normal part of aging or merely check a urinalysis. With newer undergarments and pads that better absorb and deodorize, the doctor may be unaware of the problem unless he or she asks about it.
4. **e. may not be the cause of incontinence**. It is important to realize that involuntary bladder contractions are found commonly in even continent, neurologically intact elderly; the prevalence ranges in various studies between 5% and 50%. This fact underscores the concept that such contractions are a risk factor for UI but not necessarily sufficient. Moreover, even when such contractions are the major contributor to UI, they may be due to a urethral abnormality. Over half of obstructed individuals and approximately 25% of those with stress incontinence have associated DO that usually remits with correction of the urethral abnormality alone. The proportion of elderly individuals in whom DO remits is likely lower, but clearly it is insufficient merely to identify involuntary contractions on cystometry and attribute the incontinence to them. To be considered the cause of the UI, such contractions must reproduce the patient's type of leakage and urethral abnormalities must be excluded. This is particularly important because a bladder relaxant medication prescribed for DO that is actually due to obstruction may precipitate acute retention.
5. **c. postvoid residual assessment**. Determining the PVR is essential in all incontinent older individuals, not only because retention can mimic other causes of UI but also because knowledge of the PVR will affect therapy. For instance, an older woman with DO and PVR of 250 mL would be approached differently from a woman with DO and PVR of 5 mL. The rest of the diagnostic evaluation depends on the need for diagnostic certainty. In many older adults, the empirical approach outlined in the chapter will be appropriate. However, if surgical correction is contemplated, or if the risk of empirical therapy exceeds the benefit, further testing is warranted. Cytology is indicated when bladder carcinoma is suspected and would be treated if found (i.e., not in a bed-fast, demented patient). Cystoscopy has many indications, but it is not routinely required for evaluation of incontinence, nor is it alone sufficient to detect or exclude prostatic obstruction. Palpated prostate size correlates poorly with the presence of obstruction.
6. **c. uninhibited detrusor contractions**. Incontinence is never part of normal aging; even at age 90, at least half of people are continent. Although renal function declines in most older adults, there is no change in serum creatinine concentration, owing to a balanced and concomitant decrease in muscle mass. Involuntary detrusor contractions are quite common in continent and even asymptomatic elderly but are rarely seen during routine cystometry in younger people. Bladder capacity *may decrease* in the elderly, but there is no evidence for an increase. Flow rate

declines, not only because obstruction becomes more likely in aging men but also because contractility appears to decrease in both sexes.

7. **a. behavioral**. Behavioral therapy is the cornerstone of treatment for detrusor overactivity, although the type of therapy must be tailored to the individual. Bladder retraining attempts to restore a normal voiding pattern by progressively lengthening the voiding interval. Scheduled toileting aims to reduce incontinence by frequent voiding, which reduces total bladder volume and the chance of triggering involuntary bladder contractions. Prompted voiding works by regularly and frequently reminding cognitively impaired residents of the need to void. The role of medications is to supplement behavioral therapy, but *only if needed*. By reducing bladder irritability, such agents allow the bladder to hold more urine before the spasm occurs. Even when continence is restored by these drugs, however, detrusor overactivity is still generally demonstrable. Furthermore, if the drug increases residual urine more than total bladder capacity, it may paradoxically *decrease* functional capacity, allowing the persistent involuntary contraction to occur at more frequent intervals. Thus, before deciding that drug therapy has failed, the postvoid residual should be re-measured. Except for flavoxate, each of the agents listed has been proved effective in randomized controlled trials that included a substantial number of elderly patients.

8. **c. can occur with detrusor hyperactivity with impaired contractility**. The differential diagnosis for urinary retention goes beyond urethral obstruction, particularly in the elderly. Patients with underactive detrusor or detrusor hyperactivity with impaired contractility (DHIC) also may develop urinary retention. In addition, fecal impaction, pain (e.g., after hip replacement), and medications with urinary tract side effects (e.g., anticholinergics, sedating antihistamines, decongestants, opiates) may induce acute urinary retention, particularly in patients with underlying bladder weakness or obstruction. Thus, the bladder should be decompressed for at least a week while reversible causes are addressed; the larger the PVR, the longer should be the decompression. Decompression allows some restoration of detrusor strength, which also facilitates urodynamic testing should it be necessary. α-Adrenergic blockers are effective for men with symptoms of prostatism, but clinical trials excluded patients with significant urinary retention. Bethanechol, although originally designed to improve bladder emptying in nonobstructed patients, has not proved effective for this purpose (and likely not for nonobstructed patients either). Decompression in some elderly patients can reduce but not eliminate residual urine; provided it does not cause symptoms or renal compromise, subclinical retention need not necessarily be treated in all elderly patients, even if obstruction is present.

9. **e. should be tailored to the individual**. The cost of pads is rarely covered by insurance and can easily exceed $1/day. Menstrual pads, although often employed for incontinence, are usually inappropriate. They are designed to absorb small amounts of slowly leaking viscid fluid rather than rapid gushes of urine. From among the numerous types of pads and garments, selection should be tailored to the individual's needs and comorbidity; the type of incontinence matters less than the severity.

10. **a. 5% to 10%**. Few studies have examined the issue, but the risk of developing acute urinary retention in men with prostatism appears to be quite low for at least 5 years. In the recent M-TOPS trial, for instance (mean age = 63 years at baseline), the risk of acute retention was <5% over nearly 5 years. Predictors of retention included age > 62 years, PVR 40 mL, PSA > 1.6 ng/mL, and total prostate volume > 31 mL, but these factors increased the risk only slightly (J Urol 2006;175:1422).

11. **False, False, False.** The patient's altered pattern of fluid excretion may occur for a variety of reasons. The most common one is accumulation of peripheral edema due to venous insufficiency, peripheral vascular disease, low albumin states (malnutrition, hepatic disease), drugs (e.g., NSAIDs, dihydropyridine calcium channel blockers [e.g., nifedipine], or thiazolidinediones [e.g., rosiglitazone]), or congestive heart failure. Each can be readily addressed. Before doing so, however, it is important to realize that the multiple pathologic conditions so often found in the elderly may be causal, contributory, a consequence, or unrelated to the condition for which the patient seeks help. In this individual, *daytime* leakage is the problem. Addressing the excess nocturnal excretion will not improve the daytime problem and, if it shifts the excess nocturnal excretion to the daytime (e.g., by use of pressure gradient stockings), therapy likely will *exacerbate* the daytime leakage. If the excess excretion can be eliminated entirely (e.g., by substituting a drug that does not cause fluid retention), this should be done. If, however, therapy will only shift excretion to the daytime, one may elect not to treat it if it is not dangerous (e.g., venous insufficiency).

    Daytime predominance of incontinence suggests that she has stress incontinence or DO associated with bladder neck incompetence that is exacerbated when she is upright. Once the cause is sorted out, the appropriate intervention can be prescribed, but in this individual it should not include alteration of fluid intake. This case highlights the need to tailor the evaluation and treatment to the individual patient.

12. **False**. Cystometry provides information only on the bladder, not the outlet, and only during filling, not voiding. Thus, it is insufficient to adequately characterize urinary tract dysfunction. Rather than the primary cause of this patient's leakage, the detected DO may be incidental to aging and unrelated to his incontinence; in this instance, bladder relaxants may lead only to side effects. Alternatively, if DO is due to urethral obstruction or bladder neck incompetence after prostatic resection, a bladder relaxant will likely exacerbate both. Further historical information is necessary, as is characterization of urethral function. Often, simply addressing issues outside the urinary tract—such as cognition, mobility, depression, manual dexterity, or fluid excretion and toileting—is sufficient to restore continence in an older adult. Such an approach is beneficial for other reasons: it avoids medication side effects and cost (drugs are often not covered by insurance), and it improves many of their other symptoms and quality of life.

13. **False**. Although anticholinergic agents can cause urinary incontinence, they do so by well-known mechanisms. In the absence of confusion, urinary retention, or excess fluid intake engendered by xerostomia, they should not be impugned as the cause of the leakage and the search for a cause should continue.

14. **False**. Incontinence is more common among patients with cognitive impairment than among their cognitively intact peers. The first approach should be to address all of the reversible causes, which are also more common in such patients, and to initiate a toileting regimen. If this fails, therapy with a bladder relaxant should be considered. All of the available bladder relaxants (oxybutynin, tolterodine, solifenacin, darifenacin, and trospium) have anticholinergic properties, but concern that confusion will worsen with administration of a bladder relaxant has proved to be more theoretical than real, and even trials that have included cognitively impaired nursing home patients rarely report this as a problem. Nonetheless, mental status should be carefully monitored in such patients and the drug should be stopped if mentation worsens without another identifiable cause.

15. **False.** Acetylcholine is an important neurotransmitter involved in memory. Because acetylcholinesterase inhibitors (AChEIs) are designed to increase the concentration of CNS acetylcholine, there is concern that an anticholinergic medication might attenuate or even reverse the benefit. However, AChEIs have proved to be of only modest efficacy. Improvement is experienced by only a minority of patients. Any attenuation of benefit is thereby minimal. In addition, there are only rare reports of deterioration when bladder relaxants are added to the regimen of these patients. Finally, given the impact of urge incontinence, many patients and families are willing to take the small risk. Thus, it is best to inform the patient and/or caregiver about the possible risk and, if he or she considers the expected benefit on incontinence to be worth the risk, to prescribe the drug and monitor its effect on both continence and cognition. A simple test, such as the MiniMental State Exam, can be used for this purpose. It is best to involve the primary care physician as well.

16. **b. causing/exacerbating impaired mobility.** Anticholinergic agents do not affect mobility. As noted earlier, all five of the currently available bladder relaxant medications have anticholinergic properties and thus can cause anticholinergic side effects. Confusion may result through the mechanism described in Answer No. 15. Dry mouth (xerostomia) results from the anticholinergic effect on the salivary and parotid glands. Even the M_3-specific agents have this effect because M_3 receptors are the predominant receptor in these glands as well as in the bladder. Because bladder relaxants generally do not abolish the involuntary detrusor contractions, the xerostomia-mediated increased fluid intake results in the bladder filling more often to a point at which detrusor contractions are triggered. Bladder relaxants often impair detrusor contractility and can lead to subacute retention; if the PVR increases to more than total bladder capacity, effective bladder capacity will decrease and allow involuntary contractions to occur at a lower effective volume; an increase in incontinence frequency can ensue.

17. **False.** Nocturnal incontinence is common in the elderly and it has a broad differential diagnosis. As indicated in Table 71-3, the causes of nocturia in older adults can be grouped generally into three categories: excess excretion (polyuria), conditions that disrupt sleep (including pain, anxiety, depression, CHF, and nocturnal bronchospasm), and conditions that result in impaired bladder storage. Like most geriatric symptoms, however, the causes may be multiple in a single person so evaluation and management must address each. Once this has been accomplished, the symptom may disappear or improve so substantially that the inconvenience, side effects, and cost of further therapy may not be desired. Even if the symptom does not improve, however, treatment with desmopressin is generally not warranted for several reasons. In trials that included older adults, treatment with desmopressin was associated with a significant risk of hyponatremia despite the restrictive enrollment criteria and meticulous evaluation and follow-up. The risk would be higher in clinical practice, where it is more difficult to identify contraindications and to monitor patients' renal, cardiac, and fluid status as closely. In addition, there is little evidence that desmopressin is actually effective for incontinence in older adults. Thus, given the frequency and potential seriousness of desmopressin's adverse effects, the minimal evidence of its efficacy, and the considerable associated cost, its use should be considered as a last option in an otherwise healthy patient who can be carefully assessed and followed with the help of a capable and willing internist.

72

Urinary Tract Fistula

ERIC S. ROVNER

QUESTIONS

1. The most common cause of vesicovaginal fistula (VVF) in the nonindustrialized, developing world is:
   a. caesarean section.
   b. surgical trauma during abdominal hysterectomy.
   c. surgical trauma during vaginal hysterectomy.
   d. obstructed labor.
   e. none of the above.
2. The most common type of acquired urinary fistula is:
   a. VVF.
   b. ureterovaginal fistula.
   c. colovesical fistula.
   d. rectourethral fistula.
   e. vesicouterine fistula.
3. VVFs may occur as a result of all of the following EXCEPT:
   a. locally advanced vaginal cancer.
   b. incidentally noted and repaired iatrogenic cystotomy during hysterectomy.
   c. radiation therapy for cervical cancer.
   d. cystocele repair with bladder neck suspension.
   e. ovarian cancer
4. Intraoperative consultation is requested by a gynecologist for a possible urinary tract injury during a difficult abdominal hysterectomy. There is clear fluid noted in the pelvis. The gynecologist is particularly worried about postoperative VVF formation. All of the following statements are correct with regard to counseling this gynecologist EXCEPT which one?
   a. The incidence of iatrogenic bladder injury during hysterectomy is 0.5% to 1.0%.
   b. Approximately 0.1% to 0.2% of individuals undergoing hysterectomy develop VVF.
   c. The risk of ureterovaginal fistula is greater than the risk of a VVF in this setting.
   d. The absence of blue-stained fluid in the operative field after the administration of intravenous indigo carmine does not eliminate the possibility of a urinary tract injury.
   e. Injury in this setting is most likely in the distal ureter.
5. VVFs from obstructed labor are:
   a. common in Nigeria.
   b. usually located at the vaginal apex.
   c. never associated with simultaneous rectovaginal fistula.
   d. typically found in multiparous women.
   e. usually smaller and simpler to repair than those associated with gynecologic surgery.
6. A 47-year-old woman presents with the new onset of constant urinary leakage 5 years after completing radiation therapy for locally advanced cervical carcinoma. Which of the following may be considered part of the diagnostic evaluation?
   a. cystoscopy and possible biopsy.
   b. Voiding cystourethrogram (VCUG).
   c. CT scan of the abdomen and pelvis.
   d. urodynamics.
   e. positive pressure urethrogram.
7. A 52-year-old woman with a history of an abdominal hysterectomy 2 months previously presents for the evaluation of a constant clear vaginal discharge since the surgery. The differential diagnosis includes:
   a. VVF.
   b. ureterovaginal fistula.
   c. peritoneovaginal fistula.
   d. all of the above.
   e. a and b.
8. Approximately what percentage of individuals with postsurgical VVF have an associated ureteral injury?
   a. 0.1%
   b. 10%
   c. 25%
   d. 50%
   e. 75%
9. A 68-year-old woman presents with the recent onset of vaginal leakage 6 months after completion of radiation therapy for locally advanced cervical cancer. VCUG reveals a VVF. On physical examination the fistula is irregular and indurated and approximately 3 mm in size. Cystoscopy reveals bullous edema surrounding the fistula, and biopsy of the fistula tract reveals only fibrosis without evidence of malignancy. There is no suggestion of recurrent malignancy on CT.
   a. The optimal timing for repair of this fistula may be in 5 to 6 months.
   b. The best chance to repair this fistula is with immediate surgical intervention.
   c. A vaginal approach is not indicated.
   d. The use of an adjuvant flap will not be necessary.
   e. The success rate for the repair of this fistula is similar to that of a nonirradiated VVF.

10. The abdominal approach to VVF repair:
    a. is the preferred approach in all patients with VVF.
    b. has a higher success rate than the vaginal approach.
    c. is suitable for the use of an omental interpositional flap.
    d. is associated with less morbidity and a shorter hospital stay than the vaginal approach.
    e. is more often associated with postoperative vaginal shortening and dyspareunia than the vaginal approach.
11. The vaginal approach to an uncomplicated VVF repair:
    a. is most often bolstered with use of a gracilis flap.
    b. may be accomplished with a three- or four-layer closure.
    c. requires the use of nonabsorbable suture.
    d. is not indicated for obstetric related fistula.
    e. is contraindicated if the fistula tract is within 2 cm of the ureter.
12. Principles of urinary fistula repair include all of the following EXCEPT:
    a. excision of the fistula tract.
    b. tension-free closure.
    c. use of well-vascularized tissue flaps.
    d. watertight closure.
    e. adequate postoperative urinary drainage.
13. Level I evidence (one or more randomized control trials) exists to support which of the following statements?
    a. Preoperative administration of topical estrogens improves tissue quality before the repair of VVF.
    b. Preoperative administration of topical estrogens improves the success rate of transvaginal VVF repair.
    c. Preoperative administration of broad-spectrum intravenous antibiotics improves the success rate of all types of VVF repair.
    d. Suprapubic bladder drainage is superior to urethral (Foley) catheter drainage in preventing surgical failure after VVF repair.
    e. None of the above
14. Vaginal repair of VVF is contraindicated in:
    a. multiparity.
    b. large fistulas.
    c. radiation-induced fistulas.
    d. fistulas located at the vaginal cuff.
    e. none of the above.
15. Potential complications of repair for a VVF after abdominal hysterectomy include all of the following EXCEPT:
    a. stress urinary incontinence.
    b. dyspareunia.
    c. recurrence of the fistula.
    d. urinary urgency and frequency.
    e. ureteral injury.
16. Advantages of the transabdominal approach to VVF repair as compared with the transvaginal repair include all of the following EXCEPT:
    a. ease of mobilization of the omentum as an interpositional flap.
    b. decreased rate of intraoperative ureteral injury.
    c. preservation of vaginal depth.
    d. easier access to the apical VVF in high narrow vaginal canals.
    e. ability to perform an augmentation cystoplasty through the same incision.
17. Seventeen days after a transvaginal VVF repair, a cystogram is performed. The bladder is filled to 100 mL with contrast medium and several images are taken. There is no evidence of a fistula on the filling images. The patient was unable to void during the study. A postvoid film was not obtained. This study:
    a. demonstrates successful repair of the VVF, and the catheter should be removed.
    b. is nondiagnostic because it was done too soon after repair.
    c. is nondiagnostic because there are no voiding images or postvoid images.
    d. is nondiagnostic because the bladder was not filled to an adequate volume.
    e. b, c, and d.
18. Before surgical mobilization, the blood supply to a potential Martius flap (fibrofatty labial flap) is via the:
    a. internal pudendal artery.
    b. external pudendal artery.
    c. obturator artery.
    d. a and b.
    e. all of the above.
19. A interpositional flap of greater omentum during VVF repair:
    a. may be able to reach the deep pelvis without any mobilization.
    b. is most commonly based on the superior mesenteric artery.
    c. is contraindicated in the setting of inflammation or infection.
    d. is not divided or incised vertically in the midline because this may compromise the blood supply.
    e. is most commonly utilized during a transvaginal approach.
20. A 39-year-old woman presents with constant vaginal leakage for 1 month after an abdominal hysterectomy. She describes symptoms of stress incontinence before the hysterectomy. She has no urgency and is voiding normally. Physical examination demonstrates no obvious fistula tract at the vaginal cuff. Oral phenazopyridine is given, and the bladder is filled with 100 mL of saline mixed with indigo carmine. A gauze pad is packed from the apex of the vagina proximally to the introitus distally, and the patient is told to ambulate for 90 minutes. Upon return, the pad is removed and examined. The most proximal portion of the pad is stained yellow orange, and the most distal portion is blue. This is most consistent with:
    a. ureterovaginal fistula.
    b. VVF.
    c. urethrovaginal fistula.
    d. a and b.
    e. a and c.
21. Ureterovaginal fistulas are:
    a. not associated with transvaginal hysterectomy.
    b. usually associated with normal voiding patterns.
    c. best diagnosed using VCUG.
    d. found more commonly after hysterectomy for malignancy than for benign indications.
    e. usually located in the middle third of the ureter.

22. Two weeks after an emergent cesarean section for fetal distress during labor, a 28-year-old woman reports constant leakage per vagina. Analysis of the collected fluid reveals it to have a high creatinine level consistent with urine. Physical examination including pelvic examination reveals absolutely no abnormalities or surgical trauma to suggest a urinary fistula. There is no stress incontinence elicited on physical examination. Renal ultrasound demonstrates no hydronephrosis, and the bladder is empty. The most likely diagnosis is:
    a. occult VVF.
    b. occult ureterovaginal fistula.
    c. urethrovaginal fistula.
    d. vesicouterine fistula.
    e. peritoneovaginal fistula.
23. Which of the following studies is generally unnecessary in the evaluation of vesicouterine fistula?
    a. Biopsy of the fistula tract
    b. VCUG
    c. CT cystogram
    d. Cystoscopy
    e. Intravenous urogram (IVU)
24. Potential options for therapy for vesicouterine fistula in a patient desiring long-term preservation of fertility include:
    a. observation.
    b. cystoscopy and fulguration of the fistula tract.
    c. hormonal therapy.
    d. surgical exploration and repair of the fistula with interpositional omental flap.
    e. all of the above.
25. Two months after resection of a large urethral diverticulum extending proximally beyond the bladder neck, a patient complains of urinary leakage. All of the following may be the source of this patient's symptoms EXCEPT:
    a. urethrovaginal fistula.
    b. VVF.
    c. stress urinary incontinence.
    d. recurrent urethral diverticulum.
    e. vesicouterine fistula.
26. Urethrovaginal fistulas in the distal one third of the urethra:
    a. are often asymptomatic.
    b. are associated with significant bladder overactivity.
    c. cannot be repaired using a vaginal flap technique.
    d. can result in severe stress incontinence.
    e. are usually the result of malignant infiltration.
27. The most common cause of colovesical fistula is:
    a. colon cancer.
    b. bladder cancer.
    c. prostate cancer.
    d. Crohn's disease.
    e. diverticulitis.
28. CT findings suggestive of a colovesical fistula include:
    a. intravesical mass, air in the bladder, bladder wall thickening.
    b. air in the bladder, bowel wall thickening adjacent to the bladder, clear fluid in a bowel segment adjacent to the bladder.
    c. air in the bladder, bladder wall thickening adjacent to a loop of thickened bowel wall, presence of colonic diverticula.
    d. air in the colon, colonic mass adjacent to the bladder, debris within the bladder.
    e. air in the colon, bladder wall thickening, intravesical mass.
29. In the evaluation of a possible colovesical fistula, cystoscopy:
    a. has high diagnostic accuracy.
    b. has a high yield in identifying potential fistulas.
    c. should not be performed due to the risk of sepsis.
    d. is usually normal.
    e. most commonly reveals a large connection to the bowel.
30. A 62-year-old man presents with pneumaturia and recurrent urinary tract infections. A cystoscopy is performed revealing a bullous lesion on the posterior bladder wall. Two hours later, CT is performed revealing air in the bladder. In this patient, air in the bladder:
    a. suggests colovesical fistula.
    b. may be due to a bacterial infection.
    c. may be due to instrumentation.
    d. is a nonspecific finding.
    e. all of the above.
31. The most common cause of ureterocolic fistula is:
    a. locally extensive colon cancer.
    b. appendicitis with associated abscess.
    c. diverticulitis.
    d. Crohn's disease.
    e. tuberculosis.
32. The incidence of rectal injury during radical retropubic prostatectomy is:
    a. 0.1%.
    b. 1.0%.
    c. 5.0%.
    d. 10%.
    e. 0.001%
33. Rectourethral fistula (RUF) formation after brachytherapy for prostate cancer:
    a. may require complex reconstructive surgery or urinary diversion for repair.
    b. is located at the level of the prostate.
    c. is associated with fecaluria.
    d. may be associated with recurrent malignancy.
    e. all of the above.
34. A 61-year-old otherwise healthy man returns to the office with symptoms of mild stress urinary incontinence and fecaluria 3 weeks after radical retropubic prostatectomy. A VCUG is performed and reveals a 1-mm fistula at the vesicourethral junction. PSA is immeasurable, and the final pathology reveals organ-confined disease. This patient should be counseled that:
    a. a York-Mason transsphincteric approach to this fistula is associated with a high risk of anal incontinence.
    b. a trial of indwelling catheterization may result in resolution of the fistula.
    c. immediate colostomy is indicated.
    d. stress incontinence will become more severe after repair of the fistula.
    e. urinary and fecal diversion will be necessary to repair this fistula.

35. Pyelovascular fistulas:
    a. are usually related to percutaneous procedures in the upper urinary tract.
    b. are most often due to renal malignancy.
    c. should be treated by removal of the nephrostomy tube.
    d. usually occur after radiation therapy.
    e. are uniformly fatal.

36. A 74-year-old woman with a history of colon cancer and external beam radiation therapy develops ureteral obstruction, and a stent is placed. Three months later, she presents with severe anemia and ongoing bright red gross hematuria for several hours. On examination she is pale and tachycardic with a thready pulse and a systolic blood pressure of 60 mm Hg. As resuscitation is initiated with fluids and blood transfusion, the next step in management is:
    a. CT of the abdomen and pelvis.
    b. cystoscopy, removal of the stent, and retrograde pyelography.
    c. immediate laparotomy and possible nephrectomy.
    d. angiography and possible embolization.
    e. tagged red blood cell scan to lateralize the bleeding.

ANSWERS

1. **d. obstructed labor.** In the industrialized world, the most common cause of VVF is surgical trauma during gynecologic surgery, specifically hysterectomy. In the developing world, untreated obstructed labor results in ischemic necrosis of the anterior vaginal wall and underlying lower urinary tract and VVF is the most common fistula in these geographic areas.
2. **a. VVF.** The vast majority of urinary fistulas in both the industrialized and nonindustrialized world involve the bladder and vagina. The other types of the fistulas listed are much less common.
3. **e. ovarian cancer.** Causes of VVF in the industrialized world include surgical trauma during hysterectomy, locally advanced gynecologic malignancy, anterior vaginal wall prolapse and anti-incontinence surgery, and pelvic radiation therapy. Intraoperative recognition and repair of bladder injury during hysterectomy should reduce the probability of VVF formation, but it does not eliminate the possibility.
4. **c. The risk of ureterovaginal fistula is greater than the risk of VVF in this setting.** The most common injury to the urinary tract during hysterectomy is a bladder laceration. Although ureteral injuries are not uncommon, they occur with far less frequency than bladder injuries. Furthermore, ureterovaginal fistulas are much less common than VVFs. The absence of blue-colored fluid in the pelvis does not exclude injury to the urinary tract. For example, a small bladder laceration may not be evident, especially if the bladder is decompressed with a Foley catheter.
5. **a. common in Nigeria.** VVFs in the developing world occur primarily due to obstructed labor. Typically, these occur in individuals who are young primigravidas, with a narrow bony pelvis. These fistulas are usually large, located distally in the vagina, sometimes encompassing large segments of the trigone, posterior bladder wall, and bladder neck, and often part of a larger complex of presenting signs and symptoms termed the *obstructed labor injury complex*, which includes rectovaginal fistula. Due to their size and extensive ischemia of the surrounding tissues, these fistulas are often difficult to repair.
6. **e. positive pressure urethrogram.** This individual does not have diagnosis of VVF and therefore multiple considerations are present. Nevertheless, VVF is a strong possibility given the history of radiation therapy and pelvic malignancy. A VCUG can establish the presence of a fistula. Cystoscopy and biopsy of a fistula (if present) is mandatory to rule out recurrent malignancy. CT of the abdomen and pelvis can evaluate for recurrent malignancy. Urodynamics may be helpful in evaluating for other types of incontinence as well as assessing for bladder compliance and capacity in this individual with a risk for impaired compliance due to radiation therapy.
7. **d. all of the above.** Clear fluid draining from the vagina after surgery should be properly characterized. A urinary fistula is a possible source, but urinary incontinence (e.g., stress, urge, overflow) are strong considerations as well. A peritoneovaginal fistula is a rare complication of hysterectomy in which peritoneal fluid leaks through the vaginal cuff. The fluid may be collected and analyzed for creatinine level. A creatinine level similar to that found in serum excludes urinary fistula as the source of the fluid.
8. **b. 10%.** Ten to 12 percent of individuals with VVF are found to have an associated ureteral injury.
9. **a. The optimal timing for repair of this fistula may be in 5 to 6 months.** This patient has a VVF due to radiation therapy. It is recent in onset, suggesting that the fistula is immature and has a possibility of enlarging because the radiation injury has not yet completely demarcated. The optimal timing for repair of this fistula may be in 5 to 6 months. A reevaluation at that time will be needed to assess whether the VVF is now mature and amenable to repair. Radiation fistulas can be repaired vaginally and adjuvant flaps are utilized to bolster the repair. The success rates for radiation-induced VVF are less than that associated with non–radiation-induced VVF whether they are approached vaginally or abdominally.
10. **c. is suitable for the use of an omental interpositional flap.** The choice of approach for VVF repair is generally individualized based on the patient's anatomy, clinical circumstances, and the experience of the operating surgeon. Success rates are similar between the two approaches in experienced hands. Advantages of the vaginal approach include a shorter hospital stay and less postoperative morbidity as compared with the abdominal approach; however, vaginal shortening may be an issue with some types of vaginal VVF repairs, including the Latzko operation.
11. **b. may be accomplished with a three- or four-layer closure.** Absorbable suture is preferred to avoid complications related to foreign bodies in the urinary tract, including stone formation and infection. Gracilis flaps are rarely necessary because peritoneal flaps or Martius labial fat flaps are much more convenient and local. The vaginal approach is not contraindicated in obstetric fistula nor if the ureter is near the fistula tract.
12. **a. excision of the fistula tract.** Although some authors have suggested that excision of the epithelialized portion of the fistula tract is beneficial, it is not required in all cases.

13. **e. None of the above**. There is no evidence-based medicine to support any of these statements. Although both topical estrogens and intravenous antibiotics are commonly utilized, this is on the basis of expert opinion. There is no preferred method for postoperative bladder drainage after VVF repair, although unobstructed drainage is critical in preventing disruption of the suture line.

14. **e. none of the above**. The transvaginal approach to VVF repair can be utilized in most patients with uncomplicated VVF. There are few absolute contraindications to the vaginal approach. In nulliparous individuals, VVF located at the vaginal cuff in a high narrow vagina can be challenging to repair vaginally owing to anatomic considerations, but this approach is not contraindicated.

15. **a. stress urinary incontinence**. Stress urinary incontinence may coexist with VVF, but it is usually not related to the repair. One exception is the fistula located at the bladder neck or with involvement of the proximal urethra such as obstetric fistulas. These individuals may have new-onset stress incontinence after repair owing to destruction of the sphincter from the original injury.

16. **b. decreased rate of intraoperative ureteral injury**. The transabdominal approach to VVF repair has several distinct advantages as compared with the transvaginal approach. However, there are no studies to suggest that ureteral injury is less common using a transabdominal approach than a transvaginal approach.

17. **c. is nondiagnostic because there are no voiding images or postvoid images.** A postoperative cystogram should include voiding or postvoiding images to ensure that the VVF has been adequately repaired. Voiding may marginally increase the intravesical pressure, thereby providing opacification of some VVF that otherwise would be missed on simple filling cystograms. There is no standard filling volumes for cystography. Generally, 2 or 3 weeks from surgery is an adequate time period for postoperative imaging.

18. **e. all of the above.** The blood supply to the Martius flap is provided from three sources: the internal and external pudendal arteries as well as the obturator artery. Generally, the small branches from the obturator artery supplying the flap from a lateral direction are sacrificed during mobilization. Furthermore, either the anterior (external pudendal) or posterior (internal pudendal) blood supply is divided so as to tunnel and then position the flap over the fistula.

19. **a. may be able to reach the deep pelvis without any mobilization.** Greater omentum has several favorable properties that support its use during transabdominal VVF repair. It is based on the right and left gastroepiploic arteries. Because of its rich blood supply and lymphatic properties it can be a useful adjunctive measure in the setting of infection or inflammation. The blood supply enters the omentum perpendicular to its origin off the greater curvature of the stomach, enabling vertical incisions and mobilization into the deep pelvis. Wide mobilization may be necessary to permit the omentum to reach the deep pelvis in some cases, but in many individuals the flap will reach into the deep pelvis without mobilization and without tension.

20. **a. ureterovaginal fistula.** This patient has at least a ureterovaginal fistula based on the yellow-orange staining at the proximal portion of the gauze pad. This would be consistent with the normal voiding pattern. The distal blue staining would be consistent with stress incontinence as noted by the patient preoperatively. Hysterectomy is not associated with formation of urethrovaginal fistula. VVF is less likely because the staining would tend to be green (combination of blue and yellow) and located in the midportion of the pad. A VCUG would be most helpful in definitively ruling out a VVF.

21. **b. usually associated with normal voiding patterns.** Ureterovaginal fistula involve the distal third of the ureter. They most commonly occur in the setting of hysterectomy: laparoscopic, abdominal, and vaginal hysterectomy may all result in ureterovaginal fistula. Most ureterovaginal fistulas occur after hysterectomy for benign indications. Patients often do not complain of voiding dysfunction as the contralateral upper urinary tract provides filling of the bladder. VCUG is utilized primarily to exclude a concomitant VVF.

22. **d. vesicouterine fistula**. The most common cause of vesicouterine fistula is low segment caesarean section. The normal physical examination suggests a lack of surgical trauma to the vagina, which most likely excludes a vaginal fistula. In the postpartum period, urine from a vesicouterine fistula will leak out of the incompetent cervical os, resulting in constant urinary leakage. A VCUG will confirm the diagnosis.

23. **a. Biopsy of the fistula tract.** Since the vast majority of vesicouterine fistulas are due to benign causes, biopsy of the fistula tract is usually not indicated. The other listed studies may provide useful anatomic information.

24. **e. all of the above.** All of the listed options may preserve long-term fertility in patients with vesicouterine fistula. In those not desiring preservation of fertility, hysterectomy is indicated.

25. **e. vesicouterine fistula.** It is very unlikely that a vesicouterine fistula can result from such a clinical circumstance. Stress incontinence, VVF, urethrovaginal fistula, and a recurrent diverticulum may all result in the described symptoms.

26. **a. are often asymptomatic.** Distal urethrovaginal fistulas are often asymptomatic because they originate beyond the sphincter. Vaginal voiding and pseudoincontinence may be present in some patients. A vaginal flap technique is an effective method of repair.

27. **e. diverticulitis.** Diverticulitis is the most common cause of colovesical fistula in most series. Colon cancer is the second most common cause, followed by Crohn's disease.

28. **c. air in the bladder, bladder wall thickening adjacent to a loop of thickened bowel wall, presence of colonic diverticula.** The classic triad found on CT suggestive of a colovesical fistula includes air in the bladder, bladder wall thickening adjacent to a loop of thickened bowel, and the presence of colonic diverticula.

29. **b. has a high yield in identifying potential fistulas.** The finding of bullous edema during cystoscopy is nonspecific, although, in the appropriate clinical setting, this can be very suggestive of a colovesical fistula. Eighty to 100 percent of cases of colovesical fistulas have an abnormality noted on cystoscopy. Cystoscopy and biopsy are useful to rule out a malignant fistula when this is a consideration.

30. **e. all of the above.** Air can be introduced into the bladder from instrumentation (i.e., cystoscopy or catheterization) or may be present because of infection with a gas-forming organism. Less commonly, air in the bladder results from colovesical fistula.

31. **d. Crohn's disease.** Most ureterocolic fistulas occur on the right side and occur in patients with Crohn's disease. Left-sided fistulas are much less common.

32. **b. 1.0%.** Most large series report a 1.0% to 1.5% incidence of rectal injury during radical retropubic prostatectomy. When recognized and repaired intraoperatively, very few of these injuries result in a rectourethral fistula.

33. **e. all of the above**. RUF commonly presents with fecaluria regardless of the etiology. RUF in the setting of prostatic malignancy should be sampled to evaluate for the possibility of recurrent disease.

34. **b. A trial of indwelling catheterization may result in resolution of the fistula**. This is a small fistula and as such a trial of conservative therapy is warranted. Because this fistula is not associated with signs of local infection or sepsis, immediate colostomy is not indicated. A York-Mason operation is not associated with a high rate of anal incontinence. Furthermore, a single-stage approach may be attempted (without fecal diversion) in this uncomplicated fistula if conservative measures fail. Finally, urinary incontinence may not worsen after surgical repair of the fistula.

35. **a. are usually related to percutaneous procedures in the upper urinary tract**. Pyelovascular fistulas are most often related to interventional procedures in the upper urinary tract, especially percutaneous procedures. Renal neoplasms and radiation therapy are not usually causative of these fistulas. Initial treatment consists of tamponade of the bleeding vessel. If this is unsuccessful, angiographic embolization may be necessary.

36. **d. angiography and possible embolization**. This individual is at high risk for a ureteroarterial fistula at the level of the stent. CT and retrograde pyelography will both most likely be nondiagnostic. Removal of the stent could result in an increase in bleeding and be rapidly fatal. Angiography in the setting of active bleeding will provide both the diagnosis of a ureteroarterial fistula (if present) and a possible therapeutic intervention in the form of embolization. Nephrectomy will not stop the acute hemorrhage. A red blood cell scan will be too time consuming; and although it may lateralize the side of the bleeding, it will delay a potentially lifesaving intervention.

73

Bladder and Urethral Diverticula

ERIC S. ROVNER

QUESTIONS

1. A 68-year-old man presents with hematuria. Cystoscopy reveals a 15-cm bladder diverticulum with a 1-cm papillary lesion at the base of the diverticulum. All of the following are appropriate next steps EXCEPT:
   a. urine cytology.
   b. urine culture.
   c. biopsy of the lesion.
   d. transurethral resection of the prostate (TURP).
   e. intravenous urography.
2. Acquired bladder diverticula can be related to or associated with:
   a. prostatic obstruction.
   b. calyceal diverticula.
   c. nephrogenic adenoma.
   d. perivesical gland infection.
   e. erectile dysfunction.
3. Congenital bladder diverticula are:
   a. most commonly associated with neurogenic voiding dysfunction and cellule formation.
   b. uniformly larger and more numerous than acquired bladder diverticula.
   c. usually located at the dome or anterior wall of the bladder.
   d. resected by a transvesical approach.
   e. associated with a high risk of malignant transformation.
4. The most common malignant tumor found in bladder diverticula is:
   a. adenocarcinoma.
   b. transitional cell carcinoma.
   c. carcinosarcoma.
   d. squamous cell carcinoma.
   e. none of the above.
5. A 65-year-old man with bladder outlet obstruction and a 10-cm bladder diverticulum undergoes uneventful TURP. Postoperatively, the patient's symptoms are improved, and a VCUG demonstrates satisfactory emptying of the bladder and the bladder diverticulum. Appropriate management options would include all of the following EXCEPT:
   a. ongoing surveillance with cystoscopy and urine cytology.
   b. discharge from urologic care.
   c. transvesical bladder diverticulectomy.
   d. extravesical bladder diverticulectomy.
   e. endoscopic incision of the diverticular neck.
6. Ten years after TURP in a symptomatic 71-year-old man with recurrent UTIs, a video-urodynamic study shows a 14-cm poorly emptying bladder diverticulum. The peak subtracted detrusor pressure (Pdet) during micturition is 15 cm H_2O. Which of the following statements is correct?
   a. Another TURP is needed to treat regrowth adenoma and bladder outlet obstruction.
   b. The initiation of clean intermittent self-catheterization (CIC) may improve symptoms.
   c. Bladder diverticulectomy should not be performed in this patient.
   d. A trial of bethanechol is likely to improve bladder contractility and emptying.
   e. This individual has little risk of upper urinary tract deterioration due to low pressure voiding, and therefore upper urinary tract imaging is not indicated.
7. Bladder diverticula may be associated with all of the following EXCEPT:
   a. stress urinary incontinence.
   b. vesicoureteral reflux.
   c. vesical calculi.
   d. Ehlers-Danlos syndrome.
   e. urethral stricture.
8. Endoscopic examination of the lower urinary tract in the setting of bladder diverticula:
   a. is best performed with a resectoscope.
   b. is associated with a high risk of perforation.
   c. includes examination of the entire interior of the diverticulum.
   d. is not indicated if elective submucosal bladder diverticulectomy is planned.
   e. All of the above.
9. Pathologic examination of bladder diverticulectomy specimens:
   a. most commonly reveals atypical cytologic changes.
   b. should always include samples of perivesical adipose tissue.
   c. shows four distinctly organized histologic layers: mucosa, submucosa, lamina propria, and muscularis propria.
   d. may show scattered bundles of smooth muscle.
   e. None of the above.
10. Bladder diverticula:
    a. often do not produce specific symptoms.
    b. can be associated with urinary tract infections.
    c. are commonly diagnosed incidentally during the evaluation of other symptoms or conditions.
    d. may be associated with persistent pyuria.
    e. All of the above.

11. Bladder diverticula associated with bladder outlet obstruction are:
    a. usually found in the absence of cellules and saccules.
    b. associated with a greater than 99% prevalence of ipsilateral vesicoureteral reflux.
    c. not imaged on CT.
    d. associated with medial deviation of pelvic ureter.
    e. never found in the setting of hydronephrosis.
12. Common symptoms associated with urethral diverticula include all of the following EXCEPT:
    a. vaginal pruritus.
    b. dysuria.
    c. dyspareunia.
    d. postvoid dribbling.
    e. urinary frequency.
13. The prevalence of urethral diverticula is estimated to be:
    a. 1% to 5% in the general population.
    b. up to 25% in autopsy studies.
    c. less than 1.5% in selected, highly symptomatic patients.
    d. 25-fold more common in whites than in nonwhites.
    e. None of the above.
14. The evaluation of a patient with a suspected urethral diverticulum may include all of the following EXCEPT:
    a. endoluminal MRI of the urethra.
    b. video-urodynamics.
    c. DMSA renal scan.
    d. transvaginal ultrasound.
    e. voiding cystourethrography.
15. A 1.5-cm anterior vaginal wall mass is noted in a 35-year-old woman approximately 2 cm proximal to the urethral meatus without distorting the meatus. It is nontender and stripping of the mass reveals no discharge per urethra. Urinalysis is unremarkable. This mass may represent all of the following EXCEPT:
    a. Vaginal wall cyst.
    b. Skene's gland abscess.
    c. Urethral diverticulum.
    d. Vaginal leiomyoma.
    e. Gartner's duct cyst.
16. The ostia of a urethral diverticulum is:
    a. most commonly found in the proximal third of the urethra.
    b. most commonly found dorsolaterally.
    c. usually seen on transvaginal ultrasound imaging.
    d. a and b.
    e. None of the above.
17. Two weeks after removal of a large proximal urethral diverticulum, a 48-year-old woman returns to the office with complaints of urine stains on her undergarments. Possible causes include which of the following?
    a. urethrovaginal fistula.
    b. ureterovaginal fistula.
    c. vesicovaginal fistula.
    d. a and c.
    e. All of the above.
18. During performance of a urethral diverticulectomy, the Foley catheter is suddenly noted through a 0.5-cm surgically induced defect in the urethral wall, as the specimen is removed from the operative field. Of the following, the most appropriate next step would be:
    a. mobilization of a Martius flap to buttress the urethral closure.
    b. placement of a midurethral polypropylene sling to prevent postoperative stress incontinence.
    c. primary closure of the urethra with fine absorbable suture.
    d. interposition of a biologically compatible graft such as autologous fascia to close the gap in the urethral wall.
    e. excision and utilization of a portion of the urethral diverticulectomy specimen as a free graft to close the urethra.
19. The most common malignant tumor found in urethral diverticula is:
    a. adenocarcinoma.
    b. transitional cell carcinoma.
    c. carcinosarcoma.
    d. squamous cell carcinoma.
    e. none of the above.
20. Principles of surgical urethral diverticulectomy include all of the following EXCEPT:
    a. preservation or creation of urinary continence.
    b. excision of all identifiable periurethral fascia.
    c. identification of the ostia of the urethral diverticulum.
    d. closure of periurethral fascia after removal of the urethral diverticulum.
    e. watertight closure of the urethra.
21. What is the most likely cause of urethral diverticula?
    a. Congenital lack of fusion of the urethral crest
    b. Infection of vaginal cysts
    c. Traumatic vaginal delivery
    d. Infection of the periurethral glands
    e. Dysfunctional voiding
22. All of the following may be associated with the postoperative course after urethral diverticulectomy surgery EXCEPT:
    a. apical vaginal prolapse.
    b. urethrovaginal fistula.
    c. recurrent urethral diverticula.
    d. UTI.
    e. persistent pelvic pain.

ANSWERS

1. **d. transurethral resection of the prostate (TURP)**. Urine cytology, urine culture, and biopsy are helpful in establishing a diagnosis. Intravenous urography may be helpful in assessing the cause of the hematuria and evaluating the upper urinary tract for hydronephrosis. TURP would not be indicated in this patient until a biopsy is performed, the final pathology on the papillary lesion is known, and a diagnosis of benign prostatic obstruction or other indication for TURP is established.
2. **a. prostatic obstruction**. Acquired bladder diverticula are often associated with bladder outlet obstruction. There is no well-recognized association between bladder diverticula and the other listed entities.
3. **d. resected by a transvesical approach**. When indicated, these lesions can be resected by a simple transvesical approach. The majority of congenital bladder diverticula are not associated with lower urinary tract voiding dysfunction. The pathogenesis of this lesion is believed to be a result of an anatomic weakness at the level of the ureterovesical junction. Congenital bladder diverticula are not associated with neurogenic vesicourethral dysfunction, are usually small and solitary, and are found in smooth-walled bladders without significant cellule formation.
4. **b. transitional cell carcinoma**. The most common malignant tumor found in bladder diverticula is transitional cell carcinoma in over 70% of cases. The remaining histologic types are much less common.
5. **b. discharge from urologic care**. Both ongoing surveillance and operative intervention are possible treatment options in this individual. Because the diverticulum empties satisfactorily and the patient has had significant improvement in symptomatology, ongoing surveillance is an option for the patient who elects nonoperative therapy. However, the potential risk of malignant transformation remains and, therefore, discharge from urologic care would not be appropriate.
6. **b. The initiation of clean intermittent self-catheterization (CIC) may improve symptoms.** CIC will likely result in complete emptying of the lower urinary tract and reduce both the patient's symptoms and his propensity for UTIs. The diagnosis of recurrent obstruction has not been established in this patient with relatively poor contractility and therefore TURP may not be indicated. Bladder diverticulectomy may be helpful in restoring satisfactory bladder emptying in this individual even though bladder contractility is suboptimal. The apparent poor contractility may be due to a venting of intravesical pressure into the bladder diverticulum with micturition. Bethanechol is unlikely to significantly improve emptying of the bladder diverticulum. Hydronephrosis in the setting of the bladder diverticula may be due to ureteral obstruction, perivesical inflammation, and vesicoureteral reflux among other possibilities. Therefore, upper tract imaging is indicated in this patient.
7. **a. stress urinary incontinence**. Bladder diverticula are not associated with stress urinary incontinence. The remaining choices may be associated with bladder diverticula.
8. **c. includes examination of the entire interior of the diverticulum.** Endoscopic examination should include visualization of the entire surface of the diverticulum. If this is not possible with rigid instrumentation, then a flexible cystoscope can be utilized. Biopsy of the interior of a bladder diverticulum is associated with an increased risk of perforation due to the relatively thin wall, but simple endoscopic examination is not necessarily associated with an increased risk of perforation.
9. **d. may show scattered bundles of smooth muscle**. The adventitial layer of an excised bladder diverticulum may show scattered disorganized bundles of smooth muscle. Although atypia may be present, it is rare. In a true bladder diverticulum, there is usually a lack of the muscularis propria layer. Perivesical adipose tissue may or may not be present in the final pathologic specimen depending on the type of bladder diverticulectomy performed.
10. **e. All of the above.**
11. **d. associated with medial deviation of pelvic ureter.** Cellules and saccules are commonly found in patients with long-standing bladder outlet obstruction and are considered by some authors to be on a continuum with bladder diverticula. Although ipsilateral reflux may be present in patients with bladder diverticula, this is not a common finding. CT is an excellent modality for visualization and characterization of bladder diverticula, especially those with a narrow or obstructed neck. Medial deviation of the ureter is more common than lateral deviation of the ureter in the setting of bladder diverticula.
12. **a. vaginal pruritus.** Urethral diverticula may present with a variety of symptoms, but vaginal pruritus is not commonly reported in the setting of urethral diverticula.
13. **a. 1% to 5% in the general population.** Although it is difficult to accurately quantitate the prevalence of urethral diverticula due to several factors, it is generally estimated at between 1% and 5% of the general population. The reported prevalence in autopsy studies is much lower than 25%, and the reported prevalence in highly symptomatic patients is much higher than 1.5%. Historically, the prevalence of urethral diverticula in African Americans has been reportedly higher than that in whites, but this may be inaccurate owing to reporting bias at urban academic medical centers.
14. **c. DMSA renal scan.** Radiographic imaging of the urethra in the setting of a suspected urethral diverticulum can be helpful in confirming the diagnosis as well as providing information regarding relevant anatomy. The ultimate choice of imaging depends on many factors, including availability, cost, and expertise. DMSA renal scan is not indicated in the evaluation of suspected urethral diverticula.
15. **b. Skene's gland abscess.** It is unlikely that this mass represents Skene's gland abscess because it is nontender and is not located distally in the region of the urethral meatus. The remaining choices are all possible. Urethral diverticulum do not uniformly result in a discharge per urethra upon stripping of the anterior vaginal wall and may not be tender in some patients.
16. **e. None of the above.** The ostia or neck of a urethral diverticulum is usually found posterolaterally in the middle third of the urethra. The ostia is often very difficult to visualize on any type of imaging, including ultrasound.
17. **e. All of the above.** Proximal urethral diverticula may extend beneath the bladder neck and trigone of the bladder. Therefore, surgical excision of these lesions can risk injury to not only the urethra but also the bladder and distal ureter. Fortunately, these occurrences are quite rare.
18. **c. primary closure of the urethra with fine absorbable suture.** The Foley catheter is almost always seen during excision of a urethral diverticulum especially as the ostia is identified. The urethral defect can be closed primarily over as small as a 14-French Foley catheter. The other choices are either not indicated or unnecessary in the setting of an uncomplicated urethral diverticulectomy.

19. **a. adenocarcinoma.** As opposed to bladder diverticula, the most common tumor found in association with urethral diverticula is adenocarcinoma. Transitional cell carcinoma and squamous cell carcinoma are less common.

20. **b. excision of all identifiable periurethral fascia.** The periurethral fascia should be preserved during dissection of the urethral diverticulum. This tissue is utilized to buttress the urethral closure and close dead space remaining from urethral diverticulectomy.

21. **d. Infection of the periurethral glands.** The most likely etiology of urethral diverticula in the female is infection of the periurethral glands.

22. **a. apical vaginal prolapse.** Apical vaginal prolapse is not associated with urethral diverticulectomy. Persistent pelvic pain and/or UTI may occur despite a technically successful operation, but a recurrent UD should be considered in the setting of these symptoms. Urethrovaginal fistula is a potential complication of urethral diverticulectomy.

74

Surgical Treatment of Male Sphincteric Urinary Incontinence: The Male Perineal Sling and Artificial Urinary Sphincter

DAVID R. STASKIN • CRAIG V. COMITER

QUESTIONS

1. All of the following are contraindications to sling surgery EXCEPT:
   a. low volume detrusor overactivity.
   b. detrusor underactivity.
   c. diminished vesical compliance.
   d. metastatic disease.
   e. vesicourethral anastomotic stricture.
2. Which of the following sling materials is associated with the highest success rates?
   a. Silicone-coated polyester
   b. Autologous rectus fascia
   c. Porcine dermis
   d. Human dermis allograft
   e. Human fascia allograft
3. Dry/improved rates for male perineal sling surgery are approximately:
   a. 80%.
   b. 40%.
   c. 50%.
   d. 20%.
   e. 10%.
4. Which of the following is associated with a diminished success rate for the male perineal sling?
   a. Prior collagen injection
   b. Prior adjuvant radiation therapy
   c. Prior transurethral resection of the prostate
   d. Prior artificial sphincter placement
   e. Concomitant penile prosthesis surgery
5. The principle of delayed activation in artificial urinary sphincter (AUS) implantation refers to:
   a. 6- to 8-week postoperative deactivation to decrease cuff compression.
   b. time before the cuff closes after voiding.
   c. time between squeezing pump and the cuff opening.
   d. pressure transmission from pump to cuff during a cough.
   e. pressure transmission from cuff to reservoir during a cough.
6. Which is NOT a cause of urinary retention with the AUS in the immediate postoperative period?
   a. Edema
   b. Untreated urethral stricture
   c. Failure to deactivate sphincter
   d. Underactive bladder
   e. Reservoir leakage
7. Which of the following is an advantage of the penoscrotal versus perineal implantation technique?
   a. Patient is hyperflexed in the lithotomy position.
   b. Penile urethra is not stretched permitting easier dissection.
   c. It requires two incisions.
   d. Reservoir technique requires retropubic dissection.
   e. Pump can be placed on either side of scrotum.
8. Cuff erosion can be decreased by:
   a. utilizing a higher pressure reservoir.
   b. transcorporeal implanting of cuff post irradiation or trauma.
   c. leaving a large French gauge urethral catheter for drainage.
   d. immediate activating of device.
   e. placing cuff over area of inadvertent urethral entry.
9. A 12-year-old boy with myelodysplasia underwent implantation of an AUS 3 years ago. He now has recurrent incontinence. What is the next step?
   a. Physical examination to determine if pump is palpable and full
   b. Cystometry to determine function of bladder
   c. Retrograde sphincterometry to assess leak pressure of cuff
   d. Cystoscopy to rule out cuff erosion
   e. a and d only
   f. a, b, c, and d

10. A female patient has an AUS placed via the transvaginal route and after operation has continuous leakage after activation. Which is NOT a likely cause?
    a. Urinary retention
    b. Inadvertent cuff deactivation
    c. Vesicovaginal fistula
    d. Severe detrusor overactivity
    e. Grade II-III reflux

11. A patient with a functioning AUS is to undergo inflatable penile prosthesis (IPP) implantation 3 years after sphincter implantation. The proper course of action would be to:
    a. remove and replace all AUS components at time of IPP implantation.
    b. remove and then reinsert AUS cuff at time of IPP implantation in a patient with a previously placed transcorporal cuff.
    c. place IPP pump and reservoir on the same side as the AUS components and place both pumps on the side of the dominant hand.
    d. undersize the IPP to avoid the AUS cuff.
    e. replace AUS reservoir and utilize same reservoir with Y-connector for AUS and IPP.

ANSWERS

1. **d. metastatic disease**. Contraindications to surgery are similar for the male perineal sling and the artificial urinary sphincter and include those disorders that may jeopardize the upper urinary tract, such as diminished vesical compliance, as well as those abnormalities that may require future transurethral management such as anastomotic stricture or recurrent bladder tumors. In patients with untreated low-volume detrusor overactivity, symptomatic improvement may be inadequate. The perineal sling relies on a fixed resistance, unlike the artificial sphincter, which is "opened" for micturition. Therefore, detrusor underactivity is a relative contraindication for sling surgery.
2. **a. Silicone-coated polyester**. The male perineal sling relies on a constant and fixed tension, unlike the female suburethral sling, which generally prevents descent of the bladder outlet. In the male, where hypermobility is less of an issue but sphincteric incompetence is more of an issue, a permanent sling material is necessary. Synthetic slings are more successful than organic slings, which degrade over time.
3. **a. 80%**. While the definition of success may vary, the male perineal sling has proven successful in the intermediate term, as documented by several series by several different investigators. The vast majority (80%) of patients are either improved or cured of their stress incontinence postoperatively.
4. **d. Prior artificial sphincter placement**. The urethral fibrosis and diminished urethral compliance that results from prior AUS placement and explantation may prevent adequate urethral compression by the male perineal sling, which does not provide circumferential compression. Previous collagen injection, adjuvant radiation, concomitant placement of a penile prosthesis, and prior transurethral resection of the prostate do not diminish the efficacy of the sling.
5. **a. 6- to 8-week postoperative deactivation to decrease cuff compression**. The AUS is deactivated by emptying the cuff and preventing the refilling of the cuff for a period of 6 to 8 weeks after implantation. The technique of cuff "delayed activation" is performed by squeezing the pump and compressing the "deactivation button" on the pump. The pump should be palpated several minutes after "deactivation"—and should not refill—and the cuff can be visualized as empty. The AUS is activated by a forceful squeeze of the pump, which will allow fluid to flow though the system to fill the cuff. The cuff refills from the pressure of the reservoir flowing through the pump resistor until the system equilibrates, approximately 2 to 3 minutes, the cuff deflates immediately with squeezing of the pump, there is no transmission of pressure from the pump to the cuff because the pump is not intra-abdominal and there is a retrograde check valve, and there is no transmission of pressure from the reservoir to the cuff during a cough because the resistor in the pump prevents acute pressure communication.
6. **e. Reservoir leakage**. A leak in the reservoir would empty the system and the cuff would deflate without any filling pressure. The rest of the choices may contribute to decreased bladder emptying. The most common is edema of the urethra, which may be treated with a small-caliber urethral catheter. Placement of a suprapubic tube should weigh the risk and benefits of reservoir trauma and/or infection of components placed in the retropubic space.
7. **b. penile urethra is not stretched permitting easier dissection**. The penoscrotal approach does not require placement of the patient's legs in the lithotomy position and avoids "stretching" of the bulbar urethra. Advocates of this approach report a more facile dissection of the urethra from the corpora by avoiding the lithotomy position. In the penoscrotal approach the reservoir is placed through the inguinal ring. Both the penoscrotal and perineal approaches allow pump placement that favors utilization side of the dominant hand.
8. **b. transcorporeal implanting of cuff post irradiation or trauma**. Transcorporeal cuff placement avoids the dissection of the urethra from the corpora and thus provides an advantage in cases with fibrosis from prior erosion or radiation. The other choices are associated with an increase in risk for erosion, especially placement of the cuff over an area of intraoperative urethral trauma.
9. **f. a, b, c, and d.** A physical examination should be performed to determine if the pump is palpable and full—the soft portion of the pump should be firm and should refill within 2 minutes after compression if there is not a significant fluid leak. A small amount of fluid loss may not be detectable. A cystometry is recommended to determine that the bladder has remained a low-pressure reservoir without detrusor overactivity. Retrograde sphincterometry is done to assess the leak pressure of the cuff—the pressure required for retrograde flow should be the same pressure that is within the reservoir if the patient's own sphincter is relaxed. A cystoscopy is recommended to rule out cuff erosion. A plain film to determine contrast loss or an ultrasound to determine reservoir decompression may also be useful to estimate fluid loss from the system.
10. **e. grade II-III reflux**. Grade II-III reflux would not affect the patient's continence but may be a relative contraindication to sphincter implantation. The patient may be incontinent from urinary retention (overflow), inadvertent cuff deactivation (technical), a vesicovaginal fistula (trauma during surgery),

or severe detrusor overactivity (preoperative cystometry with bladder neck occlusion if necessary to prevent leakage around catheter).

11. **b. remove and then reinsert AUS cuff at time of IPP implantation with prior transcorporeal cuff.** Remove and then reinsert AUS cuff at time of IPP implantation if a transcorporeal cuff was implanted. The cuff should be removed during the time of corporeal dilation and reinserted before the gentle placement of the rear tip extenders or prosthesis (preferably by a scrotal approach). Placement of the IPP pump and reservoir on different sides is recommended.

    It would not be recommended to undersize the IPP to avoid the AUS cuff. The reservoir for the IPP is a "volume reservoir" and not a "pressure reservoir" and would not work—resulting in sphincter malfunction!

SECTION XV

BLADDER; LOWER GENITOURINARY CALCULI AND TRAUMA

75

Urothelial Tumors of the Bladder

EDWARD M. MESSING

QUESTIONS

1. Members of which of the following American demographic groups are most likely to die of bladder cancer if they contract it?
   a. White women
   b. White men
   c. African American women
   d. African American men
   e. Latina women
2. Underreporting of bladder cancer is NOT likely to explain the differences in this disease's incidence in various demographic groups in the United States for which of the following reasons?
   a. The national Surveillance, Epidemiology, and End Result database keeps very accurate statistics.
   b. There are relatively similar incidences in all geographic regions.
   c. Bladder cancer is rarely found incidentally.
   d. The disease is rare in the elderly, in whom other illnesses prove fatal before bladder cancer is diagnosed.
   e. There are many noninvasive ways to achieve an accurate diagnosis.
3. *TP53* abnormalities in bladder cancer are frequently associated with:
   a. hypermethylation of the *TP53* gene's promoter.
   b. nuclear overexpression of the TP53 protein.
   c. loss of heterozygosity of chromosome 9q.
   d. low-grade papillary superficial tumors.
   e. primarily those cancers not related to cigarette smoking.
4. Progress in identifying the early genetic abnormalities of low-grade papillary superficial bladder cancer has been hindered by which of the following?
   a. The predominance of *TP53* abnormalities in these tumors
   b. Genomic instability associated with these tumors
   c. The molecular fingerprint of smoking-related mutations
   d. The frequent loss of all of chromosome 9
   e. The slow rate of growth of these tumors in situ
5. The product of the retinoblastoma gene *(RB)* effect on the cell cycle:
   a. is associated with trisomy of chromosome 7.
   b. is mediated through *BCL2.*
   c. is controlled by *CDKN2A.*
   d. is unaltered by its phosphorylation status.
   e. acts primarily on the $G_2 \rightarrow$ M transition.
6. In former cigarette smokers, a significant decline in the risk of developing bladder cancer does not occur until smoking has been discontinued for how long?
   a. 1 year
   b. 2 to 4 years
   c. 5 to 9 years
   d. 10 to 20 years
   e. 21 to 30 years
7. Which of the following statements is TRUE of urothelial (transitional cell) cancers associated with cigarette smoking and/or industrial carcinogen exposures?
   a. They tend to be far more aggressive than those arising in patients without these exposures.
   b. They are more indolent than are those arising in patients without these exposures.
   c. They are about as likely to be as aggressive and indolent as those arising in patients without these exposures.
   d. They are less often associated with abnormalities in the *TP53* gene than are cancers arising in patients without these exposures.
   e. They are likely to be caused by the same chemical carcinogen, acrolein.

8. Which of the following is a recently documented urothelial mutagen associated with ingestion of herbal preparations used for weight reduction?
   a. 4-Aminobiphenyl
   b. Arsenic
   c. Phenacetin
   d. Aristolochic acid
   e. Acrolein
9. Which of the following is the strongest argument against there being a directly inherited form of most cases of bladder cancer?
   a. Polymorphisms in enzymes involved in mutagen activation and detoxification seem not to be important in bladder cancer development.
   b. More distant relatives have a higher likelihood of contracting bladder cancer than closer relatives.
   c. Familial clusters of bladder cancer have not been reported.
   d. Blackfoot disease-related bladder cancer has a very large male predominance.
   e. Chinese weight-reducing herb-associated urothelial cancer occurs almost exclusively in females.
10. Which of the following is a normal anatomic structure that confounds the accurate staging of bladder cancer on transurethral resection specimens?
   a. Glycosaminoglycan layer
   b. Basal lamina
   c. Lamina propria
   d. Muscularis mucosae
   e. Muscularis propria
11. What is the nonmalignant lesion associated with prior, concurrent, or subsequent bladder cancer?
   a. Overactive atypia
   b. Inverted papilloma
   c. Malacoplakia
   d. Nephrogenic adenoma
   e. Cystitis cystica
12. Abnormalities of which of the following genes or gene products often occur in carcinoma in situ?
   a. *ERBB2*
   b. RB
   c. DBCCR1
   d. *TP53*
   e. *RAS-CDKN1A*
13. Low-grade urothelial cancer in the 1998 World Health Organization (WHO) and the International Society of Urological Pathology (ISUP) classification is the same lesion as which of the following?
   a. Papillary urothelial tumor of low malignant potential
   b. Urothelial papilloma
   c. Grade 1 transitional cell carcinoma
   d. Grade 2 transitional cell carcinoma
   e. Grade 3 transitional cell carcinoma
14. Which of the following statements is TRUE regarding bilharzial squamous cell carcinoma of the bladder?
   a. It generally occurs in individuals who are older than those in whom nonbilharzial squamous cell carcinoma of the bladder occurs.
   b. It occurs more commonly in females than does nonbilharzial squamous cell carcinoma of the bladder.
   c. It less frequently has distant metastases than does nonbilharzial squamous cell carcinoma of the bladder.
   d. It is more responsive to systemic chemotherapy than is nonbilharzial squamous cell carcinoma of the bladder.
   e. It is a common sequela of infections with all species of schistosomes that are pathogenic in humans.
15. Genetic aberrations frequently occur in which of the following pairs of genes in both squamous cell and transitional cell carcinomas of the bladder?
   a. *RB* and *BCL2*
   b. *TP53* and *CDKN2A*
   c. *HRAS* and *CDKN1B*
   d. *RB* and *ERBB2*
   e. *DBCCR1* and *TP53*
16. Which of the following statements is TRUE regarding urachal carcinoma?
   a. It is usually transitional cell carcinoma.
   b. If nonmetastatic, it is best treated by partial cystectomy.
   c. It responds well to radiation therapy.
   d. It is usually adenocarcinoma.
   e. It is usually squamous cell carcinoma.
17. The existence of both clonal and multiclonal origins of urothelial cancer's occurrences and recurrences is supported by:
   a. molecular fingerprinting of tumors and remote urothelium.
   b. development of late recurrences after tumor-free intervals of more than 5 years.
   c. success of immediate postresection intravesical therapy.
   d. relative consistency between phenotypes of recurrent and initial tumors.
   e. success of intravesical bacille Calmette-Guérin started several weeks after transurethral resection.
18. Which biologic process does not enable cancer cells to invade and metastasize?
   a. Proliferation
   b. Motility
   c. Expression of proteolytic enzymes
   d. Apoptosis
   e. Neoangiogenesis
19. The normal expression of which intracellular adhesion molecule provides a barrier to invasion?
   a. Urokinase plasminogen activator
   b. Autocrine motility factor receptor
   c. Vascular endothelial growth factor
   d. E-cadherin
   e. Matrix metalloproteinase-2 (MMP-2)
20. Which of the following statements is TRUE regarding bladder cancer metastases? They:
   a. rarely develop before muscularis propria invasion occurs.
   b. involve primarily perivesical nodes.
   c. involve the liver more commonly than pelvic nodes.
   d. almost never appear in bone.
   e. frequently result from transurethral resection.
21. What proportion of newly diagnosed urothelial cancers are high-grade tumors?
   a. Less than 20%
   b. 21% to 29%
   c. 30% to 39%
   d. 40% to 49%
   e. 50% to 59%
22. Nuclear expression of *TP53* detected immunohistochemically:
   a. is a poor surrogate for abnormalities of the *TP53* gene.
   b. cannot be seen unless both alleles of *TP53* are deleted or mutated.
   c. predicts a poor response to systemic therapy with cisplatin-containing regimens.
   d. is commonly found in low-grade urothelial tumors in young adults.
   e. is not detected in formalin-fixed, paraffin-embedded specimens.

23. Increased expression of which of the following markers is not associated with a worse prognosis?

a. Endothelial growth factor receptor
b. *TP53*
c. RB
d. E-cadherin
e. MMP-2

24. Aberrations of which chromosome or chromosome segment are associated most closely with papillary low-grade, superficial urothelial tumors?

a. 17p
b. 13q
c. 9q
d. 9p
e. 7

25. Which of the following statements is TRUE of hematuria caused by bladder cancer? It:

a. is usually accompanied by discomfort and painful voiding.
b. is intermittent.
c. occurs in a minority of patients with bladder cancer.
d. commonly causes anemia.
e. occurs primarily only in the initial phase of the urinary stream when grossly visible.

26. A patient with hematuria undergoes cystoscopy, and a lesion with the typical appearance of a low-grade, superficial papillary urothelial tumor is identified. What is the chief benefit of sending a urinary or bladder wash specimen for cytologic examination? To:

a. confirm the cystoscopic impression
b. determine whether upper urinary tract imaging is needed
c. identify as yet invisible high-grade cancer
d. decide whether cystoscopic resection or biopsy is needed
e. serve as a baseline for follow-up

27. The rarity of finding urothelial cancer incidentally at autopsy indicates what?

a. That bladder cancer screening is likely to detect tumors that normally would have gone unrecognized throughout the lifetime of patients
b. That underdiagnosis is contributing to differences in the reported incidences of bladder cancer among people of different sexes, races, and ages
c. That there is a very brief presymptomatic period in which tumors are diagnosed before they cause symptoms
d. That bladder cancer screening could safely be performed once every 3 to 5 years
e. That high-grade cancers grow much more rapidly than low-grade ones

28. It is important for a bladder cancer screening instrument to be able to detect low-grade urothelial cancers with as great a sensitivity as for high-grade cancers because:

a. both of these tumors have similar likelihoods of causing morbidity.
b. low-grade cancers often become high-grade ones if their diagnosis is delayed.
c. effectiveness of a screening program depends on diagnosing more cancers in a screened than in an unscreened population.
d. confidence in the screening program will be seriously undermined if any bladder cancers are undiagnosed.
e. low-grade cancers are more readily controlled by endoscopic means than are high-grade ones.

29. Of the following, which is the diagnostic test most likely not to detect low-grade cancers?

a. Multiple Hemastix strips
b. Telomerase activity in urine
c. Lewis immunocytology
d. Bladder tumor antigen (BTA) stat
e. Immunocytology

30. Determining the specificity of all bladder cancer diagnostic tests is complicated by which of the following factors?

a. Inability to detect very small tumors
b. Detection of cancer not yet cystoscopically visible
c. Inability to detect low-grade tumors
d. Controversy about criteria for papillary urothelial tumors of low malignant potential
e. Positive results caused by inflammation

31. In individuals exposed to known bladder carcinogens, a positive "marker" test:

a. is usually less sensitive than in sporadic bladder cancer.
b. may detect molecular alterations induced by the carcinogen that are not necessarily associated with malignant transformation.
c. must be evaluated more thoroughly than nonexposed individuals.
d. has been shown to effectively reduce bladder cancer mortality in exposed individuals.
e. is not related to cumulative carcinogen exposure.

32. What is a major benefit of fluorescent cystoscopy after intravesical instillation of 5-aminolevulinic acid (ALA)? It:

a. is used to treat tumors with photodynamic therapy.
b. permits resection of endoscopically invisible tumors.
c. enables treatment of tumors with the use of local anesthesia.
d. shortens the time of transurethral resection.
e. does not require special instrumentation.

33. Which of the following statements is TRUE regarding transurethral biopsy of normal-appearing bladder urothelium? It:

a. is of value when there are multifocal low-grade superficial bladder tumors and negative urinary cytologic results.
b. is of value when there is multifocal high-grade superficial urothelial cancer.
c. helps management of multifocal invasive bladder cancer.
d. is very important preceding planned partial cystectomy.
e. is not helpful when there are positive cytologic results and low-grade papillary cancer.

34. For prognosis and planned therapy, what is the most important distinction between levels of invasiveness of a urothelial tumor? Between:

a. epithelium and lamina propria
b. superficial and deep lamina propria
c. lamina propria and muscularis propria
d. superficial and deep muscularis propria
e. muscularis propria and perivesical fat

35. Tests needed to appropriately stage and evaluate muscle-invading urothelial cancer include all of the following EXCEPT which one?

a. CT of the abdomen and pelvis
b. Chest radiograph
c. Nuclear bone scan
d. Chest CT
e. Serum creatinine assay

36. Invasion of bladder cancer into deep detrusor muscle is which of the following T stages in the 1997 American Joint Committee on Cancer Staging-International Union Against Cancer (AJC-UICC) system?
    a. T1
    b. T2a
    c. T2b
    d. T3a
    e. T3b

37. Strategies and nonprescription agents for which there are substantial data indicating efficacy in preventing urothelial cancer include which of the following?
    a. Vitamin D supplements
    b. Selenium dietary supplements
    c. Switching from unfiltered to filtered cigarettes
    d. High consumption of fluids
    e. High-fiber diet

38. Of the following uncommon bladder malignancies, which one has the most aggressive behavior and most ominous prognosis?
    a. Nonurachal adenocarcinoma
    b. Carcinosarcoma
    c. Primary bladder lymphoma
    d. Leiomyosarcoma
    e. Embryonal rhabdomyosarcoma

ANSWERS

1. **c. African American women.** There is some evidence that this increased risk in whites is primarily limited to noninvasive cancers, which implies a later diagnosis of tumors in African Americans. However, recent genetic and epidemiologic evidence indicates that African Americans may have a more aggressive form of other malignancies. Men have higher 5-year survival rates than women, with this difference in mortality being particularly impressive in African American women (5-year survival rates: white men, 84%; black men, 71%; white women, 76%; black women, 51%).

2. **c. Bladder cancer is rarely found incidentally.** Because it "always" causes symptoms or signs, bladder cancer is almost always diagnosed before patients die. Thus, it almost never goes undiagnosed as other malignancies often do.

3. **b. nuclear overexpression of the TP53 protein.** The TP53 protein exists in a multimeric form, and abnormal chains (from a mutated allele) lead to a nonfunctional protein but one that is not degraded as rapidly as is wild-type TP53. Thus, the altered form collects in the nucleus and is readily detectable by immunohistochemistry. In addition, because the wild-type TP53 protein functions as a tetramer, the altered product of a mutant allele stabilizes (permitting nuclear accumulation) but inactivates the tetrameric protein (resulting in tumorigenesis), even when the nonmutated allele is expressed normally. This dominant negative effect offers a theoretical hurdle to genetic therapeutic strategies that attempt to insert a wild-type *TP53* gene into tumors with mutated *TP53* alleles.

4. **d. The frequent loss of all of chromosome 9.** An entire copy of chromosome 9 is frequently lost, making molecular analysis of specific deleted genes on this chromosome very difficult.

5. **c. is controlled by p16.** Unphosphorylated RB binds to and inactivates the transcription factor E2F. When RB is phosphorylated, E2F is released to induce expression of genes needed for mitogenesis. CDKN2A inhibits the cyclin-dependent kinases, which phosphorylate RB.

6. **d. 10 to 20 years.** That the reduction of risk takes far longer for bladder cancer than for lung or esophageal cancer indicates that bladder cancer carcinogens in cigarette smokers are usually activated and detoxified via different mechanisms than those in patients with other cancers, in whom the carcinogen reaches the target directly, without metabolism.

7. **c. They are about as likely to be as aggressive and indolent as those arising in patients without these exposures.** However, when *TP53* mutations in bladder tumors of smokers were compared with those in bladder cancers of patients who never smoked, differences in the types or sites of mutations were not seen, although a higher number of mutations occurred in smokers. This suggests that smoking might increase the number of mutations in urothelial cells without necessarily directing the site or type of mutation that occurs. This type of analysis correlates closely with the elegant case control study of Hayes and coworkers, who found that although exposure to industrial carcinogens and smoking clearly correlated with an increased risk for developing bladder cancer, with the exception of young patients, these exposures did not correlate with any particular bladder cancer phenotype. Thus, assuming that low-grade superficial and high-grade rapidly invasive transitional cell carcinomas have different fundamental "genetic pathways," the two best described environmental carcinogenic exposures for bladder cancer predispose for developing each of these genetic alterations in similar proportions to those seen in the nonexposed population.

8. **d. Aristolochic acid.** A Chinese herb (containing *Stephania tetrandra* and *Magnolia officinalis*) that was imported into Belgium as a popular weight reduction aid used primarily by women became responsible for an epidemic of interstitial nephropathy, presumably because of contamination with *Aristolochia fangchi*, which had been substituted for *S. tetrandra.* Subsequently, patients with Chinese herb nephropathy have been reported to be at much higher risk for developing transitional cell carcinoma, primarily of the upper urinary tract but also in the bladder. A major mechanism in transitional cell cancer appears to be the development of aristolochic acid–related DNA adducts in the urothelium of both the upper urinary tract and bladder.

9. **b. More distant relatives have a higher likelihood of contracting bladder cancer than closer relatives.** Perhaps the most compelling evidence in this regard comes from the work of Kiemeney and coworkers, who studied the records of more than 12,000 relatives of 190 patients diagnosed with transitional cell cancer in Iceland between 1983 and 1992 and found that although the risk of developing transitional cell carcinoma was slightly elevated in relatives (observed-to-expected odds ratio 1.24, 95% confidence interval 0.90 to 1.67), this ratio was greater

among second- and third-degree than among first-degree relatives. This result argues strongly against a straightforward genetic mechanism being responsible.

10. **d. Muscularis mucosae.** Part of the reason for discrepancies in the interpretation of histologic sections among different pathologists assessing tumor grade and depth of infiltration is related to the smooth muscle fibers of the tunica muscularis mucosae in the lamina propria of the bladder wall, which may be confused with detrusor muscle.

11. **b. Inverted papilloma.** Rare cases of malignant transformation of inverted papillomas have been reported. However, there is a more common association of inverted papilloma occurring in patients with coexistent transitional cell carcinoma elsewhere in the bladder or with histories of such tumors.

12. **d. *TP53*.** *TP53* abnormalities occur in more than half of high-grade urothelial cancers. Its aberration in carcinoma in situ indicates that this is a precursor lesion for high-grade, but not low-grade, urothelial cancer.

13. **d. Grade 2 transitional cell carcinoma.** Moderately differentiated (grade 2) tumors (see Fig. 76-5) have a wider fibrovascular core, a greater disturbance of the base-to-surface cellular maturation, and a loss of cell polarity, compared with well-differentiated tumors. The nuclear/cytoplasmic ratio is higher, with more nuclear pleomorphism and prominent nucleoli. Mitotic figures are more frequent. These have been termed *low-grade urothelial carcinoma* in the WHO/ISUP classification.

14. **c. It less frequently has distant metastases than does nonbilharzial squamous cell carcinoma of the bladder.** These cancers occur in patients who are, on the average, 10 to 20 years younger than patients with transitional cell carcinoma. Bilharzial cancers are exophytic, nodular, fungating lesions that are usually well differentiated and have a relatively low incidence of lymph node and distant metastases. Whether the low incidence of distant metastases is due to capillary and lymphatic fibrosis resulting from chronic schistosomal infection or the relatively low histologic grade of these tumors is not clear. Nonbilharzial squamous cell cancers are usually caused by chronic irritation from urinary calculi, long-term indwelling catheters, chronic urinary infections, or bladder diverticula.

15. **b. *TP53* and *CDKN2A*.** As with aggressive urothelial (transitional cell) cancer, squamous cell cancers often have *CDKN2A* and *TP53* abnormalities, although the mechanisms of gene silencing often differ between the two tumor types.

16. **d. It is usually adenocarcinoma.** Urachal carcinomas are extremely rare tumors that arise outside the bladder and are usually adenocarcinomas, although they may be primary transitional cell or squamous cell carcinomas and, rarely, even sarcomas. They are rarely responsive to radiation therapy, and, because of their infiltrative nature under the epithelium, they often have extensions that are overlooked so that partial cystectomy is unsuccessful.

17. **a. molecular fingerprinting of tumors and remote urothelium.** The other answers primarily support either clonal (c and d) or multiclonal (b) theories or are unrelated to clonality (e).

18. **d. Apoptosis.** Apoptosis, programmed cell death in a cancer cell, impedes metastases.

19. **d. E-cadherin.** Major intracellular adhesion molecules, such as E-cadherin and the transmembrane protein family of integrins, also appear to be important barriers against invasion that can become disrupted in invasive tumors.

20. **a. They rarely develop before muscularis propria invasion occurs.** It is very unusual for patients to have metastases without concomitant or prior muscularis propria–invading cancer.

21. **d. 40% to 49%.** Forty to 45 percent of newly diagnosed bladder cancers are high-grade lesions, more than half of which are muscle invading or more extensive at the time of diagnosis.

22. **d. is commonly found in low-grade urothelial tumors in young adults.** Peculiarly, the majority of patients younger than 30 years of age with bladder cancer, despite almost all having low-grade superficial papillary cancers, have nuclear overexpression of *TP53* (which in older individuals is almost always overexpressed in only high-grade cancers).

23. **d. E-cadherin.** E-cadherin, an extracellular matrix protein connecting the environment to the cytoskeleton, is deleted or deficient in cancers likely to invade and metastasize. The other markers are all overexpressed in high-grade cancers.

24. **c. 9q.** Several loci on 9q, particularly in 9q32-34, which includes *DBCCR1*, have been best described with low-grade, superficial tumors. The other aberrations are all associated with high-grade disease.

25. **b. It is intermittent.** Often only one in three to five voidings in patients with active bladder cancer have any hematuria.

26. **c. To identify as yet invisible high-grade cancer.** High-grade cancer cells in a cytology specimen are very unlikely to come from a low-grade cancer. Thus, a high-grade cancer or carcinoma in situ producing these cells is probably somewhere in the urinary tract.

27. **c. That there is a very brief presymptomatic period in which tumors are diagnosed before they cause symptoms.** The failure to find bladder cancer incidentally implies that from the time a tumor is large enough to be diagnosed until it causes symptoms is sufficiently brief that death from unrelated causes rarely occurs in that interval. Thus, the disease is not likely to be incidentally found (symptoms or signs occur rapidly).

28. **d. confidence in the screening program will be seriously undermined if any bladder cancers are undiagnosed.** If a screening participant has a negative test result and shortly thereafter has hematuria recognized and a bladder tumor (even a low-grade superficial one) diagnosed, participants and primary care physicians who do not recognize that only high-grade cancers are likely to be lethal will lose confidence in the screening test and program and will drop their support for it. Thus, screening must detect low- and high-grade cancers equally well.

29. **d. BTA stat.** The others all detect low-grade cancers also, almost as well as high-grade cancers.

30. **b. Detection of cancer not yet cystoscopically visible.** Specificity is the number of true-negative results divided by the sum of the number of true-negative plus false-positive results. If tests can detect tumors too small to be endoscopically visible (and hence before they can be diagnosed), false-positive rates will appear to increase, enlarging the denominator and reducing specificity. Although inflammatory lesions can cause some bladder cancer detection tests (e.g., hematuria) to be positive (answer e), several tests are *not* affected by inflammation, so that this is not a generic problem in determining specificity for *all* bladder cancer tests.

31. **b. may detect molecular alterations induced by the carcinogen that are not necessarily associated with malignant transformation.** Studies have been limited because of a combination of factors, including incomplete information about previous exposures, changing production standards, and difficulties with compliance and follow-up. Additionally, the

possibility of the chemical exposures themselves causing abnormal test results without leading to diagnosable malignancy is uncertain. Even when a positive biomarker test precedes the appearance of overt malignancy, whether the positive test indicates the presence of (1) a premalignant field change that may be reversed by cessation of carcinogen exposure, (2) irreversible changes in the urothelium, or (3) true malignant transformation that was not yet clinically detectable is not clear.

32. **b. It permits resection of endoscopically invisible tumors.** ALA, when administered intravesically in conjunction with fluorescent cystoscopy using blue light at 375 to 440 nm, can enable detection of lesions invisible with white light cystoscopy. In the largest series to date, the authors claimed that this procedure increased sensitivity in detecting small tumors and carcinoma in situ from 77% with white light to nearly 98% with fluorescent cystoscopy.

33. **d. It is very important preceding planned partial cystectomy.** Regardless of the questionable wisdom of performing selected site urothelial biopsies for most bladder tumors, these biopsies are required if partial cystectomy is contemplated, or if urinary cytology indicates the presence of high-grade cancer and cystoscopically no tumors are seen or all lesions look like low-grade superficial papillary tumors.

34. **c. Between lamina propria and muscularis propria.** The first treatment decision based on tumor stage is whether the patient has a superficial or muscle invasive tumor.

35. **d. Chest CT.** Chest CT may be too sensitive in detecting small pulmonary lesions that are not metastases. Because standard films do not have the sufficient resolution to demonstrate small granulomas, but rather detect only lesions larger than 1 cm in diameter, routine chest radiographs rather than CT are usually relied on to rule out pulmonary metastases in bladder cancer patients.

36. **c. T2b.** In the AJC-UICC system, muscle-invading tumors, depending on whether there is superficial or deep muscle invasion, are classified as stage T2a or T2b, respectively.

37. **d. High consumption of fluid.** Not surprisingly, dilution of carcinogenic agents in the urine by increasing fluid ingestion protects against bladder cancer, with a relative risk of 0.51 for the highest quartile of chronic fluid ingestion compared with the lowest.

38. **b. Carcinosarcoma.** Carcinosarcomas are highly malignant tumors containing both malignant mesenchymal and epithelial elements. The common presenting symptom is gross, painless hematuria. The prognosis is uniformly poor despite aggressive treatment with cystectomy, radiation, and/or chemotherapy.

76

Non–Muscle-Invasive Bladder Cancer (Ta, T1, and Tis)

J. STEPHEN JONES • STEVEN C. CAMPBELL

QUESTIONS

1. Postoperative intravesical chemotherapy administered in the recovery room is appropriate for which of the following cases?
   a. Solitary 3.0-cm, low-grade–appearing tumor on posterior bladder wall
   b. Multifocal (n = 4) low-grade, low-stage bladder tumor, all 4 to 10 mm in diameter
   c. A 6.5-cm high-grade, broad-based tumor on the lateral wall with deep resection
   d. a and b
   e. a to c
2. Which of the following agents is contraindicated for postoperative intravesical chemotherapy administered in the recovery room?
   a. Thiotepa
   b. BCG
   c. Mitomycin C
   d. Epirubicin
   e. b and c
3. Potential advantages of tumor markers such as BTA, stat NMP-22 and UroVysion (FISH) when compared with urinary cytology for monitoring patients with bladder cancer are improved:
   a. sensitivity.
   b. specificity.
   c. positive predictive value.
   d. a and c.
   e. a to c.
4. Progression rates for low-grade Ta tumors range from:
   a. 0% to 3%.
   b. 3% to 10%.
   c. 10% to 17%.
   d. 17% to 25%.
   e. >25%.
5. General anesthesia is most important when resecting a bladder tumor in which setting?
   a. Large, mobile papillary tumor
   b. Tumor in a posterior wall diverticulum
   c. Lateral location at about 4 or 8 o'clock
   d. Extensive carcinoma in situ (CIS)
   e. Tumor at dome and along anterior bladder wall
6. An otherwise healthy 55-year-old man undergoes resection of a 2.0-cm bladder tumor in a posterior wall bladder diverticulum. Pathology demonstrates a pT1 high grade bladder tumor with associated areas of CIS. Muscularis mucosa is involved, but there is no definite muscularis propria in the specimen. Optimal management includes:
   a. repeat resection to stage the cancer.
   b. intravesical BCG therapy.
   c. partial cystectomy with excision of the diverticulum.
   d. radical cystectomy and neobladder urinary diversion.
   e. chemotherapy and radiation therapy.
7. The most important principle to follow when resecting tumor near or overlying a ureteral orifice is:
   a. stent frequently.
   b. avoid resection.
   c. avoid cautery.
   d. resect at will (a stent or nephrostomy tube can be placed later).
   e. obtain an ultrasound preoperatively and place a nephrostomy tube if hydronephrosis is found.
8. A restaging TURBT with possible postoperative intravesical chemotherapy administered in the recovery room is indicated in which of the following situations?
   a. pT1, high grade tumor with no muscularis propria identified
   b. pTa, low grade tumor that is multifocal (n = 5), for which resection appeared to be complete but postoperative intravesical therapy was not administered
   c. pT1, high grade tumor with muscularis propria identified and findings negative
   d. a and c
   e. a to c
9. The optimal laser for fulguration of bladder tumors is:
   a. CO_2.
   b. Nd:YAG.
   c. holmium.
   d. KTP.
   e. argon.

10. Intravesical mitomycin C chemotherapy for high-risk superficial bladder cancer:
    a. reduces the risk of progression.
    b. reduces the risk of recurrence.
    c. is preferred over BCG, particularly for CIS.
    d. is virtually free of side effects.
    e. is less expensive than BCG.
11. Which of the following are contraindications to BCG therapy?
    a. cirrhosis
    b. history of tuberculosis
    c. total incontinence
    d. immunosuppression
    e. all of the above
12. The combination of reduced-dose BCG and interferon-α for intravesical therapy is:
    a. more effective than BCG alone.
    b. more toxic than BCG alone.
    c. preferred first-line therapy in multifocal CIS.
    d. less expensive than BCG alone.
    e. option for BCG failure after one course of therapy.
13. Common side effects of thiotepa include:
    a. irritative voiding symptoms and fever.
    b. hematuria and irritative voiding symptoms.
    c. bladder contraction and myelosuppression.
    d. irritative voiding symptoms and myelosuppression.
    e. flu-like symptoms and fever.
14. Long-term (15 years) outcome after intravesical BCG therapy for patients with high-risk non–muscle-invasive bladder cancer include which of the following?
    a. Approximately 50% progression rate
    b. Approximately 25% alive and with bladder intact
    c. High incidence of recurrence in extravesical sites (prostatic urothelium and upper tracts)
    d. Approximately 33% cancer-related mortality rates
    e. All of the above
15. Understaging for patients with pT1 high grade bladder cancer is approximately:
    a. 5% to 10%.
    b. 10% to 20%.
    c. 20% to 30%.
    d. 30% to 50%.
    e. 50% to 70%.
16. A patient is diagnosed with a 1.0-cm pTa low grade bladder cancer. Imaging of the upper tracts is:
    a. not indicated.
    b. performed only at diagnosis.
    c. performed at diagnosis and 5 years later.
    d. performed at diagnosis and every other year thereafter.
    e. performed at diagnosis and every year thereafter.
17. For patients with stage pTa low grade bladder tumor and a negative cytology, random bladder biopsies are:
    a. more likely to be positive in the prostatic fossa than the bladder.
    b. done in a systematic manner.
    c. samples of the muscularis mucosa and preferably the muscularis propria.
    d. indicated at initial diagnosis and need not be repeated if negative.
    e. not indicated in most cases.
18. The risk of progression to muscle-invasive disease for patients with untreated CIS of the bladder is approximately:
    a. 5% to 15%.
    b. 15% to 25%.
    c. 25% to 35%.
    d. 35% to 45%.
    e. >45%.
19. Current consensus about *TP53* as a prognostic marker for bladder cancer is which of the following?
    a. Established predictive factor for response to BCG therapy
    b. Independent predictive factor of tumor progression for pT1 high grade disease
    c. Stronger predictive value than grade for pTa tumors
    d. Of no clinical value at present
    e. Prospective validation required
20. Which of the following disease entities is least common?
    a. pTa low grade
    b. pTa high grade
    c. pT1 high grade
    d. CIS of any form
    e. pT2-3

ANSWERS

1. **d. a and b.** Postoperative intravesical chemotherapy should be considered for most cases of new or recurrent non–muscle-invasive bladder cancer, because it has been shown to reduce recurrence rates and improve outcomes for this disease. One exception is the patient in whom an extensive resection has been performed or whenever there is a possible perforation. In these patients intravesical chemotherapy should be withheld due to concern about local extravasation and absorption.
2. **b. BCG.** BCG should never be given in association with known trauma to the urinary tract such as after TURBT owing to concern over systemic absorption and sepsis. All of the other agents have shown efficacy in this setting with a favorable morbidity profile.
3. **a. sensitivity.** Tumor markers such as BTA stat, NMP-22, and UroVysion (FISH) provide improved sensitivity, particularly for low-grade tumors. High specificity is the strength of urinary cytology. This approaches 90% to 100% in many series and cannot be improved on with these other markers. Positive predictive value is highest for urinary cytology because the number of false-positive results is low. Put another way, if the cytology is positive, the patient usually has active disease.
4. **b. 3% to 10%.** Recurrence is common (50% to 70%) for patients with low-grade, pTa tumors, but progression to a higher tumor stage is uncommon, occurring in 5% to 10% of patients.
5. **c. Lateral location, at about 4 or 8 o'clock.** Resection along the lateral bladder wall posterolaterally places one in proximity to the obturator nerve, and this can lead to an obturator reflex. This can predispose to bladder wall perforation. In this situation, general anesthesia with complete paralysis is indicated to allow the procedure to be performed in a safe and facile manner.

6. **d. radical cystectomy and neobladder urinary diversion.** This patient should be strongly considered for radical cystectomy. Partial cystectomy is not a good option owing to the presence of CIS, which indicates a high risk of field effect disease and subsequent recurrence. Deeper biopsies will risk perforation and would be unlikely to influence management. Understaging is common with tumors in diverticula, and high-grade invasive tumors like this are best managed with radical cystectomy to ensure local disease control and optimize outcomes on a long-term basis.
7. **c. avoid cautery.** A stent should be avoided if possible to prevent reflux of tumor cells into the upper tracts. In most cases this area can be resected and most ureters will remain unobstructed as long as the orifice is identified and cautery is not used in this area. Preoperative placement of a nephrostomy tube is often unnecessary as long a renal function is stable. Many patients with hydronephrosis will have invasive disease and will be undergoing urinary diversion in the near future, and this will relieve the obstruction. Hence, temporary nephrostomy tube placement is usually not required.
8. **d. a and c.** Patients with pT1 tumor for whom the muscularis propria was not identified are understaged about 50% of the time and a repeat resection is clearly indicated. Patients who have undergone repeat resection for pT1 high grade tumor with muscularis propria present and negative are found to have residual or invasive disease 30% of the time. A repeat TURBT is thus indicated in both of these patient populations to accurately stage the tumor and to optimize patient management.
9. **b. Nd:YAG.** The ND:YAG laser has the best properties (e.g., depth of penetration, intensity of energy for effective tumor ablation) for coagulation of bladder tumors and the greatest clinical experience demonstrating safety and efficacy in appropriately selected patients.
10. **b. reduces the risk of recurrence**. Mitomycin C (MMC) is very expensive, especially when compared with BCG. It can reduce the risk of recurrence but there is no convincing evidence that it can reduce progression rates, which is true for all forms of intravesical chemotherapy. Most comparative studies and meta-analyses suggest an advantage to BCG, particularly for CIS. MMC can lead to local bladder irritation and dermatitis and is thus far from risk free.
11. **e. all of the above.** BGC is contraindicated in patients with liver disease (isoniazid cannot be given if they develop BCG sepsis), a personal history of tuberculosis, total incontinence (they cannot retain the BCG so efficacy would be poor), and immunosuppression (BCG's mechanism of action is to stimulate an immune response). Other contraindications include disrupted urothelium, gross hematuria, or active or persistent UTI.
12. **e. option for BCG failure after one course of therapy**. Combined therapy with BCG and interferon-α has shown activity in BCG failure and is one viable option for this challenging patient population. However, it is more expensive and there are no data to suggest that it is more effective than BCG alone. BCG remains the treatment of choice for CIS. Combined BCG and interferon-α is well tolerated with a side effect profile that is better on average than BCG alone, because most of the side effects are related to the BCG and its dose is reduced in this regimen.
13. **d. irritative voiding symptoms and myelosuppression**. Irritative voiding symptoms are reported by 12% to 69% of patients receiving intravesical thiotepa. The low molecular weight of this agent (189 kD) predisposes to systemic absorption and myelosuppression. These are the two most common side effects of this agent.
14. **e. All of the above**. Data about long-term outcomes for a patient with high-risk superficial bladder cancer treated with intravesical BCG therapy is derived primarily from the experience at Memorial-Sloan Kettering (Cookson et al, 1997). In this series, 50% of patients progressed and one third died of cancer progression. Approximately one third developed disease in the prostatic fossa or upper tracts, and only 27% survived with an intact bladder. Such data should be considered when counseling patients about treatment options for high-risk disease.
15. **d. 30% to 50%**. The risk of understaging of a pT1G3 bladder tumor is about 30%, but it is even higher if there is no muscularis propria in the specimen. Altogether, the risk is 30% to 50% in this high-risk patient population.
16. **a. is not indicated.** The incidence of upper tract tumor associated with pTa low grade bladder cancer is extremely low (0.3% to 2.3%) and current consensus is that upper tract imaging is not indicated in this patient population (Oosterlinck et al, 2005).
17. **e. not indicated in most cases.** The yield of random bladder biopsy in patients with low-grade, low-stage bladder tumors and a negative cytology is very low and is not indicated unless high risk features are present.
18. **e. >45%**. Untreated CIS is very high risk (>50%) for progressing to muscle invasive disease. Even patients with a complete response to intravesical BCG will experience progression in 30% to 40% of cases on longitudinal follow-up (Sylvester et al. 2005).
19. **e. Prospective validation required**. Almost all studies of *TP53* as a prognostic marker have been retrospective to date. While promising, this marker will require prospective validation before it can be generally used for clinical decision-making. However, the balance of available data has been promising, and the use of this marker for decision-making in very challenging cases has been advocated by many in this field. Most studies suggest that BCG is not a good predictor of response to BCG therapy, and it is clearly not better than grade for predicting outcomes for pTa disease. Its ultimate role for predicting progression for pT1 high grade tumors is not well defined at present.
20. **b. pTa low grade**. pTa low grade represents 50% to 70% of all non–muscle-invasive bladder tumors and is the most common of these entities. CIS is commonly associated with high-grade tumors and, overall, is found in 10% to 20% of non–muscle-invasive bladder tumors. pT1 high grade is found in about 20% of patients with non–muscle-invasive bladder tumors. pT2-3 represents about 20% of all bladder cancer patients. pTa high grade is often misclassified and in reality only represents about 5% to 10% of all non–muscle-invasive tumors (Sylvester et al, 2005).

77

Management of Invasive and Metastatic Bladder Cancer

MARK L. GONZALGO • MARK P. SCHOENBERG

QUESTIONS

1. Which of the following statements is NOT true with regard to staging of invasive bladder cancer?
   a. Bimanual examination is highly predictive of the presence of extravesical disease if a mass is palpable after transurethral resection.
   b. CT and MRI are equivalent methods of noninvasive axial imaging for prediction of nodal involvement.
   c. Bone scanning is a useful routine staging tool for asymptomatic patients with clinically organ-confined invasive bladder cancer.
   d. Positron emission tomography is limited by concentration of the fluorodeoxyglucose agent in the lumen of the bladder.
2. Which of the following statements is TRUE regarding nerve-sparing cystoprostatectomy? It is
   a. more likely to result in local recurrence than is standard cystectomy.
   b. accomplished by high lateral ligation of the pedicles of the prostate gland adjacent to the seminal vesicles.
   c. associated with potency rates higher than 50% in men aged 75 years and older when both nerves are preserved.
   d. associated with inferior stage-for-stage disease-specific survival compared with standard cystectomy.
3. In a 34-year-old woman with T2N0Mx bladder cancer who undergoes radical cystectomy, which of the following is TRUE?
   a. Excision of the anterior vaginal wall is required.
   b. The urethra is usually involved in the tumor diathesis.
   c. Orthotopic reconstruction is not recommended if the trigone is diffusely involved by carcinoma in situ.
   d. Classic anterior exenteration does not require removal of the uterus.
4. Which of the following statements is TRUE regarding radical cystectomy? It:
   a. results in disease-free survival rates that decline with increasing stage of disease.
   b. is best for patients with moderate local nodal disease appreciated via preoperative imaging.
   c. produces overall survival rates that have been shown in prospective trials to exceed those obtained with bladder-sparing protocols.
   d. results in bowel obstruction requiring operative correction in 20% of patients.
5. Which of the following statements is TRUE regarding pelvic lymphadenectomy in the context of radical cystectomy? It:
   a. can result in long-term disease-free survival in patients with N1 bladder cancer.
   b. is routinely recommended for patients with palpable adenopathy above the aortic bifurcation.
   c. will usually identify metastatic disease contralateral to the patient's known tumor.
   d. provides limited staging information that cannot be obtained from axial imaging studies performed preoperatively.
6. Which of the following statements is TRUE regarding neoadjuvant chemotherapy for bladder cancer? It:
   a. generally relies on normal renal function.
   b. provides a relative advantage to patients with disease of T3 stage or greater.
   c. has been associated with improved disease-specific survival rates in randomized U.S. trials.
   d. All of the above.
7. Which of the following statements is TRUE regarding adjuvant chemotherapy? It:
   a. improves disease-specific outcome in patients undergoing cystectomy.
   b. is most appropriate for patients with disease of less than stage pT2.
   c. is better tolerated than neoadjuvant chemotherapy.
   d. None of the above.
8. Which of the following statements is TRUE regarding transurethral resection? It:
   a. can achieve a long-term disease-free survival rate in patients with invasive bladder cancer equivalent to that achieved with standard surgical therapy.
   b. is unlikely to achieve disease-free survival in patients with T2N0Mx bladder cancer.
   c. is most likely to be successful if residual disease is only microscopic.
   d. None of the above.

9. Which of the following statements is TRUE regarding bladder preservation protocols? They:
   a. are indicated for all stages of clinically organ-confined bladder cancer.
   b. are equally effective whether hydronephrosis is present or absent.
   c. are flawed by reliance on clinical staging.
   d. achieve 5-year disease-specific survival rates similar to those obtained with radical cystectomy.
10. Each of the following statements is TRUE of systemic chemotherapy for bladder cancer EXCEPT which one? It:
    a. is reserved for the treatment of patients with measurable metastatic bladder cancer.
    b. is usually more successful if a multiagent regimen as opposed to a single-agent protocol is used.
    c. often includes methotrexate, cisplatin, doxorubicin, and bleomycin.
    d. All of the above.
11. Salvage cystectomy is appropriate:
    a. when residual disease is limited to the true pelvis.
    b. and is most likely to achieve the greatest chance of disease-free survival when the patient's response to chemotherapy is incomplete.
    c. for patients who have received radiation to the pelvis and chemotherapy, but it is never safe to perform orthotopic reconstruction in this setting.
    d. None of the above.
12. A 41-year-old otherwise healthy male patient with T2N0Mx transitional cell carcinoma of the bladder:
    a. should have a preoperative bone scan because the alkaline phosphatase level is normal.
    b. is not a candidate for bladder preservation on the basis of age.
    c. has an approximately 5% risk of positive lymph nodes at the time of radical cystectomy.
    d. should have ureteral frozen section analysis at the time of cystectomy.
13. All of the following are TRUE with regard to the role of lymphadenectomy for treatment of bladder cancer EXCEPT:
    a. An extended lymph node dissection should include the distal para-aortic, paracaval, and presacral nodes.
    b. Among patients with lymph node positive disease, the total number of lymph nodes removed at the time of surgery has been shown to be of prognostic value.
    c. Extended PLND may yield a greater number of positive and total number of LNs compared with standard PLND.
    d. Percentage of patients with node-positive disease is higher when an extended PLND is performed compared with standard PLND.
    e. Ratio-based lymph node staging may improve stratification of lymph node positive cases by accounting for the total number of positive lymph nodes (tumor burden) and the total number of lymph nodes removed (extent of lymphadenectomy).
14. All of the following are TRUE with regard to neoadjuvant chemotherapy for bladder cancer EXCEPT:
    a. there is a modest improvement in overall survival among patients treated with neoadjuvant chemotherapy.
    b. cisplatin-based single-agent chemotherapy has been shown to improve overall survival.
    c. combination chemotherapy (MVAC) is superior to single-agent cisplatin-based chemotherapy.
    d. patients with bulky, locally advanced disease appear most likely to benefit from neoadjuvant chemotherapy.
    e. lack of definitive pathological staging associated with neoadjuvant chemotherapy may lead to overtreatment of patients with organ-confined disease.
15. General criteria for selective bladder sparing treatment for muscle-invasive disease include all of the following EXCEPT:
    a. normal CBC.
    b. absence of hydronephrosis.
    c. normal renal function.
    d. poor candidate for cystectomy.
    e. absence of metastatic disease on imaging studies.

ANSWERS

1. **c. Bone scanning is a useful routine staging tool for asymptomatic patients with clinically organ-confined invasive bladder cancer.** Several studies from the past 2 decades substantiate the impression that, in general, preoperative bone scanning is not necessary for patients with clinically organ-confined muscle invasive bladder carcinoma.
2. **b. accomplished by high lateral ligation of the pedicles of the prostate adjacent to the seminal vesicles.** A key technical point to observe intraoperatively when performing nerve-sparing cystoprostatectomy is high lateral ligation of the pedicles of the bladder and prostate, because these tissues coalesce near the seminal vesicles.
3. **c. Orthotopic reconstruction is not recommended if the trigone is diffusely involved by carcinoma in situ.** Female patients with overt cancer at the bladder neck and urethra, diffuse carcinoma in situ, or a positive margin at surgery are poor candidates for orthotopic reconstruction and should be treated by immediate en bloc urethrectomy as part of the radical cystectomy.
4. **a. results in disease-free survival rates that decline with increasing stage of disease.** Pathologic stage of disease correlates significantly with patient outcome after intervention. Nowhere is this more clearly delineated than in the contemporary literature on radical cystectomy with pelvic lymphadenectomy for clinically organ-confined bladder cancer. Long-term survival is uniformly better for patients with pathologically organ-confined disease (see Table 77-2). Although the results of radical cystectomy for patients with clinically organ-confined disease appear unimpeachable, radical cystectomy performed in the context of locoregional disease or malignant pelvic adenopathy is more controversial.
5. **a. can result in long-term disease-free survival in patients with N1 bladder cancer.** Pelvic lymphadenectomy provides insight into the local extent of disease. In addition, patients with very limited nodal burden experience unexpectedly high rates of long-term survival in the absence of additional interventions.
6. **d. All of the above.** Utilizing cisplatin-based therapy, trials have shown a trend toward improved long-term disease-specific survival rates in some younger patients and in those with lesions greater than stage T3.

7. **d. None of the above**. There is no evidence to suggest that the administration of adjuvant chemotherapy to patients with organ-confined bladder cancer (T1-T2) will provide either a survival advantage or an improvement in local control after cystectomy.

8. **a. It can achieve long-term disease-free survival in patients with invasive bladder cancer equivalent to that achieved with standard surgical therapy**. In one study, a large group of patients was treated by transurethral resection with a negative tumor bed and peripheral biopsies after complete "radical" transurethral resection. The 5-year disease-specific survival statistics were impressively similar to those reported for radical cystectomy.

9. **d. achieve 5-year disease-specific survival rates similar to those obtained with radical cystectomy**. One study treated 106 patients with T2-4NxM0 bladder cancer by transurethral resection, neoadjuvant chemotherapy (methotrexate, cisplatin, and vinblastine), and subsequent radiation therapy. Patients not responding were treated by radical cystectomy. These authors reported a 52% overall survival rate. Of the patients completing the full course of therapy, 75% retained bladders free of disease with a median follow-up of 64 months. Subsequent studies by other investigators have lent support to these conclusions.

10. **c. often includes methotrexate, cisplatin, doxorubicin, and bleomycin**. The most commonly employed agents are methotrexate, vinblastine, doxorubicin (Adriamycin), and cisplatin.

11. **d. None of the above.** Patients electing conservative or primarily nonsurgical forms of therapy for invasive or locoregionally advanced bladder cancer may require subsequent definitive surgical intervention when conservative treatment has produced a partial response and residual disease remains clinically confined to the bladder. Another study found that orthotopic reconstruction is safe and effective in selected patients undergoing salvage surgery. Resection appears to help patients who have had a complete response to systemic therapy, but surgery for residual extravesical disease confers no long-term survival advantage and is generally to be discouraged.

12. **d. should have ureteral frozen section analysis at the time of cystectomy**. Analysis of the ureteral margin at the time of cystectomy before urinary tract reconstruction is standard contemporary practice. The rationale for this procedure is that carcinoma and particularly carcinoma in situ can involve the distal ureteral margin. Urologists have historically resected positive margins to effect clearance of all documented cancer, assuming that this would provide better long-term local disease control.

13. **d. Percentage of patients with node-positive disease is higher when an extended PLND is performed compared with standard PLND**. An extended PLND may yield a greater number of positive and total number of lymph nodes compared with standard PLND, but the percentage of patients with node-positive disease who are identified is similar between these two groups (Bochner et al, 2004).

14. **b. cisplatin-based single-agent chemotherapy has been shown to improve overall survival.** Multiple trials have demonstrated no benefit to overall survival with neoadjuvant single-agent therapy (Wallace et al, 1991; Martinez-Pineiro et al, 1995).

15. **d. poor candidate for cystectomy.** General criteria for selective bladder sparing includes presence of muscle-invasive disease, absence of hydronephrosis, normal renal function, normal CBC, suitable candidate for cystectomy, and absence of metastatic disease on imaging studies.

78

Surgery of Bladder Cancer

PETER T. NIEH • FRAY F. MARSHALL

QUESTIONS

1. Which of the following statements regarding the arterial supply to the bladder is TRUE? The:
   a. inferior vesical artery arises from the posterior trunk of the internal iliac artery.
   b. superior vesical artery arises from the anterior trunk of the internal iliac artery.
   c. majority of the blood supply to the bladder is derived from the obturator artery.
   d. inferior gluteal artery sends no branches to the bladder.
   e. bladder cannot be mobilized substantially because of its tenuous blood supply.
2. Which of the following statements regarding cold-cup biopsy of bladder lesions is TRUE?
   a. It is useful for biopsy of large bladder tumors.
   b. It is most amenable to lesions on the inside of the bladder neck.
   c. It is difficult to perform through a standard cystoscope.
   d. It requires suprapubic pressure if the lesion is located on the trigone.
   e. It allows for better tissue procurement without coagulation defects when compared with standard loop resection.
3. Tumor characteristics that would allow for transurethral resection as the sole treatment for muscle-invasive disease include which of the following?
   a. High grade
   b. Multifocal
   c. Papillary
   d. Tumor base larger than 2 cm
   e. Sessile
4. A suitable bowel preparation for a radical cystectomy should include all of the following EXCEPT which one?
   a. A cathartic such as GoLYTELY
   b. Metronidazole
   c. Gentamicin
   d. Neomycin
   e. A clear liquid diet
5. What is the cephalad limit to a standard pelvic lymphadenectomy?
   a. Peritoneal reflection
   b. Bifurcation of the common iliac artery
   c. Vas deferens
   d. Median umbilical ligament
   e. Node of Cloquet
6. What is the mortality rate associated with radical cystectomy in most modern series?
   a. 0.1% to 0.2%
   b. 1% to 3%
   c. 5% to 7%
   d. 9% to 11%
   e. 15% to 17%
7. What is the incidence of urethral recurrence after radical cystoprostatectomy?
   a. 0.5% to 4%
   b. 4% to 18%
   c. 19% to 28%
   d. 29% to 37%
   e. 38% to 48%
8. Which of the following statements regarding urethrectomy is TRUE?
   a. The dissection is much easier if carried out several weeks after radical cystectomy.
   b. Drainage is not recommended after urethrectomy.
   c. The bulbar urethral arteries should be preserved throughout the dissection.
   d. When a urethrectomy is performed, the best position for the patient is the exaggerated lithotomy.
   e. It is necessary to split the glans to remove all of the transitional cell epithelium at the meatus.
9. Which of the following statements regarding urethral involvement in bladder cancer in the female patient is TRUE?
   a. Female patients have a much higher incidence of urethral involvement than do male patients.
   b. Orthotopic bladder substitution can rarely be used in the female patient because of the risk of urethral recurrence.
   c. Intraoperative frozen section is the best way to determine whether the urethra is suitable for orthotopic reconstruction.
   d. Tumor involvement at the bladder neck always signifies urethral involvement.
   e. Incidence of urethral involvement in female patients has been shown to be consistently above 15%.

10. A complete anterior exenteration in the female includes all of the following procedures EXCEPT which one?
    a. Cystectomy
    b. Hysterectomy
    c. Bilateral pelvic lymphadenectomy
    d. Pubovaginal sling
    e. Partial vaginectomy
11. All of the following can be considered indications for simple cystectomy EXCEPT which one?
    a. Pyocystis in a neurogenic bladder
    b. Colovesical fistula after urinary diversion
    c. Urachal adenocarcinoma
    d. Hemorrhagic cystitis resulting from cyclophosphamide
    e. Pain and incomplete emptying in patients with prior supravesical diversions
12. What is the advantage of partial cystectomy over total cystectomy in the management of bladder cancer?
    a. More accurate staging
    b. Improved survival
    c. Preservation of bladder and sexual function
    d. Possibility of using surveillance cystoscopy
    e. Lower recurrence rates of tumor
13. Which of the following is a contraindication to partial cystectomy?
    a. Tumor location at the dome of the bladder
    b. Grade 1 transitional cell carcinoma
    c. Tumor within a bladder diverticulum
    d. Multifocal tumor associated with multifocal carcinoma in situ
    e. Urachal adenocarcinoma
14. Which of the following statements about pelvic lymphadenectomy is NOT correct?
    a. Extended dissection to the aortic bifurcation is associated with increased incidence of lymphocele.
    b. En bloc resection yields fewer lymph nodes than dissecting separate packets.
    c. Extended lymphadenectomy improves survival in N0 patients.
    d. Extended lymphadenectomy improves survival in patients with limited lymph node metastases.
    e. The lateral extent of the dissection is the genitofemoral nerve.

ANSWERS

1. **b. superior vesical artery arises from the anterior trunk of the internal iliac artery.** The urinary bladder has a rich blood supply derived from the superior and inferior vesical branches that arise from the anterior trunk of the internal iliac artery and by smaller branches from the obturator and internal gluteal arteries.
2. **e. It allows for better tissue procurement without coagulation defects when compared with standard loop resection.** If the bladder lesion is small, it may be amenable to cold-cup biopsy and fulguration. This technique has the advantage of tissue procurement without coagulation defects from the resectoscope.
3. **c. Papillary.** No randomized studies have compared transurethral resection alone with cystectomy. However, there is probably a small subset of patients with stage T2 transitional cell carcinoma who may be candidates for resection therapy alone. These patients are likely to have tumors that are small, solitary, papillary, moderately differentiated, less than 2 cm in diameter at the tumor base, and stage T2 or minimal stage T3a.
4. **c. Gentamicin.** Clear liquids are recommended for the 2 days before surgery. Polyethylene glycol-electrolyte solution (GoLYTELY) is given on the day before surgery, and oral antibiotics containing either neomycin or erythromycin base and metronidazole are administered on the day before surgery.
5. **b. Bifurcation of the common iliac artery.** The bifurcation of the common iliac artery is the cephalad limit of the dissection.
6. **b. 1% to 3%.** The operative mortality rate for radical cystectomy has been shown to be between 1% and 3% in most modern series.
7. **b. 4% to 18%.** The incidence of urethral recurrence has been documented in prior studies to be between 4% and 18%.
8. **d. When a urethrectomy is performed, the best position for the patient is the exaggerated lithotomy.** The urethrectomy from the perineal approach is most easily performed with the patient in the exaggerated lithotomy position.
9. **c. Intraoperative frozen section is the best way to determine whether the urethra is suitable for orthotopic reconstruction.** An intraoperative frozen section of the proximal urethra should now be considered the best way to determine whether a female patient is a suitable candidate for orthotopic neobladder.
10. **d. Pubovaginal sling.** The anterior approach has advantages in that it allows for simultaneous pelvic lymphadenectomy, cystectomy, urethrectomy, hysterectomy, salpingo-oophorectomy, and partial vaginectomy if clinically indicated for extensive carcinomatous involvement.
11. **c. Urachal adenocarcinoma.** Various benign conditions that may warrant simple cystectomy include pyocystis, neurogenic bladder, severe urinary incontinence, severe urethral trauma, large vesical fistula, cyclophosphamide cystitis, and radiation cystitis after treatment of other pelvic malignancies.
12. **c. Preservation of bladder and sexual function.** The benefits of partial cystectomy include complete pathologic staging of the tumor and pelvic lymph nodes, as well as preservation of both bladder and sexual function.
13. **d. Multifocal tumor associated with multifocal carcinoma in situ.** Absolute contraindications to partial cystectomy would include multifocal carcinoma in situ.
14. **a. Extended dissection to the aortic bifurcation is associated with increased incidence of lymphocele.** An extended pelvic lymphadenectomy does increase operating time but has not been associated with increased complications, such as lymphocele, bleeding, or deep venous thrombosis. Submitting separate node packets significantly increases the yield of nodes compared with an en bloc resection. The increased number of lymph nodes resected has improved survival in patients with both negative nodes and limited lymph node metastases.

79

Laparoscopic Surgery of the Urinary Bladder

INDERBIR S. GILL

QUESTIONS

1. The preferred treatment option for a recurrent, symptomatic seminal vesicle cyst is:
   a. transrectal needle aspiration.
   b. cystoscopic TUR deroofing.
   c. laparoscopic excision.
   d. open transvesical approach.
   e. posterior transcoccygeal approach.
2. All of the following are essential surgical aspects of the Boari flap EXCEPT:
   a. an adequate-sized bladder must be present (200 to 300 mL).
   b. the contralateral vesical pedicle may need to be transected to allow adequate bladder mobilization.
   c. the bladder flap should be slightly shorter than anticipated because bladder tissue can be easily stretched.
   d. a tension-free anastomosis is important.
   e. typically, a refluxing ureteral anastomosis is created.
3. Principles of open surgical or laparoscopic repair of a vesicovaginal fistula include all of the following EXCEPT:
   a. good exposure of the fistulous tract.
   b. wide excision of the fibrous and scar tissue.
   c. tension-free repair of the vagina and bladder.
   d. interposition of a flap of peritoneum or omentum.
   e. adequate drainage.
4. Contraindications for laparoscopic enterocystoplasty include all of the following EXCEPT:
   a. diverticulosis.
   b. inflammatory bowel disease.
   c. renal failure.
   d. noncompliance..
   e. ulcerative colitis.
5. Which of the following statements is NOT correct regarding laparoscopic enterocystoplasty?
   a. Subtotal cystectomy is mandatory.
   b. Mesenteric pedicle of the selected bowel segment is wide and broad-based.
   c. Mesenteric window is closed.
   d. Reestablishment of bowel continuity is a critical step of the operation and may be performed extracorporally for added security, if necessary.
   e. Bowel to bladder anastomosis is optimally performed with interrupted serosa-to-serosa sutures.
6. Partial cystectomy can be performed in all of the following circumstances EXCEPT:
   a. tumor at the bladder dome.
   b. tumor in the bladder diverticulum.
   c. solitary invasive bladder tumor located at a distance from the ureteric orifices.
   d. history of multiple tumors or carcinoma in situ.
   e. good bladder capacity.
7. Which of the following statements is TRUE regarding partial cystectomy?
   a. Thirty to 40 percent of patients with bladder cancer are candidates for a partial cystectomy.
   b. Five-year survival rates range from 80% to 90%.
   c. Laparoscopic partial cystectomy is now an established procedure.
   d. All of the above
   e. None of the above
8. Which of the following is a contraindication for laparoscopic radical cystectomy today?
   a. Multiple bladder tumors
   b. Nonbulky, invasive bladder cancer
   c. T4 disease
   d. Moderate obesity
   e. Open pelvic surgery

9. As regards radical cystectomy, all of the following have been performed laparoscopically EXCEPT:
   a. extended pelvic lymph node dissection.
   b. uterus and vagina sparing radical cystectomy.
   c. anterior pelvic exenteration in the female.
   d. orthotopic neobladder.
   e. Indiana pouch, constructed intracorporally.
10. Contraindications for prostate-sparing radical cystectomy include all of the following EXCEPT:
   a. multifocal CIS.
   b. tumor located near the bladder neck.
   c. prostate nodule on DRE.
   d. PSA 7.2 ng/mL.
   e. tumor located at left lateral bladder wall.
11. Anatomic boundaries of extended pelvic lymph node dissection include all of the following EXCEPT:
   a. external iliac artery (lateral).
   b. obturator nerve (posterior).
   c. aortic bifurcation area (proximal).
   d. internal inguinal ring (distal).
   e. bladder (medial).
12. Future directions for laparoscopic radical cystectomy are likely to include which of the following?
   a. Careful, prospective, long-term evaluation of oncologic and functional outcomes
   b. Intracorporeal performance of radical cystectomy and extracorporeal performance of bowel work
   c. Elimination of bowel through use of novel bladder substitutes
   d. International collaboration
   e. All of the above

ANSWERS

1. **c. laparoscopic excision.** Seminal vesicle cysts are extremely rare and may occasionally be associated with ipsilateral renal dysgenesis. Management of a symptomatic cyst often involves concomitant removal of the dysgenetic renal moiety and any ectopic ureter if present. Whereas transrectal needle aspiration or cystoscopic TUR deroofing of the ejaculatory duct may be an appropriate first step in select patients, typically the significantly enlarged and inflamed seminal vesicle cyst requires complete excision, with concomitant en bloc excision of the dysgenetic renoureteral segment. Historically, such excision was performed open surgically through either a retroperitoneal, transvesical, transperineal, or posterior transcoccygeal approach. Given the deep pelvic location of the seminal vesicle cyst, these open surgical incisions were large, caused significant morbidity, and provided suboptimal surgical exposure. Laparoscopy allows excellent visualization of this deep, retrovesically located pathology and achieves the requisite surgical objectives, without compromising adjacent structures. As such, laparoscopy has emerged as the technique of choice for seminal vesicle pathology.
2. **c. the bladder flap should be slightly shorter than anticipated because bladder tissue can be easily stretched.** A tension-free anastomosis of the anterolateral bladder flap based on the ipsilateral vesical pedicle is critical. The bladder flap should be somewhat longer and wider than anticipated because the nondistended bladder shrinks in size, thus placing tension on the anastomosis. Ideally, a flap length-to-breadth ratio of 3:1 ensures good vascularity of its apex.
3. **b. wide excision of the fibrous and scar tissue.** Wide circumferential excision of the fistula and associated scar tissue is not necessary and may not even be feasible. Only the fibrotic VVF tract and its edges need to be excised. Adequate mobilization of the anterior vaginal wall and posterior bladder wall is performed to achieve a tension-free repair. Care is taken not to compromise the ureteral orifices. An interposition graft of omentum is anchored between the vagina and the bladder with a stitch.
4. **a. diverticulosis.** The presence of bowel pathology such as diverticulitis or ulcerative colitis requires the use of alternative, nondiseased bowel segments. Similar to open surgery, laparoscopic enterocystoplasty should not be performed in the presence of advanced renal or liver failure, inflammatory bowel disease, or short gut syndrome, or in a patient who is unable or noncompliant in performing intermittent catheterization reliably. Diverticulosis is not a contraindication for performing enterocystoplasty.
5. **e. Bowel to bladder anastomosis is optimally performed with interrupted serosa-to-serosa sutures.** The technical principles of enterocystoplasty are identical between open surgical and laparoscopic techniques. Generous mobilization of the bladder allows creation of an adequate anteroposterior cystotomy. Subtotal cystectomy is necessary only in patients with severely symptomatic interstitial cystitis. An optimal segment of bowel based on a broad, well-vascularized mesenteric pedicle is selected that will reach the pelvis without tension. The bowel segment is isolated and bowel continuity reestablished by either intracorporeal or extracorporeal techniques, and the mesenteric window is closed. The isolated bowel segment is detubularized, and a bowel plate is created appropriately. A tension-free, watertight, full-thickness, circumferential, running anastomosis of the bowel segment to the bladder is created. Adequate urinary drainage is established.
6. **a. tumor at the bladder dome.** Contraindications to partial cystectomy include multiple bladder tumors, tumors involving the bladder neck or posterior urethra or trigone, and concomitant carcinoma in situ. History or current evidence of multifocal TCC with or without carcinoma in situ is a contraindication for partial cystectomy. The ideal patient for partial cystectomy is one who has a solitary, organ-confined invasive bladder tumor located at the dome of a good capacity bladder, without any concomitant multifocality or CIS.
7. **e. None of the above.** In large series of patients with bladder cancer, less than 10% of the patients are candidates for a partial cystectomy. In the properly selected patient, 5-year survival ranges from 50% to 70%. Laparoscopic partial cystectomy has only been performed in a few selected cases and is currently a controversial procedure.
8. **c. T4 disease.** Laparoscopic radical cystectomy is an emerging procedure performed at centers of laparoscopic expertise. At this writing, laparoscopic radical cystectomy should be offered to nonobese patients with nonbulky, organ-confined bladder cancer without pelvic lymphadenopathy on preoperative CT. Various conditions such as morbid obesity, prior radiotherapy, or pelvic surgery are relative contraindications because of the increase in laparoscopic technical complexity. Locally advanced T4 disease should not be approached laparoscopically.
9. **e. Indiana pouch, constructed intracorporally.** Since the initial report of laparoscopic cystectomy in 1992 by Parra and colleagues, over 300 laparoscopic radical cystectomies have been performed worldwide. In the female, laparoscopic anterior pelvic exenteration and uterus, fallopian tube, vagina-sparing radical cystectomy have been performed. In the male, conventional

radical cystectomy and prostate-sparing radical cystectomy have been performed. Bilateral extended pelvic lymph node dissection with mean nodal yields of 21 lymph nodes has been reported. With regard to urinary drainage, ileal conduit, Mainz pouch, Indiana pouch (extracorporally constructed), and orthotopic neobladder have all been performed laparoscopically. However, long-term follow-up outcomes are still lacking.

10. **e. tumor located at left lateral bladder wall**. Prostate-sparing radical cystectomy is a controversial procedure, whether performed open surgically or laparoscopically. Although some initial encouraging results have been reported, widespread and long-term data are lacking. Concern about the oncologic adequacy of prostate-sparing cystectomy has been rightly raised. As such, extreme care should be taken in selecting a patient for this procedure. Patients with multifocal CIS, tumor located at the bladder neck or prostatic urethra, abnormal DRE findings, or elevated PSA have a significantly higher chance of either TCC involvement of the prostate or de novo prostate cancer. As such, these are clear contraindications for prostate-sparing radical cystectomy.

11. **a. external iliac artery (lateral)**. Laterally, the dissection is extended up to the genitofemoral nerve. At the conclusion of an extended bilateral pelvic lymph node dissection, the external and internal iliac artery and vein, the common iliac artery, the obturator nerve, the pelvic side wall, and the perivesical area should be bilaterally devoid of lymphatic fatty tissue.

12. **e. All of the above**. Laparoscopic radical cystectomy is an evolving treatment modality with increasing experience being reported from multiple centers worldwide. With earlier detection of bladder cancer, careful application of laparoscopic techniques, and meticulous long-term follow-up, laparoscopic radical cystectomy is likely to emerge as a viable treatment option for the selected patient with bladder cancer.

80

Intestinal Segments and Urinary Diversion

DOUGLAS M. DAHL • W. SCOTT MCDOUGAL

QUESTIONS

1. When a portion of stomach is to be used for augmentation it should:
   a. always be based on the right gastroepiploic artery.
   b. include only the antrum.
   c. never extend to the pylorus.
   d. include a significant portion of the lesser curve.
2. The ileum differs from jejunum in that:
   a. it has a larger diameter.
   b. the mesentery is thinner.
   c. it has multiple arcades.
   d. the vessels in the mesentery are larger.
3. When stomach is used for urinary diversion the electrolyte abnormality that may occur is what type of metabolic acidosis?
   a. Hyperchloremic
   b. Hypochloremic
   c. Hyperkalemic
   d. Hypokalemic
4. Postoperative bowel obstruction is most common when which of the following segments are used for diversion?
   a. Colon
   b. Stomach
   c. Sigmoid
   d. Ileum
5. Mechanical bowel preparation results in a reduction in:
   a. bacterial counts per gram of enteric contents.
   b. bacterial count in the jejunum.
   c. total number of bacteria in the bowel.
   d. bacterial counts in the stomach.
6. Systemic antibiotics in elective surgery should be given:
   a. before the patient is anesthetized.
   b. before the skin incision is made.
   c. intraoperatively before closure commences.
   d. does not make a difference as long as they are given in the perioperative period.
7. The most common cause of a lethal bowel complication is:
   a. use of prior irradiated bowel.
   b. lack of mechanical bowel prep.
   c. lack of antibiotic bowel prep.
   d. placement of a drain adjacent to the anastomosis.
8. The difference between stapled anastomoses and sutured anastomoses is:
   a. less leaks.
   b. less compatible with urine.
   c. reduced overall operative time.
   d. lesser incidence of bowel obstruction.
9. The use of a nasogastric tube in the postoperative period:
   a. hastens return of intestinal motility.
   b. reduces incidence of bowel leak.
   c. reduces postoperative vomiting.
   d. increases the risk of aspiration.
10. The abdominal stoma for a conduit should be:
    a. flush with the skin.
    b. placed through the belly of the rectus muscle.
    c. be made as a loop to reduce parastomal hernia.
    d. made with colon for the least complication rate.
11. The loop end ileostomy is best used in:
    a. the obese patient.
    b. the thin patient.
    c. when a stoma is revised.
    d. in female patients.
12. Ureteral strictures occurring after an ileal conduit not associated with the ureteral intestinal anastomosis most frequently occur:
    a. at the ureteral pelvic junction.
    b. in the right ureter several centimeters proximal to the ureteral intestinal anastomosis.
    c. on the left side where the ureter crosses the aorta.
    d. in the mid ureter.
13. Renal deterioration after a conduit diversion with normal kidneys occurs in what percent of renal units?
    a. 20%
    b. 40%
    c. 60%
    d. 80%

14. The most common cause of death in patients with ureterosigmoidostomies over the long term is:
    a. cancer.
    b. renal failure.
    c. electrolyte abnormalities.
    d. the primary disease.
15. The minimal GFR in mL/min necessary for a continent diversion is:
    a. 70.
    b. 50.
    c. 35.
    d. 25.
16. The urinary diversion with the least number of interoperative and immediate postoperative complications is:
    a. ileal conduit.
    b. colon conduit.
    c. Koch pouch.
    d. Indiana pouch.
17. The jejunal conduit syndrome is manifested by:
    a. hyperchloremic metabolic acidosis.
    b. hypochloremic metabolic alkalosis.
    c. hyperkalemic, hyponatremic metabolic acidosis.
    d. hypokalemic, hyponatremic metabolic alkalosis.
18. The primary advantage of a transverse colon conduit is:
    a. its ease of construction.
    b. the ability to perform a nonrefluxing anastomosis.
    c. less likely to be injured by radiation.
    d. reduced electrolyte problems.
19. Total body potassium depletion is most common in:
    a. ureterosigmoidostomy.
    b. ileal conduit.
    c. colon conduit.
    d. sigmoid conduit.
20. In urinary intestinal diversion serum creatinine may not be an accurate reflection of renal function because of:
    a. interfering substances.
    b. tubule secretion.
    c. tubule reabsorption.
    d. bowel reabsorption.
21. Patients with urinary diversions who have a hyperchloremic metabolic acidosis over time:
    a. retain the ability to maintain the acidosis.
    b. lose the ability for electrolyte transport in the intestinal segments.
    c. compensate for the metabolic acidosis, thus eliminating risk.
    d. intermittently absorb ammonia when infection is present.
22. Bone density abnormalities:
    a. are unlikely to occur with ileum.
    b. are most likely to occur with colon.
    c. are more common in hyperchloremic metabolic acidosis.
    d. are common in total body potassium depletion.
23. Urinary intestinal diversion's effect on growth in children:
    a. is unknown.
    b. is not a problem.
    c. has been shown to adversely affect it.
    d. accelerates growth.
24. Cancer occurring in urinary intestinal diversion is most likely to occur in:
    a. augmentations.
    b. colon conduits.
    c. ileal conduits.
    d. ureterosigmoidostomies.
25. Reconfiguring the bowel over the long term:
    a. results in decreased motor activity.
    b. increased volume.
    c. decreased metabolic complications.
    d. decreased absorption of solutes.
26. The syndrome of severe metabolic alkalosis is most prone to occur in patients who have:
    a. decreased aldosterone levels.
    b. jejunum interposed in the urinary tract.
    c. total body potassium depletion.
    d. elevated gastrin levels.

ANSWERS

1. **c. never extend to the pylorus.** When a wedge of fundus is employed, it should not include a significant portion of the antrum and should never extend to the pylorus or all the way to the lesser curve of the stomach.
2. **c. it has multiple arcades.** The ileum, being more distal in location, has a smaller diameter. It has multiple arterial arcades, and the vessels in the arcades are smaller than those in the jejunum.
3. **b. Hypochloremic.** Complications specific to the use of stomach include the hematuria-dysuria syndrome and uncontrollable metabolic alkalosis in some patients. When stomach is used, a hypochloremic, hypokalemic metabolic alkalosis may ensue.
4. **d. ileum.** The incidence of postoperative bowel obstruction is 4% to 10%. Colon, stomach, and sigmoid result in a 4% incidence, less than that occurring with ileum.
5. **c. total number of bacteria in the bowel.** The mechanical preparation reduces the amount of feces, whereas the antibiotic preparation reduces the bacterial count. A mechanical bowel preparation reduces the total number of bacteria but not their concentration.
6. **a. before the patient is anesthetized.** Systemic antibiotics must be given before the operative event if they are to be effective.
7. **a. use of prior irradiated bowel.** In one study of urinary intestinal diversion, 75% of the lethal complications that occurred in the postoperative period were related to the bowel. Eighty percent of these patients had received radiation before the intestinal surgery.
8. **b. less compatible with urine.** In general, sutured anastomoses are preferable for intestinal segments that are exposed to urine.

9. **c. reduces postoperative vomiting.** There was no significant difference in major intestinal complications between the two study groups; however, those who did not have gastric decompression showed a much greater incidence of abdominal distention, nausea, and vomiting.
10. **b. placed through the belly of the rectus muscle.** All stomas should be placed through the belly of the rectus muscle and be located at the peak of the infraumbilical fat roll.
11. **a. the obese patient.** The loop end ileostomy obviates some of these problems and is usually easier to perform than the ileal end stoma in the patient who is obese.
12. **c. on the left side where the ureter crosses the aorta.** It is important to note that ureteral strictures also occur away from the ureterointestinal anastomosis. This stricture is most common in the left ureter and is usually found as the ureter crosses over the aorta beneath the inferior mesenteric artery.
13. **a. 20%.** Patients who are studied over the long term show a significant degree of renal deterioration. Indeed, 20% of renal units have shown significant anatomic deterioration.
14. **b. renal failure.** The most common cause of death in patients who have had a ureterosigmoidostomy for more than 15 years is acquired renal disease (i.e., sepsis or renal failure).
15. **c. 35 mL/min.** If the patient is able to achieve a urine pH of 5.8 or less after an ammonium chloride load, has a urine osmolality of 600 mOsm/kg or greater in response to water deprivation, has a glomerular filtration rate that exceeds 35 mL/min, and has minimal protein in the urine, the patient may be considered for a retentive diversion.
16. **a. ileal conduit.** It is the simplest type of conduit diversion to perform and is associated with the fewest number of intraoperative and immediately postoperative complications.
17. **c. hyperkalemic, hyponatremic metabolic acidosis.** The early and long-term complications are similar to those listed for ileal conduit except that the electrolyte abnormality that occurs is hyperkalemic, hyponatremic metabolic acidosis instead of the hyperchloremic metabolic acidosis of ileal diversion.
18. **c. less likely to be injured by radiation.** The transverse colon is used when one wants to be sure that the segment of conduit employed has not been irradiated in individuals who have received extensive pelvic irradiation.
19. **a. ureterosigmoidostomy.** Hypokalemia and total body depletion of potassium may occur in patients with urinary intestinal diversion. This is more common in patients with ureterosigmoidostomies than it is with patients who have other types of urinary intestinal diversion.
20. **d. bowel reabsorption.** Because urea and creatinine are reabsorbed by both the ileum and the colon, serum concentrations of urea and creatinine do not necessarily accurately reflect renal function.
21. **a. retain the ability to maintain the acidosis.** The ability to establish a hyperchloremic metabolic acidosis, however, appears to be retained by most segments of ileum and colon over time.
22. **c. are more common in persistent hyperchloremic metabolic acidosis.** Osteomalacia in urinary intestinal diversion may be due to persistent acidosis, vitamin D resistance, and excessive calcium loss by the kidney. It appears that the degree to which each of these contributes to the syndrome may vary from patient to patient.
23. **c. has been shown to adversely affect it.** There is considerable evidence to suggest that urinary intestinal diversion has a detrimental effect on growth and development.
24. **d. ureterosigmoidostomies.** The highest incidence of cancer occurs when the transitional epithelium is juxtaposed to the colonic epithelium and both are bathed by feces.
25. **b. increased volume.** Reconfiguring bowel usually increases the volume, but its effect on motor activity and wall tension over the long term is unclear at this time.
26. **d. elevated gastrin levels.** The syndrome of severe metabolic alkalosis is most likely to occur in patients with high resting gastrin levels who are dehydrated and fail to empty their pouch in a timely manner.

81

Cutaneous Continent Urinary Diversion

MITCHELL C. BENSON • JAMES M. McKIERNAN • CARL A. OLSSON

QUESTIONS

1. A 45-year-old man underwent ileal conduit diversion as a child for bladder exstrophy. He reports requesting continent diversion. Serum creatinine is 2.0 mg/dL. Loopogram shows bilaterally thin ureters with small kidneys. Which is the best procedure?
   a. Ureterosigmoidostomy
   b. T-pouch utilizing the ileal conduit
   c. Abandon continent diversion
   d. Penn pouch utilizing the ileal conduit
2. A 45-year-old man underwent ileal conduit urinary diversion as a child for bladder exstrophy. He presents requesting continent diversion. Serum creatinine is 2.0 mg/dL. Loopogram shows bilateral hydronephrosis and a pipe-stem conduit. What is the best course of action?
   a. Mainz II to avoid problems with dilated ureters
   b. T-pouch abandoning the disease conduit
   c. No continent diversion
   d. Drain the upper tracts and reassess renal function
3. A patient undergoing cystectomy and attempted continent cutaneous diversion has positive ureteral margin biopsies up to 2 cm above each iliac artery, at which point negative biopsies are seen. What is the best course of action?
   a. Utilize the terminal ileum for ureteral implantation and a Mitrofanoff continence mechanism
   b. No continent diversion
   c. Mobilize the kidneys and stretch the ureters to the reservoir
   d. Use a T-pouch with a long chimney
4. Preservation of the ileocecal valve can be maintained with which catheterizable pouch?
   a. T-pouch or Kock pouch
   b. LeBag
   c. Indiana pouch
   d. Mainz I or II
5. In which procedure to repair a nipple valve would resection of additional bowel be required routinely?
   a. Stones on exposed staples
   b. Nipple valve slippage
   c. Nipple valve atrophy
   d. Pin-hole leak
6. A 10-year-old child has undergone urinary diversion by ileal conduit for myelomeningocele. The conduit was replaced on two occasions for pipe-stem conduit development. The conduit is again affected by the same process. The patient's family wishes a continent diversion. Which is the best procedure?
   a. Ureterosigmoidostomy
   b. Revise the conduit
   c. T-pouch utilizing the ileal conduit
   d. Penn pouch utilizing the ileal conduit
7. A patient with chronic active hepatitis and invasive bladder cancer associated with intravesical carcinoma in situ reports for treatment. The serum creatinine concentration is 1.0 mg/dL. Prostatic urethral biopsy shows mild atypia. What is the best approach? Cysoprostatectomy and
   a. T-pouch
   b. ileal conduit
   c. right colon reservoir
   d. Mainz II
8. The highest reoperation rate in catheterizable pouches occurs with what type of sphincter?
   a. In situ appendix
   b. Imbricated terminal ileum
   c. Plicated terminal ileum
   d. Nipple valves
9. Which of the Mitrofanoff sphincter deficiencies can be corrected surgically?
   a. Length of the appendix
   b. Absence of the appendix
   c. Stenosis of the appendix
   d. All of the above
10. Hematuria and skin breakdown may occur with what type of pouch?
    a. T
    b. Gastric
    c. Mainz
    d. Right colon

11. Preoperative colonoscopy is indicated in candidates for which reservoir procedures?
    a. Small intestinal
    b. Gastric
    c. Rectal
    d. All of the above

12. What condition may complicate absorbable stapled ileal pouches?
    a. Urine leaks
    b. Valve failure
    c. Hydronephrosis
    d. Ischemic pouch contraction

13. Anastomotic transitional cell carcinoma develops in a patient who has undergone cystectomy and continent cutaneous urinary diversion. What is the best treatment?
    a. Distal ureterectomy and reimplant
    b. Conversion to ileal conduit
    c. Ileal ureter interposition
    d. Nephroureterectomy

14. Drainage of mucus is hardest with which sphincteric mechanism?
    a. Kock valve
    b. In situ appendix
    c. Imbricated ileum
    d. Plicated ileum

15. Which continent cutaneous diversion allows for a refluxing ureteroenteric anastomosis?
    a. Mitrofanoff with implantation of the ureters into terminal ileum
    b. Mitrofanoff with implantation of the ureters into the colon
    c. T-pouch
    d. Kock pouch

16. Three years after radical cystectomy and construction of a Kock pouch, a patient presents with right lower quadrant discomfort and associated spurts of urinary leakage. What is the most important diagnostic test?
    a. CT
    b. IVP
    c. Urine culture and sensitivity
    d. Cystogram of pouch

17. Three years after cystectomy and Kock pouch for bladder cancer, a patient presents with recurrent episodes of bilateral pyelonephritis. What is the most important diagnostic test?
    a. CT
    b. IVP
    c. Urine culture and sensitivity
    d. Cystogram of pouch

18. What is the most important feature in preventing nipple valve slippage?
    a. Absorbable staples
    b. Length of the intussusception
    c. Resecting adequate mesentery
    d. Attaching the nipple valve to the side wall of the reservoir

19. In a patient with pipe-stem conduit and bilateral hydronephrosis requesting conversion to continent urinary diversion, nephrostomy drainage results in clearance values of 40 mL/min on the right and 10 mL/min on the left. Serum creatinine is 1.8 mg/dL. What should the surgeon do?
    a. Mainz II to avoid problems with his dilated ureters
    b. T-pouch abandoning the disease conduit
    c. No continent diversion
    d. Ureterosigmoidostomy

20. A patient with squamous cell cancer of the bladder desires cystectomy and continent diversion. He has lost 10 pounds in the month before surgery. Which procedure is helpful in his management?
    a. Increase oral intake
    b. Preoperative hyperalimentation
    c. Postoperative hyperalimentation
    d. Proceed directly with surgery

21. Preoperative evaluation with an oatmeal enema is required in which procedure?
    a. Right colon reservoir
    b. Mainz I pouch
    c. Mainz II procedure
    d. LeBag pouch

22. Follow-up urinary cytology and colonoscopy should be employed in which type of continent diversion?
    a. Ureterosigmoidostomy
    b. Mainz II procedure
    c. Right colon reservoir
    d. All of the above

23. Nocturnal emptying of the patient's reservoir is required in which type of diversion?
    a. Ureterosigmoidostomy
    b. T-pouch
    c. Right colon reservoir
    d. Penn pouch

24. The appendix is sacrificed in patients undergoing which pouch construction?
    a. Indiana
    b. LeBag
    c. Mainz I
    d. All of the above

25. Pouch stone development occurs most commonly with which pouch operation?
    a. T-pouch
    b. Kock pouch
    c. Penn pouch
    d. Gastric-ileal composite pouch

26. What is the typical catheter used for appendiceal sphincters?
    a. 22-Fr straight-tipped
    b. 22-Fr coudé-tipped
    c. 14-Fr straight-tipped
    d. 14-Fr coudé-tipped

27. Urinary retention resulting from continent diversion occurs most commonly with what type of sphincter?
    a. Appendiceal stoma
    b. Benchekroun hydraulic valve
    c. Nipple valve sphincter
    d. Imbricated Indiana mechanism

28. Immediate postoperative initial pouch capacity is least in which pouch?
    a. T- or Kock ileal
    b. Right colon
    c. Gastric
    d. Mainz I

29. Elevated pouch pressures would potentially facilitate the continence mechanism seen with which valve or sphincter?
    a. Benchekroun ileal valve
    b. Kock valve
    c. Appendiceal tunnel
    d. All of the above

30. The long-term failure rate of continence mechanisms is greatest with which mechanism?
    a. T-pouch valve
    b. Appendiceal tunnel
    c. Benchekroun hydraulic valve
    d. Imbricated terminal ileum
31. Absorbable staples in continent urinary diversion is best suited to what type of reservoir pouch?
    a. Ileal
    b. Right colon
    c. Gastric-ileal composite
    d. None of the above
32. When creating a large intestinal reservoir from absorbable staples, why is bowel eversion necessary?
    a. Staples should not be utilized in reservoir construction
    b. To inspect the inside of the reservoir
    c. To avoid injury to the mesenteric blood supply
    d. To allow application of the second row of staples
33. Which of the following patients may not be suitable candidates for continent urinary diversion? Those with
    a. Multiple sclerosis
    b. Quadriplegia
    c. Mental impairment or fraility
    d. All of the above
34. Which of the following sutures should not be used in the construction of a reservoir?
    a. Chromic catgut
    b. Plain catgut
    c. Silk
    d. Polyglycolic acid (Dexon)
35. Which of the following diversions places the patient at risk for the development of a late malignancy?
    a. Ureterosigmoidostomy
    b. T-pouch
    c. Mainz II
    d. All of the above
36. Which of the following diversions places the patient at greatest risk for the development of a late malignancy?
    a. Ureterosigmoidostomy
    b. T-pouch
    c. Mainz II
    d. Indiana reservoir
37. Continent urinary diversion has which of the following effects?
    a. Results in a psychotic depression
    b. Results in an improved psychosocial adjustment
    c. Results in violent behavior
    d. None of the above
38. Which of the following is NOT true of continent urinary diversion?
    a. The gold standard of urinary diversion
    b. A safe and reliable urinary diversion
    c. Associated with an increased complication rate.
    d. Appropriate for selected individuals
39. Which of the following circumstances would contraindicate a rectal bladder?
    a. Prior pelvic irradiation
    b. Dilated ureters
    c. Lax anal sphincter tone
    d. All of the above
40. During the construction of a continent cutaneous urinary diversion, the surgeon should do what?
    a. Not be concerned about the continence mechanism since the mechanism will mold to the catheter
    b. Not test the continence mechanism for ease of catheterization.
    c. Not be concerned about pouch integrity, the pouch will seal itself
    d. None of the above
41. If the urine in a continent cutaneous reservoir is found to be infected, what should be done?
    a. Nothing needs to be done in the absence of symptoms.
    b. The urine should always be sterilized with appropriate antibiotics.
    c. The infection should be eradicated and prophylactic antibiotics prescribed.
    d. IVP to check for upper tract damage.
42. The most appropriate and conservative care for pouch rupture is which of the following?
    a. Broad-spectrum antibiotic therapy
    b. Careful radiologic imaging and antibiotic therapy
    c. Surgical exploration for repair of the rupture and broad-spectrum antibiotic therapy
    d. Pouch drainage and broad-spectrum antibiotic therapy
43. The first pouch to employ the Mitrofanoff principle was the:
    a. Mainz I.
    b. Penn.
    c. Kock.
    d. Indiana.
44. Which of the following represents the advantage of the gastric pouch?
    a. Electrolyte reabsorption is reduced
    b. Absorptive malabsorption is avoided
    c. Acid urine may reduce the risk of infection
    d. All of the above
45. When converting from an ileal conduit to a continent diversion, what should be done with the conduit? It should be:
    a. discarded because it is older and subject to higher complications.
    b. preserved for the ureteroileal anastomosis.
    c. incorporated into the continent diversion when possible.
    d. None of the above
46. Which of the following is true of absorbable staples?
    a. Their use has been shown to shorten operative time.
    b. They are safe and reliable.
    c. Unlike nonabsorbable staples, they must not be overlapped.
    d. All of the above.

ANSWERS

1. **c. Abandon continent diversion**. A creatinine level greater than 1.8 mg/dL indicates a level of renal function insufficient for continent diversion.
2. **d. Drain the upper tracts and reassess renal function**. The best course of action is to place ureteral cutaneous stents bilaterally (bypassing the pipe-stem segment) and reassess urinary function. In evaluating the hydronephrotic patient with impaired renal function for continent diversion, upper tract drainage is advised. If necessary, bilateral nephrostomy tubes can be employed.
3. **a. Utilize the terminal ileum for ureteral implantation and a Mitrofanoff continence mechanism**. The best course of action is to perform a right colon reservoir with anastomosis of the ureters to the terminal ileum. The appendix or other pseudo-appendiceal (Mitrofanoff) mechanisms can be used for continence. The terminal ileum can accommodate short ureters.
4. **a. T-pouch or Kock pouch**. Preservation of the ileocecal valve can be maintained with the T- or Kock pouch. All other pouches are of right colon, so that the ileocecal valve is sacrificed.
5. **c. Nipple valve atrophy**. Nipple valve atrophy requires that a new nipple valve be made of additional bowel.
6. **b. Revise the conduit**. With significant small bowel compromise as well as loss of the ileocecal valve in a neurogenic bladder patient, severe diarrhea may ensue.
7. **b. cystoprostatectomy and an ileal conduit**. The best approach is cystoprostatectomy and a conduit. Normal hepatic function is mandated in any patient undergoing continent diversion.
8. **d. Nipple valves**. The highest reoperation rate is associated with nipple valve sphincter failure.
9. **d. All of the above**. The caliber of Mitrofanoff mechanisms, the length of the appendix, stenosis, and even absence of the appendix can be resolved by surgical variations.
10. **b. Gastric pouch**. Hematuria and cutaneous skin erosion may occur with a gastric pouch. With gastric reservoirs or composite reservoirs, the low pH of the urine may lead to hematuria and cutaneous breakdown.
11. **c. Rectal reservoirs.** Preoperative colonoscopy is relatively indicated in candidates for any pouch. Any pouch utilizing colon mandates preoperative colonic evaluation.
12. **d. Ischemic pouch contraction.** Because of the overlap of staple lines in absorbable stapled ileal pouches, ischemic pouch contraction may occur.
13. **a. Distal ureterectomy and reimplant**. An additional segment of ileum can serve as a proximal limb to the reservoir. If nephrectomy is necessary, careful attention must be paid to the residual renal function.
14. **b. In-situ appendix**. The small-diameter catheter used in draining appendiceal sphincter pouches allows for less effective mucus drainage.
15. **a. Mitrofanoff with implantation of the ureters into terminal ileum**. The implantation of the ureters into the terminal ileum may allow for reflux. The ileal cecal valve and the isoperistaltic ileal segment may either prevent or diminish reflux.
16. **c. Urine culture and sensitivity**. The most important diagnostic test is urine culture. The symptoms described are those of pouchitis. This is treated by appropriate antibiotic therapy.
17. **d. Pouch-o-gram**. The proximal nipple valve may have failed, leading to reflux and pyelonephritis. This is tested by the pouch-o-gram.
18. **d. Attaching the nipple valve to the side wall of the reservoir**. This results in a relative lengthening of the valve rather than a foreshortening of the valve with pouch filling.
19. **c. No continent diversion**. In this case, although the serum creatinine level returns to 1.8 mg/dL, the clearance value measured is less than the 60 mL/min required for continent diversion. Continent diversion should be abandoned, and simple replacement of the conduit considered.
20. **b. Preoperative hyperalimentation**. The 10-pound weight loss indicates a potential for nutritional depletion or metastatic disease. A careful search for metastatic disease should be undertaken. For the patient with nutritional depletion, preoperative hyperalimentation is suggested to be of value.
21. **c. Mainz II procedure.** Any procedure that relies on the intact anal sphincter for continence (i.e., the Mainz II pouch) requires an assessment of the sphincter before carrying out the operation. This can be assessed by an oatmeal enema, which mimics the constitution of a combination of the urinary and fecal streams.
22. **d. All of the above.** Follow-up urinary cytology and colonoscopy is mandatory with any procedure that combines urinary and fecal streams. Because of an increased risk of malignancy even in the absence of admixture of urine and stool, all large intestinal pouches should be subjected to annual investigation by pouchoscopy as well as cytology.
23. **a. Ureterosigmoidostomy.** Nocturnal reservoir emptying may be required with any of the continent cutaneous reservoirs to prevent overdistention and possible rupture but is mandatory with ureterosigmoidostomy owing to the additional risk of metabolic acidosis.
24. **d. All of the above**. The appendix is sacrificed in patients undergoing Indiana, LeBag, and Mainz I pouch reconstruction because it can serve as a nidus for infection and abscess formation.
25. **b. Kock**. Pouch stone development occurs most commonly with the Kock pouch. Despite the exclusion of distal staples, the stapling techniques used to secure nipple valves will lead to a higher potential for stone development than in pouches not requiring nipple valves.
26. **d. 14-Fr coudé-tipped.** Larger catheters will not fit into the appendix. A straight catheter is more difficult to pass.
27. **c. Nipple valve sphincter.** Urinary retention occurs most commonly with nipple valve sphincters. If the chimney of the nipple valve is not near the surface of the abdomen, the catheter can be misdirected into folds of bowel rather than through the nipple valve.
28. **a. T- or Kock ileal.** Immediate postoperative initial pouch capacity is least in ileal reservoirs (i.e., the T- or Kock pouch). Small bowel pouches have initial capacities that are much lower than right colon pouches.
29. **a. Benchekroun ileal valve**. Because the Benchekroun ileal valve is hydraulic, higher pouch pressures would facilitate continence, whereas lower pouch pressures might lead to incontinence.

30. **c. Benchekroun hydraulic valve.** The long-term outcome of Benchekroun hydraulic ileal valve mechanisms is possibly the worst of all reported sphincteric mechanisms.

31. **b. Right colon reservoir.** The use of absorbable staples is best suited to large bowel pouches. With large bowel pouches there is no problem with staple lines causing subsequent bowel ischemia.

32. **d. To allow application of the second row of staples.** In an absorbable-stapled right colon pouch, bowel eversion is required to allow for the application of the second row of staples. Staple lines must not cross because this will prevent the bulky, absorbable staples from seating properly. The bowel is everted, a cut is made beyond the end of the staple line, and the next line of staples is applied.

33. **d. All of the above.** Patients with multiple sclerosis, quadriplegic individuals, and the very frail or mentally impaired patient will at some point in their lives require the care of members of the family or visiting nurse attendance; and we view such patients as poor candidates for any form of continent diversion.

34. **c. Silk.** All sutures utilized in the urinary tract should be absorbable.

35. **d. All of the above.** Late malignancy has been reported in all bowel segments exposed to the urinary stream, whether or not there is a commingling with feces.

36. **a. Ureterosigmoidostomy.** Although late malignancy has been reported in all bowel segments exposed to the urinary stream, whether or not there is a commingling with feces, the mixture of urothelium, urine, and feces poses the greatest risk.

37. **b. Results in an improved psychosocial adjustment.** Many studies from throughout the world have suggested an improved psychosocial adjustment of the patient undergoing continent urinary and fecal diversion compared with those patients with diversions requiring collecting appliances.

38. **a. The gold standard of urinary diversion.** Ileal conduit should be considered the "gold standard" of urinary diversion.

39. **d. All of the above.** Dilated ureters, pelvic irradiation, and lax anal sphincteric tone are all contraindications to the procedure.

40. **d. None of the above.** The continence mechanism must be catheterized to ensure ease of catheter passage. This is an extremely important and crucial maneuver since the inability to catheterize is a serious complication that will often result in the need for reoperation.

41. **a. Nothing needs to be done in the absence of symptoms.** Most authors would suggest that bacteriuria in the absence of symptomatology does not warrant antibiotic treatment.

42. **c. Surgical exploration for repair of the rupture and broad-spectrum antibiotic therapy.** In general, these patients require immediate pouch decompression, radiologic pouch studies, and surgical exploration with pouch repair. If the amount of urinary extravasation is small and the patient does not have a surgical abdomen, catheter drainage and antibiotic administration may suffice in treating intraperitoneal rupture of a pouch. Patients managed with this conservative approach require careful monitoring.

43. **b. Penn pouch.** The Penn pouch was the first continent diversion employing the Mitrofanoff principle wherein the appendix served as the continence mechanism.

44. **d. All of the above.** Electrolyte reabsorption is greatly diminished, shortening of the absorptive bowel does not occur, and the acid urine may decrease the likelihood of reservoir colonization.

45. **c. It should be incorporated into the continent diversion when possible.** We prefer to utilize the conduit in some form whenever possible. The use of an existing bowel segment has the potential to diminish metabolic sequelae and may result in a lower complication rate.

46. **d. All of the above.** The use of absorbable staplers has substantially reduced the time required to fashion bowel reservoirs and has demonstrated short-term and long-term reliability with respect to reservoir integrity and volume. They must not be overlapped because overlapping will prevent the proper close of the staple.

82

Orthotopic Urinary Diversion

JOHN P. STEIN • DONALD G. SKINNER

QUESTIONS

1. Before 1950, what was the most common form of urinary diversion performed?
   a. Colon conduit
   b. Orthotopic neobladder
   c. Ileal conduit
   d. Ureterosigmoidostomy
2. What long-term complication is NOT commonly associated with ureterosigmoidostomy urinary diversion?
   a. Renal deterioration
   b. Hyperchloremic metabolic acidosis
   c. Hypercalcemia
   d. Secondary malignancy
3. What is the most common long-term complication associated with the ileal conduit?
   a. Ureteroileal stenosis
   b. Pyelonephritis
   c. Stomal stenosis
   d. Nephrolithiasis
4. With regard to orthotopic urinary diversion, all the following statements are true EXCEPT which one?
   a. Voiding is accomplished by a Valsalva maneuver and relaxation of the external sphincter.
   b. Most patients are continent.
   c. The rhabdosphincter complex is responsible for the continent mechanism.
   d. Most patients require intermittent catheterization to empty their neobladder.
5. With regard to renal function before continent urinary diversion, which of the following statements is TRUE?
   a. A minimum creatinine clearance of 60 mL/min should be documented.
   b. A serum creatinine value of 2.0 mg/dL or less should be documented.
   c. Patients with ureteral obstruction should first undergo decompression to determine the true baseline level.
   d. All of the above.
6. Patients with borderline renal function may be best served with what form of orthotopic diversion?
   a. Gastric neobladder
   b. Ileal neobladder
   c. Colonic neobladder
   d. Ileal colonic neobladder
7. Regarding patient age and orthotopic diversion, which of the following statements is TRUE?
   a. Orthotopic diversion should not be performed in patients older than 80 years of age.
   b. Orthotopic diversion should not be performed in patients younger than 30 years of age.
   c. Differentiation between physiologic and chronologic age should be made.
   d. Advanced age is an absolute contraindication to orthotopic diversion.
8. Which of the following is an absolute contraindication to an orthotopic bladder substitute?
   a. An obese patient
   b. A patient with lymph node–positive bladder cancer after cystectomy
   c. A female with bladder neck tumor involvement with an uninvolved urethra
   d. A male with an intraoperative positive distal surgical margin at the proximal urethra
9. Which orthotopic bladder substitute shape will accommodate the largest volume with the lowest pressures?
   a. Tube structure
   b. Cylindrical structure
   c. Spherical structure
   d. U-shaped structure
10. Innervation of the striated rhabdosphincter complex, which is crucial in the continence mechanism in patients undergoing orthotopic diversion, is from which of the following?
    a. The parasympathetic fibers from the sacral segments
    b. The sympathetic fibers from the superior hypogastric plexus
    c. A combination of both the parasympathetic and sympathetic fibers
    d. The pudendal innervation
11. To best preserve the pudendal innervation and the continence mechanism in patients undergoing cystectomy and orthotopic diversion, one should perform:
    a. minimal dissection along the pelvic floor.
    b. minimal dissection along the lateral aspect of the rectum.
    c. nerve-sparing cystectomy.
    d. minimal dissection along the lateral aspect of the vagina.

12. The ultimate decision to perform an orthotopic bladder substitution after cystectomy for bladder cancer can be made:
    a. preoperatively at the time of consultation with the patient.
    b. only if there is not gross evidence of extravesical tumor extension.
    c. if the urethra is palpably normal.
    d. if the intraoperative frozen section analysis of the distal surgical margin (urethra) is normal.

13. In women who have a penetrating posterior bladder wall tumor, it is best to:
    a. never perform an orthotopic bladder substitution.
    b. remove the anterior vaginal wall en bloc with the bladder.
    c. remove the entire vagina en bloc with the bladder.
    d. strip the bladder off the anterior bladder wall.

14. Options for vaginal reconstruction in women at the time of anterior exenteration for bladder cancer include which of the following?
    a. Myocutaneous flap
    b. Detubularized bowel
    c. Omental flap
    d. All of the above

15. With regard to urethral recurrence after cystectomy for transitional cell carcinoma of the bladder, which of the following statements is TRUE?
    a. Overall risk for men of a urethral recurrence after cystectomy is approximately 10%.
    b. Urethral recurrence is not thought to represent a failure of definitive treatment of the primary tumor but rather a manifestation of the multicentric defect of transitional cell carcinoma.
    c. Prostatic tumor involvement with the primary tumor is a risk factor for a urethra recurrence in the retained urethra after cystectomy.
    d. All of the above.

16. What is the greatest risk factor for a urethral tumor recurrence after cystectomy for bladder cancer?
    a. Lymph node tumor involvement
    b. Carcinoma in situ
    c. Tumor multifocality
    d. Prostatic stroma involvement

17. Which of the following statements is TRUE in patients undergoing cystectomy with the intent for orthotopic reconstruction for bladder cancer?
    a. Preoperative prostate biopsies are mandatory in all patients considering orthotopic diversion to exclude prostatic tumor involvement.
    b. Intraoperative frozen section analysis of the urethra (distal surgical margin) is mandatory in all patients considering orthotopic diversion.
    c. Patients with a history of prostatic mucosa tumor involvement must be excluded from orthotopic diversion.
    d. Intraoperative frozen section analysis of the urethra is an unreliable method to evaluate for tumor involvement.

18. Which of the following statements is TRUE regarding urethral tumor involvement in women with bladder cancer?
    a. Bladder neck tumor involvement is the most significant risk factor for urethral tumor involvement.
    b. Urethra is the most common site of tumor involvement.
    c. Concomitant urethral tumor involvement is found.
    d. Lymph node–positive disease is found.

19. Which of the following statements is TRUE regarding a woman with a history of transitional cell carcinoma of the bladder and with bladder neck tumor involvement? She has:
    a. approximately an 80% chance of having tumor in the urethra.
    b. approximately a 50% chance of having tumor in the urethra.
    c. approximately a 20% chance of having tumor in the urethra.
    d. an extremely low (<5%) chance of having tumor in the urethra.

20. Which of the following statements is TRUE regarding urethral tumor involvement in women with bladder cancer?
    a. They will almost always have bladder neck tumor involvement.
    b. Approximately 50% with bladder neck or anterior vaginal wall involvement will have concomitant urethral tumor involvement.
    c. Anterior vaginal wall tumor involvement is a significant risk factor for urethral tumor involvement.
    d. All of the above.

21. Intraoperative frozen section analysis of the proximal urethra in women considered for orthotopic diversion and who are undergoing cystectomy for bladder cancer is:
    a. an unreliable means of evaluating the proximal urethra.
    b. not performed in women with bladder neck tumor involvement.
    c. mandatory to exclude tumor in all women considered for an orthotopic bladder substitution.
    d. necessary only in those with a history of multifocal carcinoma in situ.

22. Which of the following statements is TRUE regarding intraoperative frozen section analysis of the proximal urethra in patients considered for orthotopic diversion? It is:
    a. mandatory in all women.
    b. mandatory in all men.
    c. a reliable method for evaluating the urethra.
    d. All of the above.

23. Which of the following statements is TRUE regarding local pelvic recurrence after radical cystectomy for bladder cancer? It:
    a. occurs in less than 10% of all patients.
    b. has a rate of approximately 50% in patients with lymph node–positive disease.
    c. has a rate of approximately 30% in patients with extravesical, lymph node–negative disease.
    d. has a rate that does not relate to the pathologic subgroup.

24. Patients who develop a local pelvic tumor recurrence after radical cystectomy and orthotopic diversion should in general:
    a. expect involvement with the neobladder.
    b. undergo conversion to a cutaneous form of diversion.
    c. expect normal neobladder function.
    d. have bilateral percutaneous nephrostomy tubes placed.

25. Orthotopic urinary diversion after definitive radiation therapy:
    a. is an absolute contraindication.
    b. is performed in properly selected individuals.
    c. is associated with a significantly higher incidence of urinary retention rate.
    d. requires intermittent catheterization in most patients.

26. Male patients undergoing orthotopic diversion after definitive radiation therapy should be counseled that they may:
    a. require placement of an artificial urinary sphincter.
    b. have a significantly high incidence of urinary retention rate.
    c. require intermittent catheterization.
    d. All of the above.

27. Which of the following statements concerning reflux prevention is TRUE? It is:
    a. controversial only in those undergoing a continent cutaneous form of urinary diversion.
    b. not controversial in those undergoing an orthotopic form of urinary diversion.
    c. clearly shown in randomized studies not to be a crucial issue in patients undergoing an orthotopic form of urinary diversion.
    d. None of the above.
28. Which of the following statements concerning patients undergoing an orthotopic bladder substitution is TRUE? They may:
    a. generally have infected urine.
    b. always require intermittent catheterization to empty the neobladder.
    c. should have an antireflux mechanism incorporated regardless of the incidence of obstruction associated with the antireflux technique.
    d. All of the above.
29. Which of the following statements is TRUE regarding renal deterioration in patients undergoing an ileal conduit? It may:
    a. occur even in the presence of normal radiographic studies.
    b. take 20 years to occur.
    c. be related to the combination of obstruction and reflux of infected urinary constituents.
    d. All of the above.
30. Complications associated with the antireflux intussuscepted nipple valve of the Kock ileal reservoir occur in what percent of patients?
    a. 10%
    b. 30%
    c. 80%
    d. 90%
31. What is the most common complication associated with the antireflux intussuscepted nipple valve of the Kock ileal reservoir?
    a. Afferent nipple stenosis
    b. Prolapse of the afferent nipple (extussusception)
    c. Stones
    d. None of the above
32. Which of the following statements is TRUE regarding the "serous-lined tunnel" technique to create an antireflux mechanism?
    a. This is a flap-valve technique.
    b. This requires an isoperistaltic afferent limb.
    c. This requires the use of staples to create.
    d. Only ileum can be used to construct this antireflux mechanism.
33. Which of the following statements is TRUE regarding the T-mechanism as described by Stein and Skinner? It:
    a. is a flap-valve technique.
    b. can be incorporated into an antireflux (afferent) and a continent catheterizable (efferent) limb.
    c. can be applied in cases in which there are dilated and or shortened ureters.
    d. All of the above.
34. Which of the following statements is TRUE regarding the orthotopic T-pouch ileal neobladder?
    a. This reservoir maintains the same geometric configuration as the Kock ileal neobladder.
    b. Vascular arcades are preserved to the afferent limb to maintain the blood supply.
    c. No staples are required in the construction of this neobladder.
    d. All of the above.
35. The etiology of Kock pouch stones in the orthotopic ileal neobladder is thought to be related primarily to which of the following?
    a. Infected urine
    b. Retained mucus
    c. Exposed metallic staples
    d. Prolapse of the intussuscepted nipple
36. Which of the following statements is FALSE when comparing an orthotopic neobladder with an ileal conduit?
    a. There is definitely an increased complication rate with an orthotopic form of diversion over an ileal conduit.
    b. The orthotopic reservoir may provide an improved cosmetic result compared with an ileal conduit.
    c. The operative time required to create an orthotopic neobladder is similar to that for an ileal conduit.
    d. The hospitalization required for those receiving an orthotopic neobladder is similar to those receiving an ileal conduit.
37. Which of the following statements is FALSE regarding the application of absorbable stapling techniques to orthotopic diversions?
    a. The application decreases operative time.
    b. Detubularization and folding of the bowel are still required.
    c. The staple line is usually watertight.
    d. Recent advancements have decreased the bulk of the stapler and facilitated the application of this technique.
38. Which of the following statements is TRUE regarding quality of life assessment after cystectomy and urinary diversion?
    a. It is becoming more important.
    b. A well-validated measurement is important in this evaluation.
    c. Methodologic problems limited their conclusions in the past.
    d. All of the above.
39. Which of the following statements is TRUE regarding an orthotopic bladder substitute?
    a. Most patients are continent and volitionally void per urethra.
    b. There is an increased complication rate compared with other forms of diversion.
    c. Quality of life studies clearly favor this diversion.
    d. All of the above.

ANSWERS

1. **d. Ureterosigmoidostomy**. Ureterosigmoidostomy remained the diversion of choice until the late 1950s.
2. **c. Hypercalcemia**. Electrolyte imbalances, renal problems, and secondary malignancies arising at the ureteral implantation site were described.
3. **b. Pyelonephritis**. Problems with stomal stenosis, pyelonephritis, calculus formation, ureteral obstruction, and renal deterioration became more apparent with longer follow-up times (see Table 82-1).
4. **d. Most patients require intermittent catheterization to empty their neobladder**. This form of lower urinary tract reconstruction relies on the intact rhabdosphincter continence mechanism, eliminating the need for intermittent catheterization. Voiding is accomplished by concomitantly increasing intra-abdominal pressure (the Valsalva maneuver), with relaxation of the pelvic floor. The majority of patients undergoing orthotopic reconstruction are continent.
5. **d. All of the above**. Permanently compromised renal function (serum creatinine level greater than 2.0 mg/dL) should be considered a contraindication to continent urinary diversion. A minimum creatinine clearance of 60 mL/min should be documented before orthotopic diversion. Patients with an elevated serum creatinine value secondary to ureteral obstruction should undergo upper urinary tract decompression (via percutaneous nephrostomy) allowing recovery and re-determination of the true baseline renal function before the decision to perform the particular urinary diversion.
6. **a. Gastric neobladder.** Patients with borderline renal function, who otherwise would be candidates for lower urinary tract reconstruction, may be more appropriate candidates for a gastric form of neobladder.
7. **c. Differentiation between physiologic and chronologic age should be made.** Although controversial, the patient's age alone should not necessarily be a contraindication to orthotopic diversion. Therefore, a differentiation between physiologic and chronologic age should be made.
8. **d. A male with an intraoperative positive distal surgical margin at the proximal urethra.** A contraindication to orthotopic diversion in male and female patients includes those patients demonstrating carcinoma in situ or overt carcinoma of the urethral margin detected on intraoperative frozen section analysis.
9. **c. Spherical structure**. The increase of volume capacity achieved in the intestinal segment depends on its shape; volume is almost double in a U-shaped pouch and is still greater in an S-shaped, a W-shaped, or a Kock pouch, closely resembling that of a sphere.
10. **d. The pudendal innervation**. Most interested investigators agree that the rhabdosphincter is probably supplied by the branches of the pudendal nerve.
11. **a. minimal dissection along the pelvic floor**. In any pelvic surgery that involves maintaining the rhabdosphincter innervation and ultimate function, excessive dissection along the pelvic floor should be avoided, where the branches of the pudendal nerve course to the sphincteric complex. Therefore, minimal dissection should be performed, during any pelvic surgery, along the pelvic floor levator musculature to avoid injury to the rhabdosphincter innervation.
12. **d. if the intraoperative frozen section analysis of the distal surgical margin (urethra) is normal**. Regardless of the technique, frozen section analysis of the distal urethral margin (prostatic apex) on the cystectomy specimen is performed to exclude tumor involvement. The decision to perform an orthotopic bladder substitution is ultimately made at this time.
13. **b. remove the anterior vaginal wall en bloc with the bladder.** Alternatively, in the case of a deeply invasive posterior bladder tumor, with concern for an adequate surgical margin, the anterior vaginal wall may be removed en bloc with the cystectomy specimen.
14. **d. All of the above.** Vaginal reconstruction by a clam-shell (horizontal) or side-to-side (vertical) technique is required. Other means of vaginal reconstruction may include a rectus myocutaneous flap, a detubularized cylinder of ileum, a peritoneal flap, and an omental flap.
15. **d. All of the above.** It is generally believed that urethral tumors in patients with a history of bladder cancer represent a second manifestation of the multicentric defect of the primary transitional cell mucosa that led to the original bladder tumor. The overall risk of a urethral recurrence for transitional cell carcinoma after cystectomy is approximately 10%. There is a growing body of data to suggest that, by far, the most ominous criterion for a urethral tumor recurrence is prostatic urethral involvement.
16. **d. Prostatic stroma involvement.** Collectively, these studies suggest that prostatic stromal invasion is the strongest single predictor for subsequent recurrence in the anterior urethra after cystectomy for bladder cancer.
17. **b. Intraoperative frozen section analysis of the urethra (distal surgical margin) is mandatory in all patients considering orthotopic diversion.** Data are emerging to suggest that it may be reasonable to abandon the preoperative prostatic biopsies and perform frozen section analysis on the prostatic urethral apex at the time of surgery to determine appropriate patients for orthotopic urinary diversion in men.
18. **a. Bladder neck tumor involvement is the most significant risk factor for urethral tumor involvement.** The authors emphasized that the only consistent risk factor found for urethral tumor involvement was concurrent tumor at the bladder neck.
19. **b. approximately a 50% chance of having tumor in the urethra.** All patients with an uninvolved bladder neck also had an uninvolved urethra, whereas approximately 50% of patients with a bladder neck tumor had concomitant urethral tumor involvement.
20. **d. All of the above.** Patients with urethral involvement also had concomitant bladder neck involvement regardless of the presence or absence of carcinoma in situ. In addition to bladder neck involvement, one study identified anterior vaginal wall tumor involvement (P4) as a major risk factor for simultaneous urethral tumor, and 50% of these patients also demonstrated urethral tumors.
21. **c. mandatory to exclude tumor in all women considered for an orthotopic bladder substitution.** These data suggest that intraoperative frozen section analysis of the distal surgical margin may provide an accurate and reliable means of evaluating the proximal urethra and should determine which female patients would be appropriate candidates to undergo orthotopic diversion.
22. **d. All of the above.** Intraoperative frozen section analysis of the distal surgical margin in both men (apical prostatic urethra) and women (proximal urethra) provides an accurate

assessment of the urethra and may appropriately determine candidacy for orthotopic diversion.

23. **a. occurs in less than 10% of all patients.** In this large series, an overall local pelvic recurrence rate of 7% was observed for the entire group of patients.

24. **c. expect normal neobladder function.** One study concluded that most patients may anticipate normal neobladder function even in the presence of recurrent disease or until death. Local recurrence rates after cystectomy are low even in high-risk patients and seldom affect the function of the neobladder or the ability to deliver therapy.

25. **b. is performed in properly selected individuals.** It is becoming more clear that in carefully selected patients, orthotopic lower urinary tract reconstruction can be performed after definitive, full-dose pelvic irradiation.

26. **a. require placement of an artificial urinary sphincter.** All patients should be informed that incontinence rates after salvage cystectomy and orthotopic diversion are significant and in nearly 25% of subjects may require the need for an artificial urinary sphincter placement.

27. **d. None of the above.** Controversy exists regarding the need to incorporate an antireflux mechanism in patients undergoing an orthotopic form of urinary diversion. First, it must be emphasized that it will be only after well-designed, prospective, randomized studies with appropriate patient numbers and with long-term follow-up that a convincing answer can be obtained. To date, this study has not been performed.

28. **a. generally have infected urine.** These data suggest that a significant number of patients with an orthotopic bladder substitute will have chronically infected urinary constituents.

29. **d. All of the above.** Upper tract urinary deterioration may not become clinically apparent until as long as 10 to 20 years after urinary diversion. In addition, deterioration of renal function may occur even in the presence of normal radiographic findings. The development of renal insufficiency was thought to be related to or a combination of high pressures, obstruction, and chronically infected urine.

30. **a. 10%.** An overall complication rate of 10% was observed with the intussuscepted antireflux nipple in more than 800 patients (undergoing either a continent cutaneous or an orthotopic Kock ileal reservoir) with long-term follow-up (median, 6 years).

31. **c. Stones.** The three most common complications related to the intussuscepted afferent nipple included the formation of calculi (usually on exposed staples that secure the afferent nipple valve) in 5%, afferent nipple stenosis (thought to be caused by ischemic changes resulting from the mesenteric stripping required to maintain the intussuscepted limb) in 4%, and extussusception (prolapse of the afferent limb) in 1% of patients.

32. **a. This is a flap-valve technique.** If a tubular structure (ureter, appendix, or intestine) is laid in this trough, the incised intestinal mucosa on either side can be sutured together (covering the tubular structure) and transform the trough into a serous-lined tunnel—an effective flap-valve technique.

33. **d. All of the above.** Stein and Skinner subsequently developed and described a modification of this technique, which has been called the T-mechanism. This flap-valve T-mechanism is a versatile technique that can easily be applied as an antireflux mechanism, as well as a continent cutaneous mechanism. Advantages of this technique include application even in the presence of grossly dilated ureters and/or in the presence of concomitant pathology of the distal ureters that may result in shortened ureteral length.

34. **d. All of the above.** The orthotopic T-pouch ileal neobladder maintains exactly the same geometric configuration as the Kock ileal neobladder, the only difference being the antireflux technique. The unique aspect of the T-pouch is maintaining the vascular arcades by opening the windows of Deaver, which then allows permanent fixation of a segment of ileum within a serous-lined ileal trough to create an effective flap-valve technique.

35. **c. Exposed metallic staples.** Because no exposed staples exist within the reservoir, pouch stones typically associated with exposed metallic staples used to maintain the intussuscepted nipple should not develop.

36. **a. There is definitely an increased complication rate with an orthotopic form of diversion over an ileal conduit.** There was no significant difference in the perioperative mortality and complication rates when comparing these different forms (conduit vs. continent) of urinary diversion. These findings were similar to those from a previous study that found no difference in hospitalization stay, complication rate, and reoperation rate when comparing patients undergoing an ileal conduit and various forms of orthotopic diversion.

37. **c. The staple line is usually watertight.** To reduce the operative time, the use of absorbable staples has been applied in the construction of the urinary reservoir. The initial application of this technology was hampered by the fact that the stapler was bulky and difficult to manipulate. Improvements in the staples and the applicators (absorbable staplers) have now facilitated the application to continent diversion. This technique allows for a secure, watertight staple line.

38. **d. All of the above.** Quality of life issues are becoming increasingly important in the selection of the type of urinary diversion and are likely to play a larger role in future management of patients undergoing lower urinary tract reconstruction after cystectomy. Most of the aforementioned studies, evaluating and comparing quality of life issues in patients undergoing various forms of urinary diversion, have been criticized for the methodologic problems that may limit their conclusions. In the future, large, well-designed, randomized, prospective studies will be required to better understand and evaluate quality of life issues in patients undergoing various forms of urinary diversion. Furthermore, these studies must incorporate well-validated measures or surveys to evaluate patients.

39. **a. Most patients are continent and volitionally void per urethra.** Overall, most patients undergoing orthotopic diversion are continent, have the luxury of voiding every 4 to 6 hours with excellent voided volumes, retain a more routine micturition pattern, and avoid the need for a cutaneous stoma or external urostomy appliance. There is a similar complication rate of orthotopic reservoirs compared with ileal conduits. However, quality of life studies do not sufficiently suggest that the orthotopic neobladder is superior to other forms of diversion.

83

Genital and Lower Urinary Tract Trauma

ALLEN F. MOREY • THOMAS A. ROZANSKI

QUESTIONS

1. Which of the following is an absolute indication for open repair of blunt bladder rupture injury?
   a. Significant extraperitoneal bladder rupture with extravasation of contrast into the scrotum
   b. Significant extraperitoneal bladder rupture with gross hematuria
   c. Significant extraperitoneal bladder rupture that has not healed after 3 weeks of Foley catheter drainage
   d. Intraperitoneal bladder rupture
   e. Significant extraperitoneal bladder rupture associated with pelvic fracture requiring treatment by external fixation
2. Which of the following is TRUE regarding cystography for diagnosis of bladder injury?
   a. If the patient is already undergoing CT for evaluation of associated injuries, CT cystography should be performed via antegrade filling of the bladder after intravenous administration of radiographic contrast material and clamping the Foley catheter.
   b. If plain film cystograms are obtained, oblique films are also obtained.
   c. CT cystogram is best performed with undiluted contrast.
   d. An absolute indication for immediate cystography is the presence of pelvic fracture and microhematuria.
   e. None of the above.
3. Which of the following is TRUE about blunt bladder rupture injuries?
   a. They are present in 90% of patients presenting with pelvic fractures.
   b. They coexist with urethral disruption in 50% of cases.
   c. Extraperitoneal ruptures are always amenable to nonoperative treatment.
   d. High mortality rate is primarily related to nonurologic comorbidities.
   e. They are associated with microhematuria or no hematuria in 40% of cases.
4. The risk of complications from nonoperative treatment of extraperitoneal bladder rupture is increased by associated:
   a. orthopedic injury.
   b. vaginal injury.
   c. urethral injury.
   d. rectal injury.
   e. all of the above.
5. Three months after a urethral distraction injury, a patient develops a 2-cm posterior urethral obliterative stricture. Which of the following is TRUE about the repair?
   a. One-stage, open, perineal anastomotic urethroplasty is preferred.
   b. Orthopedic hardware in the pubic symphysis area is a contraindication to open posterior urethroplasty.
   c. Buccal mucosa graft urethroplasty is recommended.
   d. Urolume stent placement is recommended.
   e. Incontinence is likely after posterior urethral reconstruction surgery.
6. In a blunt trauma patient with pelvic fracture in whom no urine is returned after catheter placement, what is the best method to evaluate urethral injury?
   a. Retrograde urethrography
   b. CT of abdomen and pelvis
   c. Filiforms and followers.
   d. Bladder sonogram
   e. None of the above
7. What is the best method to evaluate suspected penile rupture?
   a. Exploration of the penile corpora through a circumcision incision
   b. Ultrasonography of the penis
   c. Exploration of the penile corpora through a midline scrotal incision
   d. MRI of the penis
   e. Cavernosography

8. During exploration after scrotal gunshot wound, 20% of the left testicular capsule is found to be destroyed. What should the next approach be?
   a. Left orchiectomy
   b. Wet dressings and delayed testicular surgery
   c. Left testicular reconstruction with dermal graft
   d. Close the scrotal laceration and follow with ultrasound
   e. Immediate primary repair of the left testis
9. An 80% transection of the anterior urethra is confirmed after a gunshot wound with a 22-caliber pistol. What is the most appropriate therapy?
   a. Nonsurgical
   b. Spatulated, stented, tensionless, watertight repair of the urethra with absorbable sutures
   c. Suprapubic tube placement
   d. Urethral catheterization alone
   e. Perineal urethrostomy
10. If a patient gets his penis caught in his zipper, what should the first step be?
    a. Local anesthetic block, lubrication, and a single attempt at opening the zipper
    b. Dismantle zipper one tooth at a time
    c. Utilize a bone cutter to disrupt the median bar of the zipper slide
    d. Excise the attached zipper and associated skin and subcutaneous tissue
    e. All children should be examined and treated using anesthesia in the OR
11. The blood in a hematocele is contained in which of the following?
    a. Tunica albuginea
    b. Tunica vaginalis
    c. Dartos muscle
    d. Camper's fascia
    e. Spermatic cord
12. Blunt scrotal trauma that results in testis rupture:
    a. is usually a bilateral process.
    b. is reliably diagnosed by presence of intratesticular hypoechoic areas on ultrasound.
    c. has a degree of hematoma that correlates with the extent of injury.
    d. requires conservative management that results in acceptable viability and function.
    e. is definitively diagnosed during physical examination alone in most cases.
13. Which of the following is TRUE regarding penile amputation injury?
    a. It usually results from aggravated assault.
    b. The severed phallus should be placed directly on ice during transport.
    c. Microvascular reanastomosis is the best method of repair.
    d. Reanastomosis invariably results in erectile dysfunction.
    e. Skin loss is rarely a problem after macroscopic repair.
14. What is the best option for coverage of acute penile skin loss?
    a. Foreskin flap for small distal lesions
    b. Meshed skin graft in a young child
    c. Wet-to-dry dressings
    d. Thigh flaps
    e. Burying penile shaft in scrotal skin tunnel
15. Advantages of open suprapubic tube placement after posterior urethral disruption injuries include:
    a. inspection of bladder.
    b. provision of an opportunity for urethral realignment.
    c. allowance for large-bore catheter insertion.
    d. not jeopardizing continence or potency rates.
    e. all of the above.

ANSWERS

1. **d. Intraperitoneal bladder rupture.** When intraperitoneal bladder laceration occurs after blunt trauma, a large laceration of the bladder dome is usually produced that predisposes to urinary ascites and/or peritonitis if not repaired promptly.
2. **e. None of the above.** The CT cystogram must be performed via retrograde distention of the bladder with dilute contrast. Most bladder lacerations are associated with gross hematuria, not microhematuria.
3. **d. High mortality rate is primarily related to nonurologic comorbidities.** Bladder lacerations occur in roughly 10% of pelvic fractures and often occur in the context of multisystem trauma.
4. **e. All of the above.** All of the above concomitant injuries increase the risk of complications such as abscess, fistula, or incontinence.
5. **a. One-stage, open, perineal anastomotic urethroplasty is preferred.** Posterior urethral reconstruction including excision of the fibrotic segment with distal urethral mobilization and primary anastomosis is associated with the best long-term outcomes after urethral disruption. Incontinence occurs in less than 5% of patients.
6. **a. Retrograde urethrography.** Retrograde urethrography is the most reliable imaging study for urethral evaluation.
7. **a. Exploration of the penile corpora through a circumcision incision.** Penile exploration via a circumcision incision should be performed when a clinical diagnosis of penile rupture is suspected. Whereas MRI has been found to provide accurate imaging, its routine use is not justified in this setting owing to cost and availability constraints.
8. **e. Immediate primary repair of the left testis.** Immediate primary repair should be attempted in the setting of subtotal injury to an otherwise viable testis.
9. **b. Spatulated, stented, tensionless, watertight repair of the urethra with absorbable sutures.** Immediate urethral repair with fine absorbable suture over a Foley catheter is associated with superior outcomes after penetrating injury.
10. **a. Local anesthetic block, lubrication, and a single attempt at opening the zipper.** Local block with lubrication and an attempt at opening the zipper is a simple and often effective solution.
11. **b. Tunica vaginalis.** Blood fills the space between the visceral and parietal layers of the tunica vaginalis.
12. **b. is reliably diagnosed by presence of intratesticular hypoechoic areas on ultrasound.** Testicular rupture is often difficult to detect clinically. Ultrasonic evaluation usually shows intratesticular heterogeneity as a sentinel finding.
13. **c. Microvascular reanastomosis is the best method of repair.** Microvascular reanastomosis is suggested as the preferred treatment modality whenever possible.
14. **a. Foreskin flap for small distal lesions.** Redundant foreskin provides excellent closure when ample viable tissue exists.
15. **e. all of the above.** Antegrade urethral realignment may simplify treatment of the defect, and a large-bore suprapubic catheter will promote identification of the prostatic apex while preventing tube encrustation or obstruction.

84

Lower Urinary Tract Calculi

KHAI-LINH V. HO • JOSEPH W. SEGURA

QUESTIONS

1. Vesical calculus disease is usually associated with what condition in the United States?
   a. Foreign bodies
   b. Urinary tract infections
   c. Catheterization
   d. Bladder outlet obstruction
   e. None of the above
2. Magnesium ammonium phosphate stones are most often formed in association with infection with what bacteria?
   a. *Pseudomonas*
   b. *Providencia*
   c. *Klebsiella*
   d. *Staphylococcus*
   e. *Proteus*
3. Urease-producing bacteria hydrolyze urea into which of the following?
   a. Uric acid
   b. Carbon monoxide
   c. Carbon dioxide
   d. Ammonium
   e. Carbon dioxide and ammonium
4. Which continent diversion has the highest risk of stone formation?
   a. Mainz pouch
   b. Kock pouch
   c. Orthotopic hemi-Kock pouch
   d. Indiana pouch
   e. Cecal reservoir
5. Risk factors for the formation of stones in patients with urinary diversions include all of the following EXCEPT which one?
   a. Hypocitruria
   b. Hyperchloremic metabolic acidosis
   c. Hypercalciuria
   d. Hyperoxaluria
   e. Urinary tract infection
6. What is the single most accurate examination to document the presence of a bladder stone?
   a. Ultrasound
   b. Excretory urogram
   c. CT
   d. Cystoscopy
   e. Plain radiograph (KUB)
7. Appropriate treatment options for bladder calculi include all of the following EXCEPT which one?
   a. Irrigation with Suby solution G
   b. Shockwave lithotripsy
   c. Electrohydraulic lithotripsy
   d. Ultrasonic lithotripsy
   e. Holmium laser lithotripsy
8. Urethral calculi in women are associated with which of the following?
   a. Metabolic disturbances
   b. Urethral stricture
   c. Urethral diverticulum
   d. Foreign bodies
   e. None of the above

ANSWERS

1. **d. Bladder outlet obstruction.** Bladder outlet obstruction may be an etiologic factor in over 75% of bladder calculi cases and is most often related to benign prostatic hyperplasia.
2. **e. *Proteus*.** Whereas all these organisms produce urease, infection with *Proteus* species is most commonly associated with bladder calculi.
3. **e. Carbon dioxide and ammonium.** The urease hydrolyzes urea forming ammonium and carbon dioxide, which increases urinary pH. Alkaline urine promotes supersaturation and precipitation of crystals of magnesium ammonium phosphate and carbonate apatite.
4. **b. Kock pouch.** The Kock pouch has a 4% to 43% incidence of stone formation. The predominant location of calculi in the Kock pouch is along staple lines of the afferent nipple valve. Substituting polyglycolic mesh for Marlex mesh in collar construction and limiting the number of staples reduced the incidence of pouch calculi.
5. **d. Hyperoxaluria.** Patients with augments and diversions often have reabsorption of urinary solutes, especially sulfate and ammonium, through the intestinal segment with resultant metabolic disturbances. Chronic hyperchloremic metabolic acidosis may develop that in turn can result in hypercalciuria, hyperphosphaturia, hypermagnesuria, and hypocitraturia, predisposing the patient to urinary tract calculi.

6. **d. Cystoscopy.** Cystoscopy is the single most accurate examination to document the presence of a bladder calculus. Cystoscopy also assists in surgical planning by identifying prostatic enlargement, bladder diverticulum, or urethral stricture that may need correction before or in conjunction with the treatment of the stone.
7. **a. Irrigation with Suby solution G.** Dissolution as primary treatment for bladder calculi can be protracted and is, now, rarely employed.
8. **c. Urethral diverticulum.** Urethral calculi in females are exceptionally rare due to low rates of bladder calculi and a short urethra that permits passage of many smaller calculi. Calculi in the female urethra are typically associated with urethral diverticulum or urethrocele.

SECTION XVI
PROSTATE

85

Molecular Biology, Endocrinology, and Physiology of the Prostate Gland and Seminal Vesicles

ROBERT VELTRI • RONALD RODRIGUEZ

QUESTIONS

1. Which of the following is not considered a sex accessory tissue?
   a. Prostate gland
   b. Seminal vesicles
   c. Tunica albuginea
   d. Ampullae
   e. Bulbourethral gland
2. Which of the following biologic substances does not appear in the seminal plasma?
   a. Tyrosine kinase
   b. Fructose
   c. Citric acid
   d. Spermine
   e. Prostaglandins
3. Which fetal hormone stimulates the development of the wolffian ducts?
   a. Estradiol
   b. Dihydrotestosterone (DHT)
   c. Estrone
   d. Testosterone
   e. Inhibin
4. Which fetal hormone stimulates the growth of the prostate during development?
   a. Estradiol
   b. DHT
   c. Estrone
   d. Testosterone
   e. Inhibin
5. Which biologic substance is responsible for regression of the müllerian ductal system?
   a. Insulin
   b. Glucagon
   c. Cholesterol
   d. Müllerian-inhibiting substance
   e. All of the above.
6. At what point in neonatal development time does the neonatal surge of testosterone occur?
   a. 1 week
   b. 6 months
   c. 2 months
   d. 5 months
   e. 8 months
7. Which of the following is TRUE regarding neuroendocrine cells found within the prostate?
   a. The major secretory product is somatostatin.
   b. A minor component of the secretory products is serotonin.
   c. Another name for them is AFUD.
   d. A major secretory product of the neuroendocrine cells is thyroid-stimulating hormone (TSH).
   e. Insulin is the major stimulator of secretion in the neuroendocrine cell system within the prostate.
8. Which of the following secretory products is not known to be expressed by mature terminally differentiated prostate epithelial cells?
   a. PSA
   b. Prostate acid phosphatase
   c. Androgen receptor
   d. Telomerase
   e. 15-Lipoxygenase

9. Which of the following biomarkers is not characteristic of prostate stem cells?
   a. Telomerase
   b. a6-Integrin
   c. Keratins 5/14
   d. CDKN1A^{Kip1}
   e. *TP53*
10. Which α_1-adrenergic receptor subtype is linked to smooth muscle contraction in the prostate?
    a. α_{1d}
    b. α_{1a}
    c. α_{1b}
    d. α_2
    e. α_{2b}
11. Which of the following is TRUE regarding testosterone?
    a. Testosterone is synthesized by the Sertoli cells of the testes.
    b. Testosterone is synthesized by the Leydig cells of the testes.
    c. Testosterone is a direct precursor of pregnenolone.
    d. 5α-Reductase is an enzyme that converts DHT into testosterone.
    e. Aromatase converts estrogens into testosterone.
12. The role of prolactin within the prostate is thought to:
    a. enhance the synthesis of fructose.
    b. enhance the uptake of androgens into the prostate through an effect on the synthesis of citric acid.
    c. enhance the conversion of testosterone to DHT.
    d. enhance the conversion of estrogen to DHT.
    e. stimulate secretion of the neuroendocrine cells through its effect on somatostatin.
13. The normal concentration of DHT in the plasma of normal males is:
    a. 100 ng/dL.
    b. 300 ng/dL.
    c. 400 ng/dL.
    d. 50 ng/dL.
    e. 20 ng/dL.
14. Dehydroepiandrosterone has been suggested as a major source of testosterone within the plasma. What percentage of total testosterone has been determined to be derived from dehydroepiandrosterone?
    a. 1%
    b. 2%
    c. 5%
    d. 15%
    e. 20%
15. To what is the majority of testosterone found in the plasma bound?
    a. Insulin
    b. Cholesterol
    c. Prostaglandins
    d. TP53
    e. Testosterone-estradiol-binding globulin (TeBG)
16. Which of the following is not a well-recognized type of growth control regulating the prostate?
    a. Endocrine factors
    b. Neuroendocrine factors
    c. Anabolic factors
    d. Autocrine factors
    e. Extracellular matrix factors
17. Which of the following is TRUE regarding androgen receptor intracellular event?
    a. DHT or testosterone binding to specific nucleotide receptors in the cytoplasm
    b. Dimerization and activation of the steroid receptor
    c. Endocytosis of native androgen
    d. Transport of the active receptor and androgen from the nucleus to the cell membrane
    e. Release of coactivators from the androgen receptor elements
18. How many isoenzymes of 5α-reductase exist?
    a. 1
    b. 4
    c. 2
    d. 7
    e. 3
19. Which 5α-reductase isoenzyme predominates in the prostate gland?
    a. Type I
    b. Type II
    c. Type III
    d. Type IV
    e. Type V
20. Which hormone has been determined to cause squamous cell metaplasia in prostatic growth?
    a. Androgen
    b. Insulin
    c. TSH
    d. Estrogen
    e. Inhibin
21. Which growth factor has been determined to play the most important role in maintaining the structure and functional integrity of prostatic growth?
    a. Fibroblast growth factor (FGF)
    b. Transforming growth factor (TGF)-β
    c. Epidermal growth factor (EGF)
    d. FGF-7
    e. FGF-1
22. Which biologic peptide has a profound effect on regulating the muscular tone of the prostate as well as constriction of blood vessels and elevation of blood pressure?
    a. Acetylcholine
    b. Epinephrine
    c. Insulin
    d. Endothelin
    e. Fructose
23. Which of the following characteristics has not been found to be indicative of a prostate transit amplifying cell (TAC)?
    a. Keratin 5/14
    b. Keratin 8/18
    c. High levels of androgen receptor
    d. TP53
    e. c-Met
24. The expression of which protein is thought to be induced after castration and is directly associated with epithelial cell involution?
    a. TP53
    b. PTEN
    c. TURP-7
    d. trpm-2
    e. PROS-1

25. Which of the following biologic functions is not regulated by the laminins?
    a. Cell adhesion
    b. Proliferation
    c. Differentiation
    d. Chromatin remodeling
    e. Migration
26. What proportion of the total human ejaculate comes from the prostate?
    a. 1/2
    b. 1/6
    c. 1/4
    d. 1/8
    e. 1/16
27. Seminal plasma has unusually high concentrations of all of the following EXCEPT:
    a. citric acid.
    b. insulin.
    c. fructose.
    d. spermine.
    e. prostaglandin.
28. What is the source of fructose in seminal plasma?
    a. Prostate gland
    b. Bulbourethral gland
    c. Vas deferens
    d. Seminal vesicles
    e. Tissue thromboplastin
29. All of the following are secretory products of the prostate EXCEPT which one?
    a. hK17
    b. Prostate-specific transglutaminase
    c. KLK-L1
    d. Prostatic acid phosphatase (PAP)
    e. PSP-94
30. For chromatin remodeling and activation of transcription all but which one of these molecular components is required?
    a. CPB/p300
    b. SWI-SNF
    c. Histone 1A (H1A)
    d. Androgen receptor (AR)
    e. TRAP/DRIP

ANSWERS

1. **c. Tunica albuginea.** Sex accessory tissues include the prostate gland, seminal vesicles, ampullae, and bulbourethral glands, and they are believed to play a major, but unknown, role in the reproductive process.
2. **a. Tyrosine kinase.** In the human, the sex accessory tissues produce extremely high concentrations of many important and potent biologic substances that appear in the seminal plasma, such as fructose (2 mg/mL), citric acid (4 mg/mL), spermine (3 mg/mL), and prostaglandins (200 μg/mL); extremely high concentrations of zinc (150 μg/mL); proteins (40 mg/mL); and specific proteins such as immunoglobulins, proteases, esterases, and phosphatases.
3. **d. Testosterone.** The wolffian ducts develop into the seminal vesicles, epididymis, vas deferens, ampulla, and ejaculatory duct; and the developmental growth of this group of glands is stimulated by fetal testosterone and not DHT.
4. **b. DHT.** In contrast, the prostate first appears and starts its development from the urogenital sinus during the third month of fetal growth, and development is directed primarily by DHT, not testosterone.
5. **d. Müllerian-inhibiting substance.** Growth factors will be discussed later, but it is important to note that the müllerian-inhibiting substance, which is expressed early in gonadal differentiation in the male, causes the regression of the müllerian duct as a prerequisite for virilization in the male.
6. **c. 2 months.** In the human male, neonatal surges in testosterone are observed to peak between 2 and 3 months of age. During this period, serum testosterone levels rise to 60 times that of normal prepubertal levels and often reach the adult serum testosterone range of about 400 ng/dL.
7. **d. A major secretory product of the neuroendocrine cells is thyroid-stimulating hormone (TSH).** There are three types of prostate neuroendocrine cells, with the major type containing both serotonin and TSH. The two minor cell types contain calcitonin and somatostatin. Neuroendocrine cells are also termed APUD, for amine precursor uptake decarboxylase cells, and bring about their regulatory activity by the secretion of hormonal polypeptides or biogenic amines such as serotonin (5-hydroxytryptamine), which is a common marker for these cells.
8. **d. Telomerase.** Numerous proteins have been identified as being expressed in terminally differentiated epithelial cells. Secretory cells stain abundantly with PSA, acid phosphatase, androgen receptor (AR), leucine amino peptidase, and 15-lipoxygenase (LOX-s). They are also rich in keratins (subtypes 8 and 19). Telomerase is expressed primarily in germ cells stem cells and transit amplifying cells (TACs) as well as in most cancer cells. Stem cells overcome this "Hayflick limit" via an enzyme telomerase (a ribonucleoprotein with reverse transcriptase activity), which adds TTAGGG repeats back to the telomere, preventing telomere shortening and subsequent crises.
9. **e. TP53.** Several biomarkers have been demonstrated in stem cells of the prostate: prostate stem cell antigen (PSCA), stem cell antigen-1 (Sca-1), α_6-integrin, $\alpha_2\beta_1$-integrin, $p27^{Kip1}$, keratins 5/14, telomerase, pp32, p63, glutathione transferase Pi (GSTPi), cluster determinant (CD133), and BCL-2. However, *TP53* like the *RB* gene is a tumor suppressor gene, that is, its activity stops the formation of tumors. If a person inherits only one functional copy of the *TP53* gene from his or her parents, the person is predisposed to cancer and usually develops several independent tumors in a variety of tissues in early adulthood. This condition is rare and is known as Li-Fraumeni syndrome. However, mutations in *TP53* are found in most tumor types and so contribute to the complex network of molecular events leading to tumor formation. The *TP53* gene has been mapped to chromosome 17. In the cell, TP53 protein binds DNA, which in turn stimulates another gene to produce a protein called CDKN1A that interacts with a cell division-stimulating protein (cdk2). When CDKN1A is complexed with cdk2 the cell cannot pass through to the next stage of cell division. Mutant *TP53* can no longer bind DNA in an effective way, and, as a consequence, the CDKN1A protein is not made available to act as the "stop signal" for cell division.
10. **b. α_{1a}.** Research work has demonstrated three subtypes of the α_1-adrenergic receptor (α1a, α1b, and α1d), of which the α1a receptor appears to be linked to contraction.

11. **b. Testosterone is synthesized by the Leydig cells of the testes.** Foremost among the hormones and growth factors that stimulate the prostate is the prohormone testosterone, which must be converted within the prostate into the active androgen DHT. Testosterone is synthesized in the Leydig cells of the testes from pregnenolone by a series of reversible reactions; however, once testosterone is reduced by 5α-reductase into DHT or to estrogens by aromatase, the process is irreversible. In other words, whereas testosterone can be converted into DHT and into estrogens, estrogens and DHT cannot be converted into testosterone.

12. **b. enhance the uptake of androgens into the prostate through an effect on the synthesis of citric acid.** Prolactin is believed to enhance the uptake of androgens into the prostate and to affect the synthesis of citric acid.

13. **d. 50 ng/dL.** The concentration of DHT in the plasma of normal men is very low, 50 ng/dL, in comparison to testosterone.

14. **a. 1%.** Less than 1% of the total testosterone in the plasma is derived from dehydroepiandrosterone.

15. **e. Testosterone-estradiol-binding globulin (TeBG).** The majority of testosterone bound to plasma protein is associated with TeBG.

16. **c. Anabolic factors.** These interactive types of growth control are usually accomplished by several generalized systems (see Fig. 85-6) and include (1) endocrine factors or long-range signals arriving at the prostate by serum transport of hormone originating from the secretions of distant organs (this would include serum hormone-like steroids such as testosterone, estrogens, and serum endocrine polypeptide hormones such as prolactin and gonadotropins); (2) neuroendocrine signals originating from neural stimulation such as 5-hydroxytryptamine, acetylcholine, and norepinephrine; (3) paracrine factors or soluble tissue growth factors that stimulate or inhibit growth and are elaborated over short ranges between neighboring cells within the prostate tissue compartment such as β-fibroblast growth factor and epidermal growth factor; (4) autocrine factors or growth factors such as autocrine motility factor, produced and released by a cell and then fed back on the same cell's external membrane receptors to regulate its own growth or function; (5) intracrine factors, factors that share structural and regulatory features with autocrine factors but that work inside the cell; (6) extracellular matrix factors, insoluble tissue matrix systems that make direct and coupled contact by being attached through integrins and adhesion molecules of the basal membrane to couple cytoskeleton organization with the extracellular matrix components that include the glycosaminoglycans such as heparin sulfate; and (7) cell-cell interactions.

17. **b. dimerization and activation of the steroid receptor.** A simplified schematic of the temporal sequence of intracellular events is depicted in Figures 85-10 and 85-11 and includes (1) cellular uptake of testosterone; (2) testosterone converted to DHT by metabolism of 5α-reductase; (3) DHT or testosterone binding to specific androgen receptors in the cytoplasm; (4) dimerization and activation of the steroid receptor by a variety of post-translational steps including, for instance, phosphorylation; (5) active nuclear transportation of the activated androgen receptor in an ATP-dependent manner; (6) chromatin remodeling via interaction with co-regulatory molecules; (7) transactivation or transrepression, via interactions with other coactivators or corepressors, in a histone acetyl transferase–dependent process; (8) binding of the activated receptor/co-activator complex to androgen receptor elements that are short, specific sequences of DNA recognized by androgen receptor dimers; and (9) gene regulation, in which the receptor acts as a transcription factor and, when bound to the DNA and matrix in proximity to androgen target genes, increases the RNA polymerase (Pol II) transcription of the DNA into messenger RNA.

18. **c. 2.** In the human, rat, and monkey, there are two isozymes of 5α-reductase.

19. **b. Type II.** The type II enzyme is mutated in 5α-reductase deficiency and is the dominant isoform present in the prostate gland.

20. **d. Estrogen.** Estrogens can cause a florid squamous cell metaplasia in prostatic growth that can be offset by androgens.

21. **c. Epidermal growth factor (EGF).** A comparison of EGF and TGF-α concluded that EGF appears to be the predominant EGF-related growth factor in both normal prostate and benign prostatic hyperplasia (BPH). It is believed that these two growth factors are important for maintaining the structural and functional integrity of BPH.

22. **d. Endothelin.** There has been increased interest in the biologic properties of the peptide endothelins, of which there are three kinds: endothelin-1, -2, and -3. The most potent activity of these peptides is in constricting blood vessels and elevating blood pressure in mammals, and they may have profound effects on the muscular tone of the prostate as well as its growth.

23. **c. High levels of androgen receptor.** The TACs tend to be AR negative and also possess high-molecular-weight keratins K5 and K14 as well as K8 and K18, which are secretory biomarkers for differentiated secretory epithelial cells. Additionally, these TACs produce TP53-related p63 mRNA, c-Met, plasma receptor for hepatocyte growth factor (HGF), and BCL-2 (a pro-survival protein).

    Castration causes a 90% loss in the total number of prostatic epithelial cells and a slower, but less complete, reduction of approximately 40% in the number of stromal cells.

24. **d. trpm-2.** It has been reported that a temporal series of proteins is induced in the prostate gland after castration, and the most actively studied was trpm-2, in the work of Tenniswood and colleagues. This was followed by the cloning of the gene. This trpm-2 protein was dramatically increased 48 hours after castration and was associated with epithelial cell involution in the prostate gland. The trpm-2 protein now appears to be a secondary marker associated with, but not causing, involution. This protein has been shown to be similar to clusterin, a sulfated glycoprotein-2 normally found in Sertoli cells and present in human seminal plasma, and is suggested to be important in fertility.

25. **d. Chromatin remodeling.** The key functional properties of the laminins include cell adhesion, proliferation, differentiation, growth, and migration. Laminin surrounds the basement membrane of prostate acinar epithelial cells, capillaries, smooth muscle, and nerve fibers but not lymphatics, lymphocytes, or fibroblasts; and the laminin's structure and its distribution is disrupted in BPH and higher-grade prostatic intrepithelial neoplasia (PIN) and higher-grade prostate neoplasms.

26. **b. 1/6.** The major contribution to the volume of seminal plasma (average 3 mL) comes from the seminal vesicles (1.5 to 2 mL); from the prostate (0.5 mL); and from Cowper's gland and glands of Littre (0.1 to 0.2 mL).

27. **b. insulin.** In relation to other body fluids, the seminal plasma is unusual because of its very high concentrations of potassium, zinc, citric acid, fructose, phosphorylcholine, spermine, free amino acids, prostaglandins, and enzymes, most notably acid phosphatase, diamine oxidase, β-glucuronidase,

lactate dehydrogenase, α-amylase, prostate-specific antigen, and seminal proteinase.

28. **d. Seminal vesicles.** The source of fructose in human seminal plasma is the seminal vesicles. Patients with congenital absence of the seminal vesicles also have an associated absence of fructose in their ejaculates.

29. **a. hK17.** Major secretory protein markers that are found in abundance and have clinical significance include (1) prostate-specific antigen (human kallikrein 3 [hK3 (protein) or *KLK3* (gene)]; (2) human kallikrein 2 (hK2 or KLK2); (3) prostate KLK-L1; (4) prostatic acid phosphatase (PAP); and (5) prostate-specific protein (PSP-94), also termed β-microseminoprotein or β-MSP.

30. **c. Histone 1A (H1A).** To achieve such coordinate regulation, the protective packaging of DNA is engineered through an elegant system of tightly wound DNA around an eight-component histone core called a nucleosome. This core consists of dimers of H2A, H2B, H3, and H4, whose ability to compact DNA is directly regulated by post-translational modifications. The selective regulation of such post-translational histone modification constitutes a major regulatory mechanism for gene expression and is referred to as the "histone code" (see Fig. 85-10). Histone modifications include acetylation, phosphorylation, ubiquinization, and methylation.

86

Benign Prostatic Hyperplasia: Etiology, Pathophysiology, Epidemiology, and Natural History

CLAUS G. ROEHRBORN • JOHN D. MCCONNELL

QUESTIONS

1. The prevalence of a disease is defined as the number of:
   a. diseased people per 100,000 population per year.
   b. existing cases per 100,000 population at a distinct target date.
   c. deaths per 100,000 population per year.
   d. deaths per number of diseased.
2. Concerning the autopsy prevalence of benign prostatic hperplasia (BPH) or stromoglandular hyperplasia, which of the following statements is TRUE?
   a. No adequate studies have been done to date.
   b. It is commonly found in men of all ages.
   c. It is very uncommon in men younger than the age of 30 years.
   d. It is found in 100% of men starting at the age of 40 years.
   e. International comparisons are impossible due to a lack of its definition.
3. Which of the following statements regarding the I-PSS symptom frequency score is TRUE?
   a. Moderate symptom severity is defined as a score from 10 to 20 points.
   b. The I-PSS score addresses irritative and obstructive symptoms and issues of incontinence.
   c. Quantitative symptom scores in BPH are not as important as are objective measures such as a flow rate recording.
   d. The I-PSS score has been translated and validated in many languages.
4. Which statement is correct regarding prostate volume?
   a. International studies show significant similarity in prostate volume in white, age-stratified men.
   b. Prostate volume assessment by digital rectal examination is reproducible across examiners.
   c. Although there is a steady increase in total prostate volume with age, the transition zone volume increases only marginally.
   d. MRI measurements are in general smaller compared with transrectal ultrasound measurements.
5. Concerning liver diseases and BPH which of the following statements is TRUE?
   a. EtOH consumption increases circulating levels of estrogens.
   b. The risk of having surgery for BPH is increased in heavy drinkers.
   c. The intake of EtOH can decrease serum testosterone levels by a variety of mechanisms.
   d. Most autopsy studies find a higher prevalence of BPH in men with liver cirrhosis.
6. How do medications influence symptoms and flow rate?
   a. There is no documented influence of any medication on symptoms or flow rate.
   b. Antihistamines and bronchodilators significantly decrease urinary flow rates.
   c. Calcium channel blockers and β-adrenergic blockers reduce urinary flow rates significantly.
   d. Antidepressants, antihistamines, and bronchodilators increase the symptom score by several points.
7. Concerning correlations between baseline parameters which statement is TRUE?
   a. A clinically useful correlation exists between prostate volume and serum PSA.
   b. Many studies have shown a significant correlation between the transition zone volume and symptom severity.
   c. Correlation of symptoms, bother, interference, and quality of life are poor.
   d. Urinary flow rate and prostate volume correlate highly with serum PSA.
8. Which statement is correct regarding the study of the natural history of BPH?
   a. Placebo groups from treatment trials are useful because they do not have treatment biases.
   b. A longitudinal population-based study has the fewest biases and is the most useful type of study.
   c. Control groups from intervention or medical therapy trials reflect the natural history of the disease in unselected community dwelling men.
   d. Placebo groups have fewer selection biases compared with population-based studies.

9. Regarding the magnitude of the placebo response and its perception, which of the following statements is TRUE?
   a. Placebo response is not dependent of the baseline severity score.
   b. Most patients report subjective improvement when the drop from baseline is > 30%.
   c. The higher the baseline score, the more of a drop is required for patients to subjectively feel improved.
   d. Perception of improvement is independent of baseline score.
10. Descriptive studies of the incidence rates (IR) of acute urinary retention (AUR) have demonstrated that:
   a. depending on the population studied incidence rates between < 5 to > 130 cases/1000 person-years have been reported.
   b. the IR reported do not differ significantly between various studies and populations.
   c. AUR has been poorly defined, and therefore no IR can be calculated.
   d. IR of < 10/1000 person-years have been reported in all watchful waiting studies.
11. What is the most significant finding regarding analytical epidemiology of AUR?
   a. Serum PSA is a more powerful predictor of AUR compared with age.
   b. Serum PSA and prostate volume have limited ability to predict episodes of AUR.
   c. Urinary flow rates in placebo control groups are strong predictors of AUR episodes.
   d. Age has been found to be the most significant risk factor for AUR in population-based studies.
12. Which statement regarding surgery for BPH is TRUE?
   a. The incidence rates of surgery are similar across wide geographic regions and ethnic backgrounds.
   b. Compared with AUR, surgery is a softer endpoint.
   c. Surgery is a less common endpoint compared with AUR.
   d. Most patients with BPH eventually require surgery for their condition.

ANSWERS

1. **b. existing cases per 100,000 population per year.** When studying diseases by descriptive or analytical epidemiologic methods, it is important to have a good understanding of the definitions that apply. Most epidemiologic terms are expressed as rates, which are a number of cases for persons expressed over the population. The definitions that are of relevance are incidence rates = the number of diseased people/100,000 population/year; prevalence= the number of existing cases of the disease of interest/100,000 *at a distinct target date;* mortality rate, which is the number of deaths/100,000 population/year; and fatality, which equals the number of deaths due to the disease/number of diseased people.
2. **c. It is very uncommon in men younger than the age of 30 years.** The autopsy prevalence of BPH has been studied as early as 1984 by Berry and colleagues. Since then, many studies have been done on virtually all continence in many ethnic groups. It is astonishing that these studies find a very significant agreement in terms of the actual prevalence of histologic BPH or stromoglandular hyperplasia around the world. Stromoglandular hyperplasia or BPH is very uncommon in men younger than the age of 30 but then increases steadily and in an almost linear manner. In fact, approximately 90% of men in their 80s have evidence of stromoglandular hyperplasia.
3. **d. The I-PSS score has been translated and validated in many languages.** The I-PSS symptom score is a 7-question self-administered questionnaire that yields a total score ranging from 0 to 35 points. Men who score 0 to 7 points are classified as mildly symptomatic, those scoring from 8 to 19 points as moderately symptomatic, and those from 20 to 35 points as severely symptomatic. The I-PSS score addresses irritative and obstructive but no incontinence symptomatology. It is widely accepted that quantitative symptom scores are far more important than, for example, urinary flow rate recordings. Fortunately, the I-PSS score, the most widely utilized instrument, has been translated and culturally validated in many languages.
4. **a. International studies show significant similarity in prostate volume between white age-stratified men.** Prostate volume can relatively easily be assessed by transrectal ultrasonography. Transrectal ultrasonography has been found to be a reliable measure that is reproducible across examiners in contrast to digital rectal examination, which is only poorly reproducible. MRI is very expensive and it yields in general a larger volume compared with transrectal ultrasound measurements. Of note is the fact that international studies show significant similarity in regard to total and transitional zone prostate volume in Caucasian age-stratified men.
5. **c. The intake of EtOH can decrease serum testosterone levels by a variety of mechanisms.** It is known that alcohol intake may decrease plasma testosterone levels by reducing production of and increasing clearance of testosterone. However, despite this hypothetical reason for a lower incidence, an inverse relationship has been described. The age-adjusted multivariant relative risks for undergoing surgery for BPH in men drinking more than three or four glasses of alcohol per day is lower than in age-matched controls. Of course, this could be due to a bias against surgery in patients who are heavy drinkers and therefore in poor health. It is interesting to note, however, that in the majority of studies, namely, four of five, a lower prevalence of BPH is found in men with cirrhosis compared with those without cirrhosis.
6. **d. Antidepressants, antihistamines, and bronchodilators increase the symptom score by several points.** There is only one study that systematically assessed the effect of medications on urinary symptoms and flow rate. Cold medications containing α-sympathomimetics tend to exacerbate lower urinary tract symptoms by the expected effect on the smooth muscle of the bladder outlet. Data from the Olmsted County MN study show that daily use of antidepressants, antihistamines, or bronchodilators are associated with a 2- to 3-point increase in the symptom score. However, only the daily use of antidepressants is associated with a decrease in the age-adjusted urinary flow rate.
7. **a. A clinical useful correlation exists between prostate volume and serum PSA.** In general, there is an absence of useful baseline correlations between subjective and objective parameters such as symptoms, frequency, quality of life, and urinary flow rate measures of obstruction and prostate volume. However, symptom, bother, and interference with quality of life show excellent correlation with each other, and a clinically useful

correlation exists between total and transition zone prostate volume and serum PSA in men with BPH.

8. **b. A longitudinal population-based study has the fewest biases and is the most useful type of study.** There are several ways to study the natural history of BPH. One can look at watchful waiting cohorts, placebo-controlled groups of medication trials, or study population-based groups of men longitudinally over time. The latter is clearly the best way of studying the natural history of the disease because it incurs the fewest biases. However, it is also the most tedious and most expensive way to study this. Placebo groups in medication trials clearly suffer from enrollment biases but do provide useful information.

9. **c. The higher the baseline score, the more of a drop is required for patients to subjectively feel improved.** The placebo response is partially a regression to the mean and partially an effect induced by the interaction between patient and doctor. The response is clearly dependent on the baseline severity score with patients' higher scores having a larger decrease from baseline. Barry and colleagues have shown that the perception of subjective improvement is dependent on the drop from baseline as well as the baseline itself. For example, the higher the baseline score, the more of a drop from baseline is required for patients to have a subjective perception of improvement. Overall, a 3-point decrease is associated with a subjective perception of improvement.

10. **a. depending on the population studied incidence rates between < 5 to > 130 cases/1000 person-years have been reported.** Acute urinary retention has been studied over the past few years in population-based studies as well as in placebo-control groups from long-term treatment trials. The incidence rates vary greatly from < 5 to > 130 cases/1000 person-years. They do differ significantly between different studies owing to the inclusion and exclusion criteria and selection biases. Fortunately, acute urinary retention is a very clearly defined outcome and, thus, incidence rates can easily be calculated and compared.

11. **d. Age has been found to be the most significant risk factor for AUR in population-based studies.** In population-based studies such as the Olmsted County study, age is the most significant predictor of acute urinary retention. Data from placebo groups of long-term medical treatment trials demonstrate that serum PSA is the most powerful predictor of acute urinary retention together with prostate volume. Although this appears to be on the surface a contradiction, it can be relatively easily explained by the fact that in BPH treatment trials, elderly men with already an existing diagnosis of BPH are enrolled. Thus, age plays a lesser factor in terms of predicting AUR. In population-based studies in which men stratified by age are followed over long periods of time, age plays a more significant factor compared with PSA.

12. **b. Compared with AUR, surgery is a softer endpoint.** Incidence rates of surgery vary significantly across geographic regions and patients with different ethnic backgrounds. This is the reason that surgery is a softer endpoint compared with AUR. Depending on the interaction between patient and physician, the physician can convince the patient to undergo surgery or, based on the patient's comorbidities, talk him out of surgery. The same cannot be said for urinary retention. It is clear that a vast majority of patients do not require surgery in the course of their disease but, rather, can be treated effectively with reassurance alone or medication.

87

Evaluation and Nonsurgical Management of Benign Prostatic Hyperplasia

ROGER KIRBY • HERBERT LEPOR

QUESTIONS

1. Where does benign prostatic hyperplasia (BPH) originate? In the:
   a. transition zone
   b. peripheral zone
   c. periurethral glands
   d. transition zone and periurethral zone
2. A strong correlation exists between prostate volume and:
   a. serum prostate-specific antigen (PSA).
   b. American Urological Association (AUA) symptom score.
   c. peak urinary flow rate.
   d. postvoid residual.
3. Medications that may exacerbate lower urinary tract symptoms (LUTS) include:
   a. α-adrenergic antagonists.
   b. α-adrenergic agonists.
   c. β-adrenergic agonists.
   d. muscarinic agonists.
4. What is the primary objective of the digital rectal examination (DRE) in evaluation of men with LUTS? To:
   a. estimate prostate volume
   b. obtain prostatic secretions
   c. identify prostate nodules
   d. determine rectal tone
5. In older men with LUTS, which test should be routinely performed to obtain the differential diagnosis?
   a. Urinalysis
   b. Peak flow rate
   c. Serum creatinine assay
   d. Renal ultrasonography
6. It is advisable in a man with BPH and a slightly elevated creatinine level to perform:
   a. transurethral resection of the prostate (TURP).
   b. intravenous pyelogram.
   c. renal sonogram.
   d. urodynamic study.
7. What percentage of men have histologically proven BPH with a serum PSA value of 4.0 ng/mL or greater?
   a. 5%
   b. 15%
   c. 30%
   d. 50%
8. An AUA symptom score of 20 indicates severe:
   a. LUTS.
   b. BPH.
   c. bladder outlet obstruction.
   d. bladder dysfunction.
9. An absolute indication for surgery (TURP or open prostatectomy) is:
   a. severe symptoms.
   b. postvoid residual (PVR) urine of 300 mL or more.
   c. single episodes of acute urinary retention.
   d. refractory gross hematuria secondary to BPH.
10. A low peak flow rate suggests:
    a. severe symptoms.
    b. bladder outlet obstruction.
    c. impaired detrusor contractility.
    d. b or c.
11. What is the next step for a man with a PVR of 300 mL?
    a. Repeat the PVR assay
    b. Upper urinary tract imaging
    c. Urodynamic testing
    d. TURP
12. The probability that a urodynamic study helps to decrease the failure rate of TURP in men with a peak flow rate of 15 mL/s is approximately:
    a. 10%.
    b. 25%.
    c. 50%.
    d. 75%.

13. What is the percentage of men with LUTS who have uninhibited contraction?
    a. 10%
    b. 30%
    c. 60%
    d. 80%
14. What is the likelihood that uninhibited detrusor contractions (UDCs) in men with BPH will resolve after TURP?
    a. Never
    b. Unlikely
    c. Likely
    d. Always
15. The finding of bladder trabeculation suggests:
    a. high-grade obstruction.
    b. high successful rate after TURP.
    c. high PVR.
    d. none of the above.
16. Imaging of the upper tract is indicated for:
    a. prostate glands weighing more than 50 g.
    b. urinalysis demonstrating hematuria.
    c. bladder trabeculation.
    d. severe LUTS.
17. An improvement in the AUA symptom score of 5 units correlates with which level of symptoms improved?
    a. Marked
    b. Moderate
    c. Slight
    d. None
18. Urodynamic testing reliably predicts response after:
    a. TURP.
    b. α-adrenergic blockers.
    c. 5α-reductase inhibitors.
    d. none of the above.
19. There is compelling evidence that PVR is:
    a. related to symptom severity.
    b. associated with the risk for urinary tract infection (UTI).
    c. both a and b.
    d. neither a nor b.
20. The definition of detrusor instability is bladder pressure greater than which level at a bladder volume of 300 mL or less?
    a. 5 cm H_2O.
    b. 15 cm H_2O.
    c. 40 cm H_2O.
    d. 60 cm H_2O.
21. The likelihood that a man with acute urinary retention will develop a subsequent episode of urinary retention within 1 week is approximately:
    a. 20%.
    b. 40%.
    c. 60%.
    d. 80%.
22. The incidence of developing acute urinary retention is related to:
    a. prostate size.
    b. age.
    c. severity of symptoms.
    d. all of the above.
23. The best way to eliminate bias in a clinical study is to use:
    a. honest investigators.
    b. placebo-controlled double-blind design.
    c. randomization.
    d. large sample size.
24. The larger the sample size, the:
    a. less treatment effect required to achieve statistical significance.
    b. better the study.
    c. greater the treatment effect required to achieve statistical significance.
    d. none of the above.
25. Which of the following is the attractive feature of medical therapy relative to TURP?
    a. Fewer side effects.
    b. Reversible side effects.
    c. Less serious side effects.
    d. All of the above.
26. During the past decade, the incidence of TURP in the United States has decreased by approximately:
    a. 10%.
    b. 50%.
    c. 100%.
    d. 200%.
27. Which of the following percentages of men older than 50 years of age have moderate or severe LUTS?
    a. 2%
    b. 5%
    c. 30%
    d. 50%
28. The ideal candidate for medical therapy should have which type of symptoms?
    a. Severe
    b. Moderate
    c. Minimal
    d. Bothersome
29. Smooth muscle accounts for what percentage of the area density of the prostate?
    a. 5%.
    b. 10%.
    c. 20%.
    d. 40%.
30. The tension of prostate smooth muscle is mediated by the:
    a. α_1 receptor.
    b. α_2 receptor.
    c. β_2 receptor.
    d. muscarinic cholinergic receptor.
31. What is the advantage of terazosin over prazosin?
    a. Its longer half-life
    b. Its better absorption
    c. Its greater α_1-receptor selectivity
    d. None of the above.
32. Which α_1 receptor subtype mediates prostate smooth muscle tension?
    a. α_{1a}
    b. α_{1b}
    c. α_{1c}
    d. α_{1d}

33. The improvement in AUA symptom score after terazosin administration depends on baseline:
    a. age.
    b. prostate size.
    c. PVR.
    d. None of the above.
34. The mean treatment-related improvement in response to terazosin in AUA symptom score units is approximately:
    a. 2.
    b. 4.
    c. 6.
    d. 8.
35. The durability of the improvement in symptom scores and peak flow rates for α_1-adrenergic blockers has been reported to be up to how many months?
    a. 12.
    b. 42.
    c. 60.
    d. 92.
36. Which of the following α-adrenergic blockers does not lower blood pressure in men with uncontrolled hypertension?
    a. Terazosin
    b. Doxazosin
    c. Tamsulosin
    d. Prazosin
37. Retrograde ejaculation is most commonly seen with:
    a. terazosin.
    b. prazosin.
    c. finasteride.
    d. tamsulosin.
38. Approximately what percentage of men have both BPH and hypertension?
    a. 5%
    b. 15%
    c. 30%
    d. 50%
39. What is the likely mechanism for dizziness after α_1-adrenergic blocker therapy?
    a. Vascular
    b. Central nervous system
    c. Carotid baroreceptor
    d. None of the above
40. The major advantage of tamsulosin 0.4 mg over terazosin 10 mg is:
    a. greater efficiency.
    b. less retrograde ejaculation.
    c. no dose titration.
    d. greater lowering of blood pressure.
41. The embryologic development of the prostate is mediated primarily by:
    a. testosterone.
    b. dihydrotestosterone.
    c. androstenedione.
    d. estradiol.
42. Finasteride significantly decreases the long-term risk of:
    a. acute urinary retention.
    b. surgical intervention.
    c. all of the above.
    d. none of the above.
43. Finasteride is most effective at relieving hematuria in men with:
    a. prostatitis.
    b. enlarged prostate.
    c. transurethral prostatectomy.
    d. obstructing prostate.
44. Dutasteride:
    a. is a dual inhibitor of type 1 and type 2 5α-reductase.
    b. is more effective than finasteride.
    c. results in a 95% reduction in PSA after 6 months of therapy.
    d. is less likely than finasteride to result in loss of libido.
45. The adverse event that limits the use of flutamide as a primary treatment of BPH is:
    a. breast tenderness.
    b. diarrhea.
    c. erectile dysfunction.
    d. loss of libido.
46. A potential advantage of cetrorelix, a gonadotropin-releasing hormone antagonist, for the treatment of BPH is:
    a. lower cost.
    b. ability to titrate the level of androgen suppression.
    c. ease of administration.
    d. rapid response.
47. A Veterans Affairs study demonstrated that terazosin is more effective than finasteride at rapidly relieving symptoms in men with:
    a. small prostates.
    b. intermediate-size prostates.
    c. large prostates.
    d. all of the above.
48. In the Veterans Affairs study, finasteride was no better than placebo at:
    a. improving symptoms.
    b. lowering micturition voiding pressure.
    c. decreasing prostate size.
    d. all of the above.
49. The MTOPS study confirmed that:
    a. α-adrenergic blockers and 5α-reductase inhibitors are equivalent in relieving symptoms.
    b. α-adrenergic blockers reduce the risk of acute urinary retention over 7 years of treatment.
    c. finasteride reduces the risk of adenocarcinoma of the prostate.
    d. a combination of an α-adrenergic blocker and a 5α-reductase inhibitor is the most effective way of preventing BPH progression.
50. The amount spent on phytotherapy for the treatment of BPH is estimated to be:
    a. $10 million.
    b. $100 million.
    c. $1 billion.
    d. $10 billion.
51. The definitive mechanism of action for *Serenoa repens* is:
    a. inhibition of 5α-reductase.
    b. inhibition of cyclooxygenase.
    c. inhibition of lipoxygenase.
    d. inconclusive.

52. Potential future therapeutic avenues in BPH pharmacotherapy include:
   a. nitric oxide donors.
   b. α-adrenoceptor agonists.
   c. HMG coenzyme A inhibitors.
   d. endothelin antagonists.

53. The next major step in the treatment of LUTS will require:
   a. unraveling the pathophysiology of LUTS.
   b. more selective α_1 blockers.
   c. duel inhibitors of dihydrotestosterone.
   d. new strategies for relaxing prostate smooth muscle.

ANSWERS

1. **d. transition zone and periurethral zone.** The proliferative process originates in the transition zone and the periurethral glands.
2. **a. serum prostate-specific antigen (PSA).** A strong correlation exists between serum PSA levels and prostate volume.
3. **b. α-adrenergic agonists.** Current prescription and over-the-counter medications should be examined to determine whether the patient is taking drugs that impair bladder contractility (anticholinergics) or that increase outflow resistance (α-sympathomimetics).
4. **c. identify prostate nodules.** The DRE and neurologic examination are done to detect prostate or rectal malignancy, to evaluate anal sphincter tone, and to rule out any neurologic problems that may cause the presenting symptoms.
5. **a. Urinalysis.** In older men with BPH and a higher prevalence of serious urinary tract disorders, the benefits of an innocuous test such as urinalysis clearly outweigh the harm involved.
6. **c. renal sonogram.** An elevated serum creatinine level in a patient with BPH is an indication for imaging studies (ultrasonography) to evaluate the upper urinary tract.
7. **c. 30%.** Twenty-eight percent of men with histologically proven BPH have a serum PSA level greater than 4.0 ng/mL.
8. **a. LUTS.** The International Prostate Symptom Score (I-PSS), which is identical to the AUA Symptom Index, is recommended as the symptom scoring instrument to be used for the baseline assessment of symptom severity in men presenting with LUTS. When the I-PSS system is used, symptoms can be classified as mild (0 to 7), moderate (8 to 19), or severe (20 to 35). The I-PSS cannot be used to establish the diagnosis of BPH.
9. **d. refractory gross hematuria secondary to BPH.** Surgery is recommended if the patient has refractory urinary retention (at least one failed attempt at catheter removal) or any of the following conditions, clearly secondary to BPH: recurrent urinary tract infection, recurrent gross hematuria, bladder stones, renal insufficiency, or large bladder diverticula.
10. **d. b or c.** One study found that flow rate recording cannot distinguish between bladder outlet obstruction and impaired detrusor contractility as the cause for a low Qmax.
11. **a. Repeat the PVR assay.** Residual urine volume measurement has significant intraindividual variability that limits its clinical usefulness.
12. **a. 10%.** One study recommended invasive urodynamic testing for patients with a Qmax higher than 15 mL/s. For the population in their study, this would have resulted in an additional 9% of patients being excluded from surgery and a decrease in failure rate to 8.3%.
13. **c. 60%.** Overactive contractions are present in about 60% of men with LUTS and correlate strongly with irritative voiding symptoms.
14. **c. Likely.** UDCs resolve in most patients after surgery.
15. **d. none of the above.** Bladder trabeculation may predict a slightly higher failure rate in patients managed by watchful waiting but does not predict the success or failure of surgery.
16. **b. a urinalysis demonstrating hematuria.** Upper urinary tract imaging is not recommended for routine evaluation of men with LUTS unless they also have one or more of the following: hematuria; urinary tract infection; renal insufficiency (ultrasonography recommended); history of urolithiasis; and history of urinary tract surgery.
17. **b. Moderate.** The group mean changes in AUA Symptom Index for subjects rating their improvement as markedly, moderately, or slightly improved, unchanged, or worse were −8.8, −5.1, −3.0, −0.7, and +2.7, respectively.
18. **d. none of the above.** Urodynamic testing does not predict symptom improvement after α-adrenergic blockade, transurethral microwave thermotherapy, or prostatectomy.
19. **d. neither a nor b.** One study reported no correlation between the AUA symptom score and PVR volume. There are also no data documenting that the incidence of UTI is related to PVR volume.
20. **b. 15 cm H_2O.** The definition of detrusor instability is the development of a detrusor contraction exceeding 15 cm H_2O at a bladder volume less than or equal to 300 mL.
21. **d. 80%.** Of 59 Danish patients presenting to an emergency department with acute retention, 73% had recurrent urinary retention within 1 week after removal of the catheter.
22. **d. all of the above.** The incidence of acute urinary retention was related to age, severity of symptoms, and size of the prostate gland.
23. **b. a placebo-controlled double-blind design.** The only mechanism to ensure that the potential bias of the subject and the investigator does not influence the outcome is a randomized double-blind placebo-controlled design.
24. **a. less treatment effect required to achieve statistical significance.** The larger the number of subjects enrolled in a study, the smaller the change required to achieve statistical significance.
25. **d. All of the above.** The attractive feature of medical therapy relative to prostatectomy is that clinically significant outcomes are obtained with fewer, less serious, and reversible side effects.
26. **b. 50%.** A 55% reduction in transurethral prostatectomy has occurred despite the progressively increasing number of men enrolled in the Medicare program.
27. **c. 30%.** Approximately 30% of American men older than 50 years of age have moderate to severe symptoms.
28. **d. Bothersome.** The ideal candidate for medical therapy should have symptoms that are bothersome and have a negative impact on the quality of life.
29. **d. 40%.** Smooth muscle is one of the dominant cellular constituents of BPH, accounting for 40% of the area density of the hyperplastic prostate.

30. **a. α_1 receptor.** The tension of prostate smooth muscle is mediated by the α_1 adrenergic receptors.
31. **a. Its longer half-life.** Terazosin and doxazosin are long-acting α-adrenergic blockers that have been shown to be safe and effective for the treatment of BPH.
32. **a. α_{1a}.** Prostate smooth muscle tension has been shown to be mediated by the α_{1a} adrenergic receptors.
33. **d. None of the above.** The relationships between percent change in total symptom score and peak flow rate versus baseline age, prostate size, peak flow rate, PVR volume, and total symptom score were examined to identify clinical or urodynamic factors that predicted response to terazosin therapy. No significant association was observed between treatment effect and any of these baseline factors.
34. **b. 4.** The treatment-related improvement (terazosin minus placebo) in the AUA symptom score and urinary peak flow rate was 1.4 mL/s and 3.9 symptom units, respectively.
35. **b. 42.** The initial improvements in symptom scores and peak flow rate in 450 subjects were maintained for up to 42 months.
36. **c. Tamsulosin.** The advantage of not lowering blood pressure in men who are hypertensive at baseline is controversial.
37. **d. tamsulosin.** The treatment-related incidences of asthenia, dizziness, rhinitis, and abnormal ejaculation observed for 0.4 mg of tamsulosin were 2%, 5%, 3%, and 11%, respectively, and for 0.8 mg of tamsulosin were 3%, 8%, 9%, and 18%, respectively.
38. **c. 30%.** Approximately 30% of men treated for BPH have coexisting hypertension.
39. **b. Central nervous system.** The α_1-mediated dizziness and asthenia are likely due to effects at the level of the central nervous system.
40. **c. no dose titration.** The major advantage of 0.4 mg tamsulosin and slow-release alfuzosin is the lack of requirement for dose titration.
41. **b. dihydrotestosterone.** The embryonic development of the prostate is dependent on the androgen dihydrotestosterone.
42. **c. all of the above.** The Proscar Long-Term Efficacy and Safety Study (PLESS) represents one of the longest duration multicenter randomized double-blind placebo-controlled studies reported in the literature on medical therapy for BPH. The unique findings of PLESS were related to incidences of both acute urinary retention and surgical intervention for BPH. The risk reduction of acute urinary retention and BPH-related surgery was clinically relevant, especially in men with very large prostates.
43. **c. transurethral prostatectomy.** These preliminary observations have been confirmed by a randomized, double-blind placebo-controlled study demonstrating that finasteride prevents recurrent gross hematuria secondary to BPH after prostatectomy.
44. **a. is a dual inhibitor of type 1 and type 2 5α-reductase.** Unlike finasteride, which only inhibits the type 2 isoenzyme.
45. **a. breast tenderness.** The incidences of breast tenderness and diarrhea in the flutamide group were 53% and 11%, respectively.
46. **b. ability to titrate the level of androgen suppression.** A potential advantage of a gonadotropin-releasing hormone antagonist over the luteinizing hormone–releasing hormone agonists in the treatment of BPH is the ability to titrate the level of androgen suppression.
47. **d. all of the above.** In the study, the mean group differences between terazosin versus placebo and terazosin versus finasteride for all of the outcome measures other than prostate volume were highly statistically significant. Terazosin was more effective than finasteride in those subjects with large prostates.
48. **a. improving symptoms.** The mean group differences between finasteride and placebo were not statistically significant for AUA symptom index, symptom problem index, BPH impact index, and peak flow rate.
49. **d. a combination of an α-adrenergic blocker and a 5α-reductase inhibitor is the most effective way of preventing BPH progression.** This was the key conclusion of the important MTOPS study that looked at finasteride versus doxazosin versus a combination of both and placebo in men with symptomatic BPH.
50. **c. $1 billion.** Usage of these agents in the United States and throughout the world has escalated. It has been estimated that more than $1 billion was spent in the United States alone for these products.
51. **d. inconclusive.** Although experimental data have suggested numerous possible mechanisms of actions for the phytotherapeutic agents, it is uncertain which, if any, of these proposed mechanisms is responsible for the clinical responses.
52. **d. Endothelin antagonists.** Although currently untested, endothelin antagonists represent a possible therapeutic avenue in BPH.
53. **a. unraveling the pathophysiology of LUTS.** Our current understanding of the pathophysiology of clinical BPH is rudimentary. It is, therefore, imperative to develop a more comprehensive understanding of the pathophysiology of symptoms.

88

Minimally Invasive and Endoscopic Management of Benign Prostatic Hyperplasia

JOHN M. FITZPATRICK

QUESTIONS

1. Intraprostatic stents were developed after first being used to treat which of the following conditions?
   a. Peripheral vascular disease
   b. Coronary artery disease
   c. Urethral strictures
   d. Bronchial obstruction
   e. Lacrimal duct obstruction
2. The recognized role for the use of intraprostatic stents is:
   a. to replace transurethral resection of the prostate (TURP).
   b. in preoperative patients likely to develop retention.
   c. in patients unfit for TURP.
   d. in patients receiving anticoagulants.
   e. for temporary relief of obstruction.
3. The most common complication associated with temporary stents is:
   a. urinary retention.
   b. stent migration.
   c. clot retention.
   d. urinary incontinence.
   e. encrustation.
4. Which of the following statements is TRUE of transurethral needle ablation (TUNA)?
   a. It causes necrosis at 15 days.
   b. It induces fibrosis at 7 days.
   c. It causes damage to α-adrenergic receptors at 1 week.
   d. It affects nitric oxide synthase receptors, which are least vulnerable to damage.
   e. It does not affect prostate-specific antigen (PSA) staining.
5. The complication most commonly reported after TUNA is:
   a. hemorrhage.
   b. urinary retention.
   c. irritative voiding symptoms.
   d. urinary tract infection.
   e. urethral strictures.
6. Transurethral microwave therapy (TUMT) has been shown to:
   a. damage nerve fibers, with necrosis possible.
   b. induce apoptosis of prostatic cells.
   c. be superior to TURP in terms of clinical efficacy.
   d. cause retrograde ejaculation.
   e. induce post-treatment voiding difficulties with low-energy treatment.
7. Treating symptomatic benign prostatic hyperplasia with the laser:
   a. causes the greatest degree of tissue vaporization with the holmium laser.
   b. is most appropriate for large prostates.
   c. is associated with a low incidence of postoperative urinary infection.
   d. has a hemorrhage rate of 8%.
   e. causes erectile dysfunction in 46% of patients.
8. An absolute indication for TURP is:
   a. postvoid residual urine volume of 250 mL.
   b. recurrent urinary infections.
   c. American Urological Association symptom score of 20 or greater.
   d. detrusor pressure at a maximum flow of 65 cm H_2O.
   e. inability to use medical treatment because of side effects.
9. Postoperative complications have been related to preoperative measurement of:
   a. urinary flow rate.
   b. detrusor pressure at a maximum urinary flow rate.
   c. postvoid residual urine.
   d. prostatic size.
   e. serum creatinine value.
10. Outflow obstruction can be predicted by:
    a. serum creatinine level.
    b. urine culture results.
    c. maximum urinary flow rate.
    d. cystoscopy.
    e. pressure-flow studies.
11. TURP should commence with:
    a. incision of the bladder neck.

b. resection of the middle lobe.
c. resection of the bladder neck.
d. resection of prostatic tissue at 12 o'clock.
e. resection of prostatic tissue at 3 or 9 o'clock.

12. The most common complication after TURP is:

a. failure to void.
b. hemorrhage requiring transfusion.
c. clot retention.
d. urinary tract infection.
e. transurethral resection syndrome.

13. Transurethral vaporization of the prostate transurethral vaporization of the prostate (TUVP) results in:

a. vaporization.
b. coagulation.
c. desiccation.
d. vaporization and desiccation.
e. cauterization.

14. In short-term studies, transurethral vaporization of the prostate (TUVP) has been shown to be comparable to TURP in what area?

a. Urinary flow rate improvement
b. Incidence of postoperative hemorrhage
c. Postoperative urinary infection
d. Sexual complications
e. Improvement in postvoid residual urine

15. Which of the following statements is true of transurethral incision of the prostate (TUIP)? It:

a. is appropriate for large prostates.
b. has a high complication rate.
c. causes retrograde ejaculation in up to 37% of cases.
d. commonly results in TURP syndrome.
e. was described by Bottini in 1900.

ANSWERS

1. **b. Coronary artery disease.** Stents were first introduced as a method of treating certain cardiovascular conditions.

2. **c. in patients unfit for TURP.** Eventually it became clear that the major role for stents was likely to be found in the management of patients who were unfit for surgery, either in the short or in the long term, in whom the alternative would have been months or indeed a lifetime of indwelling urethral catheterization.

3. **d. urinary incontinence.** In the largest number of patients (318) reported from one center, complications were divided into none, moderate, and severe. In the patients who were described as having severe complications, stress or urge incontinence occurred in 63, emptying problems in 8, and frequency and/or nocturia (>3 episodes) in 57.

4. **c. It causes damage to α-adrenergic receptors at 1 week.** In studies with the TUNA system, necrosis was maximal at 7 days, with fibrosis developing by 15 days. In treated areas, there was an absence of staining for PSA, smooth muscle actin, and α-adrenergic neural tissue. Nitric oxide synthase receptors were found to be most vulnerable to thermal damage and occurred earliest, with damage to the α-adrenergic receptors maximal at 1 to 2 weeks.

5. **b. urinary retention.** By far the most common complication reported, however, is post-treatment urinary retention, occurring at a rate of 13.3% to 41.6%. It can be expected that within the first 24 hours, about 40% of patients will experience urinary retention.

6. **b. induce apoptosis of prostatic cells.** In one study, apoptosis was verified by the terminal deoxynucleotidyl nick-end labeling (TUNEL) technique in sections showing histologic changes suggestive of apoptosis, such as pyknotic nuclei and chromatin segregation. Necrotic areas were frequently seen in the prostate to a depth of 4 to 5 cm. Outside these necrotic areas, normal and apoptotic areas were interspersed, the latter confirmed by TUNEL. The area of tissue damage seen after TUMT was relatively small compared with the volume of the prostates. The heat was implicated as the cause of the apoptosis, but there was no speculation as to the exact mechanism whereby heat brought about this effect.

7. **a. causes the greatest degree of tissue vaporization with the holmium laser.** The vaporization techniques using the neodymium:yttrium-aluminum-garnet (Nd:YAG) laser with high-energy density beams at high power (60 to 100 W) at a wavelength of 1064 nm have been effective for removing small amounts of tissue immediately during the procedure. However, this is a relatively inefficient technique because of the high power required. The holmium:yttrium-aluminum-garnet (Ho:YAG) laser energy is absorbed by water (unlike the Nd:YAG) at a wavelength of 2140 nm and causes considerable tissue vaporization. The methods of using the Ho:YAG laser have evolved because of several modifications in both the technology and the methodology. The technique has passed through simple vaporization to combined endoscopic laser ablation of the prostate and is now used to resect large pieces of prostatic tissue.

8. **b. recurrent urinary infections.** Although symptoms constitute the primary reason for recommending intervention, in patients with an obstructing prostate there are some absolute indications. These are acute urinary retention, recurrent infection, recurrent hematuria, and azotemia.

9. **e. serum creatinine value.** Patients with a serum creatinine level greater than 1.5% had a 25% incidence of postoperative complications, versus an incidence of 17% in those who had a normal creatinine level.

10. **e. pressure-flow studies.** Pressure-flow studies are recommended as an optional test. This is one of the best ways to evaluate a patient's degree of obstruction and detrusor function, particularly when the diagnosis is unclear.

11. **d. resection of tissue at 12 o'clock.** The resection begins at the bladder neck, starting at the 12-o'clock position and carried down to the 9-o'clock position, in a stepwise manner.

12. **a. failure to void.** The most common complications in the immediate postoperative period were, in one study, failing to void (6.5%), bleeding requiring transfusion (3.9%), and clot retention (3.3%).

13. **d. vaporization and desiccation.** With TUVP, two electrosurgical effects are combined: vaporization and desiccation. Vaporization steams tissue away using high heat, and coagulation uses lower heat to dry out tissue.

14. **a. Urinary flow rate improvement.** One study showed that in a relatively small number of cases, TUVP was as effective as TURP in relieving urodynamically proven outflow obstruction but the overall complication rate for TUVP was 17.5%.

15. **c. causes retrograde ejaculation in up to 37% of cases.** TUIP causes a decrease in retrograde ejaculation compared with TURP. The incidence of retrograde ejaculation after TURP ranges from 50% to 95%, but after TUIP it has been reported as occurring in 0% to 37% of cases.

89

Retropubic and Suprapubic Open Prostatectomy

MISOP HAN • ALAN W. PARTIN

QUESTIONS

1. The major advantage of open prostatectomy over transurethral resection of prostate (TURP) in the management of prostatic adenoma includes:
   a. removal of the prostatic adenoma under direct vision.
   b. decreased risk of hypernatremia.
   c. shortened convalescence period.
   d. decreased perioperative hemorrhage.
   e. enhanced preservation of erectile function.
2. The suprapubic prostatectomy, in comparison to the retropubic prostatectomy, allows:
   a. a direct visualization of the prostatic adenoma during enucleation.
   b. a better visualization of the prostatic fossa after enucleation to obtain hemostasis.
   c. an easier management of a large median lobe and/or bladder calculi.
   d. an extraperitoneal approach.
   e. a possible management of concomitant ureteral calculi.
3. The suprapubic approach to the prostatectomy is ideal for the patient with a large prostatic adenoma and:
   a. multiple small bladder calculi.
   b. total PSA greater than 10.0 ng/mL.
   c. erectile dysfunction.
   d. symptomatic bladder diverticulum.
   e. presence of dilated renal pelvis.
4. The most appropriate definitive treatment options for the patient with a 120-g prostatic adenoma and a symptomatic bladder diverticulum are:
   a. retropubic open prostatectomy with the fulguration of bladder diverticulum.
   b. long-acting α-adrenergic antagonist and prophylactic antibiotics.
   c. transurethral resection of prostate (TURP) followed by bladder diverticulectomy in 3 months.
   d. TURP and partial cystectomy.
   e. suprapubic prostatectomy with bladder diverticulectomy.
5. The contraindications to open prostatectomy include:
   a. biopsy-proven prostate cancer.
   b. bladder diverticulum.
   c. large bladder calculi secondary to obstruction.
   d. recurrent urinary tract infection.
   e. acute urinary retention.
6. Both retropubic and suprapubic prostatectomies:
   a. are performed in the space of Retzius.
   b. are ideal for patients with a large, obstructive prostatic adenoma and a concomitant, small bladder tumor.
   c. allow direct visualization of prostatic adenoma during enucleation.
   d. cause no trauma to the urinary bladder.
   e. require the control of dorsal vein complex before the enucleation of an obstructive prostatic adenoma.
7. The most common adverse event of the open prostatectomy is:
   a. erectile dysfunction.
   b. bladder neck contracture.
   c. retrograde ejaculation.
   d. deep vein thrombosis.
   e. stress urinary incontinence.

ANSWERS

1. **a. removal of the prostatic adenoma under direct vision.** When compared with TURP, open prostatectomy offers the advantages of lower re-treatment rate and more complete removal of the prostatic adenoma under direct vision and avoids the risk of dilutional hyponatremia (the TURP syndrome) that occurs in approximately 2% of patients undergoing TURP. The disadvantages, as compared with TURP, include the need for a lower midline incision and a resultant longer hospitalization and convalescence period. In addition, there may be an increased potential for perioperative hemorrhage.
2. **c. easier management of a large median lobe and/or bladder calculi.** Because the suprapubic procedure allows direct visualization of the bladder neck and bladder mucosa, this operation is ideally suited for patients with a large median lobe protruding into the bladder or large bladder calculi.
3. **d. symptomatic bladder diverticulum.** The suprapubic approach is also ideal for a patient with a large prostatic adenoma and a clinically significant bladder diverticulum.
4. **e. suprapubic prostatectomy with bladder diverticulectomy.** Open prostatectomy should be considered when the obstructive tissue is estimated to weigh more than 75 g. If sizable bladder diverticula justify removal, suprapubic prostatectomy and diverticulectomy should be performed concurrently.
5. **a. biopsy-proven prostate cancer.** Contraindications to open prostatectomy include a small fibrous gland, the presence of prostate cancer, previous prostatectomy, or pelvic surgery that may obliterate access to the prostate gland.
6. **a. they are performed in the space of Retzius.** For both the retropubic prostatectomy and the suprapubic prostatectomy, a mild Trendelenburg position is used to increase the distance between the umbilicus and the pubic symphysis and give optimal exposure to the retropubic space. In both procedures, a lower midline incision from the umbilicus to the pubic symphysis permits the linea alba to be incised, allowing the rectus abdominis muscles to be separated in the midline and the transversalis fascia to be incised sharply to expose the space of Retzius.
7. **c. retrograde ejaculation.** Retrograde ejaculation occurs in 80% to 90% of patients after open prostatectomy.

90

Epidemiology, Etiology, and Prevention of Prostate Cancer

ERIC A. KLEIN • ELIZABETH A. PLATZ • IAN M. THOMPSON

QUESTIONS

1. Following the prostate-specific antigen (PSA) "cull effect," the incidence of prostate cancer in the United States is:
   a. decreasing.
   b. stable.
   c. increasing.
   d. fluctuating.
2. The declining rate of prostate cancer mortality in the United States since 1991 has been caused by:
   a. PSA-based screening.
   b. better therapies for localized disease.
   c. more aggressive hormone therapy.
   d. combination of these factors.
3. Worldwide, prostate cancer is:
   a. the leading cancer diagnosis in men.
   b. the leading cause of cancer-related mortality.
   c. more common in northern European countries than in southern European ones.
   d. entirely genetic in origin.
4. Compared with a man with no family history of prostate cancer, the risk of developing prostate cancer in a man with one affected first-degree relative is:
   a. unchanged.
   b. 1.5 times higher.
   c. 2 times higher.
   d. 5 times higher.
5. *HPC1*-associated prostate cancers are:
   a. histologically similar to sporadic prostate cancer.
   b. caused by defects in the *BRCA2* gene.
   c. deficient in DNA repair.
   d. inherited in X-linked fashion.
6. Biologic functions of known prostate cancer susceptibility genes include:
   a. control of inflammatory response.
   b. DNA repair mechanisms.
   c. susceptibility to infection.
   d. all of the above.
7. Proliferative inflammatory atrophy (PIA) of the prostate represents:
   a. prior history of a sexually transmitted disease.
   b. cellular hyperproliferation to replace damaged tissue.
   c. genetic predisposition to prostate cancer.
   d. histologic evidence of a defect in the *MSR1* gene.
8. Shorter numbers of CAG repeats in exon 1 of the androgen receptor are believed to be associated with:
   a. a higher risk of developing prostate cancer.
   b. less aggressive tumors.
   c. higher levels of intraprostatic dihydrotestosterone.
   d. worse response to androgen deprivation.
9. The direct effect of estrogen on prostate cancer is:
   a. stimulation of tumor growth.
   b. inhibition of tumor growth.
   c. variable depending on receptor status.
   d. negligible.
10. Elevated serum levels of insulin-like growth factor (IGF) have been associated with:
    a. higher serum PSA levels.
    b. lower body mass index.
    c. reduced intraprostatic inflammation.
    d. higher risk of developing prostate cancer.
11. Evidence suggesting that vitamin D affects the risk of prostate cancer includes the fact that:
    a. men living in areas with less UV exposure have lower prostate cancer mortality rates.
    b. vitamin D levels are higher in older men.
    c. a calcium-poor diet predisposes men to prostate cancer.
    d. polymorphisms conferring lower vitamin D receptor activity are associated with increased risk for prostate cancer.
12. High body mass index is associated with:
    a. protection against oxidative stress.
    b. higher circulating androgens.
    c. lower serum PSA levels.
    d. better cancer-specific survival after radical prostatectomy.
13. Tumorigenic properties of the cyclooxygenase-2 enzyme include:
    a. inhibition of apoptosis.
    b. promotion of angiogenesis.
    c. stimulation of cellular proliferation.
    d. all of the above.

14. Impaired cellular defense mechanisms against oxidative stress in human prostate cancer include:
    a. promoter methylation of the *GSTP1* gene.
    b. enhanced DNA repair due to mutations in the *OGG1* gene.
    c. tumor production of racemase (AMACR).
    d. all of the above.
15. The major goal of a chemoprevention strategy is reduction in:
    a. disease incidence and morbidity.
    b. cost associated with treatment.
    c. disease-promoting lifestyle habits.
    d. disease-related mortality.
16. The major finding of the Prostate Cancer Prevention Trial (PCPT) was:
    a. finasteride reduced the 7-year period prevalence of prostate cancer by 25%.
    b. more men who took finasteride died of prostate cancer than those who did not.
    c. finasteride biased the interpretation of the prostate biopsies.
    d. finasteride worked best in men with a positive family history.
17. In the interpretation of the PCPT, "overdetection bias" refers to:
    a. more men taking finasteride were sampled.
    b. the histologic effect of finasteride on tumor grade.
    c. more men on placebo had high-grade cancers.
    d. the effect of volume reduction on tumor detection.
18. Shared cellular effects of selenium and vitamin E include:
    a. induction of apoptosis.
    b. cell-cycle arrest.
    c. antiandrogenic action.
    d. all of the above.
19. The protective effect of lycopene against prostate cancer may best be achieved by consuming:
    a. cooked foods.
    b. pure form as oral capsules.
    c. pure form with other antioxidants.
    d. raw vegetables.
20. In the PCPT, compared with placebo finasteride use was associated with a higher incidence of:
    a. prostatitis.
    b. urinary tract infection.
    c. surgical intervention for lower urinary tract symptoms.
    d. erectile dysfunction.
21. The HPC1 enzyme ribonuclease L (RNaseL):
    a. causes apoptosis.
    b. is mutated in most men with prostate cancer.
    c. is inhibited by selenium and vitamin E.
    d. is regulated by androgens.
    e. is inactive in men with benign prostatic hyperplasia.
22. The existence of multiple prostate cancer susceptibility genes suggests:
    a. dominant inheritance pattern.
    b. common clinical features associated with all identified genes.
    c. genetic heterogeneity in the cause of prostate cancer.
    d. need for yearly screening in those with a family history.
    e. multifocal tumors in affected individuals.
23. Compared with sporadic prostate cancers, cancers in men with *HPC1* mutations:
    a. have more high-grade prostatic intraepithelial neoplasia.
    b. have less perineural invasion.
    c. are more likely to be aneuploid.
    d. are histologically similar.
    e. have an intact basal cell layer.
24. A 62-year-old man with a PSA of 5.7 and a family history of prostate cancer undergoes a radical prostatectomy for clinical stage T1c prostate cancer. Pathology reveals an organ-confined Gleason 6 (3 + 3) tumor with negative margins. Molecular analysis of this tumor reveals an inactivating mutation in *HPC1*. He should be advised:
    a. to begin immediate hormonal therapy.
    b. to undergo adjuvant radiation therapy.
    c. that he is at risk of developing a central nervous system tumor.
    d. that his mother was an *HPC1* carrier.
    e. to begin serial PSA levels.
25. Hereditary prostate cancer is defined as:
    a. family history of prostate cancer.
    b. prostate cancer in a father or brother.
    c. prostate cancer in a man under age 55.
    d. prostate cancer in three successive generations.
    e. family with two affected members.

ANSWERS

1. **c. increasing.** According to SEER estimates, the incidence of prostate cancer in the United States was rising before the introduction of PSA screening, rose and declined sharply in the first 5 years that PSA was used as a screening test, and is now rising at a rate similar to that seen before the introduction of PSA testing (see Fig. 90-1).
2. **d. combination of these factors.** The observed decline in mortality since 1991 is temporally related to increased diagnostic and treatment activity in both the pre-PSA and PSA eras. Outcomes for patients treated in the 1980s should be reflected in the mortality data of the 1990s, whereas outcomes for patients treated in the PSA era (the 1990s) have had less time to affect recent mortality data. Although the effect of PSA screening has not been fully accounted for yet, it seems likely that a combination of screening and treatment-related factors have resulted in lower mortality.
3. **c. more common in northern European countries than in southern European ones.** Prostate cancer is the fourth most common male malignancy worldwide. Scandinavian countries have a particularly high rate of prostate cancer diagnosis and death when compared with southern European countries.
4. **c. 2 times higher.** In someone with a positive family history of prostate cancer, the relative risk increases according to the number of affected family members, their degree of relatedness, and the age at which they were affected. Men with one affected first-degree relative have double the risk of someone with no family history. (See Table 90-2.)
5. **a. are histologically similar to sporadic prostate cancer.** *HPC1*-associated cancers are caused by defects in the *RNaseL* gene, which has antiviral and proapoptotic functions but does not affect DNA repair mechanisms. These tumors have

autosomal dominant inheritance and are histologically indistinguishable from sporadic cancers.

6. **d. all of the above.** All of these biologic functions are represented in genes shown to predispose men with variant gene structure to prostate cancer. (See Table 90-3.)

7. **b. cellular hyperproliferation to replace damaged tissue.** PIA is a spectrum of lesions characterized by epithelial atrophy, low apoptotic index, and an increased proliferative index, usually associated with inflammatory infiltrates. Evidence suggests that PIA is a regenerative lesion appearing as a consequence of infection or cell trauma resulting from oxidant damage, hypoxia, infection, or autoimmunity and that its hyperproliferative state leads to cancer.

8. **a. a higher risk of developing prostate cancer.** The length of the polymorphic repeat is inversely related to the transcriptional activity of the androgen receptor (AR) gene (i.e., it modulates the response of AR to androgens). For example, long CAG repeats are associated with androgen insensitivity in patients with spinobulbar muscular atrophy (Kennedy's disease). Short CAG repeat lengths are hypothesized to result in enhanced AR-mediated androgen activity and increased susceptibility to benign prostatic hyperplasia and prostate cancer but have no effect on intraprostatic DHT levels or response to androgen withdrawal.

9. **c. variable depending on receptor status.** Estrogens have been postulated to protect against prostate cancer via inhibition of prostate epithelial cell growth but alternatively to increase risk by eliciting inflammation in concert with androgens or by the production of mutagenic metabolites. Estradiol promotes prostate epithelial cell growth via binding of estrogen receptor (ER)α, and inhibits growth by effects mediated through ERβ, so its net effect will depend on the relative levels of these two receptors. ERβ expression is silenced by methylation in most human prostate cancers.

10. **d. higher risk of developing prostate cancer.** Several studies have correlated plasma IGF-1 levels with an increased risk of prostate cancer, with relative risks as high as 4.3 versus controls. Higher levels of IGF-1 are associated with higher body mass index but have not been demonstrated to affect serum PSA or intraprostatic inflammation.

11. **d. polymorphisms conferring lower vitamin D receptor activity are associated with increased risk for prostate cancer.** Interest in vitamin D as a determinant of prostate cancer risk comes from several epidemiologic observations: (1) men living in Northern latitudes with less exposure to sunlight-derived ultraviolet (UV) exposure have a higher mortality rate from prostate cancer; (2) prostate cancer occurs more frequently in older men, in whom vitamin D deficiency is more common both because of less UV exposure and age-related declines in the hydroxylases responsible for synthesis of active vitamin D; (3) African-Americans, whose skin melanin blocks UV radiation and inhibits activation of vitamin D, have the highest worldwide incidence and mortality rates for prostate cancer; (4) dietary intake of dairy products rich in calcium, which depresses serum levels of vitamin D, are associated with a higher risk of prostate cancer; and (5) native Japanese, whose diet is rich in vitamin D derived from fish, have a low incidence of prostate cancer. Finally, polymorphisms resulting in vitamin D receptors with lower activity have been associated with increased risk for prostate cancer.

12. **c. lower serum PSA levels.** Higher body mass index has been associated with increased biologic measures of oxidative stress, lower circulating androgen levels, lower serum PSA (perhaps as a consequence of lower circulating androgens), and worse cancer specific survival after radical prostatectomy.

13. **d. all of the above.** Cyclooxygenase-2 (COX-2) is an inducible enzyme that mediates acute and chronic inflammation, pain, and cellular repair mechanisms. COX-2 expression is rapidly induced in response to inflammatory or mitogenic stimuli, including bacterial lipopolysaccharides, proinflammatory cytokines (IL-1α, IL-2, and TNF-α), epidermal and platelet-derived growth factors, and androgens. Prostaglandins resulting from COX-2 expression mediate a variety of responses to tissue injury and hypoxia, including apoptosis, cellular proliferation, and angiogenesis, all of which promote tumor formation.

14. **a. promoter methylation of the *GSTP1* gene.** GSTP1 is a frontline antioxidant enzyme that is turned off in about 70% of cases of prostatic intraepithelial neoplasia and 100% of prostate cancers, leading to a defect in scavenging of reactive oxygen and nitrogen species. Mutations in *OGG1* result in defective, not enhanced, DNA repair, which also contributes to defects in fighting oxidative stress. Racemase catalyzes the oxidation of fatty acids and produces reactive oxygen species, but this is a part of normal cellular metabolism and does represent a defect in handling oxidative stress.

15. **a. disease incidence and morbidity.** As observed by Thomas Adams, "Prevention is so much better than cure, because it saves the labor of being sick." Thus, the major goal of chemoprevention is reduction in disease incidence and its attendant morbidity, with reduced cost and mortality being secondary advantages.

16. **a. finasteride reduced the 7-year period prevalence of prostate cancer by 25%.** The main findings of the PCPT were: (1) the prevalence of prostate cancer was reduced by 24.8% (HR = 0.75, 95% CI 18.6 to 30.6), from 24.4% to 18.4% in those randomized to finasteride compared with placebo; (2) the prevalence of Gleason grade 7 to 10 tumors was higher in the finasteride group than placebo (6.4 vs. 5.1%, HR= 1.27, 95% CI 1.07 to 1.50); (3) the risk reduction associated with finasteride among risk groups defined by age, family history, race, and PSA were of the same general magnitude; and (4) sexual side effects were more common with finasteride, whereas urinary symptoms were more common with placebo. There were an equal number of deaths due to prostate cancer (5) in each study arm, and finasteride worked equally well in men with and without a family history of prostate cancer.

17. **d. the effect of volume reduction on tumor detection.** A similar number of tissue cores were taken on end-of-study biopsy in both arms of the PCPT, and because the finasteride-treated glands were on average 25% smaller than those on the placebo arm, a relatively larger proportion of the gland was sampled and evaluated histologically, leading to an increased chance of detecting cancer ("overdetection bias"). This suggests the possibility that the risk reduction associated with finasteride may in fact be larger than observed.

18. **d. all of the above.** Selenium and vitamin E possess all of these biologic activities and act synergistically in in-vitro models.

19. **a. cooked foods.** Lycopene is a red-orange carotenoid found primarily in tomatoes and tomato-derived products including tomato sauce, tomato paste, and ketchup, and other red fruits and vegetables. In an in-vivo model in which male rats were treated with *N*-methyl-*N*-nitrosourea and testosterone to induce prostate cancer, a protective effect was observed both for calorie restriction and tomato powder but not pure lycopene. This observation suggests that tomato products contain compounds in addition to lycopene that modify prostate carcinogenesis and that reduced caloric consumption and a diet rich in tomato-based foods may be more beneficial than taking oral lycopene supplements in reducing the risk of prostate cancer.

20. **d. erectile dysfunction.** The incidence of erectile dysfunction and other sexually related side effects was more frequent in the finasteride arm, whereas the incidence of prostatitis, urinary tract infection, benign prostatic hyperplasia, urinary retention, and surgical intervention for lower urinary tract symptoms or retention was lower.

21. **a. causes apoptosis.** RNase L is the terminal enzyme of the 2-5A system, an RNA degradation pathway that plays an important role in mediating the biologic effects of interferons, especially in response to viral infection. Type I interferons induce a family of 2-5A synthetases that are activated by dsRNA resulting in the conversion of adenosine triphosphate to a series of short 2′ to 5′ linked oligoadenylates (2-5A). 2-5A binds with high affinity to RNase L, converting it from its inactive form as a monomer to a potent dimer that degrades single-stranded RNA, preventing viral replication, interfering with protein synthesis, and causing caspase-mediated apoptosis. (See Fig. 90-5.)

22. **c. genetic heterogeneity in the cause of prostate cancer.** Current evidence suggests that most prostate cancer is polygenic in origin.

23. **d. are histologically similar.** Cancers linked to HPC1 have been reported to present with higher grade and more advanced stages, although there are no reported histologic differences with sporadic cancers.

24. **e. to begin serial PSA levels.** The presence of a mutation in HPC1 has not been shown to be associated with adverse outcome after curative treatment, so that this patient's management should be dictated by his pathologic stage. Gleason's stage 6 disease that is organ confined has a very favorable prognosis, and the appropriate management is serial monitoring of PSA.

25. **d. prostate cancer in three successive generations.** Hereditary prostate cancer is a subset of the familial form and has been defined as nuclear families with more than three affected members, prostate cancer in three successive generations, or two affected individuals diagnosed with cancer before age 55.

91

Pathology of Prostatic Neoplasia

JONATHAN I. EPSTEIN

QUESTIONS

1. Which of the following statements regarding prostatic intraepithelial neoplasia (PIN) is FALSE?
   a. Low-grade PIN should not be commented on in diagnostic reports.
   b. PIN by itself does not give rise to elevated serum prostate-specific antigen (PSA) values.
   c. High-grade PIN predominates in the transition zone.
   d. The incidence of high-grade PIN on needle biopsy averages 5% to 10%.
   e. High-grade PIN is thought to be a precursor to many prostate cancers.
2. According to the largest studies, when high-grade PIN is found by needle biopsy, what is the approximate probability of finding carcinoma on subsequent biopsy?
   a. 0% to 5%
   b. 5% to 10%
   c. 20% to 30%
   d. 40% to 50%
   e. 70% to 80%
3. What percentage of stage T1c cancers are located predominantly in the transition zone?
   a. 5%
   b. 15%
   c. 30%
   d. 50%
   e. 70%
4. What percentage of prostate cancers are multifocal?
   a. 15%
   b. 25%
   c. 40%
   d. 60%
   e. 85%
5. The Gleason grade in a radical prostatectomy factors in the:
   a. two highest grade architectural patterns.
   b. most prevalent and second most prevalent architectural patterns and a tertiary grade if present.
   c. highest and lowest grade architectural patterns.
   d. highest architectural pattern and highest cytologic grade and tertiary grade if present.
   e. most prevalent architectural pattern and cytologic grade and tertiary grade if present.
6. Which of the following statements is FALSE regarding a needle biopsy showing a small focus of atypical glands?
   a. The average incidence of atypical glands on biopsy is less than 10%.
   b. Cases diagnosed as atypical have a relatively high likelihood of being changed upon expert review.
   c. Repeat biopsy should increase the sampling of the initial atypical site.
   d. The risk of cancer on subsequent biopsy is 40% to 50%.
   e. The level of serum PSA correlates with the risk of cancer on subsequent biopsy.
7. What percentage of tumors with positive margins progress after radical prostatectomy?
   a. 10%
   b. 30%
   c. 50%
   d. 70%
   e. 90%
8. Which of the following is least crucial to note in every radical prostatectomy pathology report?
   a. Margin status
   b. Gleason score
   c. Organ-confined status
   d. Perineural invasion
   e. Seminal vesicle invasion status
9. Which of the following subtypes of prostate cancer is associated with a worse prognosis compared with ordinary acinar carcinoma?
   a. Mucinous carcinomas
   b. Ductal adenocarcinomas
   c. Small cell carcinomas
   d. Squamous cell carcinoma
   e. All of the above
10. Which of the following immunohistochemical markers is least useful in distinguishing between prostate adenocarcinoma and transitional cell carcinoma?
    a. PSA
    b. PSAP
    c. Thrombomodulin
    d. 34BE12
    e. Cytokeratin 20

ANSWERS

1. **c. High-grade PIN predominates in the transition zone.** Several studies have noted an increase of high-grade PIN in the peripheral zone of the prostate, corresponding to the site of origin for most adenocarcinomas of the prostate.
2. **c. 20% to 30%.** The largest studies published to date on this issue report a 23% to 35% probability of cancer found on subsequent biopsy.
3. **b. 15%.** In clinical stage T2 carcinomas and in 85% of nonpalpable tumors diagnosed on needle biopsy (stage T1c), the major tumor mass is peripheral in location.
4. **e. 85%.** Adenocarcinoma of the prostate is multifocal in more than 85% of cases.
5. **b. most prevalent and second most prevalent architectural patterns and a tertiary grade if present.** It is recommended that in radical prostatectomy specimens, the routine Gleason score, consisting of the most prevalent and second most prevalent architectural patterns, should be recorded along with a note stating that there is a tertiary high-grade pattern (Pan et al, 2000).
6. **e. The level of serum PSA correlates with the risk of cancer on subsequent biopsy.** Surprisingly, in men with a prior atypical biopsy, the level of serum PSA elevation or results of digital rectal examination do not correlate with the risk of a subsequent biopsy showing carcinoma.
7. **c. 50%.** In only approximately 50% of men with positive margins does the disease progress after radical prostatectomy.
8. **d. Perineural invasion.** Perineural invasion by itself in radical prostatectomy specimens does not worsen prognosis because perineural invasion merely represents extension of tumor along a plane of decreased resistance and not invasion into lymphatics (Hassan and Maksem, 1980; Ng et al, 2004).
9. **e. All of the above.** Mucinous adenocarcinoma of the prostate gland is one of the least common morphologic variants of prostatic carcinoma. It has an aggressive biologic behavior and, like nonmucinous prostate carcinoma, has a propensity to produce bone metastases and increased serum acid phosphatase and PSA levels with advanced disease. The average survival time of patients with small cell carcinoma of the prostate is less than 1 year. Most prostatic duct adenocarcinomas are of advanced stage at presentation and have an aggressive course. Pure primary squamous carcinoma of the prostate is rare and is associated with a poor survival.
10. **e. Cytokeratin 20.** CK7 and CK20 positivities in transitional cell carcinoma are 70% to 100% and 15% to 71%, respectively. The problem with these markers is that they are not specific.

92

Ultrasonography and Biopsy of the Prostate

JOHN R. RAMEY • ETHAN J. HALPERN • LEONARD G. GOMELLA

QUESTIONS

1. The prostatic corpora amylacea are:
   a. always associated with prostate infection.
   b. most commonly seen between the transition and peripheral zone of the prostate.
   c. pathognomonic for acute prostatitis.
   d. associated with hypoechoic lesions and prostate cancer.
   e. are calcifications in the peripheral zone exclusively and are located in blood vessels.
2. Which of the following statements is TRUE about transrectal ultrasound of the seminal vesicles?
   a. Masses in the seminal vesicles are the most common lesion seen on TRUS of the prostate.
   b. The seminal vesicles are usually asymmetrical and normally measure less than 2 cm in length in the adult.
   c. Most cystic masses in the seminal vesicle are malignant and related to prostate cancer.
   d. A solid mass in the seminal vesicle is always associated with malignancy.
   e. Solid masses in the seminal vesicle can be caused by schistosomiasis in endemic regions.
3. Which of the following statements about transrectal sonography after radical prostatectomy is FALSE? It:
   a. should show a smooth tapering of the bladder neck to the urethra.
   b. often reveals a hypoechoic mass anterior to the anastomosis, which usually represents recurrent cancer.
   c. should have an intact fat plane between the bladder neck/urethra and the rectum.
   d. should always be accompanied by biopsies of the perianastomotic area and bladder neck in patients with prostate specific-antigen (PSA) recurrence.
   e. is contraindicated because of potential disruption of the anastomosis.
4. Which of the following statements concerning ultrasonographic estimates of prostate size/volume is TRUE?
   a. Only one formula (prolate ellipse) is acceptable to determine prostate volume.
   b. There is poor correlation between radical prostatectomy specimen weights and volume as measured by the TRUS.
   c. The mature average prostate is between 20 and 25 g and remains relatively constant until about age 50 when the gland enlarges in many men.
   d. Prostate cancer is always associated with an increase in overall volume of the prostate.
   e. Planimetry with a stepping device should be used for routine prostate volume determinations.
5. A hypoechoic lesion of the prostate can be caused by all of the following EXCEPT:
   a. hematologic malignancies.
   b. prostate cancer.
   c. transition zone, benign prostatic hyperplasia nodules.
   d. granulomatous prostatitis.
   e. normal urethra.
6. Which one of the following is NOT considered to be a commonly agreed upon indication for transrectal prostate biopsy?
   a. PSA velocity > 0.75 to 1.0 ng/dL/yr
   b. Nodule on digital rectal examination regardless of PSA level
   c. Routine evaluation of male infertility
   d. Free PSA of < 10% with a total PSA < 10 ng/dL
   e. Diagnosis of recurrence after radiation therapy in a rising PSA

7. Which of the following statements is TRUE about anesthesia for TRUS prostate biopsy?
   a. Intrarectal lidocaine gel is as effective as the injection of lidocaine.
   b. It is not necessary even with extended-core biopsies owing to the small size of the needle.
   c. It is best performed using direct injection of lidocaine into the prostate gland.
   d. It is typically performed using lidocaine, a long 22-gauge spinal needle, and the biopsy channel of the ultrasound probe.
   e. It is typically performed using digital guidance to ensure that the base of the prostate near the seminal vesicles is infiltrated.

8. When performing TRUS prostate biopsy:
   a. the left lateral decubitus position is most commonly used.
   b. color and power Doppler should be available to localize the malignant foci.
   c. enemas are never used before the procedure and may increase the risk of bleeding.
   d. intravenous antibiotic prophylaxis is necessary in all patients to prevent urosepsis.
   e. the dorsal lithotomy position increases the diagnostic accuracy of the prostate biopsies.

9. When performing TRUS prostate biopsy:
   a. only hypoechoic lesions should be sampled.
   b. a minimum of 8 to 10 systematic biopsies is now most commonly used.
   c. the transition zone should be included in all initial biopsies because of the high incidence of cancer in this area.
   d. sextant biopsy represents the standard of care for the diagnosis of prostate cancer today.
   e. isoechoic lesions are rarely cancerous and should not be sampled unless they are calcified.

10. Which of the following statements is TRUE concerning fine-needle aspiration of the prostate?
    a. Complications are greater than with TRUS needle biopsy techniques.
    b. Diagnostic accuracy in determining Gleason score is superior to that with core needle biopsy.
    c. It is more costly than other TRUS biopsy techniques commonly used.
    d. It is commonly used outside the United States and has a low morbidity.
    e. It is the most accurate way to diagnose and grade prostate cancer.

11. Which of the following statements about antibiotic prophylaxis for TRUS biopsy is TRUE?
    a. It eliminates the risk of any infection.
    b. It reduces the risk of febrile urinary tract infection requiring hospitalization.
    c. It is not necessary if the probe is sterilized and an enema is given.
    d. Epididymitis is the most common infection after TRUS biopsy even if antibiotics are used.
    e. Bacteriuria is the only indication for antibiotics after TRUS prostate biopsy.

12. Hematospermia after TRUS biopsy:
    a. usually requires hospitalization.
    b. is eliminated with the routine use of antibiotics.
    c. usually clears immediately after TRUS biopsy.
    d. can persist for up to 4 to 6 weeks after TRUS biopsy.
    e. is eliminated if the probe is held firmly against the prostate after the needle is passed.

13. Which of the following statements is TRUE in men with a negative prostate biopsy?
    a. They can be assured that no cancer is present.
    b. They will require repeated biopsy until the diagnosis is made.
    c. Transurethral biopsy is the next step after an initial negative biopsy.
    d. Additional biopsies demonstrate decreasing yield of detecting cancer, and the cancer tends to be of lower grade and stage.
    e. They should undergo transperineal biopsy for all future biopsies because these have been shown to be the most accurate approach in large randomized European trials.

14. Color and power Doppler examinations are being used to improve the diagnostic accuracy of TRUS needle biopsy of the prostate. Which of the following statements is FALSE?
    a. On color Doppler, red signals indicate arterial flow and blue signals indicate venous flow.
    b. These are the most accurate technologies to use to diagnose prostate cancer on TRUS-directed biopsy.
    c. Power Doppler cannot identify slow-moving blood in vessels.
    d. Ultrasonic contrast media appears to enhance the utility of color and power Doppler examinations.
    e. Doppler ultrasound may be effective in predicting Gleason grade and outcome in prostate cancer.

ANSWERS

1. **b. most commonly seen between the transition and peripheral zone of the prostate.** Corpora amylacea develop in the surgical capsule between the transition and peripheral zones of the prostate.

2. **e. Solid masses in the seminal vesicle can be caused by schistosomiasis in endemic regions.** While cystic lesions of the seminal vesicle can be presumed to be benign, solid masses represent a small chance of malignancy. Schistosomiasis should be considered in the differential diagnosis of a solid seminal vesicle mass, especially in endemic regions.

3. **b. often reveals a hypoechoic mass anterior to the anastomosis, which usually represents recurrent cancer.** Many patients will demonstrate a nodule of tissue anterior to the anastomosis, representing the ligated dorsal vein complex.

4. **c. The mature average prostate is between 20 and 25 g and remains relatively constant until about age 50 when the gland enlarges in many men.** The prostate size increases at puberty. Many men develop symptomatic enlargement of the prostate that typically begins after age 50.

5. **a. hematologic malignancies.** Many lesions can be hypoechoic and many will prove to be malignant, reinforcing the need for biopsy of these lesions if seen. Many cancers, including hematologic malignancies of the prostate, are isoechoic.

6. **c. Routine evaluation of male infertility.** Although a TRUS of the prostate may be useful to identify anatomic abnormalities of the prostate, biopsy of the prostate is not part of routine infertility evaluation.

7. **d. It is typically performed using lidocaine, a long 22-gauge spinal needle, and the biopsy channel of the ultrasound probe.** All recent studies indicate that infiltration of lidocaine around the neurovascular bundles increases tolerability of TRUS prostate biopsy.

8. **a. the left lateral decubitus position is most commonly used.** TRUS biopsy has become the gold standard to diagnose prostate cancer. It is most commonly performed with the patient in the left lateral decubitus position. Dorsal lithotomy may also be used in certain circumstances.

9. **b. a minimum of 8 to 10 systematic biopsies is now most commonly used.** Sextant biopsy revolutionized the utility of TRUS biopsy to diagnose prostate cancer. However, significant numbers of cancers were missed based on the analysis of radical prostatectomy specimens. Increasing to a minimum of 8 to 10 systematic biopsies has increased the diagnostic yield on the first biopsy session.

10. **d. It is commonly used outside the United States and has a low morbidity.** Fine-needle aspiration is associated with a low morbidity and is used extensively outside the United States. The concern about the procedure is that it requires great skill to analyze the samples and grading may not be as accurate as core sampling.

11. **b. It reduces the risk of febrile urinary tract infection requiring hospitalization.** Although the short-term use of prophylactic antibiotics can reduce the incidence of serious infections, it does not completely eliminate the risk of infection.

12. **d. can persist for up to 4 to 6 weeks after TRUS biopsy.** Patients should be counseled about the likelihood of hematospermia after TRUS biopsy.

13. **d. Additional biopsies demonstrate decreasing yield of detecting cancer and the cancers tend to be of lower grade and stage.** A large European screening study suggested that as the number of biopsy sessions increased to ultimately diagnose prostate cancer, the cancers diagnosed after several biopsy sessions were generally of lower grade and stage.

14. **a. On color Doppler, red signals indicate arterial flow and blue signals indicate venous flow.** Advanced ultrasound techniques such as color and power Doppler are being investigated to improve the diagnostic accuracy of TRUS biopsy. The color registration on routine color Doppler refers to the direction of flow relative to the transducer and is not related to specific arterial or venous flow.

93

Prostate Cancer Tumor Markers

MATTHEW B. GRETZER • ALAN W. PARTIN

QUESTIONS

1. Serum prostate-specific antigen (PSA) levels are specific for the presence of prostate:
   a. disease.
   b. cancer.
   c. enlargement.
   d. inflammation.
   e. none of the above.

2. Most detectable PSA in sera is bound to:
   a. albumin.
   b. α_1-antichymotrypsin.
   c. α_2-macroglobulin.
   d. human kallikrein.
   e. none of the above.

3. Is it TRUE or FALSE that as many as 75% of men presenting with elevated PSA levels are not found to have prostate cancer after TRUS biopsy?

4. Compared with prostatic tissue PSA levels, prostatic tissue levels of hK2 are:
   a. elevated in well-differentiated prostate cancer tissue.
   b. elevated in poorly differentiated prostate cancer tissue.
   c. depressed in well-differentiated prostate cancer tissue.
   d. depressed in poorly differentiated prostate cancer tissue.
   e. not measurable in prostatic cancer tissue.

5. The serum half-life of PSA calculated after removal of all prostate tissue is closest to:
   a. 24 hours.
   b. 36 hours.
   c. 48 hours.
   d. 60 hours.
   e. 96 hours.

6. Evaluation of tissue from prostate cancer specimens has demonstrated higher mRNA expression levels compared with normal prostate tissue, suggesting that prostate cancer cells make more PSA than normal prostatic tissue. (TRUE or FALSE)

7. A man with a PSA of 4 ng/mL on finasteride for 2 years stops this medication and begins saw palmetto. What should his PSA be on his next annual check-up?
   a. 2 ng/mL
   b. 4 ng/mL
   c. 6 ng/mL
   d. 8 ng/mL
   e. 10 ng/mL

8. In the absence of prostate cancer, serum PSA levels vary with:
   a. age alone.
   b. race alone.
   c. prostate volume alone.
   d. albumin concentration.
   e. age, race, and prostate volume.

9. The minimal length of follow-up time over which changes in PSA should be adjusted for PSA velocity to be useful in cancer detection is:
   a. 4 months.
   b. 6 months.
   c. 12 months.
   d. 18 months.
   e. 24 months.

10. Compared with men without prostate cancer, the fraction of free or unbound PSA in serum from men with prostate cancer is:
    a. equal.
    b. lower.
    c. greater.
    d. undetectable by current assays.
    e. varies depending on which assay is used.

11. The percentage of free PSA has been approved by the U.S. Food and Drug Administration (FDA) for use in improving:
    a. cancer detection in men with PSA levels < 4 ng/mL.
    b. cancer detection in men with benign digital rectal examinations and PSA levels of 4 to 10 ng/mL.
    c. the determination of prognosis.
    d. cancer detection in men found to have ASAP.
    e. cancer detection in men with a family history of prostate cancer.

12. After stopping finasteride, serum PSA should _______ and the percentage of free PSA should ________.
    a. increase, not change
    b. increase, increase
    c. decrease, not change
    d. decrease, decrease
    e. not change, not change

13. Immunohistochemical studies have demonstrated different expression patterns for hK2 and PSA in benign versus cancerous tissue and may be best described as:
    a. benign: intense PSA and minimal hK2 expression.
    b. cancer: intense PSA and minimal hK2 expression.
    c. benign: minimal PSA and hK2 expression.
    d. benign: intense PSA and hK2 expression.
    e. cancer: minimal PSA and hK2 expression.

14. The methylation status of these regions may affect gene expression and play a role in carcinogenesis.
    a. Stop codon
    b. Glycine-cytosine–rich regions
    c. Promoter region
    d. Thymine islands
    e. All of the above

15. The products of two hypermethylated genes evaluated in prostate cancer development are:
    a. UROC28 and hepsin.
    b. GSTP1 and RASSF1A.
    c. DD3 PAC and NMP 48.
    d. all of the above.

ANSWERS

1. **e. none of the above.** Although PSA is widely accepted as a prostate cancer tumor marker, it is organ specific and not disease specific. Unfortunately there is an overlap in the serum PSA levels among men with cancer and benign disease. Thus, elevated serum PSA levels may reflect alterations within the prostate secondary to tissue architectural changes such as cancer, inflammation, or benign prostatic hyperplasia (BPH).
2. **b. α_1-antichymotrypsin.** The current clinically relevant immunodetectable complexed forms of PSA are bound to ACT and, to a lesser extent, to API. The sum of these and other presently unknown PSA complexes is represented by the term complexed PSA (cPSA). The major form of cPSA in serum, PSA bound to ACT, is found in greater serum concentrations in men with cancer than in men with benign disease.
3. **True**. Although up to 30% of men presenting with an elevated PSA level may be diagnosed after this invasive procedure, as many as 75% to 80% will not be found to have cancer.
4. **b. elevated in poorly differentiated prostate cancer tissue.** Immunohistochemical studies reveal different tissue expression patterns for hK2 and PSA. In benign epithelium, PSA is intensely expressed compared with the minimal immunoreactivity of hK2. This is in contrast to cancerous tissue, in which more intense expression of hK2 is seen.
5. **d. 60 hours.** PSA is likely cleared from the blood through the liver because the size of the complexed structure is too large for glomerular filtration. The serum half-life of PSA, calculated after removal of all prostate tissue is 2 to 3 days. Thus, after surgical removal several weeks are required for PSA to become undetectable.
6. **False.** Although prostate cancer cells do not necessarily make more PSA than normal prostate cells, elevated serum levels are likely a result of cancer progression and destabilization of the prostate histologic architecture (Stamey et al, 1987). Studies have demonstrated that prostate cancer cells do not make more PSA but rather less PSA than normal prostatic tissue (Meng et al, 2002). Evaluation of tissue from prostate cancer specimens have demonstrated up to 1.5-fold lower mRNA expression levels compared with normal prostate tissue (Meng et al, 2002).
7. **d. 8 ng/mL.** Finasteride (5 mg) and other 5α-reductase inhibitors for treatment of BPH have been shown to lower PSA levels by an average of 50% after 6 months of treatment (Guess et al, 1993). Thus, one can multiply the PSA level by 2 to obtain the "expected" PSA level of a patient who has been on finasteride for 6 months or more. Although saw palmetto has not been shown to affect PSA levels, possible contamination of these unregulated supplements may contain compounds that can alter PSA levels (i.e., PC-SPES, now off the market).
8. **e. age, race, and prostate volume.** In men without BPH, the rate of change in PSA is 0.04 ng/mL/yr (Carter et al, 1992b; Oesterling et al, 1993), compared with 0.07 to 0.27 ng/mL/yr in men with BPH who are between the ages 60 and 85 years (Carter et al, 1992b). Cross-sectional data suggest that PSA increases 4% per milliliter of prostate volume and 30% and 5% of the variance in PSA can be accounted for by prostate volume and age, respectively (Oesterling et al, 1993). African-Americans without prostate cancer have higher PSA values than whites (Morgan et al, 1996; Fowler et al, 1999). Fowler and colleagues (1999) have demonstrated that on a volume/volume basis, the benign prostatic tissue of African-American men contributes more PSA to sera than does the benign prostatic tissue of white men—a difference that increases with age.
9. **d. 18 months.** The minimal length of follow-up time over which changes in PSA should be adjusted for PSA velocity to be useful in cancer detection has been calculated in separate studies to be 18 months (Smith and Catalona, 1994; Carter et al, 1995b; Kadmon et al, 1996). Furthermore, evaluation of three repeated PSA measurements, to determine an average rate of change in PSA, would appear to optimize the accuracy of PSA velocity for cancer detection (Carter et al, 1992a, 1992b; 1995b).
10. **b. lower.** Although prostate cancer cells do not produce more PSA than benign prostate epithelium, the PSA produced from malignant cells appears to escape proteolytic processing. Thus, men with prostate cancer have a greater fraction of serum PSA complexed to ACT and a lower percentage of total PSA that is free compared with men without prostate cancer (Christensson et al, 1993; Leinone et al, 1993; Lilja et al, 1993; Stenman et al, 1994).
11. **b. cancer detection in men with benign digital rectal examinations and PSA levels of 4 to 10 ng/mL.** Currently the percentage of free PSA is FDA approved for use to aid PSA testing in men with benign digital rectal examinations and minimal PSA elevations, within the diagnostic gray zone of 4 to 10 ng/mL.
12. **c. decrease, not change.** Free PSA and total PSA both decrease in men on finasteride. As both decline, the percentage of free PSA is not altered significantly by this medication (Keetch et al, 1997; Panneck et al, 1998).
13. **a. benign: intense PSA and minimal nK2 expression.** Immunohistochemical studies reveal different tissue expression patterns for hK2 and PSA. In benign epithelium, PSA is intensely expressed compared with the minimal immunoreactivity of hK2 (Tremblay et al, 1997; Darson et al, 1999). This is in contrast to cancerous tissue, in which more intense expression of hK2 is seen. Furthermore, hK2 immunohistochemically stains the different Gleason grades of prostate cancer differently than does PSA. This inverse staining relationship of hK2 is seen as intense staining in high-grade (Gleason primary grade 4 to 5) cancers and lymph node metastasis compared with minimal staining of low-grade (Gleason primary grade 1 to 3) cancers and even weaker association in benign tissue, in which PSA exhibits intense staining (Darson et al, 1997, 1999; Tremblay et al, 1997; Kwiatkowski et al, 1998).
14. **b. Glycine-cytosine–rich regions.** Segments within the gene promoter that are composed of glycine-cytosine–rich regions

are termed **CpG islands**. Alterations in the methylation status of these regions may affect gene expression and have been shown to play a role in carcinogenesis (Jones et al, 2002). Furthermore, cumulative effects of environmental exposures such as diet and stress throughout one's life may impact DNA methylation status and thus contribute to risk of cancer development (Li et al, 2003).

15. **b. GSTP1 and RASSF1A.** The products of two hypermethylated genes that have been evaluated in prostate cancer development are glutathione S-transferase P1 (GSTP1) and RAS-association domain family protein isoform A (RASSF1A). GSTP1 belongs to a family of detoxifying enzymes that are involved in metabolic reduction of electrophilic carcinogens. In addition to GSTP1, hypermethylation of RASSF1A has been noted to occur in up to 70% of prostate cancers (Kuzmin et al, 2002; Liu et al, 2002). Early findings have noted an association of this marker with more aggressive tumors and may aid in distinguishing these cancers from more indolent cancers.

94

Diagnosis and Staging of Prostate Cancer

H. BALLENTINE CARTER • MOHAMMED ALLAF • ALAN W. PARTIN

QUESTIONS

1. What is the most useful first-line test for diagnosis of prostate cancer?
   a. Digital rectal examination (DRE)
   b. Prostate-specific antigen (PSA) assay
   c. Prostatic acid phosphatase (PAP) assay
   d. Transrectal ultrasonography (TRUS)
   e. Combination of DRE and PSA
2. Most immunodetectable PSA in sera is bound to which of the following?
   a. Albumin
   b. α_1-Antichymotrypsin (ACT)
   c. α_2-Macroglobulin (MG)
   d. Human kallikrein
   e. ACT and MG
3. Serum PSA levels vary with which factor?
   a. Age
   b. Race
   c. Prostate volume
   d. ACT concentration
   e. Age, race, and prostate volume
4. Serum PSA elevations are specific for which of the following? The presence of prostate:
   a. disease
   b. cancer
   c. enlargement
   d. inflammation
   e. None of the above
5. A 60-year-old man taking finasteride (Proscar) for 2 years with a PSA value of 4 ng/mL would most likely, if he were not taking finasteride, have which PSA value?
   a. 2 ng/mL
   b. 6 ng/mL
   c. 8 ng/mL
   d. 12 ng/mL
   e. 4 ng/mL
6. Which of the following tests has the highest positive predictive value for prostate cancer?
   a. PSA
   b. DRE
   c. TRUS
   d. Combination of DRE and TRUS
   e. Human glandular kallikrein (hK2)
7. The goals of staging for prostate cancer include which of the following?
   a. To predict the prognosis
   b. To select rational therapy on the basis of predicted extent of disease
   c. To select radical retropubic or perineal prostatectomy
   d. Both a and b
   e. To predict the pathologic extent of disease
8. The currently available modalities for assessing disease extent in men with prostate cancer include which of the following?
   a. DRE
   b. Serum PSA
   c. Histologic grade
   d. Bone scan
   e. All of the above
9. Pathologic staging is superior to clinical staging because all of the following factors are known EXCEPT which one?
   a. PSA
   b. Surgical margin status
   c. Seminal vesicle involvement
   d. Tumor volume
   e. Capsular penetration
10. What pathologic finding or findings at radical prostatectomy are highly predictive of the presence of occult metastatic disease?
    a. Positive surgical margins
    b. Seminal vesicle involvement
    c. Lymph node involvement
    d. Both b and c
    e. Both a and b

11. The finding of pathologic perineural invasion of cancer (PNI) on a prostate biopsy specimen suggests:
    a. organ-confined disease.
    b. 20% likelihood of capsular penetration.
    c. 75% likelihood of capsular penetration.
    d. pelvic lymph node involvement.
    e. a bilateral nerve-sparing prostatectomy should not be considered.
12. Which staging modality provides the highest degree of understaging?
    a. Bone scan
    b. Immunoscintigraphy
    c. PSA
    d. PAP
    e. DRE
13. As general guidelines regarding PSA levels and pathologic stage, which of the following statements is TRUE?
    a. Twenty five percent of men with a PSA value less than 4.0 ng/mL have organ-confined disease.
    b. One hundred percent of men with a PSA value greater than 50 ng/mL have pelvic lymph node involvement.
    c. Ten percent of men with a PSA value greater than 10 ng/mL have extraprostatic extension.
    d. Serum PSA has no predictive value for staging.
    e. Seventy percent or more of men with a PSA value between 4.0 and 10.0 ng/mL have organ-confined disease.
14. With respect to the Gleason primary and secondary grade, all of the following statements are TRUE except which one?
    a. Primary grade ranges from 1 to 5.
    b. Secondary grade ranges from 1 to 5.
    c. Secondary grade and primary grade are summed to provide a Gleason score (2 to 10).
    d. The primary grade represents the second largest area of cancer on the biopsy specimen.
    e. The presence of a Gleason primary or secondary grade 4 or 5 on any biopsy specimen is predictive of poor prognosis.
15. On the basis of the Partin tables, a man with a PSA value of 7.4 before biopsy, a Gleason score of 3 + 4 = 7 on a biopsy specimen, and a nonsuspect (T1c) DRE before biopsy has all of the following EXCEPT:
    a. 54% likelihood of organ-confined disease.
    b. 36% likelihood of isolated capsular penetration.
    c. 2% likelihood of pelvic lymph node involvement.
    d. 97% likelihood of organ-confined disease.
    e. 8% likelihood of seminal vesicle invasion.

ANSWERS

1. **e. Combination of DRE and PSA.** The DRE and serum PSA are the most useful first-line tests for assessing the risk that prostate cancer is present in an individual.
2. **b. α_1-Antichymotrypsin (ACT).** Most detectable PSA in sera (65% to 90%) is bound to ACT.
3. **e. Age, race, and prostate volume.** In the absence of prostate cancer, serum PSA levels vary with age, race, and prostate volume.
4. **e. None of the above.** Serum PSA elevations may occur as a result of disruption of the normal prostatic architecture that allows PSA to diffuse into the prostatic tissue and gain access to the circulation. This can occur in the setting of prostate disease (benign prostatic hyperplasia [BPH], prostatitis, prostate cancer) and with prostate manipulation (prostate massage, prostate biopsy). The presence of prostate disease (prostate cancer, BPH, and prostatitis) is the most important factor affecting serum levels of PSA. PSA elevations may indicate the presence of prostate disease, but not all men with prostate disease have elevated PSA levels. Furthermore, PSA elevations are not specific for cancer.
5. **c. 8 ng/mL.** Finasteride (a 5α-reductase inhibitor for treatment of BPH) at 5 mg has been shown to lower PSA levels by 50% after 12 months of treatment. Thus, one can multiply the PSA level by 2 to obtain the "true" PSA level of a patient who has been taking finasteride for 12 months or more. Men who are to be treated with finasteride should have a baseline PSA measurement before initiation of treatment and should be followed with serial PSA measurements. If the PSA value does not decrease by 50%, or if there is a rise in the PSA value when the patient is taking finasteride, these men should be suspected of having an occult prostate cancer.
6. **a. PSA.** PSA is the single test with the highest positive predictive value for cancer.
7. **d. Both a and b.** The goals in staging of prostate cancer are twofold: (1) to predict prognosis and (2) to rationally select therapy on the basis of predicted extent of disease.
8. **e. All of the above.** The currently available modalities for assessing disease extent in men with prostate cancer are DRE, serum tumor markers, histologic grade, radiographic imaging, and pelvic lymphadenectomy.
9. **a. PSA.** Pathologic staging is more useful than clinical staging in the prediction of prognosis because tumor volume, surgical margin status, extent of extracapsular spread, and involvement of seminal vesicles and pelvic lymph nodes can be determined.
10. **d. Both b and c.** The finding of seminal vesicle invasion or lymph node metastases on pathologic evaluation after radical prostatectomy is associated with a very low probability of total eradication of tumor and a high probability of distant disease.
11. **c. 75% likelihood of capsular penetration.** PNI in a prostatectomy specimen has little independent prognostic staging value as initially reported by Byar. However, in biopsy cores, its presence is associated with a higher chance of non–organ-confined disease at prostatectomy. De la Taille and colleagues demonstrated that the presence of PNI on a biopsy specimen was closely associated with high PSA values, poorly differentiated tumor, and involvement of multiple cores with cancer, and thus a higher pathologic stage. Seventy-five percent of men with PNI on a biopsy specimen will have capsular penetration on examination of the prostatectomy specimen.
12. **e. DRE.** Histologic evaluation of surgical specimens after radical prostatectomy for presumed organ-confined disease

demonstrates a significant degree of understaging by DRE. Understaging of disease increases with increasing clinical stage.

13. **e. Seventy percent or more of men with a PSA value between 4.0 and 10.0 ng/mL have organ-confined disease.** As a general guideline, the majority of men (80%) with PSA values less than 4.0 ng/mL have pathologically organ-confined disease, two thirds of men with PSA levels between 4.0 and 10.0 ng/mL have organ-confined cancer, and more than 50% of men with PSA levels more than 10.0 ng/mL have disease beyond the prostate. Pelvic lymph node involvement is found in nearly 20% of men with PSA levels greater than 20 ng/mL and in most men (75%) with serum PSA levels greater than 50 ng/mL.

14. **d. The primary grade represents the second largest area of cancer on the biopsy specimen.** The pathologic criteria and method for determining the Gleason grade of a prostatic tumor are discussed in Chapter 86. The Gleason grading system is based on a low-power microscopic description of the architectural criteria of the cancer. A Gleason grade (or pattern) of 1 to 5 is assigned as a primary grade (the pattern occupying the greatest area of the specimen) and a secondary grade (the pattern occupying the second largest area of the specimen). A Gleason sum (2 to 10) is determined by adding the primary grade and the secondary grade. The presence of Gleason pattern 4 or greater (primary or secondary) or a Gleason sum of 7 or greater is predictive of a poorer prognosis.

15. **d. 97% likelihood of organ-confined disease.** Probability tables, based on the parameters of preoperative clinical stage, serum PSA level, and Gleason sum, have been constructed based on large numbers of men who have undergone radical prostatectomy with precise determination of the pathologic stage. In the "Partin tables," numbers within the nomogram represent the percent probability of having a given final pathologic stage based on logistic regression analyses for all three variables combined; dashes represent data categories in which insufficient data existed to calculate a probability. This information is useful in counseling men with newly diagnosed prostate cancer with respect to treatment alternatives and probability of complete eradication of tumor, keeping in mind that men with organ-confined, high-grade cancers are often not cured of prostate cancer with surgery because of early microscopic spread of disease.

95

Definitive Therapy for Localized Prostate Cancer: Overview

WILLIAM J. CATALONA • MISOP HAN

QUESTIONS

1. Prostate cancer is the cause of mortality in what percentage of U.S. men?
   a. 1%
   b. 3%
   c. 10%
   d. 16%
   e. 30%
2. An outcome comparison between different treatment modalities for localized prostate cancer is difficult because:
   a. most patients currently present with early disease with good outcomes regardless of the treatment.
   b. of lack of agreement on which outcome measures should be used.
   c. the treatment outcomes in any patient series may be influenced by the malignant potential of the tumor as well as the treatment used.
   d. there are many effective treatments for clinically localized prostate cancer.
   e. randomized clinical trials have only been performed in patients with advanced prostate cancer.
3. A suggested rationale for deferred treatment protocols for localized prostate cancer is:
   a. a prospective, randomized clinical trial demonstrated similar local cancer progression and metastasis rates for patients with clinically localized prostate cancer managed with deferred treatment and radical prostatectomy.
   b. in most deferred treatment studies, only approximately 15% of patients develop objective evidence of tumor progression within 5 years.
   c. an accurate assessment of clinically insignificant or indolent cancers is possible with biopsy results.
   d. active monitoring allows timely intervention as long as patients with localized prostate cancer are followed up semi-annually with digital rectal examination and prostate-specific antigen (PSA) levels.
   e. potential benefits of surgery do not outweigh potential complications of surgery in men with a life expectancy of less than 10 years and a low-grade prostate cancer.
4. What recent innovation has led to the wider use of radical prostatectomy?
   a. Discovery that the pudendal nerves are responsible for urinary continence.
   b. Preservation of the external sphincter muscle that yields urinary continence rates in excess of 90%.
   c. Development of saturation biopsy using general anesthesia.
   d. Minimal blood loss associated with laparoscopic prostatectomy.
   e. Decreased incidence of lymph node metastases with PSA screening.
5. What features characterize the following radical prostatectomy approach?
   a. Perineal: more blood loss and a longer operative time than the retropubic approach.
   b. Retropubic: higher risk for rectal injury and postoperative fecal incontinence.
   c. Laparoscopic: lowest complication rate.
   d. Laparoscopic: lowest positive surgical margin rate.
   e. Robotic: available three-dimensional visualization.
6. What do the Partin nomograms predict?
   a. Clinical stage
   b. Gleason score
   c. Pathologic stage
   d. Biochemical recurrence-free probability
   e. Cancer-specific survival probability
7. During the nerve-sparing portion of radical retropubic prostatectomy, a surgeon should:
   a. dissect the neurovascular bundles free of the posterolateral surface of the prostate gland.
   b. dissect the neurovascular bundles using bipolar electrocautery.
   c. perform a retrograde dissection to identify the neurovascular bundles at the bladder neck.
   d. release the endopelvic fascia after the neurovascular bundle dissection.
   e. use the harmonic scalpel to release neurovascular bundles.

8. What is the most important factor for urinary continence recovery after radical retropubic prostatectomy?
   a. Preoperative continence
   b. Pathologic stage
   c. Nerve-sparing status
   d. Patient age
   e. Bladder neck sparing dissection

9. The return of erectile function after radical retropubic prostatectomy correlates best with:
   a. preoperative hormonal therapy.
   b. postoperative radiation therapy.
   c. antihypertensive therapy.
   d. smoking history.
   e. nerve-sparing status.

10. What is true of "PSA bounce"? It:
   a. is strongly associated with an intermittent androgen ablation therapy.
   b. usually occurs within 2 years of radiation therapy.
   c. is treated immediately with combined androgen blockage therapy.
   d. is more commonly associated with external-beam radiation therapy.
   e. cannot exceed an increase of 2 ng/mL after radiation therapy.

11. What is the ASTRO (American Society of Therapeutic Radiation Oncology) definition for recurrence after radiation therapy?
   a. Three consecutive elevations of PSA after radiation therapy and back-dates the time of cancer progression to halfway between the second and third rising PSA levels.
   b. Three consecutive elevations of PSA after radiation therapy with at least one PSA bounce.
   c. Three PSA elevations measured 12 months apart and back-dates the time of cancer progression to halfway between the first and the second rising PSA levels.
   d. Three consecutive PSA elevations measured 6 months apart and back-dates the time of cancer progression to halfway between the PSA nadir and the first rising PSA level.
   e. Three consecutive PSA elevations of total 2 ng/mL after reaching a PSA nadir.

12. Which of the following parameters is predictive of favorable response to postoperative salvage radiation therapy?
   a. Preoperative PSA less than 10 ng/mL
   b. Extracapsular tumor extension
   c. PSA doubling time of more than 3 months
   d. Positive surgical margin
   e. Pre-radiation PSA less than 4 ng/mL

ANSWERS

1. **b. 3%.** About 1 in 6 men are diagnosed with prostate cancer during their lifetime. Because of effective treatment of some prostate cancers and the biologic indolence relative to the life expectancy of others, only about 16% of men diagnosed with prostate cancer ultimately die of it. As a result, prostate cancer is the cause of death in about 3% of the U.S. male population.

2. **c. the treatment outcomes in any patient series may be influenced by the malignant potential of the tumor as well as the treatment used.** Patients whose tumor has a low malignant potential are predetermined to fare better with most treatments. Therefore, the treatment outcomes in any patient series may be influenced by the malignant potential of the tumors and also by the treatment used. Accordingly, it is difficult to compare the results of different reports, because the patient populations usually are not strictly comparable.

3. **e. potential benefits of surgery do not outweigh potential complications of surgery in men with a life expectancy of less than 10 years and a low-grade prostate cancer.** Traditionally, deferred treatment has been reserved for men with a life expectancy of less than 10 years and a low-grade (Gleason score 2 to 5) prostate cancer. However, active monitoring is now being studied in younger patients with low-volume, low- or intermediate-grade tumors to avoid or delay treatment that might not be immediately necessary.

4. **b. Preservation of the external sphincter muscle that yields urinary continence rates in excess of 90%.** Recent innovations that have led to the wider use of radical prostatectomy include (1) the development of the anatomic radical retropubic prostatectomy that allows the dissection to be performed with good visualization and preservation of the cavernosal nerves responsible for erectile function and preservation of the external sphincter muscle that yields urinary continence rates in excess of 90%; (2) the development of extended ultrasound-guided biopsy regimens, performed under local anesthesia as an office procedure; and (3) the widespread use of PSA testing, which has led to the great majority of patients being diagnosed with clinically localized disease.

5. **e. Robotic: available three-dimensional visualization.** Remotely controlled, robot-assisted laparoscopic surgery recently has been popularized because of its greater technical ease for the surgeon, especially for tying sutures and performing the vesicourethral anastomosis. The availability of three-dimensional visualization is also an advantage over standard laparoscopic techniques.

6. **c. Pathologic stage.** Because imaging studies are not accurate for staging prostate cancer, preoperative clinical and pathologic parameters are used in the Partin nomograms to predict the pathologic stage and thus identify patients most likely to benefit from the operation.

7. **a. dissect the neurovascular bundles free of the posterolateral surface of the prostate gland.** Meticulous dissection is required to preserve the neurovascular bundles during the nerve-sparing radical retropubic prostatectomy. In performing nerve-sparing surgery, the neurovascular bundles are identified at the apex of the prostate and the bundles are dissected free of the posterolateral surface of the prostate gland.

8. **d. Patient age.** The return of urinary continence after radical retropubic prostatectomy is strongly associated with patient age: more than 95% of men younger than age 50 are continent after surgery; 85% of men older than age 70 regain complete continence.

9. **e. nerve-sparing status.** The return of erectile function after radical retropubic prostatectomy correlates with the age of the patient, preoperative potency status, extent of nerve-sparing surgery, and the era of surgery.

10. **b. usually occurs within 2 years of radiation therapy.** Inflammation in the prostate gland can produce transient PSA elevations, called a PSA "bounce" after radiation therapy. PSA bounce usually occurs during the first 2 years after treatment and is less common with external-beam radiation therapy than with brachytherapy.

11. **d. Three consecutive PSA elevations measured 6 months apart and back-dates the time of cancer progression to halfway between the PSA nadir and the first rising PSA level.** Currently, the most frequently used definition for recurrence after radiation therapy is the American Society of Therapeutic Radiation Oncology (ASTRO) definition. It requires three consecutive PSA increases measured 6 months apart and back-dates the time of cancer progression to halfway between the PSA nadir and the first rising PSA level. Thus, it usually takes years to determine whether progression has occurred after radiation therapy.

12. **d. Positive surgical margin.** Adjuvant radiotherapy is most likely to benefit patients with positive surgical margins or extracapsular tumor extension without seminal vesicle invasion or lymph node involvement. However, not all patients with extracapsular tumor extension or positive margins have tumor recurrence without radiotherapy, and most patients with highly adverse findings have treatment failure with distant metastases, despite adjuvant radiotherapy.

96

Expectant Management of Prostate Cancer

JAMES A. EASTHAM • PETER T. SCARDINO

QUESTIONS

1. For a man in the United States, the lifetime risk of dying of prostate cancer is currently approximately:
   a. 1.8%.
   b. 3.5%.
   c. 7.5%.
   d. 12%.
   e. 18%.
2. Watchful waiting is appropriate for men who have:
   a. high risk of developing prostate cancer.
   b. impalpable cancer not visible on MRI or transrectal ultrasound.
   c. serum prostate-specific antigen (PSA) level approximately 10 ng/mL.
   d. life expectancy approximately 10 years and well to moderately differentiated cancer.
   e. no major comorbidities.
3. Which of the following is important for monitoring men on watchful waiting?
   a. Repeat biopsy
   b. Endorectal MRI
   c. Serial transrectal ultrasound
   d. Periodic PSA testing
   e. None of the above
4. For men with well or moderately differentiated prostate cancer on watchful waiting, the 10-year cancer-specific mortality is approximately:
   a. 0.8%.
   b. 2%.
   c. 5%
   d. 15%.
   e. 30%.
5. For men with well-differentiated prostate cancer, the rate of metastases within the first 10 years of watchful waiting is approximately:
   a. 2%.
   b. 5%.
   c. 20%.
   d. 50%.
   e. 75%.
6. Compared with men treated by radical prostatectomy, men on watchful waiting have a higher risk of:
   a. obstructive voiding problems.
   b. bowel problems.
   c. metastases.
   d. death from prostate cancer.
   e. all of the above.
7. The best way to select men for active surveillance is:
   a. age.
   b. life expectancy.
   c. PSA level.
   d. results of transrectal ultrasound or endorectal MRI.
   e. assessment by multiple variables, such as Epstein's risk assessment or nomogram.
8. The most important procedure for following men who have chosen active surveillance with selective delayed definitive therapy is:
   a. biopsy.
   b. endorectal MRI.
   c. serial transrectal ultrasound.
   d. periodic PSA testing.
   e. bone scan.
9. The strongest predictor that a prostate cancer will not progress is:
   a. no cancer on repeat biopsy.
   b. no cancer on TRUS.
   c. patient age.
   d. negative digital rectal examination (DRE).
   e. long PSA doubling time.
10. During follow-up of men on active surveillance, DRE is most valuable as:
    a. a predictor of cancer progression.
    b. an indicator that a repeat biopsy is warranted.
    c. an indicator to order an imaging study such as transrectal ultrasound or an endorectal MRI.
    d. a means to assess prostate size as an indication for TURP.
    e. DRE has no value apparent value in this setting.

ANSWERS

1. **b. 3.5%.** The lifetime risk that an American man will die of prostate cancer is 3.6%.
2. **d. life expectancy 10 years and well to moderately differentiated cancer.** Watchful waiting is a reasonable option in patients with a life expectancy of 10 years and clinically localized, well or moderately differentiated prostate cancer.
3. **e. none of the above.** Because the goal of watchful waiting is to limit morbidity, not to administer potentially curative treatment, PSA testing, repeat biopsy, and imaging studies are unimportant.
4. **d. 15%.** According to a study by Bill-Axelson and coworkers, men who were managed conservatively had a 14% cancer-specific mortality rate at 10 years after diagnosis.
5. **c. 20%.** Chodak and colleagues found that, for men with well-differentiated, clinical stage T1 to T2 cancer managed conservatively, the risk of metastasis at 10 years was 19%.
6. **e. all of the above.** In a randomized comparison of watchful waiting and radical prostatectomy in Sweden, men on watchful waiting experienced significantly more obstructive voiding complaints, bowel problems, metastases, and death from prostate cancer.
7. **e. assessment by multiple variables, such as Epstein's risk assessment or nomogram.** Models that incorporate multiple factors have proven to be better predictors of indolent prostate cancer than any single factor.
8. **a. biopsy.** Repeat prostate biopsies are considered an important aspect of continued evaluation of men managed with active surveillance. In contrast, imaging studies and bone scans are unlikely to yield positive results in men with low-risk disease and PSA has not yet proven to be helpful in determining the need for therapy.
9. **a. no cancer on repeat biopsy.** In a study of men on active surveillance, Patel and colleagues found that positive second biopsy was the most significant prognostic factor for progression.
10. **b. an indicator that a repeat biopsy is warranted.** None of the current active surveillance studies has found DRE to be an independent predictor of cancer progression, although it can be useful in determining that a repeat biopsy should be taken.

97

Anatomic Radical Retropubic Prostatectomy

PATRICK C. WALSH • ALAN W. PARTIN

QUESTIONS

1. What is the arterial blood supply to the prostate?
   a. The pudendal artery
   b. The superior vesical artery
   c. The inferior vesical artery
   d. The external iliac artery
2. What vessels are located in the neurovascular bundle?
   a. Capsular arteries and veins
   b. Pudendal artery and vein
   c. Hemorrhoidal artery and vein
   d. Santorini's plexus
3. A radical prostatectomy may compromise the arterial blood supply to the penis by injuring the aberrant blood supply from which artery?
   a. The obturator artery
   b. The inferior vesical artery
   c. The superior vesical artery
   d. All of the above
4. The main parasympathetic efferent innervation to the pelvic plexus arises from:
   a. S1.
   b. S2-S4.
   c. T11-L2.
   d. L3-S1.
5. What is the relationship of the neurovascular bundle to the prostatic fascia?
   a. Inside Denonvilliers' fascia
   b. Outside the lateral pelvic fascia
   c. Inside the prostatic fascia
   d. Between the layers of the prostatic fascia and the levator fascia
6. Why is there less blood loss during radical perineal prostatectomy?
   a. It is easier to ligate the dorsal vein complex through the perineal approach than through the retropubic approach.
   b. There is no need to divide the puboprostatic ligaments.
   c. The dorsal vein complex is not divided because the dissection occurs beneath the lateral fascia and anterior pelvic fascia.
   d. Because the perineum is elevated, there is lower venous pressure.
7. What anatomic structure is responsible for the maintenance of passive urinary control after radical prostatectomy?
   a. Bladder neck
   b. Levator ani musculature
   c. Preprostatic sphincter
   d. Striated urethral sphincter
8. What is the major nerve supply to the striated sphincter and levator ani?
   a. The neurovascular bundle
   b. The sympathetic fibers from T11 to L2
   c. The pudendal nerve
   d. The obturator nerve
9. What is the posterior extent of the pelvic lymph node dissection?
   a. The hypogastric veins
   b. The obturator nerve
   c. The obturator vessels
   d. The sacral foramen
10. In opening the endopelvic fascia, there are often small branches traveling from the prostate to the pelvic sidewall. What are these branches? Tributaries from the:
    a. obturator artery
    b. external iliac artery
    c. inferior vesical artery
    d. pudendal artery and veins
11. How extensively should the puboprostatic ligaments be divided?
    a. Superficially, with just enough excised to expose the junction between the anterior apex of the prostate and the dorsal vein complex
    b. Extensively, down to the pelvic floor, including the pubourethral component
    c. Not at all; the puboprostatic ligaments should be left intact
    d. Widely enough to permit a right angle to be placed around the dorsal vein complex

12. When the dorsal vein complex is divided anteriorly, what is the most common major structure that can be damaged, and what is the most common adverse outcome?
    a. Aberrant pudendal arteries; impotence
    b. Neurovascular bundle; impotence
    c. Striated urethral sphincter; incontinence
    d. Levator ani musculature; incontinence
13. What is the most common site for a positive surgical margin and when does this occur?
    a. Posterolateral; during release of the neurovascular bundle
    b. Posterior; when the prostate is dissected from the rectum
    c. Apex; during division of the striated urethral sphincter-dorsal vein complex
    d. Bladder neck; during separation of the prostate from the bladder
14. How should the back-bleeders from the dorsal vein complex on the anterior surface of the prostate be oversewn and why?
    a. The edges should be pulled together in the midline to avoid bleeding.
    b. Bunching sutures should be used to avoid excising too much striated sphincter.
    c. The edges should be oversewn in the shape of a **V** to avoid advancing the neurovascular bundles too far anteriorly on the prostate.
    d. They should be oversewn horizontally to avoid a positive surgical margin.
15. After the dorsal vein complex has been ligated and the urethra has been divided, what posterior structure, other than the neurovascular bundles, attaches the prostate to the pelvic floor?
    a. Rectourethralis
    b. Denonvilliers' fascia
    c. Rectal fascia
    d. Posterior portion of the striated sphincter complex
16. What are the advantages of releasing the levator fascia higher at the apex?
    a. More soft tissue on the prostate
    b. Less traction on the neurovascular bundles as they are released
    c. Preservation of anterior nerve fibers
    d. Less blood loss
17. Once the apex of the prostate has been released, what is the best way to retract the prostate for exposure of the neurovascular bundle?
    a. Traction on the catheter, producing upward rotation of the apex of the prostate
    b. Use of a sponge stick to roll the prostate on its side
    c. Downward displacement of the prostate with a sponge stick
    d. Use of finger dissection to release the prostate posteriorly
18. To avoid a positive surgical margin, what is the best way to release the neurovascular bundle?
    a. Right-angle dissection beginning on the posterior surface of the prostate and dissecting anterolaterally
    b. Using sharp dissection, laterally dissecting toward the rectum
    c. Using finger dissection to fracture the neurovascular bundle from the prostate
    d. Using electrocautery to separate the neurovascular bundle from the prostate
19. What is the latest point at which a decision can be made regarding preservation or excision of the neurovascular bundle?
    a. When perineural invasion is identified on the needle biopsy specimen
    b. When the neurovascular bundle is being released from the prostate and fixation is identified
    c. When the prostate has been removed and tissue covering the posterolateral surface of the prostate is thought to be inadequate
    d. When the patient is found to have a positive biopsy result at the apex
20. Before the lateral pedicles are divided, what is the last major branch of the neurovascular bundle that must be identified and released?
    a. Apical branch
    b. Posterior branch
    c. Capsular branch
    d. Bladder neck branch
21. When the vesicourethral anastomosis sutures are being tied, if tension is found, what is the best way to release it?
    a. Creating an anterior bladder neck flap
    b. Placing the Foley catheter on traction postoperatively
    c. Releasing attachments of the bladder to the peritoneum
    d. Using vest sutures
22. If there is excessive bleeding from the dorsal vein complex while it is being divided, what should the surgeon do?
    a. Abandon the operation and close the incision
    b. Ligate the hypogastric arteries
    c. Inflate a Foley balloon and place traction on it
    d. Divide the dorsal vein complex completely over the urethra and oversew the end
23. If a rectal injury occurs during the operation, what is the most certain way to avoid the development of a fistula with the fewest side effects?
    a. Loop colostomy
    b. End colostomy
    c. Hartman's pouch
    d. Interposition of omentum
24. In postoperative patients who require transfusions of blood for hypotension, what is the correct approach and why?
    a. Avoid re-exploration because it might damage the anastomosis
    b. Perform re-exploration
    c. Place the Foley catheter on traction
    d. Administer fresh frozen plasma
25. What is the best way to ensure good coaptation of the anastomotic mucosal surfaces to avoid a bladder neck contracture?
    a. Hold the catheter on traction while tying the sutures
    b. Use a sponge stick in the perineum
    c. Use a Babcock clamp to hold the bladder down
    d. Vest sutures
26. What is the most common cause of incontinence after radical prostatectomy?
    a. Intrinsic sphincter deficiency
    b. Detrusor instability
    c. Failure to reconstruct the bladder neck
    d. Injury to the neurovascular bundles

27. Preservation of the seminal vesicles during radical prostatectomy has demonstrated:
    a. improved erectile function in the majority of men.
    b. no increase in biochemical recurrence.
    c. improved early and late urinary control.
    d. increased rate of pelvic abscess.
    e. none of the above.
28. Preservation of the bladder neck during radical prostatectomy has demonstrated:
    a. improved erectile function.
    b. improved long-term urinary control.
    c. decreased surgical margins.
    d. improved anastomotic stricture rate.
    e. none of the above.
29. What percentage of men who had bilateral sural nerve grafting demonstrated full erections sufficient for penetration?
    a. 9%
    b. 13%
    c. 26%
    d. 38%
    e. 57%
30. Sural nerve grafts are placed:
    a. end to end on the ipsilateral side from the tumor.
    b. above the bladder neck and below the pubic arch.
    c. in reverse to the natural position (proximal to distal) and (distal to proximal).
    d. in a circle to enhance nerve growth factor release.
    e. Next to the prostatectomy specimen in the pelvis until time for anastomosis.
31. Which complication has changed dramatically with experience with salvage prostatectomy?
    a. Overall urinary incontinence
    b. Potency
    c. Blood loss
    d. Rectal injury
    e. Stricture rate

ANSWERS

1. **c. The inferior vesical artery.** The prostate receives arterial blood supply from the inferior vesical artery.
2. **a. Capsular arteries and veins.** The capsular branches run along the pelvic sidewall in the lateral pelvic fascia posterolateral to the prostate, providing branches that course ventrally and dorsally to supply the outer portion of the prostate. Histologically, the capsular arteries and veins are surrounded by an extensive network of nerves. These capsular vessels provide the macroscopic landmark that aids in the identification of the microscopic branches of the pelvic plexus that innervate the corpora cavernosa.
3. **d. All of the above.** The major arterial supply to the corpora cavernosa is derived from the internal pudendal artery. However, pudendal arteries can arise from the obturator, inferior vesical, and superior vesical arteries. Because these aberrant branches travel along the lower part of the bladder and anterolateral surface of the prostate, they are divided during radical prostatectomy. This may compromise arterial supply to the penis, especially in older patients with borderline penile blood flow.
4. **b. S2-S4.** The autonomic innervation of the pelvic organs and external genitalia arises from the pelvic plexus, which is formed by parasympathetic visceral efferent preganglionic fibers that arise from the sacral center (S2 to S4).
5. **d. Between the layers of the prostatic fascia and the levator fascia.** The neurovascular bundles are located in the lateral pelvic fascia *between* the prostatic and levator fasciae (see Fig. 97-6).
6. **c. The dorsal vein complex is not divided because the dissection occurs beneath the lateral fascia and anterior pelvic fascia.** In an effort to avoid injury to the dorsal vein of the penis and Santorini's plexus during radical perineal prostatectomy, the lateral fascia and anterior pelvic fascia are reflected off the prostate. This accounts for the reduced blood loss associated with radical perineal prostatectomy.
7. **d. Striated urethral sphincter.** The striated sphincter contains fatigue-resistant, slow-twitch fibers that are responsible for passive urinary control.
8. **c. The pudendal nerve.** The pudendal nerve provides the major nerve supply to the striated sphincter and levator ani.
9. **a. The hypogastric vein.** The obturator artery and vein are skeletonized but are usually left undisturbed and are not ligated unless excessive bleeding occurs. The dissection then continues down to the pelvic floor exposing the hypogastric veins.
10. **d. pudendal artery and veins.** The incision in the endopelvic fascia is carefully extended in an anteromedial direction toward the puboprostatic ligaments. At this point, one often encounters small arterial and venous branches from the pudendal vessels, which perforate the pelvic musculature to supply the prostate. These vessels should be ligated with clips to avoid coagulation injury to the pudendal artery and nerve, which are located just deep to this muscle as they travel along the pubic ramus.
11. **a. Superficially, with just enough excised to expose the junction between the anterior apex of the prostate and the dorsal vein complex.** The dissection should continue down far enough to expose the juncture between the apex of the prostate and the anterior surface of the dorsal vein complex at the point where it will be divided. The pubourethral component of the complex must remain intact to preserve the anterior fixation of the striated urethral sphincter to the pubis.
12. **c. Striated urethral sphincter; incontinence.** The goal is to divide the complex with minimal blood loss while avoiding damage to the striated sphincter.
13. **c. Apex; during division of the striated urethral sphincter-dorsal vein complex.** The exact plane on the anterior surface of the prostate can be visualized, avoiding inadvertent entry into the anterior prostate and ensuring minimal excision of the striated sphincter musculature. This is the most common site for positive surgical margins, because it can be difficult to identify the anterior apical surface of the prostate.
14. **c. The edges should be oversewn in the shape of a V to avoid advancing the neurovascular bundles too far anteriorly on the prostate.** To avoid back-bleeding from the anterior surface of the prostate, the edges of the proximal dorsal vein complex on the anterior surface of the prostate are sewn in the shape of a **V** with a running 2-0 absorbable suture (see Fig. 97-16). If one tries to pull these edges together in the midline, the neurovascular bundles can be advanced too far anteriorly on the prostate.

15. **d. Posterior portion of the striated sphincter complex.** The posterior band of urethra is now divided to expose the posterior portion of the striated urethral sphincter complex. The posterior sphincter complex is composed of skeletal muscle and fibrous tissue.

16. **b. Less traction on the neurovascular bundles as they are released and c. Preservation of anterior nerve fibers.** The purpose of this technique is to speed up recovery of sexual function by reducing traction on the branches of the nerves to the cavernous bodies and striated sphincter and/or avoiding inadvertent transection of the small branches that travel anteriorly. However, because there is less soft tissue at the apex the risk of positive margins may be increased.

17. **b. Use of a sponge stick to roll the prostate on its side.** When the surgeon releases the neurovascular bundle, there should be no upward traction on the prostate. Rather, the prostate should be rolled from side to side.

18. **a. Right-angle dissection beginning on the posterior surface of the prostate and dissecting anterolaterally.** After the plane between the rectum and prostate in the midline has been developed, it is possible to release the neurovascular bundle from the prostate, beginning at the apex and moving toward the base, by using the sponge stick to roll the prostate over on its side. Beginning on the rectal surface, the bundle is released from the prostate by spreading a right angle gently. With use of this plane, Denonvilliers' fascia and the prostatic fascia remain on the prostate; only the residual fragments of the levator fascia are released from the prostate laterally.

19. **c. When the prostate has been removed and tissue covering the posterolateral surface of the prostate is thought to be inadequate.** Clues that indicate that wide excision of the neurovascular bundle is necessary include inadequate tissue covering the posterolateral surface of the prostate once the prostate had been removed, leading to secondary wide excision of the neurovascular bundle. This last point is very important to understand. You do not have to make the decision about whether to excise or preserve the neurovascular bundle until the prostate is removed, and, if there is not enough soft tissue covering the prostate, you can excise the neurovascular bundle then.

20. **b. Posterior branch.** The surgeon should look for a prominent arterial branch traveling from the neurovascular bundle over the seminal vesicles to supply the base of the prostate. This posterior vessel should be ligated on each side and divided. By this method, the neurovascular bundles are no longer tethered to the prostate and fall posteriorly.

21. **c. Releasing attachments of the bladder to the peritoneum.** The anterior suture is tied initially. There should be no tension. If there is, the bladder should be released from the peritoneum.

22. **d. Divide the dorsal vein complex completely over the urethra and oversew the end.** If there is troublesome bleeding from the dorsal vein complex at any point, the surgeon should completely divide the dorsal vein complex over the urethra and oversew the end. This is the single best means to control bleeding from the dorsal vein complex. Any maneuver short of this will only worsen the bleeding. To gain exposure for the prostatectomy, one must put traction on the prostate. If the dorsal vein is not completely divided, traction opens the partially transected veins and usually worsens the bleeding.

23. **d. Interposition of omentum.** It is wise to interpose omentum between the rectal closure and the vesicourethral anastomosis to reduce the possibility of a rectourethral fistula.

24. **b. Perform re-exploration.** These results suggest that patients requiring acute transfusions for hypotension after radical prostatectomy should undergo exploration to evacuate the pelvic hematoma in an effort to decrease the likelihood of bladder neck contracture and incontinence.

25. **c. Use a Babcock clamp to hold the bladder down.** We have found that the use of a Babcock clamp to approximate the bladder neck and urethra while the anastomotic sutures are tied has virtually eliminated bladder neck contractures in our practice.

26. **a. Intrinsic sphincter deficiency.** After radical prostatectomy, incontinence is usually secondary to intrinsic sphincter deficiency.

27. **e. none of the above.** Sparing of the seminal vesicles has not improved incontinence, potency, nor margin status; and there have been no reported cases of pelvic abscess.

28. **e. none of the above.** Sparing of the bladder neck has not improved incontinence, potency, margin status, nor stricture rates.

29. **c. 26%.** The percentage of men who had bilateral sural nerve grafting and demonstrated full erections (sufficient for penetration) was 26%.

30. **c. in reverse to the natural position (proximal to distal) and (distal to proximal).** Sural nerve grafts are placed in reverse to the natural position (proximal to distal) and (distal to proximal).

31. **d. Rectal injury.** Only rectal injury rates have dramatically changed.

98

Radical Perineal Prostatectomy

DAVID M. HARTKE • MATIN I. RESNICK

QUESTIONS

1. Which of the following statements about perineal prostatectomy is FALSE?
   a. The pathologic outcomes are similar to those of radical retropubic prostatectomy and proven over considerable time.
   b. It has experienced a resurgence of interest as a result of its low morbidity and rapid convalescence.
   c. It fell out of favor as the principle technique in the 1970s secondary to high intraoperative blood loss.
   d. Nerve-sparing techniques have been applied to the approach allowing for postoperative potency.
   e. Partin tables allow for relatively accurate predictions of pathologic stage, forfeiting the need for staging lymphadenectomy in many patients.
2. With regard to postoperative neurapraxia, which of the following statements is TRUE?
   a. The literature supports that is almost always transient.
   b. It usually results in a motor deficit that is transient.
   c. Most studies show that a self-limited neurapraxia occurs in approximately 25% of patients.
   d. The same rates of neurapraxia tend to occur in retropubic prostatectomy as well.
   e. This is a major source of morbidity and the reason many surgeons do not utilize this approach.
3. Which of the following statements with regard to rectal injury associated with perineal prostatectomy is FALSE?
   a. If unrecognized it may result in the occurrence of a rectocutaneous or urethrocutaneous fistula.
   b. Despite the close proximity of the rectum in the initial dissection, the incidence is fairly low.
   c. It can be avoided when an assistant places gentle downward pressure on the Lowsley tractor while the rectourethralis muscle is divided.
   d. If repaired with a two-layer closure, most clinical sequelae are avoided.
   e. After repair with a two-layer closure, the operation can continue without a problem.
4. When selecting a patient for radical perineal prostatectomy, which of the following must always be considered?
   a. Gleason score of biopsy specimen.
   b. Preoperative serum prostatic-specific antigen (PSA).
   c. Mild degenerative lumbar disk disease.
   d. a and b only.
   e. All of the above.
5. Which of the following is TRUE regarding the radical perineal prostatectomy?
   a. Patients who require lymph node sampling for staging purposes must should undergo a radical retropubic prostatectomy because the radical perineal prostatectomy, when combined with a laparoscopic lymph node dissection, yields much higher morbidity and is not cost effective.
   b. Patients with ankylosis of the hips or spine may not tolerate a radical perineal prostatectomy.
   c. Patients with a prior history of renal transplant surgery with the allograft in the right iliac fossa are not candidates for a radical perineal prostatectomy.
   d. Morbid obesity is becoming a common contraindication to a radical perineal prostatectomy.
   e. None of the above.
6. Which of the following statements regarding blood loss during radical perineal prostatectomy is TRUE?
   a. Although transfusion rates are low, a blood type and crossmatch is recommended before starting the case.
   b. Unlike a radical retropubic prostatectomy, the dorsal venous complex is not usually encountered and blood loss is significantly reduced.
   c. Transfusion rate in most reports is approximately 15%.
   d. The dorsal venous complex is ligated early, resulting in reduced blood loss.
   e. Rates of transfusion are generally greater than those in the retropubic literature.
7. Which of the following statements concerning postoperative care is TRUE?
   a. The diet is rapidly advanced to a regular diet.
   b. Most patients are discharged from the hospital by postoperative day 2.
   c. A rectal suppository is administered on a scheduled basis while in the hospital to minimize Foley catheter discomfort except in cases of intraoperative rectal injury.
   d. a and b only.
   e. All of the above.
8. Which of the following statements is FALSE with regard to potency outcomes of the radical perineal prostatectomy?
   a. Using a nerve-sparing technique, potency is shown to return in up to 70% of men.
   b. Older patients are as likely to be as potent as younger patients if a nerve-sparing technique is employed.
   c. Pharmacotherapy is demonstrated to improve postoperative potency status.
   d. All of the above.
   e. a and c only.

9. Exposure of the urethra is facilitated by:
   a. encircling the urethra with umbilical tape.
   b. the Lowsley retractor.
   c. division of the puboprostatic ligaments.
   d. division of the dorsal venous complex.
   e. retraction of the neurovascular bundles medially.

10. Which of the following statements concerning the technique of urethral anastomosis is TRUE?
    a. The presence of the Lowsley retractor assists in identifying the membranous urethral stump for the initial placement of interrupted sutures.
    b. A running suture technique is advocated for a watertight anastomosis.
    c. The visualization of the anastomosis is difficult, one of the few disadvantages of the radical perineal prostatectomy.
    d. The sutures are interrupted in a tennis racquet fashion.
    e. The indwelling Foley catheter is not passed until after the anterior vesicourethral anastomotic sutures are placed and tied down.

ANSWERS

1. **c. It fell out of favor as the principle technique in the 1970s secondary to high intraoperative blood loss.** In the 1970s, the procedure fell out of favor because the importance of pelvic lymphadenectomy was understood for the purposes of staging. However, with advent of Partin tables, surgeons could accurately predict the chances of lymph node involvement, obviating the need for staging lymphadenectomy. Furthermore, laparoscopic lymphadenectomy has gained favor and allows for radical perineal prostatectomy and lymph node dissection in one operative setting in those where it is required. Pathologic outcomes are not significantly different for either procedure. It offers shorter hospital stays and lower costs than the retropubic prostatectomy. Blood loss is significantly lower than with the retropubic approach. A nerve-sparing technique can be accomplished through the perineal approach.
2. **a. The literature supports it is almost always transient.** Sensory neurapraxia of the lower extremity is reported to occur in approximately 2% of radical perineal prostatectomy cases. However, one study did report an incidence of 25%. This is reported significantly more often than with retropubic prostatectomy. True motor deficits are rare. Because of the transient nature, this is not a major source of morbidity.
3. **c. It can be avoided when an assistant places gentle downward pressure on the Lowsley tractor while the rectourethralis muscle is divided.** Traction on the Lowsley tractor during division of the rectourethralis muscle tents the rectum upward and increases the likelihood of injury. Traction should not be placed until after the rectourethralis muscle is divided. When unrecognized, a fistula may ensue. Although one report showed an incidence of rectal injury in 11% of cases, most series recognize an incidence of 1% to 5%. When recognized and repaired at the time of injury, the operation can continue without problem.
4. **d. a and b only.** The patient's Gleason score and PSA value help determine the likelihood of organ-confined disease and, thus, the candidacy for a radical perineal prostatectomy. A history of degenerative disk disease is not a contraindication to surgery.
5. **b. Patients with ankylosis of the hips or spine may not tolerate a radical perineal prostatectomy.** Because of the necessity of either an exaggerated lithotomy or modified exaggerated lithotomy position, ankylosis of the hips or spine may be a contraindication to the procedure. Concomitant radical perineal prostatectomy and laparoscopic lymph node dissection results in little increased morbidity and remains cost effective when compared with radical retropubic prostatectomy. Patients with prior renal transplantation or morbid obesity are often better candidates for a perineal approach than the retropubic approach.
6. **b. Unlike a radical retropubic prostatectomy, the dorsal venous complex is not usually encountered and blood loss is significantly reduced.** The dorsal venous complex is usually not encountered, resulting in relatively lower blood loss when compared with the retropubic approach. A blood type and antibody screen are performed in the days or hours before surgery, but a crossmatch is generally unnecessary. Transfusion rates are generally around 5%.
7. **d. a and b only.** Postoperatively, the diet is advanced rapidly as tolerated, patients ambulate early, and the overwhelming majority of patients are discharged by the second postoperative day. However, rectal stimulation or manipulation is prohibited in the postoperative period.
8. **e. a and c only.** In a series by Weldon and associates, up to 70% of the patients were potent postoperatively. Furthermore, pharmacotherapy has been demonstrated to improve potency outcomes. However, older age has been demonstrated to be a risk factor for postoperative impotency.
9. **b. the Lowsley retractor.** The apex of the prostate and adjacent urethra can be palpated easily due to the presence of the Lowsley retractor.
10. **e. The indwelling Foley catheter is not passed until after the anterior vesicourethral anastomotic sutures are placed and tied down.** During placement of the anterior vesicourethral anastomotic sutures, a red rubber catheter is placed transurethrally and used to identify the membranous urethral stump and also provide traction on the urethra to assist in placement of the sutures. The red rubber catheter is then removed and the indwelling Foley catheter is then placed retrograde into the bladder. Simple interrupted sutures are placed for the anastomosis. A tennis racquet technique is utilized for bladder neck reconstruction should it be deemed necessary.

99

Laparoscopic and Robotic-Assisted Laparoscopic Radical Prostatectomy and Pelvic Lymphadenectomy

LI-MING SU • JOSEPH A. SMITH JR.

QUESTIONS

1. With laparoscopic/robotic prostatectomy (LRP/RALP), a continuous suture for the vesicourethral anastomosis:
   a. avoids incontinence.
   b. has a high rate of bladder neck contracture.
   c. can be performed with the need for only a single knot.
   d. requires an indwelling catheter for at least 2 weeks.
   e. eliminates the need for a pelvic drain.
2. With LRP/RALP, positive margin status is not influenced by:
   a. surgical technique.
   b. patient selection.
   c. pathologic analysis.
   d. transperitoneal versus extraperitoneal exposure.
   e. tumor grade and stage.
3. Compared with open surgical approaches, LRP/RALP has been consistently shown to decrease:
   a. postoperative pain.
   b. urinary incontinence.
   c. bleeding.
   d. erectile dysfunction.
   e. positive margins.
4. Positive surgical margins with LRP/RALP:
   a. decrease as technical experience is gained.
   b. are rare at the prostatic apex.
   c. occur only in extracapsular disease.
   d. are seen most commonly at the prostate base.
   e. can be avoided by using a robotic-assisted approach.
5. Laparoscopic pelvic lymph node dissection (PLND):
   a. is difficult to perform along with robotic radical prostatectomy.
   b. should always be performed intraperitoneally.
   c. has an increased risk of thromboembolic complication compared with open approaches.
   d. should only be performed for tumors Gleason grade 7.
   e. can be performed as a staging operation or at prostatectomy.
6. Compared with open surgery, intraperitoneal laparoscopic lymph node dissection has a lower risk of:
   a. bleeding.
   b. lymphocele.
   c. ureteral injury.
   d. obturator nerve transaction.
   e. infection.
7. Rectal injury with LRP/RALP:
   a. is best avoided by antegrade release of the rectum from the posterior prostate.
   b. usually is from trocar placement.
   c. is avoided by bluntly dividing Denonvilliers' fascia.
   d. is treated with an immediate diverting colostomy.
   e. often is unrecognized and heals spontaneously.
8. Bleeding during LRP/RALP is usually minimal because the:
   a. plane of periprostatic tissue dissection is different than with open surgery.
   b. dorsal vein complex does not have to be divided.
   c. pneumoperitoneum tamponades venous bleeding.
   d. suturing is easier than with open surgery.
   e. Trendelenburg positioning decreases venous pressure.
9. Robotic assistance with laparoscopy is most useful in:
   a. trocar insertion and removal.
   b. maintaining a steady insufflation pressure.
   c. decreasing operating room costs.
   d. facilitating suturing.
   e. eliminating the need for a table-side assistant.
10. The neurovascular bundle lies within which two periprostatic fascial planes:
    a. prostate capsule and prostatic fascia.
    b. prostate capsule and levator fascia.
    c. prostatic fascia and levator fascia.
    d. Denonvilliers' fascia and prostate capsule.
    e. Denonvilliers' fascia and endopelvic fascia.

11. Antegrade laparoscopic dissection of the prostate results in less blood loss as compared with the retrograde approach owing to:
    a. early division of the dorsal venous complex and prostatic pedicles.
    b. early division of the prostatic pedicles and late division of the dorsal venous complex.
    c. less tissue manipulation.
    d. better visualization.
    e. late division of the dorsal venous complex and prostatic pedicles.
12. The higher cost of LRP/RALP as compared with open radical prostatectomy is mostly a consequence of:
    a. higher blood loss and transfusion rate.
    b. higher complication rate.
    c. longer operative time and disposable equipment.
    d. longer hospital stays.
    e. higher surgical and anesthesia costs.
13. As a consequence of the CO_2 pneumoperitoneum used during minimally invasive prostatectomy, the anesthesia team must be most aware of the potential for:
    a. bleeding and hypotension.
    b. hypoxia and acidosis.
    c. tachycardia and hypertension.
    d. bradycardia and hypotension.
    e. hypercarbia and oliguria.
14. Positive margins at the prostatic apex:
    a. are more common with the robotic-assisted technique as compared with open surgery.
    b. can occur due to protrusion of the posterior prostatic apex beneath the urethra.
    c. can occur more commonly with retrograde versus antegrade dissection of the prostate.
    d. are less common in laparoscopic versus open surgery.
    e. are less common than at the prostatic base.
15. Men who are NOT candidates for LRP/RALP include those with:
    a. palpable tumors.
    b. history of pelvic surgery.
    c. morbid obesity.
    d. uncorrectable bleeding diatheses.
    e. prior neoadjuvant hormonal therapy.

ANSWERS

1. **c. can be performed with the need for only a single knot.** The vesicourethral anastomosis may be accomplished using either an interrupted closure or a running continuous suture with a single knot (van Velthoven et al, 2003).
2. **d. transperitoneal versus extraperitoneal exposure.** Comparison of margin status between high-volume centers with the operations performed by experienced surgeons has shown no definitive advantage for one surgical approach over the other in achieving negative surgical margins (Brown JA et al, 2003; Khan et al, 2005).
3. **c. bleeding.** Because most of the blood loss that occurs during radical prostatectomy is from venous sinuses, the tamponade effect from the pneumoperitoneum helps diminish ongoing blood loss during LRP/RALP. Blood loss of less than a few hundred milliliters is routinely reported (Guillonneau et al, 2001; Hoznek et al, 2002).
4. **a. decrease as technical experience is gained.** In most series of LRP and RALP, positive margin percentages decrease as greater familiarity with the procedure is obtained (Ahlering et al, 2004b; Salomon et al, 2004; Rassweiler et al, 2005).
5. **e. can be performed as a staging operation or at prostatectomy.** Staging PLND may have a role in some patients in whom radical perineal prostatectomy is planned. With radical retropubic prostatectomy, LRP, or RALP, PLND usually is performed simultaneous with the radical prostatectomy.
6. **b. lymphocele.** With laparoscopic PLND, postoperative lymphoceles are less common (Kavoussi et al, 1993; Kerble, et al, 1993; Chow, et al, 1994). A transperitoneal laparoscopic approach allows continuous egress and absorption of lymphatic fluid by the peritoneum in the event of a lymphatic leak.
7. **a. is best avoided by antegrade release of the rectum from the posterior prostate.** Thorough dissection of the rectum off of the posterior prostate is critical to minimize the risk of rectal injury during subsequent steps such as division of the urethra and dissection of the prostatic apex. With LRP and RALP, sharp and complete incision of the posterior layer of Denonvilliers' fascia is necessary after seminal vesicle dissection to allow adequate mobilization of the rectum.
8. **c. pneumoperitoneum tamponades venous bleeding.** Because most of the blood loss that occurs during radical prostatectomy is from venous sinuses, the tamponade effect from the pneumoperitoneum helps diminish ongoing blood loss during LRP/RALP. Blood loss of less than a few hundred milliliters is routinely reported (Guillonneau et al, 2001; Hoznek et al, 2002).
9. **d. facilitating suturing.** Most surgeons, however, believe that the robotic technology significantly facilitates suturing (especially for the vesicourethral anastomosis) and other aspects of the surgical dissection (Dasgupta, 2005).
10. **c. prostatic fascia and levator fascia.** The neurovascular bundle travels between two distinct fascial planes that surround the prostate, namely, the prostatic fascia and levator fascia.
11. **b. early division of the prostatic pedicles and late division of the dorsal venous complex.** Because the dorsal venous complex is divided early in the operation and the prostatic pedicles late, there is potentially a greater risk of ongoing bleeding with the retrograde technique (Rassweiler et al, 2001). In contrast, during the antegrade neurovascular bundle dissection, the arterial blood supply to the prostate (via the prostatic pedicles) is divided early and the dorsal venous complex is divided near the end of the operation, thus reducing blood loss during the operation.
12. **c. longer operative time and disposable equipment.** In the study by Link and colleagues (2004), the factors that most influenced overall cost in order of importance included

operative time, length of hospital stay, and consumable items (e.g., disposable laparoscopic equipment and trocars).

13. **e. hypercarbia and oliguria.** The anesthesiologist must be aware of the potential consequences of CO_2 insufflation and pneumoperitoneum, including oliguria and hypercarbia.

14. **b. can occur due to protrusion of the posterior prostatic apex beneath the urethra.** Before division of the posterior urethra, great care must be taken to inspect the contour of the posterior prostatic apex. In some patients, the posterior prostatic apex can protrude beneath the urethra, resulting in an iatrogenic positive margin if not identified.

15. **d. uncorrectable bleeding diatheses.** Contraindications to minimally invasive laparoscopic prostatectomy include uncorrectable bleeding diatheses or the inability to undergo general anesthesia due to severe cardiopulmonary compromise.

100

Radiation Therapy for Prostate Cancer

ANTHONY V. D'AMICO • JUANITA CROOK • CLAIR J. BEARD • THEODORE L. DEWEESE • MARK HURWITZ • IRVING KAPLAN

QUESTIONS

1. An advance in the radiotherapeutic management of prostate cancer includes which of the following?
   a. Three-dimensional conformal technique and image guidance for radioactive source placement in the prostate gland
   b. The ability to remove all uncertainty related to patient set-up
   c. The ability to deliver three-dimensional conformal radiation therapy with no risk of side effects
   d. The ability to cure all patients with prostate cancer
   e. The ability to identify who has clinically significant prostate cancer
2. What are four important predictors of prostate-cancer specific mortality after external-beam radiation therapy?
   a. Patient's age, performance status, height, and weight
   b. Biopsy Gleason score, age, weight, and height
   c. Biopsy Gleason score, age, height, and weight
   d. Biopsy Gleason score, PSA level, percentage of prostate biopsies, and clinical stage
   e. Biopsy Gleason score, PSA level, clinical stage, and height
3. The percentage of positive prostate biopsies is:
   a. not an important predictor of PSA failure-free survival after external-beam radiation therapy.
   b. equal to the number of cores sampled divided by 100.
   c. not an important predictor of prostate cancer–specific mortality after external-beam radiation therapy in low-risk patients.
   d. able to identify the patients at higher risk of prostate cancer–specific mortality despite having low-risk disease.
   e. equal to the PSA value divided by the biopsy Gleason score.
4. Which of the following statements is TRUE regarding local control after radiation therapy for prostate cancer?
   a. It is an unimportant endpoint because it does not predict for survival.
   b. Local control improves with higher radiation doses.
   c. Local control is associated with a longer time to PSA nadir and lower nadir.
   d. a and b.
   e. b and c.
5. Which of the following statements is TRUE regarding the PSA bounce phenomenon after prostate brachytherapy?
   a. It is seen in 25% to 30% of prostate brachytherapy cases using permanent seed implant monotherapy.
   b. It may occur anytime between 8 and 30 months after implant.
   c. Patient may be asymptomatic.
   d. It may be associated with a positive biopsy showing treatment effect.
   e. All of the above.
6. What are the three most important predictors of prostate-specific antigen (PSA) failure-free survival after external-beam radiation therapy?
   a. Patient's age, performance status, and weight
   b. Patient's age, PSA level, and weight
   c. PSA value, biopsy Gleason score, and clinical T stage
   d. PSA value, biopsy Gleason score, and age
   e. Biopsy Gleason score, age, and weight
7. Two years after definitive radiotherapy for prostate cancer, what should the serum PSA level be?
   a. Undetectable
   b. <0.5 ng/mL
   c. Stable and not rising
   d. Normal
   e. None of the above
8. One year after radiotherapy, the serum PSA value has fallen to within the "normal range" (2.5 ng/mL) but then starts to rise, with subsequent readings of 3.5 and 5.1 ng/mL over a 6-month period. What would appropriate management be?
   a. Tell the patient that radiation therapy has not worked and discuss salvage prostatectomy and cryosurgery.
   b. Tell the patient that the PSA value is still normal and not to worry.
   c. Tell the patient that he likely has a recurrence and that rising PSA may indicate a distant component to the failure.
   d. None of the above
   e. Both a and b

9. With regard to the PSA nadir after radiation therapy, which of the following statements is TRUE?
   a. An early nadir is good.
   b. Patients showing distant failure reach a nadir later.
   c. Patients who are cured may take 24 to 30 months to reach a nadir.
   d. A nadir greater than 0.5 ng/mL means that treatment has failed.
   e. None of the above.

10. Prostate biopsy samples should be negative for disease by what time after radiation therapy?
    a. 6 months
    b. 12 months
    c. 18 months
    d. 30 months
    e. None of the above

11. Which of the following statements is TRUE regarding local control after radiation therapy for prostate cancer?
    a. It is an unimportant endpoint because it does not predict for survival.
    b. It is lower in patients with early disease because they receive lower doses of radiation.
    c. It is equal for all types of radiation treatment.
    d. It is associated with treatment technique and dose of radiation.
    e. None of the above.

12. Which of the following statements is TRUE regarding conformal radiation therapy?
    a. It is available in almost all radiation centers.
    b. It is more accurate than conventional radiation.
    c. It is unassociated with improved outcomes in prostate cancer patients.
    d. It is a form of particle therapy.
    e. None of the above.

13. Which of the following statements is TRUE regarding complications after radiation therapy?
    a. They are related to treatment technique, type of radiation used, and total dose given.
    b. They are identifiable in the majority of treated patients.
    c. They are higher with dose escalation protocols.
    d. They are lower with particle beam therapy.
    e. None of the above.

14. Dose escalation trials using conformal radiation show improved outcomes at which of the following doses?
    a. 60 Gy
    b. 66 Gy
    c. 70 Gy
    d. Above 75 Gy
    e. None of the above

15. Dose escalation trials show a benefit for all of the following groups except which one?
    a. Patients with favorable tumors (T1 or T2, Gleason score of < 7) and PSA levels < 10
    b. Patients with favorable tumors (T1 or T2, Gleason score of < 7) and PSA levels > 20
    c. Patients with unfavorable tumors (T2b or T3, Gleason score of > 7) and PSA levels < 10
    d. Patients with unfavorable tumors (T2b or T3, Gleason score of ≥ 7) and PSA levels > 4
    e. None of the above

16. Which of the following statements is TRUE regarding particle beam therapy?
    a. It has a theoretical advantage over photon therapy.
    b. It has been shown to be more effective than photon therapy.
    c. It is less expensive than photon therapy.
    d. It is less toxic than photon therapy.
    e. None of the above.

17. Which of the following statements is TRUE regarding intensity-modulated radiation therapy?
    a. It is a form of particle therapy.
    b. It has been proved to improve treatment outcome.
    c. It gives equal emphasis to the target tissue (prostate) and normal tissue (bladder and rectum) during treatment planning.
    d. It can be delivered inexpensively because of software improvements.
    e. None of the above

18. With regard to complications of permanent implant brachytherapy, which of the following statements is TRUE?
    a. There is a higher rate of urinary toxicity than with external-beam irradiation.
    b. There is a higher rate of rectal toxicity than with external-beam irradiation.
    c. There is a higher rate of impotence than in radical prostatectomy.
    d. There is a higher rate of impotence than in external-beam irradiation.
    e. None of the above.

19. Which of the following statements is TRUE regarding high-dose-rate brachytherapy?
    a. It is usually delivered as monotherapy for advanced prostate cancer.
    b. It uses high-activity iodine-103 or paladium-103 (^{103}Pd) as the source.
    c. It does not require a surgical procedure.
    d. It is generally delivered in several fractions as a boost to external-beam irradiation.
    e. None of the above.

20. When comparing iodine-125 (^{125}I) to ^{103}Pd, which of the following statements is TRUE?
    a. ^{125}I has a shorter half-life than ^{103}Pd.
    b. ^{125}I delivers a significantly higher dose to the rectum when compared with ^{103}Pd.
    c. ^{125}I delivers a significantly higher dose to the urethra when compared with ^{103}Pd.
    d. The dose prescribed for a ^{125}I implant is higher than the dose for a ^{103}Pd implant.
    e. None of the above.

21. When prostate brachytherapy monotherapy is compared with a brachytherapy boost, which of the following statements is TRUE?
    a. A higher implant dose is used with monotherapy than with the boost.
    b. Brachytherapy monotherapy is associated with a higher rate of rectal complications than is brachytherapy boost.
    c. Brachytherapy monotherapy is preferred for patients with preexisting urinary outlet obstruction.
    d. Brachytherapy monotherapy is preferred for larger glands.
    e. None of the above.

22. Prostate brachytherapy monotherapy is appropriate for which group of patients? Patients with
    a. T3 cancer
    b. T1c prostate cancer
    c. a high probability of organ-confined disease
    d. a high probability of organ-confined disease, prostates weighing < 60 g, and low American Urological Association (AUA) symptom scores
    e. None of the above

23. MRI-guided prostate brachytherapy is able to provide optimal placement of the radioactive sources within the prostate gland for what reason?
    a. A real-time imaging mechanism permits the physician to verify that the trajectory of the catheter containing the radioactive sources is in the ideal location when compared with the pre-plan.
    b. The magnetic field aligns the sources perfectly.
    c. The procedure can be done under local anesthesia.
    d. A Foley catheter is not needed.
    e. a and b.
24. With MRI-guided prostate brachytherapy, patients with large prostate glands (>60 g) can have implants and still have very low acute urinary retention rates (4%) for what reason?
    a. MRI guidance allows for urethral sparing.
    b. MRI guidance allows for fewer sources.
    c. A Foley catheter is not needed with MRI-guided brachytherapy.
    d. A cystoscopy is not performed with MRI-guided brachytherapy.
    e. The procedure can be performed using local anesthesia.
25. What is the principal reason for neoadjuvant androgen suppression before initiation of radiation therapy?
    a. To prevent early development of metastatic disease
    b. To reduce prostate size, thus minimizing the field size and side effects of external beam treatment
    c. To reduce the tumor burden requiring eradication with radiation
    d. To delay the need for radiation
    e. To improve overall survival
26. For a patient with a Gleason score of 8, which of the following statements is best supported by the findings of phase III studies? Androgen suppression:
    a. is always used with radiation.
    b. improves overall survival when used with radiation.
    c. improves biochemical freedom from failure (bNED) survival when given in addition to standard dose radiation.
    d. has no role in treatment based on this factor alone.
    e. is given for 4 months before radiation.
27. The findings of RTOG 92-02 indicate that when given in combination with radiation for T3 Gleason score 7 disease:
    a. prolonged adjuvant androgen deprivation provides added benefit as compared with neoadjuvant therapy alone.
    b. the optimal duration of androgen suppression with radiation is now defined.
    c. prolonged androgen deprivation results in improved overall survival.
    d. neoadjuvant androgen deprivation is sufficient.
    e. radiation alone is suboptimal therapy.
28. A patient has a history of hormone-refractory metastatic prostate cancer. He now has a new painful lesion of his upper femoral shaft. What is a typical course of palliative radiation therapy for this man?
    a. One fraction of radiation at 3000 cGy
    b. 7 weeks of daily radiation to 7000 cGy
    c. 10 fractions of daily radiation to 3000 cGy
    d. One fraction of daily radiation to 7000 cGy
    e. None of the above
29. A patient with a history of metastatic prostate cancer, under treatment with a luteinizing hormone–releasing hormone agonist and a nonsteroidal antiandrogen, presents to your office with a 3-week history of increasing middle to low back pain and 2 days of leg weakness. What is the most appropriate first step at this point?
    a. Increasing the dose of nonsteroidal antiandrogen
    b. MRI of the thoracic and lumbar spine
    c. Radiation therapy with a systemic radionuclide such as strontium-89
    d. Treatment with a selective cyclooxygenase-2 inhibitor for 5 to 7 days and reevaluation
    e. None of the above
30. What is the most common toxicity of systemic radionuclide therapy with strontium-89 and samarium-153?
    a. Hematologic toxicity, particularly with a decrement in the platelet count
    b. Neurologic toxicity, including tinnitus
    c. Genitourinary toxicity, particularly azotemia
    d. Hepatic toxicity associated with an elevation of transaminase levels
    e. None of the above
31. What would be an attractive gene therapy approach that could be combined with radiation for the treatment of prostatecancer?
    a. One that requires prolonged transgene expression
    b. One that kills cells by a mechanism that complements and does not overlap with radiation-induced cell death
    c. One that requires all prostate cancer cells to be transduced
    d. a and c
    e. None of the above

ANSWERS

1. **a. Three-dimensional conformal technique and image guidance for radioactive source placement in the prostate gland.** The first advance has been the generation of linear accelerators and conformal techniques capable of delivering high doses of radiation deep within the pelvis while simultaneously respecting the normal tissue tolerance of the anterior rectal wall, prostatic urethra, femoral heads, and bladder neck. The second advance was made when image-guided techniques were introduced for use during the insertion of radioactive sources directly into the prostate gland.
2. **d. Biopsy Gleason score, PSA level, percentage of prostate biopsies, and clinical stage.** The pretreatment prognostic factors that have established roles in predicting recurrence include the PSA value, biopsy Gleason score, and the 1992 American Joint Committee on Cancer Staging (AJCC) clinical stage.
3. **d. able to identify the patients at higher risk of prostate cancer-specific mortality despite having low-risk disease.** Of particular importance is that the majority of patients (158/207 [76%]) in the intermediate-risk group could be classified into either a 30% or an 85% 5-year PSA control high- or low-risk cohort, respectively, by using the preoperative prostate biopsy data.
4. **e. b and c.**
5. **e. All of the above.**
6. **c. PSA value, biopsy Gleason score, and clinical T stage.** The pretreatment prognostic factors that have established roles in predicting recurrence include the PSA value, biopsy Gleason score, and the 1992 American Joint Committee on Cancer Staging (AJCC) clinical stage.
7. **c. Stable and not rising.** It is clear that there is no distinct PSA threshold that defines successful treatment but that PSA stability after the nadir is important.
8. **c. Tell the patient that he likely has a recurrence and that rising PSA may indicate a distant component to the failure.** The level of PSA nadir achieved to some extent reflects the type of failure. The median PSA nadir for patients exhibiting local failure is 2 to 3 ng/mL and for those exhibiting distant failure it is 5 to 10 ng/mL. The postnadir doubling time of the PSA value also correlates with the type of failure, with distant failures having shorter PSA doubling times of 3 to 6 months and local failures having longer PSA doubling times of 11 to 13 months.
9. **c. Patients who are cured may take 24 to 30 months to reach a nadir.** The time to nadir has been shown to be inversely proportional to disease-free survival. The median time to nadir in patients who remain free from failure is 22 to 33 months, with 92% of men whose PSA value reached a nadir at 36 months or longer remaining disease free.
10. **d. 30 months.** In a series of 498 men followed with sequential systematic postirradiation biopsies, biopsy samples cleared at a mean time of 30 months after radiation therapy.
11. **d. It is associated with treatment technique and dose of radiation.** Tumor control was better in patients who received higher doses of radiation to larger fields, at the expense of increased complications.
12. **b. It is more accurate than conventional radiation.** The result is loosely described as *conformal* radiation therapy because the radiation beams conform to the shape of the treatment target.
13. **a. They are related to treatment technique, type of radiation used, and total dose given.** The percentage of patients who experience side effects and the severity of the side effects differ somewhat from series to series depending on the morbidity scale used and also on whether the assessment is physician or patient based.
14. **d. Above 75 Gy.** Dose escalation therapy, to doses greater than 75 Gy, is still experimental, but the early data appear to be highly favorable.
15. **a. Patients with favorable tumors (T1 or T2, Gleason score of < 7) and PSA levels of < 10.** Patients with favorable tumors (Gleason score of < 6, T1 or T2a) who also had a PSA level < 10 ng/mL derived no benefit from dose escalation because all patients in this group did well. Patients with unfavorable tumors (Gleason score of 7 to 10 and T2b or T3) who also had a PSA level > 20 ng/mL also derived no benefit from dose escalation.
16. **a. It has a theoretical advantage over photon therapy.** The heavy particle beams are difficult to produce and to control but have certain theoretical advantages over conventional x-ray and electron beams.
17. **c. It gives equal emphasis to the target tissue (prostate) and normal tissue (bladder and rectum) during treatment planning.** The goal of this method of treatment planning and delivery is to maximize treatment to the target, for example, the prostate, while minimizing treatment to the surrounding tissues to a degree that is not possible with conformal therapy.
18. **a. There is a higher rate of urinary toxicity than with external-beam irradiation.** One study showed that 37% of patients report grade I urinary toxicity (symptoms not requiring medical intervention) within the first 60 days after implantation. Grade II urinary toxicity (requiring medical intervention), with a mean duration of 19 months after implantation and with a likelihood of resolution of 68% at 36 months, has been reported. Significant continued obstruction requiring self-catheterization occurs in 1% to 5% of patients.
19. **d. It is generally delivered in several fractions as a boost to external-beam irradiation.** This therapy is delivered as a boost in two to four applications, either before or after external-beam irradiation.
20. **d. The dose prescribed for a ^{125}I implant is higher than the dose for a ^{103}Pd implant.** Higher activity seeds are required for ^{103}Pd versus ^{125}I to deliver a similar tumoricidal dose (i.e., 1.3 mCi per palladium seed vs. 0.4 mCi per iodine seed).
21. **b. Brachytherapy monotherapy is associated with a higher rate of rectal complications than is brachytherapy boost.** There is relatively little radiation delivered to the rectum with brachytherapy alone. However, the prostatic urethra receives a full dose. When an implant is combined with external-beam therapy the dosage to the urethra is less but increased radiation is received by the rectum.
22. **d. a high probability of organ-confined disease, prostates weighing < 60 g, and low American Urological Association (AUA) symptom scores.** Larger prostatic volumes—specifically glands > 60 g—were associated with urinary toxicities. Other investigators reported that transurethral prostatic resection in the distant past is not a contraindication to implantation. Patients with a pretreatment AUA score > 20 demonstrated a 29% risk of developing urinary retention, whereas a pretreatment score < 10 was associated with a 2% risk.
23. **a. A real-time imaging mechanism permits the physician to verify that the trajectory of the catheter containing the radioactive sources is in the ideal location when compared with the pre-plan.** By using this technique, the three-dimensional trajectory that the catheter containing the

radioactive sources traverses can be checked intraoperatively and compared, within a few seconds, with the ideal location based on the pre-plan using real-time MRI.

24. **a. MRI guidance allows for urethral sparing.** Therefore, despite implanting 45 men with glands > 60 g, the acute urinary retention rate was 4% and the need for prolonged use of oral α_{1a}-adrenergic blockers was 5%, consistent with a urethral sparing technique.

25. **c. To reduce the tumor burden requiring eradication with radiation.** Short-duration neoadjuvant androgen suppression therapy may be used with the goal of reducing the local tumor burden requiring eradication by subsequent radiation.

26. **c. Androgen suppression improves biochemical freedom from failure (bNED) survival when given in addition to standard dose radiation.** Among strategies to improve outcome for patients with locally advanced prostate cancer, hormonal manipulation in combination with radiation therapy has consistently demonstrated improvement in treatment outcome as compared with standard-dose radiation alone. A meta-analysis of both retrospective and prospective trials of androgen deprivation in combination with radiation therapy demonstrated near-universal benefit in regard to local/regional control, disease-free survival, and bNED survival.

27. **a. prolonged adjuvant androgen deprivation provides added benefit as compared with neoadjuvant therapy alone.** The optimal type, timing, and duration of androgen suppression in combination with radiation therapy remains to be defined. In RTOG 92-02, patients with T2c-T4, N0-1, M0 disease were randomized to receive a total of 4 months of total androgen suppression with radiation administered after 2 months or the same regimen followed by an additional 2 years of goserelin. Subgroup analysis revealed significant improvement in overall survival for patients with Gleason scores 8 to 10.

28. **c. 10 fractions of daily radiation to 3000 cGy.** A frequently used regimen in the United States is to give 3000 cGy in 10 divided fractions.

29. **b. MRI of the thoracic and lumbar spine.** The diagnostic tool of choice to evaluate a spinal cord compression is MRI.

30. **a. Hematologic toxicity, particularly with a decrement in the platelet count.** Toxicity of strontium-89 is mainly hematologic. Platelet depression is dose dependent.

31. **b. One that kills cells by a mechanism that complements and does not overlap with radiation-induced cell death.** A rational combination of one of these approaches with a more standard cytotoxic therapy such as radiation may provide superior cell killing as a result of nonoverlapping modes of cell death.

101

Cryotherapy for Prostate Cancer

JOHN S. LAM • LOUIS L. PISTERS • ARIE S. BELLDEGRUN

QUESTIONS

1. Technical innovations improving cryotherapy for prostate cancer include all EXCEPT the use of:

   a. transrectal ultrasound.
   b. urethral warming catheters.
   c. warming of neurovascular bundles.
   d. thermocouples placed in critical areas of the prostate.
   e. smaller-diameter cryoprobes allowing percutaneous insertion.

2. Which of the following statements concerning open cryotherapy of the prostate performed in the 1970s is TRUE?

   a. It was performed through the retropubic approach.
   b. It resulted in a low complication rate.
   c. It used ultrasound and thermocouples to monitor the freezing process.
   d. It was later reported to have a local recurrence rate of 15%.
   e. It achieved favorable results in terms of survival.

3. What is the most clinically important parameter of tissue ablation other than lowest temperature achieved by cryotherapy?

   a. The diameter of the cryoprobe
   b. The number of freeze/thaw cycles
   c. The velocity of tissue thawing
   d. The velocity of tissue freezing
   e. The duration of freezing

4. Typically, the cryoprobes that are activated first in cryotherapy for prostate cancer are located:

   a. anteriorly.
   b. posteriorly.
   c. laterally.
   d. anteriorly.
   e. periurethrally.

5. What is the characteristic appearance of frozen tissue on ultrasound?

   a. Mixed echogenicity
   b. Hyperechogenicity
   c. Anechogenicity
   d. Hypoechogenicity
   e. None of the above

6. Prostate cell death is likely to occur completely in a single freeze cycle when tissue temperature reaches:

   a. 20°C.
   b. 0°C.
   c. −20°C.
   d. −40°C.
   e. none of the above.

7. A patient with Gleason's grade 3+4, clinical stage T1c prostate cancer associated with a serum prostate-specific antigen (PSA) value of 8.6 ng/mL is noted to have a prostate gland volume of 70 mL and an American Urological Association (AUA) Symptom Score of 18. Which of the following statements is TRUE?

   a. This patient is best treated with cryotherapy.
   b. This patient requires microwave therapy of the prostate before cryotherapy.
   c. This patient will likely develop urinary tract obstruction after cryotherapy.
   d. This patient should undergo neoadjuvant hormone therapy to reduce the gland before cryotherapy.
   e. This patient cannot undergo cryotherapy.

8. Failure after prostate cryotherapy may be defined as:

   a. failure to reach PSA nadir by 2 months.
   b. PSA cut-off greater than 0.1 ng/mL.
   c. 3 consecutive elevations in PSA after nadir.
   d. 2 consecutive elevations in PSA after nadir.
   e. PSA nadir greater than 0.2 ng/mL.

9. Two years after cryosurgery for clinical stage T2a, PSA 7.0, Gleason's grade 3+4 cancer, a patient is found to have benign glands on a prostate biopsy specimen from the right apex. No malignancy is detected. The PSA level is detectable at 0.2 ng/mL. What is the next step in management?

   a. Repeat cryoablation of the left lobe
   b. Radiation therapy
   c. Surveillance
   d. Androgen deprivation
   e. Repeat biopsy

10. Which clinical parameter most accurately predicts for cancer control after cryotherapy?

   a. PSA nadir < 0.1 ng/mL
   b. Preoperative Gleason score < 6
   c. Preoperative serum PSA level < 15 ng/mL
   d. A prostate volume < 40 mL
   e. Preoperative T stage

11. Several potential advantages that primary cryotherapy for prostate cancer offers over other local therapies include all EXCEPT:
    a. capable of destroying a biologically heterogeneous population of cancer cells, including cell populations that are resistant to radiation therapy and hormonal therapy.
    b. freezing process can extend beyond the capsule of the prostate, potentially eradicating extracapsular disease.
    c. proven benefit with adjuvant therapies.
    d. can be repeated with minimal morbidity.
    e. can treat high Gleason score prostate cancer.
12. Salvage cryotherapy for radiorecurrent prostate cancer:
    a. will not reduce the PSA below 0.4 ng/mL.
    b. may be useful in the control of local spread in the face of distant metastases.
    c. has the same incidence of incontinence and fistula rates as primary cryotherapy.
    d. may be performed on all patients for whom irradiation fails.
    e. is unlikely to cure high-risk disease (PSA >10 ng/nL and Gleason score > 7).
13. Clinical pretreatment factors associated with early treatment failure after salvage cryotherapy include:
    a. PSA level > 10 ng/mL.
    b. Prostate volume > 50 mL.
    c. Gleason score ≥ 9.
    d. Failure to reach PSA nadir in 3 months.
    e. a and c.
14. The most common complication after cryotherapy for prostate cancer is:
    a. rectourethral fistula.
    b. incontinence.
    c. erectile dysfunction.
    d. urethral sloughing.
    e. pelvic pain.
15. Two months after cryotherapy, a patient complains of urinary frequency and dysuria. Urinalysis reveals pyuria. What is the most likely diagnosis?
    a. Pelvic abscess
    b. Urethral sloughing
    c. Extravasation of urine
    d. Rectourethral fistula
    e. Bladder neck contraction

ANSWERS

1. **c. warming of neurovascular bundles.** Use of TRUS for real-time monitoring of the freezing process, use of a urethral warming catheter, use of thermocouples placed in critical areas of the prostate, and improved cryoprobes allowing percutaneous insertion are technical innovations that have all contributed to improving cryotherapy for prostate cancer.
2. **e. It achieved favorable results in terms of survival.** In an early report on the open transperineal approach to treat patients with various stages of prostate cancer, approximately 41% of patients eventually had evidence of persistent or recurrent disease. Although the technique compared favorably with other treatment modalities with respect to survival, morbidity was significant. Sloughing of urethral tissue was common. Urethrorectal or urethrocutaneous fistulas developed in 13% of patients, bladder neck obstruction in 2.3%, and urinary incontinence in 6.5%. This early experience was reviewed more recently: cancer recurrence was documented in 78.4% of the men, and 47.1% died of prostate cancer. Local recurrence was documented in at least 67% of those undergoing the procedure.
3. **b. The number of freeze/thaw cycles.** In a clinical setting, the number of freezing cycles, the lowest temperature achieved, and the existence of any regional "heat sinks" may be more important factors relating to cancer destruction. Repeating a freeze/thaw cycle results in more extensive tissue damage compared with a single cycle.
4. **d. anteriorly.** To maintain TRUS visibility, the freezing is started at the anterior probe layer and continued posteriorly. Uncovered areas may be visualized and a correcting maneuver may be used. If the freezing is started posteriorly, the acoustic shadowing would prevent visualization of tissue beyond the ice.
5. **d. Hypoechogenicity.** Frozen tissue is significantly different from unfrozen tissue in sound impedance, resulting in strong echo reflection at the interface of frozen and normal tissue.
   The frozen area could be seen as a well-marginated hyperechoic rim with acoustic shadowing by ultrasonography. Sonography provides no information about the temperature distribution within the ice nor does it show the extent of freezing at the lateral or anterior aspects of the prostate.
6. **d. −40°C.** Complete cell death is unlikely to occur at temperatures higher than −20°C, and temperatures lower than −40°C are required to completely destroy cells.
7. **d. This patient should undergo neoadjuvant hormone therapy to reduce the gland before cryotherapy.** A gland in excess of 50 mL may be treated best with neoadjuvant androgen deprivation to reduce target volume and allow for more effective cryoablation.
8. **c. 3 consecutive elevations in PSA after nadir.** There is no established definition of biochemical failure after cryotherapy and different PSA cutoff levels of 0.3, 0.4, 0.5, and 1.0 ng/mL have been used in numerous studies. The American Society for Therapeutic Radiology and Oncology (ASTRO) definition of failure of three consecutive rises in the PSA level has also been used.
9. **c. Surveillance.** Benign epithelium, often very focal, has been seen in up to 71% of patients after cryotherapy. The significance of benign epithelium is unknown, and such findings may represent areas of the prostate not frozen to low temperatures, perhaps in the area of the urethral warmer.
10. **a. PSA nadir < 0.1 ng/mL.** Biochemical failure (subsequent rise in PSA > 0.2 ng/mL) was lowest in those who achieved PSA nadirs less than 0.1 ng/mL (21%), but was common in those with higher nadir values. Biopsy failure was lowest in those with nadirs less than 0.1 ng/m (1.5%), followed by those with nadirs less than 0.4 ng/mL (10%).
11. **c. proven benefit with adjuvant therapies.** Potential advantages that primary cryotherapy for prostate cancer offers over other local therapies include the capability of destroying a biologically heterogeneous population of cancer cells, including cell populations that are resistant to radiation therapy and hormonal therapy, extension of the freezing process beyond the capsule of the prostate, potentially eradicating extracapsular disease, repeat of treatment with minimal morbidity, and treatment of high Gleason score prostate cancer.
12. **e. is unlikely to cure high-risk disease (PSA > 10 ng/mL and Gleason score > 7).** In patients who have experienced radiation

therapy failure for prostate cancer, those with a PSA greater than 10 ng/mL and Gleason score of the recurrent cancer greater than or equal to 9 are unlikely to be successfully salvaged. The incidence of incontinence and fistulas is higher in salvage cryotherapy.

13. **e. a and c.** Clinical pretreatment factors associated with early treatment failure after salvage cryotherapy for radiorecurrent prostate cancer include a PSA level greater than 10 ng/mL and Gleason score greater than or equal to 9.

14. **c. erectile dysfunction.** The most common complication after cryotherapy for prostate cancer is erectile dysfunction. Rectourethral fistula, incontinence, urethral sloughing, and pelvic pain are complications that can occur after cryotherapy. More contemporary series report higher impotence rates of 80% or more. This is probably because of the use of multiple freeze/thaw cycles and extension of the ice ball beyond the prostate into the area of the neurovascular bundles.

15. **b. Urethral sloughing.** Tissue sloughing is manifested by irritative and obstructive voiding symptoms. Pyuria is noted as well. Urinary retention is not uncommon. This condition typically occurs 3 to 8 weeks after the procedure. Initial management consists of antibiotics.

102

Treatment of Locally Advanced Prostate Cancer

MAXWELL V. MENG • PETER R. CARROLL

QUESTIONS

1. Identification of patients with locally advanced prostate cancer is best achieved by:
   a. transrectal ultrasonography.
   b. serum PSA.
   c. digital rectal examination.
   d. serum PSA, biopsy grade, clinical stage.
   e. PSA kinetics.
2. Using the Kattan postoperative nomogram, which of the following contributes most to the risk of biochemical recurrence after radical prostatectomy?
   a. Positive surgical margin
   b. Pre-treatment serum PSA of 17 ng/mL
   c. Gleason 4+3 disease
   d. Established capsular penetration
   e. Seminal vesicle invasion
3. Neoadjuvant androgen deprivation before radical prostatectomy leads to:
   a. improved biochemical-free survival.
   b. improved overall survival.
   c. reduced positive surgical margins.
   d. reduced local recurrence.
   e. increased operative morbidity.
4. In men with locally advanced prostate cancer undergoing prostatectomy, clinical overstaging (i.e., pathologically organ confined disease) occurs in:
   a. <10%.
   b. 15% to 30%.
   c. 40% to 60%.
   d. 70% to 80%.
   e. >90%.
5. The use of high-dose antiandrogen monotherapy after prostatectomy in men with locally advanced disease:
   a. reduces disease progression.
   b. increases cardiac morbidity.
   c. does not have an impact on sexual function.
   d. improves overall survival.
   e. improves local disease control.
6. In men with locally advanced/high risk prostate cancer, the most effective treatment among the following options is:
   a. brachytherapy + external-beam radiation therapy.
   b. neoadjuvant AD + external-beam radiation therapy.
   c. neoadjuvant AD + external-beam radiation therapy + adjuvant AD.
   d. concurrent AD + external-beam radiation therapy.
   e. long-term AD alone.
7. Risk assessment schemes for prostate cancer are most accurate for patients with:
   a. low-risk disease.
   b. high-risk disease.
   c. the disease.
   d. metastatic disease.
   e. locally advanced cancers
8. The current appropriate dose for adjuvant radiation therapy after radical prostatectomy is:
   a. <45 Gy.
   b. 45 to 50 Gy.
   c. 51 to 55 Gy.
   d. 56 to 60 Gy.
   e. >60 Gy.
9. The use of androgen deprivation in combination with radiation therapy for those with high-risk cancers is associated with all of the following EXCEPT:
   a. improved local control.
   b. improved biochemical-free survival.
   c. less gastrointestinal toxicity.
   d. worsened sexual function.
   e. more urinary frequency.

ANSWERS

1. **d. serum PSA, biopsy grade, clinical stage.** Although clinical stage, serum PSA, and Gleason score all individually predict pathologic stage and prognosis, the combination of these three variables increases the accuracy of this assessment.
2. **b. pre-treatment serum PSA of 17 ng/mL.** Despite the trend toward lower serum PSA at the time of diagnosis, PSA remains an important predictor of treatment failure and greater elevations (>8 ng/mL) of PSA contribute significantly to calculated biochemical recurrence.
3. **c. reduced positive surgical margins.** The randomized and nonrandomized studies of neoadjuvant androgen deprivation in men with lower clinical stage (cT1-T2) clearly demonstrate a reduction in the rate of positive surgical margins; however, this advantage has not been observed in men with cT3c and has not translated into improved long-term PSA-free survival.
4. **b. 15% to 30%.** Recent data suggest that clinical overstaging occurs in approximately 27% of men with clinical stage T3 disease undergoing prostatectomy, consistent with the range in the literature of 7% to 26%.
5. **a. reduces disease progression.** Bicalutamide at greater dose (150 mg) appears to have a positive effect in those men with locally advanced disease, with 43% reduction in disease progression and potential benefit of improved survival; however, it should be remembered that high-dose bicalutamide given to men with *localized* prostate cancer is associated with increased risk of death (hazard ratio: 1.23).
6. **c. neoadjuvant AD + external-beam radiation therapy + adjuvant AD.** The accumulated data from multiple RTOG and EORTC trials suggests that improved outcomes are achieved with greater duration of administration of androgen deprivation in combination with external-beam radiation therapy, with apparent benefit of both neoadjuvant and adjuvant therapy.
7. **a. low-risk disease.** Validation has confirmed the general accuracy of the available risk assessment tools, but there is a tendency to overestimate the risk of cancer recurrence in men with high-risk disease features.
8. **e. >60 Gy.** There is a trend to improve response to adjuvant radiation therapy and, most contemporary series report doses greater than 60 Gy, with potential threshold of either 61.2 or 64 Gy.
9. **c. less gastrointestinal toxicity.** The longer application (>6 to 9 months) of androgen deprivation in conjunction with radiation therapy may be associated with increased rectal morbidity as well as sexual dysfunction.

103

Clinical State of the Rising PSA after Definitive Local Therapy: A Practical Approach

MICHAEL J. MORRIS • HOWARD I. SCHER

QUESTIONS

1. The most appropriate therapeutic approach for a patient with a rising PSA after definitive local therapy is which of the following?
   a. He should be started on hormonal therapy because he is destined to relapse systemically.
   b. He should undergo salvage local procedures, such as radiation or cryotherapy or prostatectomy, before undergoing any systemic treatment.
   c. He should undergo neither systemic nor local treatments, because the only appropriate context in which to begin any intervention is when radiographically proven metastases have developed.
   d. He should be risk stratified and treated with a modality of therapy that matches his risk of relapse, risk of developing local vs. systemic disease, and risk of dying of other causes.
2. Which of the following best describes the state of knowledge of systemic treatment for patients with a rising PSA?
   a. Randomized prospective data have demonstrated that patients with a rising PSA live longer if they are started on hormones as soon as the PSA is detectable rather than waiting until they have radiographically proven metastases.
   b. There have been no randomized trials performed in this population demonstrating that any therapy is superior to observation. Therefore, the most appropriate treatment for these patients is to place them on a clinical trial, if a reasonable and appropriate study is available in the community.
   c. Clinical trials that have shown an improvement in survival when hormones are used for early node-positive cases and as adjuvant therapy after radiation as opposed to deferred strategies are clearly applicable to patients with a rising PSA, and therefore early hormonal therapy is the standard of care.
   d. Bicalutamide at 150 mg daily will prolong survival and preserve quality of life.
3. The PSA doubling time can be used as part of prognosticating for:
   a. time to metastatic disease.
   b. overall survival.
   c. likelihood of remaining free of evidence of disease after salvage radiation therapy.
   d. all of the above.
   e. a and c only.
4. The PSA is used in clinical trials involving patients with a rising PSA in which of the following ways?
   a. The post-treatment PSA decline is a surrogate for survival.
   b. A post-treatment PSA decline of 50% is the means by which experimental therapies should be judged as either a success or failure.
   c. The patient's PSA kinetics can be used to assess the patient's risk of a clinical event such as developing metastases, progression-free survival, or overall survival to help formulate eligibility criteria.
   d. A rising PSA on therapy is a universally accepted indicator that the patient has progressed on therapy.
5. Which of the following characterizes the clinical state of "rising PSA"?
   a. Postoperative patients enter it when the PSA is detectable.
   b. Postradiation patients enter it when the PSA is 0.1 ng/mL.
   c. Patients who have not received definitive therapy enter it when their PSA rises.
   d. Patients enter it when they have consistently rising PSAs in accordance with an indication of treatment failure for their primary therapy and who have negative imaging studies.
6. Salvage radiation therapy should be used:
   a. in patients whose PSA kinetics and other prognostic features either predict for a low likelihood of developing metastatic disease and/or a high likelihood of deriving a durable remission after radiation therapy.
   b. as a supplement to or in lieu of hormones in selected patients with palpable masses in the prostate bed.
   c. to a dose of 66 Gy in all patients.
   d. for all patients who have a positive margin.

7. High-dose bicalutamide (150 mg) as monotherapy for patients with a rising PSA:
   a. is standard treatment for patients with a rising PSA.
   b. has risks and benefits that have not yet been fully elucidated.
   c. has a proven survival advantage over standard treatment with a GnRH agonist.
   d. has all of the benefits of a GnRH agonist and none of the drawbacks.

ANSWERS

1. **d. He should be risk stratified and treated with a modality of therapy that matches his risk of relapse, risk of developing local vs. systemic disease, and risk of dying of other causes.** A critical question is what is the probability that a patient with systemic disease will develop metastases that are detectable on imaging studies, a point in the disease where death from prostate cancer exceeds that of death from other causes, or that he will develop symptoms and ultimately die of the disease rather than with it? Once this is addressed, and the need for treatment is determined, consideration can be given to what options are available and their likelihood of success in controlling the disease or, preferentially, eliminating it completely.
2. **b. There have been no randomized trials performed in this population demonstrating that any therapy is superior to observation. Therefore, the most appropriate treatment for these patients is to place them on a clinical trial, if a reasonable and appropriate study is available in the community.** An issue that has long been debated is what is the optimal time to begin androgen deprivation therapy, because there have been no clinical trials to compare hormones with expectant observation specifically in the rising PSA population. Indeed, the American Society of Clinical Oncology Clinical Practice Guidelines argue formally against an "early" treatment policy (Loblaw, 2004). In spite of this, there is a significant body of literature to suggest that early hormonal therapy has the potential to confer a survival advantage in selected patients relative to hormones that have been deferred to the point of having radiographically evident metastases. Most are randomized trials of androgen deprivation applied before, during, and after radiation therapy for variable amounts of time from 6 months to continuous, which show improvements in disease-free and overall survival compared with either no hormonal therapy or hormonal therapy that has been deferred until the time of metastatic disease (Lawton, 2001; Pilepich, 2001; Bolla, 2002; Pilepich, 2003; D'Amico, 2004). The caveat is that the patients in the state of localized disease enrolled in these trials may not be directly comparable to those in the clinical state of rising PSA who have already failed either local or combined modality treatments and are now at risk of developing radiographic metastases as the next point in the natural history.
3. **d. All of the above.** *Predicting local vs. systemic relapse:* In general, low pretreatment PSA levels, lower grade tumors, low clinical or pathologic staging, late time from definitive local therapy to PSA relapse, and long PSA doubling times generally prognosticate for a low likelihood of developing distant radiographically apparent metastases (Pound, 1999).

   Risk of developing metastatic disease: High-grade disease, short time intervals to biochemical relapse (<2 years vs. >2 years), and a PSA doubling time of < 10 months vs. > 10 months predicted for a shorter time to radiographic progression (Pound, 1999). In an updated analysis, time to PSA failure was no longer predictive when PSADT was considered (Eisenberger, 2003). In numerous studies, PSADT is the dominant factor used to assess the risk of developing metastasis-free survival (Roberts, 2001; Kwan, 2003; Sandler, 2003). In one study, a PSADT < 6 months was associated with a 5-year progression-free survival of 64% versus 93% of patients who had a longer PSADT (Roberts, 2001).

   Risk of disease-specific and all cause risk death: Data now exist that demonstrates an association between PSADT and disease-specific survival after radiation therapy (Lee, 1997; Zagars, 1997; Sandler, 2000; D'Amico, 2002, 2003), and the post-treatment PSADT with time to prostate cancer-specific and all-cause mortality (all $P<.001$).
4. **c. The patient's PSA kinetics can be used to assess the patient's risk of a clinical event such as developing metastases, progression-free survival, or overall survival to help formulate eligibility criteria.** Patients with unfavorable PSA kinetics who are at a high risk of metastases or death from disease are a group who not only need systemic therapy but are most likely to benefit.

   Based on this we can divide this patient group into three groups based on prognosis: low-risk patients who are unlikely to develop metastases, symptoms, or death from disease and who should be managed expectantly; intermediate-risk patients can be considered for investigational approaches designed to slow the disease to the point where the patient dies of other causes (tantamount to cure) or receive androgen deprivation; and high-risk patients (those with PSA doubling times of 6 months or less) can be considered for androgen deprivation or, ideally, enrolled in a clinical trial.

   Outcome Measures for the Patient with a Rising PSA: There are several useful endpoints for trials in this clinical state. The most immediate of these is the post-therapy change in PSA. The attraction of measuring serial PSA levels is that these assays can be obtained simply and frequently with minimal inconvenience to the patient. Ease of use and mathematical objectivity should not be confused with true surrogacy for clinical benefit. Time to PSA progression can be defined by an increase to a predetermined number, or an increase by an absolute percentage, or a change in the post-intervention rate of rise. The definition must also vary for drugs that produce "no change," those that produce a decline, or those that produced an undetectable PSA.

   As noted previously, the demonstration of an association does not equate with surrogacy, and there remains a large proportion of the association between PSA-based metrics and clinical outcomes that are yet unexplained.

5. **d. Patients enter it when they have consistently rising PSAs in accordance with an indication of treatment failure for their primary therapy and who have negative imaging studies.** When a patient has entered the clinical state of a "rising PSA" depends on the primary therapy he has received and the sensitivity of the assay used to measure PSA.

6. **a. in patients whose PSA kinetics and other prognostic features either predict for a low likelihood of developing metastatic disease and/or a high likelihood of deriving a durable remission after radiation therapy.** The majority of patients in this clinical state do not have clinically evident disease in conjunction with a rise in PSA. It is for these patients that models were developed to help assess the likelihood of durable PSA control after salvage radiation therapy. Although many models have been reported, the recurring factors associated with a favorable outcome are Gleason scores < 8, long PSADT (>6 to 12 months, depending on the trial), and positive margin status. An additional factor is the so-called trigger PSA above which the chance of durable control is reduced. A consensus report from the American Society of Therapeutic Radiology and Oncology recommends a trigger PSA of 1.5 (Cox, 1999). Other authors have suggested that this threshold is set too high, however.

   Although salvage radiation therapy can benefit a clear subset of patients, the downside of applying such a strategy to all patients is the risk of side effects. The ASTRO consensus report suggests the highest dose that can be given without significant morbidity, which it specifies as at least 64 Gy (Cox, 1999). Most studies have shown that salvage radiation therapy is well tolerated, in spite of the fact that patients may be suffering from the side effects of their previous surgical procedures.

7. **b. has risks and benefits that have not yet been fully elucidated.** The demand that hormones not be considered a standard of care in such patients until phase III data is available has erroneously gained support from the results of the Early Prostate Cancer trial that enrolled 8113 men with T1-4, M0, any N (though N0 in one study), who were randomized to receive either 150 mg of bicalutamide or placebo in addition to standard care, which was either surgery, radiation, or observation. No survival difference between the two arms was seen in the overall population (HR 1.03, 95% CI 0.92, 1.15, P=.582), although the patients with localized disease on observation appeared to have a survival decrement if they received bicalutamide (HR 1.23, 95% CI 1, 1.5, P=.05) (Iversen, 2004; Wirth, 2004). The use, however, of a non–testosterone-lowering form of androgen deprivation in a patient population where the primary tumor was not treated cannot be extrapolated to a rising PSA group with treated primary tumors who are placed on testosterone-lowering therapy.

104

Hormone Therapy for Prostate Cancer

JOEL B. NELSON

QUESTIONS

1. The effectiveness of estrogen as a hormone therapy for prostate cancer is primarily based on:
   a. direct cytotoxic effects of estrogen on prostate cancer cells.
   b. competitive binding of estrogen to the androgen receptor.
   c. inhibition of the conversion of cholesterol to pregnenolone.
   d. desensitizing LH-RH receptors in the anterior pituitary.
   e. negative feedback on LH secretion by the pituitary.
2. The expected response of a man to the administration of the nonsteroidal antiandrogens is:
   a. LH increases, testosterone decreases, estrogen decreases.
   b. LH increases, testosterone increases, estrogen decreases.
   c. LH increases, testosterone increases, estrogen increases.
   d. LH decreases, testosterone decreases, estrogen increases.
   e. LH decreases, testosterone increases, estrogen increases.
3. All of the following therapeutic approaches for androgen axis blockade are in current clinical use EXCEPT:
   a. inhibition of androgen synthesis.
   b. blocking androgen action by binding to the androgen receptor in a competitive fashion.
   c. ablating the source of androgens.
   d. direct inhibition of androgen receptor–mediated pathways.
   e. inhibition of LH-RH and LH release.
4. Nonsteroidal antiandrogens:
   a. do not act as agonists for prostate cancer cells when used in combination with LH-RH agonists.
   b. allow long-term maintenance of erectile function and sexual activity at rates similar to men undergoing surgical castration.
   c. commonly induce gastrointestinal toxicity, manifest as constipation leading, on occasion, to fecal impaction.
   d. cause pancreatic toxicity, ranging from reversible mild to fulminant, life-threatening suppurative pancreatitis requiring periodic monitoring of serum amylase and lipase.
   e. cause fluid retention and thromboembolism in the majority of patients.
5. Which of the following nonsteroidal antiandrogens is associated with a delayed adaptation to darkness after exposure to bright illumination and interstitial pneumonitis?
   a. Bicalutamide
   b. Flutamide
   c. Hydroxyflutamide
   d. Nilutamide
   e. Cyproterone acetate
6. Concerning LH-RH agonists:
   a. based on a review of 24 trials, involving more than 6600 patients, survival after therapy with an LH-RH agonist was significantly better than surgical castration.
   b. although depot preparations and osmotic pump devices allow dosing to extend from 28 days to 1 year, the most effective dosing regimen is daily.
   c. current LH-RH agonists are based on analogs of the native LH-RH decapeptide by amino acid substitutions, particularly position 6 of the peptide.
   d. widespread use of orally effective LH-RH agonists has been limited by severe allergic reactions in some patients, even after previously uneventful treatment.
   e. use of LH-RH agonists is limited to combined androgen blockade.
7. Each of the following has been associated with a favorable initial response to androgen deprivation therapy (ADT) EXCEPT the:
   a. magnitude of the PSA decline.
   b. rapidity of the PSA decline.
   c. PSA doubling time before initiating ADT.
   d. Gleason score of the primary tumor.
   e. maintenance of a detectable PSA.
8. Which of the following statements about the complications of ADT is TRUE?
   a. Most men undergoing ADT have normal bone mineral density before initiating therapy, and it usually takes at least a decade of treatment before the average man will develop osteopenia.
   b. Hot flashes occur in about one fourth of men on ADT but should always be treated because of the associated rare but life-threatening cardiovascular side effects.
   c. Erectile dysfunction after surgical castration or use of an LHRH is common but not inevitable: although 1 in 5 men maintain some sexual activity, only 1 in 20 maintain high levels of sexual interest (libido).
   d. Because most men on ADT maintain lean muscle mass the increase in weight is due to increases in adipose tissue.
   e. Gynecomastia and mastodynia are common with estrogenic compounds and antiandrogens but are effectively treated by external-beam radiation therapy after they occur.

9. Which of the following statements about the combination of 3 months of neoadjuvant ADT before radical prostatectomy is TRUE?
   a. Positive surgical margin rates are significantly reduced with ADT-treated patients.
   b. There is a significant reduction in biochemical (PSA) progression with ADT-treated patients.
   c. The benefit of neoadjuvant ADT appears to be in men with locally advanced disease and/or those with high-grade disease.
   d. Antiandrogen monotherapy has not shown a significant reduction of biochemical failure, but LH-RH agonists have demonstrated this reduction.
   e. Although the results of prospective randomized studies of this combination are mixed, the overall body of evidence supports the use of ADT in this setting.
10. Combined androgen blockade:
    a. is designed to address the low levels of testicular androgens remaining after the use of LH-RH agonists or antagonists.
    b. typically uses antiandrogens at the time of PSA rise after treatment with an LH-RH agonist.
    c. has not shown a survival advantage compared with an LH-RH agonist alone.
    d. significantly benefits men with minimally metastatic disease when used in combination with surgical castration.
    e. using cyproterone acetate has a slightly worse outcome.
11. Compared with deferred ADT, early ADT instituted before the development of objective metastatic disease:
    a. provides an overall survival advantage in all clinical disease states.
    b. has an equivalent quality of life.
    c. does not increase overall death rates.
    d. does not prevent the emergence of hormone-refractory prostate cancer.
    e. should be offered to men with PSA recurrence after radical prostatectomy because of the rapid disease progression in this clinical setting.
12. In men with lymph node metastatic prostate cancer discovered at the time of radical prostatectomy a significant overall survival benefit of immediate ADT:
    a. is limited to those with extrapelvic positive nodes.
    b. has been demonstrated in men who have also undergone subsequent radical prostatectomy.
    c. has been demonstrated in men who have not undergone subsequent radical prostatectomy.
    d. b and c are correct.
    e. a, b, and c are correct.
13. From a strictly financial point of view, which of the following forms of ADT is the least expensive?
    a. Scrotal orchiectomy
    b. LH-RH agonist
    c. DES
    d. Antiandrogen monotherapy
    e. LH-RH antagonist
14. Compared with continuous ADT, intermittent ADT has been shown in randomized prospective studies to:
    a. delay progression to hormone-refractory prostate cancer.
    b. improve quality of life.
    c. improve cancer-specific survival.
    d. All of the above.
    e. None of the above.
15. There is general consensus that ADT should always be initiated in a hormonally intact patient in which of the following clinical settings?
    a. Before radical prostatectomy with a clinical T2 tumor
    b. In all clinical stages when undergoing external-beam radiation therapy
    c. In one with clinically localized prostate cancer who does not want local treatment
    d. In one with symptomatic metastatic disease
    e. In one with high-grade prostatic intraepithelial neoplasia on needle biopsy who refuses a subsequent biopsy

ANSWERS

1. **e. negative feedback on LH secretion by the pituitary.** After the success of surgical castration in treating prostate cancer, the first central inhibition of the hypothalamic-pituitary-gonadal axis exploited the potent negative feedback of estrogen on LH secretion. Estradiol is 1000-fold more potent at suppressing LH and FSH secretion by the pituitary compared with testosterone. Although estrogen has some direct cytotoxic effects on prostate cancer cells, this is not its primary mode of action. All antiandrogens competitively bind to the androgen receptor. Aminoglutethimide inhibits the conversion of cholesterol to pregnenolone, an early step in steroidogenesis. The LH-RH agonists desensitize LH-RH receptors in the anterior pituitary.
2. **c. LH increases, testosterone increases, estrogen increases.** Unlike the steroidal antiandrogens, such as cyproterone acetate, which have central progestational inhibitory effects, the nonsteroidal antiandrogens simply block androgen receptors, including those in the hypothalamic-pituitary axis. Because those central androgen receptors no longer sense the normal negative feedback exerted by testosterone, both LH levels and the normal testicular response to increased LH-testosterone levels increase. Peripheral conversion of this excessive testosterone also increases estrogen levels, leading to the gynecomastia and mastodynia associated with the nonsteroidal antiandrogens.
3. **d. direct inhibition of androgen receptor–mediated pathways.** There are four therapeutic approaches for androgen axis blockade in current clinical use (see Table 104-2). All current forms of ADT function by reducing the ability of androgen to activate the androgen receptor, whether through lowering levels of androgen or by blocking androgen-androgen receptor binding. Therefore, the androgen receptor is not directly affected by ADT, leading many to hypothesize that hormone-refractory prostate cancer is a reactivation of androgen receptor–mediated pathways.
4. **b. allow long-term maintenance of erectile function and sexual activity at rates similar to men undergoing surgical castration.** By blocking testosterone feedback centrally, the nonsteroidal antiandrogens cause LH and testosterone levels to increase, allowing antiandrogen activity without inducing hypogonadism, and potency can be preserved. In clinical trials specifically examining erectile function and sexual activity in men on antiandrogen monotherapy, however, long-term preservation of those domains was 20% and not significantly different than men undergoing surgical castration. All antiandrogens can act agonistically on prostate cancer cells and, when used in combination with LH-RH agonists, withdrawal of the antiandrogen can lead to declines in PSA and even objective responses. The common gastrointestinal toxicity is diarrhea,

most often seen with flutamide. Liver toxicity, ranging from reversible hepatitis to fulminate hepatic failure is associated with all nonsteroidal antiandrogens and requires periodic monitoring of liver function tests. The steroidal antiandrogen cyproterone acetate is associated with fluid retention and thromboembolism.

5. **d. Nilutamide.** About one fourth of men on nilutamide therapy will note a delayed adaptation to darkness after exposure to bright illumination, and nilutamide is also associated with interstitial pneumonitis in approximately 1% of patients that can progress to pulmonary fibrosis. Hydroxyflutamide is the active metabolite of flutamide. Cyproterone acetate is a steroidal antiandrogen.
6. **c. current LH-RH agonists are based on analogs of the native LH-RH decapeptide by amino acid substitutions, particularly position 6 of the peptide.** The LH-RH agonists exploit the desensitization of LH-RH receptors in the anterior pituitary after chronic exposure to LH-RH, thereby shutting down the production of LH and, ultimately, testosterone. Analogs of native LH-RH increase their potency and half-lives (see Table 104-3). The initial flare in LH and testosterone may last 10 to 20 days, and co-administration of an antiandrogen is required for only 21 to 28 days. Survival after therapy with an LH-RH agonist was equivalent to that of orchiectomy. The clinical utility of the first LH-RH agonists was hampered by their short-half lives, requiring daily dosing. The LH-RH antagonist abarelix has been associated with severe allergic reactions: all LH-RH agonists are administered either intramuscularly or subcutaneously. LH-RH can be used without combination with an antiandrogen.
7. **e. the maintenance of a detectable PSA.** The odds ratio of progressing to androgen-refractory progression at 24 months of starting ADT was 15-fold higher in those who did not achieve an undetectable PSA. The magnitude and rapidity of PSA decline, the pre-ADT PSA doubling time, and pretreatment testosterone levels are all associated with the response to ADT. For each unit increase in Gleason score the cumulative hazard of androgen-refractory progression was nearly 70%.
8. **c. Erectile dysfunction after surgical castration or use of an LH-RH is common but not inevitable: although 1 in 5 men maintain some sexual activity, only 1 in 20 maintain high levels of sexual interest (libido).** The loss of sexual functioning is not inevitable with surgical or chemical castration, with up to 20% of men able to maintain some sexual activity. Libido is more severely compromised, with approximately 5% maintaining a high level of sexual interest. More than half of men undergoing ADT meet the bone mineral density criteria for osteopenia or osteoporosis; it is estimated that osteopenia will develop in the average man within 4 years of initiating ADT. Hot flashes are among the most common side effects of ADT, affecting between 50% and 80% of patients. Hot flashes should be treated only in those who find them bothersome. Loss of muscle mass and increase in percent fat body mass are common in men undergoing ADT. Prophylactic radiation therapy (10 Gy) has been used to prevent or reduce gynecomastia and mastodynia, but it has no benefit once these side effects have already occurred.
9. **a. Positive surgical margin rates are significantly reduced with ADT-treated patients.** In both nonrandomized and randomized clinical trials, the pathologic positive surgical margin rate is significantly reduced. In one study, the positive surgical margin rate fell from nearly 50% in hormonally intact patients to 15% in ADT-treated patients. Despite this improvement, there has not been a corresponding significant reduction in biochemical (PSA) progression in ADT-treatment patients, a finding in four separate prospective randomized studies. The benefit of ADT in men with locally advanced disease and/or high-grade disease has been in combination with external-beam radiation therapy. There is no evidence any form of 3-month neoadjuvant ADT before radical prostatectomy reduces biochemical failure rates.
10. **e. using cyproterone acetate has a slightly worse outcome.** In studies of combined androgen blockade using the steroidal antiandrogen cyproterone acetate compared with LH-RH agonists alone, the outcomes were slightly worse with the combination, suggesting increased nonprostate cancer deaths with this agent. Combined androgen blockade is designed to block the possible contribution of adrenal androgens to prostate cancer progression. Combined androgen blockade uses an antiandrogen along with an LH-RH agonist: addition of an antiandrogen at the time of PSA rise (evidence of hormone-refractory disease) is considered secondary hormonal manipulation. There are several clinical trials that have shown a slight but significant survival advantage for combined androgen blockade. A landmark randomized clinical trial comparing surgical castration alone to surgical castration combined with flutamide did not show a significant benefit in men with minimal metastatic disease.
11. **d. does not prevent the emergence of hormone-refractory prostate cancer.** The timing of the initiation of ADT has not prevented the development of hormone-refractory prostate cancer. Although early ADT may provide an overall survival advantage in certain clinical disease states, in most studies there is no significant overall survival advantage. Indeed, in localized, low-risk prostate cancer, early ADT is associated with an increase in overall death rates. The natural history of disease progression after biochemical failure after radical prostatectomy is protracted: median time to bone metastases is 8 years.
12. **b. has been demonstrated in men who have also undergone subsequent radical prostatectomy.** A randomized prospective study of men with positive regional, pelvic lymph nodes discovered at the time of radical prostatectomy showed an overall survival advantage to immediate ADT. In that study, all men also underwent the radical prostatectomy. A similar study, performed by the EORTC, in men who did not undergo radical prostatectomy if positive nodes were discovered did not show a significant survival advantage to immediate ADT.
13. **c. DES.** At a dose of 1 to 3 mg/day with no prophylactic breast irradiation, DES is the least expensive form of ADT. LH-RH agonists would be less expensive than scrotal orchiectomy only if the patient lived a few months after the administration of ADT. Combined androgen blockade is the most expensive form of ADT.
14. **e. none of the above.** Randomized prospective studies of intermittent ADT are ongoing and no results are yet available. The possible benefits of intermittent ADT listed have not been demonstrated.
15. **d. In one with symptomatic metastatic disease.** In hormonally intact men with symptomatic metastatic prostate cancer, ADT is always indicated. There is no significant biochemical (PSA) disease-free advantage in men treated with neoadjuvant ADT. The benefits of ADT in combination with external-beam radiation therapy are in men with locally advanced and/or high grade disease. The use of ADT in men with low-risk, localized prostate cancer is associated with a significantly lower overall survival. There is no indication for ADT in the management of prostatic intraepithelial neoplasia.

105

Treatment of Hormone-Refractory Prostate Cancer

MARIO A. EISENBERGER • MICHAEL CARDUCCI

QUESTIONS

1. All of the following represent appropriate management in a patient with evidence of prostate cancer progression after initial hormonal therapy EXCEPT:
   a. obtain a serum testosterone level to evaluate adequate gonadal suppression, restage the disease with radiographs and scans, discontinue the antiandrogen, maintain gonadal suppression, and plan the next therapeutic step.
   b. as above; if the patient is on antiandrogen therapy, discontinue treatment for 4 weeks in the case of flutamide and nilutamide and 8 weeks in the case of bicalutamide.
   c. if the patient has no symptoms, the workup shows that he has adequate gonadal suppression (serum testosterone < 50 ng/mL), and the only evidence of disease progression is a rising prostate-specific antigen (PSA) (scans are unchanged) try a second-line hormonal therapy before chemotherapy is offered.
   d. if the patient experiences severe focal bone pain that requires regular use of narcotic analgesics, consider palliative radiation therapy.
   e. restage with radiographs and scans, evaluate serum testosterone level if < 50 ng/mL, and discontinue all hormonal therapy for 4 to 8 weeks before planning the next therapeutic step.
2. A patient has a rising PSA after 24 months of treatment with a luteinizing-hormone–releasing hormone (LHRH) analog; the workup shows no evidence of metastasis (as prior to initiation of hormonal therapy). Which of the following constitutes the most reasonable approach?
   a. Send the patient to an oncologist for initiation of chemotherapy.
   b. Continue follow-up with regular PSA tests and restage when the patient becomes symptomatic.
   c. Radiate the prostatic bed or even the entire pelvis.
   d. Assess the PSADT (PSA doubling time): if < 6 months, consider treatment as soon as possible; otherwise, watch.
   e. Evaluate adequacy of gonadal suppression and plan for second-line endocrine manipulations.
3. A patient with bone metastasis shows evidence of rising serum PSA levels while on LHRH analog treatment. Bone scan indicates slow progression, and he has no symptoms. Which of the following constitutes part of the appropriate management?
   a. Plan for next treatment approach, including the infusion of zoledronic acid given 3 times yearly.
   b. Docetaxel, 75 mg/m^2 every 3 weeks, and zoledronic acid, 4 mg monthly.
   c. Administer a radiopharmaceutical.
   d. He should be treated aggressively with high-dose bicalutamide, calcium, and vitamin D.
   e. Wait until he becomes symptomatic.
4. A patient with diffuse bone metastasis develops severe back pain. PSA is stable. Which is the most appropriate type of approach?
   a. Give analgesics as needed and consider a workup when PSA rises.
   b. Add zoledronic acid to management.
   c. Consider radiation therapy.
   d. Same as c followed by docetaxel.
   e. MRI of the spine to rule out cord compression.
5. A patient who is stable on hormonal therapy for many years develops a rapid deterioration with perirectal pain, liver metastasis, and weight loss. PSA is undetectable. CT scan of the pelvis shows a large pelvic mass. Which of the following is the next step?
   a. He has hormone-refractory prostate cancer (HRPC), and you offer him docetaxel.
   b. Radiation to the pelvis followed by docetaxel.
   c. Bicalutamide because the PSA is still low.
   d. Biopsy of the pelvic mass to rule out the neuroendocrine subtype.
   e. Because he probably has another cancer since the PSA is negative, send him for a colonoscopy.

6. The above patient's pelvic mass is sampled, and the pathology report shows a small cell carcinoma. The best approach now is:
   a. radiation therapy followed by second-line hormonal therapy until progression; then offer chemotherapy.
   b. docetaxel combined with zoledronic acid.
   c. chemotherapy with carboplatin + etoposide preceded or followed by irradiation.
   d. because of the histology (small cell), send the patient for a bronchoscopy.
   e. radiation to the pelvis followed by ketoconazole + hydrocortisone.
7. Results of the phase III TAX-327 trial showed significant improvements in which of the following outcomes in patients with HRPC with docetaxel versus mitoxantrone?
   a. Overall survival
   b. PSA response
   c. Pain response
   d. Quality of life
   e. All of the above
8. Which of the following is TRUE for estramustine phosphate?
   a. It is critical to use it combined with docetaxel.
   b. It has significant single-agent activity.
   c. It has no activity in HRPC.
   d. Thromboembolic effects are usually prevented by prophylactic anticoagulation.
   e. It adds significant toxicity to docetaxel without apparent survival benefit.
9. The following are all true regarding toxicity of docetaxel chemotherapy EXCEPT:
   a. myelosuppression.
   b. grade 2 fatigue and neurotoxicity.
   c. edema.
   d. modest elevation of liver function tests.
   e. toxicity overrides quality of life benefits.
10. Bone loss associated with androgen deprivation is characterized by:
    a. proliferation of osteoblasts.
    b. hypocalcemia.
    c. depletion of osteoclasts.
    d. a, b, and c.
    e. increased osteoclastic activity.
11. In prostate cancer which of the following is TRUE about bone metastasis?
    a. It is always osteoblastic because of a growth factor effect.
    b. Pathologic fractures are common.
    c. Hypercalcemia is common.
    d. It is mostly lytic associated with a predominant osteoclastic effect associated with treatment.
    e. There is increasing evidence that growth factors, cytokines, and other proteins may play a role in the development of bone metastasis.
12. Which of the following is TRUE about zoledronic acid?
    a. Side effects include anemia and renal dysfunction.
    b. It may cause osteonecrosis of the jaw in patients who are undergoing dental work.
    c. It reduces the increase in osteoclastic activity associated with androgen deprivation.
    d. It is approved for the treatment of hypercalcemia.
    e. All of the above.
13. A decline in PSA associated with chemotherapy represents evidence indicating the following EXCEPT that it is:
    a. of therapeutic benefit but not necessarily an indication of a longer survival.
    b. seen in about 50% of patients receiving docetaxel treatment.
    c. usually seen in the first 3 months of treatment.
    d. All of the above.
14. Which of the following is TRUE about brain metastasis in prostate cancer?
    a. It is seen in about 25% of HRPC patients.
    b. It is common in patients progressing rapidly on hormonal therapy.
    c. Routine MRI of the brain is considered in all HRPC patients.
    d. It is seen in less than 1% of patients except when they demonstrate the neuroendocrine phenotype.
    e. Brain metastasis associated with small cells should be treated surgically.
15. Taxanes, including docetaxel, have which of the following clinical and biological properties?
    a. Antimitotic agent
    b. Induces a BCL2 phosphorylation
    c. Is associated with an increased accumulation of cells in the G_2M phase
    d. Causes radiosensitization in vitro
    e. All of the above
16. Which of the following is a target for the development of new chemotherapeutic approaches in prostate cancer?
    a. Microtubules
    b. PTEN-associated signaling pathways
    c. Endothelin axis
    d. RANK-ligand overexpression in bone metastasis
    e. All of the above
17. All of the following are true about the androgen receptor (AR) in prostate cancer progression to the androgen independent phenotype EXCEPT:
    a. wild-type AR remains active after testosterone suppression.
    b. aberrant function is not an uncommon feature as the disease progresses toward the androgen-independent state. This is clinically manifested by responses to withdrawal of antiandrogens.
    c. transcriptional activity can be seen without ligand activation.
    d. ligand-independent activation can be seen via growth factors pathways.
    e. it can never be found in the hormone-refractory state.
18. Which of the following is TRUE about vitamin D analogs in prostate cancer?
    a. They have significant single-agent activity.
    b. They have differentiating and antiproliferative activity in vitro.
    c. Encouraging results were seen with docetaxel in combination.
    d. None of the above.
    e. b and c.

ANSWERS

1. **e. restage with radiographs and scans, evaluate serum testosterone level if < 50 ng/mL, and discontinue all hormonal therapy for 4 to 8 weeks before planning the next therapeutic step.** Discontinuation of antiandrogens (both steroidal and nonsteroidal) can result in short-term clinical responses expressed by decreases in PSA levels, symptomatic benefits, and, less frequently, objective improvements in soft tissue and bone metastasis in a small proportion of these patients. Because of this we recommend that in patients treated with antiandrogens in combination with other forms of androgen deprivation, the first step should involve the discontinuation of these agents and provide careful observation, including serial monitoring of PSA levels for a period 4 to 8 weeks before embarking on the next therapeutic maneuver.
2. **e. Evaluate adequacy of gonadal suppression and plan for second-line endocrine manipulations.** Patients with evidence of inadequate suppression of testosterone may respond with readjustment of gonadal suppressive treatment. Second-line endocrine maneuvers are effective in 20% to 60% of these patients and certainly much less toxic. Furthermore, the benefits of chemotherapy in this setting (androgen independent, nonmetastatic disease) have not been demonstrated. Given the major difference in terms of incidence and type of toxicities seen with sequential hormonal therapy versus cytotoxic chemotherapy, in the absence of data, we recommend implementing the least toxic approach first. Clinical trials are clearly recommended.
3. **b. Docetaxel, 75 mg/m^2 every 3 weeks, and zoledronic acid, 4 mg given monthly.** Docetaxel has become the agent of choice as of 2004, based on a large phase III randomized trial, TAX-327 (see Figs. 105-3 through 105-5 and Tables 105-6 through 105-8), which demonstrated its superiority to the past standard, mitoxantrone and prednisone (Tannock, 2004). TAX-327 enrolled 1006 patients with no prior chemotherapy, and stable pain scores to one of three arms, all with concomitant prednisone at 5 mg PO bid: mitoxantrone, 12 mg/m^2 IV q 21 days; docetaxel, 75 mg/m^2 IV q 21 days; and docetaxel, 30 mg/m^2 IV weekly. Patients remained on gonadal suppression but had all other hormonal agents discontinued within 4 to 6 weeks. Treatment duration was 30 weeks in all arms, or a maximum of 10 cycles in the every-3-week arms, with more patients completing treatment in the every-3-week docetaxel arm than the mitoxantrone arm, owing mostly to differences in disease progression (46% vs. 25%). After a median 20.7-month follow-up, overall survival in the every-3-week docetaxel arm was 18.9 months with a pain response rate of 35% and a PSA response of 45%, contrasted to weekly docetaxel at 17.3 months, 31%, and 48%, respectively. This translated into a 24% relative risk reduction in death (95% CI 6% to 48%, P =.0005) with every-3-week docetaxel (see Fig. 105-4). Patients on the mitoxantrone arm had a median survival of 16.4 months, a pain response of 22%, and a PSA response of 32%.

   Bisphosphonates have become an integral part in the management of metastatic prostate cancer to the bones. These compounds reduce bone resorption by inhibiting osteoclastic activity and proliferation. Zoledronic acid is a potent intravenous bisphosphonate approved for the treatment of hypercalcemia and the treatment of decreased bone mineral density in postmenopausal women (Green, 2002). Recent experience in patients with progressive HRPC with bone metastasis showed zoledronic acid reduced the incidence of skeletal-related events compared with placebo in a prospective randomized trial. In addition, it has also been shown to increase mineral bone density in patients with prostate cancer receiving long-term androgen deprivation (Saad, 2002, 2004; Smith, 2003). At the present time this compound is indicated for the treatment of patients with progressive prostate cancer with evidence of bone metastasis at doses of 4 mg given by short intravenous infusion repeated at intervals of 3 to 4 weeks for several months. Side effects include fatigue, myalgias, fever, anemia, and mild elevations of serum creatinine.
4. **e. MRI of the spine to rule out cord compression.** Spinal MRI is routinely used to exclude the possibility of significant epidural disease, and it has almost entirely replaced other methodology such as CT myelography and conventional myelograms. Cancer-related pain is undoubtedly the most debilitating symptom associated with metastatic prostatic carcinoma. Prompt recognition of the various pain syndromes associated with this disease is critical to accomplish effective control of this devastating symptom. Table 105-9 describes the most common pain syndromes and their respective therapeutic considerations.
5. **d. Biopsy the pelvic mass to rule out the neuroendocrine subtype.** Laboratory and clinical evidence indicate that alterations in the differentiation pathway (neuroendocrine transformation) of prostate cancer can be seen in a variable proportion of patients with primarily advanced disease (Logothetis, 1994; diSant'Agnese, 1995). The therapeutic implications of this finding are of significance because tumors demonstrating the neuroendocrine phenotype usually represent an inherently endocrine-resistant disease, and in view of their different clinical and biologic properties compared with the usual adenocarcinoma of the prostate phenotype these tumors usually require separate therapeutic considerations.
6. **c. chemotherapy with carboplatin + etoposide preceded or followed by irradiation.** Treatment is usually similar to that in patients with other neuroendocrine tumors, such as small cell carcinoma of the lung, and include combinations of cisplatin or carboplatin and etoposide (Frank, 1995), taxol or docetaxel (Taxotere), and topotecan. Radiation is very effective and should be considered in cases with bulky disease and brain metastasis and when local disease control in critical areas will have a positive impact in quality of life (pain, potential pathologic fractures, and bladder outlet obstruction). Combined chemo/radiation approach is frequently necessary to accomplish maximal control of disease.
7. **e. All of the above.** TAX-327 and SWOG 9916 are the two seminal studies that demonstrate a survival advantage for docetaxel in HRPC over mitoxantrone and prednisone and establish docetaxel as the standard chemotherapy treatment for this disease.
8. **e. It adds significant toxicity to docetaxel without apparent survival benefit.**
9. **e. toxicity overrides quality of life benefits.** Toxicity in the every-3-week versus weekly docetaxel arms was notable for more hematologic toxicity in the every-3-week arm (3% neutropenic fever vs. 0%, and 32% grade 3/4 neutropenia vs. 1.5%) (see Table 105-8) but slightly lower rates of nausea and vomiting, fatigue, nail changes, hyperlacrimation, and diarrhea. Neuropathy was slightly more common in the every-3-week arm (grade 3/4 in 1.8% vs. 0.9%). Quality of life as measured by the FACT-P scores did not differ significantly among the docetaxel schedules but were more favorable than the mitoxantrone arm.
10. **e. increased osteoclastic activity.** Bone loss associated with prostate cancer can result from an enhanced osteoclastic

activity associated with long-term androgen suppression, which in turn will cause excessive resorption of bone mineral and organic matrix.

11. **e. There is increasing evidence that growth factors, cytokines, and other proteins may play a role in the development of bone metastasis.** Bone loss associated with prostate cancer can result from an enhanced osteoclastic activity associated with long-term androgen suppression, which in turn will cause excessive resorption of bone mineral and organic matrix. Tumor cells may also cause mineral release and matrix resorption in the areas involved by metastatic disease (Galasko, 1986). In addition to various cytokines, growth factors, tumor necrosis factors, as well as bone morphogenic proteins have been shown in preclinical studies to play a major role in the induction of both osteoclastic and osteoblastic activity (Galasko, 1986; Reddi, 1990). In prostate cancer bone metastases are predominantly blastic, which reflects a predominance of osteoblastic activity in the process of bone remodeling (Averbush, 1993).

12. **e. All of the above.** Zoledronic acid is a potent intravenous bisphosphonate approved for the treatment of hypercalcemia and the treatment of decreased bone mineral density in postmenopausal women (Green, 2002). At the present time this compound is indicated for the treatment of patients with progressive prostate cancer with evidence of bone metastasis at doses of 4 mg given by short intravenous infusion repeated at intervals of 3 to 4 weeks for several months. Side effects include fatigue, myalgias, fever, anemia, and mild elevations of serum creatinine. Hypocalcemia has been described, and concomitant use of oral calcium supplements (1500 mg/day) and vitamin D (400 units/day) is recommended. An unusual complication is the development of severe jaw pain associated with osteonecrosis of the mandibular bone.

13. **d. All of the above.**

14. **d. It is seen in less than 1% of patients except when they demonstrate the neuroendocrine phenotype.**

15. **e. All of the above.** Docetaxel (Taxotere) is a cytotoxic agent and member of the taxoid family. It induces apoptosis in cancer cells through TP53-independent mechanisms that are believed to be due to its inhibition of microtubule depolymerization and inhibition of antiapoptotic signaling. The induction of microtubule stabilization intracellularly through β-tubulin interactions causes guanosine triphosphate–independent polymerization and cell cycle arrest at G_2M, and some have reported a twofold greater microtubule affinity compared with paclitaxel. Additionally, docetaxel has been found to induce BCL2 phosphorylation in vitro, a process that has been correlated with caspase activation and loss of its normal antiapoptotic activity. Unable to inhibit the proapoptotic molecule BAX, phosphorylated BCL2 may also induce apoptosis through this independent mechanism. However, additional mechanisms may be important, such as $CDKN1B^{kip1}$ induction and repression of BCLxl.

16. **e. All of the above.**

17. **e. it can never be found in the hormone-refractory state.** In prostate cancer, the AR is one potential target. Various molecular changes in the AR have been shown to parallel disease progression in castrate patients and in some situations may provide the explanation for the responses associated with some therapeutic maneuvers (antiandrogen withdrawal syndrome, responses to secondary endocrine manipulations with compounds designed to bind to the receptor). Despite this, a precise role of the AR in the pathogenesis of disease progression remains to be better elucidated.

18. **e. b and c.** Vitamin D analogs may have differentiation, antiproliferation, and chemosensitizing properties. A phase II trial of weekly docetaxel and high-dose calcitriol demonstrated PSA responses in 30 of 37 patients (80%) and measurable responses in 8 of 15 (53%), with a median time to progression of 11.4 months and median survival of 19.4 months. A randomized study with a total of 250 patients (125 per arm) comparing the combination to docetaxel alone resulted in > 50% PSA declines in 63% of the patients receiving the combination compared with 52% with docetaxel alone (P =.07, not significant); however, interestingly the authors reported a survival difference in favor of the combination (23.4 months vs. 16.4 months, adjusted P value of 0.03).

SECTION XVII

PEDIATRIC UROLOGY

106

Normal Development of the Urogenital System

JOHN M. PARK

QUESTIONS

1. The fetal kidneys develop from which of the following embryonic structures?
   a. Paraxial (somite) mesoderm
   b. Intermediate mesoderm
   c. Neural tube
   d. Lateral mesoderm
2. Which of the following statements is FALSE regarding the mesonephros?
   a. It serves as a transient excretory organ during the development of the definitive kidneys, the metanephros.
   b. Certain elements persist as part of the reproductive tract.
   c. The excretory portion begins to degenerate during the first year of life.
   d. Development of the nephric ducts (also called wolffian ducts) precedes that of the mesonephric tubules.
3. At what gestational time point does the metanephros development begin?
   a. 20th day
   b. 24th day
   c. 28th day
   d. 32nd day
4. Which of the following statements is TRUE of the metanephric development?
   a. It requires the reciprocal inductive interaction between müllerian duct and metanephric mesenchyme.
   b. The calyces, pelvis, and ureter derive from the differentiation of the metanephric mesenchyme.
   c. Older, more differentiated nephrons are located at the periphery of the developing kidney, whereas newer, less differentiated nephrons are found near the juxtamedullary region.
   d. Although renal maturation continues postnatally, nephrogenesis is completed by birth.
5. The fused lower pole of the horseshoe kidney is trapped by which of the following structures during the ascent?
   a. Inferior mesenteric artery
   b. Superior mesenteric artery
   c. Celiac artery
   d. Common iliac artery
6. The homozygous gene disruption (gene knock-out) in which of the following molecules does NOT lead to a significant renal maldevelopment in mice?
   a. *Wt-1*
   b. *Pax-2*
   c. Glial cell line–derived neurotrophic factor (GDNF)
   d. *p53*
7. Which of the following statements is FALSE regarding GDNF?
   a. It is a ligand for the RET receptor tyrosine kinase.
   b. GDNF gene knock-out mice demonstrate an abnormal renal development.
   c. It is expressed in the metanephric mesenchyme but not in the ureteric bud.
   d. GDNF arrests the ureteric bud growth in vitro.
8. Which of the following statements is FALSE regarding the renin-angiotensin system during renal and ureteral development?
   a. The embryonic kidney is able to produce all components of the renin-angiotensin system.
   b. Both subtypes of angiotensin II receptor, AT1 and AT2, are expressed in the developing metanephros.
   c. *At1* gene knock-out mice demonstrate a spectrum of congenital urinary tract abnormalities, including ureteropelvic junction obstruction and vesicoureteral reflux.
   d. Infants born to mothers treated with angiotensin-converting enzyme inhibitors during pregnancy have increased rates of oligohydramnios, hypotension, and anuria.

9. The bladder trigone develops from which of the following structures?
   a. Mesonephric ducts
   b. Müllerian ducts
   c. Urogenital sinus
   d. Metanephric mesenchyme
10. The urachus involutes to become:
   a. verumontanum.
   b. median umbilical ligament.
   c. appendix testis.
   d. Epoöphoron.
11. Which of the following statements is FALSE regarding bladder development?
   a. The bladder body is derived from the urogenital sinus whereas the trigone develops from the terminal portion of the mesonephric ducts.
   b. Bladder compliance seems to be low during early gestation, and it gradually increases thereafter.
   c. Epithelial-mesenchymal inductive interactions appear to be necessary for proper bladder development.
   d. Histologic evidence of smooth muscle differentiation begins near the bladder neck and proceeds toward the bladder dome.
12. The primordial germ cell migration and the formation of the genital ridges begin at which time point during gestation?
   a. Third week
   b. Fifth week
   c. Seventh week
   d. Ninth week
13. Which of the following statements is FALSE regarding the paramesonephric (müllerian) ducts?
   a. Both male and female embryos form paramesonephric (müllerian) ducts.
   b. In male embryos, the paramesonephric ducts degenerate under the influence of the müllerian-inhibiting substance (MIS) produced by the Leydig cells.
   c. In male embryos, the paramesonephric ducts become the appendix testis and the prostatic utricle.
   d. In female embryos, the paramesonephric ducts form the female reproductive tract, including fallopian tubes, uterus, and upper vagina.
14. Which of the following structures in the male reproductive tract develops from the urogenital sinus?
   a. Vas deferens
   b. Seminal vesicles
   c. Prostate
   d. Appendix epididymis
15. Which of the following statements is FALSE regarding normal prostate development?
   a. It requires the conversion of testosterone into dihydrotestosterone by 5α-reductase.
   b. It is dependent on epithelial-mesenchymal interactions under the influence of androgens.
   c. It is first seen at the 10th to 12th week of gestation.
   d. It requires the effects of MIS.
16. In female embryos, the remnants of the mesonephric ducts persist as the following structures EXCEPT:
   a. epoöphoron.
   b. paroöphoron.
   c. hymen.
   d. Gartner's duct cysts.
17. Which of the following statements is FALSE regarding the external genitalia development?
   a. The appearance of the external genitalia is similar in male and female embryos until the 12th week.
   b. The external genital appearance of males who are deficient in 5α-reductase is similar to that of females.
   c. In males, the formation of the distal glandular urethra may occur by the fusion of urethral folds proximally and the ingrowth of ectodermal cells distally.
   d. In females, the urethral folds become the labia majora and the labioscrotal folds become the labia minora.
18. The testes descend to the level of internal inguinal ring by which time point during gestation?
   a. Sixth week
   b. Third month
   c. Sixth month
   d. Ninth month
19. Which of the following statements is FALSE regarding the *SRY* (the sex-determining region of the Y chromosome)?
   a. Its expression triggers the primitive sex cord cells to differentiate into the Sertoli cells.
   b. Approximately 25% of sex reversal conditions in humans are attributable to *SRY* mutations.
   c. It is located on the short arm of the Y chromosome.
   d. It causes the regression of mesonephric ducts.

ANSWERS

1. **b. Intermediate mesoderm.** Mammals develop three kidneys in the course of intrauterine life. The embryonic kidneys are, in order of their appearance, the pronephros, the mesonephros, and the metanephros. The first two kidneys regress in utero, and the third becomes the permanent kidney. In terms of embryology, all three kidneys develop from the intermediate mesoderm.
2. **c. The excretory portion begins to degenerate during the first year of life.** Like pronephros, mesonephros is also transient but in mammals it serves as an excretory organ for the embryo while the definitive kidney, metanephros, begins its development. Development of the nephric ducts (also called wolffian ducts) precedes the development of the mesonephric tubules. Soon after the appearance of the nephric ducts during the fourth week, mesonephric vesicles begin to form. Initially, several spherical masses of cells are found along the medial side of the nephrogenic cords at the cranial end. This differentiation progresses caudally and results in the formation of 40 to 42 pairs of mesonephric tubules, but only about 30 pairs are seen at any one time, because the cranially located tubules start to degenerate starting at about the fifth week. By the fourth month, the human mesonephros has almost completely disappeared, except for a few elements that persist into maturity. Certain elements of the mesonephros are retained in the mature urogenital system as part of the reproductive tract.

3. **c. 28th day.** The definitive kidney, metanephros, forms in the sacral region as a pair of new structures, called the ureteric buds, sprouts from the distal portion of the nephric duct, and comes in contact with the blastema of metanephric mesenchyme at about the 28th day.

4. **d. Although renal maturation continues postnatally, nephrogenesis is completed by birth.** It requires the inductive interaction between the ureteric bud and metanephric mesenchyme. The calyces, pelvis, and ureter derive from the ureteric bud. Older, more differentiated nephrons are located in the inner part of the kidney near the juxtamedullary region. In humans, although renal maturation continues to take place postnatally, nephrogenesis is completed before birth.

5. **a. Inferior mesenteric artery.** The inferior poles of the kidneys may fuse, forming a horseshoe kidney that crosses over the ventral side of the aorta. During ascent, the fused lower pole becomes trapped under the inferior mesenteric artery and thus does not reach its normal site.

6. **d. *Tp53*.** Mutant *Wt-1* mice do not form ureteric buds, and in *Pax*-2 gene knock-out mice, no nephric ducts, müllerian ducts, ureteric buds, or metanephric mesenchyme form, and the animals die within 1 day of birth because of renal failure. Ureteric bud formation is impaired in GDNF knock-out mice, but *p53* gene knock-out mice do not demonstrate significant renal developmental anomaly.

7. **d. GDNF arrests the ureteric bud growth in vitro.** GDNF promotes ureteric bud growth in vitro. Although the importance of RET in kidney development was clearly demonstrated, it is only recently that its ligand, GDNF, has been identified. GDNF is a secreted glycoprotein that possesses a cystine-knot motif. GDNF is expressed within the metanephric mesenchyme prior to ureteric bud invasion, and ureteric bud formation is impaired in GDNF knock-out mice.

8. **c. *At1* gene knock-out mice demonstrate a spectrum of congenital urinary tract abnormalities, including ureteropelvic junction obstruction and vesicoureteral reflux.** *At2* gene knock-out mice demonstrate a spectrum of congenital urinary tract abnormalities, including ureteropelvic junction obstruction, multicystic dysplastic kidney, megaureter, vesicoureteral reflux, and renal hypoplasia.

9. **a. Mesonephric ducts.** The terminal portion of the mesonephric duct, called the common excretory ducts, becomes incorporated into the developing bladder and forms the trigone.

10. **b. median umbilical ligament.** By the 12th week, the urachus involutes to become a fibrous cord, which becomes the median umbilical ligament.

11. **d. Histologic evidence of smooth muscle differentiation begins near the bladder neck and proceeds toward the bladder dome.** Between the 7th and 12th weeks, the surrounding connective tissues condense and smooth muscle fibers begin to appear, first at the region of the bladder dome and later proceeding toward the bladder neck.

12. **b. Fifth week.** During the fifth week, primordial germ cells migrate from the yolk sac along the dorsal mesentery to populate the mesenchyme of the posterior body wall near the 10th thoracic level. In both sexes, the arrival of primordial germ cells in the area of future gonads serves as the signal for the existing cells of the mesonephros and the adjacent coelomic epithelium to proliferate and form a pair of genital ridges just medial to the developing mesonephros.

13. **b. In male embryos, the paramesonephric ducts degenerate under the influence of the müllerian-inhibiting substance (MIS) produced by the Leydig cells.** A new pair of ducts, called the paramesonephric (müllerian) ducts, begins to form just lateral to the mesonephric ducts in both male and female embryos. These ducts arise by the craniocaudal invagination of thickened coelomic epithelium, extending all the way from the third thoracic segment to the posterior wall of the developing urogenital sinus. The caudal tips of the paramesonephric ducts adhere to each other as they connect with the urogenital sinus between the openings of the right and left mesonephric ducts. The cranial ends of the paramesonephric ducts form funnel-shaped openings into the coelomic cavity (the future peritoneum). As developing Sertoli cells begin their differentiation in response to the SRY (sex-determining region of the Y chromosome), they begin to secrete MIS, which causes the paramesonephric (müllerian) ducts to regress rapidly between the 8th and 10th weeks. Small müllerian duct remnants can be detected in the developed male as a small tissue protrusion at the superior pole of the testis, called the appendix testis, and as a posterior expansion of the prostatic urethra, called the prostatic utricle. In female embryos, MIS is absent, so the müllerian ducts do not regress and instead give rise to the fallopian tubes, uterus, and vagina.

14. **c. Prostate.** Vas deferens, seminal vesicles, and appendix epididymis all develop from the mesonephric ducts. The prostate and bulbourethral glands develop from the urogenital sinus.

15. **d. It requires the hormonal effects of MIS.** The prostate gland begins to develop during the 10th to 12th week as a cluster of endodermal evaginations budding from the pelvic urethra (derived from the urogenital sinus). These presumptive prostatic outgrowths are induced by the surrounding mesenchyme, and this process depends on the conversion of testosterone into dihydrotestosterone by 5α-reductase. Similar to renal and bladder development, prostatic development depends on mesenchymal-epithelial interactions but under the influence of androgens. There is no evidence that MIS plays a direct role in prostate development.

16. **c. hymen.** In the absence of MIS and androgens, the mesonephric (wolffian) ducts degenerate and the paramesonephric (müllerian) ducts give rise to the fallopian tubes, uterus, and upper two thirds of the vagina. The remnants of mesonephric ducts are found in the mesentery of the ovary as the epoöphoron and paroöphoron and near the vaginal introitus and anterolateral vaginal wall as Gartner's duct cysts. The hymen develops from the endodermal membrane located at the junction between the vaginal plate and the definitive urogenital sinus, which is the future vestibule of the vagina.

17. **d. In females, the urethral folds become the labia majora and the labioscrotal folds become the labia minora.** The early development of the external genital organ is similar in both sexes until the 12th week. Early in the 5th week, a pair of swellings called cloacal folds develops on either side of the cloacal membrane. These folds meet just anterior to the cloacal membrane to form a midline swelling called the genital tubercle. During the cloacal division into the anterior urogenital sinus and the posterior anorectal canal, the portion of the cloacal folds flanking the opening of the urogenital sinus becomes the urogenital folds and the portion flanking the opening of the anorectal canal becomes the anal folds. A new pair of swellings, called the labioscrotal folds, then appears on either side of the urogenital folds. In the absence of dihydrotestosterone, the primitive perineum does not lengthen and the labioscrotal and urethral folds do not fuse across the midline in the female embryos. The phallus bends inferiorly, becoming the clitoris, and the definitive urogenital sinus

becomes the vestibule of the vagina. The urethral folds become the labia minora, and the labioscrotal folds become the labia majora. The external genital organ develops in a similar manner in genetic males who are deficient in 5α-reductase and therefore lack dihydrotestosterone.

18. **b. Third month.** The testis reaches the level of internal inguinal ring by the third month and passes through the inguinal canal to reach the scrotum between the seventh and ninth months.

19. **d. It causes the regression of mesonephric ducts.** When the Y-linked master regulatory gene, called *SRY*, is expressed in the male, the epithelial cells of the primitive sex cords differentiate into Sertoli cells, and this critical morphogenetic event triggers subsequent testicular development. Analysis of DNA narrowed the location of *SRY* to a relatively small region within the short arm of the chromosome. It is now clear that only about 25% of sex reversals in humans can be attributed to disabling mutations of *SRY*.

107

Renal Function in the Fetus, Neonate, and Child

ROBERT L. CHEVALIER • JONATHAN A. ROTH

QUESTIONS

1. In the human, nephrogenesis is completed by:
   a. 20 weeks.
   b. 24 to 28 weeks.
   c. 30 to 32 weeks.
   d. 34 to 36 weeks.
   e. the postnatal period.
2. When does urine production begin in the human fetus?
   a. 6 to 8 weeks
   b. 10 to 12 weeks
   c. 14 to 16 weeks
   d. 18 to 20 weeks
   e. 22 weeks
3. During the first 24 hours of life:
   a. less than 50% of infants void, regardless of gestational age.
   b. 60% of term infants void, whereas 40% of preterm infants void.
   c. 40% of term infants void, whereas 60% of preterm infants void.
   d. 90% of infants void, regardless of gestational age.
   e. 100% of infants void.
4. The glomerular filtration rate (GFR) doubles during the first 2 weeks of life, regardless of gestational age because of:
   a. diminished renal vasculature resistance, increasing glomerular permeability and filtration surface.
   b. increased renal vasculature resistance, decreasing glomerular permeability and filtration surface.
   c. the neonate's limited concentrating ability.
   d. decreasing serum creatinine.
   e. increasing oral intake.
5. Serum creatinine:
   a. decreases by 10% in the first week of life.
   b. decreases by 25% in the first week of life.
   c. decreases by 50% in the first week of life.
   d. does not decrease in the first week of life.
   e. does not reflect maternal levels at birth.
6. Acid-base regulation in the neonate is characterized by a reduced threshold for:
   a. bicarbonate reabsorption.
   b. bicarbonate excretion.
   c. acid reabsorption.
   d. acid excretion.
   e. an immediate ability to respond to an acid load.
7. The most common etiology of hypercalciuria in neonates is:
   a. prematurity.
   b. diet.
   c. dehydration.
   d. calciuric medications.
   e. nephrolithiasis.
8. What are the normal values for the ratio of calcium to creatinine in the urine of term infants and older children? Less than:
   a. 0.4 and 0.2
   b. 0.4 and 0.8
   c. 0.8 and 0.4
   d. 0.2 and 0.4
   e. Greater than 0.4 and 0.8, respectively
9. Significant risks to overhydration of the neonate include:
   a. hyperglycemia and hyperbilirubinemia.
   b. hypoglycemia and hyperbilirubinemia.
   c. hypertension and necrotizing enterocolitis.
   d. cerebral intraventricular hemorrhage and necrotizing enterocolitis.
   e. cerebral intraventricular hemorrhage and hyperosmolality.
10. When does compensatory renal growth in the child with a solitary kidney begin?
    a. In utero
    b. At 3 months of age
    c. At 6 months of age
    d. At 1 year of age
    e. At 2 years of age

ANSWERS

1. **d. 34 to 36 weeks.** The metanephros begins its inductive phase after 5 weeks of gestation; and, in the human, nephrogenesis follows a sigmoidal curve, with most rapid increase in mid gestation, and is completed by 34 to 36 weeks.
2. **b. 10 to 12 weeks.** Urine production in the human kidney is known to begin around 10 to 12 weeks. The placenta throughout gestation, however, primarily handles salt and water homeostasis.
3. **e. 100% of infants void.** In a study of 500 normal neonates, Clark found that every infant voided within the first 24 hours of life regardless of gestational age. After the first 2 days of life, oliguria is generally defined as a urine flow rate less than 1 mL/kg/hr.
4. **a. diminished renal vasculature resistance, increasing glomerular permeability and filtration surface.** After birth, GFR doubles during the first 2 weeks regardless of gestational age. Factors responsible for this rapid rise include diminished renal vascular resistance, increasing perfusion pressure, glomerular permeability, and filtration surface.
5. **c. decreases by 50% in the first week of life.** Serum creatinine, which reflects maternal levels at birth, also decreases by 50% in the first week of life in term or near-term infants. Moreover, in very low birth weight infants, GFR does not catch up to that of age-matched term infants of the same postconceptional age until after 9 months of age.
6. **a. bicarbonate reabsorption.** Acid-base regulation in the neonate is characterized by a reduced threshold for bicarbonate reabsorption. Bicarbonate reabsorption is gradually increased with increasing GFR. There is also an inability to respond to an acid load. This improves by 4 to 6 weeks postnatally and is accentuated in the premature infant who tends to be slightly acidotic, by comparison to the adult.
7. **d. calciuric medications.** The most common etiology of hypercalciuria in neonates is administration of calciuric drugs, such as furosemide and glucocorticoids, which are used in the management of bronchopulmonary dysplasia. Such patients may be at risk for development of nephrocalcinosis or nephrolithiasis. This, in turn, may lead to renal dysfunction later in childhood. Although it may not be feasible to discontinue glucocorticoids, substitution of chlorothiazide for furosemide may reduce urinary calcium excretion.
8. **a. 0.4 and 0.2.** Urinary calcium excretion in the neonate is most easily assessed by determination of the calcium/creatinine ratio (mg/mg) in a random urine sample. In contrast to the older child, in whom a ratio exceeding 0.2 should be considered abnormal, the ratio in the infant receiving breast milk can rise to 0.4 in the term infant and to 0.8 in the preterm neonate.
9. **d. cerebral intraventricular hemorrhage and necrotizing enterocolitis.** There are significant hazards to overhydration of the neonate, including the opening of a symptomatic patent ductus arteriosus, cerebral intraventricular hemorrhage, and necrotizing enterocolitis. Severe underhydration, on the other hand, may lead to hypoglycemia, hyperbilirubinemia, and hyperosmolality. To replace the usual urinary losses, 50 to 80 mL/100 kcal of formula is a reasonable starting point.
10. **a. In utero.** A reduction in the number of functioning nephrons in early development is most often the result of a congenital malformation or a perinatal vascular accident such as a renal embolus or renal vein thrombosis. Unilateral ureteral occlusion in the fetal lamb at midtrimester results in a 50% increase in contralateral kidney weight by 1 month. These findings are corroborated by two prenatal ultrasound studies of human fetuses with unilateral renal agenesis or multicystic kidney. In both reports, the single functioning kidneys were significantly longer than those in the control patients. Such studies demonstrate unequivocally that compensatory renal growth can begin prenatally.

108

Congenital Urinary Obstruction: Pathophysiology

CRAIG A. PETERS • ROBERT L. CHEVALIER

QUESTIONS

1. After relief of a unilateral obstructing lesion, continued loss of renal function is most likely due to:
   a. glomerular hyperfiltration.
   b. asymmetrical renal growth.
   c. established renal tubular fibrosis.
   d. neural imbalance.
   e. compensatory hypertrophy.
2. Congenital obstruction differs from acquired obstruction in that it:
   a. affects glomerular development.
   b. induces interstitial fibrosis.
   c. affects tubular function.
   d. causes renal atrophy.
   e. alters renal homeostasis.
3. Renal dysplasia associated with obstruction is characterized by:
   a. renal atrophy.
   b. glomerular cysts.
   c. fibromuscular collars.
   d. heterotopic bone formation.
   e. excess production of afferent arteriole renin.
4. In a unilaterally hydronephrotic kidney, supranormal function on a renal scan is indicative of:
   a. renal hyperplasia.
   b. vascular recruitment due to obstruction.
   c. artifactual increased tubular uptake.
   d. uncertain prognosis.
   e. significant obstructive effect.
5. In the obstructed kidney, epidermal growth factor (EGF) has been shown to:
   a. reduce glomerular sclerosis.
   b. accelerate interstitial fibrosis.
   c. reduce renin recruitment in the afferent arteriole.
   d. improve collecting duct function.
   e. reduce renal apoptosis.
6. Epithelial to mesenchymal transformation in the developing kidney is:
   a. seen only in the setting of obstruction.
   b. integral to glomerular development.
   c. the basis for glomerular sclerosis.
   d. reflected in the presence of α-smooth muscle actin.
   e. a one-way process.
7. Regulation of the extracellular matrix in the kidney:
   a. depends on normal expression of EGF.
   b. depends on balanced activity of TIMPs and MMPs.
   c. depends entirely on collagen synthesis.
   d. is not related to angiotensin expression.
   e. is independent of transforming growth factor-β activity.
8. Inflammatory changes in the congenitally obstructed kidney:
   a. are similar to that seen in postnatally obstructed kidneys.
   b. are mediated by the renin-angiotensin system.
   c. are minimal in the absence of overt infection.
   d. are the key element in glomerular damage.
   e. affect renal interstitial fibrosis.
9. In the fetal kidney, angiotensin activity:
   a. is tightly regulated by EGF.
   b. acts predominantly through the AT-1 receptor.
   c. affects epithelial mesenchymal transformations.
   d. is an important regulator of renal growth.
   e. is unaffected by renal obstruction.

ANSWERS

1. **b. asymmetrical renal growth.** When renal function appears to decline after relief of obstruction, it is often due to different growth and functional development rates of the two kidneys, when the affected kidney cannot increase its absolute function as rapidly as the other intact kidney. This produces a progressive differential functional uptake on nuclear imaging that gives the impression of functional loss that is relative and not absolute.
2. **a. affects glomerular development.** Only congenital obstruction will change glomerular development, whereas acquired obstruction can produce all of the other changes indicated. As it occurs during development, congenital obstruction can produce an altered developmental pattern whereas acquired obstruction cannot change an already established pattern.
3. **c. fibromuscular collars.** One of the histologic hallmarks of dysplasia are fibromuscular collars, so-called primitive ducts reflecting abnormal differentiation of the peritubular mesenchyme. Renal growth impairment is common with dysplasia, but this is not atrophy but growth failure. Glomerular cysts are not characteristic of dysplasia. Heterotopic cartilage may be seen but not bone. Excess renin expression may be seen in obstruction without dysplasia.
4. **d. uncertain prognosis.** It remains controversial as to the basis for supranormal function on renal scan in the setting of hydronephrosis. In some cases it is thought to be artifactual but may also reflect a compensatory mechanism that reflects obstructive effects. There is no evidence that it reflects vascular recruitment, but it may be mediated by vascular factors.
5. **e. reduce renal apoptosis.** Administration of EGF to the congenitally obstructed kidney can reduce renal apoptosis and reduce the effects of growth impairment. The other effects have not been reported.
6. **d. reflected in the presence of α-smooth muscle actin.** Epithelial to mesenchymal transformations are an important part of renal development but have not been shown to be part of normal glomerular development. It is the presumed basis for the presence of α-smooth muscle actin in the obstructed kidney. It is bidirectional.
7. **b. depends on balanced activity of TIMPs and MMPs.** Extracellular membrane (ECM) regulation is due to collagen synthesis rates as well as to the rate of ECM breakdown. The latter is determined by the balanced activities of the TIMPs and MMPs; these are regulated by TGF-β and the renin-angiotensin system.
8. **c. are minimal in the absence of overt infection.** In contrast to acquired obstruction, congenital obstruction is not characterized by a significant inflammatory infiltrate, except when complicated by infection.
9. **d. is an important regulator of renal growth.** In the developing kidney, angiotensin is an important growth regulator, as well as mediator of fibrosis, and is altered significantly by obstruction. Fetal angiotensin acts predominantly through the AT2 receptor until late in gestation when the AT1 receptor begins to exert a greater role.

109

Perinatal Urology

CRAIG A. PETERS

QUESTIONS

1. When does compensatory renal growth in the child with a solitary kidney begin?
   a. In utero
   b. At birth
   c. At 2 weeks
   d. At 1 month
   e. At 3 months
2. A neonate is reported to have a single cyst on the upper pole of the left kidney. What does this most likely represent?
   a. Benign simple cyst
   b. Cystic neuroblastoma
   c. Duplication anomaly with upper pole dilatation
   d. Upper pole dilatation caused by reflux
   e. Neurenteric cyst
3. During gestation, the makeup of the amniotic fluid (AF) becomes increasingly:
   a. like fetal plasma.
   b. the product of fetal urine output.
   c. an ultrafiltrate from the placenta.
   d. hyperosmotic to fetal plasma.
   e. a product of gastrointestinal secretions.
4. What is the most reliable predictor of vesicoureteral reflux in the fetus?
   a. Pelvic dilatation greater than 7 mm at 30 weeks
   b. Intermittent ureteral dilatation
   c. Calyceal dilatation
   d. Echogenic renal parenchyma
   e. There are no reliable predictors of reflux
5. A 24-week fetus is found to have evidence of a ureterocele and bilateral moderately severe hydronephrosis of all renal units. What is the likely cause?
   a. Concomitant posterior urethral valves
   b. Bilateral ectopic ureters
   c. Obstruction of the ureteral orifices by the ureterocele
   d. Bladder outlet obstruction by the ureterocele
   e. Associated neurogenic bladder dysfunction
6. The characteristic ultrasonographic appearance of a multicystic dysplastic kidney (MCDK) in utero is multiple noncommunicating cysts and:
   a. absence of a large central cyst with minimal parenchyma.
   b. presence of a large central cyst with echogenic parenchyma.
   c. presence of a large central cyst without parenchyma.
   d. absence of a large central cyst with thick echogenic parenchyma.
   e. a peripheral array around a large central cyst.
7. A 34-week fetus has bilateral, large echogenic kidneys without recognizable cysts. There is little amniotic fluid. What is the likely diagnosis?
   a. Bilateral MCDK
   b. Bilateral congenital mesoblastic nephromas
   c. Congenital medullary nephronophthisis
   d. Bilateral fetal renal vein thrombosis
   e. Autosomal recessive polycystic kidneys
8. A fetus with intracardiac masses consistent with rhabdomyosarcomas should be screened for:
   a. Down syndrome.
   b. Beckwith-Wiedemann syndrome.
   c. trisomy 14.
   d. tuberous sclerosis.
   e. Denys-Drash syndrome.
9. A fetus with apparent obstructive uropathy has had adequate amniotic fluid until about 32 weeks' gestation. The kidneys are dilated and nonechogenic. What is the likely outcome?
   a. Early neonatal respiratory death
   b. Pulmonary insufficiency and death by 4 months of age
   c. Early neonatal death because of renal failure
   d. Moderate renal insufficiency
   e. Normal renal and pulmonary function
10. What is the most compelling reason for in utero urinary tract shunting for obstructive uropathy?
    a. Severe bilateral hydronephrosis
    b. Echogenic kidneys at 24 weeks' gestation
    c. Decreasing amniotic fluid volume after 28 weeks
    d. Absence of bladder refilling on percutaneous aspiration
    e. Oligohydramnios at 21 weeks associated with severe hydronephrosis

11. A neonatal boy with prenatal hydronephrosis is found to have bilateral grade 5 reflux and a bladder capacity of 200 mL. There is no trabeculation. What is the best explanation for the large bladder capacity?
    a. Recycling of refluxed urine
    b. Bladder outlet obstruction from valves
    c. Neurogenic bladder
    d. Prune-belly variant
    e. Impaired bladder emptying
12. A neonatal boy with bilateral grade 4 reflux may be expected to have which pattern on urodynamic studies?
    a. Normal bladder
    b. Impaired contractility
    c. Bladder outlet obstruction
    d. Small capacity, high pressure
    e. Hypertonicity and instability
13. A 7-day-old boy with hypospadias and undescended testes is seen in the emergency department with hypotension, hyponatremia, hyperkalemia, and dehydration. The most appropriate management is intravenous fluid resuscitation and:
    a. intravenous antibiotics.
    b. hypertonic saline.
    c. parenteral corticosteroids.
    d. abdominal CT.
    e. voiding cystourethrogram.
14. A newborn boy has a penile abnormality. The surface of the penis closest to the abdomen appears to be mucosal, with the defect extending from the pubis to the glans. The foreskin is dangling from the opposite side of the glans. The scrotum is normal. The pubic bones feel more widely spaced than normal. What is this condition, most likely?
    a. Penoscrotal hypospadias
    b. Superior vesical fissure
    c. Classic bladder exstrophy
    d. Congenital urethrocutaneous fistula
    e. Epispadias
15. A 5-month-old child undergoes a KUB (kidney, ureter, bladder) study for abdominal distention. There are calcifications in the left upper quadrant in a peripheral, eggshell pattern. What is the most likely cause?
    a. Neuroblastoma
    b. Renal vein thrombosis
    c. Renal artery stenosis
    d. Adrenal hemorrhage
    e. Wilms' tumor
16. When should newborn boys with bilateral, moderately severe hydronephrosis be evaluated?
    a. Within a week after referral
    b. Immediately after delivery
    c. At the time of discharge from the newborn nursery
    d. At the first well-baby visit
    e. At the family's convenience

ANSWERS

1. **a. In utero.** Compensatory renal hypertrophy has been shown in animal and human studies to occur prenatally, although at a lesser pace than seen postnatally. The mechanisms remain undefined.
2. **c. Duplication anomaly with upper pole dilatation.** A true renal cyst is rare in the neonate while the likelihood is that this represents a duplication anomaly associated with an ectopic ureter or ureterocele, causing upper pole hydronephrosis, often with thin parenchyma
3. **b. the product of fetal urine output.** Starting about 16 weeks, the amniotic fluid becomes progressively made up of fetal urine. This accounts for the progression of oligohydramnios with fetal bladder outlet obstruction or renal dysfunction.
4. **e. There are no reliable predictors of reflux.** Whereas most of these elements may be seen with fetal reflux, none is specific enough to either make the diagnosis or rule it out through their absence.
5. **d. Bladder outlet obstruction by the ureterocele.** When all renal units are affected in the setting of a ureterocele, consideration for bladder outlet obstruction from the prolapsing ureterocele is important. Rarely, this will cause severe obstruction and oligohydramnios.
6. **a. absence of a large central cyst with minimal parenchyma.** The classic MCDK will have no central cystic structure that might be a dilated renal pelvis and will have minimal echogenic renal parenchyma.
7. **e. Autosomal recessive polycystic kidneys.** Fetal ARPKD appears as bilaterally enlarged bright kidneys without macrocysts. There is rarely hydronephrosis. Amniotic fluid may be declining.
8. **d. tuberous sclerosis.** The association of an intracardiac mass with tuberous sclerosis should prompt a search for renal masses and the extrarenal manifestations of tuberous sclerosis.
9. **e. Normal renal and pulmonary function.** While it cannot be predicted with certainty, the absence of echogenic changes and adequate amniotic fluid would suggest a good prognosis for an infant in this situation. There is very low risk of pulmonary insufficiency since the effect of oligohydramnios occurs earlier than 30 weeks' gestation.
10. **e. Oligohydramnios at 21 weeks associated with severe hydronephrosis.** The fetus with oligohydramnios at 20 to 21 weeks is at the highest risk for pulmonary insufficiency due to pulmonary hypoplasia and has the most to benefit from in-utero shunting.
11. **a. Recycling of refluxed urine.** Boys with high-grade reflux may empty their bladders, but they are quickly refilled from draining urine that had been refluxed into the upper tracts. This has the effect of slowly dilating the bladders without bladder wall thickening.
12. **e. Hypertonicity and instability.** Many boys with high-grade neonatal reflux have been found to have hypertonic and unstable bladders with urodynamic testing. The etiology is unclear, and the pattern tends to settle down in the first 2 years. Its impact on renal injury is unclear.
13. **c. parenteral corticosteroids.** This clinical scenario suggests the possibility of congenital adrenal hyperplasia with adrenal insufficiency. It may have the appearance of urosepsis, and appropriate evaluation for that possibility should be undertaken, but the possibility of congenital adrenal hyperplasia must be considered and acted upon.

14. **e. Epispadias.** This description is typical for epispadias with the open urethra on the upper, dorsal side of the penis and an upward curve to the penis. The degree of pubic diastasis is related to the severity of the bladder neck abnormality.

15. **a. Neuroblastoma.** This radiographic pattern is typical for adrenal hemorrhage; although neuroblastoma can have residual calcifications, they are in a more central arrangement. Renal artery stenosis might have renal calcifications.

16. **b. Immediately after delivery.** In the setting of a boy with significant hydronephrosis, the possibility of posterior urethral valves must be considered and acted upon. In this case an ultrasound will nearly always detect significant pathology if present and intervention may be instituted.

110

Evaluation of the Pediatric Urology Patient

DOUGLAS A. CANNING • MICHAEL T. NGUYEN

QUESTIONS

1. Which one of the following patients does NOT need to be seen emergently?
   a. A newborn with hydronephrosis in a solitary kidney
   b. A 4-year-old boy with acute right scrotal pain
   c. A 12-year-old girl with microscopic hematuria during a routine examination
   d. An 8-year-old boy with sickle-cell anemia and a 5-hour history of priapism
   e. A male newborn with a distended bladder, bilateral hydronephrosis, and respiratory insufficiency
2. Which of the following is a potential complication of neonatal circumcision?
   a. Wound infection
   b. Meatal stenosis
   c. Death
   d. Penile curvature
   e. All of the above
3. Current limitations of the routine use of magnetic resonance urography (MRU) in pediatric urology include:
   a. ionizing radiation.
   b. high cost.
   c. sedation/anesthesia.
   d. both b and c.
   e. none of the above.
4. The optimal timing of spinal ultrasound during screening for occult spinal dysraphism is:
   a. after puberty.
   b. before 6 months of age.
   c. between 1 year and 6 years.
   d. none of the above.
   e. all of the above.
5. All the following are true about sexual assault victims EXCEPT:
   a. 12% to 38% of adult women were sexually abused by age 18.
   b. the incidence of sexual abuse in males is less than 1%.
   c. of females presenting to an urban sexual assault clinic, 43% were adolescents.
   d. approximately 75% of pediatric patients with sexually transmitted diseases had histories/signs of sexual abuse.
   e. All of the above.
6. Findings associated with the Beckwith-Wiedemann syndrome include:
   a. macroglossia.
   b. hepatosplenomegaly.
   c. nephromegaly.
   d. all of the above.
   e. only a and b.
7. All the following are true of "failure to thrive" EXCEPT:
   a. It is often associated with poor developmental and socioemotional functioning.
   b. a parent fails to offer adequate calories.
   c. family discord, maternal depression, and neonatal problems other than low birth weight are associated.
   d. All of the above are true.
   e. None of the above is true.
8. When should a newborn with suspected congenital adrenal hyperplasia be tested?
   a. At the first well-baby visit
   b. Before discharge from the nursery
   c. No testing is required
   d. None of the above
   e. Both a and b
9. All of the following statements about the pediatric abdominal examination are true EXCEPT:
   a. renal pathology is the source of up to two thirds of neonatal abdominal masses.
   b. abdominal distention at birth or shortly afterward suggests either obstruction or perforation of the gastrointestinal tract.
   c. the abdominal wall is normally strong, especially in premature infants.
   d. a solid flank mass may be due to renal vein thrombosis.
   e. All of the above.

10. Which of the following statements is true about cutaneous markers of occult spinal dysraphism?
    a. Forty percent of patients with atypical presacral dimples have associated occult spinal dysraphism.
    b. A combination of two or more congenital midline skin lesions is the strongest marker of occult spinal dysraphism.
    c. An "atypical" presacral dimple as defined may indicate spina bifida or cord tethering if the dimple is in the midline, less than 2.5 cm from the anal verge at birth, or shallower than 0.5 cm.
    d. All of the above.
    e. Both a and b.
11. What is genitourinary sinography used for?
    a. To identify the presence of a cervix in a patient with ambiguous genitalia
    b. To provide details about the relative positions of the urethra, vagina, and distal hindgut in a patient with a cloaca
    c. To assess the distance between the perineum and the point of confluence between the vagina and the urethra
    d. a and c
    e. a, b, and c
12. Urethral meatal stenosis occurs in the newborn:
    a. as a result of birth trauma.
    b. after urinary tract infection.
    c. after a newborn physical examination.
    d. after healing of the inflamed, denuded glans after circumcision.
    e. from undergarment irritation.
13. In newborns with ambiguous genitalia, what does a symmetrical gonadal examination suggest?
    a. Congenital adrenal hyperplasia or true hermaphroditism
    b. Mixed gonadal dysgenesis or androgen insensitivity syndrome
    c. Congenital adrenal hyperplasia or mixed gonadal dysgenesis
    d. Congenital adrenal hyperplasia or androgen insensitivity syndrome
    e. True hermaphroditism or mixed gonadal dysgenesis
14. Common urologic sources of failure to thrive include which of the following?
    a. Urinary tract infection
    b. Renal tubular acidosis
    c. Diabetes insipidus
    d. Chronic renal insufficiency
    e. All of the above
15. A newborn should have a hydrocele surgically corrected in the newborn period if:
    a. it is large.
    b. it is changing in volume.
    c. it accompanies a symptomatic hernia.
    d. a, b, and c.
    e. b and c.

ANSWERS

1. **c. A 12-year-old girl with microscopic hematuria during a routine examination.** In the absence of other symptoms, microscopic hematuria in children is not an emergency. Bilateral hydronephrosis or hydronephrosis in a solitary kidney both represent emergencies and should be evaluated as soon as possible. Acute scrotal pain should always be considered testicular torsion until proven otherwise. Boys with sickle cell anemia are at increased risk for priapism and should always be treated immediately to decrease the long-term sequela associated with priapism.
2. **e. All of the above.** Wound infections, meatal stenosis, death, and removal of insufficient foreskin are all potential complications of neonatal circumcision.
3. **d. both b and c.** As an individual test, MRU provides the best information of anatomy and function of the genitourinary tract. It avoids the use of ionizing radiation. However, current limitations include its high cost and the requirement of sedation or anesthesia in some children.
4. **b. before 6 months of age.** Ossification of the posterior elements after 6 months of age prevents an acoustic ultrasound window. After 6 months, a spinal MRI is recommended when an occult spinal dysraphism is suspected.
5. **b. the incidence of sexual abuse in males is less than 1%.** Abuse of children is surprisingly common. The incidence of sexual abuse in males ranges from 3% to 9% of the population.
6. **d. all of the above.** Beckwith-Wiedemann syndrome is caused by a mutation on chromosome 11p15.5. Clinical features include exomphalos, macroglossia, and gigantism in the neonate. Many of the affected infants have hypoglycemia in the first few days of life. Patients are at increased risk of developing specific tumors (e.g., adrenal carcinoma, Wilms' tumors, hepatoblastoma, and rhabdomyosarcoma).
7. **d. All of the above are true.** "Failure to thrive" may be used to describe an infant or child whose physical growth is significantly less than that of his or her peers.
8. **b. Before discharge from the nursery.** Because congenital adrenal hyperplasia may result in salt wasting, infants with ambiguous genitalia must be quickly evaluated and stabilized.
9. **c. the abdominal wall is normally strong, especially in premature infants.** Renal pathology accounts for approximately two thirds of abdominal masses found in the neonate. Solid masses include neuroblastoma, congenital mesoblastic nephroma, teratoma, and renal enlargement due to renal vein thrombosis. The abdominal wall is normally weak, especially in premature infants.
10. **e. Both a and b.** The lower back should be examined for any evidence of cutaneous markers of occult spinal dysraphisms that may account for abnormal bladder function. In a series of 207 neonates with sacral and presacral cutaneous stigmata, 40% of patients with atypical dimples were found to have occult spinal dysraphism. An "atypical" presacral dimple is defined as a dimple that is off center, more than 2.5 cm from the anal verge at birth, or deeper than 0.5 cm.
11. **e. a, b, and c.** The genitourinary sinogram will help to differentiate a cervix from a prostatic utricle. If a cloaca is present, the sinogram will provide details about the positions of the rectum, vagina, and urethra and about the point of confluence and the distance to the perineum.
12. **d. after healing of the inflamed, denuded glans after circumcision.** Meatal stenosis is common after circumcision. It may result from contraction of the meatus after healing of the inflamed, denuded glans tissue that occurs after retraction of the foreskin or from damage to the frenular artery at the time of circumcision.

13. **d. Congenital adrenal hyperplasia or androgen insensitivity syndrome.** Particular attention to the symmetry of the examination is important if intersex conditions are thought to exist. A symmetrical gonadal examination (gonads palpable on each side or impalpable on both sides) suggests a global disorder such as congenital adrenal hyperplasia or androgen insensitivity.

14. **e. All of the above.** As urologists, we must be alert to common urologic sources of failure to thrive such as urinary tract infection, renal tubular acidosis, diabetes insipidus, and chronic renal insufficiency.

15. **e. b and c.** A hydrocele that changes in volume suggests a patent processus vaginalis. These infants are at risk for inguinal hernia. The processus vaginalis is not likely to close after birth. If a hernia has been symptomatic, the processus vaginalis should be corrected in the newborn period.

Renal Disease in Childhood

H. NORMAN NOE • DEBORAH P. JONES

QUESTIONS

1. A 3-year-old African-American boy presents to the emergency department with swelling and decreased urine output. He has had eyelid edema on awakening for the past week. His BP is 90/50 mm Hg, and he has marked eyelid edema, distended abdomen, and pitting edema of the legs and feet. Urinalysis showed a specific gravity of 1.030, pH 5, 3+ protein, and trace amount of blood. Blood sent for a comprehensive metabolic panel showed sodium level of 131 mEq/L, BUN value of 30 mg/dL, creatinine level of 0.3 mg/dL, and albumin level of 1.6 g/dL. The appropriate next step in management is:
   a. admission to inpatient unit for quantitation of urinary protein excretion.
   b. renal imaging.
   c. initiation of oral diuretics, and asking parents to collect a timed urine for protein at home, with outpatient follow-up.
   d. workup for occult malignancy.
2. A 6-year-old white girl is seen for a school physical. She has been well, without urinary tract complaints or systemic illness. Urinalysis has a specific gravity of 1.020, pH 6, trace protein, and moderate amount of blood on dipstick testing. The microscopic test shows 5-6 RBCs/HPF. The LEAST appropriate next step is:
   a. renal ultrasound
   b. random urine calcium and creatinine
   c. clean catch urine culture
   d. empirical 10-day course of antibiotics
   e. repeat urinalysis in 2 weeks
3. Each of the following forms of glomerulonephritis is associated with hypocomplementemia EXCEPT:
   a. membranoproliferative glomerulonephritis
   b. diffuse proliferative lupus nephritis
   c. acute post-streptococcal glomerulonephritic
   d. IgA nephropathy
4. An 8-year-old boy is referred because a urinalysis at the primary care physician's office showed specific gravity 1.030, pH 5, trace protein, and moderate amount of blood. He has a normal physical examination including BP of 96/56 mm Hg. On further history, you discover that he was hospitalized 2 months ago during the early summer when he was visiting his grandparents and was diagnosed with post-streptococcal glomerulonephritis. The most appropriate course of action is:
   a. schedule cystoscopy.
   b. renal ultrasound.
   c. a course of antibiotics after obtaining a urine culture.
   d. reassure his family and obtain records from the outside institution.
5. A 6-year-old boy presents to the emergency department with right-sided flank pain and gross hematuria. He has been previously well and without urologic complaints until the day prior. He has no dysuria or fever but has vomited three times. His BP is 120/70 mm Hg, and the physical examination reveals right costovertebral angle tenderness. The urinalysis shows brown urine with a specific gravity of 1.030, pH 7, large amount of blood, and 2+ protein. The next step in diagnostic evaluation might include all of the following EXCEPT:
   a. high-resolution CT of abdomen/pelvis without contrast.
   b. microscopic examination of the urine.
   c. cystoscopy.
   d. renal ultrasound.
6. In the child described in Question 5, urine microscopy revealed TNTC eumorphic RBCs and no casts or WBCs. A 3-mm renal calculus was identified on CT. The stone was recovered by straining the urine. It was sent for analysis, which revealed calcium oxalate. The next step is to:
   a. start a thiazide diuretic.
   b. obtain a 24-hour urine collection to test for calcium, creatinine, oxalate, and citrate.
   c. start potassium citrate.
   d. restrict dietary calcium.

7. A 6-year-old boy presents to the emergency department with a headache and gross hematuria. He has been previously well and without urologic complaints until the day prior. He has no dysuria or fever but has vomited three times. He had a sore throat the week before, but it has resolved. BP is 140/90 mm Hg, and physical examination reveals a heart murmur. The urinalysis shows brown urine with a specific gravity of 1.030, pH 7, large amount of blood, and 2+ protein. The next step in the diagnostic evaluation might include all of the following EXCEPT:
   a. CT scan of the abdomen and pelvis.
   b. comprehensive metabolic panel.
   c. C3.
   d. anti–streptolysin O titer.
   e. microscopic examination of the urine.

8. A 3-year-old boy presents to the emergency department with a respiratory problem and gross hematuria. He has been previously well and without urologic complaints until the day prior to onset of the upper respiratory tract infection. He has no dysuria or abdominal pain but has fever, rhinorrhea, and cough. BP is 120/70 mm Hg, and physical examination shows rhinorrhea, mild pharyngeal erythema, and no edema or abdominal tenderness. The urinalysis shows brown urine with a specific gravity of 1.030, pH 7, large amount of blood, and 2+ protein. (His mother also has had hematuria in the past, and his maternal uncle is deaf and on hemodialysis.) The next step in diagnostic evaluation might include all of the following EXCEPT:
   a. CT scan of the abdomen and pelvis.
   b. comprehensive metabolic panel.
   c. renal biopsy.
   d. anti–streptolysin O titer and C3.
   e. microscopic examination of the urine.

ANSWERS

1. **a. admission to inpatient unit for quantitation of urinary protein excretion.** The patient has hypoalbuminemia, edema, and proteinuria and most likely has nephrotic syndrome. The initial illness is best treated with inpatient admission to complete the diagnostic studies (quantitate urinary protein, measure plasma lipids) and education of the family including a low salt diet. Oral prednisone is started because a renal biopsy is rarely indicated. Oral diuretics are not commonly prescribed unless careful observation is possible due to poor response and the potential for thromboses. Malignancy is rarely associated with nephrotic syndrome in children, and therefore a workup is not indicated. Imaging of the urinary tract is rarely indicated in children with nephrotic syndrome. Fortunately, most children with primary nephrotic syndrome respond to corticosteroids within 14 days and have spontaneous diuresis with loss of edema and proteinuria.
2. **d. empirical 10-day course of antibiotics.** Although asymptomatic hematuria may be caused by occult urinary tract infection, empirical treatment without culture is never the correct approach. Unfortunately, this scenario happens far too often in the primary care world. It is reasonable to repeat the urinalysis before proceeding with diagnostic evaluation. If the hematuria persists, then imaging the kidneys and urinary tract and screening for hypercalciuria is a reasonable approach.
3. **d. IgA nephropathy.** Hypocomplementemia is commonly seen in three forms of glomerulonephritis: acute postinfectious, proliferative lupus nephritis, and a rare cause of immune-complex–mediated glomerulonephritis called membranoproliferative glomerulonephritis. IgA nephropathy is the most common chronic nephropathy of children and adults and is not accompanied by hypocomplementemia.
4. **d. reassure the family and obtain records from the outside institution.** Given the previous history of postinfectious glomerulonephritis (in his case due to a preceding streptococcal infection), the most likely cause of microscopic hematuria is resolving nephritis. The microhematuria may persist for up to 1 year, while the proteinuria and macroscopic hematuria usually resolve within the 2-week acute phase. It would be helpful to confirm the diagnosis by review of medical records.
5. **c. cystoscopy.** The clinical picture is that of a child presenting with a renal calculus. Cystoscopy is rarely indicated in the diagnostic evaluation, although it might be included during the treatment phase of nephrolithiasis in children. A high-resolution CT without contrast is the test of choice, but one cannot argue with ultrasonography as a first test. Examination of the urine is also a viable first step because children with nephritis occasionally complain of flank pain.
6. **b. obtain a 24-hour urine collection to test for calcium, creatinine, oxalate, and citrate.** A metabolic evaluation for the cause of calcium oxalate nephrolithiasis should be initiated because the differential diagnosis included hyperoxaluria, hypercalciuria, renal tubular acidosis, or idiopathic calcium stones. In children, preventative treatment is rarely initiated without attempts to diagnose the underlying metabolic disturbance. Dietary calcium restriction is never a treatment for children with calcium stones with or without hypercalciuria.
7. **a. CT scan of the abdomen and pelvis.** With symptomatic hypertension and gross hematuria, one must entertain the possibility of acute glomerulonephritis. The prior history of pharyngitis is consistent with post-streptococcal associated disease. Examination of the urine sediment for signs of glomerulonephritis (cellular casts) and documentation of renal function and electrolytes as well as elevated anti–streptolysin O titer and decreased C3 are the usual steps taken to confirm the diagnosis. Hypertension is treated aggressively with salt restriction, loop diuretics, and antihypertensive agents. Resolution of the hypertension parallels resolution of the acute phase.
8. **a. CT scan of the abdomen and pelvis.** The presentation of gross hematuria during a respiratory tract infection is not characteristic of postinfectious glomerulonephritis because the onset of nephritis usually follows the infection. The positive family history is important because the onset of macroscopic hematuria during a respiratory tract infection is characteristic of two forms of chronic glomerulonephritis: IgA nephropathy and Alport's hereditary nephritis. Imaging is usually not indicated if glomerulonephritis can be confirmed by microscopic examination of the urine. Patients with both IgA and hereditary nephritis would be expected to have normal C3. A renal biopsy is needed for diagnosis of IgA and is usually needed for diagnosis of hereditary nephritis except in the case where the affected relative has already undergone biopsy.

112

Infection and Inflammation of the Pediatric Genitourinary Tract

LINDA M. DAIRIKI SHORTLIFFE

QUESTIONS

1. Boys have more urinary tract infections (UTIs) than girls:
   a. during the first year of life.
   b. when they become sexually active.
   c. during elementary school years.
   d. if they are uncircumcised toddlers.
   e. at puberty.
2. Characteristics of bacteria more likely to infect the kidney include:
   a. growth in mannose.
   b. hemolysis.
   c. p-fimbriae.
   d. KOH staining.
   e. urease production.
3. Intracellular bacterial pods may allow microbial adaptation and protection via:
   a. uroplakins.
   b. bacterial clonal genes.
   c. Toll-like receptors.
   d. Tamm-Horsfall protein.
   e. biofilm.
4. Risk factors for recurrent UTI in young women include:
   a. age at first UTI and UTI in mother.
   b. other congenital abnormalities.
   c. vesicoureteral reflux.
   d. recent antimicrobial usage.
   e. encopresis and voiding history.
5. Incidence of vesicoureteral reflux differs by:
   a. circumcision status.
   b. ethnicity or race.
   c. gene polymorphisms.
   d. bacterial colonization.
   e. blood group antigen.
6. The best urinary indicators of infection on urinalysis are positive:
   a. pyuria, leukocyte esterase, and catalase.
   b. nitrite, microscopic RBC and WBC casts.
   c. glitter cells in spun urine.
   d. microscopic bacteria, leukocyte esterase, nitrite.
   e. Gram stain and nitrite.
7. A source of bacterial persistence is:
   a. sexual activity.
   b. prepuce.
   c. struvite calculus.
   d. fecal colonization.
   e. increased postvoid residual.
8. A radiologic finding of pyelonephritis is:
   a. hot spot on DMSA nuclear renogram.
   b. focal renal wedge lesion on intravenous pyelogram.
   c. hypoechogenicity on renal ultrasonography.
   d. ureteral dilation.
   e. renal pelvic debris levels.
9. Renal scarring in association with vesicoureteral reflux is caused by:
   a. "water hammer" effect of vesicoureteral reflux.
   b. intrarenal reflux with pyelotubular backflow.
   c. bacteriuria and vesicoureteral reflux.
   d. compound calyces.
   e. elevated bladder pressure.
10. In children the likelihood of renal scarring correlates with:
    a. number of occurrences of UTI.
    b. severity of fever.
    c. intrapelvic pressure.
    d. renal dysplasia.
    e. duration of vesicoureteral reflux.
11. Nocturnal enuresis accompanies recurrent UTIs in children and:
    a. treatment is associated with decreased UTIs.
    b. these are independent findings.
    c. vesicoureteral reflux may be involved.
    d. both findings are likely to resolve spontaneously by puberty.
    e. dysfunctional voiding is likely.
12. Increased periurethral bacterial colonization is present:
    a. in children who experience recurrent UTIs.
    b. on the foreskin of boys age 5 and older.
    c. when children are constipated.
    d. during antimicrobial therapy.
    e. in children with vesicoureteral reflux.

13. During pregnancy what is more likely to occur?
    a. UTIs
    b. renal scarring
    c. bacteriuria progressing to pyelonephritis
    d. vesicoureteral reflux
    e. asymptomatic bacteriuria
14. During pregnancy, females who have had surgically corrected vesicoureteral reflux for breakthrough UTIs:
    a. will be protected from UTIs.
    b. do *not* need urinary tract antimicrobial prophylaxis.
    c. do *not* have accelerated renal insufficiency.
    d. do need the urine screened for bacteriuria.
    e. risk increased fetal complications.
15. Evaluation and management of the first UTI in a 2-year-old should include:
    a. DMSA scan.
    b. parenteral antimicrobial agents.
    c. WBC count and nitrite test.
    d. ESR and creatinine.
    e. prophylactic antimicrobial agents until imaging.
16. When a child does not appear to improve after 2 to 3 days of appropriate antimicrobial therapy for the first UTI, one should:
    a. perform a DMSA scan.
    b. obtain CBC and blood cultures.
    c. perform renal and bladder ultrasonography.
    d. perform voiding cystourethrography.
    e. change antimicrobial therapy.
17. A characteristic sign of mature renal scarring on a DMSA renogram is:
    a. focal circular area of diminished uptake.
    b. diffuse renal enlargement.
    c. wedged-shaped areas of increased uptake.
    d. polar areas of diminished uptake.
    e. areas of increased focal cortical activity.
18. When an asymptomatic UTI is diagnosed:
    a. it should be treated to prevent recurrence.
    b. about a third clear spontaneously.
    c. the infecting bacteria is commonly p-piliated.
    d. imaging evaluation is not needed unless it is the second UTI.
    e. monthly urinary specimens are needed to check for UTI.
19. Appropriate treatment of children with UTI includes:
    a. follow-up culture after 48 hours.
    b. hospitalization of all infants younger than age 6 months.
    c. single dose oral treatment for most schoolage children.
    d. "switch" therapy for febrile children with UTI.
    e. radiologic evaluation after the second febrile UTI.
20. In a 6-year-old girl with recurrent UTIs, occasional diurnal incontinence, and normal genitourinary tract by renal and bladder ultrasonography and voiding cystourethrogram:
    a. monthly screening cultures should be performed.
    b. annual renal and bladder ultrasonography is warranted.
    c. urodynamics should be performed.
    d. constipation should be suspected.
    e. daily perineal hygiene should be initiated.
21. Good practice to lower incidence of surgical site infections excludes:
    a. short hospitalization.
    b. preoperative antimicrobial agents 60 minutes before open operations.
    c. bowel preparation before bowel surgery with mechanical preparation and nonabsorbable oral and intravenous antibiotics.
    d. clipping hair in the operating room if hair needs removal.
    e. vancomycin 120 minutes before surgery when required because of allergies.
22. An 8-year-old boy recovering from a bone marrow transplant has frequency, urgency, and dysuria with hematuria and is treated for a UTI. The cultures return in 48 hours showing no growth so the antimicrobial treatment is stopped, but the symptoms continue. The next step should be:
    a. renal arteriography.
    b. cystoscopy.
    c. interferon and acyclovir.
    d. reculture urine.
    e. renal and bladder ultrasonography and voiding cystourethrography.
23. A 12-year-old boy is explored for possible testicular torsion, but epididymitis is found, and urine cultures show growth. The next step should be:
    a. antimicrobial treatment, renal and bladder ultrasonography, voiding cystourethrogram.
    b. antimicrobial treatment and testicular color flow Doppler ultrasonography in 3 months.
    c. no further treatment.
    d. intravenous pyelogram.
    e. testicular biopsy, special cultures, and testes ultrasonography.
24. After 10 days of urethral catheter drainage, the urine from a 5-year-old child with multiple traumatic injuries grows 10,000 cfu/mL of *Candida glabrata*. The next step is to:
    a. administer parenteral amphotericin before catheter removal.
    b. change the catheter.
    c. give intravesical amphotericin irrigation before catheter removal.
    d. change the indwelling catheter and alkalinize the urine.
    e. perform renal and bladder ultrasonography.
25. After an acute UTI, when selecting a drug for low-dose urinary tract antimicrobial prophylaxis:
    a. the same drug that was used for treatment should be optimal.
    b. serum concentrations of drug should be high.
    c. urinary excretion should be rapid.
    d. there should be minimal effect on the fecal flora.
    e. drug dosage should be higher for the first few weeks.
26. Nitrofurantoin is useful for treating recurrent UTIs because it:
    a. has high serum and tissue concentrating levels.
    b. has a hemolytic effect.
    c. affects the bacterial biofilm.
    d. diffuses into the vagina and decreases bacterial colonization.
    e. has lower systemic absorption and may generate less microbial resistance.
27. In CT evaluation of a possible renal abscess:
    a. cortical attenuation is diagnostic.
    b. striations are characteristic.
    c. delayed renal views 2 to 3 hours later may be needed.
    d. wedge defects are helpful.
    e. vascular phase is most important.

ANSWERS

1. **a. during the first year of life.** Only during the first year of life do males get more UTIs than females, and during that period uncircumcised boys have up to 10 times the risk of circumcised boys of having a UTI.

2. **c. p-fimbriae.** Two important markers for *Escherichia coli* virulence are MRHA characteristics and P blood group–specific adhesins (P-fimbriae or P-pili).

3. **e. biofilm.** Biofilms appear to allow microbial adaptation to variable environments and then allow aggregate detachment that will cause systemic infection, antimicrobial resistance via plasmid exchange, endotoxin production, and overall increased resistance to host immune systems.

4. **a. age at first UTI and UTI in mother.** Two distinct risks for recurrent UTI in young women (age 18 to 30 years) are age at first UTI (UTI < age 15; odds ratio [OR] 3.9) and UTI in the mother (OR 2.3).

5. **b. ethnicity or race.** Several studies show that African-Americans have fewer UTIs, lower incidence of vesicoureteral reflux, and perhaps less likelihood of reflux nephropathy than Hispanics or whites.

6. **d. microscopic bacteria, leukocyte esterase, nitrite.** The combination of positive leukocyte esterase and nitrite testing and microscopic confirmation of bacteria has almost 100% sensitivity for detection of UTI, and when all (or leukocyte esterase and nitrite tests) are negative the negative predictive value approaches 100%.

7. **c. a struvite calculus.** Sources of urinary tract bacterial persistence are usually found early in children, because imaging is performed after the first UTI. The discovery of surgically correctable sources of bacterial persistence is obviously important. The majority of recurrent UTI is, however, reinfection with the same or different organism that ascends from the bowel and is not surgically correctable.

8. **d. ureteral dilation.** Focal or general renal enlargement or swollen kidneys may be found in acute pyelonephritis; other findings on ultrasonography include thickening of the renal pelvis, hypoechogenicity, focal or diffuse hyperechogenicity, and ureteral dilation.

9. **c. bacteriuria and vesicoureteral reflux.** Renal scarring in association with vesicoureteral reflux occurs when bacteriuria is present.

10. **a. number of occurrences of UTI.** The likelihood of renal scarring directly correlates, moreover, with the number of UTI occurrences.

11. **b. these are independent findings.** Epidemiologic investigations show monosymptomatic nocturnal enuresis is unassociated with UTI, but diurnal enuresis or a combination of diurnal and nocturnal enuresis even if as infrequent as once a week may be associated with pediatric UTI.

12. **a. in children who experience recurrent UTIs.** Women and children who suffer repeated UTIs remain more colonized by periurethral gram-negative bacteria than those who do not. Times and conditions of increased periurethral colonization are, therefore, associated with increased risk of UTI.

13. **c. bacteriuria progressing to pyelonephritis.** The likelihood that the bacteriuria may progress to pyelonephritis is greatly increased. Thirteen and a half to 65% of pregnant women who are bacteriuric on a screening urinary culture will develop subsequent pyelonephritis during pregnancy if untreated, whereas pyelonephritis is rarely the consequence of uncomplicated cystitis in a nonpregnant woman.

14. **d. do need the urine screened for bacteriuria.** If vesicoureteral reflux is surgically corrected, these patients should not be assured that pyelonephritis during pregnancy is impossible or even unlikely. The urine of these pregnant women must still be screened routinely for bacteriuria.

15. **e. prophylactic antimicrobial agents until imaging.** After the therapeutic regimen for acute UTI, the child should be started on a daily prophylactic antimicrobial agent until full radiologic evaluation of the urinary tract may be conveniently performed in the next days to weeks.

16. **c. perform renal and bladder ultrasonography.** Early urinary tract imaging is important in a seriously ill and/or febrile child in whom the site of infection is unclear or who has unusual circumstances. Circumstances include newly diagnosed azotemia or a poor response to appropriate antimicrobial drugs after 3 to 4 days.

17. **d. Polar areas of diminished uptake.** Later after the acute episode heals scans will show (1) normal pattern; (2) generally diminished uptake and small kidney volume; (3) diminished uptake in the medial kidney; or (4) polar defects with diminished uptake in the renal poles.

18. **b. about a third clear spontaneously.** A majority of infants who have covert bacteriuria may clear their bacteriuria without treatment; others state that only about 30% of asymptomatic school-age girls with asymptomatic UTI clear spontaneously without treatment.

19. **d. "switch" therapy for febrile children with UTI.** A large series of children from 3 months to 5 years had successful treatment of febrile UTI with intravenous gentamicin, 5 mg/kg/day once daily, until afebrile (2 to 4 days) given in a day treatment center of a tertiary care hospital, followed by an oral antibiotic for a total of 10 days.

20. **d. constipation should be suspected.** Girls with recurrent UTI are more likely to have a family history of UTI, infrequent voiding, poor fluid intake, and stool retention.

21. **b. preoperative antimicrobial agents 60 minutes before open operations.** The most recent published Centers for Disease Control and Prevention guidelines related to surgical site infections were published in 1999 and summarized by Nichols. None is specific for children nor includes genitourinary operations. The CDC recommends (1) not removing hair unless it will interfere with the operation and, if removed, clipping immediately before operation; (2) identifying and treating all remote infections; (3) maintaining as short a hospitalization as possible; (4) administering antimicrobial agents only when indicated, based on published recommendations for a specific operation; (5) administering antimicrobial agents intravenously to ensure bactericidal serum and tissue levels when the incision is made (60 minutes before most and 120 minutes before vancomycin) and maintaining these levels for a few hours after closure with discontinuation no later than 24 hours after surgery, even if drainage catheters are left in place; (6) preparing bowel for elective operations with mechanical bowel preparation including enemas and cathartic agents and nonabsorbable oral antimicrobial agents the day before surgery in addition to the intravenous drugs; and (7) withholding routine vancomycin usage.

22. **e. renal and bladder ultrasonography and voiding cystourethrography.** BK virus, a DNA virus of the polyomavirus genus, has been found in the urine of bone marrow transplantation and other immunosuppressed patients having hemorrhagic cystitis (2 weeks to 5 months after

transplantation) causing both symptomatic (hematuria and dysuria) and asymptomatic infections.

23. **a. antimicrobial treatment, renal and bladder ultrasonography, voiding cystourethrogram.** During or after treatment of the acute bacterial urinary and epididymal infections, radiologic evaluation of the urinary tract should be performed as with any UTI. In young boys and infants, epididymitis is more likely to be related to genitourinary abnormalities (abnormal connections) or systemic hematogenous dissemination than in older males. Urethral and urinary cultures from the prepubertal male are likely to show either nothing or gram-negative organisms and thus be referred to as "nonspecific epididymitis," whereas in the postpubertal sexually active boys the cause may involve sexually transmitted organisms *(Neisseria gonorrhoeae, Chlamydia trachomatis)*.

24. **c. give intravesical amphotericin irrigation before catheter removal.** Although stopping unnecessary antimicrobial agents, changing or removing the indwelling catheter, and urinary alkalinization may be helpful, these means do not clear many cases of funguria. Recent prospective studies with intravesical amphotericin B bladder irrigation and oral fluconazole appear to show that both may clear funguria, although fungal recurrences are common.

25. **d. there should be minimal effect on the fecal flora.** The ideal prophylactic agent should have low serum and high urinary concentrations, have minimal effect on the normal fecal flora, be easily administered and tolerated, and be cost effective.

26. **e. has lower systemic absorption and may generate less microbial resistance.** Nitrofurantoin is an effective urinary prophylactic agent because its serum levels are low, its urinary levels are high, and it produces minimal effect on the fecal flora.

27. **c. delayed renal views 2 to 3 hours later may be needed.** Scans delayed 3 or more hours may help in differentiating renal abscess from hypofunctioning parenchyma in severe pyelonephritis.

113

Anomalies of the Upper Urinary Tract

STUART B. BAUER

QUESTIONS

1. "Potter facies" is a typical appearance for which kidney abnormality?
   a. Bilateral renal agenesis
   b. Unilateral renal agenesis
   c. Bilateral renal ectopia
   d. Horseshoe kidney
   e. Megacalycosis
2. Pulmonary development during gestation requires which factor for maturation?
   a. Surfactant
   b. Amniotic fluid
   c. Proline
   d. Acetylcholine
   e. Epinephrine
3. The absence of a kidney probably occurred during which week of development?
   a. Third week
   b. Fourth week
   c. Fifth week
   d. Seventh week
   e. Eighth week
4. In girls with unilateral renal agenesis, which condition is likely to be seen after the onset of puberty?
   a. Hydrocolpos
   b. Gartner's duct cyst
   c. Contralateral reflux
   d. Cystocele
   e. Ectopic pregnancy
5. Which of the following findings on a physical examination suggest unilateral renal agenesis?
   a. Absent testis
   b. Communicating hydrocele
   c. Undescended testis
   d. Absent vas
   e. Hypospadias
6. Renal ectopia is the result of abnormal migration of the metanephric tissue during which week of gestation?
   a. Fourth week
   b. Sixth week
   c. Eighth week
   d. Tenth week
   e. Twelfth week
7. Which of the following statements is TRUE regarding renal ectopia?
   a. Boys are more likely than girls to have an associated genital anomaly.
   b. The arterial tree to the ectopic kidney derives from its normal location.
   c. The ectopic kidney is more prone to disease than the normally positioned organ.
   d. Despite the ectopic kidney, the adrenal gland is usually in the normal location.
   e. The left colonic flexure does not reside in the renal fossa with a left ectopic kidney.
8. Which of the following statements is TRUE regarding horseshoe kidney?
   a. The two kidneys usually join at their superior poles.
   b. The isthmus functions almost as well as the remainder of the kidneys.
   c. The horseshoe kidneys are usually in their normal location.
   d. The majority of patients with Turner's syndrome have horseshoe kidneys.
   e. Patients with horseshoe kidneys rarely have other anomalies.
9. The most common tumor associated with a horseshoe kidney is:
   a. renal pelvic tumor.
   b. Wilms' tumor.
   c. renal cell carcinoma.
   d. neuroblastoma.
   e. transitional cell carcinoma of the bladder.
10. The posterior branch of the main renal artery supplies which segment of the kidney?
    a. Upper
    b. Middle
    c. Anterior
    d. Posterior
    e. Renal pelvis
11. Renal artery aneurysms should be excised if the patient exhibits each of the following characteristics EXCEPT:
    a. incomplete ring-like calcification.
    b. aneurysm greater than 2.5 cm.
    c. increase in size with time.
    d. postmenopause.
    e. hypertension.

12. Which of the following statements is TRUE with regard to calyceal diverticula?
    a. The diagnosis is best made by using renal ultrasonography.
    b. Diverticula tend to collect milk-of-calcium stones.
    c. The diverticula communicate with the renal pelvis.
    d. Vesicoureteral reflux is rarely associated with these diverticula.
    e. Calyceal diverticula begin as cysts and then rupture into the collecting system.

13. Megacalycosis has which of the following characteristics?
    a. This entity is more likely in females.
    b. It is associated with an increased number of calyces that are dilated.
    c. The ureter is usually dilated as well.
    d. It has an autosomal recessive pattern of inheritance.
    e. The renal scan reveals an obstructive pattern.

ANSWERS

1. **a. Bilateral renal agenesis.** Infants with bilateral renal agenesis generally look prematurely senile and have "a prominent fold of skin that begins over each eye, swings down in a semi-circle over the inner canthus and extends onto the cheek."
2. **c. Proline.** Hislop and colleagues in 1979 suggested that the anephric fetus fails to produce proline, which is needed for collagen formation in the bronchiolar tree. The kidney is the primary source of proline. Thus, pulmonary hypoplasia may result from absence of renal parenchyma and not from diminished amniotic fluid.
3. **b. Fourth week.** The abnormality most likely occurs no later than the fourth or fifth week of gestation.
4. **a. Hydrocolpos.** Obstruction of one side of a duplicated system is not uncommon, and unilateral hematocolpos or hydrocolpos has been described.
5. **d. Absent vas.** The diagnosis should be suspected during a physical examination when the vas deferens or body and tail of the epididymis are missing or when an absent, septate, or hypoplastic vagina is associated with a unicornuate or bicornuate uterus.
6. **c. Eighth week.** This process of migration and rotation is completed by the end of the eighth week of gestation.
7. **d. Despite the ectopic kidney, the adrenal gland is usually in the normal location.** Rarely, the adrenal gland is absent or is abnormally positioned.
8. **d. The majority of patients with Turner's syndrome have horseshoe kidneys.** Horseshoe kidney may also be seen in as many as 60% of female patients with Turner's syndrome.
9. **c. renal cell carcinoma.** One hundred fourteen cases of renal carcinoma within a horseshoe kidney have been reported; more than half of these cancers were hypernephromas.
10. **d. Posterior.** The main renal artery divides initially into anterior and posterior branches. The anterior branch almost always supplies the upper, middle, and lower segments of the kidney. The posterior branch invariably nourishes the posterior and lower segments.
11. **d. postmenopause.** Excision is recommended if (1) the hypertension cannot be easily controlled; (2) an incomplete ring-like calcification is present; (3) the aneurysm is larger than 2.5 cm; (4) the patient is female and likely to become pregnant because rupture during pregnancy is a likely possibility; (5) the aneurysm increases in size on serial angiograms; or (6) an arteriovenous fistula is present.
12. **b. Diverticula tend to collect milk-of-calcium stones.** Over time, these diverticula tend to progressively distend with trapped urine. Infection, milk-of-calcium stones, and true stone formation are complications of stasis or obstruction that can produce symptoms.
13. **b. It is associated with an increased number of calyces that are dilated.** Megacalycosis is best defined as nonobstructive enlargement of calyces because of malformation of the renal papillae. The calyces that are generally dilated may be increased in number. The ureteropelvic junction is normally funneled, without evidence of obstruction.

114

Renal Dysgenesis and Cystic Disease of the Kidney

KENNETH I. GLASSBERG

QUESTIONS

1. Which of the following is a correct match?
   a. Von Hippel-Lindau disease—adenoma sebaceum
   b. Tuberous sclerosis—angiomyolipoma
   c. Autosomal dominant polycystic kidney disease (ADPKD)—salt-losing nephropathy
   d. Congenital nephrosis (Finnish type)—medullary cysts
   e. Autosomal recessive polycystic kidney disease (ARPKD)—colonic diverticulosis
2. What is the most likely event to precede the development of renal cell carcinoma in von Hippel-Lindau disease?
   a. Hypertension
   b. Chronic renal failure
   c. Angiomyolipoma
   d. *VHL* gene heterozygosity loss
   e. Adenoma sebaceum
3. The development of acquired renal cystic disease (ARCD) is most related to which factor?
   a. Age of the patient
   b. Duration of renal failure
   c. Recent initiation of hemodialysis
   d. *Escherichia coli* infection
   e. Genetic defect on chromosome 16
4. Which of the following statements regarding ADPKD is most correct?
   a. Manifests with clinical symptoms in almost all patients possessing the genetic defect by age 40 years.
   b. Approximately 50% of patients have cysts by 30 years of age.
   c. Approximately 25% of offspring have the disease.
   d. Associated with a high incidence of diverticulosis and mitral valve prolapse.
   e. Associated with a high incidence of portal hypertension.
5. What is the characteristic ultrasonographic appearance of the bilateral kidneys in a newborn with ARPKD?
   a. Large kidneys with large cysts
   b. Large, homogeneous, hyperechogenic kidneys
   c. Large, homogeneous, hypoechoic kidneys
   d. Small kidneys with large cysts
   e. Small kidneys with absent pyramids
6. Which of the following statements is most correct about ADPKD?
   a. The genetic defect is located on chromosome 6.
   b. Most affected infants have congenital hepatic fibrosis.
   c. Renal cysts are infrequently seen on ultrasonographic scans of affected patients before 30 years of age.
   d. Glomerular cysts are sometimes found in the kidneys of newborns diagnosed with ADPKD.
   e. The incidence of renal cell carcinoma in ADPKD is twice that in the normal population.
7. All of the following conditions frequently have cysts with epithelial hyperplasia EXCEPT which one?
   a. Tuberous sclerosis
   b. Acquired renal cystic disease
   c. Simple cysts
   d. von Hippel-Lindau disease
   e. ADPKD
8. Which of the following statements is FALSE regarding unilateral multicystic dysplastic kidneys?
   a. The majority of multicystic dysplastic kidneys become smaller or sonographically undetectable with time.
   b. There is an absence of communication between cysts on ultrasonographic scans.
   c. Cysts are usually found in communication with each other when injected intracystically with contrast material.
   d. The sine qua non for diagnosis of a multicystic dysplastic kidney is the presence of primitive ducts.
   e. Multicystic dysplastic kidneys appear more often in females and more often on the right side.
9. Which signaling molecule is most likely responsible for inducing renal epithelial cells to align into simple tubules?
   a. p Wnt-11
   b. p Wnt-4
   c. p VHL
   d. GDNF (glial cell line–derived neurotrophic factor)
   e. PAX-2
10. Which gene is associated with a multiple malformation syndrome and clear cell renal cell carcinoma?
    a. *PDK1*
    b. *PDK2*
    c. *TG737*
    d. Wnt-2
    e. *VHL*

11. A benign multilocular cyst is seen most often:
    a. in males younger than 4 years of age and in females older than 30 years of age.
    b. in females younger than 4 years of age and in males older than 30 years of age.
    c. in males between 4 and 30 years of age.
    d. equally in both sexes before 4 years of age and in females after 30 years of age.
    e. equally in both sexes before 4 years of age and in males after 30 years of age.
12. Which of the following pairs of genes is an example of a contiguous gene syndrome?
    a. *TSC1* and *VHL*
    b. *TSC2* and *PKD1*
    c. *PKD2* and *TSC1*
    d. *VHL* and *PKD1*
    e. *TSC2* and *PKD2*
13. Unilateral renal cystic disease is:
    a. an autosomal polycystic kidney disease.
    b. an inherited disease.
    c. a condition associated with hemodialysis.
    d. multiple simple cysts clustered together.
    e. most often diagnosed in children.
14. A high-density lesion is recognized with a postcontrast CT scan. No precontrast record was obtained. To help diagnose this high-density lesion as a possible neoplasm versus a benign cyst, what should first be considered?
    a. Evaluating for further enhancement on a CT scan 15 to 30 minutes later
    b. Repeating the study without contrast enhancement at another visit
    c. Obtaining a renal angiogram
    d. Injecting a second bolus of contrast material
    e. Looking for de-enhancement on a CT scan 15 to 30 minutes later
15. A patient with which of the following entities has the highest likelihood of having a renal cell carcinoma develop?
    a. ADPKD
    b. Tuberous sclerosis
    c. von Hippel-Lindau disease
    d. Acquired renal cystic disease
    e. Medullary sponge kidney
16. What is the best study to help determine renal function when trying to differentiate severe hydronephrosis from multicystic renal dysplastic kidney?
    a. Dimercaptosuccinic acid (DMSA) renal scan
    b. Intravenous urogram
    c. Mercaptoacetyltriglycine (MAG3) renal scan
    d. Diethylenetriaminepentaacetic acid (DTPA) renal scan
    e. Furosemide (Lasix) washout renal scan
17. Which one of the following criteria helps confirm the diagnosis of unilateral renal cystic disease?
    a. Absence of contralateral renal cysts; siblings with similar findings.
    b. Absence of cysts in the contralateral kidney; absence of cysts in family members.
    c. Absence of cysts in the contralateral kidney; diffuse, noncontiguous unilateral renal cysts.
    d. Genetic linkage studies; gross hematuria.
    e. Hypertension; absence of contralateral renal cysts.
18. Renal sinus cysts are most likely derived from:
    a. vascular elements.
    b. renal parenchyma.
    c. renal pelvis.
    d. lymphatic system.
    e. nephrogenic rests.
19. Most simple renal cysts identified in utero represent:
    a. the first sign of a multicystic kidney.
    b. the first sign of ARPKD.
    c. the first sign of ADPKD.
    d. a calyceal diverticulum.
    e. resolve before birth.
20. Approximately what percentage of individuals older than 60 years will have an identifiable renal cyst by CT?
    a. 1% to 5%
    b. 10%
    c. 33%
    d. 75%
    e. 90%
21. Which term best describes an entity that appears with renal agenesis, renal dysplasia, or multicystic dysplasia and is seen in multiple family members?
    a. Oligomeganephronia
    b. Familial hypodysplasia
    c. Renal aplasia
    d. Familial adysplasia
    e. Mayer-Rokitansky-Küster-Hauser syndrome
22. Which of the following group of antibiotics includes the best choice for treating an infected renal cyst in a patient with ADPKD?
    a. Trimethoprim-sulfamethoxazole, chloramphenicol, fluoroquinolones
    b. Cephalosporins, trimethoprim-sulfamethoxazole, doxycycline
    c. Gentamicin, cephalosporins, vancomycin
    d. Fluoroquinolones, metronidazole (Flagyl), vancomycin
    e. Doxycycline, amoxicillin, gentamicin
23. In what is laparoscopic unroofing of renal cysts in patients with ADPKD most useful?
    a. Managing hypertension
    b. Improving renal function
    c. Relieving pain
    d. Treating an infected cyst
    e. Diagnosing disease
24. In neonates with a unilateral multicystic kidney, what is the incidence of contralateral vesicoureteral reflux?
    a. 0% to 7%
    b. 18% to 43%
    c. 50% to 67%
    d. 75%
    e. 7% to 15%
25. What consequence does the identification of the defective *VHL* gene have?
    a. One has to screen all siblings with an ophthalmologic examination.
    b. One has to obtain renal sonographic monitoring of those with a defect in both VHL genes.
    c. Follow-up of siblings has not changed.
    d. The incidence of angiomyolipoma can more readily be determined.
    e. Only those siblings identified with the gene defect require routine screening and follow-up.

26. What is the most likely cause of loin pain and hematuria in a 50-year-old patient with end-stage renal disease who has been undergoing dialysis for 5 years?
    a. Acute renal vein thrombosis
    b. Acute renal artery thrombosis
    c. Renal cell carcinoma
    d. ARCD
    e. Uric acid stones
27. When patients with ARCD undergo renal transplantation, what happens?
    a. The cysts usually continue to grow.
    b. The cysts usually get smaller, and the risk of renal cell carcinoma dramatically falls.
    c. The cysts usually get smaller, but a significant risk for renal cell carcinoma persists.
    d. There is a significantly increased incidence of hematuria.
    e. The cysts calcify.
28. Major theories on the etiology of cyst development in ADPKD include which one of the following?
    a. Calcification of tubular basement membrane
    b. Increased number of epidermal growth factor receptors at the base (i.e., nonluminal side) of renal tubular epithelial cells
    c. Increased apoptosis of renal tubular cells
    d. Apical (i.e., luminal side) location of Na^+, K^+-ATPase and epidermal growth factor receptors in renal tubular epithelial cells
    e. Fusion of podocytes
29. What is the main difference between a newborn with ADPKD with glomerular cysts and a newborn with sporadic glomerulocystic kidney disease?
    a. Absence of biliary dysgenesis in ADPKD
    b. Retinal angiomas in sporadic glomerulocystic disease
    c. Presence of liver cysts in ADPKD
    d. Presence of more severely compromised kidneys in ADPKD
    e. Absence of affected family members in sporadic glomerulocystic disease
30. Which group of three findings best describes the typical ultrasonographic image of a multicystic dysplastic kidney?
    a. The cysts are organized around a central large cyst; there is no identifiable renal sinus; there are communications between the cysts.
    b. The cysts have a haphazard distribution; there is absence of a central or medial large cyst; there are no obvious communications between the cysts.
    c. The cysts have a haphazard distribution; there is no obvious renal sinus; there is a large central cyst.
    d. Connections exist between the cysts; a medial cyst is present; a renal sinus is usually present.
    e. The cysts are organized at the periphery; the largest is the central one; there is an identifiable renal sinus.
31. The Mayer-Rokitansky-Küster-Hauser syndrome refers to which group of associated findings?
    a. Wilms' tumor, nephrotic syndrome, ambiguous genitalia
    b. Caudad ureteric budding, lateral orifice position, lower pole dysplasia
    c. Hypertension, vesicoureteral reflux, deep cortical depression over an area of the kidney with "thyroidization" of tubules
    d. Bilateral renal agenesis, respiratory failure, oligohydramnios
    e. Unilateral renal agenesis or renal ectopia, ipsilateral müllerian defects, vaginal agenesis
32. Which one of the following conditions is most representative of a neoplastic growth?
    a. Benign multilocular cyst
    b. Oligomeganephronia
    c. Multicystic dysplastic kidney
    d. Calyceal diverticulum
    e. Ask-Upmark kidney
33. Which of the following is the best match?
    a. ARPKD—congenital hepatic fibrosis
    b. Medullary sponge kidney—predominance of glomerular cysts
    c. Juvenile nephronophthisis—cortical cysts
    d. Ask-Upmark kidney—hypotension
    e. von-Hippel-Lindau disease—adenoma sebaceum
34. Which of the following matches is correct?
    a. ARPKD—chromosome 2
    b. ADPKD—chromosomes 4 and 16
    c. Tuberous sclerosis— chromosomes 9 and 15
    d. von Hippel-Lindau disease—chromosome 4
    e. Juvenile nephronophthisis—chromosome 6
35. A renal cyst with increased number of septa and prominent calcification in a nonenhancing cyst wall does not require exploration. According to the Bosniak grading system this cyst would be categorized as:
    a. I
    b. II
    c. II F
    d. III
    e. IV

ANSWERS

1. **b. Tuberous sclerosis—angiomyolipoma.** Angiomyolipomas occur in 40% to 80% of patients.
2. **d. *VHL* gene heterozygosity loss.** In kidney cells of individuals with von Hippel-Lindau disease, for example, once the wild-type allele mutates, heterozygosity is lost and there is a propensity to develop a clear cell renal cell carcinoma.
3. **b. Duration of renal failure.** At first, ARCD was thought to be confined to patients receiving hemodialysis. However, it shortly became apparent that the disorder is almost as common in patients receiving peritoneal dialysis and that it may develop in patients with chronic renal failure who are being managed medically without any type of dialysis. Thus, ARCD appears to be a feature of end-stage kidney disease rather than a response to dialysis.
4. **d. Associated with a high incidence of diverticulosis and mitral valve prolapse.** A number of associated anomalies are common: cysts of the liver, pancreas, spleen, and lungs; aneurysms of the circle of Willis (berry aneurysms); colonic diverticula; and mitral valve prolapse.

5. **b. Large, homogeneous, hyperechogenic kidneys.** Sonography identifies very enlarged, homogeneously hyperechogenic kidneys, especially compared with the echogenicity of the liver. The increased echogenicity is a result of the return of sound waves from the enormous number of interfaces created by tightly compacted, dilated collecting ducts.

6. **d. Glomerular cysts are sometimes found in the kidneys of newborns diagnosed with ADPKD.** A variant form of ADPKD probably exists in which the renal cysts are located primarily in Bowman's space. One cytogenetic study provided evidence that such a condition is a form of ADPKD. The authors found that a fetus with cystic disease predominantly of the glomeruli had the same genetic linkages on chromosome 16 as did its ADPKD-affected mother. Another study suggested that glomerulocystic kidneys in members of families with ADPKD are variants; the glomerular cysts may be an early stage of polycystic kidney disease gene expression.

7. **c. Simple cysts.** That the incidence of renal cell carcinoma is not increased in ADPKD is also surprising in view of the frequent finding of epithelial hyperplasia. For example, two other conditions, tuberous sclerosis and von Hippel-Lindau disease, are associated with epithelial hyperplasia. The cyst lining is a single layer of flattened or cuboidal epithelium. The hyperplastic lining in the cyst is thought by some workers to be a precursor of renal tumors.

8. **e. Multicystic dysplastic kidneys appear more often in females and more often on the right side.** At any age, the condition is more likely to be found on the left. Males are more likely to have unilateral multicystic dysplastic kidneys (2.4:1).

9. **b. p Wnt-4.** Wnt-4 stimulates transcription processes within epithelial cells as well as the development of cell adhesion molecules, which allow the kidney epithelial cells to adhere to one another in such a manner as to take on the shape of a tubule.

10. **e. *VHL*.** The gene associated with the transmission of von Hippel-Lindau disease is located on chromosome 3. In non–von Hippel-Lindau patients with sporadic clear cell renal cell carcinoma, 50% of cell lines are associated with a mutational form of the *VHL* gene.

11. **a. in males younger than 4 years of age and in females older than 30 years of age.** The great majority of patients present before the age of 4 years or after the age of 30 years. Five percent present between 4 and 30 years of age. The patient is twice as likely to be male if younger than 4 years and eight times as likely to be female if older than 30 years of age.

12. **b. *TSC2* and *PKD1*.** When severe polycystic kidneys are present in patients, particularly infants with tuberous sclerosis, they likely represent a contiguous gene syndrome, that is, defects in both *TSC2* and *PKD1*.

13. **d. multiple simple cysts clustered together.** Large renal cysts of varying size appearing side by side, often more numerous at one pole, have been referred to as unilateral renal cystic disease. Because the entity seems to represent nothing more than multiple simple cysts lying side by side within a kidney, for the present the author prefers to include it as a variation of the presentation of simple cysts.

14. **e. Looking for de-enhancement on a CT scan 15 to 30 minutes later.** Occasionally, a high-density (>30 HU), well-marginated lesion may be noticed on a postcontrast CT scan when no record of density of the previously unrecognized lesion was obtained. In such situations, one can look for "de-enhancement," a finding that occurs after the initial flow of contrast material to an organ and that offers proof of vascularity—that is, neoplasm. One study found 15 minutes to be a sufficient period of delay to detect de-enhancement. If there is still a question of de-enhancement, the patient can be taken off the table and returned 30 or more minutes later.

15. **c. von Hippel-Lindau disease.** Tuberous sclerosis and von Hippel-Lindau disease are associated with epithelial hyperplasia (and adenomas as well) and have an increased incidence of renal cell carcinoma (tuberous sclerosis, 2%, and von Hippel-Lindau disease, 35% to 38%).

16. **a. Dimercaptosuccinic acid (DMSA) renal scan.** In these difficult cases, radioisotope studies may be helpful. Hydronephrotic kidneys generally show some function on a DMSA scan, whereas renal concentration is seldom seen with multicystic kidneys.

17. **b. Absence of cysts in the contralateral kidney; absence of cysts in family members.** Such a diagnosis requires long-term follow-up demonstrating absence of cyst development in the contralateral kidney and no family members with cystic disease.

18. **d. lymphatic system.** The predominant type of renal sinus cyst appears to be one derived from the lymphatics.

19. **e. resolve before birth.** In 28 of 11,000 fetuses with renal cysts, 25 fetuses had the cysts resolve before birth. Of two cysts that remained postnatally, in one it was the first sign of a multicystic kidney.

20. **c. 33%.** In adults, the frequency of renal cyst occurrence increases with age. Using CT, one group demonstrated a 20% incidence of cysts by 40 years of age and approximately 33% incidence of cysts after 60 years of age.

21. **d. Familial adysplasia.** Renal agenesis, renal dysplasia, multicystic dysplasia, and renal aplasia usually appear as isolated sporadic occurrences. On rare occasions, this group of anomalies may appear in many family members, but heterogeneously. In other words, one family member may have renal agenesis whereas another has renal dysplasia and still another has a multicystic dysplastic or aplastic kidney. When all or part of this group of anomalies is seen in one family, an encompassing term for these four entities is used: familial renal adysplasia.

22. **a. Trimethoprim-sulfamethoxazole, chloramphenicol, fluoroquinolones.** In the experience of one group of researchers, the only dependable antibiotics were those that were lipid soluble, namely, trimethoprim-sulfamethoxazole and chloramphenicol. Chloramphenicol produced better results. The fluoroquinolones, which are also lipid soluble, are proving useful. If a patient with suspected pyelonephritis does not respond to an antibiotic and if the antibiotic used is not lipid soluble, one must consider whether the infection may be present in a noncommunicating cyst.

23. **c. Relieving pain.** At a mean follow-up of 2.2 years, subjective pain was reduced by 62% in 11 of 15 patients, and those who had bilateral unroofing faired better. The remaining 4 had less impressive results. Unfortunately, the effect of laparoscopic unroofing in those with hypertension was quite variable.

24. **b. 18% to 43%.** Contralateral vesicoureteral reflux is seen even more often than contralateral ureteropelvic junction obstruction, being identified in 18% to 43% of infants.

25. **e. Only those siblings identified with the gene defect require routine screening and follow-up.** Recommendations by Levine and colleagues published in 1990 for all asymptomatic relatives now apply only to those with genetic evidence of the disease.

26. **d. ARCD.** The most common presentation of ARCD is loin pain, hematuria, or both. Bleeding occurs in as many as 50% of patients.

27. **c. The cysts usually get smaller, but a significant risk for renal cell carcinoma persists.** A number of investigators have found that the cysts of ARCD regress after renal transplantation

(see Fig. 114-32). One study found improvement in the number and size of cysts in 16 of 25 (64%) ARCD patients 1 year after transplantation. Therefore, it was considered that the incidence of renal cell carcinoma might fall after transplantation as well. However, another group found that although the majority of cysts either disappear or become smaller, 18% of patients develop new cysts after transplantation, and a more recent report of four cases of renal carcinoma occurring in the native kidney 3 to 8 years after transplantation suggested that the risk of carcinoma does not lessen after transplantation. In a different series of 96 transplant patients, renal cell carcinoma had developed in 6 patients and 5 of the 6 had associated ARCD. The authors suggested that the malignant potential of ARCD persists for many years after transplantation. They also found a higher incidence of renal cell carcinoma in older transplant patients and in men. We must keep in mind that although the native kidneys may become smaller after transplantation and although the cysts may disappear from view on ultrasonographic follow-up, it does not necessarily mean that the cells that previously surrounded these cysts have disappeared.

28. **d. Apical (i.e., luminal side) location of Na^+, K^+-ATPase and epidermal growth factor receptors in renal tubular epithelial cells.** The receptors for epidermal growth factor have been identified ectopically on the apical side of cells adjacent to the cyst fluid. Na^+, K^+-ATPase in polycystic epithelial cells was located in the apical position in cells lining the cyst rather than in the usual basolateral position. If this is the case, fluid would preferably enter the cyst lumen rather than leave it.

29. **e. Absence of affected family members in sporadic glomerulocystic disease.** ADPKD should not be referred to as glomerulocystic kidney disease to avoid confusing it with sporadic glomerulocystic kidney disease, a condition that seems to be histologically identical to ADPKD in infants except for the absence of affected family members.

30. **b. The cysts have a haphazard distribution; there is absence of a central or medial large cyst; there are no obvious communications between the cysts.** Renal masses in infants most often represent either multicystic kidney disease or hydronephrosis, and it is important to distinguish the two, especially if the surgeon wishes to remove a nonfunctioning hydronephrotic kidney or repair a ureteropelvic junction obstruction while leaving a multicystic organ in situ. In newborns, ultrasonography is generally the first study performed. In a few cases, it is difficult to distinguish multicystic kidney disease from severe hydronephrosis. In general, however, the multicystic kidney has a haphazard distribution of cysts of various sizes without a larger central or medial cyst and without visible communications between the cysts. Frequently, very small cysts appear in between the large cysts. In comparison, in ureteropelvic junction obstruction, the cysts or calyces are organized around the periphery of the kidney, connections can usually be demonstrated between the peripheral cysts and a central or medial cyst that represents the renal pelvis, and there is absence of small cysts between the larger cysts (see Fig. 114-20). When there is an identifiable renal sinus, the diagnosis is more likely to be hydronephrosis than multicystic kidney.

31. **e. Unilateral renal agenesis or renal ectopia, ipsilateral müllerian defects, vaginal agenesis.** The term *Mayer-Rokitansky-Küster-Hauser syndrome* refers to a group of associated findings that include unilateral renal agenesis or renal ectopia, ipsilateral müllerian defects, and vaginal agenesis. *Drash syndrome* includes Wilms' tumor, nephrotic syndrome, and ambiguous genitalia; the findings of caudad ureteric budding, lateral orifice position, and lower pole dysplasia follow *the bud theory;* the grouping of hypertension, vesicoureteral reflux, and deep cortical depression over an area of the kidney with "thyroidization" of tubules defines the *Ask-Upmark kidney;* and the grouping of bilateral renal agenesis, respiratory failure, and oligohydramnios can lead the fetus to be born with *Potter's syndrome* and *Potter facies.*

32. **a. Benign multilocular cyst.** For the benign multilocular cystic lesion, certain authors prefer the term *cystic nephroma* because this term implies a benign but neoplastic lesion.

33. **a. ARPKD—congenital hepatic fibrosis.** All patients with ARPKD have varying degrees of congenital hepatic fibrosis.

34. **b. ADPKD—chromosomes 4 and 16.** For the genetic cystic disease ADPKD, the chromosomal defect is on chromosome 16 for *PKD1* and 4 for *PKD2; PKD3* has not been mapped. Autosomal recessive polycystic kidney disease involves chromosome 6; tuberous sclerosis involves chromosomes 9 and 16; von Hippel-Lindau disease involves chromosome 3; and juvenile nephronophthisis involves chromosome 2.

35. **c. II F.** The Bosniak classification has recently been updated to include category II F as defined in the answer.

115

Anomalies and Surgery of the Ureteropelvic Junction in Children

MICHAEL C. CARR • ALAA EL-GHONEIMI

QUESTIONS

1. Obstruction at the ureteropelvic junction (UPJ) can be due to all of the following EXCEPT:
   a. interruptions in development of circular musculature.
   b. persistent fetal convolutions.
   c. Ostling's folds.
   d. upper ureteral polyps.
   e. lower pole crossing vessels.
2. The surgical approach that is most likely to improve a secondary UPJ obstruction is:
   a. retrograde endopyelotomy (Acucise).
   b. dismembered pyeloplasty.
   c. extravesical ureteral reimplantation.
   d. endoscopic approach (Deflux) to the refluxing ureter.
   e. antegrade endopyelotomy.
3. Congenital malformations seen in association with UPJ obstructions include all of the following EXCEPT:
   a. contralateral UPJ.
   b. multicystic dysplastic kidney.
   c. renal agenesis.
   d. renal dysplasia.
   e. autosomal dominant polycystic kidney disease.
4. Which radiographic modality provides the most useful information to assess a UPJ obstruction?
   a. Renal ultrasonography
   b. Intravenous urography
   c. Mercaptoacetyltriglycine (MAG3)-furosemide (Lasix) renography
   d. Nuclear voiding cystourethrography
   e. Doppler ultrasonography
5. Variables that have been shown to affect washout of the renal pelvis after furosemide administration include all of the following EXCEPT:
   a. hydrational status.
   b. timing of furosemide administration.
   c. size of renal pelvis.
   d. drainage of the bladder.
   e. radionuclide agent.
6. Magnetic resonance urography provides information about all of the following issues EXCEPT:
   a. differential renal function.
   b. anatomic imaging comparable to intravenous urography.
   c. washout curve after furosemide administration.
   d. renal transit time.
   e. visualization of cortical and medullary phases after administration of gadolinium-enhanced DTPA.
7. Which surgical repair for UPJ obstruction yields the greatest likelihood of success if there is a long segment of ureteral stenosis?
   a. Dismembered pyeloplasty
   b. Endopyelotomy
   c. Laparoscopic Anderson-Hynes pyeloplasty
   d. Spiral flap (Culp-deWeerd) pyeloplasty
   e. Davis intubated ureterotomy
8. The key steps in performing a dismembered pyeloplasty include all of the following EXCEPT:
   a. spatulating the ureter on the lateral margin an adequate distance.
   b. excising as much redundant renal pelvis as possible.
   c. ensuring that a tension-free anastomosis exists.
   d. placing a feeding tube into the ureter during the suturing of the anastomosis.
   e. placing a Penrose drain adjacent to the repair.
9. The laparoscopic approach for the repair of a UPJ obstruction includes all of the following benefits EXCEPT:
   a. mean hospital stay less than with conventional open pyeloplasty.
   b. exclusively via the retroperitoneum or transperitonally.
   c. less analgesia than with conventional pyeloplasty.
   d. repair without internal (JJ) stenting.
   e. improved cosmesis.
10. Surgical options in the repair of a failed pyeloplasty include all of the following EXCEPT:
    a. endopyelotomy.
    b. ureterocalicostomy.
    c. redo pyeloplasty.
    d. transureteroureterostomy.
    e. nephrectomy.

ANSWERS

1. **c. Ostling's folds.** Ostling's folds are now considered folds that are not obstructive and disappear with linear growth. They are rarely seen in an older child.
2. **b. dismembered pyeloplasty.** In the face of a secondary UPJ obstruction, the obstructive lesion needs to be corrected initially, which could best be accomplished with a dismembered pyeloplasty. The success rate of a dismembered pyeloplasty is greater than that of an antegrade or retrograde endopyelotomy, and correcting the reflux alone may not alter the pathophysiology at the UPJ. A pyeloplasty can be done in conjunction with an endoscopic approach to the refluxing ureter, which should alleviate both the obstructive component as well as the refluxing component.
3. **e. autosomal dominant polycystic kidney disease.** UPJ obstruction is the most common anomaly encountered in the opposite kidney; it occurs in 10% to 40% of cases. Renal dysplasia and multicystic dysplastic kidney are the next most frequently observed contralateral lesions. In addition, unilateral renal agenesis has been noted in almost 5% of children.
4. **c. Mercaptoacetyltriglycine (MAG3)-furosemide (Lasix) renography.** Intravenous urography was previously the primary radiographic study used to define UPJ obstruction. In most institutions, this has been supplanted with radionuclide renography, because this study can provide differential renal function and an assessment of washout from the individual kidney.
5. **e. radionuclide agent.** A number of parameters have been shown to effect the washout after furosemide administration, including such factors as renal maturation, body proportion, differential renal function, pelvic capacity, tubular reabsorption, timing and effect of the diuretic, drainage from the bladder, and hydrational status of the patient. Various radionuclide agents have been used in the past, including Hippurate, DTPA, and, most recently, mercaptoacetyltriglycine (MAG3), which is cleared by the kidneys by secretion in the proximal tubules with a higher extraction fraction than DTPA. This provides an improved background ratio and a good image quality, but the choice of the agent will not affect the washout.
6. **c. washout curve after furosemide administration.** Magnetic resonance urography holds the promise of supplanting radionuclide renography but as yet there is no way to determine washout after furosemide administration. Renal transit time has been substituted for the half-life time after furosemide administration and seems to correlate with this parameter.
7. **d. spiral flap (Culp-deWeerd) pyeloplasty.** The Culp-deWeerd spiral flap is created from the renal pelvis and is used to repair the defect at the UPJ. Such a flap is able to bridge the gap between the pelvis and healthy ureter over a distance of several centimeters.
8. **b. excising as much redundant renal pelvis as possible.** The portion of pelvis is excised and is generally a diamond-shaped segment that is present within the traction sutures that were placed in the renal pelvis. It is better to leave too much renal pelvis than too little, especially when resecting along the medial aspect of the renal pelvis. Infundibula can be encountered if one is not careful.
9. **d. repair without internal** (JJ) **stenting.** Laparoscopic pyeloplasties have not yet been performed without the use of internal stenting, which either necessitates a subsequent brief anesthetic procedure to remove the double-J stent or the placement of an internal-external stent that does not require subsequent removal in the operating room.
10. **d. transureteroureterostomy.** Lack of drainage for a prolonged period would necessitate further intervention, including an endopyelotomy, redo pyeloplasty, or even ureterocalicostomy.

116

Ectopic Ureter, Ureterocele, and Other Anomalies of the Ureter

RICHARD N. SCHLUSSEL • ALAN B. RETIK

QUESTIONS

1. All of the following are possible drainage sites for an ectopic ureter in a female EXCEPT which one?
   a. Fallopian tube
   b. Uterus
   c. Ovary
   d. Vagina
2. Inadequate interaction between the ureteral bud and metanephric blastema will most likely lead to which of the following conditions?
   a. Dysplasia
   b. Hydronephrosis
   c. Reflux
   d. Ureteral ectopia
3. How is the relationship between the upper and lower pole orifices in a complete ureteral duplication best described? The upper pole:
   a. orifice is cephalad and lateral to the lower orifice.
   b. ureter joins the lower pole ureter just before entry into the bladder.
   c. orifice is caudal and medial to the lower pole orifice.
   d. orifice and lower pole orifice sit transversely side by side.
4. All of the following are contribute to vesicoureteral reflux EXCEPT:
   a. lateral ureteral insertion.
   b. lax bladder neck.
   c. poorly developed trigone.
   d. gaping ureteral orifice.
5. What is the most common site of drainage of an ectopic ureter in a male?
   a. Vas deferens
   b. Anterior urethra
   c. Seminal vesicle
   d. Posterior urethra
6. Which voiding pattern is most often seen in a girl with an ectopic ureter?
   a. Urge incontinence
   b. Stress incontinence
   c. Continuous incontinence
   d. Interrupted urinary stream
7. Which of the following findings is most likely present on an excretory urogram in a patient with an ectopic ureter in a duplicated system?
   a. Nonvisualization of the lower pole of the kidney
   b. Medially displaced lower pole of the kidney
   c. Filling defect in the bladder
   d. Tortuous lower pole ureter
8. Which of the following anatomic derangements will NOT be seen in a patient with single-system ectopic ureters?
   a. Poorly developed bladder neck
   b. Decreased bladder capacity
   c. Hutch diverticulum
   d. Trigone underdevelopment
9. Ureteroceles are most often associated with all of the following EXCEPT:
   a. smoking during pregnancy.
   b. white race.
   c. female gender.
   d. duplicated kidneys.
10. All of the following can be caused by a ureterocele. Which is the least likely?
    a. Bladder outlet obstruction
    b. Upper pole obstruction
    c. Ipsilateral lower pole reflux
    d. Contralateral reflux
11. Which cystographic finding is most likely seen in a child with a ureterocele?
    a. Ureterocele eversion
    b. Reflux
    c. Midline filling defect
    d. Bilateral ureteroceles
12. A girl undergoes open resection of a large ectopic ureterocele. After removal of the catheter, she has high postvoid residuals demonstrated on a sonogram. Which complication is most likely responsible?
    a. Persistent reflux
    b. Residual flap of the ureterocele in the urethra
    c. Neurapraxia secondary to bladder retraction
    d. Excessive buttressing of deficient detrusor at the bladder neck

13. What is the preferred method of endoscopic treatment of a ureterocele?
    a. Resection of the roof of the ureterocele
    b. Puncture of the ureterocele's urethral extension
    c. Puncture of the roof of the ureterocele
    d. Transverse incision at the base of the ureterocele
14. An adult is evaluated as a possible kidney donor. An excretory urogram demonstrates a round contrast agent–filled area at the bladder base with a thin radiolucent rim around it. What is the most likely finding?
    a. Single-system kidney
    b. Marked opacification delay of the kidney
    c. Extension of a ureterocele to the bladder neck and urethra
    d. Reflux
15. A white infant is found to have a smooth interlabial mass on the posterior aspect of the urethra. What would be the most appropriate initial management?
    a. Chemotherapy
    b. Puncture of the mass
    c. Topical estrogen cream
    d. Observation
16. Which of the following areas of the ureter is least prone to stenosis?
    a. Immediately proximal to the ureterovesical junction
    b. At the level of the pelvic brim
    c. At the ureteropelvic junction
    d. All are equal in incidence
17. Which of the following statements is TRUE regarding ureteral duplications?
    a. The right side predominates.
    b. The left side predominates.
    c. Unilateral duplications outnumber bilateral duplications by a 6:1 ratio.
    d. Most commonly they have associated upper pole obstruction.
18. Which of the following statements regarding duplex kidneys is TRUE?
    a. Duplex kidneys are the same size as single-system kidneys.
    b. The upper pole moiety is the more likely of the two to have a ureteropelvic junction obstruction.
    c. The duplex kidney arises as a consequence of two separate ureteric buds.
    d. The duplex kidney arises as a consequence of two separate metanephric blastemal entities arising near the mesonephric duct.
19. Anastomosis of an upper pole and lower pole ureter should NOT be done at the distal segments because of:
    a. injury to the ureteral nerve supply.
    b. to-and-fro peristalsis of urine into the bifid ureters.
    c. injury to the adjacent vas deferens.
    d. vesicoureteral reflux.
20. Which of the following abnormalities is associated with inverted-Y ureteral duplications?
    a. Urachal abnormalities
    b. Ectopic ureters
    c. Horseshoe kidneys
    d. Posterior urethral valves
21. What is the most common form of ureteral triplication?
    a. All three ureters joining to terminate in a single bladder orifice
    b. Three ureters joining to form two ureteral orifices
    c. Three ureters draining as three separate orifices
    d. One of the three ureters terminating ectopically, the other two draining orthotopically
22. Which of the following ureters is involved in preureteral vena cava and at which level?
    a. Right ureter at level L3-L4
    b. Right ureter at level L1
    c. Left ureter at level L3-L4
    d. Left ureter at level L1
23. Failure of atrophy of which vein leads to the formation of a preureteral vena cava?
    a. Posterior cardinal vein
    b. Subcardinal vein
    c. Supracardinal vein
    d. Umbilical artery
24. Which of the following types of ureterocele is associated with the lowest incidence of secondary procedures after endoscopic treatment?
    a. Ectopic ureterocele
    b. Ureterocele in a female patient
    c. Intravesical ureterocele
    d. Ureterocele associated with a duplicated system
25. What is the most common method of presentation of a ureterocele?
    a. Incontinence
    b. Urinary tract infection
    c. Failure to thrive
    d. Stranguria
26. In what percentage of cases is reflux associated with a ureterocele?
    a. 10% to 25%
    b. 25% to 40%
    c. 50% to 65%
    d. 65% to 80%
27. A patient with a suspected ectopic ureter has a renal moiety that is difficult to visualize on an ultrasonographic study. Which of the following tests is a sensitive method of detecting this moiety?
    a. Diethylenetriaminepentaacetic acid (DTPA) renal scanning
    b. MRI of the abdomen and pelvis
    c. Nuclear voiding cystourethrography
    d. Positron emission tomography
28. Voiding cystourethrography is performed on a patient with a known ureterocele. Which of the following images will most likely fail to depict the ureterocele?
    a. Beginning of the first cycle of filling
    b. Beginning of the second cycle of filling
    c. The lateral image
    d. Bladder filled to capacity

29. Which of the following factors is most likely associated with the need for a second operative procedure in ectopic ureteroceles?
    a. Single-system ureterocele
    b. Male sex
    c. Left-sided position
    d. Preoperative high-grade reflux

30. What is the incidence of reflux into a ureterocele after its endoscopic incision?
    a. 10%
    b. 30%
    c. 65%
    d. 90%

ANSWERS

1. **c. Ovary.** An ectopic ureter draining into any of the female structures can rupture into the adjoining fallopian tube, uterus, upper vagina, or vestibule.
2. **a. Dysplasia.** These clinical and experimental observations combine to support the commonly held notion that dysplasia is the product of inadequate ureteric bud-to-blastema interaction.
3. **c. orifice is caudal and medial to the lower pole orifice.** The lower pole orifice is more cranial and lateral to the caudad medial upper pole orifice.
4. **b. lax bladder neck.** It is owing to the combined effects of the lateral ureteral orifice position, the ureter's shortened submucosal course, the poorly developed trigone, and the abnormal morphology of the ureteral orifice that primary vesicoureteral reflux develops.
5. **d. Posterior urethra.** In the male, the posterior urethra is the most common site of the termination of the ectopic ureter.
6. **c. Continuous incontinence.** Continuous incontinence in a girl with an otherwise normal voiding pattern after toilet training is the classic symptom of an ectopic ureteral orifice.
7. **d. Tortuous lower pole ureter.** The upper pole displaces the lower pole downward and outward, the so-called drooping lily appearance. When the upper pole does not excrete contrast material and make the duplicated system readily apparent, there are several other clues to suggest that a duplicated system is present. First, the calyces of a lower pole are fewer in number than in the normal kidney. Second, the axis of the lowest to uppermost calyx does not point toward the midline. Third, the uppermost calyx of the lower pole unit is usually farther from the upper pole border than is the lowest calyx from the corresponding lower pole limit. In addition, the lower pole pelvis and the upper portion of its ureter may be farther from the spine than on the contralateral side, and the lower pole ureter may also be scalloped and tortuous secondary to its wrapping around a markedly dilated upper pole ureter (similar to the findings of upper pole hydroureteronephrosis seen in the child with a ureterocele in Fig. 116-30).
8. **c. Hutch diverticulum.** Because there is no formation of the trigone and base plate, a very wide, poorly defined, incompetent vesical neck results. In rare instances, bilateral single ectopic ureters are associated with agenesis of the bladder and urethra. This condition is usually, but not always, incompatible with life. Commonly, the involved kidneys are dysplastic or display varying degrees of hydronephrosis (see Fig. 116-23). The ureters are usually dilated, and reflux is often present. The bladder neck is incompetent; therefore, the child dribbles continuously. Because there is poor resistance, the bladder does not have the opportunity to distend with urine and therefore has a small capacity (see Fig. 116-24).
9. **a. smoking during pregnancy.** They occur most frequently in females (4:1 ratio) and almost exclusively in whites. Approximately 10% are bilateral. Eighty percent of all ureteroceles arise from the upper poles of duplicated systems.
10. **a. Bladder outlet obstruction.** Ultrasonographic study shows a dilated ureter emanating from a hydronephrotic upper pole (see Fig. 116-26). This finding should signal the examiner to image the bladder to determine whether a ureterocele is present. If the lower pole is associated with reflux, or if the ureterocele has caused delayed emptying from the ipsilateral lower pole, this lower pole may likewise be hydronephrotic. Similarly, the ureterocele may impinge on the contralateral ureteral orifice or obstruct the bladder neck and cause hydronephrosis in the opposite kidney. The upper pole parenchyma drained by the ureterocele will exhibit varying degrees of thickness and echogenicity. Increased echogenicity correlates with dysplastic changes. The bladder frequently displays a thin-walled cyst that is the ureterocele (see Fig. 116-27). Reflux may also be seen in the contralateral system if the ureterocele is large enough to distort the trigone and the opposite ureteral submucosal tunnel. In one series, 35 of 127 patients (28%) had reflux in the contralateral unit.
11. **b. Reflux.** Voiding cystourethrography can demonstrate the size and location of the ureterocele as well as the presence or absence of vesicoureteral reflux. Assessing the severity of such reflux is crucial to future management. Reflux into the ipsilateral lower pole is common.
12. **b. Residual flap of the ureterocele in the urethra.** The authors of one study emphasized the need for passing a large catheter antegrade through the bladder neck to ascertain that all mucosal lips that might act as obstructing valves have been removed.
13. **d. Transverse incision at the base of the ureterocele.** Our preferred method of incising the ureterocele is similar to the one described by Rich and colleagues in 1990, that is, a transverse incision through the full thickness of the ureterocele wall using the cutting current. Making the incision as distally on the ureterocele and as close to the bladder floor as possible lessens the chance of postoperative reflux into the ureterocele.
14. **a. Single-system kidney.** Excretory urography often demonstrates the characteristic cobra-head (or spring-onion) deformity: an area of increased density similar to the head of a cobra with a halo or less dense shadow around it (see Fig. 116-39). The halo represents a filling defect, which is the ureterocele wall, and the oval density is contrast material excreted into the ureterocele from the functioning kidney.
15. **b. Puncture of the mass.** A ureterocele that extends through the bladder neck and the urethra and presents as a vaginal mass in girls is termed a *prolapsing ureterocele*. This mass can be distinguished from other interlabial masses (e.g., rhabdomyosarcoma, urethral prolapse, hydrometrocolpos, and periurethral cysts) by virtue of its appearance and location. The prolapsed ureterocele has a smooth round wall, as compared with the grapelike cluster that typifies rhabdomyosarcoma (see Fig. 116-25). The color may vary from pink to bright red to the necrotic shades of blue, purple, or brown. The ureterocele usually slides down the posterior wall of the urethra and, hence, the urethra can be demonstrated anterior to the mass and can be catheterized. The short-term goal is to decompress the ureterocele. The prolapsing ureterocele may be

manually reduced back into the bladder; however, even if this is successful, the prolapse is likely to recur. Upper pole nephrectomy (as previously described) combined with aspiration of the ureterocele from above is usually effective in achieving decompression.

16. **b. At the level of the pelvic brim.** Three areas of the ureter are particularly liable to ureteral stenosis. They are, in order of decreasing frequency, the distal ureter just above the extravesical junction, the ureteropelvic junction, and, rarely, the mid ureter at the pelvic brim.
17. **c. Unilateral duplications outnumber bilateral duplications by a 6:1 ratio.** Unilateral duplication occurs about six times more often than bilateral duplication, with the right and left sides being involved about equally.
18. **c. The duplex kidney arises as a consequence of two separate ureteric buds.** If two separate ureteric buds originate from the mesonephric duct, two complete and separate interactions will develop between the ureter and the metanephric blastema. The result is two separate renal units and collecting systems, ureters, and ureteral orifices.
19. **b. to-and-fro peristalsis of urine into the bifid ureters.** Bifid ureter is often clinically unimportant, but stasis and pyelonephritis do occur. When the Y junction is extravesical, free to-and-fro peristalsis of urine from one collecting system to the other may appear, with preferential retrograde waves passing into slightly dilated limbs instead of down the common stem.
20. **b. Ectopic ureters.** One of the distal ureteral limbs not uncommonly ends in an ectopic ureter or ureterocele.
21. **a. All three ureters joining to terminate in a single bladder orifice.** In the classification used by most investigators, there are four varieties of triplicate ureter. In one variety, all three ureters unite and drain through a single orifice. This appears to be the most common form encountered.
22. **a. The right ureter at level L3-L4.** This disorder involves the right ureter, which typically deviates medially behind (dorsal to) the inferior vena cava, winding about and crossing in front of it from a medial to a lateral direction, to resume a normal course distally, to the bladder. Excretory urography often fails to visualize the portion of the ureter beyond the J hook (i.e., extending behind the vena cava), but retrograde ureteropyelography demonstrates an S curve to the point of obstruction (see Fig. 116-48), with the retrocaval segment lying at the level of L3 or L4.
23. **b. Subcardinal vein.** If the subcardinal vein in the lumbar portion fails to atrophy and becomes the primary right-sided vein, the ureter is trapped dorsal to it.
24. **c. Intravesical ureterocele.** One study concluded that intravesical ureteroceles fared better than ectopic ureteroceles with regard to decompression (93% vs. 75%), preservation of upper pole function (96% vs. 47%), newly created reflux (18% vs. 47%), and need for secondary procedures (7% vs. 50%).
25. **b. Urinary tract infection.** Many ureteroceles are still diagnosed clinically. The most common presentation is that of an infant who has a urinary tract infection or urosepsis.
26. **c. 50% to 65%.** In various series, the incidences of reflux reported were 49%, 59%, 67%, 54%, and 65%.
27. **b. MRI of the abdomen and pelvis.** Occasionally, the renal parenchyma is difficult to locate and may be identified only by alternative imaging studies. In such cases in which an ectopic ureter is strongly suspected because of incontinence yet no definite evidence of the upper pole renal segment is found, CT or MRI has demonstrated the small, poorly functioning upper pole segment (see Fig. 116-18).
28. **d. Bladder filled to capacity.** Images should be obtained from early in the filling phase because some ureteroceles may efface later in filling and may not be seen.
29. **d. Preoperative high-grade reflux.** One study noted that infants who will likely need a secondary procedure include those with high-grade reflux or a prolapsed ureterocele. Another study found that the reoperation rate varied on the basis of the degree of preoperative reflux. If there was no reflux, only 20% required reoperation. If there was low-grade reflux versus high-grade reflux, 30% versus 53% required reoperation, respectively.
30. **b. 30%.** In one study, incision of the ectopic ureterocele appeared to be mostly successful with regard to decompression, but it did not achieve the goal of correcting preexisting reflux and resulted in a significant incidence of reflux into the ureterocele itself (30%).

117

Reflux and Megaureter

ANTOINE KHOURY • DARIUS J. BÄGLI

QUESTIONS

1. The estimated prevalence of vesicoureteral reflux in children with a urinary tract infection (UTI) is best estimated at:
   a. 1%.
   b. 3%.
   c. 5%.
   d. 10%.
   e. 30%.
2. Which of the following statements regarding reflux is FALSE?
   a. Antenatally detected reflux is associated with a male preponderance.
   b. Antenatally detected reflux is usually low grade in boys when compared with that in girls.
   c. Antenatally detected reflux is usually bilateral in boys when compared with that in girls.
   d. When reflux is detected antenatally, renal impairment is frequently present at birth and is likely due to congenital dysplasia.
   e. The majority of reflux detected later in life occurs in females.
3. Which one of the following statements regarding vesicoureteral reflux in regard to patient's race is TRUE?
   a. The incidence of vesicoureteral reflux is equal in children of all races.
   b. The disparity in the incidence of vesicoureteral reflux with respect to race becomes clearer in adulthood.
   c. The frequency of detected vesicoureteral reflux is lower in female children of African descent.
   d. African infants and white infants have a similar incidence of reflux diagnosed based on antenatal hydronephrosis.
   e. There is a clear understanding regarding the predisposition of reflux because many of the studies have included patients from different countries around the world.
4. Which of the following statements is FALSE in regard to the diagnosis and treatment of sibling vesicoureteral reflux?
   a. Based on clinical judgment and the presence or absence of UTI the patient's age should be taken into account in regard to the decision to proceed with diagnostic intervention to diagnose sibling reflux.
   b. It is reasonable to prescribe antibiotic prophylaxis while the decision to diagnose sibling reflux or not takes place.
   c. Once sibling reflux is diagnosed the indications for correction are different from the indications for treating reflux in the general pediatric population diagnosed after UTI.
   d. Siblings who are younger than 5 years of age with normal imaging studies of the kidneys can be managed based on clinical judgment and it is not absolutely necessary to obtain a voiding cystogram.
   e. Siblings younger than 5 years of age who present with cortical renal defects have the most to lose by febrile UTIs in the presence of vesicoureteral reflux.
5. Primary reflux is a congenital anomaly of the ureterovesical junction with which of the following characteristics? A deficiency of the:
   a. longitudinal muscle of the extravesical ureter results in an inadequate valvular mechanism.
   b. longitudinal muscle of the intravesical ureter results in an inadequate valvular mechanism.
   c. circumferential muscle of the extravesical ureter results in an inadequate valvular mechanism.
   d. circumferential muscle of the intravesical ureter results in an inadequate valvular mechanism.
   e. longitudinal and circumferential muscles of the intravesical ureter results in an inadequate valvular mechanism.
6. What is the ratio of tunnel length to ureteral diameter found in normal children without reflux?
   a. 5:1
   b. 4:1
   c. 3:1
   d. 2:1
   e. 1:1

7. Which of the following is TRUE regarding children with non-neurogenic neurogenic bladders?
   a. Constriction of the urinary sphincter occurs during voiding in a voluntary form of detrusor-sphincter dyssynergia.
   b. Gradual bladder decompensation and myogenic failure result from incomplete emptying.
   c. Gradual bladder decompensation and myogenic failure result from increasing amounts of residual urine.
   d. All of the above.
   e. None of the above.

8. Which of the following statements is TRUE in regard to secondary vesicoureteral reflux?
   a. The most common cause of anatomic bladder obstruction in the pediatric population is posterior urethral valves, and vesicoureteral reflux is present in a great majority of these children.
   b. Anatomic obstruction of the bladder is a common cause of secondary vesicoureteral reflux in female patients.
   c. Patients with neurofunctional etiology for secondary vesicoureteral reflux benefit from immediate surgical intervention to try to correct vesicoureteral reflux.
   d. A sacral dimple or hairy patch on the lower back is *not* a significant finding in regard to evaluation and treatment of vesicoureteral reflux.
   e. The most common structural obstruction in male and female patients is the presence of a ureterocele at the bladder neck.

9. The complex anatomic relationships required of the ureterovesical junction may be gradually damaged by which of the following?
   a. Decreases in bladder wall compliance
   b. Detrusor decompensation
   c. Incomplete emptying
   d. All of the above
   e. None of the above

10. What does the initial management of functional causes of reflux involve?
    a. Surgical treatment
    b. Medical treatment
    c. Observation only
    d. All of the above
    e. None of the above

11. Signs or symptoms of voiding dysfunction include:
    a. dribbling.
    b. urgency.
    c. incontinence.
    d. "curtseying" behavior in girls.
    e. all of the above.

12. Treatment of bladder dysfunction and instability, regardless of its severity or cause, is directed at:
    a. damping uninhibited bladder contractions.
    b. dilating the urethral sphincter.
    c. lowering intravesical pressures.
    d. all of the above.
    e. a and c only.

13. There is a strong association between the presence of reflux in patients with neuropathic bladders and intravesical pressures of greater than:
    a. 10 cm H_2O.
    b. 20 cm H_2O.
    c. 40 cm H_2O.
    d. 60 cm H_2O.
    e. 80 cm H_2O.

14. Bladder infections and their accompanying inflammation can also cause reflux by what mechanism?
    a. Lessening compliance
    b. Elevating intravesical pressures
    c. Distorting and weakening the ureterovesical junction
    d. All of the above
    e. None of the above

15. Which system provides the current standard for grading reflux based on the appearance of contrast in the ureter and upper collecting system during voiding cystourethrography?
    a. The Heikel and Parkkulainen system
    b. The International Classification system
    c. The Dwoskin and Perlmutter system
    d. The National Classification system
    e. The Dwoskin and Parkkulainen system

16. Which of the following is TRUE regarding accurately grading reflux with coexistent ipsilateral obstruction?
    a. It is not possible.
    b. It is facilitated by obtaining a renal scan.
    c. It is facilitated by obtaining an ultrasonographic scan.
    d. It is facilitated by obtaining an excretory urogram.
    e. It is facilitated by obtaining a radionuclide cystogram.

17. Which of the following is TRUE regarding the presence of fever?
    a. It may be an indicator of upper urinary tract involvement.
    b. It may *not* always be a reliable sign of upper urinary tract involvement.
    c. It increases the likelihood of discovering vesicoureteral reflux.
    d. All of the above.
    e. None of the above.

18. Complete evaluation including a voiding cystourethrogram and ultrasound are required for which of the following patients?
    a. An uncircumcised male infant with a febrile illness and a positive urine culture obtained through a bagged specimen
    b. A 3-year-old girl admitted to the hospital with pneumonia and found to have *Escherichia coli* on a urine culture without pyuria detected by microscopic analysis.
    c. A female patient with recurrent culture and urinalysis proven to have afebrile UTIs and later found to have scarring on a DMSA scan.
    d. Any child older than 5 years of age with documented UTIs.
    e. None of the above.

19. Which of the following statements is TRUE regarding screening of older children who present with asymptomatic bacteriuria? They can be screened initially with:
    a. ultrasonography.
    b. cystography.
    c. excretory urography.
    d. renal scan.
    e. They do *not* require any screening studies.

20. Which of the following is TRUE regarding cystography?
    a. Cystography performed with a Foley catheter or while the patient is under anesthesia produces static studies that inaccurately screen for reflux or sometimes exaggerate its degree because of bladder overfilling.
    b. Cystography performed in the presence of excessive hydration may mask low grades of reflux because diuresis can blunt the retrograde flow of urine.
    c. Cystograms may show reflux only during active infections when cystitis weakens the ureterovesical junction with edema or by increasing intravesical pressures.
    d. Cystograms obtained during active infections can overestimate the grade of reflux because the endotoxins produced by some gram-negative organisms can paralyze ureteral smooth muscle and exaggerate ureteral dilatation.
    e. All of the above.

21. Which of the following statements is TRUE regarding radionuclide cystography?
    a. It provides similar anatomic detail to that obtained with fluoroscopic cystography.
    b. It is an accurate method for detecting and following reflux.
    c. It is associated with more radiation exposure than is fluoroscopic cystography.
    d. It is a less sensitive test than fluoroscopic cystography.
    e. It provides more anatomic detail than fluoroscopic cystography.

22. Which of the following statements is TRUE regarding ultrasonography?
    a. It is the diagnostic study of choice to initially evaluate the upper urinary tracts of patients with suspected or proven vesicoureteral reflux.
    b. It can effectively rule out reflux.
    c. It should be performed every 2 to 3 years in patients with reflux who are medically managed.
    d. It is the study of choice for assessing renal function.
    e. An ultrasonogram showing intermittent dilatation of the renal pelvis or ureter confirms the presence of reflux.

23. What is the best study for the detection of pyelonephritis and cortical renal scarring?
    a. Diethylenetriaminepentaacetic acid (DTPA) renal scan
    b. Dimercaptosuccinic acid (DMSA) renal scan
    c. Mercaptoacetyltriglycine (MAG3) renal scan
    d. Pyelogram
    e. Renal ultrasonographic scan

24. Which of the following is TRUE regarding urodynamic studies?
    a. They may be indicated in any child suspected of having a secondary cause for reflux (valves, neurogenic bladder, non-neurogenic neurogenic bladder, voiding dysfunction).
    b. They should be performed without the use of prophylactic antibiotics in children with secondary reflux.
    c. They help direct therapy in patients with secondary reflux.
    d. All of the above.
    e. a and c only.

25. Which of the following is TRUE in regard to evaluation of vesicoureteral reflux?
    a. Routine cystoscopy is indicated in the workup of patients with vesicoureteral reflux.
    b. The radiation doses with modern digital techniques have improved the anatomic detail but the radiation dose with voiding cystourethrogram remains drastically higher than that of a radionuclide cystogram.
    c. Grading of reflux by voiding cystourethrogram and radionuclide cystogram is similar and comparable between the two imaging modalities.
    d. Ultrasonography provides an alternative means to evaluate the presence or absence of vesicoureteral reflux.
    e. Uroflowmetry is a valuable tool in the workup of a patient with vesicoureteral reflux.

26. Which of the following accurately describes what happens during ureteral development? A ureteral bud that:
    a. is medially (caudally) positioned from a normal takeoff at the trigone offers an embryologic explanation for primary reflux.
    b. is laterally (cranially) positioned from a normal takeoff at the trigone offers an embryologic explanation for primary reflux.
    c. fails to meet with the renal blastema offers an embryologic explanation for primary reflux.
    d. is laterally (cranially) positioned is often obstructed.
    e. fails to meet with the renal blastema is often obstructed.

27. In regard to the diagnosis of renal scars based on renal scintigraphy which of the following is TRUE?
    a. An area of photopenia detected during an acute episode of pyelonephritis always represents renal scar.
    b. Photopenic areas may result from postinfection renal scarring as well as some renal dysplasia.
    c. Ultrasound is a sensitive and accurate diagnostic modality for renal scarring.
    d. Areas for photopenia detected during an acute episode of pyelonephritis that later resolve on a subsequent renal scan represent resolution of renal scarring.
    e. All of the above.

28. Which of the following is TRUE regarding hypertension?
    a. In children and young adults it is most commonly caused by reflux nephropathy.
    b. It is not related to the grade of reflux or severity of scarring.
    c. It is not associated with abnormalities of Na^+,K^+-ATPase activity.
    d. All of the above.
    e. None of the above.

29. Which of the following factors might contribute to the effects of reflux on renal growth?
    a. The congenital dysmorphism often associated with, but not caused by, reflux
    b. The number and type of urinary infections and their resultant nephropathy
    c. The quality of the contralateral kidney and its implications for compensatory hypertrophy
    d. The grade of reflux in the affected kidney
    e. All of the above.

30. With regard to renal growth and reflux, which of the following is TRUE?
    a. With the exception of those kidneys that are developmentally arrested, most studies implicate infection as the cause for altered renal growth.
    b. Successful antireflux surgery can accelerate renal growth.
    c. Successful antireflux surgery may not allow the affected kidneys to return to normal size.
    d. All of the above.
    e. None of the above.
31. The anatomy of patients with ureteral duplication typically follows the Weigert-Meyer rule, in which the upper pole ureter enters the bladder:
    a. distally and medially and the lower pole ureter enters the bladder proximally and laterally.
    b. proximally and medially and the lower pole ureter enters the bladder distally and laterally.
    c. distally and laterally and the lower pole ureter enters the bladder proximally and medially.
    d. proximally and laterally and the lower pole ureter enters the bladder distally and medially.
    e. superior to the lower pole ureter.
32. Which of the following is TRUE regarding vesicoureteral reflux?
    a. It is infrequently associated with complete ureteral duplications.
    b. It may occur into either ureter of a duplicated system.
    c. It more often involves the ureter from the upper pole in a duplicated system.
    d. It resolves less frequently in patients with double ureters.
    e. All of the above.
33. Which of the following regarding reflux is true?
    a. The reflux associated with small paraureteral diverticula resolves at rates similar to those of primary reflux and can be managed accordingly.
    b. The reflux associated with paraureteral large diverticula is less likely to resolve and usually requires surgical correction.
    c. The reflux associated with diverticula, in which the ureter enters the diverticulum, regardless of size, should be corrected surgically.
    d. All of the above.
    e. None of the above.
34. Which of the following accurately describes the state of the bladder during pregnancy?
    a. Urine volume decreases in the upper collecting system as the physiologic dilatation of pregnancy evolves.
    b. Bladder tone increases because of edema and hyperemia.
    c. Bladder changes predispose the patient to bacteriuria.
    d. All of the above.
    e. None of the above.
35. During pregnancy, the presence of vesicoureteral reflux in a system already prone to bacteriuria may lead to increased morbidity. What is an additional risk factor?
    a. Renal scarring
    b. Tendency to get urinary infections
    c. Hypertension
    d. Renal insufficiency
    e. All of the above
36. Which of the following is considered to be TRUE regarding reflux management?
    a. Spontaneous resolution of vesicoureteral reflux is common.
    b. Higher grades of vesicoureteral reflux are less likely to resolve than lower grades.
    c. Reflux of sterile urine is a benign process that does not lead to significant renal damage.
    d. Prolonged use of antibiotic prophylaxis has no known health consequences.
    e. All of the above.
37. Regarding surgical correction of vesicoureteral reflux, which of the following is currently accepted?
    a. Extravesical ureteral reimplantation
    b. Intravesical ureteral reimplantation
    c. Endoscopic injection of bulking agent
    d. All of the above.
    e. None of the above.
38. Common to each type of open surgical repair for reflux is the creation of a:
    a. valvular mechanism that enables ureteral compression with bladder filling and contraction.
    b. mucosal tunnel for reimplantation having adequate muscular backing.
    c. tunnel length of three times the ureteral diameter.
    d. all of the above.
    e. none of the above.
39. How can complete ureteral duplications with reflux be best managed surgically? By:
    a. separating the ureters and reimplanting them separately
    b. a common sheath repair in which both ureters are mobilized with one mucosal cuff
    c. performing an upper to lower ureteroureterostomy and reimplanting the lower ureter
    d. performing a lower to upper ureteroureterostomy and reimplanting the upper ureter
    e. None of the above
40. Early postoperative obstruction can occur after a ureteral reimplant due to:
    a. edema.
    b. subtrigonal bleeding.
    c. mucus plugs.
    d. blood clots.
    e. all of the above.
41. If early postoperative obstruction occurs after a ureteral reimplant, what would the best management involve?
    a. Immediate nephrostomy tube placement
    b. Immediate placement of a ureteral stent
    c. Initial observation and diversion for unabating symptoms
    d. Placement of both a nephrostomy tube and a ureteral stent
    e. Reoperation
42. Which of the following is TRUE regarding persistent reflux after ureteral reimplantation?
    a. It may be due to unrecognized secondary causes of reflux, such as neuropathic bladder and severe voiding dysfunction.
    b. It seldom results from a failure to provide adequate muscular backing for the ureter within its tunnel.
    c. It may be repaired surgically using minor submucosal advancements.
    d. All of the above.
    e. None of the above.

43. Which of the following is TRUE regarding the treatment of vesicoureteral reflux?
    a. Since the widespread acceptance of endoscopic treatment the indications for surgical correction differ between open endoscopic and laparoscopic approach.
    b. Long-term follow-up data support the durability of endoscopic injection therapy.
    c. All injection materials provide a similar success rate and are just as easily injected under similar circumstances.
    d. The accuracy of the needle entry point during endoscopic injection as well as the needle placement are important components for the success of the surgical procedure.
    e. The learning curve for endoscopic injection is similar to the learning curve for open surgical reimplantation.

44. Which of the following is TRUE regarding the laparoscopic approach for ureteral reimplantation?
    a. The advantages of this approach over open surgery include smaller incisions, less discomfort, brief hospitalizations, and quicker convalescence.
    b. As with other laparoscopic procedures, experience is essential to the success of this approach.
    c. Costs may be increased because of lengthier surgery and the expense of disposable equipment.
    d. All of the above.
    e. None of the above.

45. Which of the following is TRUE regarding primary obstructive megaureter?
    a. It is caused by an aperistaltic juxtavesical segment that is unable to propagate urine at acceptable rates of flow.
    b. It most commonly occurs with neurogenic and non-neurogenic voiding dysfunction or infravesical obstructions such as posterior urethral valves.
    c. It may be due to acute infections, nephropathies, and other medical conditions that cause significant increases in urinary output that overwhelm maximal peristalsis.
    d. It is diagnosed when reflux, obstruction, and secondary causes of dilatation are ruled out.
    e. None of the above.

46. Which of the following is TRUE regarding secondary obstructive megaureter?
    a. It is caused by an aperistaltic juxtavesical segment that is unable to propagate urine at acceptable rates of flow.
    b. It most commonly occurs with neurogenic and non-neurogenic voiding dysfunction or infravesical obstructions such as posterior urethral valves.
    c. It may be due to acute infections, nephropathies, and other medical conditions that cause significant increases in urinary output that overwhelm maximal peristalsis.
    d. It is diagnosed once reflux, obstruction, and secondary causes of dilatation are ruled out.
    e. None of the above.

47. Which of the following is TRUE regarding secondary nonobstructive, nonrefluxing megaureter?
    a. It is caused by an aperistaltic juxtavesical segment that is unable to propagate urine at acceptable rates of flow.
    b. It most commonly occurs with neurogenic and non-neurogenic voiding dysfunction or infravesical obstructions such as posterior urethral valves.
    c. It may be due to acute infections, nephropathies, and other medical conditions that cause significant increases in urinary output that overwhelm maximal peristalsis.
    d. It is diagnosed once reflux, obstruction, and secondary causes of dilatation are ruled out.
    e. None of the above.

48. Which of the following is TRUE regarding primary nonobstructive, nonrefluxing megaureter?
    a. It is caused by an aperistaltic juxtavesical segment that is unable to propagate urine at acceptable rates of flow.
    b. It most commonly occurs with neurogenic and non-neurogenic voiding dysfunction or infravesical obstructions such as posterior urethral valves.
    c. It may be due to acute infections, nephropathies, and other medical conditions that cause significant increases in urinary output that overwhelm maximal peristalsis.
    d. It is diagnosed once reflux, obstruction, and secondary causes of dilatation are ruled out.
    e. None of the above.

49. Which of the following is TRUE regarding primary obstructive, nonrefluxing megaureters?
    a. As long as renal function is not significantly affected and urinary infections do not become a problem, expectant management is preferred.
    b. Antibiotic suppression is appropriate in most cases.
    c. Close radiographic surveillance is appropriate in most cases.
    d. All of the above.
    e. None of the above.

50. Which of the following is TRUE regarding the surgical management of megaureters?
    a. Ureteral tailoring is usually necessary to achieve the proper length-diameter ratio required of successful reimplants.
    b. Plication or infolding is useful for the more severely dilated ureter.
    c. Excisional tapering is preferred for the moderately dilated ureter.
    d. Narrowing the ureter may theoretically lead to less effective peristalsis.
    e. Patients usually have such massively dilated and tortuous ureters that straightening with removal of excess length and proximal revision become necessary.

ANSWERS

1. **e. 30%.** A meta-analysis of studies of children undergoing cystography for various indications has indicated that the prevalence of vesicoureteral reflux has estimated to be 30% for children with UTIs and about 17% in children without infection.
2. **b. Antenatally detected reflux is usually low grade in boys when compared with that in girls.** The reflux is usually high grade and bilateral in boys when compared with reflux in girls.
3. **c. The frequency of detected vesicoureteral reflux is lower in female children of African descent.** One of the clear differences that has been established over several studies is the relative tenfold lower frequency of vesicoureteral reflux in female children of African descent.
4. **c. Once sibling reflux is diagnosed the indications for correction are different from the indications for treating reflux in the general pediatric population diagnosed after UTI.** By taking into account the imaging of the kidneys first as well as the patient's age and history of UTI, a rational top-down approach to sibling reflux screening emerges. In any sibling, however, in which reflux is diagnosed the indications for treatment remain the same as for general reflux in the pediatric population.
5. **b. longitudinal muscle of the intravesical ureter results in an inadequate valvular mechanism.** Primary reflux is a congenital anomaly of the ureterovesical junction in which a deficiency of the longitudinal muscle of the intravesical ureter results in an inadequate valvular mechanism.
6. **a. 5:1.** In Paquin's novel study, a 5:1 tunnel length-ureteral diameter ratio was found in normal children without reflux.
7. **d. All of the above.** On the far end of this spectrum are children with non-neurogenic neurogenic bladders. Here, constriction of the urinary sphincter occurs during voiding in a voluntary form of detrusor-sphincter dyssynergia. Gradual bladder decompensation and myogenic failure result from incomplete emptying and increasing amounts of residual urine.
8. **a. The most common cause of anatomic bladder obstruction in the pediatric population is posterior urethral valves, and vesicoureteral reflux is present in a great majority of these children.** This diagnosis is obviously limited to male patients; consequently, female patients have a lower incidence of anatomic bladder obstruction. The most common structural obstruction in female patients is the presence of a ureterocele that prolapses and obstructs the bladder neck. Between 48% and 70% of patients with posterior urethral valves have vesicoureteral reflux, and relief of obstruction appears to be responsible for resolution of the reflux in a good number of those patients. The presence of a neurologic disorder should prompt the clinician to treat based on the primary etiology as opposed to proceeding with immediate surgical correction. One important aspect of the physical examination in children who present with vesicoureteral reflux is detection of potential occult spinal dysraphism, and this includes a thorough physical examination looking for sacral dimples, hairy patches, or gluteal cleft abnormalities.
9. **d. All of the above.** Decreases in bladder wall compliance, detrusor decompensation, and incomplete emptying gradually damage the complex anatomic relationships required of the ureterovesical junction.
10. **b. Medical treatment.** The initial management of functional causes of reflux is medical. It is imperative that clinicians inquire about, and determine, the voiding patterns of children with reflux.
11. **e. all of the above.** In addition to a careful physical examination, signs or symptoms of voiding dysfunction include dribbling, urgency, and incontinence. Girls often exhibit curtseying behavior, and boys will squeeze the penis in an attempt to suppress bladder contractions.
12. **e. a and c only.** Treatment of bladder dysfunction and instability, regardless of its severity or cause, is directed at dampening uninhibited contractions and lowering intravesical pressures.
13. **c. 40 cm H_2O.** There is a strong association between intravesical pressures of greater than 40 cm H_2O and the presence of reflux in patients with myelodysplasia and neuropathic bladders.
14. **d. All of the above.** Bladder infections (UTIs) and their accompanying inflammation can also cause reflux by lessening compliance, elevating intravesical pressures, and distorting and weakening the ureterovesical junction.
15. **b. The International Classification System.** The Heikel and Parkkulainen system gained popularity in Europe a few years before the Dwoskin and Perlmutter system became widely accepted in the United States. The International Classification System devised in 1981 by the International Reflux Study represents a melding of the two. It provides the current standard for grading reflux based on the appearance of contrast in the ureter and upper collecting system during voiding cystourethrography.
16. **a. It is not possible.** Accurately grading reflux is impossible with coexistent ipsilateral obstruction.
17. **d. All of the above.** The presence of fever may be an indicator of upper urinary tract involvement but is not always a reliable sign. However, if fever (and presumably pyelonephritis) is present, the likelihood of discovering vesicoureteral reflux is significantly increased.
18. **c. A female patient with recurrent culture and urinalysis proven to have afebrile UTIs and later found to have scarring on a DMSA scan.** The presence of culture-proven UTIs in the setting of an abnormal renal scan should raise the question of vesicoureteral reflux, and it is reasonable to proceed with a VCUG and ultrasound in those patients. The other clinical scenarios include a patient without pyuria and a clear alternative source for her fever as well as an infant diagnosed with UTI with a specimen obtained through a bagged collection. In those children the diagnosis of UTI should be questioned before proceeding with evaluation through cystogram and renal ultrasonography. Patients older than 5 years of age should not undergo immediate voiding cystourethrogram just based on the presence of a UTI.
19. **a. ultrasonography.** Older children who present with asymptomatic bacteriuria or UTIs that manifest solely with lower tract symptoms can be screened initially with ultrasonography alone, reserving cystography for those with abnormal upper tracts or recalcitrant infections.
20. **e. All of the above.** Excessive hydration may mask low grades of reflux because diuresis can blunt the retrograde flow of urine. Some reflux is demonstrated only during active infections when cystitis weakens the ureterovesical junction with edema or by increasing intravesical pressures. In addition, cystograms obtained during active infections can overestimate the grade of reflux because the endotoxins produced by some gram-negative organisms can paralyze ureteral smooth muscle and exaggerate ureteral dilatation.

21. **b. It is an accurate method for detecting and following reflux.** Nuclear cystography is the scintigraphic equivalent of conventional cystography. Although the technique does not provide the anatomic detail of fluoroscopic studies, it is an accurate method for detecting and following reflux.

22. **a. It is the diagnostic study of choice to initially evaluate the upper urinary tracts of patients with suspected or proven vesicoureteral reflux.** Ultrasonography has replaced the excretory urogram (intravenous pyelogram) as the diagnostic study of choice to initially evaluate the upper urinary tracts of patients with suspected or proven vesicoureteral reflux.

23. **b. Dimercaptosuccinic acid (DMSA) renal scan.** Renal scintigraphy with technetium 99m-labeled DMSA is the best study for detection of pyelonephritis and the cortical renal scarring that sometimes results.

24. **e. a and c only.** Urodynamic studies may be indicated in any child suspected of having a secondary cause for reflux (e.g., valves, neurogenic bladder, non-neurogenic neurogenic bladder, voiding dysfunction), and they help direct therapy.

25. **e. Uroflowmetry is a valuable tool in the workup of a patient with vesicoureteral reflux.** Evaluation of the lower urinary tract cannot solely rely on imaging studies since reflux is considered to be a dynamic phenomenon. Urethrometry provides valuable information in the clinical assessment of these patients. Modern management of reflux does not include the routine evaluation through cystoscopy. The radionuclide cystogram has historically been described as a technique that requires a significant lower dose of radiation than a regular voiding cystourethrogram, but the requirements with modern digital techniques have significantly narrowed the difference between these two imaging modalities. Unfortunately, ultrasound cannot reliably detect between the presence or absence of vesicoureteral reflux.

26. **b. A ureteral bud that is laterally (cranially) positioned from a normal takeoff at the trigone offers an embryologic explanation for primary reflux.** As Mackie and Stevens have suggested, a ureteral bud that is laterally (cranially) positioned from a normal takeoff at the trigone offers an embryologic explanation for primary reflux whereas those inferiorly (caudally) positioned are often obstructed.

27. **b. Photopenic areas may result from postinfection renal scarring as well as some renal dysplasia.** Vesicoureteral reflux, particularly reflux of higher grades, may result in renal dysplasia, which often appears scintigraphically identical to postinfection pyelonephritic scars. During an episode of active pyelonephritis the renal scan may show an area of photopenia that later on if it persists represents renal scarring secondary to the infection. Neither renal scan nor ultrasonography can differentiate accurately between renal dysplasia and renal scarring.

28. **a. In children and young adults it is most commonly caused by reflux nephropathy.** Reflux nephropathy is the most common cause of severe hypertension in children and young adults, although the actual incidence is unknown.

29. **e. All of the above.** Factors that might contribute to the effects of reflux on renal growth include the congenital dysmorphism often associated with (30% of cases), but not caused by, reflux; the number and type of urinary infections and their resultant nephropathy; the quality of the contralateral kidney and its implications for compensatory hypertrophy; and the grade of reflux in the affected kidney.

30. **d. All of the above.** With the exception of those kidneys that are developmentally arrested, most studies implicate infection as the cause for altered renal growth. Successful antireflux surgery can accelerate renal growth but may not allow affected kidneys to return to normal size.

31. **a. distally and medially and the lower pole ureter enters the bladder proximally and laterally.** The anatomy of patients with ureteral duplication typically follows the Weigert-Meyer rule wherein the upper pole ureter enters the bladder distally and medially and the lower pole ureter enters the bladder proximally and laterally.

32. **b. It may occur into either ureter of a duplicated system.** Although urine may reflux into either ureter, it more commonly involves the ureter from the lower pole because of its lateral position and shorter submucosal tunnel.

33. **d. All of the above.** Reflux associated with small diverticula resolves at rates similar to those of primary reflux and can be managed accordingly. In contrast, reflux found with paraureteral large diverticula is less likely to resolve and usually requires surgical correction. In any case, when the ureter enters the diverticulum, regardless of size, surgery is recommended.

34. **c. Bladder changes predispose the patient to bacteriuria.** Bladder tone decreases because of edema and hyperemia, which are changes that predispose the patient to bacteriuria. In addition, urine volume increases in the upper collecting system as the physiologic dilatation of pregnancy evolves.

35. **e. All of the above.** It seems logical to assume that during pregnancy the presence of vesicoureteral reflux in a system already prone to bacteriuria would lead to increased morbidity. Maternal history also becomes a factor if past reflux, renal scarring, and a tendency to get urinary infections are included. Women with hypertension and an element of renal failure are particularly at risk.

36. **e. All of the above.** As summarized by Walker in 1994, vesicoureteral reflux resolves spontaneously in many cases but is less likely to resolve in patients with a higher grade of reflux. The reflux of sterile urine is considered to be benign as well as the extended use of prophylactic antibiotics. Surgical open correction has a very high success rate.

37. **d. All of the above.** Extravesical and intravesical ureteral reimplantation are all options for treatment of vesicoureteral reflux. In the past decade, we have seen widespread enthusiasm for endoscopic treatment and different bulking agents have been used to correct vesicoureteral reflux utilizing minimal invasive techniques.

38. **a. valvular mechanism that enables ureteral compression with bladder filling and contraction.** Common to each technique is the creation of a valvular mechanism that enables ureteral compression with bladder filling and contraction, thus re-enacting normal anatomy and function. A successful ureteroneocystostomy provides a submucosal tunnel for reimplantation having sufficient length and adequate muscular backing. A tunnel length of five times the ureteral diameter is cited as necessary for eliminating reflux.

39. **b. a common a sheath repair in which both ureters are mobilized with one mucosal cuff.** Approximately 10% of children undergoing antireflux surgery have an element of ureteral duplication. The most common configuration is a complete duplication that results in two separate orifices. This is best managed by preserving a cuff of bladder mucosa that encompasses both orifices. Because the pair typically share blood supply along their adjoining wall, mobilization as one unit with a "common sheath" preserves vascularity and minimizes trauma.

40. **e. all of the above.** Early after surgery, various degrees of obstruction can be expected of the reimplanted ureter. Edema, subtrigonal bleeding, and bladder spasms all possibly contribute. Mucus plugs and blood clots are other causes. Most postoperative obstructions are mild and asymptomatic and resolve spontaneously. More significant obstructions are

usually symptomatic. Affected children typically present 1 to 2 weeks after surgery with acute abdominal pain, nausea, and vomiting.

41. **c. Initial observation and diversion for unabating symptoms.** The large majority of perioperative obstructions subside spontaneously, but placement of a nephrostomy tube or ureteral stent sometimes becomes necessary for unabating symptoms.

42. **a. It may be due to unrecognized secondary causes of reflux, such as neuropathic bladder and severe voiding dysfunction.** Other than technical errors, failure to identify and treat secondary causes of reflux is a common cause of the reappearance of reflux. Foremost among these secondary causes are unrecognized neuropathic bladder and severe voiding dysfunction.

43. **d. The accuracy of the needle entry point during endoscopic injection as well as the needle placement are important components for the success of the surgical procedure.** The learning curve for endoscopic injection is believed to be different from that of open surgical reimplantation, but studies have not been carried out comparing these two surgical approaches for correction of vesicoureteral reflux. Treatment is currently based on the same indications, and these indications do not differ between the different types of intervention.

44. **d. All of the above.** The advantages of this approach over open surgery include smaller incisions, less discomfort, brief hospitalizations, and quicker convalescence. As with other laparoscopic procedures, a learning curve needs to be broached and experience is essential to the success of this approach. Laparoscopic reimplantation requires a team with at least two surgeons; the repair is converted from an extraperitoneal to an intraperitoneal approach; many of the available instruments are less than ideal for use in children; operative time is greater than with open techniques; and cost is increased because of lengthier surgery and the expense of disposable equipment.

45. **a. It is caused by an aperistaltic juxtavesical segment that is unable to propagate urine at acceptable rates of flow.** It is generally agreed that the cause of primary obstructive megaureter is an aperistaltic juxtavesical segment 3 to 4 cm long that is unable to propagate urine at acceptable rates of flow.

46. **b. It most commonly occurs with neurogenic and non-neurogenic voiding dysfunction or infravesical obstructions such as posterior urethral valves.** This form of megaureter most commonly occurs with neurogenic and non-neurogenic voiding dysfunction or infravesical obstructions such as posterior urethral valves.

47. **c. It may be due to acute infections, nephropathies, and other medical conditions that cause significant increases in urinary output that overwhelm maximal peristalsis.** Significant ureteral dilatation can result from acute UTIs accompanied by bacterial endotoxins that inhibit peristalsis. Resolution is expected with appropriate antibiotic therapy. Nephropathies and other medical conditions that cause significant increases in urinary output that overwhelm maximal peristalsis can also lead to progressive ureteral dilatation as collecting systems comply to handle the output from above. These include lithium toxicity, diabetes insipidus or mellitus, sickle cell nephropathy, and psychogenic polydipsia.

48. **d. It is diagnosed once reflux, obstruction, and secondary causes of dilatation are ruled out.** Once reflux, obstruction, and secondary causes of dilatation are ruled out, the designation of primary nonrefluxing, nonobstructed megaureter is appropriate.

49. **d. All of the above.** Most clinicians now believe that as long as renal function is not significantly affected and urinary infections do not become a problem, expectant management is preferred. Antibiotic suppression and close radiologic surveillance are appropriate in most cases.

50. **a. Ureteral tailoring is usually necessary to achieve the proper length-diameter ratio required of successful reimplants.** Ureteral tailoring (excision or plication) is usually necessary. Narrowing the ureter also theoretically enables its walls to coapt properly, leading to more effective peristalsis. Revising the distal segment intended for reimplantation is all that is usually required.

118

Prune-Belly Syndrome

ANTHONY A. CALDAMONE • JOHN R. WOODARD

QUESTIONS

1. Common findings in the prune-belly syndrome include all but which of the following?
   a. Deficiency of abdominal wall musculature
   b. Urinary tract dilatation
   c. Palpable undescended testes
   d. Urachal pseudodiverticulum
   e. Vesicoureteral reflux
2. Which of the following statements regarding the prognosis of patients with prune-belly syndrome is FALSE?
   a. The patient will likely be infertile.
   b. A substantial risk of renal failure exists.
   c. Testicular descent will not occur spontaneously.
   d. The male "pseudo-prune" phenotype is protected from renal failure.
   e. Chronic constipation and ineffective cough may result from abdominal wall laxity.
3. Complications involving which of the following organ systems are most likely to threaten the early survival of an infant with prune-belly syndrome?
   a. Cardiac
   b. Renal
   c. Pulmonary
   d. Gastrointestinal
   e. Endocrine
4. Ureteral dysfunction in prune-belly syndrome is related to all of the following EXCEPT:
   a. ureteral dilatation with failure of luminal coaptation during peristalsis.
   b. reduced smooth muscle tissue.
   c. failure of propagation of an electrical conduction due to increased fibrous connective tissue.
   d. more severe proximal ureteral dysfunction with failure to conduct a urinary bolus from the renal pelvis.
   e. abnormal myofilament content in smooth muscle cells.
5. Urodynamic bladder evaluation in prune-belly syndrome is primarily characterized by bladder enlargement with:
   a. elevated voiding pressures and detrusor-sphincter dyssynergia.
   b. high-amplitude uninhibited contractions.
   c. poorly contractile detrusor or myogenic failure.
   d. poor compliance.
   e. absent sensation.
6. The classic findings on prenatal ultrasound on prune-belly syndrome include all of the following EXCEPT:
   a. ambiguous genitalia.
   b. hydroureteronephrosis.
   c. distended bladder.
   d. early fetal ascites.
   e. irregular abdominal wall circumferences.
7. A management strategy of observation in the prune-belly syndrome is strongly supported by which finding?
   a. That spontaneous improvement in dilatation of the urinary tract generally occurs after puberty
   b. That vesicoureteral reflux occurs at low pressures and does not represent a threat to renal parenchyma
   c. That the risk of obstruction after ureteral reimplantation always outweighs the benefit
   d. That operative risks in this patient population are excessive
   e. None of the above
8. Which statement is most accurate when considering management of the lower urinary tract in the patient with prune-belly syndrome?
   a. Reduction cystoplasty is indicated when bladder capacity becomes greater than expected for age.
   b. Internal urethrotomy improves postvoid residual urine volumes without risk of incontinence.
   c. Reduction cystoplasty permanently improves bladder dynamics.
   d. Internal urethrotomy should be specifically based on pressure-flow studies.
   e. Routine intermittent catheterization should be used to improve postvoid residual urine volumes in all patients.
9. Which statement regarding orchiopexy in the patient with prune-belly syndrome is TRUE?
   a. It requires a microvascular testicular autotransplantation due to the high intra-abdominal position.
   b. It maintains endocrine function but has no potential to preserve spermatogenesis.
   c. It can be best accomplished by transperitoneal mobilization before 1 year of age.
   d. It should never involve the use of the Fowler-Stephens technique because of the unreliability of collateral testicular blood supply.
   e. It is performed if spontaneous descent fails to occur by 2 years of age.

10. The most appropriate indication for prenatal intervention in suspected prune-belly syndrome is:
    a. oligohydramnios.
    b. urinary ascites.
    c. urethral atresia and progressive oligohydramnios.
    d. pulmonary hypoplasia.
    e. distended bladder.
11. The most appropriate initial management of the newborn with prune-belly syndrome includes:
    a. percutaneous drainage of the upper urinary tract after stabilization.
    b. stabilization and then vesicostomy if anesthetic risk permits.
    c. stabilization and then bilateral cutaneous ureterostomy if anesthetic risk permits.
    d. evaluation of pulmonary status and voiding cystourethrogram to rule out posterior urethral valves and reflux.
    e. evaluation of pulmonary status, renal ultrasonographic study, and prophylactic antibiotics.
12. The prostatic urethra in prune-belly syndrome:
    a. is dilated and associated with bladder neck hypertrophy on a voiding cystogram.
    b. is sometimes associated with congenital urethral obstruction resulting in megalourethra.
    c. is associated with a hypoplastic prostate with decreased epithelium and increased smooth muscle.
    d. results in retrograde ejaculation.
    e. None of the above.

ANSWERS

1. **c. Palpable undescended testes.** Bilateral cryptorchidism is a central feature of the syndrome, and in most patients both testes are intra-abdominal, overlying the ureters at the pelvic brim near the sacroiliac level.
2. **d. The male "pseudo-prune" phenotype is protected from renal failure.** Although it is exceptionally rare to encounter a normal urinary tract in association with the characteristic abdominal wall defect in a male, the converse is not unusual. Some patients (with pseudo–prune-belly syndrome) with a normal or relatively normal abdominal wall exhibit many or all of the internal urologic features. These features may include dysplastic or dysmorphic kidneys or dilated and tortuous ureters. One report noted eight boys with relatively mild external features of the syndrome, five of whom progressed to renal failure, evidence that these children remain vulnerable to renal deterioration.
3. **c. Pulmonary.** The most urgent matters are actually those concerned with cardiopulmonary function. Pulmonary complications including pulmonary hypoplasia, pneumomediastinum, pneumothorax, and cardiac abnormalities must be excluded.
4. **d. more severe proximal ureteral dysfunction with failure to conduct a urinary bolus from the renal pelvis.** The proximal ureter usually displays a more normal appearance, an important feature when considering corrective surgery.
5. **c. poorly contractile detrusor or myogenic failure.** Usually, the cystometrogram reveals excellent detrusor compliance; the end-filling pressure assumes a normal value; and the bladder functions well as a reservoir. However, bladder sensation during filling is shifted to the right with a delayed first sensation to void and bladder capacity may be more than double the normal volume. Less consistent and less favorable results are seen with the voiding profile. The compressor capabilities of the detrusor are diminished by the frequent presence of vesicoureteral reflux and reduced detrusor contractility.
6. **a. Ambiguous genitalia.** The findings on prenatal ultrasound in prune-belly syndrome may not be diagnosed in all cases but would include hydronephrosis, an enlarged bladder, ascites presenting in the second trimester, and irregular abdominal wall circumference. While external genital anomalies such as bilaterally undescended testes and megalourethra occur with prune-belly syndrome, these would not be detected on prenatal ultrasound as abnormalities of external genital development.
7. **e. None of the above.** The obvious implication of different studies was that a more aggressive approach was necessary to improve the fate of the infant with prune-belly syndrome. With the recognition that infection and progressive renal insufficiency are the factors that most often pose the greatest threat to quality of life and survival, surgical reconstruction to normalize the anatomy and function of the genitourinary tract was advocated. Early re-tailoring of the urinary system to reduce stasis and eliminate reflux or obstruction has included ureteral shortening, tapering and vesicoureteral reimplantation, and reduction cystoplasty. Reconstruction is best delayed until the child is approximately 3 months old, to allow for pulmonary maturation. This approach has been successful in achieving anatomic and functional improvement.
8. **d. Internal urethrotomy should be specifically based on pressure-flow studies.** Some initial improvement in voiding dynamics can be achieved by aggressive bladder remodeling. However, with long-term follow-up, there has been no evidence that this improvement is maintained and excessive bladder volumes tend to recur with time. Internal urethrotomy is indicated in the rare patient with true anatomic urethral obstruction or in patients with urodynamic evidence of urethral obstruction by pressure-flow studies.
9. **c. It can be best accomplished by transperitoneal mobilization before 1 year of age.** Orchiopexy in all patients is now generally performed during infancy in an effort to maintain the germ cell population and protect spermatogenesis. In the neonate and in patients up to at least 6 months of age, transabdominal complete mobilization of the spermatic cord almost always allows the testis to be positioned in the dependent portion of the scrotum without dividing the vascular portion of the spermatic cord. The Fowler-Stephens technique for performing orchiopexy in patients with intra-abdominal testes has become part of the standard urologic armamentarium.
10. **c. urethral atresia and progressive oligohydramnios.** Because most hydronephrosis in prune belly syndrome is well tolerated, its presence alone is not an indication for intervention. Similarly, oligohydramnios, pulmonary hypoplasia, distended bladder, and urinary ascites do not independently warrant prenatal intervention. The only situation with prune-belly syndrome that is potentially reversible is the pulmonary hypoplasia that is seen from urethral atresia and due to

progressive oligohydramnios. Oligohydramnios that occurs early in the second trimester is generally indicative of severe renal dysplasia.

11. **e. evaluation of pulmonary status, renal ultrasonographic study, and prophylactic antibiotics.** The most urgent matters are those concerned with cardiopulmonary function. After stabilization, urologic evaluation proceeds with physical examination and ultrasonography. Imaging requiring catheterization and the potential for introduction of bacteria should be avoided unless the results are needed for immediate clinical decision-making. Attention to sterile technique is crucial if invasive studies are performed. Once introduced, infection in a static system may be difficult to eradicate.

12. **d. results in retrograde ejaculation.** The characteristically wide bladder neck merges with a grossly dilated prostatic urethra, so that the junction is nearly imperceptible both radiographically and by gross inspection. The prostatic urethra does, however, taper to a relatively narrow membranous urethra at the urogenital diaphragm. Retrograde ejaculation is common.

119

Exstrophy–Epispadias Complex

JOHN P. GEARHART • RANJIV MATHEWS

QUESTIONS

1. What is the live birth incidence of classic bladder exstrophy?
   a. 1 in 100,000
   b. 1 in 60,000
   c. 1 in 50,000
   d. 1 in 70,000
   e. 1 in 90,000
2. What is the live birth risk of bladder exstrophy in the offspring of individuals with bladder exstrophy and epispadias?
   a. 1 in 70
   b. 1 in 300
   c. 1 in 500
   d. 1 in 700
   e. 1 in 450
3. The main theory of embryologic maldevelopment in exstrophy is that of abnormal:
   a. underdevelopment of the cloacal membrane, preventing medial migration of the mesoderm tissue and proper lower abdominal wall development.
   b. overdevelopment of the cloacal membrane, preventing medial migration of the mesodermal tissue and proper lower abdominal wall development.
   c. infiltration of ectoderm into the cloacal membrane.
   d. infiltration of mesoderm into the cloacal membrane.
   e. invasion of endoderm into the cloacal membrane.
4. In evaluation of the skeletal defects of bladder exstrophy, Sponseller and colleagues found that with classic bladder exstrophy there are changes in the orientation of the pelvic bones. These include which of the following?
   a. External rotation of the posterior aspect of the pelvis of 12 degrees on each side
   b. Retroversion of the acetabulum
   c. An 18-degree rotation of the anterior pelvis
   d. A 30% shortening of the pubic rami in addition to a significant pubic symphyseal diastasis
   e. All of the above
5. Which of the following statements is TRUE regarding hernias in children with exstrophy?
   a. Identification at the time of initial closure is not possible.
   b. They are usually unilateral
   c. They are noted in 80% of boys and 10% of girls.
   d. The orientation of the pelvic bones makes them infrequent.
   e. A patent processus vaginalis is rarely noted.
6. Which of the following statements is TRUE regarding the male genital defect in exstrophy?
   a. The posterior length of the corporeal bodies was 30% shorter than normal controls.
   b. The diameter of the posterior corporeal segments was less than normal controls.
   c. The shortening of the penis was due entirely to the pubic diastasis.
   d. The anterior corporeal segments are 50% shorter than that of normal control subjects.
   e. The angle between the corpora cavernosa is markedly reduced in boys with exstrophy.
7. Which of the following statements best describes findings regarding the prostate in exstrophy?
   a. Volume weight and cross-sectional area appeared normal compared with published results from control subjects.
   b. Prostate extended circumferentially around the urethra in all patients with exstrophy.
   c. Free PSA values were greater than in normal controls, indicating recurrent injury from infection.
   d. Vas deferens and seminal vesicles were abnormal due to the effect of the exstrophic bladder.
   e. Total PSA values were not measurable in men with exstrophy.
8. Which of the following accurately describes the vagina in the female patient with bladder exstrophy?
   a. Shorter than normal and of smaller caliber
   b. Vaginal orifice is displaced posteriorly due to the anterior exstrophic bladder
   c. Shorter than normal but of normal caliber
   d. Longer than normal and of wider caliber
   e. Cervix enters the posterior vaginal wall
9. Findings regarding the structure and innervation of the exstrophic bladder include:
   a. density and binding affinity of the muscarinic receptors were similar to norms.
   b. decreased ratio of collagen to muscle in the exstrophic bladder.
   c. increased myelinated nerve profiles indicating a later developmental stage.
   d. threefold increase in the amount of type I collagen.
   e. study of VIP, PGP 9.5, and CGRP indicated the presence of dysinnervation.

10. Which of the following statements best describes bladder function in patients with bladder exstrophy?
    a. In patients continent after reconstruction normal cystometrograms are noted in 10% to 25%.
    b. Eighty percent of patients had compliant and stable bladders before bladder neck reconstruction.
    c. Involuntary contractions were noted infrequently after bladder neck reconstruction.
    d. After bladder neck reconstruction, 90% maintained normal bladder compliance.
    e. After successful closure, ultrastructure remains abnormal in the majority.
11. The characteristic prenatal appearance of bladder exstrophy includes which of the following?
    a. Absence of bladder filling
    b. Low-set umbilicus
    c. Widening of the pubic ramus
    d. Diminutive genitalia
    e. All of the above
12. Newborn patient selection for immediate reconstruction is based on:
    a. examination of the bladder in the nursery without anesthesia.
    b. complete lack of any surface defects on examination.
    c. indentation of the bladder using anesthesia or outward bulging when the child cries.
    d. size of the phallus at birth.
    e. extent of the pubic diastasis.
13. Fundamental steps in the modern staged reconstruction of bladder exstrophy include all of the following EXCEPT:
    a. early bladder, posterior urethral and abdominal wall closure.
    b. early epispadias repair around age 1.
    c. conversion of the bladder exstrophy to complete epispadias.
    d. bladder neck reconstruction prior to the epispadias repair to provide early continence.
    e. ureteral reimplantation at the time of bladder neck reconstruction.
14. What is the best treatment option at the time of birth in a child whose bladder template is judged to be too small to undergo closure?
    a. Excision of the bladder with a nonrefluxing colon conduit
    b. Immediate closure with epispadias repair to provide resistance and allow the bladder to grow
    c. Delaying closure by 4 to 6 months with reassessment to see if the bladder will grow
    d. Bladder closure, augmentation, ureteral reimplantation, and a continence procedure
    e. Improve the potential for successful closure with an osteotomy
15. Combined osteotomy was developed for all of the following reasons EXCEPT:
    a. approach allows the placement of an external fixator device.
    b. superior cosmesis provided by this approach.
    c. need to turn the patient to perform the osteotomy.
    d. better ease of pubic approximation.
    e. reduced risk of malunion of the iliac wing and reduction of blood loss.
16. Complications that are associated with osteotomy and immobilization techniques include all of the following EXCEPT:
    a. skin ulceration associated with use of mummy wrapping.
    b. failure of the bladder and abdominal wall closure associated with the use of spica casting.
    c. high rates of failure of reconstruction associated with the use of osteotomy and external fixation.
    d. transient femoral nerve palsy with the use of osteotomy.
    e. delayed union of the iliac wings after use of posterior osteotomy.
17. Other options have been described for reconstruction in bladder exstrophy. Which of the following statements is TRUE regarding the other described approaches?
    a. The Warsaw approach includes bladder neck reconstruction at the time of initial bladder closure.
    b. The Erlangen approach includes all of the features of reconstruction of the exstrophy in a single procedure.
    c. The Seattle approach (CPRE) includes bladder neck reconstruction as part of the complete reconstruction of exstrophy.
    d. Combined bladder closure and epispadias repair is performed in cases of primary exstrophy repair at birth.
    e. The Warsaw approach uses the Young repair as the preferred method for epispadias reconstruction.
18. After initial primary bladder closure in the newborn, what should be done if recurrent urinary tract infections occur?
    a. VCUG
    b. Bladder CT
    c. Ureteral reimplantation
    d. Prophylaxis modified
    e. Cystoscopy
19. After successful bladder closure, management should include all the following EXCEPT:
    a. calibration of the urethral outlet 4 weeks after closure to ensure free drainage.
    b. ultrasound evaluation of the kidneys and bladder.
    c. intermittent antibiotics for urinary tract infections.
    d. complete bladder drainage by suprapubic tube clamping.
    e. yearly cystoscopic evaluation.
20. In a patient with bladder exstrophy who undergoes more than one closure of the bladder and urethral defect, what is the chance of having adequate bladder capacity for later bladder neck reconstruction?
    a. 60%
    b. 70%
    c. 20%
    d. 30%
    e. 10%
21. The key concepts in the reconstruction of epispadias include all of the following EXCEPT:
    a. correction of ventral chordee.
    b. urethral reconstruction.
    c. glans reconstruction.
    d. penile skin coverage.
    e. penile lengthening.
22. Information gleaned from most major series of bladder neck reconstruction indicates that the most important factor to predict success and eventual continence after bladder neck reconstruction is:
    a. age of the child.
    b. number of prior bladder infections.
    c. number of attempts at bladder closure
    d. bladder capacity.
    e. vesicoureteral reflux.

23. After bladder neck reconstruction, within what time period do the majority of patients achieve daytime continence?

a. 2 years
b. 1 year
c. 2 months
d. 6 months
e. 4 years

24. After a failed bladder closure in the newborn period, an appropriate time period should elapse before attempting a secondary repair. What should this time period be?

a. 2 months
b. 18 months
c. 2 years
d. 6 months
e. 15 months

25. All of the following are TRUE regarding the results of modern staged reconstruction of exstrophy EXCEPT:

a. onset of eventual continence and continence rates were unchanged in those who had initial successful closure.
b. modified Cantwell-Ransley repair has replaced the Young technique because there is less urethral tortuosity and lower fistula rates.
c. incidence of fistula formation was 12% at 3 months after epispadias repair.
d. continence is more likely in those patients undergoing initial closure before 72 hours of age or those who have closure after 72 hours of age with osteotomy.
e. continence rates are higher in those who have capacities of 85 mL or more at the time of bladder neck reconstruction.

26. Which of the following is TRUE regarding exstrophy failures?

a. After successful secondary closure 90% of patients develop dryness and voided continence.
b. Dehiscence after complete primary repair may be associated with corporeal, urethral, and other major soft tissue loss.
c. Bladder prolapse can be managed with minimal outlet procedures because this is considered a mild failure.
d. Because the results of re-closure are poor, immediate resection of the bladder plate followed by neobladder construction is the preferred management.
e. Posterior urethral stricture usually is a late complication occurring 4 to 6 years after initial closure.

27. Bladder neck reconstruction is designated as a failure if a 3-hour dry interval is not achieved within 2 years after surgery. Management of such failure is with the use of:

a. collagen can lead to dryness.
b. artificial urinary sphincter small bladder capacities.
c. bladder neck transection, augmentation cystoplasty, and continent diversion.
d. repeat bladder neck in relatively tight bladder necks.
e. repeat bladder neck reconstruction in bladder instability.

28. The risks of ureterosigmoidostomy in the exstrophy population include:

a. pyelonephritis and hyperkalemic acidosis.
b. pyelonephritis, hyponatremia, and rectal incontinence.
c. low incidence for eventual development of cancer.
d. poor outcomes with upper tract deterioration.
e. prolapse of the abdominal stoma.

29. What is the live births incidence of cloacal exstrophy?

a. 1 in 400,000
b. 1 in 20,000
c. 1 in 750,000
d. 1 in 1,000,000
e. 1 in 500,000

30. Neurospinal abnormalities are noted in the majority of patients with cloacal exstrophy. All of the following are true EXCEPT:

a. Thoracic defects may be noted in 10% of patients.
b. The embryologic basis for the neurospinal defect has been identified to be failure of neural tube closure.
c. Autonomic bladder innervation is derived from a more medial location.
d. Innervation of the duplicated corporeal bodies arises from the sacral plexus and courses medial to the hemibladders.
e. Functional defects can include minimal lower extremity function.

31. Cloacal exstrophy is a multisystem abnormality. Which of the following is TRUE regarding cloacal exstrophy?

a. The bones in a child with cloacal exstrophy were microscopically, markedly different from normal controls.
b. In the presence of a normal bowel length, there is low probability for the development of short-gut syndrome.
c. The most common müllerian anomaly noted was partial uterine duplication.
d. Cardiovascular and pulmonary anomalies are frequently noted.
e. The most common upper urinary tract anomaly noted was multicystic dysplastic kidney.

32. What is the incidence of omphalocele associated with cloacal exstrophy?

a. 40%
b. 70%
c. 95%
d. 20%
e. 60%

33. In the patient with cloacal exstrophy, hindgut remnants should be preserved to:

a. enlarge the bladder.
b. permit vaginal reconstruction.
c. allow either bladder augmentation or vaginal reconstruction.
d. provide additional length of bowel for fluid absorption.
e. allow later anal pull-through.

34. Gender assignment continues to remain a controversial aspect of cloacal exstrophy management. Current research indicates which of the following?

a. Psychosexual evaluation indicates that patients have marked female shift in development.
b. Patients have feminine childhood behavior but developed masculine gender identity.
c. Histology of the testis at birth is abnormal, and therefore removal has been recommended.
d. Most recommend that gender be assigned based on ability for functional reconstruction rather than on karyotype.
e. A functional and cosmetically acceptable phallus can now be constructed.

35. What is the live birth incidence of male epispadias?

a. 1 in 150,000
b. 1 in 200,000
c. 1 in 400,000
d. 1 in 117,000
e. 1 in 250,000

36. What is the incidence of reflux in patients with complete epispadias?

a. 10% to 20%
b. 90%
c. 70%
d. 50%
e. 30% to 40%

37. In the complete epispadias group, what is the predominant indicator of eventual continence?
    a. Length of the urethral groove
    b. Lack of spinal abnormalities
    c. Bladder capacity at the time of bladder neck reconstruction
    d. Age at bladder neck reconstruction
    e. Age at epispadias repair and degree of resistance provided

38. Many variations in anatomy have been reported in the exstrophy-epispadias complex. All of the following are true regarding exstrophy variants EXCEPT:
    a. presence of musculoskeletal defects characteristic of the complex, with a normal urinary tract, is termed *pseudoexstrophy*.
    b. the bladder is completely exstrophied in the superior vesical fissure variant.
    c. with "covered" exstrophy an isolated ectopic bowel segment has been frequently noted.
    d. an isolated segment of bladder is left on the abdominal wall, with a complete urinary tract within the bladder in duplicate exstrophy.
    e. a common embryologic origin has been postulated for developments of all of the variants.

39. Sexual function and libido in male and female exstrophy patients are:
    a. normal in males, abnormal in females.
    b. normal only in males.
    c. normal in both males and females.
    d. normal only in females.
    e. abnormal in both males and females.

40. What is the most common complication after pregnancy in female exstrophy patients?
    a. Premature labor
    b. Rectal prolapse
    c. Preeclampsia
    d. Cervical and uterine prolapse
    e. Oligohydramnios

41. Psychological studies of male and female children with bladder exstrophy find that:
    a. all have clinical psychopathology.
    b. they do not have clinical psychopathology.
    c. most have significant depression due to the condition.
    d. many children have gender dysphoria.
    e. half of males and half of females have clinical psychopathology.

ANSWERS

1. **c. 1 in 50,000 live births.** The incidence of bladder exstrophy has been estimated as being between 1 in 10,000 and 1 in 50,000.
2. **a. 1 in 70 live births.** Shapiro determined that the risk of bladder exstrophy in the offspring of individuals with bladder exstrophy and epispadias is 1 in 70 live births, a 500-fold greater incidence than in the general population.
3. **b. overdevelopment of the cloacal membrane, preventing medial migration of the mesodermal tissue and proper lower abdominal wall development.** The theory of embryonic maldevelopment in exstrophy held by Marshall and Muecke is that the basic defect is an abnormal overdevelopment of the cloacal membrane, preventing medial migration of the mesenchymal tissue and proper lower abdominal wall development.
4. **e. All of the above.** Sponseller and colleagues found that patients with classic bladder exstrophy have a mean external rotation of the posterior aspect of the pelvis of 12 degrees on each side, retroversion of the acetabulum, and a mean 18-degree external rotation of the anterior pelvis, along with 30% shortening of the pubic rami.
5. **c. They are noted in 80% of boys and 10% of girls.** Connelly and colleagues, in a review of 181 children with bladder exstrophy, reported inguinal hernias in 81.8% of boys and 10.5% of girls.
6. **d. The anterior corporeal segments are 50% shorter than that of normal control subjects.** With the use of MRI to examine adult men with bladder exstrophy and comparison of this result with that from age- and race-matched control subjects, it was found that the anterior corporeal length in male patients with bladder exstrophy is almost 50% shorter than that of normal control subjects.
7. **a. Volume weight and cross-sectional area appeared normal compared with published results from control subjects.** The volume, weight, and maximum cross-sectional area of the prostate appeared normal compared with published results from control subjects.
8. **c. Shorter than normal but of normal caliber.** The vagina is shorter than normal, hardly greater than 6 cm in depth, but of normal caliber.
9. **a. density and binding affinity of the muscarinic receptors were similar to norms.** Muscarinic cholinergic receptor density and binding affinity were measured in control subjects and in patients with classic bladder exstrophy. The density of the muscarinic cholinergic receptors in both the control and exstrophy groups were similar, as was the binding affinity of the muscarinic receptor. Therefore, it was thought by the authors that the neurophysiologic composition of the exstrophied bladder is not grossly altered during its anomalous development.
10. **b. Eighty percent of patients had compliant and stable bladders before bladder neck reconstruction.** Diamond and associates (1999), looking at 30 patients with bladder exstrophy at various stages of reconstruction, found that 80% of patients had compliant and stable bladders before bladder neck reconstruction.
11. **e. All of the above.** In a review of 25 prenatal ultrasonographic examinations with the resulting birth of a newborn with classic bladder exstrophy, several observations were made: (1) absence of bladder filling; (2) a low-set umbilicus; (3) widening pubis ramus; (4) diminutive genitalia; and (5) a lower abdominal mass that increases in size as the pregnancy progresses and as the intra-abdominal viscera increase in size.
12. **c. indentation of the bladder under anesthesia or outward bulging when the child cries.** In minor grades of exstrophy that approach the condition of complete epispadias with incontinence, the bladder may be small yet may demonstrate acceptable capacity, either by bulging when the baby cries or by indenting easily when touched by a sterile gloved finger in the operating room with the child under anesthesia.
13. **d. bladder neck reconstruction prior to the epispadias repair to provide early continence.** The most significant changes in the management of bladder exstrophy have been (1) early bladder, posterior urethral, and abdominal wall closure, usually with osteotomy; (2) early epispadias repair; (3) reconstruction

of a continent bladder neck and reimplantation of the ureters; and, most importantly, (4) definition of strict criteria for the selection of patients suitable for this approach. Bladder neck repair usually occurs when the child is 4 to 5 years of age, has an adequate bladder capacity, and, most important, is ready to participate in a postoperative voiding program.

14. **c. Delaying closure by 4 to 6 months with reassessment to see if the bladder will grow.** Ideally, waiting for the bladder template to grow for 4 to 6 months in the child with a small bladder is not as risky as submitting a small bladder template to closure in an inappropriate setting, resulting in dehiscence and allowing the fate of the bladder to be sealed at that point.

15. **c. need to turn the patient to perform the osteotomy.** Combined osteotomy was developed for three reasons: (1) osteotomy is performed with the patient in the supine position, as is the urologic repair, thereby avoiding the need to turn the patient; (2) the anterior approach to this osteotomy allows placement of an external fixator device and intrafragmentary pins under direct vision; and (3) the cosmetic appearance of this osteotomy is superior to that of the posterior iliac approach.

16. **c. high rates of failure of reconstruction associated with the use of osteotomy and external fixation.** Successful closure was noted in 97% of those immobilized with an external fixator and modified Buck's traction.

17. **b. The Erlangen approach includes all of the features of reconstruction of the exstrophy in a single procedure.** This method is truly a "complete repair" because it accomplishes all of the facets of exstrophy reconstruction in a single procedure. Surgical repair is, however, performed at 8 to 10 weeks of age when the infant is larger and has had the opportunity to be medically stabilized.

18. **e. Cystoscopy.** An important caveat is that if there are recurrent urinary tract infections, or if the bladder is distended on an ultrasonographic study, cystoscopy should be performed and the posterior urethra should be carefully examined anteriorly for erosion of the intrapubic stitch, which may be the cause of the recurrent infections.

19. **c. intermittent antibiotics for urinary tract infections.** Before removal of the suprapubic tube, 4 weeks after surgery, the bladder outlet is calibrated by a urethral catheter or a urethral sound to ensure free drainage. A complete ultrasound examination is obtained to ascertain the status of the renal pelves and ureters, and appropriate urinary antibiotics are administered because all patients will have reflux post closure. Residual urine is estimated by clamping the suprapubic tube, and specimens for culture are obtained before the patient leaves the hospital and at subsequent intervals to detect infection and ensure that the bladder is empty.

20. **a. 60%.** In one study, if a patient underwent two closures, the chance of having an adequate bladder capacity for bladder neck reconstruction was 60%.

21. **a. correction of ventral chordee.** Regardless of the surgical technique chosen for reconstruction of the penis in bladder exstrophy, four key concerns must be addressed to ensure a functional and cosmetically pleasing penis: (1) correction of dorsal chordee, (2) urethral reconstruction, (3) glandular reconstruction, and (4) penile skin closure.

22. **d. bladder capacity.** The most important long-term factor gleaned from a review of all these series is the fact that bladder capacity at the time of bladder neck reconstruction is a very important determinant of eventual success.

23. **b. 1 year.** The vast majority of patients achieve daytime continence in the first year after bladder neck reconstruction.

24. **d. 6 months.** Dehiscence, which may be precipitated by incomplete mobilization of the pelvic diaphragm, and inadequate pelvic immobilization postoperatively, wound infection, abdominal distention, or urinary tube malfunction, necessitates a 6-month recovery period before a second attempt at closure.

25. **a. onset of eventual continence and continence rates were unchanged in those who had initial successful closure.** The importance of a successful initial closure is emphasized by Oesterling and Jeffs (1987) and by Husmann and colleagues (1989a), who found that the onset of eventual continence was quicker and the continence rate higher in those who underwent a successful initial closure with or without osteotomy.

26. **b. Dehiscence after complete primary repair may be associated with corporeal, urethral, and other major soft tissue loss.** Dehiscence and prolapse have also been reported after the "complete repair" and may be associated with glandular, corporeal, urethral plate, and other major soft tissue loss.

27. **c. bladder neck transection, augmentation cystoplasty, and continent diversion.** A majority of bladder neck failures require eventual augmentation or continent diversion. The artificial urinary sphincter has been used with some success in patients who have a good bladder capacity. However, in most of these failures the bladder capacity is small and augmentation will be required. At the time of reoperative surgery, either the bladder neck is transected proximal to the prostate with a Mitrofanoff substitution or a continence procedure is performed, such as an artificial sphincter or collagen injection, or both. In our extensive experience with failed bladder neck reconstructions, most of the patients have had several surgeries and need to be dry. In such cases, the most suitable alternative is bladder neck transection, augmentation, and a continent urinary stoma (Gearhart et al, 1995b; Hensle et al, 1995).

28. **a. pyelonephritis and hyperkalemic acidosis.** However, this form of diversion should not be offered until one is certain that anal continence is normal and after the family has been made aware of the potential serious complications, including pyelonephritis, hyperkalemic acidosis, rectal incontinence, ureteral obstruction, and delayed development of malignancy.

29. **a. 1 in 400,000 live births.** Fortunately, cloacal exstrophy is exceedingly rare, occurring in 1 in 200,000 to 400,000 live births.

30. **b. The embryologic basis for the neurospinal defect has been identified to be failure of neural tube closure.** The embryologic basis for the neurospinal defects associated with cloacal exstrophy have been postulated to be secondary to problems with the disruption of the tissue of the dorsal mesenchyme rather than failure of neural tube closure (McLaughlin et al, 1995). Alternatively, it has been suggested that the defects that lead to the formation of cloacal exstrophy may lead to the developing spinal cord and vertebrae being pulled apart (Cohen, 1991).

31. **c. The most common müllerian anomaly noted was partial uterine duplication.** The most commonly reported müllerian anomaly was uterine duplication, seen in 95% of patients (Diamond, 1990). The vast majority of these patients had partial uterine duplication, predominantly a bicornate uterus.

32. **c. 95%.** In Diamond's series, the incidence of omphalocele was 88%, with a majority of all series reporting 95% or greater.

33. **d. provide additional length of bowel for fluid absorption.** With the recognition of the metabolic changes in patients with ileostomy, an attempt is always made to use the hindgut remnant to provide additional length of bowel for fluid absorption.

34. **e. A functional and cosmetically acceptable phallus can now be constructed.** Most authors recommend assigning gender that is consistent with karyotypic makeup of the individual if at all possible (see Fig. 61-26). This policy can be supported

by a report indicating that the histology of the testis at birth is normal (Mathews et al, 1999a). Furthermore, with evolution of techniques for phallic reconstruction, a functional and cosmetically acceptable phallus can now be constructed (Husmann et al, 1989b).

35. **d. 1 in 117,000 live births.** Male epispadias is a rare anomaly, with a reported incidence of 1 in 117,000 males.

36. **e. 30% to 40%.** The ureterovesical junction is inherently deficient in complete epispadias, and reflux has been reported between 30% and 40% in a number of series.

37. **c. Bladder capacity at the time of bladder neck reconstruction.** In the epispadias group, much as in the exstrophy group, bladder capacity is the predominant indicator of eventual continence.

38. **b. the bladder is completely exstrophied in the superior vesical fissure variant.** In the superior vesical fissure variant of the exstrophy complex, the musculature and skeletal defects are exactly the same as those in classic exstrophy; however, the persistent cloacal membrane ruptures only at the uppermost portion, and a superior vesical fistula results that actually resembles a vesicostomy. Bladder extrusion is minimal and is present only over the normal umbilicus.

39. **c. normal in both males and females.** Sexual function and libido in exstrophy patients are normal.

40. **d. Cervical and uterine prolapse.** The main complication after pregnancy was cervical and uterine prolapse, which occurred frequently.

41. **b. they do not have clinical psychopathology.** The conclusions of this long-term study were that children with exstrophy do not have clinical psychopathology.

120

Surgical Techniques for One-Stage Reconstruction of the Exstrophy-Epispadias Complex

RICHARD W. GRADY • MICHAEL E. MITCHELL

QUESTIONS

1. Single-stage reconstruction using the complete primary exstrophy repair technique offers several advantages over staged reconstruction EXCEPT:
   a. the possibility to correct the penile, bladder, and bladder neck abnormalities of bladder exstrophy with one operation.
   b. the ability to achieve urinary continence without bladder neck reconstruction.
   c. correction of vesicoureteral reflux at the time of surgery.
   d. lower complication rates than previous attempts at single-stage reconstruction.
   e. initiation of bladder cycling early in life.
2. Single-stage reconstruction using the complete primary exstrophy repair technique relies on which of the following to achieve continence?
   a. Reestablishment of normal anatomic relationships
   b. Bladder neck reconstruction at the time of primary surgery
   c. Osteotomy at the time of single-stage reconstruction
   d. Simultaneous epispadias repair
   e. None of the above
3. The following postoperative factors have been shown to increase the success of reconstruction for bladder exstrophy EXCEPT:
   a. immobilization with external fixators, Buck's traction, a spica cast, or a mummy wrap.
   b. antibiotic therapy.
   c. prolonged NPO status to avoid abdominal distention.
   d. urinary diversion through ureteral stenting and suprapubic urinary drainage.
   e. adequate nutritional support.
4. Single-stage reconstruction using the complete primary exstrophy repair technique can be safely performed because:
   a. the neurovascular bundles of the corporeal bodies lie laterally rather than dorsally on the corporeal bodies.
   b. the cavernosal bodies and urethral wedge are not actually separated from each other in this technique.
   c. the blood supply to the corporeal bodies and that to the urethral wedge are independent of each other.
   d. the blood supply is quickly reestablished once the components are "reassembled."
   e. the distal vascular communications between the corpora and urethral wedge are preserved.
5. The proximal limits of dissection using the complete primary exstrophy repair technique are:
   a. the intersymphyseal band.
   b. the muscles of the pelvic floor.
   c. the rectum.
   d. the corpora spongiosa.
   e. the endopelvic fascia.
6. Factors that mitigate against using a single-stage reconstruction technique for cloacal exstrophy include the presence of:
   a. a large omphalocele.
   b. a wide pubic diastasis.
   c. a concomitant myelomeningocele.
   d. small bladder plate.
   e. all of the above.
7. Complications of the complete primary exstrophy repair technique include:
   a. myogenic bladder failure.
   b. testicular atrophy.
   c. urethrocutaneous fistula.
   d. hip dislocation.
   e. epispadias.

ANSWERS

1. **c. correction of vesicoureteral reflux at the time of surgery.** In most applications of the primary exstrophy repair technique, correction of vesicoureteral reflux is not performed, although some have reported performing ureteral reimplantation. All of the other elements are considered advantages of the primary repair.
2. **a. Reestablishment of normal anatomic relationships.** The fundamental basis of the primary repair technique is to reposition the bladder neck and urethral complex into the normal pelvic position more posteriorly than at birth. This permits more normal function of the pelvic floor in maintenance of continence. The other factors do not contribute as significantly to continence.
3. **c. prolonged NPO status to avoid abdominal distention.** It is not necessary to maintain an NPO status after primary repair, because this will compromise nutrition. If an ileus develops, appropriate decompression and management are necessary because abdominal distention strains the repair. All other factors contribute to a successful outcome.
4. **c. the blood supply to the corporeal bodies and that to the urethral wedge are independent of each other.** Because the three elements of the penis, the two corpora and the urethral wedge, are fully separated in the penile disassembly, their vasculature must be proximal, which it is; and this is the reason this method is successful. Nevertheless, preservation of these proximal vascular supplies is essential.
5. **b. the muscles of the pelvic floor.** The limit of dissection along the penile structures is the pelvic floor, which is then split to permit repositioning of the bladder neck complex posteriorly.
6. **e. All of the above.** All of these factors would indicate that an attempt to perform a primary repair would be at high risk for failure, predominantly by dehiscence. Several of these factors may be present at one time.
7. **c. urethrocutaneous fistula.** The most common complication after primary repair is development of a urethrocutaneous fistula on the ventrum of the penis. Other complications can include corporeal devascularization, hydronephrosis, and hypospadias.

121

Bladder Anomalies in Children

DOMINIC FRIMBERGER • BRADLEY KROPP

QUESTIONS

1. At which time point can the fetal bladder be first detected on ultrasound?
   a. At the 10th week of gestation
   b. At the 12th week of gestation
   c. Not before the third trimester
   d. The bladder can only be seen when anomalies are present
2. What are important features on prenatal bladder ultrasound?
   a. Urine cycling
   b. Size of bladder
   c. Amniotic fluid levels
   d. All of the above
3. Which of the following bladder dilatations is caused by obstruction?
   a. Posterior urethral valves
   b. Prune-belly syndrome
   c. Congenital megacystis
   d. a and b
   e. All of the above
4. Which of the following statements concerning the urachus is incorrect?
   a. The urachus is positioned intraperitoneally.
   b. The urachus is lined by the obliterated umbilical arteries.
   c. The urachal length varies from 3 to 10 cm.
   d. Four different urachal anomalies have been described.
5. Primary paraureteral diverticula are seen in trabeculated bladders as one of many diverticula in the bladder and happen in children with infravesical obstruction.
   a. True
   b. False
6. Which other condition has to be considered in the workup of a patent urachus?
   a. The presence of vesicoureteral reflux
   b. Association with bladder outlet obstruction
   c. The presence of a patent omphalomesenteric tract
   d. The presence of bladder diverticula
7. Which congenital syndrome is not associated with bladder diverticula?
   a. Ehlers-Danlos
   b. Klippel-Trenaunay
   c. Williams' elfin facies
   d. Menkes' syndrome
8. Which statement concerning bladder duplication is NOT true?
   a. Duplication anomalies of the external genitalia are present in up to 90% of patients.
   b. Duplication anomalies of the lower gastrointestinal tract are present in up to 80% of patients.
   c. Other abnormalities such as vesicoureteral reflux, renal ectopia, or dysplasia are commonly found.
   d. Duplications can occur in the coronal or sagittal plane.

ANSWERS

1. **a. At the 10th week of gestation.** The bladder can be visualized in about 50% of cases in the fetal pelvis at the 10th week of gestation, concurrent with the onset of urine production. The detection rate increases with fetal age to 78% at 11 weeks, 88% at 12 weeks, and almost 100% at 13 weeks.
2. **d. All of the above.** The fetal bladder empties every 15 to 20 minutes; therefore, a second ultrasound in the same setting is mandatory in case of nonvisualization of the bladder. The fetal bladder can appear either dilated, hypoplastic, or absent on ultrasound and therefore give clues about maldevelopment of the urinary tract. Until 16 weeks of gestation, the amniotic fluid is mainly consistent with placental transudate, at which time it changes to predominantly fetal urine.
3. **a. Posterior urethral valves.** Prune-belly syndrome and congenital megacystis are characterized by nonobstructive dilatation of the urinary bladder. Posterior urethral valves cause obstructive dilatation of the bladder and upper urinary tract.
4. **a. The urachus is positioned intraperitoneally.** The urachus is preperitoneal in the center of a pyramid-shaped space. This space is lined by the obliterated umbilical arteries, with its base on the anterior dome of the bladder and the tip directed toward the umbilicus.

5. **b. False.** Primary paraureteral diverticula are seen in smooth-walled bladders, occur isolated with no other diverticula, are intermittent in presentation, and happen in children with no infravesical obstruction.
6. **c. The presence of a patent omphalomesenteric tract.** It is important to differentiate a patent urachus from a patent omphalomesenteric duct. The presence of both anomalies in the same patient is rare. Urachal patency is often absent even with severely obstructed bladders in utero.
7. **b. Klippel-Trenaunay.** Congenital diverticula are often found in children with generalized connective tissue diseases such as Ehlers-Danlos, Williams' elfin facies, or Menkes' syndromes.
8. **b. Duplication anomalies of the lower gastrointestinal tract are present in up to 80% of patients.** Associated duplication anomalies of the external genitalia have been reported in up to 90% of cases; associated duplication anomalies of the lower gastrointestinal tract occur only in up to 42% of cases. Association with other nonurologic congenital anomalies is more frequent in sagittal than coronal duplications.

122

Posterior Urethral Valves

ANTHONY J. CASALE

QUESTIONS

1. Most patients with posterior urethral valves are diagnosed:
   a. using antenatal ultrasound screening.
   b. as neonates with failure to thrive.
   c. in the first year of life with urinary tract infections.
   d. in mid childhood with voiding dysfunction.
   e. in adolescence with renal insufficiency.
2. The major cause of mortality today in boys with posterior urethral valves is:
   a. renal failure in the newborn period.
   b. renal failure in mid childhood.
   c. urinary sepsis in infancy.
   d. pulmonary insufficiency in the newborn period.
   e. renal insufficiency in adolescence.
3. The most important determining factor in long-term renal function in posterior urethral valves is the:
   a. degree of bladder damage.
   b. severity of hydronephrosis.
   c. ability to control infection.
   d. degree of renal dysplasia.
   e. ability to concentrate urine.
4. The valve bladder syndrome can cause the most damage by:
   a. resulting incontinence.
   b. leading to recurrent infection.
   c. preventing adequate upper tract drainage.
   d. leading to hypertension.
   e. causing renal tubular damage.
5. Urinary ascites, VURD, and bladder diverticula all offer what advantage to patients with posterior urethral valves?
   a. promoting urinary drainage.
   b. providing a pressure pop-off valve.
   c. allowing free upper tract drainage through the ureterovesical junction.
   d. promoting bladder emptying.
   e. allowing early diagnosis.
6. The most important feature in managing bladder dysfunction in patients with posterior urethral valves is that it:
   a. seldom causes persistent problems.
   b. is affected by renal function.
   c. causes intermittent incontinence.
   d. causes persistent reflux.
   e. is variable and changes during life.
7. In patients with posterior urethral valves and persistent reflux it is most important to:
   a. document that the bladder can empty effectively.
   b. evaluate upper tract drainage.
   c. measure upper tract pressures.
   d. control incontinence.
   e. surgically correct the reflux in early childhood.
8. A 2-kg premature infant with posterior urethral valves and multiple medical problems is stable at 2 weeks of age. Infant cystoscopes are not available. The next step in management is:
   a. catheter drainage.
   b. cutaneous vesicostomy.
   c. cutaneous pyelostomies.
   d. cutaneous ureterostomies.
   e. percutaneous nephrostomies.
9. Antenatal intervention with a vesicoamniotic shunt is most likely to help the fetus by:
   a. improving early renal function.
   b. improving long-term renal function.
   c. preventing pulmonary hypoplasia.
   d. improving bladder function.
   e. allowing full-term delivery.
10. Ultrasound in infants with posterior urethral valves may help to predict long-term renal function by demonstrating:
    a. degree of hydronephrosis.
    b. bladder wall thickness.
    c. degree of renal dysplasia.
    d. grade of reflux.
    e. type of urethral valve.
11. Anterior urethral valves differ from posterior urethral valves in that they may appear as:
    a. bilateral hydronephrosis.
    b. urosepsis.
    c. failure to thrive.
    d. intermittent penis mass.
    e. voiding dysfunction.
12. The accuracy of diagnosing posterior urethral valves on antenatal ultrasound screening is affected by:
    a. amniotic fluid.
    b. fetal age.
    c. maternal age.
    d. fetal size.
    e. maternal hydration.

ANSWERS

1. **a. using antenatal ultrasound screening.** The diagnosis of patients with posterior urethral valves is most often made using antenatal ultrasound screening.
2. **d. pulmonary insufficiency in the newborn period.** The major cause of mortality today in posterior urethral valves is from pulmonary hypoplasia. Infants with renal failure can be dialyzed but pulmonary insufficiency may still be fatal.
3. **d. degree of renal dysplasia.** The degree of renal dysplasia is the most important factor in determining long-term renal function. Renal dysplasia develops early in fetal life and cannot be reversed. It limits renal growth and development.
4. **c. preventing adequate upper tract drainage.** The valve bladder syndrome is the greatest threat in preventing adequate upper tract drainage. It may also contribute to infection and incontinence.
5. **b. providing a pressure pop-off valve.** Urinary ascites, VURD, and bladder diverticula all offer relative protection to the valve patient by acting as pressure pop-off valves. In this way they may spare the kidney high pressures and may protect renal function.
6. **e. is variable and changes during life.** The most important feature to remember in managing bladder dysfunction in patients with posterior urethral valves is that it is variable and changes during life. Urodynamic monitoring is necessary in managing patients with posterior urethral valves.
7. **a. document that the bladder can empty effectively.** In patients with posterior urethral valves and persistent reflux it is most important to document that the bladder can empty effectively. Both valve remnants and bladder dysfunction can contribute to persistent reflux.
8. **b. cutaneous vesicostomy.** Cutaneous vesicostomy is the best initial option to establish long-term bladder drainage in a small infant with posterior urethral valves when valve ablation may be technically difficult.
9. **c. preventing pulmonary hypoplasia.** Antenatal intervention with a vesicoamniotic shunt is most likely to help the fetus by helping prevent pulmonary hypoplasia. There is no evidence that antenatal intervention will improve renal or bladder function.
10. **c. degree of renal dysplasia.** Ultrasound in infants with posterior urethral valves may help to predict long-term renal function by demonstrating the degree of renal dysplasia. Renal dysplasia is evident on ultrasound by increased echogenicity.
11. **d. intermittent penis mass.** Anterior urethral valves differ from posterior urethral valves in that they may present as an intermittent penile mass. Anterior urethral valves are often in the form of a diverticulum that fills with urine during voiding and may be visible along the shaft of the penis.
12. **b. fetal age.** The accuracy of diagnosing posterior urethral valves on antenatal ultrasound screening is affected by fetal age. Ultrasound done when the fetus is younger than 24 weeks' gestation may miss the diagnosis of posterior urethral valves.

123

Voiding Dysfunction in Children: Non-Neurogenic and Neurogenic

Non-Neurogenic Dysfunction

C. K. YEUNG • JENNIFER D. Y. SIHOE • STUART B. BAUER

QUESTIONS (PART A)

1. Development of normal bladder function involves which of the following changes?
   a. Decrease in urine production and increase in bladder capacity
   b. Increase in urine production and increase in voiding frequency
   c. Increase in bladder capacity and decrease in voiding frequency
   d. Decrease in voided volume and increase in voiding frequency
   e. Increase in bladder capacity and no change in voided volume
2. Which of the following statements best describes urodynamic findings of maximum detrusor pressures with micturition (Pdetmax) in infants with normal lower urinary tracts?
   a. There is no difference compared with adults.
   b. Lower Pdetmax is observed in infants compared with adults.
   c. Higher Pdetmax is observed in male infants only.
   d. Higher Pdetmax is observed in female infants only.
   e. Higher Pdetmax is observed in both male and female infants.
3. Which of the following statements on neurologic control of normal micturition is FALSE?
   a. Innervation of the bladder involves both the central somatic and the autonomic nervous system.
   b. Micturition is initiated with a full bladder by a simple spinal cord reflex.
   c. Micturition does not occur during sleep.
   d. Development of direct volitional control over the bladder-sphincter complex occurs.
   e. Neurologic control occurs at different levels of the central nervous system from spinal cord to brainstem.
4. Which of the following is characteristic of children with urge syndrome?
   a. Vincent's curtsy sign
   b. Hold maneuver
   c. Urgency
   d. Small bladder capacity
   e. All of the above
5. Involuntary leakage of urine on standing after voiding in a toilet-trained girl is suggestive of:
   a. vesicoureteral reflux (VUR).
   b. vesicovaginal reflux.
   c. stress incontinence.
   d. urge syndrome.
   e. Hinman's syndrome.
6. Which of the following best characterizes a decompensated bladder?
   a. Large bladder capacity with poor bladder emptying
   b. Small bladder capacity with incontinence
   c. Hyperreflexic bladder with reduced bladder capacity
   d. Small bladder capacity with frequent voiding
   e. None of the above
7. Fecal retention and constipation are often associated with which of the following urinary tract abnormalities?
   a. Urinary tract infection (UTI)
   b. VUR
   c. Hydronephrosis
   d. Enuresis
   e. All of the above
8. A 3-year-old boy presented with symptomatic UTI. Micturating cystourethrography confirmed bilateral grade 4 VUR, and prophylactic antibiotic therapy has been started. Which of the following statements is correct?
   a. There is a high rate of spontaneous resolution of the VUR.
   b. The risk of breakthrough UTI is minimal on prophylactic antibiotic therapy.
   c. Surgical intervention is a consideration when the child is older.
   d. A urodynamic study is warranted for appropriate management of any underlying bladder dysfunction.
   e. Radiologic studies of the upper urinary tract are not necessary.

9. A 6-year-old girl presents with symptoms of urge syndrome. Which of the following investigations should be done first?
   a. Micturating cystourethrogram
   b. Voiding diary
   c. Radiograph of lumbar spine
   d. Urine culture
   e. Ambulatory urodynamic study
10. Which of the following statements about urodynamic studies is correct?
    a. Natural fill urodynamics can only be performed via a suprapubic catheter.
    b. Conventional fill studies are performed during ambulatory urodynamics.
    c. Detrusor response may be inhibited during conventional fill urodynamic studies.
    d. During video-urodynamics the child is allowed to run freely within a private cubicle.
    e. Urodynamic studies are used to describe the physiologic parameters involved in the bladder mechanics during voiding only.
11. Treatment of a child with primary nocturnal enuresis may involve the following modalities EXCEPT:
    a. antibiotic prophylaxis.
    b. acupuncture.
    c. bowel management.
    d. pelvic floor rehabilitation.
    e. antimuscarinics.
12. Urodynamic studies in children with primary nocturnal enuresis commonly exhibit which of the following?
    a. Normal findings
    b. Marked reduction in bladder emptying efficiency
    c. Low leak-point pressure
    d. Poor bladder compliance
    e. Reduced functional bladder capacity

Neurogenic Dysfunction

STUART B. BAUER

QUESTIONS (PART B)

13. Urinary incontinence or voiding dysfunction in children without obvious neurologic disease is related to which of the following?
    a. Excessive urine production from nephrogenic diabetes insipidus
    b. Delayed maturation of the nervous system
    c. An ectopic ectopia
    d. All of the above
    e. b and c only
14. Rectal pressure monitoring during a cystometrogram allows for which of the following parameters?
    a. It provides a way of detecting an overactive detrusor.
    b. It determines true detrusor compliance.
    c. It differentiates detrusor from abdominal leak-point pressure.
    d. All of the above.
    e. None of the above.
15. Eliciting an overactive detrusor is easiest to diagnose during a cystometrogram under which of the following conditions?
    a. Rapid infusion of warm saline
    b. Slow infusion of cold saline
    c. Slow infusion of warm saline
    d. Rapid infusion of cold saline
    e. Having the child cough during the examination
16. Which vitamin plays a major role in the prevention of neural tube defects?
    a. Niacin
    b. Riboflavin
    c. Folic acid
    d. B_{12}
    e. Carotene
17. Which statement is TRUE about children with a thoracic level myelomeningocele?
    a. Leg function is usually normal.
    b. Infants with this level lesion often have detrusor sphincter dyssynergia.
    c. Infants with this level lesion have an underactive detrusor.
    d. Older children tend to have a normal upper urinary tract by ultrasound.
    e. Older children tend to easily achieve urinary continence with just clean intermittent catheterization alone.

18. What percent of newborns with a myelomeningocele have a normal upper urinary appearance on ultrasound within the first month of life?

    a. 45%
    b. 60%
    c. 75%
    d. 85%
    e. 95%

19. Secondary tethering of the spinal cord in infants who have had closure of the myelomeningocele in the first days of life occurs in what percentage of children?

    a. 5%
    b. 10%
    c. 15%
    d. 20%
    e. 25%

20. Credé voiding is best avoided in which of the following conditions?

    a. VUR with a severely denervated urethral sphincter
    b. VUR with a fully innervated urethral sphincter
    c. A poorly compliant bladder with a low leak-point pressure
    d. An overactive detrusor with a low leak-point pressure
    e. A compliant bladder with a low leak-point pressure

21. When considering an antireflux operation in a child with a myelomeningocele, treating which urodynamic parameter beforehand is thought to be most important for achieving a successful result?

    a. Poor compliance
    b. Presence of detrusor overactivity
    c. a and b
    d. Neither a nor b
    e. A high leak-point pressure

22. Which of the following anticholinergic medications is most potent in reducing detrusor overactivity?

    a. Hyoscyamine
    b. Propantheline bromide
    c. Oxybutynin
    d. Glycopyrrolate
    e. Tolterodine

23. After a gastrocystoplasty to enlarge the bladder and counteract a poorly compliant bladder which metabolic derangement can occur if the patient is not monitored carefully?

    a. Hyponatremic hypochloremic metabolic alkalosis
    b. Hypernatremic hyperkalemic metabolic acidosis
    c. Hypokalemic hyperchloremic metabolic alkalosis
    d. Hypernatremic hypochloremic metabolic acidosis
    e. Hyponatremic hyperchloremic metabolic acidosis

24. Which of the following statements is FALSE regarding sexual function in patients with myelodysplasia?

    a. Females are unable to bear children in 50% of the cases.
    b. Males may have normal sperm production but are unable to have adequate ejaculatory function.
    c. Females have regular menses.
    d. Pubertal changes tend to occur earlier in myelodysplastic children compared with normal children.
    e. Incontinence of urine has little effect on the sexual behavior of males or females.

25. All of the following may be an outward physical sign of an occult spinal dysraphism EXCEPT:

    a. a subcutaneous mass overlying the thoracic spine.
    b. an asymmetrical gluteal cleft.
    c. a draining pilonidal dimple.
    d. one leg slightly longer than the other.
    e. a spinal scoliosis.

26. The conus medullaris normally resides opposite which vertebral body at puberty?

    a. T11
    b. T12
    c. L1
    d. L2
    e. L3

27. Which of the following maternal factors may be responsible for sacral agenesis in a newborn?

    a. Exposure to progestational agents early in the pregnancy
    b. Insulin-dependent diabetes early in the early gestational period
    c. Insulin dependency later in the pregnancy
    d. Exposure to progestational agents later in the pregnancy
    e. None of the above

28. Which of the following statements is TRUE regarding sacral agenesis?

    a. Motor function in the lower extremities and sacral area is normal.
    b. Motor function in the lower extremities and sacral area is impaired.
    c. The abnormality can be diagnosed in the newborn due to an abnormal gluteal cleft.
    d. Sensation in the lower extremities and sacral area is normal.
    e. Sensation in the lower extremities and sacral area is impaired.

29. Which statement is TRUE regarding neurogenic bladder dysfunction in children with imperforate anus?

    a. An injury to the pelvic nerves during the pull-through procedure leads to the lesion.
    b. A injury to the pelvic floor muscles while separating the rectourethral fistula may cause the lesion.
    c. Neurogenic bladder dysfunction is almost never seen in supralevator level lesions.
    d. Neurogenic bladder dysfunction is fairly common in infralevator level lesion.
    e. A spinal cord abnormality in association with imperforate anal lesions can be seen in 30% of imperforate anus cases.

30. Most children with cerebral palsy have what type of lower urinary tract function on urodynamic testing?

    a. A hyperactive bladder with denervation in the external urethral sphincter
    b. A hyperactive bladder with bladder sphincter dyssynergy during voiding
    c. An underactive bladder with denervation in the external urethral sphincter
    d. An underactive bladder with a normally innervated external urethral sphincter
    e. A normally reflexic bladder with bladder sphincter synergy during voiding

31. The most common cause of a traumatic spinal cord injury in infants is:

    a. a motor vehicle accident.
    b. an accidental fall from a high place.
    c. a hyperextension injury to the cervical spine during delivery.
    d. spinal column surgery to correct either an intraspinal process or scoliosis.
    e. a sports-related injury.

ANSWERS (PART A)

1. **c. Increase in bladder capacity and decrease in voiding frequency.** Development of normal bladder function involves an increase in bladder capacity in response to an increase in urine production. The voiding frequency decreases whereas the voided volume of each micturition increases with age.
2. **e. Higher Pdetmax is observed in both male and female infants.** Urodynamic studies of infants with normal lower urinary tracts have documented significantly higher Pdetmax in both male and female infants compared with adults, although it was also noted that male infants had significantly higher Pdetmax compared with female infants.
3. **b. Micturition is initiated with a full bladder by a simple spinal cord reflex.** Studies have shown that even in full-term fetuses and newborns, micturition is modulated by higher centers.
4. **e. All of the above.** Detrusor overactivity during filling causes frequent attacks of sudden and imperative sensations of urge (urgency) that are often counteracted by voluntary contraction of the pelvic floor muscles in an attempt to compress the urethra (hold maneuver) exhibited as squatting (Vincent's curtsey sign). Children with urge syndrome have small bladder capacities for age.
5. **b. vesicovaginal reflux.** This best describes post-void dribbling, which is typically when urine gets trapped in the vagina during voiding and dribbles out soon after standing in otherwise normal toilet-trained girls with no other associated urinary symptoms.
6. **a. Large bladder capacity with poor bladder emptying.** A decompensated bladder can result from chronic functional bladder outflow obstruction resulting in deterioration in detrusor contractility and emptying efficiency, which eventually leads to development of a large, floppy bladder.
7. **e. All of the above.** The close proximity of the rectum to the posterior wall of the bladder makes it possible that any gross distention of the rectum can result in mechanical compression of the bladder and bladder neck, leading to urinary obstruction. Fecal impaction may also induce bladder dysfunction, which may manifest with VUR, enuresis, or UTI.
8. **d. A urodynamic study is warranted for appropriate management of any underlying bladder dysfunction.** Infants with UTI and VUR (especially boys) have a high prevalence of high maximum voiding pressures associated with detrusor overactivity. Bladder dysfunction has a powerful relationship with nonresolution of high-grade VUR. Treatment of the bladder dysfunction, however, was shown to result in a marked increase in the rate of spontaneous resolution and reduction in recurrent UTIs.
9. **b. Voiding diary.** A daily record of fluid intake and urine output at home under normal conditions would be most informative as a noninvasive first-line investigation to suggest any underlying bladder dysfunction and identify those issues that warrant further investigations.
10. **c. Detrusor response may be inhibited during conventional fill urodynamic studies.** Nonphysiologic filling of the bladder during conventional fill urodynamics, even at low filling rates, can lead to misinterpretation of true bladder activity during normal situations. Artificial filling may inhibit detrusor response and attenuate its maximum contractile potential, rendering detrusor instability less pronounced and undetectable.
11. **a. antibiotic prophylaxis.** A significant proportion of children with severe nocturnal enuresis have been shown to have underlying bladder dysfunction that may respond to the different treatment modalities listed. There is no role in long-term antibiotic prophylaxis in these children because recurrent UTI is seldom a problem when other associated urologic anomalies are excluded.
12. **e. Reduced functional bladder capacity.** A significant proportion of children with severe nocturnal enuresis shows a marked reduction in functional bladder capacity when compared with age-matched normal controls. This may be related to the high prevalence of underlying bladder dysfunction, particularly of detrusor overactivity at night, in enuretic children.

ANSWERS (PART B)

13. **d. All of the above.** One has to consider multiple, other, possibly unrelated causes of urinary incontinence when the diagnosis is not evidently the result of a neurologic lesion.
14. **d. All of the above.** It is a mandatory parameter to accurately measure actual detrusor function (compliance, contractility, and leak-point pressure) that is free of artifacts of movement.
15. **b. Slow infusion of cold saline.** A slow infusion allows the detrusor muscle to accommodate to the increasing volume in at best a reproducible physiologic way. The cold solution may stimulate the detrusor to elicit overactive contraction during filling in patients with an overactive detrusor.
16. **c. Folic acid.** Folic acid has been shown to reduce the incidence of neural tube defects in several large populations of people when given to women of child-bearing age before pregnancy is achieved.
17. **b. Infants with this level lesion often have detrusor sphincter dyssynergia.** Seventy-four percent of newborns and 54% of older children have intact sacral cord function with absence of pontine micturition center coordination of the detrusor and urethral sphincter.
18. **d. 85%.** Fifteen to 20 percent of newborns have an abnormal urinary tract on radiologic examination when first evaluated consisting of hydroureteronephrosis secondary to spinal shock, probably from the spinal canal closure, or abnormalities that developed in utero as a result of abnormal lower urinary tract function in the form of outlet obstruction.
19. **e. 25%.** The neurologic lesion in myelodysplasia is a dynamic disease process in which changes take place throughout childhood. The exact number is variable, depending on the level of the original lesion, the thoroughness with which the children were followed, and the criteria used for diagnosing a change.
20. **b. VUR with a fully innervated urethral sphincter.** When the sacral reflex arc is intact the Credè maneuver results in a reflex response in the external sphincter that increases urethral resistance and raises the pressure needed to expel urine from the bladder. This, in turn, leads to high-pressure "voiding" that can aggravate the degree of reflux present and its effect on the kidney.
21. **c. a and b.** Lowering detrusor pressure and reducing overactivity of the muscle ensure that the bladder remains a favorable organ for a successful antireflux operation.

22. **d. Glycopyrrolate.** Glycopyrrolate is the most potent oral anticholinergic drug available today, but it may have the typical belladonna-like side effects common to all these drugs (see Table 123-1).

23. **a. Hyponatremic hypochloremic metabolic alkalosis.** A gastric segment removed from the gastrointestinal system can cause hyponatremic hypochloremic metabolic alkalosis because its secretory surface involves an active H^+ and Cl^- pump that is not regulated by endogenous hormones. There is no absorptive surface in the remaining sections of the bladder that can resorb these ions, and thus a metabolic derangement can rapidly occur.

24. **a. Females are unable to bear children in 50% of the cases.** Several studies have revealed that 70% to 80% of myelodysplastic women are able to become pregnant and have uneventful pregnancies and deliveries.

25. **a. a subcutaneous mass overlying the thoracic spine.** In more than 90% of children with an occult spinal dysraphism there is a cutaneous abnormality overlying the *lower* spine in the lower lumbar or upper sacral areas.

26. **c. L1.** Under normal circumstances, the conus medullaris ends just above the L2 vertebra at birth and recedes upward to T12 by adulthood because the spinal cord grows at a slower rate than the increasing height of the vertebral bodies.

27. **b. Insulin-dependent diabetes early in the early gestational period.** Teratogenic factors may play a role in the pathogenesis of sacral agenesis because insulin-dependent diabetic mothers have a 1% chance of giving birth to a child with this disorder.

28. **c. The abnormality can be diagnosed in the newborn due to an abnormal gluteal cleft.** The only clue to the diagnosis of sacral agenesis, besides a high index of suspicion, is flattened buttocks and a low, short gluteal cleft, because sensation and lower extremity motor function is usually normal.

29. **e. A spinal cord abnormality in association with imperforate anal lesions can be seen in 30% of imperforate anus cases.** Spinal cord abnormalities including a tethered cord, thickened or fatty filum terminale, and a lipoma have been noted in 18% to 50% of patients with an imperforate anus, with the incidence varying proportionately in relation to the height of the rectal lesion.

30. **e. A normally reflexic bladder with bladder sphincter synergy during voiding.** Most children with cerebral palsy develop total urinary control. Detrusor overactivity is seen in 80%, but dyssynergy between the bladder and sphincter has only been noted in 5%, and 11% have evidence of lower motor neuron denervation in the sphincter.

31. **c. a hyperextension injury to the cervical spine during delivery.** Newborns are particularly prone to a hyperextension injury of the cervical spine during high forceps delivery.

124

Urinary Tract Reconstruction in Children

MARK C. ADAMS • DAVID B. JOSEPH

QUESTIONS

1. Children with significant bladder or sphincter dysfunction requiring reconstructive surgery most likely have:
   a. bladder exstrophy or epispadias.
   b. posterior urethral valves.
   c. cloacal anomalies.
   d. prune-belly syndrome.
   e. spinal dysraphism.
2. The most important contribution to the field of pediatric reconstructive surgery has been:
   a. Mitrofanoff's description of a continent abdominal wall stoma using appendix.
   b. Lapides' introduction of clean intermittent catheterization (CIC).
   c. Goodwin's description of ileal reconfiguration.
   d. development of several effective means to increase bladder outlet resistance.
   e. recognition that a dilated ureter could be used for bladder augmentation.
3. Normal bladder compliance is based on:
   a. ample collagen type II.
   b. inverse relationship of bladder volume and bladder pressure.
   c. bladder unfolding, elasticity, and viscoelasticity.
   d. subepithelial matrix bridges associated with collagen.
   e. hypertrophic bladder bundles interspersed with collagen.
4. Chronically elevated bladder filling pressures may cause hydronephrosis, vesicoureteral reflux, and impaired renal function. The lowest pressure threshold most often reported to cause problems is:
   a. 20 cm H_2O.
   b. 30 cm H_2O.
   c. 40 cm H_2O.
   d. 50 cm H_2O.
   e. 60 cm H_2O.
5. Upper urinary tract changes associated with a poorly compliant, hyperreflexic bladder are initially treated by:
   a. autoaugmentation.
   b. pharmacologic management and intermittent catheterization.
   c. ileal augmentation.
   d. sigmoid augmentation.
   e. gastric augmentation.
6. Preoperative bladder capacity and compliance are best determined by urodynamics using:
   a. carbon dioxide as an irrigant at a slow fill rate (10% of capacity per minute).
   b. room temperature saline at a slow fill rate (10% of capacity per minute).
   c. body temperature saline at a fast fill rate (30% of capacity per minute).
   d. cooled saline at a slow fill rate (10% of capacity per minute).
   e. cooled saline at a fast fill rate (30% of capacity per minute).
7. Urinary tract reconstruction for urinary continence requires:
   a. confirmation of a normal upper urinary tract.
   b. identification of a highly compliant bladder.
   c. documentation of the presence or absence of vesicoureteral reflux.
   d. acceptance and compliance with intermittent catheterization.
   e. documentation of a serum creatinine value less than 1.4 mg/dL.
8. Mechanical bowel preparation is performed in patients undergoing:
   a. ileocystoplasty.
   b. sigmoid cystoplasty.
   c. gastrocystoplasty.
   d. ureterocystoplasty.
   e. all of the above.
9. A urinary stricture after transureteroureterostomy (TUU) is most likely due to:
   a. mobilization of the crossing ureter with periureteral tissue.
   b. mobilization of the crossing ureter without angulation beneath the inferior mesenteric artery.
   c. mobilization of the recipient ureter to meet the crossing one.
   d. wide anastomosis of the crossing ureter to the posteromedial aspect of the recipient.
   e. watertight anastomosis.
10. Creating an antireflux mechanism is most difficult with anastomosis to the:
    a. stomach.
    b. ileum.
    c. cecum.
    d. transverse colon.
    e. sigmoid colon.

11. The Young-Dees-Leadbetter bladder neck repair in children with neurogenic sphincter deficiency:
    a. results in limited success because of a lack of muscle tone and activity of the native bladder neck.
    b. can achieve successful continence results similar to those noted in children with bladder exstrophy.
    c. does not often require bladder augmentation or intermittent catheterization.
    d. is best performed in association with a Silastic sling.
    e. limits the necessity for intermittent catheterization in children who could empty by a Valsalva maneuver preoperatively.
12. An ambulatory 15-year-old girl with lumbosacral myelomeningocele voids to completion with a low-pressure detrusor contraction and the Valsalva maneuver. She remains incontinent due to bladder neck and intrinsic sphincter deficiency refractory to pharmacologic management. To limit the risk of intermittent catheterization, the next step is:
    a. Young-Dees-Leadbetter bladder neck repair.
    b. artificial urinary sphincter placement.
    c. fascial bladder neck sling placement.
    d. Kropp bladder neck repair.
    e. Pippi-Salle bladder neck repair.
13. One side effect associated with bladder neck repair that can be decreased with good preoperative evaluation is:
    a. recurrent urolithiasis.
    b. recurrent cystitis.
    c. inability to spontaneously void.
    d. associated need for augmentation cystoplasty.
    e. unmasking of detrusor hostility, resulting in upper urinary tract changes.
14. Fascial slings used for increasing outlet resistance in children with neurogenic sphincteric incompetence:
    a. are more effective in girls than in boys.
    b. are dependent on the type of fascial or cadaveric tissue used.
    c. are dependent on the configuration of the sling and wrap used.
    d. rarely result in the need for bladder augmentation and intermittent catheterization.
    e. frequently result in urethral erosion.
15. The least favorable indication for an artificial urinary sphincter is:
    a. neurogenic bladder dysfunction.
    b. bladder exstrophy or epispadias.
    c. inability to empty the bladder by spontaneous voiding.
    d. associated need for bladder augmentation.
    e. prepubertal age.
16. The most common limitation of a Kropp urethral lengthening for continence is:
    a. fistula from the urethra to the bladder, resulting in incontinence.
    b. inability to spontaneously void, resulting in urinary retention.
    c. difficulty with intermittent catheterization, particularly in boys.
    d. new vesicoureteral reflux.
    e. distal ureteral obstruction.
17. Urinary continence is most definitively achieved after:
    a. Young-Dees-Leadbetter bladder repair.
    b. placement of an artificial urinary sphincter.
    c. placement of a circumferential fascial wrap.
    d. urethral lengthening and reimplantation.
    e. bladder neck division.
18. To avoid uninhibited pressure contractions during an enterocystoplasty:
    a. large bowel should be used.
    b. the intestinal segment should be reconfigured.
    c. the majority of the diseased bladder should be excised.
    d. a stellate incision into the bladder should be created to increase the circumference of the bowel anastomosis.
    e. small mesenteric windows are created in the bowel segment.
19. Potential ways to prevent reflux when using ileum for continent diversion include:
    a. intussuscepted nipple valve.
    b. split nipple cuff of ureter.
    c. placement of the spatulated ureter into an incised mucosal trough.
    d. flap valve created beneath a tenia.
    e. placement of the ureter within a serosa-lined tunnel between two limbs of ileum.
20. The gastrointestinal segment that most often causes permanent gastrointestinal side effects when used in children with a neurogenic bladder is the:
    a. stomach.
    b. jejunum.
    c. ileum.
    d. ileocecal segment.
    e. sigmoid colon.
21. The most likely problem after gastrointestinal bladder augmentation is:
    a. early satiety.
    b. hyperchloremic metabolic acidosis.
    c. small bowel obstruction.
    d. chronic diarrhea.
    e. vitamin B_{12} deficiency with megaloblastic anemia.
22. The gastrointestinal segment resulting in the best long-term capacity and compliance after augmentation cytoplasty is the:
    a. gastric body.
    b. gastric antrum.
    c. ileum.
    d. cecum.
    e. sigmoid colon.
23. The risk of failure to achieve appropriate capacity and compliance after augmentation cystoplasty is:
    a. $< 5\%$.
    b. 5% to 10%.
    c. 11% to 15%.
    d. 16% to 20%.
    e. $> 20\%$.
24. The serum metabolic pattern that occurs most often after an ileo- or colocystoplasty is:
    a. hypochloremic metabolic acidosis.
    b. hyperchloremic metabolic acidosis.
    c. hypochloremic metabolic alkalosis.
    d. hyperchloremic metabolic alkalosis.
    e. hyponatremic metabolic acidosis.
25. The serum metabolic pattern that occurs most often after gastrocystoplasty is:
    a. hypochloremic metabolic acidosis.
    b. hyperchloremic metabolic acidosis.
    c. hypochloremic metabolic alkalosis.
    d. hyperchloremic metabolic alkalosis.
    e. hyponatremic metabolic acidosis.

26. The risk of intermittent hematuria and dysuria after gastrocystoplasty is influenced by:

    a. gastric segment used.
    b. persistent urinary incontinence.
    c. decreased renal function.
    d. diagnosis of bladder exstrophy.
    e. neurogenic bladder dysfunction.

27. Bacteriuria should be treated after bladder augmentation when:

    a. associated with CIC.
    b. urinalysis demonstrates microscopic hematuria.
    c. there is increased mucus production.
    d. etiology is posterior urethral valves.
    e. urine culture reveals growth of a urea-splitting organism.

28. The gastrointestinal segment associated with the lowest incident of stone formation is:

    a. stomach.
    b. jejunum.
    c. ileum.
    d. cecum.
    e. sigmoid colon.

29. Adenocarcinoma of the bladder after augmentation cystoplasty can occur after:

    a. 2 years.
    b. 4 years.
    c. 8 years.
    d. 16 years.
    e. 26 years.

30. The risk of perforation after bladder augmentation includes all but:

    a. high outflow resistance.
    b. persistent hyperreflexia or uninhibited bladder contractions.
    c. use of sigmoid colon.
    d. bladder exstrophy.
    e. neurogenic bladder dysfunction.

31. The initial management of a spontaneous perforation of an augmented bladder in a child with a neurogenic bladder is:

    a. placement of a large-bore urethral catheter for drainage.
    b. placement of a large-bore suprapubic cystotomy tube for drainage.
    c. immediate surgical exploration and repair.
    d. serial abdominal examinations.
    e. urine culture.

32. Pregnancy associated with urinary reconstruction:

    a. is reasonable after urinary diversion but is contraindicated after augmentation cystoplasty.
    b. results in the mesenteric pedicle positioned directly anterior to the uterus.
    c. results in the mesenteric pedicle deflected laterally without vascular compromise to the augmented segment.
    d. is avoided due to mechanical compression of the pedicle and ischemia with loss of the augmented segment.
    e. is contraindicated because of increased risk of systemic sepsis complicating the hydronephrosis.

33. Ureterocystoplasty is limited because:

    a. it requires an intraperitoneal approach.
    b. complete mobilization of the ureter may result in vascular compromise.
    c. dilated ureter is not as compliant as a similar-sized bowel segment.
    d. dilated ureter is not available in many patients.
    e. ureterocystoplasty precludes spontaneous voiding.

34. Autoaugmentation is contraindicated with:

    a. serum creatinine value greater than 1.4 ng/dL.
    b. CIC.
    c. vesicoureteral reflux.
    d. uninhibited bladder contractions.
    e. small bladder capacity.

35. A ureterosigmoidostomy should not be undertaken with a history of:

    a. dilated ureters.
    b. anteriorly placed rectum associated with bladder exstrophy.
    c. recurrent pyelonephritis.
    d. fecal incontinence.
    e. constipation.

36. The use of efferent nipple valves for continence in the children:

    a. has not approached the results achieved in adults.
    b. has a higher complication and reoperation rate than a flap valve.
    c. is equivalent to any other continence mechanism.
    d. is often associated with difficulty in catheterization.
    e. often results in stomal stenosis.

37. The least important factor when creating an appendicovesicostomy is:

    a. taking a wide cecal cuff to decrease the risk of stomal stenosis.
    b. creating a tunnel of 4 cm, at least > 5:1 ratio of tunnel length to diameter, to achieve continence.
    c. small, uniform lumen allowing for easy catheterization.
    d. mobilizing the right colon to adequately free the appendix.
    e. tubularizing a small portion of the cecum in continuity with the appendix to increase length.

38. A frequent occurrence after an appendicovesicostomy is:

    a. urinary incontinence due to inadequate length of the flap valve mechanism.
    b. urinary incontinence due to persistently elevated reservoir pressure.
    c. appendiceal perforation often occurs due to catheterization.
    d. appendiceal stricture or necrosis.
    e. stomal stenosis.

39. A 12-year-old obese girl with spina bifida undergoes appendicocecostomy, bladder neck sling, bladder augmentation, and continent catheterizable bladder channel. The upper urinary tract is normal. The best source of tissue for the bladder channel is:

    a. distal right ureter after right-to-left TUU.
    b. tapered segment of small bowel of adequate length.
    c. right fallopian tube.
    d. gastric tube.
    e. tubularized bladder flap.

40. In complex pediatric urinary undiversion procedures, it is most difficult to:

    a. provide adequate outflow resistance.
    b. create a compliant urinary reservoir.
    c. achieve an effective antireflux mechanism without upper tract obstruction.
    d. provide a reliable access for intermittent catheterization.
    e. achieve urinary and fecal continence.

ANSWERS

1. **e. spinal dysraphism.** Most pediatric reconstructive procedures are undertaken to correct a problem of the native urinary tract causing progressive hydronephrosis, urinary incontinence unresponsive to medical management, or temporary diversion. Children with bladder and sphincteric dysfunction represent the most complex reconstructive cases seen in pediatric urology; children with the diagnoses of exstrophy, persistent cloaca and urogenital sinus, posterior urethral valves, bilateral single ectopic ureters, and prune-belly syndrome may be involved. However, children with a neurogenic bladder due to a myelomeningocele make up the vast majority of patients requiring this type of surgical intervention.

2. **b. Lapides' introduction of clean intermittent catheterization (CIC).** One of the most important contributions in the care of children with bladder dysfunction came with the acceptance of CIC described by Lapides and colleagues in 1972 and 1976, based on the work of Guttmann and Frankel. The effective use of CIC has allowed the application of augmentation and lower tract reconstruction to groups of patients who had not previously been candidates. The principle of intermittent catheterization allows the reconstructive surgeon to aggressively correct storage problems by providing an adequate reservoir and good outflow resistance. Spontaneous voiding, although a goal, is not imperative because catheterization can be used for emptying.

3. **c. bladder unfolding, elasticity, and viscoelasticity.** Multiple factors contribute to the property of compliance. Initially the bladder is in a collapsed state, which allows for the storage of urine at low pressure by simply unfolding. As it expands, detrusor properties of elasticity and viscoelasticity take effect. Elasticity allows the detrusor muscle to stretch without an increase in tension until it reaches a critical volume. When filling is slow, as in a natural state, or stops, there is a rapid decay in this pressure known as stress relaxation. Normally, stress relaxation is in balance with the filling rate and prevents an increase in detrusor pressure.

4. **c. 40 cm H_2O.** Elevated passive filling pressure becomes clinically pathogenic when a pressure greater than 40 cm H_2O is chronically reached. Pressure at this level sustained over a prolonged period of time impairs ureteral drainage and can result in acquired vesicoureteral reflux, pyelocaliceal changes, hydroureteronephrosis, and decreased glomerular filtration rate.

5. **b. pharmacologic management and intermittent catheterization.** Pharmacologic management can play a role in decreasing filling pressure, particularly when hyperreflexic detrusor contractions are present. A combination of medications and intermittent catheterization has a positive impact, particularly in children with neurogenic dysfunction.

6. **b. room temperature saline at a slow fill rate (10% of capacity per minute).** The testing medium and infusion rate can influence the results. Carbon dioxide is not as reliable as fluid infusion, particularly when evaluating bladder compliance and capacity. The most common fluids used for testing are saline and iodinated contrast material; both provide reproducible results. Use of testing media at body temperature is also appropriate, but room temperature has also been shown to be acceptable. End filling pressure, and bladder compliance, can be dramatically affected by simply changing the filling rate. The cystometrogram should be performed at a fill rate of 10% per minute of the predicted bladder capacity for age.

7. **d. acceptance and compliance with intermittent catheterization.** No test ensures that a patient will be able to void spontaneously and empty well after bladder augmentation or other reconstruction. Therefore, all patients must be prepared to perform CIC postoperatively. The native urethra should be examined for the ease of catheterization. Ideally, the patient should learn CIC and practice it preoperatively until the patient, family, and surgeon are comfortable that catheterization can and will be performed reliably. In spite of a technically perfect operation, failure to catheterize and empty the bladder after reconstruction can result in upper tract deterioration, urinary tract infection, or bladder perforation.

8. **e. all of the above.** Each patient undergoes preoperative bowel preparation to minimize the potential risk of surgery if the use of any bowel is contemplated. Even when ureterocystoplasty or other alternatives are planned, intraoperative findings may dictate the need for use of a bowel segment.

9. **c. mobilization of the recipient ureter to meet the crossing one.** If the native urinary bladder is small and adequate for only a single ureteral tunnel, TUU and a single reimplant may be helpful. Typically, the better ureter should be implanted into the bladder. The contralateral ureter drains into the reimplanted ureter via a TUU. The crossing ureter should follow a smooth path and remain tension free. It should be carefully mobilized with all of its adventitia and as much periureteral tissue as possible to preserve blood supply. Care must be taken not to angulate the crossing ureter beneath the inferior mesenteric artery. The crossing ureter should be widely anastomosed to the posteromedial aspect of the recipient ureter. The recipient ureter should not be mobilized or brought medially to meet the contralateral ureter in order to minimize devascularization.

10. **b. ileum.** The necessity of ureteral reimplantation into an intestinal segment may occasionally determine the segment to be used for bladder augmentation or replacement. Long-term experience with ureterosigmoidostomy and colon conduit diversion has established an effective means of creating a nonrefluxing ureteral implant. If a gastric segment is used for bladder augmentation or replacement, the ureters may be implanted into the stomach in a manner remarkably similar to that used in the native bladder. Creating an effective antireflux mechanism into an ileal segment is more difficult. The split nipple technique described by Griffith may prevent reflux at least at low reservoir pressure.

11. **a. results in limited success because of a lack of muscle tone and activity of the native bladder neck.** Reports of success with the Young-Dees-Leadbetter bladder neck reconstruction in children with neurogenic sphincter dysfunction are limited, not only in the number of series but in overall improvement of incontinence. Independent reviews of long-term results of this repair showed minimal success in individuals with neurogenic dysfunction. These authors speculated that the lack of success was due to a lack of muscle tone and activity in the wrapped muscle related to the neurogenic problem.

12. **b. artificial urinary sphincter placement.** The artificial urinary sphincter has been recognized as the only procedure that can result in prompt continence in selected children while preserving their ability to void spontaneously.

13. **e. unmasking of detrusor hostility, resulting in upper urinary tract changes.** It is now recognized that occlusion of the bladder neck in children with neurogenic sphincter incompetence can result in the unmasking or development of detrusor hostility manifest by a decrease in bladder compliance or increase in detrusor hyperreflexia. Careful preoperative urodynamic assessment helps to identify some of the children who are at risk.

14. **a. are more effective in girls than in boys.** Fascial slings have been used more extensively and with better results in girls with neurogenic sphincter incompetence, although recently some success has been reported in boys. Overall long-term success with fascial slings in the neurogenic population has varied greatly from 40% to 100%.

15. **c. inability to empty the bladder by spontaneous voiding.** The ultimate benefits of the artificial urinary sphincter include its ability to achieve a high rate of continence while maintaining the potential for spontaneous voiding. For practical purposes, when intermittent catheterization is required along with augmentation cystoplasty, using native tissue for continence eliminates the long-term concern for infection/erosion and the risk of mechanical failure.

16. **c. difficulty with intermittent catheterization, particularly in boys.** One study examined the results in 23 children, 22 of whom had neurogenic sphincter incompetence, and noted continence in more than 90% of the children. The most common complication was difficult catheterization, particularly in boys. Less than half of the boys in this series were catheterized through the native urethra; the majority were catheterized via an abdominal wall stoma.

17. **e. bladder neck division.** The ultimate procedure to increase bladder outlet resistance is to divide the bladder neck so that it is no longer in continuity with the urethra. This must be accompanied by creation of a continent abdominal wall stoma and should be performed only in patients who will reliably be able to perform catheterization.

18. **b. the intestinal segment should be reconfigured.** Two studies demonstrated the advantages of opening a bowel segment on its antimesenteric border, which allows detubularization and reconfiguration of that intestinal segment. Reconfiguration into a spherical shape provides multiple advantages, including maximization of the volume achieved for any given surface area, blunting of bowel contractions, and improvement of overall capacity and compliance.

19. **d. flap valve created beneath a tenia.** The split nipple technique described by Griffith may prevent reflux at least at low reservoir pressure. LeDuc and colleagues in 1987 described a technique in which the ureter is brought through a hiatus in the ileal wall. From that hiatus, the ileal mucosa is incised and the edges are mobilized so as to create a trough for the ureter. It may also be possible to create antireflux mechanism using a serosal-lined tunnel created between two limbs of ileum as described by Abol-Enein and Ghoneim in 1999. Reinforced nipple valves of ileum have been used extensively to prevent reflux with the Kock pouch. Good long-term results have been achieved by Skinner after several modifications.

20. **d. ileocecal segment.** Chronic diarrhea after bladder augmentation alone is rare. Diarrhea can occur after removal of large segments of ileum from the gastrointestinal tract, although the length of the segments typically used for augmentation is rarely problematic unless other problems coexist. Removal of the ileum and ileocecal valve from the gastrointestinal tract may cause diarrhea. One study noted that 10% of patients with neurogenic dysfunction have significant diarrhea after such displacement.

21. **b. hyperchloremic metabolic acidosis.** Postoperative bowel obstruction is uncommon after augmentation cystoplasty, occurring in approximately 3% of patients after augmentation. The rate of obstruction is equivalent to that noted after conduit diversion or continent urinary diversion. Removal of the distal ileum from the gastrointestinal tract may result in vitamin B_{12} deficiency and megaloblastic anemia. The terminal 15 to 20 cm of ileum should not be used for augmentation, although problems may arise even if that segment is preserved. Early satiety may occur after gastrocystoplasty but usually resolves with time. Disorders of gastric emptying should be extremely rare, particularly when using the body of the stomach.

22. **c. ileum.** Ileal reservoirs have been noted to have lower basal pressures and less motor activity when created for continent urinary diversion. Problems with pressure after augmentation cystoplasty usually occur from uninhibited contractions caused by the bowel segment. It is extremely rare not to achieve an adequate capacity or flat tonus limb unless a technical error has occurred with use of the bowel segment. Rhythmic contractions have been noted postoperatively with all bowel segments, particularly the stomach, although ileum is the least likely to demonstrate a remarkable urodynamic abnormality.

23. **b. 5% to 10%.** Hollensbe and associates at Indiana University reported on one of the largest experiences with pediatric bladder augmentation and found that approximately 5% of patients had significant uninhibited contractions causing clinical problems. Another study found that 6% required secondary augmentation of a previously augmented bladder for similar problems in long-term follow-up.

24. **b. hyperchloremic metabolic acidosis.** The first recognized metabolic complication related to storage of urine within intestinal segments was the occasional development of hyperchloremic metabolic acidosis after ureterosigmoidostomy. Another study demonstrated the mechanisms by which acid is absorbed from urine in contact with intestinal mucosa. A later report noted that essentially every patient after augmentation with an intestinal segment had an increase in serum chloride and a decrease in serum bicarbonate levels, although clinically significant acidosis was rare if renal function was normal.

25. **c. hypochloremic metabolic alkalosis.** Gastric mucosa is a barrier to chloride and acid resorption and, in fact, secretes hydrochloric acid. The secretory nature of gastric mucosa may at times be detrimental to the patient and can result in two unique complications of gastrocystoplasty. Severe episodes of hypokalemic hypochloremic metabolic alkalosis after acute gastrointestinal illnesses have been noted after gastrocystoplasty.

26. **e. neurogenic bladder dysfunction.** Virtually all patients with normal sensation have occasional hematuria or dysuria with voiding or catheterization after gastrocystoplasty beyond that which is expected with other intestinal segments. All patients should be warned of this potential problem, although in most patients these symptoms are intermittent and mild and do not require treatment. The dysuria is less problematic in patients with limited sensation due to neurogenic dysfunction. Patients who are incontinent or have decreased renal function may be at increased risk. These problems occur less frequently after antral gastric cystoplasty in which there is a smaller load of parietal cells.

27. **e. urine culture reveals growth of a urea-splitting organism.** It appears that the use of CIC is a prominent factor in the development of bacteriuria in patients after augmentation cystoplasty. Every episode of asymptomatic bacteriuria does not require treatment in patients performing CIC. Bacteriuria should be treated when significant symptoms occur such as fever, suprapubic pain, incontinence, and gross hematuria. Bacteriuria should also be treated when the urine culture demonstrates growth of a urea-splitting organism that may lead to stone formation.

28. **a. stomach.** Most bladder stones in the augmented child are of a struvite composition. Bacteriuria has been thought to be an important risk factor. Stones have been noted after the use of all intestinal segments with no significant difference appreciated between small and large intestine. Struvite stones are less likely after gastrocystoplasty.

29. **b. 4 years.** Patients undergoing augmentation cystoplasty should be made aware of a potential increased risk of tumor development. Yearly surveillance of the augmented bladder with endoscopy should eventually be performed; the latency period until such procedures are necessary is not well defined. The earliest reported tumor after augmentation was found only 4 years after cystoplasty.

30. **d. bladder exstrophy.** The cause of delayed perforations after bladder augmentation is unknown. Perforations may occur in bladders with significant uninhibited contractions after augmentation. High outflow resistance may maintain bladder pressure rather than allowing urinary leakage and venting of the pressure, potentially increasing ischemia. The majority of patients suffering perforations after augmentation cystoplasty have a neurogenic etiology. At Indiana University, perforations were noted in 32 of 330 patients undergoing cystoplasty an average of 4.3 years after augmentation. Analysis of this experience suggested that the use of sigmoid colon was the only significant increased risk.

31. **c. immediate surgical exploration and repair.** The standard treatment of spontaneous perforation of the augmented bladder is surgical repair, as it is for intraperitoneal rupture of the bladder after trauma. The majority of patients with perforations have myelodysplasia and present late in the course of the disease because of impaired sensation. Increasing sepsis and death of the patient may result from a delay in diagnosis or treatment.

32. **c. results in the mesenteric pedicle deflected laterally without vascular compromise to the augmented segment.** Experience is limited regarding what is known about the changes to the pedicle of a bladder augmentation during pregnancy. It has been reported that the mesenteric pedicle to bladder augmentations is not stretched over the uterus at the time of cesarean section. The pedicle has been found to be deflected laterally. Urinary tract infections may be problematic in women who have undergone urinary reconstruction, including bladder augmentation. Ureteral dilatation, increased residual urine, and diminished tone to the upper tract may all be important risk factors.

33. **d. a dilated ureter is not available in many patients.** Several series have reported good results after ureteral augmentation with a follow-up as long as 8 years. The upper urinary tract has remained stable or improved in virtually all patients. Complications are uncommon. The main disadvantage to ureterocystoplasty is the limited patient population with a poorly functioning kidney drained by a megaureter.

34. **e. small bladder capacity.** Although autoaugmentation can improve compliance, an increase in volume is "modest at best." In a report of 12 children who had undergone a detrusorotomy, 5 were considered to have excellent results, 2 had acceptable results, and 1 was lost to follow-up. The main disadvantage of autoaugmentation is a limited increase in bladder capacity such that adequate preoperative volume may be the most important predictor of success.

35. **d. fecal incontinence.** Before ureterosigmoidostomy is considered, anal sphincter competence must be ensured. Tests used to assess sphincter integrity include manometry, electromyography, and practical evaluation of the ability to retain an oatmeal enema in the upright position for a time period without soilage. Incontinence of a mixture of stool and urine results in foul soilage and must be avoided.

36. **b. has a higher complication and reoperation rate than a flap valve.** The greatest experience with nipple valves for achieving urinary continence has been with the Kock pouch. Skinner and associates made a series of modifications to aid in maintenance of the efferent nipple. Even with experience and these modifications, a failure rate of 15% or higher can be expected. Equivalent results with the nipple valve and a Kock pouch have been achieved in children.

37. **b. creating a tunnel of 4 cm, at least > 5:1 ratio of tunnel length to diameter, to achieve continence.** The appendix is an ideal natural tubular structure that can be safely removed from the gastrointestinal tract without significant morbidity. The small caliber of the appendix facilitates creation of a short functional tunnel with the bladder wall. Experience has shown that continence can be achieved with only a 2-cm appendiceal tunnel.

38. **e. stomal stenosis.** Incontinence is rare with the Mitrofanoff principle and may result from inadequate length of the flap valve mechanism or persistently elevated reservoir pressure. The most common complication has been stomal stenosis and occurs in 10% to 20% of patients. Stenosis resulting in difficult catheterization may occur early in the postoperative course and requires formal revision.

39. **b. tapered segment of small bowel of adequate length.** When the appendix is unavailable for use, other tubular structures can provide a similar mechanism for catheterization and continence. Mitrofanoff, in 1980, described a similar technique using ureter. Woodhouse and MacNeily, in 1994, as well as others, have used the fallopian tube, which can accommodate catheterization. Monti and Yang have been credited with a novel modification of the tapered intestinal segment, which can be reimplanted according to the Mitrofanoff principle.

40. **c. achieve an effective antireflux mechanism without upper tract obstruction.** The key to urinary undiversion is understanding the original pathologic condition that led to diversion. One report described a 26-year experience with urinary undiversion in 216 patients. In that series, management of the bladder was relatively straightforward and effective with bladder augmentation as necessary. In that series inadequate outflow resistance was usually treated with Young-Dees-Ledbetter bladder neck repair. Most complications were related to the ureters; 23 patients required reoperation for persistent reflux, whereas 10 did so for partial obstruction of the ureter. Those reoperation rates are indicative of the difficulty one faces in dealing with short, dilated, and scarred ureters, which may be present after urinary diversion.

125

Hypospadias

JOSEPH G. BORER • ALAN B. RETIK

QUESTIONS

1. Components of hypospadias typically include which of the following?
   a. An underdeveloped foreskin with dorsal penile curvature
   b. A urethral meatus location below the general area of the distal tip of the glans penis
   c. A universal absence of hypospadias in females
   d. A penopubic location for the urethral meatus
   e. One or more associated anomalies in an organ system other than the genitourinary tract
2. The level of the hypospadia defect is most appropriately defined at what point?
   a. At diagnosis, in the absence of penile curvature
   b. After correction of penile curvature (orthoplasty), when necessary
   c. Before repair
   d. After repair
   e. a and b
3. Regarding urethral development, which of the following is correct?
   a. The urethral groove forms between the urethral folds at an early stage in urethral development.
   b. During the 11th week of fetal life the urethral folds fuse to form the urethra.
   c. Preputial skin development is completed before development of the urethra is complete, and this sequential development explains the dorsal hood foreskin commonly seen in boys with hypospadias.
   d. a and b.
   e. b and c.
4. Embryologically, the endodermal differentiation theory purports that which of the following means "... forms the distal glanular portion of the urethra"?
   a. Differentiation of ectodermal tissue into stratified squamous epithelium
   b. Invagination of surface epithelium of ectodermal origin
   c. Differentiation of endodermal tissue into stratified squamous epithelium
   d. Closure of urethral folds in the dorsal midline
   e. Closure of primary urethral groove
5. An accurate concept of penile innervation is described by which of the following?
   a. The pattern of penile innervation does not have a significant impact on the choice of technique for treatment of penile curvature.
   b. The nerve bundles remain as two well-defined structures on the dorsal aspect of the penis.
   c. The pattern of innervation allows for reliable analgesia via a well-placed dorsal penile nerve block.
   d. The pattern of innervation permits the safe use of the dorsal plication technique for orthoplasty, when the sutures are confined to the midline.
   e. c and d.
6. Which of the following support disruption of the normal endocrine milieu as a possible cause of hypospadias?
   a. Maternal progestin intake during pregnancy
   b. Increased rate of hypospadias in male offspring conceived by in-vitro fertilization
   c. An 8.5-fold higher rate of hypospadias in one of monozygotic male twins compared with singleton live male births
   d. All of the above
7. Which of the following is an accurate explanation for the associated hypospadias seen in individuals with Reifenstein's syndrome?
   a. An end-organ androgen receptor abnormality as is the case for any of the partial androgen insensitivity syndromes
   b. Reifenstein's syndrome is a manifestation of an abnormality in the hypothalamic-pituitary-testosterone axis.
   c. Testicular Leydig cell dysfunction
   d. Testicular Sertoli cell dysfunction
   e. Maternal exogenous progestin intake in the first trimester of pregnancy
8. Recent developments regarding the etiology of penile curvature noted on histologic evaluation of boys with hypospadias include which of the following?
   a. Subepithelial biopsy of the urethral plate revealing well-vascularized smooth muscle and collagen
   b. Findings that differ from that of a fetus with hypospadias
   c. Band of dense fibrous tissue composed of abortive corpus spongiosum
   d. Scar tissue of epithelial origin

9. All of the following are causes of penile curvature without hypospadias. The least common of these is believed to be which of the following?
   a. Skin tethering
   b. Fibrotic dartos tissue
   c. Congenitally short urethra
   d. Corporeal disproportion
   e. Fibrotic Buck's fascia
10. Two independent and well-established congenital anomaly registries in the United States have shown recent trends in hypospadias prevalence that are best summarized in which of the following?
   a. A near doubling of hypospadias rates in the most recent compared with immediately preceding decades
   b. The prevalence for hypospadias of approximately 1 in every 250 live male births
   c. A three- to five-fold increase in severe hypospadias
   d. All of the above
11. The true prevalence of hypospadias at birth may be underestimated because of which of the following?
   a. Postnatal development of the genitalia in some boys
   b. Incomplete physical examination in the newborn, highlighting the need for clear visualization of the urethral meatus position at the newborn examination
   c. Environmental endocrine disruptor exposure in the newborn
   d. Underreporting of this poorly recognized anomaly
12. In which of the following settings should karyotype analysis be considered?
   a. When hypospadias is associated with hernia or hydrocele
   b. In all individuals with hypospadias of any degree of severity
   c. In individuals with hypospadias and cryptorchidism
   d. Karyotypic analysis in the setting of hypospadias is rarely indicated and is of little benefit in future care of the individual
13. Which of the following findings on physical examination should raise the suspicion of an intersex state in a presumed male with hypospadias?
   a. Mid–penile shaft hypospadias with an otherwise normal examination
   b. Bilateral cryptorchidism without hypospadias
   c. Either unilateral or bilateral cryptorchidism with any degree of hypospadias
   d. Distal hypospadias with descended, palpably normal gonads and a normal-appearing scrotum
14. Regarding the association of hypospadias, cryptorchidism, and intersex states, which of the following is correct?
   a. Approximately 15% of individuals with hypospadias and a palpable undescended gonad will have an intersex condition.
   b. Approximately 50% of individuals with hypospadias and a unilateral nonpalpable gonad will have an intersex condition.
   c. A chromosomal abnormality may be present in 20% of individuals with hypospadias and cryptorchidism.
   d. All of the above.
15. If not repaired, isolated glanular or coronal hypospadias will eventually result in which of the following?
   a. Difficulty with micturition
   b. Inability to inseminate during sexual intercourse
   c. Clinically significant meatal stenosis
   d. None of the above
16. Which of the following are TRUE regarding imaging in patients with hypospadias?
   a. Voiding cystourethrography may aid in management of severe hypospadias.
   b. A "genitogram" is indicated in severe hypospadias and nonpalpable gonads.
   c. Radiologic evaluation of the upper urinary tract is needed.
   d. Renal ultrasonography is recommended in hypospadias.
   e. a and b.
17. Preoperative androgen stimulation or administration in patients with severe hypospadias has resulted in all of the following EXCEPT:
   a. decreased penile size (relative to normal) in adulthood.
   b. 50% increase in penile size compared with preadministration measurement.
   c. hormonal levels that return to normal shortly after cessation of treatment.
   d. no appreciable lasting undesirable side effects of treatment.
18. Reliable methods for orthoplasty include which of the following?
   a. Interposition dermal graft for severe penile curvature in a short penis
   b. Several variations of multi-ply, small intestinal submucosa
   c. Tunica albuginea plication
   d. Dorsal plicating sutures at the 11 o'clock and 1 o'clock positions on the penile shaft
19. Preferably, local tissue flaps used for urethral reconstruction have all of the listed characteristics EXCEPT:
   a. axial blood supply preserved within dartos fascia.
   b. thin, nonhirsute, and reliably tailored tissue.
   c. blood supply and drainage via the internal iliac vessels.
   d. island flap type, with maintenance of vascular, but division of cutaneous, continuity.
20. Which of the following is an accurate general principle regarding tissue grafts?
   a. They rely on inosculation, defined as the diffusion of nutrient material from the adjacent graft host bed into the graft during the first 48 hours after placement.
   b. They rely on imbibition, defined as the formation of new and permanent vascularization of the graft.
   c. They survive in a graft host bed after successful completion of a process called "take."
   d. They are transferred with an intact blood supply and drainage.
21. In various forms, perhaps the single most important adjunctive measure to urethroplasty that decreases the risk of postoperative urethrocutaneous fistula formation is the use of which of the following?
   a. Compressive penile dressing
   b. Autologous dermal graft for orthoplasty
   c. Postoperative urinary diversion with an indwelling urethral catheter
   d. Subcutaneous (dartos) tissue second-layer neourethral coverage
   e. Routine postoperative immobilization
22. Factors that have led to the 6- to 12-month age range as the recommended ideal time for hypospadias repair include which of the following?
   a. Increased complication rates in older patients
   b. Psychosocial factors
   c. Amnesia
   d. Elimination of possible interference with toilet training
   e. All of the above

23. Appropriate statements regarding intraoperative hemostasis include all of the following EXCEPT:
    a. liberal use of monopolar electrocautery is encouraged in the well-vascularized glans and other penile tissues.
    b. intermittent use of a tourniquet at the base of the penis may optimize visualization of tissues during urethroplasty.
    c. bipolar electrocautery may have advantages over monopolar technology.
    d. in general, methods of achieving hemostasis without causing permanent tissue devitalization are preferred.
24. General principles with proven positive impact on outcome of hypospadias repair include which of the following?
    a. Temporary use of a soft urethral catheter in the early postoperative period after distal hypospadias repair to decrease the incidence of meatal stenosis
    b. A compressive penile dressing as a useful adjunct to distal hypospadias repair
    c. Perioperative and postoperative antibiotic administration to decrease the risk of urinary tract infection
    d. Liberal use of electrocautery to decrease the risk of postoperative complications such as bleeding
    e. Delicate handling of tissue, approximation of tissue without tension, and sterile meticulous technique
25. Ketoconazole may be used to eliminate postoperative penile erections in adolescents and adults after hypospadias repair. Which of the following best describes the method of action for ketoconazole?
    a. Decreases production of cholesterol
    b. Inhibits conversion of androstenedione to testosterone
    c. Reduces both adrenal and testicular androgen production through the inhibition of the enzyme 17,20 desmolase
    d. Directly inhibits 5α-reductase enzyme activity
    e. Competitively and irreversibly binds to the androgen receptor
26. When performing hypospadias repair, the surgeon should do which of the following?
    a. Carefully evaluate the anatomy and the tissue available before making any incision
    b. Entertain all possible options for repair
    c. Precede with complete circumferential incision approximately 5 mm proximal and parallel to the corona of the glans
    d. Begin each repair with either pharmacologic or artificial erection to assess penile curvature
    e. a and b
27. Ideal conditions for the MAGPI (meatoplasty and glanuloplasty) hypospadias repair technique include:
    a. glanular hypospadias with adequate urethral mobility and no penile curvature.
    b. distal hypospadias with or without mild penile curvature, regardless of urethral characteristics.
    c. middle and distal hypospadias with no penile curvature.
    d. all distal hypospadias not amenable to repair by tubularization techniques.
28. The principle of deep incision of the glans wings is important in almost all hypospadias repairs on what grounds?
    a. It allows for ease of neourethral closure.
    b. It secures the meatus at the tip of the glans and decreases the likelihood of meatal stenosis.
    c. It allows for approximation of the glans tissue in the ventral midline over the distal neourethra without tension.
    d. It decreased incidence of urethrocutaneous fistula.
    e. a and c.
29. Characteristics of the tubularized incised plate (TIP) urethroplasty technique for hypospadias repair include which of the following?
    a. It is a modification of the Thiersch-Duplay technique of hypospadias repair.
    b. It incorporates a longitudinal urethral plate "relaxing incision" to allow tension-free tubularization of the neourethra.
    c. It is applicable only to distal hypospadias defects.
    d. a and b
30. Factors that may limit appropriate usage of the Mathieu technique include all of the following EXCEPT:
    a. level of the hypospadias defect.
    b. less than optimal appearance of the urethral meatus.
    c. need to transect the urethral plate.
    d. mild to moderate ventral penile curvature.
31. Which of the following statements best summarizes the onlay island flap technique for hypospadias repair?
    a. It is limited to middle and anterior hypospadias.
    b. It has expanded to include proximal hypospadias defects.
    c. A high complication rate has prohibited generalized use.
    d. Popularity of this technique and its excellent results are due to a highly efficient "take" process.
32. Although controversial, indications for a "two-stage" hypospadias repair may include which of the following?
    a. Parental request
    b. Penoscrotal hypospadias with mild to moderate curvature
    c. Middle hypospadias with a previously failed hypospadias repair
    d. Scrotal or perineal hypospadias, severe curvature, and a small penis
33. All of the following statements regarding urethral stricture as a complication of hypospadias repair are true EXCEPT:
    a. stricture of the urethra may be noted distal to and may, in part, be responsible for development of a urethral diverticulum.
    b. it may present with decreased force of stream and/or straining at urination.
    c. urethral stricture after hypospadias repair is often successfully treated with endoscopic incision.
    d. urethral stricture is more common at the distal versus the proximal extent of the neourethral after transverse preputial island flap repair.
    e. Both c and d are false.

34. An accurate statement regarding general principles of reoperative hypospadias repair includes which of the following?
   a. Attempts at reoperative hypospadias surgery should not be undertaken less than approximately 6 months after previous failure.
   b. The first choice of method for repeat hypospadias repair involves use of extragenital tissue as a free graft.
   c. No attempt at repair should be entertained until all edema, infection, and inflammation has resolved, and healing is complete.
   d. a and c.
   e. a, b, and c.

35. Postoperative uroflowmetry may be useful by which of the following?
   a. It will ensure long-term patency of the repair if normal parameters are documented in the immediate postoperative period.
   b. It will identify an asymptomatic urethral stricture in some patients.
   c. It will be helpful in determining viability of tissue after complex hypospadias repair.
   d. Postoperative uroflowmetry results should be compared with routine preoperative uroflowmetry for all patients who undergo hypospadias repair.

ANSWERS

1. **b. A urethral meatus location below the general area of the distal tip of the glans penis.** Ventral penile curvature of varying degree is common in hypospadias. Hypospadias is found in females but much less commonly compared with males. The penopubic variant refers to epispadias. Hypospadias is most often an isolated finding.

2. **e. a and b.** Culp, in 1959, was perhaps the first to classify the level of hypospadias after any necessary treatment of penile curvature (orthoplasty) and to realize the importance of this method. In 1973, Barcat more formally proposed designating the location of the hypospadiac meatus, and thus the true extent of the urethral defect requiring repair, after orthoplasty.

3. **d. a and b.** The typical sequence is that of urethral closure followed by completion of foreskin development. This may explain why a later defect or interruption in development may result in a urethral meatus at the tip of the glans and an underdeveloped ventral foreskin.

4. **c. Differentiation of endodermal tissue into stratified squamous epithelium.** One study provided further support for the endodermal differentiation theory using tissue recombinant grafting techniques, which suggest that under the correct cellular signaling conditions endodermally derived epithelium (urethral plate) differentiates into the stratified squamous epithelial phenotype present in the fully developed distal glanular urethra.

5. **e. c and d.** The nerves that innervate the penis originate proximally as two well-defined bundles under the pubic rami superior and slightly lateral to the urethra. Nervous tissue then fans out laterally from the 11- and 1-o'clock positions all along the penis and does not remain confined to two well-defined bundles. The absence of neuronal structures at the 12 o'clock position along the entire shaft of the penis has also been noted and allows for treatment of ventral penile curvature in some patients by placement of dorsal midline plicating suture(s).

6. **d. All of the above.** A study investigating pathogenetic mechanisms that might have interfered with fetal testicular differentiation and/or function found a history of maternal progestin intake early in pregnancy, either for treatment of threatened abortion or in combination with estrogen for pregnancy testing. When the position of the urethral meatus was compared with the week of gestation at which progestin therapy was begun, a positive correlation was noted for more proximal hypospadias in mothers treated in the first month of pregnancy. Further support of an endocrine disruptor origin for hypospadias may be provided by markedly increased rates of hypospadias in male offspring conceived by in-vitro fertilization (progesterone given early for pregnancy support). Also, another group noted an 8.5-fold higher rate of hypospadias in one of monozygotic male twins compared with singleton live male births. These authors suggested that this strong association of monozygotic twinning and hypospadias may be due to an inability of a single placenta and reduced human chorionic gonadotropin levels to meet the requirements of two developing male fetuses.

7. **a. An end-organ androgen receptor abnormality as is the case for any of the partial androgen insensitivity syndromes.** Reifenstein's syndrome is one of several diagnoses in the spectrum of entities with partial androgen insensitivity as the etiology of hypospadias. These are some of the most difficult causes to treat, often requiring supraphysiologic doses of testosterone to elicit a growth response in genital tissues.

8. **a. Subepithelial biopsy of the urethral plate revealing well-vascularized smooth muscle and collagen.** A report has challenged most of the historical tenets that typically vilified the urethral plate as the sole source or a contributing factor in chordee or penile curvature. Using light microscopy and routine staining techniques, these investigators showed that subepithelial biopsy of the urethral plate in 17 boys with hypospadias, including 5 with curvature and 4 with penoscrotal defects, revealed well-vascularized smooth muscle and collagen without fibrous bands or dysplastic tissue. These results were consistent with histologic findings at autopsy in a boy with proximal hypospadias and a fetus with distal hypospadias.

9. **c. Congenitally short urethra.** One report evenly divided the cause of congenital penile curvature without hypospadias in a series of 87 patients into three categories: (1) skin tethering, (2) fibrotic dartos and Buck's fasciae, and (3) corporeal disproportion. According to these authors, a congenitally short urethra was a rare cause of isolated curvature.

10. **d. All of the above.** In 1997, two independent and well-established surveillance systems in the United States, the Metropolitan Atlanta Congenital Defects Program (MACDP) and the nationwide Birth Defects Monitoring Program (BDMP), reported near-doubling of hypospadias rates in the most recent decade compared with immediately preceding decades. As measured by the BDMP, hypospadias rates increased from 2.02 per 1000 male births in 1970 to 3.97 per 1000 male births in 1993. In other words, approximately 1 in every 250 live male births involved hypospadias. The rate of severe hypospadias increased three- to five-fold from 0.11 per 1000 male births in 1968 to between 0.27 and 0.55 per 1000 male births per year from 1990 to 1993 as recorded by the MACDP.

11. **b. Incomplete physical examination in the newborn, highlighting the need for clear visualization of the urethral meatus position at the newborn examination.** When complete reduction of the foreskin and full visualization of the glans and meatal position is delayed, and not performed at newborn examination, registries that depend on prevalence in the newborn will underestimate the true prevalence of hypospadias. Often it is

the megameatus intact prepuce variant of hypospadias that goes without detection in the newborn.

12. **c. In individuals with hypospadias and cryptorchidism.** A high index of suspicion for an intersex state should accompany presumed males with any degree of hypospadias and cryptorchidism. An intersex state may be present in up to one third of these patients or more if the gonad is nonpalpable.

13. **c. Either unilateral or bilateral cryptorchidism with any degree of hypospadias.** A high index of suspicion for an intersex state is important for a finding of a presumed male with any degree of hypospadias and cryptorchidism.

14. **d. All of the above.** The prevalence of an intersex state varies from 15% to 30% for individuals with hypospadias and a palpable undescended gonad. When hypospadias is associated with a nonpalpable gonad the prevalence of an intersex state increases to 50%.

15. **d. None of the above.** Given a normal caliber of the urethral meatus and absence of ventral penile curvature, there are likely to be no clinically significant negative ramifications of glanular or perhaps even coronal hypospadias. Granted, this has not been scientifically studied.

16. **e. a and b.** In general, the literature does not support routine imaging of the urinary tract with either ultrasonography or intravenous urography for evaluation of children with isolated hypospadias, particularly when the hypospadiac meatus is middle or anterior in location. Retrograde injection of radiographic contrast material into the presumed urethral meatus (genitogram) is an essential component of the intersex evaluation when such an evaluation is deemed appropriate. Preoperative evaluation is more extensive in patients with posterior hypospadias and at our institution includes voiding cystourethrography in those with a scrotal or perineal defect to evaluate the frequent presence and extent of a prostatic utricle.

17. **a. decreased penile size (relative to normal) in adulthood.** In one report, testosterone enanthate was administered intramuscularly (2 mg/kg), 5 and 2 weeks before reconstructive penile surgery. The authors noted a 50% increase in penile size and an increase in available skin and local vascularity in all patients. A near-doubling (from 3 to 5 cm) of the mean transverse length of the inner prepuce was also noted in some patients. In addition, the authors reported minimal side effects and a return of plasma testosterone levels to within the normal range for age within 6 months after therapy. Others have employed variations in the total dose and schedule of testosterone enanthate administration, using 25 mg intramuscularly once weekly for a total of either two or three injections. Other investigators have employed a 4-week period of local penile stimulation with daily application of dihydrotestosterone cream before hypospadias or epispadias repair. These authors reported a mean increase in penile circumference and length by 50% of pretreatment measurements, without any lasting side effects or gonadotropin level perturbation or effects in the pubertal or postpubertal period. Hormonal manipulation, at any age, is not without risk. Caution must be exercised with regard to neonatal administration of human chorionic gonadotropin in that evidence obtained from an experimental rat micropenis model supports delaying hormonal therapy until the pubertal period. However, in one study of boys with congenital hypogonadotropic hypogonadism and micropenis it was concluded that one or two short courses of testosterone therapy in infancy and childhood (puberty) augmented adult penile size into the normal range. These results refute the theoretical concern, and experimental evidence, that testosterone treatment in infancy or childhood impairs penile growth in adolescence and compromises adult penile length. The conclusion that prepubertal exogenous testosterone administration does not adversely affect ultimate penile growth has been supported by the study of men with true precocious puberty or congenital adrenal hyperplasia and by the study of growth and androgen receptor status of testosterone-stimulated human fetal penile tissue in vitro.

18. **a. Interposition dermal graft for severe penile curvature in a short penis.** Reliable methods of ventral penile curvature management include ventral interposition graft of dermis for severe forms and dorsal midline plicating suture(s) for mild to moderate manifestations of ventral penile curvature.

19. **c. blood supply and drainage via the internal iliac vessels.** Local tissue flaps used for urethral reconstruction must be thin, nonhirsute, and reliably tailored. These flaps are properly termed *fasciocutaneous flaps*, and the extended fascial system is called the dartos fascia. The vessels of the fasciocutaneous flap are preserved within the fascia, which provides a conduit for smaller arteries and veins. Axial blood supply and drainage are typically provided by branches of the deep and superficial external pudendal vessels, which are medial branches of the femoral vessels. The term *island flap* implies maintenance of vascular and division of cutaneous continuity.

20. **c. They survive in a graft host bed after successful completion of a process called "take."** The term *graft* implies that tissue has been excised from one location and transferred to a graft host bed, where a new blood supply develops by a process called take. As with all free grafts, a well-vascularized recipient site is crucial for optimal graft survival. The initial phase of take, called imbibition, relies on diffusion of nutrient material from the adjacent graft host bed into the graft and requires approximately 48 hours. This is followed by the second phase of take, inosculation, which is the formation of new and permanent vascularization of the graft, also requiring approximately 48 hours.

21. **d. Subcutaneous (dartos) tissue second-layer neourethral coverage.** Second-layer coverage of the neourethra with the use of various vascularized flaps has significantly decreased urethrocutaneous fistula as a complication of hypospadias repair.

22. **e. All of the above.** A combination of factors, including an improved understanding of the psychological implications of genital surgery in children, improvement in the technical aspects of surgery for hypospadias, and advances in pediatric anesthesia, has suggested that the best time for surgery for hypospadias is between 6 and 12 months of age.

23. **a. liberal use of monopolar electrocautery is encouraged in the well-vascularized glans and other penile tissues.** On the basis of the hypothesis that some complications such as urethrocutaneous fistula and repair breakdown are, in part, a result of ischemic tissue necrosis, use of electrocautery should be limited, if it is used at all, during hypospadias repair. The current of monopolar cautery is dispersed to the remote grounding site, generally along the vessels, and in this way may irreparably damage tissue microvasculature. Other practitioners employing electrocautery may prefer the bipolar variant and the use of fine-point neurologic forceps. We favor injection of a vasoconstrictive agent (epinephrine diluted 1:200,000 with lidocaine [Xylocaine]) deep to proposed glanular incision(s), as well as intermittent use of a tourniquet at the base of the penis during urethroplasty. Other options for effective temporary hemostasis without permanent tissue devitalization include intermittent compression with gauze soaked in iced saline and/or epinephrine solution.

24. **e. Delicate handling of tissue, approximation of tissue without tension, and sterile meticulous technique.** Delicate tissue handling and neourethral closure and glans wing approximation without tension increase the likelihood of

successful hypospadias repair. Limiting the use of electrocautery for the purpose of hemostasis should only enhance successful healing of the repair.

25. **c. Reduces both adrenal and testicular androgen production through the inhibition of the enzyme 17,20 desmolase.** Ketoconazole reduces adrenal and testicular androgen production through the inhibition of 17,20-desmolase, thereby preventing the conversion of cholesterol to testosterone.
26. **e. a and b.** All options for repair of a specific hypospadias defect should be entertained before any skin incision. The urethral plate should be spared and used for the neourethra either as a tube itself or as a base for an onlay technique if at all possible. Complete circumferential incision including transection of the urethral plate would eliminate these possibilities from the outset of the repair.
27. **a. glanular hypospadias with adequate urethral mobility and no penile curvature.** Glanular and some coronal hypospadias defects are amenable to the meatoplasty and glanuloplasty (MAGPI) technique, with excellent functional and cosmetic results, provided that there is adequate urethral mobility and no penile curvature.
28. **c. It allows for approximation of the glans tissue in the ventral midline over the distal neourethra without tension.** Adequate depth of longitudinal incisions in the glans placed on either side of the urethral plate facilitate neourethral closure and, perhaps, more importantly allow for approximation of the glans wings over the closed neourethra and dartos and for subcutaneous second-layer coverage without tension.
29. **d. a and b.** A modification of the Thiersch-Duplay technique has been described by Snodgrass. The tubularized incised plate (TIP) urethroplasty combines modifications of the previously described techniques of urethral plate incision and tubularization. The concept of a urethral plate "relaxing incision" as an adjunct to hypospadias repair to allow tension-free neourethral tubularization was also described simultaneously by Pervovic.
30. **c. need to transect the urethral plate.** Mid-penile shaft and more proximal hypospadias defects may incorporate tissue from the base of the penis or scrotum that is hair-bearing and thus suboptimal for inclusion in the flap used for the Mathieu repair. Mild to moderate ventral penile curvature can typically be treated adequately with a plication procedure on the dorsal aspect of the penis.
31. **b. It has expanded to include proximal hypospadias defects.** Among the most commonly used techniques for repair of middle hypospadias is the onlay island flap (onlay, OIF) technique. Since its introduction for the repair of subcoronal and midshaft hypospadias, use of this technique has expanded in frequency and for indications to include more proximal defects as well. One 1994 study reported use of the technique in 374 (33%) of the total hypospadias repairs during a 5-year period. Complications requiring reoperation occurred in 32 (8.6%) of 374 patients. Twenty-three (6%) of the patients developed a urethrocutaneous fistula.
32. **d. Scrotal or perineal hypospadias, severe curvature, and a small penis.** Because the majority of hypospadias can be repaired with a one-stage procedure, the use of two-stage techniques for repair of posterior hypospadias is controversial. In the setting of scrotal or perineal hypospadias, severe curvature, and a small penis, we prefer to perform a two-stage repair.
33. **e. Both c and d are false.** Urethral stricture after hypospadias repair may present as decreased force of stream or dribbling. Optimal repair of what is typically an anterior urethral stricture is often a pedicled flap onlay technique using penile shaft skin.
34. **d. a and c.** In general, attempts at reoperative hypospadias surgery should not be undertaken less than 6 months after the previous failure of repair. Certainly, no attempt at repair should be considered until all edema, infection, and/or inflammation have resolved and healing is complete. When possible, the use of immediately adjacent or local pedicled, well-vascularized tissue is preferred for reoperative hypospadias surgery.
35. **b. It will identify an asymptomatic urethral stricture in some patients.** At some centers, this noninvasive study is a postoperative evaluation routine and has been of value in identifying asymptomatic urethral stricture in some patients.

126

Abnormalities of the Genitalia in Boys and Surgical Management

JACK S. ELDER

QUESTIONS

1. In the male, development of the external genitalia is stimulated by which substance?
   a. Testosterone
   b. Dihydrotestosterone (DHT)
   c. Human chorionic gonadotropin
   d. Luteinizing hormone and follicle-stimulating hormone
   e. Maternal progesterone
2. In the male, what do the genital swellings become?
   a. Glans penis
   b. Urethra
   c. Penile shaft
   d. Scrotum
   e. Penis and scrotum
3. In a term male neonate, approximately how long is the mean stretched penile length?
   a. 2.5 cm
   b. 3.0 cm
   c. 3.5 cm
   d. 4.0 cm
   e. 4.5 cm
4. What is the approximate incidence of hypospadias?
   a. 1:50
   b. 1:125
   c. 1:250
   d. 1:500
   e. 1:1000
5. An 8-year-old boy is unable to retract the foreskin. He has not had balanitis or balanoposthitis but does experience mild penile discomfort during erections. What is the most appropriate management?
   a. Application of topical corticosteroid cream
   b. Forceful retraction of the foreskin
   c. "Preputioplasty" (dorsal slit)
   d. Circumcision
   e. Observation
6. In a newborn undergoing circumcision, what risk is associated with EMLA cream for local anesthesia?
   a. Hepatic toxicity
   b. Cardiac arrhythmia
   c. Allergic reaction
   d. Prolonged bleeding time
   e. Methemoglobinemia
7. A newborn male undergoes circumcision and nearly all of the penile skin and foreskin is removed. What is the most appropriate therapy?
   a. Suture the skin edges together
   b. Split-thickness skin graft
   c. Full-thickness skin graft
   d. Application of adherent gauze and antibiotic ointment
   e. Application of small intestine submucosa graft
8. During a newborn circumcision, half of the glans is amputated and the urethra is transected. What is the most appropriate treatment?
   a. Split-thickness skin graft
   b. Application of adherent gauze and antibiotic ointment and insertion of a Foley catheter
   c. Suturing of excised tissue to penis, a nonmicroscopic repair
   d. Suturing of excised tissue to penis, a microscopic repair
   e. Coverage of raw glans with penile shaft skin
9. What is the normal size of the urethral meatus of a 2-year-old boy usually?
   a. 6 Fr
   b. 8 Fr
   c. 10 Fr
   d. 12 Fr
   e. 14 Fr
10. Which of the following statements is TRUE regarding a micropenis in a term male newborn?
    a. It increases the likelihood of urinary tract infection.
    b. It is best managed by gender reassignment.
    c. It has a normal circumference but short length.
    d. It is less than 1.9 cm stretched length.
    e. It is unlikely to respond to testosterone stimulation until puberty.

11. What is the most common cause of micropenis?
    a. Hypogonadotropic hypogonadism
    b. Growth hormone deficiency
    c. Primary testicular failure
    d. Androgen insensitivity syndrome
    e. Inadequate human chorionic gonadotropin in utero

12. Micropenis is associated with:
    a. ear anomalies.
    b. cardiac anomalies.
    c. midline brain defects.
    d. myelodysplasia.
    e. VATER syndrome.

13. If a newborn male with a micropenis is given three monthly intramuscular injections of testosterone enanthate of 25 mg each, what is the result?
    a. The penis will be unlikely to increase in size.
    b. Bone age will be higher than normal.
    c. Puberty will still occur at an earlier age.
    d. The penis will still increase in size at puberty.
    e. The adult body habitus will probably be eunuchoid.

14. A male newborn with a complete penoscrotal transposition and a normal scrotum commonly has which additional condition?
    a. Urinary tract abnormality
    b. Cardiac abnormality
    c. Sex chromosome abnormality
    d. Non–sex chromosome abnormality
    e. Tethered spinal cord

15. A newborn male has a strawberry hemangioma of the scrotum. At 6 months, the lesion is noted to have doubled in size. What is the appropriate management?
    a. Observation
    b. Surgical excision
    c. Neodymium:yttrium-aluminum-garnet laser therapy
    d. Argon laser therapy
    e. KTP laser therapy

ANSWERS

1. **b. Dihydrotestosterone (DHT).** In the male embryo, differentiation of the external genitalia occurs between weeks 9 and 13 of gestation and requires production of testosterone by the testes as well as conversion of testosterone into DHT under the enzymatic influence of 5α-reductase in the genital anlagen.

2. **d. Scrotum.** Under the influence of DHT, the genital tubercle differentiates into the glans penis, the genital folds become the shaft of the penis, and the genital swellings migrate inferomedially, fusing in the midline to become the scrotum.

3. **c. 3.5 cm.** In a normal term male neonate, the penis is 3.5 ± 0.7 cm in stretched length and 1.1 ± 0.2 cm in diameter.

4. **c. 1:250.** A urethral deformity such as hypospadias or epispadias occurs in approximately 1 in 250 males.

5. **a. Application of topical corticosteroid cream.** In boys older than 4 or 5 years of age and those who develop balanitis or balanoposthitis, application of a topical corticosteroid cream (e.g., 0.1% dexamethasone) to the foreskin three or four times daily for 6 weeks loosens the phimotic ring in two thirds of the boys and usually allows the foreskin to be retracted manually.

6. **e. Methemoglobinemia.** The prilocaine in EMLA cream poses a risk for methemoglobinemia, although the risk is quite low.

7. **d. Application of adherent gauze and antibiotic ointment.** If too much penile shaft skin is removed, application of antibiotic ointment and adherent gauze to the open wound usually yields a satisfactory result. Typically, most of the skin will grow back and bridge the defect.

8. **c. Suturing of excised tissue to penis, a nonmicroscopic repair.** The most serious circumcision complications include urethral injury and removal of part of the glans or part or all of the penile shaft. Partial glans removal has been reported to occur with a Mogen clamp; in these cases, the excised tissue should be preserved and immediately sutured back to the penis. A microscopic repair is unnecessary.

9. **c. 10 Fr.**

10. **d. It is less than 1.9 cm stretched length.** Micropenis is defined as a normally formed penis that is at least 2.5 standard deviations below the mean in size. Typically, the ratio of the length of the penile shaft to its circumference is normal. In general, the penis of a term newborn should be at least 1.9 cm long. Stretched penile length is used because it correlates more closely with erectile length than the relaxed length of the penis.

11. **a. Hypogonadotropic hypogonadism.** The most common cause of micropenis is failure of the hypothalamus to produce an adequate amount of gonadotropin-releasing hormone. This condition, termed *hypogonadotropic hypogonadism*, may result from hypothalamic dysfunction, such as Kallmann's syndrome (genito-olfactory dysplasia), Prader-Willi syndrome, Lawrence-Moon-Biedl syndrome, and the CHARGE association.

12. **c. midline brain defects.** Other major causes include congenital pituitary aplasia and midline brain defects such as agenesis of the corpus callosum and occipital encephalocele.

13. **d. The penis will still increase in size at puberty.** A report on eight boys with micropenis who were treated with androgens both at birth and at puberty showed that the final penile stretched length averaged 10.3 cm, and all were in the normal range.

14. **a. Urinary tract abnormality.** When there is complete penoscrotal transposition and a normal scrotum, as many as 75% of infants have a significant urinary tract abnormality, and a renal sonogram and voiding cystourethrogram should be obtained.

15. **a. Observation.** Strawberry hemangiomas, the most common type of genital hemangioma, result from proliferation of immature capillary vessels. Although the lesions may undergo a period of rapid growth lasting 3 to 6 months, gradual involution is common and most lesions require no treatment.

127

Abnormalities of the Testes and Scrotum and Their Surgical Management

FRANCIS X. SCHNECK • MARK F. BELLINGER

QUESTIONS

1. Most adolescent varicoceles evaluated by urologists are:
   a. painful.
   b. a cosmetic concern.
   c. asymptomatic.
   d. associated with an ipsilateral hydrocele.
   e. bilateral.
2. What is the most likely cause of testicular injury from varicocele?
   a. Elevated scrotal temperature
   b. Testicular hypoxia
   c. Effect of adrenal metabolites
   d. Altered levels of spermatic vein testosterone
   e. Testicular hypertension
3. What is the upper limit of difference in testis volume between right and left?
   a. 1 mL
   b. 2 mL
   c. 3 mL
   d. 4 mL
   e. 5 mL
4. Hydrocele formation after varicocele ligation is least likely to occur after which of the following procedures?
   a. Retroperitoneal ligation
   b. Subinguinal ligation
   c. Laparoscopic ligation
   d. Microscopic inguinal ligation
   e. Transvenous embolization
5. Irreversible ischemic injury of the testicular parenchyma begins how soon after torsion of the spermatic cord?
   a. 1 hour
   b. 2 hours
   c. 4 hours
   d. 6 hours
   e. 8 hours
6. One of the best physical findings indicative of torsion of the spermatic cord is:
   a. high-riding testis.
   b. absence of the cremasteric reflex.
   c. transverse lie of the testis.
   d. absent Doppler sounds.
   e. inflammatory hydrocele.
7. After manual detorsion of the spermatic cord, which of the following is appropriate management?
   a. Color Doppler ultrasonographic examination
   b. Radionuclide scan
   c. Doppler examination of the testis and spermatic cord
   d. Discharge from the hospital and arrangement for an office reevaluation in 1 week
   e. Immediate scrotal exploration
8. An adolescent is evaluated for a history of self-limited, intermittent episodes of severe unilateral scrotal pain. Physical examination findings are normal. What is the most appropriate course of action?
   a. Color Doppler ultrasonographic examination
   b. Reassessment in 6 months
   c. Elective scrotal exploration
   d. Radionuclide scrotal imaging
   e. Immediate scrotal exploration
9. When diagnosis of a torsion of the appendix epididymis is made, which of the following is optimal management?
   a. Observation
   b. Color Doppler ultrasonographic examination
   c. Radionuclide scrotal imaging
   d. Immediate scrotal exploration
   e. Cord block and manual detorsion
10. Most boys with sterile urine and a clinical diagnosis of epididymitis will be found to have which of the following conditions?
    a. Unilateral renal agenesis
    b. Large prostatic utricle
    c. Urethral stricture disease
    d. Persistent vasoureteral fusion
    e. Radiographically normal urinary tracts

11. If the cause of neonatal scrotal swelling appears to be an acute postnatal event, what is the most appropriate course of action in an otherwise healthy neonate?

    a. Prompt surgical exploration of the affected testis
    b. Prompt surgical exploration of the affected testis with contralateral scrotal exploration
    c. Color Doppler imaging of the scrotum
    d. Radionuclide testicular scan
    e. Observation

12. What is the major gene responsible for male sexual differentiation?

    a. *TDF*
    b. *SOX*
    c. *WT1*
    d. *SRY*
    e. *ZFY*

13. During male sexual development, androgens mediate the differentiation of all of these structures EXCEPT:

    a. seminal vesicles.
    b. ureter.
    c. epididymis.
    d. vas deferens.
    e. ejaculatory ducts.

14. Testosterone and müllerian-inhibiting substance are produced by the fetal testis at what gestational week?

    a. 5th
    b. 8th
    c. 10th
    d. 12th
    e. 23rd

15. What is the incidence of cryptorchidism at 1 year of age?

    a. 10%
    b. 3%
    c. 1%
    d. 0.3%
    e. 0.1%

16. What is the most important determining factor of cryptorchidism at 1 year of age?

    a. Gestational age at delivery
    b. Birth weight
    c. Maternal smoking history
    d. Family history of cryptorchidism
    e. Asian descent

17. In utero testosterone deficiency can be due to all of the following EXCEPT:

    a. loss of function mutations involved with testosterone biosynthesis.
    b. impaired gonadotropin-releasing hormone receptor function.
    c. decreased luteinizing hormone (LH).
    d. increased inhibin B.
    e. impaired LH receptor function.

18. Patients with cryptorchidism demonstrate impaired biosynthesis of which of the following hormones in the first year of life?

    a. Follicle-stimulating hormone
    b. Testosterone
    c. Müllerian-inhibiting substance
    d. Gonadotropin-releasing hormone
    e. Inhibin A

19. All of the following structures have been theorized to aid in testicular descent EXCEPT:

    a. gubernaculum.
    b. genitofemoral nerve.
    c. epididymis.
    d. processus vaginalis.
    e. scrotum.

20. Histologic findings in cryptorchid testes include all of the following EXCEPT:

    a. decreased number of Leydig cells.
    b. delayed appearance of adult dark spermatogonia.
    c. early disappearance of gonocytes.
    d. degeneration of Sertoli cells.
    e. reduced total germ cell counts.

21. What percentage of undescended testes are nonpalpable at presentation?

    a. 1%
    b. 3%
    c. 10%
    d. 20%
    e. 30%

22. Factors most likely associated with risk for diminished paternity rates include:

    a. monorchidism.
    b. unilateral cryptorchidism.
    c. increased FSH level.
    d. age at orchidopexy.
    e. increased inhibin B level.

23. During laparoscopy, spermatic cord structures exiting the internal ring ipsilateral to a nonpalpable testis implies:

    a. vanishing testis, inguinal exploration unnecessary.
    b. vanishing testis, inguinal exploration necessary.
    c. intracanalicular atrophic testis, inguinal exploration unnecessary.
    d. intracanalicular testis, inguinal exploration necessary.
    e. further exploration unnecessary if contralateral testicular hypertrophy is present.

24. Advantages of laparoscopic management of an intra-abdominal testis include all of the following EXCEPT:

    a. more accurately assesses the presence or absence, viability, and anatomy of the testis compared with radiographic imaging.
    b. allows for laparoscopic repair of the ipsilateral inguinal hernia when present.
    c. enhances surgical exposure, lighting, and magnification.
    d. allows a greater degree of proximal dissection of the spermatic vessels.
    e. avoids more extensive inguinal exploration or laparotomy in approximately 50% of cases.

25. Which statement is FALSE regarding Fowler-Stephens orchidopexy?

    a. It has a higher success rate if performed as a single or non-staged procedure.
    b. It has a lower success rate in patients who have undergone previous inguinal surgery.
    c. Blood supply is based on the deferential artery and collateral peritoneal vessels.
    d. It should be performed at a similar age as a standard inguinal orchidopexy.
    e. It should be considered if the testis is beyond 4 cm from the internal ring.

ANSWERS

1. **c. asymptomatic.** Most adolescent varicoceles are asymptomatic.
2. **a. Elevated scrotal temperature.** The presence of varicosities impedes this countercurrent exchange mechanism, perhaps a crucial alteration in normal homeostasis because it is considered that elevated scrotal temperature associated with varicocele formation can inhibit spermatogenesis.
3. **b. 2 mL.** In adults and adolescents, testis size (volume) should be approximately equal bilaterally, with the normal differential not being more than 2 mL or 20% volume.
4. **e. Transvenous embolization.** Hydrocele formation is related to failure to preserve spermatic vessels associated with the spermatic cord and its vessels. Hydrocele formation seems most common after retroperitoneal ligation, especially when a mass ligation technique is used, and is least likely to occur after transvenous embolization.
5. **c. 4 hours.** Irreversible ischemic injury to the testicular parenchyma may begin as soon as 4 hours after occlusion of the cord.
6. **b. absence of the cremasteric reflex.** The absence of a cremasteric reflex is a good indicator of torsion of the cord.
7. **e. Immediate scrotal exploration.** It should always be kept in mind that manual detorsion may not totally correct the rotation that has occurred and prompt exploration is usually still indicated.
8. **c. Elective scrotal exploration.** If the suspicion is strong that episodes of intermittent torsion and spontaneous detorsion have occurred, our experience has been that the finding of a bellclapper deformity at exploration can be expected. Elective scrotal exploration should be performed, with scrotal fixation of both testes.
9. **a. Observation.** When the diagnosis of a torsed appendage is confirmed clinically or by imaging, nonoperative management will allow most cases to resolve spontaneously.
10. **e. Radiographically normal urinary tracts.** The majority of boys with epididymitis have sterile urine and apparently radiographically normal urinary tracts.
11. **b. Prompt surgical exploration of the affected testis with contralateral scrotal exploration.** Clearly, if the cause of scrotal swelling appears to be related to an acute postnatal event, all efforts should be made to pursue prompt surgical intervention. Exploration, when elected, should be carried out through an inguinal incision to allow for the most efficacious treatment of other potential or unexpected causes of scrotal swelling. If torsion is confirmed, contralateral scrotal exploration with testicular fixation should be carried out.
12. **d. *SRY*.** Although the *SRY* gene appears to be primarily responsible for male sexual differentiation through complex interactions involving both activation and repression of other male-specific genes, little is known about its mode of action or downstream target genes, which convert the bipotential gonad into the testis.
13. **b. ureter.** Androgens (testosterone, dihydrotestosterone) mediate the differentiation of the paired wolffian ducts into the seminal vesicles, epididymis, vas deferens, and ejaculatory ducts.
14. **b. 8th.** During the 8th week, the fetal testis begins to secrete testosterone and müllerian-inhibiting substance independent of pituitary hormonal regulation.
15. **c. 1%.** By 1 year of age, the incidence of cryptorchidism declines to about 1% and remains constant throughout adulthood.
16. **b. Birth weight.** Accurate analysis of data concludes that birth weight alone is the principal determinant of cryptorchidism at birth and at 1 year of life, independent of the length of gestation.
17. **d. increased inhibin B.** In-utero testosterone deficiency can be due to decreased LH, impaired function of the gonadotropin-releasing hormone or LH receptors, and loss of function mutations in the proteins involved in testosterone biosynthesis.
18. **c. Müllerian-inhibiting substance.** One report found that patients with cryptorchidism do not demonstrate a surge in the first year of life and that mean müllerian-inhibiting substance serum concentrations in cryptorchid boys are significantly lower than those in control subjects.
19. **e. scrotum.** The testes lie dormant within the abdomen until about the 23rd week of gestation, during which time the processus vaginalis continues its elongation into the scrotum. The testis, epididymis, and gubernaculum have been observed to descend en masse through the inguinal canal posterior to the patent processus vaginalis. The theoretical association uniting normal testicular descent to epididymal function is based on the observations that epididymal abnormalities often accompany cryptorchidism. Data have also been presented that the genitofemoral nerve induced testicular descent and gubernacular differentiation.
20. **c. early disappearance of gonocytes.** The histopathologic hallmarks associated with cryptorchidism are evident between 1 and 2 years of age and include decreased numbers of Leydig cells, degeneration of Sertoli cells, delayed disappearance of gonocytes, delayed appearance of adult dark (Ad) spermatogonia, failure of primary spermatocytes to develop, and reduced total germ cell counts. The earliest postnatal histologic abnormality in cryptorchid testes was hypoplasia of the Leydig cells, which was observed from the first month of life.
21. **d. 20%.** Twenty percent of undescended testes are nonpalpable at presentation.
22. **c. increased FSH level.** Increases in serum FSH and LH levels have been correlated with decreased paternity rates and correlate inversely with lower sperm counts and inhibin B levels. Therefore, increased FSH and low sperm count may be weighed as risks for infertility in formerly cryptorchid men.
23. **d. intracanalicular testis, inguinal exploration necessary.** An intracanalicular testis, whether normal or atrophic, needs to be confirmed with exploration. If atrophic remnant is found it needs to be removed because of the potential of viable testicular elements present in up to 13% of specimens. Blind-ending intraabdominal spermatic vessels is sine qua non of a vanishing testis, and further exploration is unnecessary if this anatomy is found. Hypertrophy of a normally descended contralateral testis may connote monorchia.
24. **b. allows for laparoscopic repair of the ipsilateral inguinal hernia when present.** Repair of the inguinal hernia or patent processus vaginalis does not require formal repair at the time of laparoscopic orchidopexy.
25. **a. It has a higher success rate if performed as a single or nonstaged procedure.** A single or nonstaged open Fowler-Stephens orchidopexy has the highest reported testicular atrophy rates compared with staged orchidopexy. The other statements are all true.

128

Sexual Differentiation: Normal and Abnormal

DAVID A. DIAMOND

QUESTIONS

1. What is the testis-determining factor (TDF)?
   a. It is synonymous with the H-Y antigen.
   b. It is located on the short arm of the Y chromosome adjacent to the pseudoautosomal boundary.
   c. It is a zinc finger gene on the Y chromosome known as *ZFY*.
   d. It was genetically mapped by the study of patients with Klinefelter's and Turner's syndrome.
   e. It is synonymous with *SRY* in humans.
2. Which of the following statements is TRUE regarding müllerian-inhibiting substance (MIS)?
   a. It acts systemically to produce müllerian regression.
   b. It is secreted by the fetal Leydig cells.
   c. It functions normally in patients with hernia uteri inguinale.
   d. It is secreted at 7 to 8 weeks of gestation, representing the initial endocrine function of the fetal testis.
   e. It is secreted by the fetal testis at 10 weeks of gestation, after testosterone production has begun.
3. Which of the following statements is TRUE regarding fetal testosterone?
   a. It results in regression of the müllerian ducts.
   b. It is produced primarily by the adrenal gland.
   c. It acts locally to virilize the urogenital sinus and genital tubercle.
   d. It acts locally to virilize the internal wolffian duct structures.
   e. It enters target tissue by active diffusion.
4. Which of the following statements is TRUE regarding dihydrotestosterone (DHT)?
   a. It produces virilization of wolffian duct structures.
   b. It is converted by 5α-reductase to testosterone in target tissues.
   c. It produces virilization of the urogenital sinus.
   d. It acts locally to produce regression of müllerian structures.
   e. It is secreted in large quantities by the fetal testis.
5. Which of the following statements is TRUE regarding patients with Klinefelter's syndrome?
   a. They have at least one X and two Y chromosomes.
   b. They are at increased risk for development of adenocarcinoma of the breast.
   c. They undergo replacement of Leydig cells with hyaline.
   d. They are characteristically fertile.
   e. They bear little resemblance to XX males.
6. The streak gonad of Turner's syndrome:
   a. can descend to the scrotum.
   b. has a reduced number of oocytes.
   c. in the presence of a Y chromosome results in increased risk for development of seminoma.
   d. is located in the round ligament.
   e. in the presence of a Y chromosome results in risk for development of gonadoblastoma.
7. Which of the following statements is TRUE regarding patients with "pure" gonadal dysgenesis?
   a. They frequently have chromosomal anomalies.
   b. They are at lesser risk for gonadal tumors than are patients with Turner's syndrome.
   c. They lack the somatic defects associated with Turner's syndrome.
   d. They have gonadal histology different from that of patient's with Turner's syndrome.
   e. They derive similar benefit from synthetic growth hormone as do patients with Turner's syndrome.
8. What is the common denominator in all cases of Denys-Drash syndrome?
   a. Gonadoblastoma
   b. Nephropathy with early-onset proteinuria
   c. Wilms' tumor
   d. Caliceal blunting
   e. Progressive renal failure
9. Which of the following statements is TRUE regarding patients with embryonic testicular regression or bilateral vanishing testes syndromes? They have:
   a. normal testosterone and elevated estradiol levels.
   b. normal testosterone but decreased DHT levels.
   c. castrate testosterone and elevated gonadotropin levels.
   d. castrate testosterone and normal gonadotropin levels.
   e. normal follicle-stimulating hormone but decreased luteinizing hormone levels.
10. Which of the following statements is TRUE regarding the ovotestis in true hermaphroditism?
    a. It cannot descend from the retroperitoneum.
    b. It is found in the minority of patients.
    c. It can be unilateral or bilateral.
    d. It has testicular and ovarian elements randomly distributed.
    e. It is impossible to cleave surgically.

11. An important consideration for gender assignment in the true hermaphrodite is:

    a. the potential for fertility.
    b. the impossibility of precisely dividing an ovotestis surgically.
    c. that malignant degeneration of gonads does not occur.
    d. the familial pattern of inheritance of the disorder.
    e. the unresponsiveness of the external genitalia to testosterone.

12. Which of the following statements is TRUE regarding the 21-hydroxylase deficiency in congenital adrenal hyperplasia (CAH)?

    a. It accounts for 99% of CAH cases.
    b. It occurs as a result of gene inactivation in the majority of cases.
    c. It occurs with simple virilization in 75% of cases and salt wasting in 25% of cases.
    d. It occurs with a predictable phenotype.
    e. It is transmitted in an autosomal dominant pattern.

13. Prenatal treatment of patients with CAH with dexamethasone:

    a. is appropriate therapy in seven of eight at-risk fetuses.
    b. is initiated after a diagnosis of CAH is confirmed.
    c. is no risk to the fetus.
    d. is demonstrated to be effective.
    e. acts by suppressing maternal corticotropin.

14. Which of the following statements is TRUE regarding enzymatic disorders of testosterone biosynthesis?

    a. They are transmitted in an autosomal dominant pattern.
    b. They are associated with persistent müllerian structures.
    c. They appear clinically with a predictable phenotype.
    d. They may involve impaired glucocorticoid and mineralocorticoid synthesis.
    e. They may be associated with fertility.

15. Which of the following statements is TRUE regarding patients with complete androgen insensitivity?

    a. They are appropriately raised as female.
    b. They have normal wolffian duct structures.
    c. They have persistent müllerian duct structures.
    d. They should undergo orchiectomy as early as possible.
    e. They have a 2% incidence of inguinal hernia.

16. What is Reifenstein's syndrome?

    a. The group of defects in testosterone biosynthesis that results in male pseudohermaphroditism
    b. A form of 5α-reductase deficiency
    c. Defects of MIS elaboration in utero
    d. A disorder of androgen receptor quantity or function
    e. An autosomal recessively transmitted disorder

17. Which of the following statements is TRUE regarding patients with 5α-reductase deficiency?

    a. Fertility is an important issue in gender assignment.
    b. Isoenzymes I and II are abnormal.
    c. Serum testosterone levels are normal, but there is a decreased testosterone/DHT ratio.
    d. Masculinization occurs at puberty.
    e. Prostatic enlargement occurs at puberty.

18. Which of the following statements is TRUE regarding patients with persistent müllerian duct syndrome?

    a. They have absent wolffian duct structures.
    b. They represent a homogeneous disorder of MIS receptor.
    c. They should undergo routine removal of müllerian structures.
    d. They experience a high incidence of transverse testicular ectopia.
    e. They are uniformly infertile.

19. Which of the following statements is TRUE regarding Mayer-Rokitansky-Küster-Hauser syndrome?

    a. It presents most commonly with infertility.
    b. It is a homogeneous disorder entailing congenital absence of the uterus and vagina.
    c. It is associated with a spectrum of ovarian abnormalities.
    d. It has associated upper urinary tract anomalies, primarily with the atypical disorder.
    e. It is associated with persistent wolffian duct structures.

20. In an unambiguous newborn with hypospadias and a unilateral cryptorchid testis:

    a. midshaft location of the urethral meatus is an important risk factor for an intersex disorder.
    b. impalpability of the cryptorchid testis carries a 50% risk of intersex disorder.
    c. palpability of the cryptorchid testis effectively rules out an intersex disorder.
    d. perineal hypospadias is not a risk factor for an intersex disorder.
    e. difference in tissue texture of the poles of the cryptorchid gonad is suggestive of tumor.

ANSWERS

1. **b. It is located on the short arm of the Y chromosome adjacent to the pseudoautosomal boundary.** Deletion maps based on the genomes of these individuals were constructed by a number of laboratories, and TDF was mapped to the most distal aspect of the Y-unique region of the short arm of the Y chromosome, adjacent to the pseudoautosomal boundary.
2. **d. It is secreted at 7 to 8 weeks of gestation, representing the initial endocrine function of the fetal testis.** The initial endocrine function of the fetal testes is the secretion of MIS by the Sertoli cells at 7 to 8 weeks of gestation.
3. **d. It acts locally to virilize the internal wolffian duct structures.** It was clearly demonstrated that androgen is essential for virilization of wolffian duct structures, the urogenital sinus, and genital tubercle. Testosterone, the major androgen secreted by the testes, enters target tissues by passive diffusion. The local source of androgen is important for wolffian duct development, which does not occur if testosterone is supplied only via the peripheral circulation.
4. **c. It produces virilization of the urogenital sinus.** In some cells, such as those in the urogenital sinus, testosterone is converted to DHT by intracellular 5α-reductase. Testosterone or DHT then binds to a high-affinity intracellular receptor protein, and this

complex enters the nucleus where it binds to acceptor sites on DNA, resulting in new messenger RNA and protein synthesis. Therefore, in tissues equipped with 5α-reductase at the time of sexual differentiation, such as prostate, urogenital sinus, and external genitalia, DHT is the active androgen.

5. **b. They are at increased risk for development of adenocarcinoma of the breast.** Gynecomastia, which can be quite marked, is a common pubertal development in patients with Klinefelter's syndrome. As a result, these patients are at eight times the risk for developing breast carcinoma relative to normal males.
6. **e. in the presence of a Y chromosome results in risk for development of gonadoblastoma.** In patients with occult Y chromosomal material, the risk of gonadoblastoma, an in situ germ cell cancer, is approximately 30%.
7. **c. They lack the somatic defects associated with Turner's syndrome.** Patients with 46,XX "pure" gonadal dysgenesis are closely related to those with Turner's syndrome. Because these subjects exhibit none of the somatic stigmata associated with Turner's syndrome and their condition entails gonadal dysgenesis only, it has been regarded by some authors as pure.
8. **b. Nephropathy with early-onset proteinuria.** The full triad of the syndrome includes nephropathy, characterized by the early onset of proteinuria, and hypertension and progressive renal failure in the majority. Because incomplete forms of the syndrome may occur, the nephropathy has become regarded as the common denominator of the syndrome.
9. **c. castrate testosterone and elevated gonadotropin levels.** The diagnosis can be made on the basis of a 46,XY karyotype and castrate levels of testosterone despite persistently elevated serum luteinizing hormone and follicle-stimulating hormone levels.
10. **c. It can be unilateral or bilateral.** True hermaphrodites are individuals having both testicular tissue with well-developed seminiferous tubules and ovarian tissue with primordial follicles, which may take the form of one ovary and one testis or, more commonly, one or two ovotestes.
11. **a. the potential for fertility.** The most important aspect of management in true hermaphroditism is gender assignment.
12. **b. It occurs as a result of gene inactivation in the majority of cases.** Mutations leading to gene conversion of the active *CYP21* gene into the inactive gene occur in 65% to 90% of cases of the classic disorder (salt wasting and simple virilizing) and all cases of nonclassic 21-hydroxylase deficiency.
13. **d. is demonstrated to be effective.** A number of series have established the effectiveness of prenatal treatment of CAH with dexamethasone.
14. **d. They may involve impaired glucocorticoid and mineralocorticoid synthesis.** A defect in any of the five enzymes required for the conversion of cholesterol to testosterone can cause incomplete (or absent) virilization of the male fetus during embryogenesis. The first three enzymes (cholesterol side chain cleavage enzyme, 3β-hydroxysteroid dehydrogenase, and 17α-hydroxylase) are present in both the adrenals and the testes. Therefore, their deficiency results in impaired synthesis of glucocorticoids and mineralocorticoids in addition to testosterone.
15. **a. They are appropriately raised as female.** It is of great interest that, currently, all studies of patients with complete androgen insensitivity support an unequivocal female gender identity, consistent with androgen resistance of brain tissue as well. To date, there has been no report of a patient raised as a female who needed gender reassignment to male.
16. **d. A disorder of androgen receptor quantity or function.** Androgen receptor studies in cultured fibroblasts have demonstrated two forms of receptor defect in the partial androgen insensitivity syndrome. These include a reduced number of normally functioning androgen receptors and normal receptor number but decreased binding affinity.
17. **d. Masculinization occurs at puberty.** At puberty, partial masculinization occurs with an increase in muscle mass, development of male body habitus, increase in phallic size, and onset of erections.
18. **d. They experience a high incidence of transverse testicular ectopia.** Persistent müllerian duct syndrome is thought to be etiologically important in transverse testicular ectopia, occurring in 30% to 50% of cases.
19. **d. It has associated upper urinary tract anomalies, primarily with the atypical disorder.** Urinary tract anomalies occur more commonly in patients with the atypical form of the disorder than in patients with the typical syndrome.
20. **b. impalpability of the cryptorchid testis carries a 50% risk of intersex disorder.** With a unilateral cryptorchid testis, the incidence of intersex was 30% overall—15% if the undescended testis was palpable and 50% if impalpable.

129

Surgical Management of Intersexuality, Cloacal Malformation, and Other Abnormalities of the Genitalia in Girls

RICHARD RINK • MARTIN KAEFER

QUESTIONS

1. Which of the following statements is TRUE regarding Mayer-Rokitansky-Küster-Hauser syndrome?
   a. It presents most commonly with infertility.
   b. It is a homogeneous disorder entailing congenital absence of the uterus and vagina.
   c. It is associated with a spectrum of ovarian abnormalities.
   d. It is associated with upper urinary tract anomalies, primarily with the atypical disorder.
   e. It is associated with persistent wolffian duct structures.
2. What is the crucial period in embryogenesis for the formation of the terminal bowel, kidney, paramesonephric ductal system, and lumbosacral spine?
   a. 4 to 6 weeks
   b. 8 to 10 weeks
   c. 10 to 14 weeks
   d. 14 to 18 weeks
   e. >18 weeks
3. Which of the following is FALSE regarding vaginal agenesis (müllerian aplasia)?
   a. It occurs with an incidence of approximately 1 in 5000 live female births.
   b. Serum follicle-stimulating hormone and luteinizing hormone levels can be expected to be abnormally high.
   c. It results from a failure of the sinovaginal bulbs to develop and form the vaginal plate.
   d. It is a condition associated with renal abnormalities.
   e. It is a condition associated with skeletal abnormalities.
4. Skeletal anomalies are found in what percentage of patients with Meyer-Rokitansky-Küster-Hauser syndrome?
   a. 10% to 20%
   b. 25% to 35%
   c. 40% to 60%
   d. 70% to 90%
   e. 0%
5. What is the most common cause of primary amenorrhea?
   a. Testicular feminization
   b. Vaginal agenesis
   c. Mixed gonadal dysgenesis
   d. Imperforate hymen
   e. Transverse vaginal septum
6. Which of the following statements is FALSE regarding the genitalia of women with Meyer-Rokitansky-Küster-Hauser syndrome?
   a. In approximately 10% of patients, a normal but obstructed uterus or rudimentary uterus with functional endometrium is present.
   b. Normal fallopian tubes are seen in approximately 35% of patients.
   c. The ovaries are not functional in the majority of patients.
   d. The hymenal fringe is usually present along with a small vaginal pouch.
   e. The labia majora are typically normal in appearance.
7. Which of the following is FALSE regarding the construction of a bowel vagina?
   a. Failure to develop an adequate space between the rectum and bladder can result in compromised blood flow to the segment used for vaginal construction.
   b. In general, colon is preferred over ileum because of its lower incidence of associated postoperative stenosis.
   c. When compared with the McIndoe procedure, the bowel vagina suffers from a higher incidence of postoperative stenosis.
   d. An advantage of a bowel vagina over the McIndoe procedure includes the lubricating properties of mucus which may help to facilitate intercourse.
   e. One specific indication for the use of ileum is a previous history of pelvic radiation.

8. Uterus didelphys with unilateral imperforate vagina most commonly occurs with which condition?
   a. Primary amenorrhea
   b. Cyclical abdominal pain associated with normal cyclical menstruation
   c. Renal anomalies contralateral to the side of the obstruction
   d. Anomalies of the axial skeleton
   e. Constipation
9. Urethral prolapse is most commonly seen in young females of which ethnic background?
   a. African-American
   b. White
   c. Asian
   d. Hispanic
   e. American Indian
10. In most cases of labial adhesions, which of the following is TRUE?
    a. They are believed to occur because of a relative state of hyperestrogenism.
    b. They should be treated with surgical lysis.
    c. They require no treatment.
    d. They occur secondary to sexual abuse.
    e. They have associated renal anomalies.
11. What is the mean age of a child with vaginal rhabdomyosarcoma?
    a. <2 years
    b. 2 to 4 years
    c. 4 to 8 years
    d. 8 to 12 years
    e. >12 years
12. Urogenital sinus anomalies are most often seen in intersex states, most commonly in association with which condition?
    a. Congenital adrenal hyperplasia
    b. Mixed gonadal dysgenesis
    c. True hermaphroditism
    d. Cloacal anomalies
13. Cloacal anomalies have been diagnosed by antenatal ultrasonography. What is the common finding in all reports?
    a. Ascites
    b. Distended rectum
    c. Distended bladder
    d. Distended vagina
    e. Hydronephrosis
14. What is the most common vaginal anatomy in cloacal malformation?
    a. Single vagina, single uterus
    b. Single vagina, double uterus
    c. Two vaginas, two uteri
    d. Two vaginas, one uterus
15. Which of the following is not part of the normal evaluation of a child born with a cloacal anomaly?
    a. Genitography
    b. MRI of the head
    c. Echocardiography
    d. MRI of the spine
16. Neonatal vaginoplasty combined with clitoroplasty and labioplasty has all of the following advantages EXCEPT which one?
    a. It allows phallic skin for vaginal reconstruction.
    b. Maternal estrogens increase vaginal thickness and vascularity.
    c. Tissues are less scarred.
    d. Vaginal stenosis is clearly less.
17. The cut-back vaginoplasty is appropriate for which condition?
    a. Labial fusion
    b. Low vaginal confluence
    c. High vaginal confluence
    d. Vaginal atresia
18. Surgical management of cloacal malformations involves all of the following steps EXCEPT which one?
    a. Decompression of the gastrointestinal tract
    b. Decompression of the genitourinary tract
    c. Vaginostomy
    d. Definitive repair of the cloaca
19. Fecal continence after cloacal reconstruction is most closely related to:
    a. level of rectal confluence.
    b. associated urinary anomalies.
    c. neurologic status.
    d. type of repair.

ANSWERS

1. **d. It is associated with upper urinary tract anomalies, primarily with the atypical disorder.** Urinary tract anomalies occur more commonly in patients with the atypical form of the disorder than in patients with the typical syndrome.
2. **a. 4 to 6 weeks.** Laboratory data with teratogens support the concept of a key event occurring between the 4th and 5th weeks of gestation that results in an error in the simultaneous development of the terminal bowel, kidney, bladder, paramesonephric ductal system, and lumbosacral spine.
3. **b. Serum follicle-stimulating hormone and luteinizing hormone levels can be expected to be abnormally high.** Vaginal agenesis, which occurs with an incidence of approximately 1 in 5000 live female births, is the congenital absence of the proximal portion of the vagina in an otherwise phenotypically (i.e., normal secondary sexual characteristics), chromosomally (i.e., 46,XX), and hormonally (i.e., normal luteinizing hormone and follicle-stimulating hormone levels) intact female. It results from a failure of the sinovaginal bulbs to develop and form the vaginal plate. Hauser brought further attention to the frequent association of renal and skeletal anomalies in these patients and stressed the differences between patients with these findings and those with testicular feminization.
4. **a. 10% to 20%.** Associated congenital abnormalities of the skeletal system have been described in 10% to 20% of cases.
5. **c. Mixed gonadal dysgenesis.** Meyer-Rokitansky-Küster-Hauser syndrome is in fact secondary only to gonadal dysgenesis as a cause of primary amenorrhea.

6. **c. The ovaries are not functional in the majority of patients.** Although occasionally cystic, the ovaries were almost always present and functional.
7. **c. When compared with the McIndoe procedure, the bowel vagina suffers from a higher incidence of postoperative stenosis.** A high incidence of postoperative vaginal stenosis necessitates postoperative vaginal dilatation.
8. **b. Cyclical abdominal pain associated with normal cyclical menstruation.** As with other obstructive disorders, the patient may present with cyclical or chronic abdominal pain. However, unlike other obstructive processes, duplication anomalies with unilateral obstruction are not associated with primary amenorrhea.
9. **a. African-American.** This entity, which was first described by Solinger in 1732, occurs most often in prepubertal black girls and postmenopausal white women.
10. **c. They require no treatment.** Most children do not require treatment unless one of the aforementioned symptoms (urine pooling within the vagina, which may lead to postvoid dribbling; perineal irritation; physical findings of sexual abuse) occurs.
11. **a. <2 years.** The mean age of patients with primary vaginal tumors is younger than 2 years.
12. **a. Congenital adrenal hyperplasia.** Urogenital sinus abnormalities are most often seen in intersex states, most commonly in association with congenital adrenal hyperplasia, which has been noted to have an incidence as frequent as 1 in 500 in the nonclassic mild forms.
13. **d. Distended vagina.** The common finding in all reports has been a cystic pelvic mass between the bladder and rectum, representing a distended vagina.
14. **c. Two vaginas, two uteri.** In Hendren's report on 154 patients with cloacal anomalies, 66 patients had one vagina, 68 had two vaginas, and the vagina was absent in 20. The incidence of vaginal duplication is even higher in our own patient population. The uterus anomaly generally is similar to the vaginal, that is, two vaginas with two uteri.
15. **b. MRI of the head.** The frequency of associated organ system abnormalities requires further radiographic evaluation. Echocardiography should always be done. MRI to evaluate the lumbosacral spine and to evaluate pelvic anatomy and musculature is necessary.
16. **d. Vaginal stenosis is clearly less.** Other investigators, including our group, have thought that vaginoplasty, regardless of the vaginal location, is best combined with clitoroplasty in a single stage. This allows the redundant phallic skin to be used in the reconstruction, adding flexibility for the surgeon, which is compromised when the skin has been previously mobilized. Furthermore, we and others have noted that maternal estrogen stimulation of the child's genitalia results in thicker vaginal tissue, which is better vascularized, making vaginal mobilization more easily performed.
17. **a. Labial fusion.** The cut-back vaginoplasty is rarely used and is appropriate only for simple labial fusion
18. **c. Vaginostomy.** Surgical management now involves four basic steps: (1) decompression of the gastrointestinal tract, (2) decompression of the genitourinary tract, (3) correction of nephron destructive or potentially lethal urinary anomalies, and (4) definitive repair of the cloaca.
19. **c. neurologic status.** Fecal continence is directly related to neurologic status.

130

Pediatric Urologic Oncology

MICHAEL L. RITCHEY • ROBERT C. SHAMBERGER

QUESTIONS

1. A chromosomal abnormality associated with an adverse prognosis in neuroblastoma is:
   a. mutation of chromosome 11p15.
   b. absence of the *MDR* gene.
   c. mutation of the *TP53* gene.
   d. deletion of the short arm of chromosome 1.
   e. loss of heterozygosity (LOH) for chromosome 11p13.
2. In situ neuroblastoma:
   a. invariably progresses to clinical neuroblastoma.
   b. usually regresses spontaneously.
   c. is associated with deletion of chromosome 11.
   d. is usually detected on newborn screening.
   e. is frequently associated with amplification of the N-*MYC* oncogene.
3. Ganglioneuroma is:
   a. a stroma-rich tumor by the Shimada classification.
   b. most commonly located in the adrenal gland.
   c. often found secondary to symptoms from metastatic disease.
   d. associated with acute myoclonic encephalopathy.
   e. associated with an unfavorable prognosis.
4. Screening for neuroblastoma:
   a. has improved survival in patients with neuroblastoma.
   b. has decreased the number of children older than 1 year of age with advanced staged disease.
   c. has identified more tumors with amplified N-*MYC* oncogene expression.
   d. discovers tumors with an improved prognosis.
   e. is widely performed in the United States.
5. A clinical feature associated with a favorable prognosis in neuroblastoma is:
   a. age > 2 years.
   b. thoracic location of the primary tumor.
   c. N-*MYC* amplification.
   d. chromosome 1p deletion.
   e. stroma-poor histology
6. A month-old girl is found to have a right suprarenal mass on abdominal ultrasound. The mass measures 4 cm in diameter. Imaging evaluation detects liver metastases. A skeletal survey is normal. Physical examination reveals multiple subcutaneous skin nodules. The mass is removed and confirmed to be neuroblastoma. Analysis of the tumor reveals no N-*MYC* amplification. The next best step is:
   a. observation.
   b. irradiation to the tumor bed.
   c. vincristine, cyclophosphamide, and doxorubicin.
   d. vincristine, cyclophosphamide, and irradiation to the tumor bed.
   e. autologous bone marrow transplantation after chemotherapy and total-body irradiation.
7. A 3-year-old girl has vaginal rhabdomyosarcoma. Her mother has a history of breast cancer. This patient most likely has:
   a. Beckwith-Wiedemann syndrome (BWS).
   b. Li-Fraumeni syndrome.
   c. Perlmann syndrome.
   d. Fragile X syndrome.
   e. Soto syndrome.
8. A 3-year-old boy has prostatic rhabdomyosarcoma. An unfavorable prognostic feature of this tumor is:
   a. alveolar histologic type.
   b. embryonal histology.
   c. LOH for chromosome 11p15.
   d. botryoid pattern.
   e. spindle cell variant.
9. A 1-year-old girl previously had partial cystectomy for rhabdomyosarcoma of the bladder. After completion of VAC chemotherapy, biopsy of the bladder reveals rhabdomyoblasts. Abdominal and chest CT are negative. The next step is:
   a. radiation therapy.
   b. continue chemotherapy.
   c. cystectomy with diversion.
   d. observation.
   e. change in chemotherapy regimen.
10. A 4-year-old boy has paratesticular rhabdomyosarcoma noted on biopsy of the spermatic cord lesion. The best next step is radical orchiectomy and:
    a. vincristine, dactinomycin, and cyclophosphamide.
    b. retroperitoneal lymph node dissection.
    c. retroperitoneal lymph node sampling.
    d. radiation therapy to the retroperitoneum.
    e. cisplatin, etoposide, and vincristine.

11. The WAGR syndrome is most frequently associated with:
    a. deletion of chromosome 15.
    b. advanced stage Wilms' tumor.
    c. neonatal presentation of Wilms' tumor.
    d. renal insufficiency.
    e. familial predisposition to Wilms' tumor.
12. A 3-year-old boy had undergone treatment for hypospadias and undescended testis as an infant. He develops renal insufficiency. Renal biopsy is consistent with a membranoproliferative glomerulonephritis. Appropriate management before renal transplantation is:
    a. Voiding cystourethrogram.
    b. gonadal biopsy.
    c. observation.
    d. bilateral nephrectomy.
    e. serial renal ultrasounds.
13. A 2-year-old boy has a palpable right-sided abdominal mass. CT shows this to be a solid lesion. On physical examination the patient's right arm and leg are noted to be slightly longer in length. Her diagnosis is most probably:
    a. Wilms' tumor.
    b. neuroblastoma.
    c. angiomyolipoma.
    d. nephroblastomatosis.
    e. renal call carcinoma.
14. A newborn is identified with Beckwith-Wiedemann syndrome. A renal ultrasound is obtained. Which clinical finding most predicts the risk of subsequent Wilms' tumor development?
    a. Hepatomegaly
    b. Hemihypertrophy
    c. Nephromegaly
    d. Mutation at chromosome 11p13
    e. Family history of Wilms' tumor
15. A 6-month-old girl is diagnosed with aniridia. Ultrasounds are done every 3 months. This will result in:
    a. increased survival.
    b. detection of lower-stage renal tumor.
    c. decreased incidence of bilateral tumors.
    d. decreased surgical morbidity.
    e. detection of tumors smaller than 3 cm in diameter.
16. A deletion of chromosome 11 has been found most frequently in Wilms' tumor patients with:
    a. aniridia.
    b. bilateral tumors.
    c. hemihypertrophy.
    d. Denys-Drash syndrome.
    e. Beckwith-Wiedemann syndrome.
17. A 5-year-old boy undergoes nephrectomy for a solid renal mass. Pathology reveals stage 1 favorable histology Wilms' tumor. An increased risk for tumor relapse is associated with:
    a. tumor aneuploidy on flow cytometry.
    b. deletion of chromosome 11p13.
    c. duplication of chromosome 1.
    d. LOH for chromosome 16q.
    e. elevated serum ferritin level.
18. A 2-year-old girl undergoes left nephrectomy for Wilms' tumor. A solitary left pulmonary lesion is noted on chest CT. The pathology shows favorable histology but with capsular penetration. The most important prognostic feature is:
    a. capsular presentation.
    b. histologic subtype.
    c. absence of lymph node involvement.
    d. age at presentation.
    e. presence of pulmonary metastasis.
19. The feature associated with the worse survival in children with Wilms' tumor is:
    a. diffuse anaplasia.
    b. diffuse tumor spill.
    c. incomplete tumor resection.
    d. tumor spread to periaortic lymph nodes.
    e. lung metastasis.
20. An increased risk for metachronous Wilms' tumor is associated with:
    a. anaplastic histology.
    b. clear cell sarcoma.
    c. blastemal predominant pattern.
    d. renal sinus invasion.
    e. nephrogenic rests.
21. A 6-year-old boy has a solid abdominal mass noted on ultrasound. A right-sided varicocele is present on physical examination. The next best step is:
    a. abdominal CT.
    b. MRI of the abdomen.
    c. chest CT.
    d. intravenous pyelogram.
    e. arteriogram.
22. A 1-year-old boy undergoes nephrectomy for Wilms' tumor. The finding that has the most adverse impact on survival is:
    a. hilar lymph node involvement.
    b. renal sinus invasion.
    c. capsular penetration.
    d. local tumor spill.
    e. renal vein thrombus.
23. One factor not predictive of local tumor relapse in children with Wilms' tumor is:
    a. local tumor spill.
    b. unfavorable histology.
    c. incomplete tumor removal.
    d. absence of lymph node sampling.
    e. capsular penetration.
24. A 4-year-old girl undergoes removal of a Wilms tumor although of favorable histology. Imaging evaluation reveals multiple pulmonary metastases. Treatment should include vincristine, dactinomycin, and:
    a. chest irradiation.
    b. doxorubicin.
    c. doxorubicin and chest irradiation.
    d. doxorubicin, cyclophosphamide, and irradiation.
    e. doxorubicin and etoposide.

25. A 3-month-old boy undergoes removal of a 300-g Wilms' tumor of the right kidney. The pathology shows diffuse anaplasia and tumor confined to the kidney. Lymph nodes were negative. The next step is:
   a. observation.
   b. vincristine and dactinomycin.
   c. vincristine, dactinomycin, and irradiation tumor beds.
   d. doxorubicin, vincristine, dactinomycin, and irradiation to the tumor bed.
   e. ifosfamide, etoposide, and doxorubicin.

26. A 5-year-old girl presents with hematuria. CT reveals a right abdominal mass with extension of tumor thrombus into the suprahepatic vena cava. The best next step is:
   a. chemotherapy.
   b. irradiation.
   c. open biopsy followed by chemotherapy.
   d. preoperative chemotherapy and radiation therapy.
   e. primary surgical removal of the kidney and tumor thrombus.

27. A 2-year-old boy is found to have bilateral Wilms' tumor. There is a tumor occupying more than 50% of the left kidney and a 4.0-cm tumor in the upper pole of the right kidney. The best next step is:
   a. left nephrectomy and right renal biopsy.
   b. bilateral partial nephrectomy.
   c. right partial nephrectomy and left renal biopsy.
   d. bilateral nephrectomies.
   e. chemotherapy.

28. A 1-year-old girl has a stage III Wilms tumor. During the course of chemotherapy she develops an enlarged heart and evidence of congestive heart failure. The drug responsible for these findings is most likely:
   a. dactinomycin.
   b. etoposide.
   c. vincristine.
   d. cyclophosphamide.
   e. doxorubicin.

29. A 2-year-old boy undergoes left orchiectomy. Pathology reveals a yolk sac tumor combined to the testis. CT findings of the chest and abdomen are negative. No preoperative tumor markers were done. At 4 weeks after surgery tumor markers are negative. The next step is:
   a. lymph node dissection.
   b. observation.
   c. chemotherapy.
   d. staining of the tumor for α-fetoprotein.
   e. retroperitoneal lymph node sampling.

30. A 1-year-old boy undergoes left radical nephrectomy for a large renal mass. The pathologic features associated with the worst prognosis are:
   a. diffuse anaplasia stage I.
   b. focal anaplasia stage III.
   c. rhabdoid tumor of the kidney stage III.
   d. clear cell sarcoma of the kidney stage III.
   e. favorable histology stage IV.

31. A newborn boy was noted to have a left renal mass on prenatal ultrasound. Postnatal evaluation confirms a 5-cm solid mass in the lower pole of the left kidney. The right kidney is normal. Chest radiography and CT of the chest are negative for metastatic disease. The mass was completely removed by a radical nephrectomy. The tumor was confined to the kidney. The next step in treatment is:
   a. 1200-cGy abdominal irradiation to the left flank.
   b. observation only.
   c. dactinomycin and vincristine for 10 weeks.
   d. dactinomycin and vincristine for 18 weeks.
   e. 2000-cGy abdominal irradiation plus dactinomycin and vincristine for 18 weeks.

32. A 6-year-old, phenotypic boy with hypospadias and bilateral cryptorchism has a 3-cm lower abdominal mass. Karyotype is XO/XY. At abdominal exploration, a tumor is found in the right gonad. Right orchiectomy is performed. Frozen section reveals gonadoblastoma. The best next step is:
   a. left orchiopexy
   b. retroperitoneal lymphadenectomy node sampling
   c. left orchiectomy
   d. chemotherapy
   e. observation.

33. A 2-year-old boy has a left upper pole testicular mass that is cystic on ultrasound. Excision of the lesion is done via an inguinal approach leaving the lower half of the testis. Frozen section demonstrates clear margins. Final pathology reveals teratoma, and the margins are negative for tumor. Serum α-fetoprotein and βHCG are negative. Chest and abdominal CT are negative. The next step is:
   a. radical orchiectomy and modified retroperitoneal lymph node dissection.
   b. observation.
   c. radical orchiectomy and combination chemotherapy.
   d. radical orchiectomy.
   e. radical orchiectomy and abdominal irradiation.

34. The tuberous sclerosis complex is associated with the development of angiomyolipoma and cystic renal disease. The patients so affected have been found to have an abnormality on which chromosome?
   a. 1
   b. 7
   c. 9
   d. 12
   e. 14

35. A 3-month-old boy undergoes removal of a solid yolk-sac tumor. The margins of resection are negative for tumor. Chest and abdominal CT results show no signs of metastatic disease. Two weeks postoperatively, the serum α-fetoprotein value is 35 ng/dL. What is the next step?
   a. Chemotherapy
   b. Retroperitoneal lymph node dissection
   c. Observation
   d. Retroperitoneal lymph node sampling
   e. Abdominal radiation

ANSWERS

1. **d. deletion of the short arm of chromosome 1.** Deletion of the short arm of chromosome 1 is found in 70% to 80% of neuroblastomas and is an adverse prognostic marker. The deletions are of different size, but in a series of eight cases a consensus deletion included the segment 1p36.1-2, suggesting that genetic information related to neuroblastoma tumorigenesis is located in this segment.

2. **b. usually regresses spontaneously.** In 1963, Beckwith and Perrin coined the term *in-situ neuroblastoma* for small nodules of neuroblastoma cells found incidentally within the adrenal gland, which are histologically indistinguishable from neuroblastoma. In infants younger than 3 months of age undergoing postmortem examination, neuroblastoma in-situ was found in 1 of 224 infants. This represents an incidence of in-situ neuroblastoma 40 to 45 times greater than the incidence of clinical tumors, suggesting that these small tumors regress spontaneously in most cases. However, more recent studies have shown that these neuroblastic nodules are found in all fetuses studied and generally regress.

3. **a. a stroma-rich tumor by the Shimada classification.** The Shimada classification is an age-linked histopathologic classification. One of the important aspects of the Shimada classification is determining whether the tumor is stroma poor or stroma rich. Patients with stroma-poor tumors with unfavorable histopathologic features have a very poor prognosis (less than 10% survival). Stroma-rich tumors can be separated into three subgroups: nodular, intermixed, and well differentiated. Tumors in the last two categories more closely resemble ganglioneuroblastoma or immature ganglioneuroma and have a higher rate of survival.

4. **d. discovers tumors with an improved prognosis.** The goal of screening programs is to detect disease at an earlier stage and decrease the number of older children with advanced stage disease and thus improve survival. An increased number of infants younger than 1 year of age have been diagnosed with the mass screening program, and most of these patients have lower-stage tumors. Regrettably, the number of children older than 1 year of age with advanced stage disease has not decreased.

5. **b. thoracic location of the primary tumor.** The site of origin is of significance, with a better survival rate noted for nonadrenal primary tumors. Most children with thoracic neuroblastoma present at a younger age with localized disease and have improved survival even when corrected for age and stage.

6. **a. observation.** The generally favorable behavior of stage IV-S disease has been explained with the development of biologic markers. The vast majority of these infants have tumors with entirely favorable markers explaining their nonmalignant behavior. A small percentage, however, have adverse markers, and it is these children who have progressive disease to which they often succumb. Resection of the primary tumor is not mandatory. Although excellent survival has been reported after surgery, information regarding histologic prognostic factors was not available for all of these patients. A more recent review was performed of a large cohort of 110 infants with stage IV-S disease. The entire cohort of infants had an estimated 3-year survival rate of 85% ± 4%. This survival rate was significantly decreased, however, to 68% ± 12% for infants who were diploid, 44% ± 33% for those who were N-*MYC* amplified, and 33% ± 19% for those with unfavorable histology tumors. Of note, there was no statistical difference in survival rate for infants who underwent complete resection of their primary tumor compared with those with partial resection or only biopsy. Patients with extensive metastatic disease who are N-*MYC*–positive represent a high-risk group. These patients should be considered for a more aggressive treatment with multimodal therapy as per the risk group classification.

7. **b. Li-Fraumeni syndrome.** Subgroups of children with a genetic predisposition to the development of rhabdomyosarcoma have been identified. The Li-Fraumeni syndrome associates childhood sarcomas with mothers who have an excess of premenopausal breast cancer and with siblings who have an increased risk of cancer. A mutation of the *TP53* tumor suppressor gene was found in the tumors in all patients with this syndrome.

8. **a. alveolar histologic type.** The second most common form is alveolar, which occurs more commonly in the trunk and extremity than in genitourinary sites and has a worse prognosis. Alveolar rhabdomyosarcoma also has a higher rate of local recurrence and spread to regional lymph nodes, bone marrow, and distant sites.

9. **d. observation.** If tumor is shrinking during chemotherapy, and another biopsy after completing radiotherapy shows maturing rhabdomyoblasts without frank tumor cells, total cystectomy can be postponed or avoided altogether.

10. **a. vincristine, dactinomycin, and cyclophosphamide.** Before effective chemotherapy, surgery alone produced a 50% 2-year relapse-free survival rate. With current multimodal treatment, survival rates of 90% are expected. Currently, the Intergroup Rhabdomyosarcoma Study Group recommends that children 10 years of age and older undergo ipsilateral retroperitoneal lymph node dissection before chemotherapy.

11. **d. renal insufficiency.** Patients with the WAGR syndrome have a germline deletion at 11p13. *WT1* mutations and deletions predispose patients to renal insufficiency. Both the Denys-Drash and WAGR syndrome are associated with an increased risk of renal failure. This occurs later in the WAGR syndrome, often in the second decade of life after treatment of the Wilms tumor.

12. **d. bilateral nephrectomy.** One specific association of male pseudohermaphroditism, renal mesangial sclerosis, and nephroblastoma is the Denys-Drash syndrome. The majority of these patients progress to end-stage renal disease. A specific mutation of the 11p13 Wilms tumor gene has been identified in these children. Although XY individuals have been reported most often, the syndrome has been reported in genotypic/phenotypic females. One should have a high index of suspicion for the development of renal failure and Wilms' tumor in patients with male pseudohermaphroditism.

13. **a. Wilms' tumor.** BWS is characterized by excess growth at the cellular, organ (macroglossia, nephromegaly, hepatomegaly), or body segment (hemihypertrophy) levels. Most cases of BWS are sporadic, but up to 15% exhibit heritable characteristics with apparent autosomal dominant inheritance. The risk of nephroblastoma in children with BWS and hemihypertrophy is 4% to 10%.

14. **c. Nephromegaly.** Children with BWS found to have nephromegaly (kidneys ≥ the 95th percentile of age-adjusted renal length) are at the greatest risk for the development of Wilms' tumor.

15. **b. detection of lower stage renal tumor.** Screening with serial renal ultrasonographic scans has been recommended in children with aniridia, hemihypertrophy, and BWS. Review of most studies suggests that 3 to 4 months is the appropriate screening interval. Tumors detected by screening will generally be at a lower stage.

16. **a. aniridia.** Approximately 50% of patients with WAGR syndrome and a constitutional deletion on chromosome 11 will develop Wilms' tumor.

17. **d. LOH for chromosome 16q.** LOH for a portion of chromosome 16q has been noted in 20% of Wilms' tumors. A study of 232 patients registered on the National Wilms Tumor Study Group (NWTSG) found LOH for 16q in 17% of the tumors. Patients with tumor-specific LOH for chromosome 16q had a statistically significantly poorer 2-year relapse-free and overall survival rate than did those patients without LOH for chromosome 16q.

18. **b. histologic subtype.** Markers associated with unfavorable outcome include nuclear atypia (anaplasia), focal or diffuse, and sarcomatous tumors (rhabdoid and clear cell type). The latter two tumor types, however, are tumor categories distinct from Wilms' tumor. These unfavorable features occurred in approximately 10% of patients but accounted for almost half of the tumor deaths in early NWTSG studies.

19. **a. diffuse anaplasia.** Anaplasia is associated with resistance to chemotherapy. This is evidenced by the similar incidence of anaplasia (5%) in the NWTSG and International Society of Paediatric Oncology studies. Although the presence of anaplasia has clearly been demonstrated to carry a poor prognosis, patients with stage I anaplastic Wilms' tumor as well as those with higher stages and focal rather than diffuse anaplasia seem to have a more favorable outcome. This confirms the observation that anaplasia is more a marker of chemoresistance than inherent aggressiveness of the tumor.

20. **e. nephrogenic rests.** NWTSG investigators demonstrated the clinical importance of nephrogenic rests. Multiple rests in one kidney usually imply that nephrogenic rests are present in the other kidney. Children younger than 12 months of age diagnosed with Wilms' tumor who also have nephrogenic rests, in particular perilobar nephrogenic rests, have a markedly increased risk of developing contralateral disease and require frequent and regular surveillance for several years.

21. **b. MRI of the abdomen.** Compression or invasion of adjacent structures may result in an atypical presentation. Extension of Wilms' tumor into the renal vein and inferior vena cava (IVC) can cause varicocele, hepatomegaly due to hepatic vein obstruction, ascites, and congestive heart failure. Such symptoms are found in less than 10% of patients with intracaval or atrial tumor extension.

22. **a. hilar lymph node involvement.** The most important determinants of outcome in children with Wilms' tumor are histopathology and tumor stage. Accurate staging of Wilms' tumor allows treatment results to be evaluated and enables universal comparisons of outcomes. The staging system used by the NWTSG is based primarily on the surgical and histopathologic findings. Examination for extension through the capsule, residual disease, vascular involvement, and lymph node involvement is essential to properly assess the extent of the tumor.

23. **e. capsular penetration.** One study identified risk factors for local tumor recurrence as tumor spillage, unfavorable histology, incomplete tumor removal, and absence of any lymph node sampling. The 2-year survival rate after abdominal recurrence was 43%, emphasizing the importance of the surgeon in performing careful and complete tumor resection.

24. **c. doxorubicin and chest irradiation.** Patients with stage III favorable histologic type tumors and stage II-III focal anaplasia are treated with dactinomycin, vincristine, and doxorubicin and 10.8-Gy abdominal irradiation. Patients with stage IV favorable histologic type tumors receive abdominal irradiation based on the local tumor stage and 12 Gy to both lungs.

25. **d. doxorubicin, vincristine, dactinomycin, and irradiation to the tumor bed.** Anaplasia tumors are resistant to chemotherapy. However, if the tumor is confined to the kidney and completely resected the prognosis is good. They do require more intense treatment than children with stage I, favorable histology tumors.

26. **c. open biopsy followed by chemotherapy.** The current recommendations from the NWTSG are that preoperative chemotherapy is of benefit in patients with bilateral involvement, inoperable at surgical exploration, and IVC extension above the hepatic veins. All other patients should undergo primary nephrectomy.

27. **e. chemotherapy.** Patients with bilateral Wilms' tumor have an increased risk for renal failure. These patients should receive preoperative chemotherapy without attempts at initial surgery. Repeat imaging after 6 weeks of chemotherapy can assess response to treatment.

28. **e. doxorubicin.** In recent years, there has been increasing concern regarding the risk of congestive heart failure in children who receive treatment with anthracyclines such as doxorubicin. In addition to the acute cardiotoxicity, cardiac failure can develop many years after treatment.

29. **b. observation.** The initial treatment for yolk-sac tumor is radical inguinal orchiectomy. This treatment is curative in most children. Routine retroperitoneal lymph node dissection and adjuvant chemotherapy are not indicated.

30. **c. rhabdoid tumor of the kidney stage III.** Typical clinical features include early age at diagnosis (median age of <16 months), resistance to chemotherapy, and high mortality rate. Unlike Wilms' tumor, which typically metastasizes to the lungs, abdomen/flank, and liver, rhabdoid tumor of the kidney, which also metastasizes to these sites, is distinguished by its propensity to metastasize to the brain.

31. **b. observation only.** The most common renal tumor in a newborn is congenital mesoblastic nephroma. The important aspect of the recognition of these tumors as a separate entity is the usually excellent outcome with radical surgery only.

32. **c. left orchiectomy.** Early gonadectomy is advocated, as tumors have been reported in children younger than 5 years of age. In patients with mixed gonadal dysgenesis who are reared as males, all streak gonads and undescended testes should be removed. Scrotal testes can be preserved because they are less prone to tumor development.

33. **b. observation.** Prepubertal mature teratomas have a benign clinical course, which contrasts to the clinical behavior of teratomas in adults, which have the propensity to metastasize. This benign behavior has led to the consideration of testicular-sparing procedures rather than radical orchiectomy.

34. **c. 9.** Two genes have been identified in the tuberous sclerosis complex on chromosome 9 (TSC1) and chromosome 16 (TSC2). It has been postulated that these genes act as tumor suppressor genes and that the LOH of TSC1 or TSC2 may explain the progressive growth pattern of renal lesions seen in these patients.

35. **c. Observation.** It is important to note that an elevated α-fetoprotein level after orchiectomy for yolk-sac tumor in an infant does not always represent persistent disease. Normal adult reference laboratory values for α-fetoprotein cannot be used in young children, because α-fetoprotein synthesis continues after birth. Normal adult levels (<10 mg/mL) are not reached until 8 months of age.

131

Pediatric Endourology and Laparoscopy

STEVEN G. DOCIMO • CRAIG A. PETERS

QUESTIONS

1. Routine follow-up after a retrograde ureteroscopic stone removal in a 5-year-old girl should include which examination?
   a. Intravenous pyelography (IVP)
   b. Voiding cystourethrography
   c. Renal ultrasonography
   d. Dimercaptosuccinic acid (DMSA) scan
   e. Mercaptoacetyltriglycine (MAG3) diuretic renography
2. In a 12-month-old child, what is the most appropriate irrigating fluid to use during percutaneous nephrolithotripsy with electrohydraulic lithotripsy?
   a. Glycine
   b. Warmed glycine
   c. Warmed water
   d. Warmed saline
   e. Either warmed glycine or warmed water
3. A 4-year-old boy with a family history of calcium oxalate stone disease is found to have a 12-mm calculus in the left renal pelvis with no hydronephrosis. He has had no urinary tract surgery. What would be the first-line approach to this stone?
   a. Shockwave lithotripsy
   b. Shockwave lithotripsy with a ureteral stent
   c. Minipercutaneous nephrolithotomy
   d. Ureteroscopy after "pre-stenting" to dilate the ureter
   e. Posterior lumbotomy approach to pyelolithotomy
4. A 2-year-old boy has had pyeloplasty and now, 3 months later, has a nephrostomy tube in place for poor drainage. Which of the following is considered an absolute contraindication to percutaneous endopyelotomy?
   a. Differential renal function less than 20%
   b. Inability to cannulate the lumen of the ureteropelvic junction
   c. Renal pelvis greater than 50 mL
   d. Suspected crossing vessel
   e. None of the above
5. An 8-year-old boy with persistent right flank pain is found to have a 4-cm cystic structure containing a calcification in the lateral upper pole of the right kidney. It fills with contrast material on IVP. What is the best management?
   a. Open marsupialization
   b. Retrograde incision of diverticular neck and stone removal
   c. Observation
   d. Percutaneous stone removal and diverticular ablation
   e. Upper pole nephrectomy
6. What is the principal goal of diagnostic laparoscopy for a nonpalpable testis?
   a. Confirmation of the absence of the testis
   b. Documentation of the location and presence of the testis
   c. Preparation for a first-stage laparoscopic orchiopexy
   d. Preparation for a one-stage laparoscopic orchiopexy
   e. Documentation of the passage of the testis through the internal inguinal ring
7. The role of laparoscopy in children with intersex conditions is principally when:
   a. gonadal development may be abnormal or discordant with sex of rearing.
   b. müllerian structures are present.
   c. external genitalia suggest the presence of 5α-reductase deficiency.
   d. congenital adrenal hyperplasia is suspected.
   e. gonadal function is deficient.
8. Which of the following is a significant functional consequence of pneumoperitoneum in children compared with adults?
   a. Increased cardiac output
   b. Reduced oxygen reserve
   c. Increased urine output
   d. Reduced CO_2 absorption
   e. Increased cardiac irritability
9. During transperitoneal laparoscopic nephrectomy, a 2-year-old child's urine output falls to less than 0.2 mL/kg/hr. What is the most appropriate management?
   a. Immediate bolus of isotonic saline, 10 mL/kg
   b. Emergency treatment for CO_2 embolus
   c. Cessation of the procedure and conversion to open nephrectomy
   d. Continuation of the procedure and monitoring of postoperative urine output
   e. Increasing the intravenous fluid rate to 100 mL/hr

10. Initial performance of a transperitoneal laparoscopic right nephrectomy includes:
    a. upper pole mobilization and control of the hilum.
    b. direct control of the hilar vessels.
    c. duodenal mobilization and hilar control.
    d. placement of a ureteral stent.
    e. lateral mobilization of the colon and medial reflection.

11. Which of the following is considered an absolute contraindication to laparoscopic surgery in a 10-year-old child?
    a. Ventriculoperitoneal shunt
    b. Previous abdominal surgery
    c. Peritoneal dialysis
    d. Renal insufficiency
    e. None of the above

ANSWERS

1. **c. Renal ultrasonography.** After stent removal, ultrasonography is used to monitor upper tract dilatation, which may occur with ureteral obstruction. The timing of follow-up should be based on the complexity of the case but should not be delayed for more than 4 weeks after the stent is removed. If there is no hydronephrosis, IVP, MAG3, and DMSA scans are not needed. If significant dilatation is present, or if the child develops symptoms of obstruction, IVP is used to define the functional anatomy of the ureter. Vesicoureteral reflux is a theoretical complication of ureteral dilatation and manipulation but has not been reported to be a significant clinical issue. Routine cystography is not recommended.
2. **d. Warmed saline.** Irrigation solutions must be warmed to prevent hypothermia, which can occur quickly in young children. Saline should be used as an irrigant in all cases to avoid dilutional hyponatremia, which can also develop quickly in the small child if extravasation should occur.
3. **a. Shockwave lithotripsy.** Percutaneous access in children is used most commonly for stone removal. Because the ureter in the child is very distensible, allowing passage of relatively large stone fragments, extracorporeal shockwave lithotripsy (ESWL) is the first-line treatment for most renal calculi in children. There is no strict upper limit of stone burden that can be managed with ESWL in children, as there is in adults, although the larger the burden is, the less likely it is that success will be achieved with one procedure.
4. **b. Inability to cannulate the lumen of the ureteropelvic junction.** Endopyelotomy is considered to be an appropriate procedure option after failed pyeloplasty in the adult and has a reasonable success rate. The same may be true in the pediatric population, although fewer cases have been reported. Endopyelotomy should be attempted only when a lumen is recognizable and can be cannulated. Considering the difficulty and morbidity of reoperative pyeloplasty, an attempt at endopyelotomy in most cases is reasonable.
5. **d. Percutaneous stone removal and diverticular ablation.** Because there are symptoms, treatment is needed. Open marsupialization and retrograde drainage are possible options but are more invasive and not always as effective as percutaneous ablation. Percutaneous intervention in children is based on obliteration and scarification of the epithelial lining of the diverticulum, rather than inducing drainage through opening of the neck of the diverticulum, as is often performed in adults. Any procedure intending to establish free drainage requires temporary indwelling stents and runs the risk of reclosure of the neck. The impact of each of these elements in the child is greater than in the adult. Laparoscopic marsupialization may be another option, although there is little experience with it. Upper pole nephrectomy would not be reasonable.
6. **b. Documentation of the location and presence of the testis.** The primary aims of diagnostic laparoscopy are to identify the presence or absence, location, and anatomy of the nonpalpable testis.
7. **a. gonadal development may be abnormal or discordant with sex of rearing.** The principal use of diagnostic laparoscopy for intersex is for conditions in which gonadal development may be abnormal or discordant with the sex of rearing, including gonadal dysgenesis and hermaphroditism. It is of little benefit in cases of congenital adrenal hyperplasia. When persistent müllerian ductal structures should be removed, laparoscopy may be useful as well, although it is not universally so.
8. **b. Reduced oxygen reserve.** Intra-abdominal pressure is increased significantly, and with the common use of CO_2 as the insufflating agent there is absorption of CO_2 across the peritoneum. There are also risks of CO_2 embolus. In children, the key differences from an anesthetic standpoint, relative to adults, is their decreased pulmonary reserve because of a relatively low functional residual capacity and lower oxygen reserve.
9. **d. Continuation of the procedure and monitoring of postoperative urine output.** As with adults, increased intra-abdominal pressure in children reduces urine output, although this is transient and has not been observed to cause any permanent renal injury. There is no need to increase normal fluid management, nor is there any reason to stop the procedure. A CO_2 embolus would present with acutely altered cardiorespiratory function.
10. **e. lateral mobilization of the colon and medial reflection.** In transperitoneal nephrectomy, the colon is first reflected from the kidney by incision of the lateral line of Toldt. In most cases, the ureter can be identified and used as a handle to lift the lower pole of the kidney. This facilitates access to the hilar vessels, which are then dissected free and independently ligated.
11. **e. None of the above.** Laparoscopically assisted surgery is widely applicable in patients who require bladder reconstruction and/or antegrade continence enema stoma. The majority of patients reported have had prior abdominal surgery, including ventriculoperitoneal shunt placement and bladder exstrophy closure. The benefit of laparoscopic mobilization is not just cosmetic; in theory, one would expect more rapid recovery and decreased intra-abdominal adhesions. Therefore, even patients with a prior midline incision might benefit. The presence of a ventriculoperitoneal shunt is not a contraindication to laparoscopic surgery and requires no special precautions or monitoring.

132

Pediatric Genitourinary Trauma

DOUGLAS HUSMANN

QUESTIONS

1. Which of the following signs or symptoms noted after a traumatic insult is suggestive of a pre-existing renal abnormality?
   a. Microscopic hematuria with shock
   b. Gross hematuria with shock
   c. Gross hematuria with clot formation
   d. Hematuria disproportionate to severity of trauma
   e. Hematuria in the absence of coexisting injuries to the thorax, spine, pelvis/femur, or intra-abdominal organs
2. The radiographic study that is the most sensitive for the presence of a renal injury is:
   a. IVP.
   b. MRI of abdomen.
   c. FAST ultrasound.
   d. triphasic abdominal CT.
   e. monophasic abdominal CT.
3. After a traumatic injury, a CT of the abdomen reveals a renal laceration that extends into the collecting system with urinary extravasation. If the injury is associated with a devitalized fragment, the grade of renal injury is:
   a. grade 1.
   b. grade 2.
   c. grade 3.
   d. grade 4.
   e. grade 5.
4. An 11-year-old boy had sustained a renal laceration that had extended into the collecting system 2 weeks previously. He has been at home for the past week with grossly clear urine. His mother contacts you due to the sudden onset of gross hematuria with clots. Your next step is:
   a. reassurance and continued observation.
   b. recommend bed rest, force fluids, and phone follow-up tomorrow.
   c. recommend continued observation and arrange for follow-up CT in the morning.
   d. bring patient by car to your office for evaluation.
   e. transportation to the emergency department by ambulance.
5. A 9-year-old boy sustained a renal laceration associated with a functional renal fragment that was completely dissociated from the kidney. He has a persistent symptomatic urinary fistula despite combined treatment with a nephrostomy tube, double-J stent, and urethral catheter. The next step is:
   a. angiographic embolization of functional renal fragment.
   b. RFA of functional renal fragment.
   c. cryotherapy of functional renal fragment.
   d. laparoscopic partial nephrectomy.
   e. open partial nephrectomy.
6. A 8-year-old boy on IV prophylaxis with cefazolin undergoes angiographic embolization of a traumatic AV fistula associated with a grade 4 traumatic renal injury. The urine is clear, but on postembolization day 1 and 2 he is having febrile temperature spikes to 40°C. Blood pressure is stable. Acetaminophen for fever and cultures for blood and urine are recommended, and:
   a. continued observation.
   b. change in antibiotic coverage to piperacillin.
   c. addition of metronidazole.
   d. CT of abdomen and aspiration of perinephric hematoma/urinoma.
   e. percutaneous nephrostomy drainage of urinoma.
7. A 2-year-old boy sustains a major renal laceration with a tear into the collecting system secondary to child abuse. He has persistent gross hematuria with clots and ileus 5 days after injury. CT done today reveals clot filling the renal pelvis; there is a significant perinephric urinoma, but good flow of contrast is seen into the patient's ipsilateral distal ureter, findings essentially unchanged from the CT scan done 48 hours previously. Vital signs and hemoglobin are normal and stable. The next step is:
   a. continued observation.
   b. angiography.
   c. percutaneous nephrostomy.
   d. cystoscopy, retrograde pyelogram, and stent placement.
   e. surgical exploration and renorrhaphy.
8. Follow-up CT for a grade 2 renal injury should be performed:
   a. only if a patient develops increased severity of localized signs or systemic symptoms.
   b. 2 to 3 days after traumatic injury.
   c. 3 to 4 weeks after traumatic injury.
   d. 3 months after traumatic injury.
   e. 1 year after traumatic injury.

9. Retroperitoneal (renal) exploration is recommended when:
   a. a stab wound to the flank results in a grade 2 renal injury.
   b. a 38-caliber gunshot wound results in a grade 2 renal injury.
   c. a motor vehicle accident results in an isolated grade 4 renal injury.
   d. a nonhemorrhagic retroperitoneal mass is found on surgical exploration after a gunshot wound.
   e. a motor vehicle accident results in need for emergent laparotomy due to vascular instability evident as retroperitoneal hemorrhage found on exploration.
10. A 12-year-old girl is involved in a bicycle-vehicular accident. A CT scan taken 1 hour after trauma reveals an isolated renal injury with no perfusion and subsequently no function of the left kidney; the right kidney function is within normal limits. Vital signs are stable and hemoglobin is normal. Your next step is:
    a. observation.
    b. angiography with stenting of left renal artery.
    c. angiographic infusion of streptokinase into left renal artery.
    d. systemic heparinization.
    e. surgical exploration.
11. In a patient with a preexisting ureteropelvic junction (UPJ) obstruction, gross hematuria after trauma is usually due to:
    a. coexisting renal lithiasis.
    b. renal contusion.
    c. laceration through the thinned renal cortex.
    d. rupture of the renal pelvis.
    e. UPJ disruption.
12. Which of the following is an absolute indication for CT cystography after blunt trauma?
    a. Gross hematuria
    b. Abdominal wall bruising
    c. Pelvic fracture
    d. Lumbar spinal fracture
    e. Inability to void
13. In the presence of an extraperitoneal bladder injury consideration for open surgical intervention should be given if:
    a. gross hematuria with clots is present.
    b. the pubic ramus is fractured.
    c. a vaginal laceration is present.
    d. a coexisting rectal injury is present.
    e. the bladder neck appears incompetent.
14. While assessing bladder function for a delayed urethroplasty, a static cystogram reveals contrast in the posterior urethra. The next step is:
    a. video-urodynamics.
    b. pudendal nerve electromyography.
    c. MRI of the pelvis and perineum.
    d. MRI of the lumbosacral spinal cord.
    e. combined cystoscopy per SP tube tract and urethroscopy per meatus.
15. A newborn has excess skin excised during circumcision leaving a 7-mm gap between the residual penile shaft skin and the mucosal collar. Your next step is to:
    a. apply wet-to-dry dressings and antibiotic ointment.
    b. mobilize and suture penile shaft skin to mucosal collar.
    c. bury the phallus in scrotal skin with planned second-stage release.
    d. perform a split-thickness skin graft from the thigh.
    e. perform a full-thickness skin graft from the thigh.

ANSWERS

1. **d. Hematuria disproportionate to severity of trauma.** The classic patient history that should make the physician think of a preexisting renal anomaly is that the degree of hematuria present is disproportionate to the severity of trauma. None of the other distracters have been found to be related to the presence of a preexisting renal abnormality during the evaluation of trauma.
2. **d. triphasic abdominal CT.** A triphasic CT study (precontrast study, followed by a study immediately following injection and then a 15- to 20-minute delayed study) is the most sensitive method for diagnosis and classification of renal trauma. A single-phase CT study is beneficial in determining renal perfusion and major renal fractures but may on occasion miss the presence of urinary extravasation and will miss the vast majority of ureteral injuries. FAST sonographic evaluations are operator and experience dependent and will miss 5% to 10% of clinically significant renal injuries. It is noteworthy, however, that a normal FAST sonographic evaluation coupled with a serial normal physical examination over 24 hours will reliably detect all clinically significant genitourinary injuries.
3. **d. grade 4.** A grade 4 renal injury is a laceration extending into the collecting system with urinary extravasation, with viable or devitalized renal fragments, or is an injury to the main renal vasculature with contained hemorrhage (see Table 132-1).
4. **e. transportation to the emergency department by ambulance.** Approximately 25% of patients with grade 3-4 renal trauma, managed in a nonoperative fashion, will have persistent or delayed hemorrhage. Classically, delayed hemorrhage will present 10 to 14 days after injury but may occur up to 1 month after the insult. Delayed hemorrhage arises from the development of arteriovenous fistulas, will not spontaneously resolve, and may be associated with life-threatening hemorrhage. Management should be by ambulance transportation; remember shock in a child may be one of the later signs of severe bleeding. Intravenous access should be obtained by emergency medical technicians and the patient immediately returned to the hospital for angiographic evaluation and embolization of the bleeding site.
5. **a. angiographic embolization of functional renal fragment.** Persistent urinary fistulas associated with a viable renal fragment that is separate from the remaining portions of traumatically injured kidney are initially managed with percutaneous nephrostomy tube drainage and double-J stent placement; if persistent fistula drainage remains, management by angiographic infarction of the isolated functional segment will prevent the need for open surgical excision of the functional segment.
6. **a. continued observation.** Postembolization syndrome is well recognized and self-limiting. It is manifested by pyrexia up to 40°C, flank pain, and adynamic ileus. Symptoms should resolve in 96 hours after the embolization. When pyrexia develops, blood and urine cultures to rule out bacterial

seeding of the necrotic tissue are necessary. Consideration for a repeat CT with possible aspiration, culture, and drainage of a perinephric hematoma/urinoma should be given if febrile response persists for more than 96 hours or if the patient's clinical course should rapidly worsen.

7. **c. percutaneous nephrostomy.** Most post-traumatic urinomas are asymptomatic and have a spontaneous resolution rate approaching 85%; they will occasionally persist and be associated with continued flank pain, adynamic ileus, and/or low-grade temperature. Frequently we will manage these patients via endoscopic intervention, with cystoscopy, retrograde pyelography, and placement of a ureteral stent. Both percutaneous nephrostomy drainage and internal stenting are equally efficacious. The advantage of an internal stent is that it prevents possible dislodgement of the draining tube and the need for external drainage devices. The two major disadvantages of internal drainage are that both stent placement and removal, in the pediatric patient population, require general anesthesia. In addition, the small size ureteral stents (4 to 5 Fr) placed in young children may become blocked with blood clots from the dissolving hematoma, resulting in persistence of the urinoma. In this young infant with large clots in the renal pelvis the best way to manage the problem is with percutaneous nephrostomy. This will allow the physician to externally irrigate the system if the tube becomes blocked with clots.

8. **a. only if a patient develops increased severity of localized signs or systemic symptoms.** Follow-up renal imaging is not recommended for grade 1 to 2 renal injuries and for grade 3 lacerations where all fragments are viable. In patients with grade 3 renal lacerations associated with devitalized fragments, grade 4, and salvaged grade 5 renal injuries, a repeat CT with delayed images should be obtained 2 to 3 days after the traumatic insult. This study serves the purpose of assessing the extent of the hematoma/urinoma and will serve as a baseline evaluation in case secondary hemorrhage or infection should occur. Irrespective of the grade of the injury, repeat imaging with a triphasic CT is recommended for patients with a history of renal trauma who have a persistent and/or increased fever, worsening flank pain, or persistent gross hematuria more than 72 hours after the traumatic insult. We recommend a 3-month follow-up triphasic CT in all grade 3 renal lacerations associated with a devitalized fragment, grade 4, and salvaged grade 5 renal injuries. This latter study is obtained to verify resolution of any perinephric urinoma and to define the anatomic configuration of the residual functioning renal parenchyma.

9. **e. a motor vehicle accident results in need for emergent laparotomy due to vascular instability, evident as retroperitoneal hemorrhage found on exploration.** Retroperitoneal exploration is recommended in the setting of blunt trauma when abdominal exploration is performed for vascular instability and retroperitoneal hemorrhage is identified, even when there has not been adequate preoperative imaging. In these cases, assessment of contralateral function is necessary as well (see Table 132-2).

10. **a. observation.** In a patient sustaining renal arterial trauma, the clinical triad of hemodynamic instability, inadequate collateral blood flow, and warm ischemic time almost invariably results in the inability to salvage renal function. Because of these facts, no attempt to repair injuries to segmental renal vessels should be considered, and repair of the traumatically injured main renal artery is seldom indicated when a normal contralateral kidney is present. In essence, reconstruction of the main renal artery after trauma is only a primary consideration in patients who are hemodynamically stable with an injury to a solitary kidney or in patients with bilateral renal arterial injuries. The infrequent exception to this rule is the presence of an incomplete arterial injury where perfusion to the kidney has been maintained by flow of blood through either the partially occluded main renal artery or via collateral vessels.

11. **b. renal contusion.** Although it has been reported that preexisting hydronephrosis or a congenital UPJ obstruction renders the patient more susceptible to a UPJ disruption, this is controversial. The vast majority of patients with a history of trauma and preexisting UPJ or hydronephrosis will be found to have a renal contusion or grade 1 renal injury on evaluation. When urinary extravasation is seen, rupture of the renal pelvis or a major laceration extending through a thinned renal cortex into the collecting system (grade 3 renal injury) is the most common finding, not a UPJ disruption.

12. **e. Inability to void.** Absolute indications for bladder imaging after blunt abdominal trauma are currently limited to two indications: (1) the presence of gross hematuria coexisting with a pelvic fracture and (2) inability to void. Neither gross hematuria alone nor pelvic fracture alone is an absolute indication for screening. Relative indications for bladder imaging after blunt abdominal trauma are urinary clot retention, perineal hematoma, and history of a prior bladder augmentation. Bladder imaging after penetrating trauma should be performed any time concern exists that the missile could have punctured the bladder.

13. **e. the bladder neck appears incompetent.** If concern for a bladder neck injury is present, the patient should undergo surgical exploration with opening of the bladder at the dome. Repair of the bladder neck should be via an intravesical approach with a multilayered closure. Great care should be given not to dislodge the pelvic hematoma to help prevent blood loss. The surgeon should be aware that anterior bladder neck lacerations are frequently associated with urethral injuries, and retrograde urethrography or cystoscopy to rule out this possibility should be considered. If a bladder neck laceration is repaired, a voiding cystourethrogram is necessary at the time of catheter removal to adequately visualize the bladder neck and confirm healing.

14. **a. video-urodynamics.** If the posterior urethra fills with contrast on the static cystogram this could be due to either a poorly felt or described detrusor contraction or an incompetent bladder neck. Because of the significant impact the latter has on the surgical prognosis, if contrast agent is seen in the posterior urethra, a video-urodynamic study is necessary. If the study documents an incompetent bladder neck, or if the patient was unable to open up the bladder neck to see the posterior urethra during the voiding cystourethrogram, we perform a simultaneous flexible cystoscopy and urethroscopy. (On occasion, the physician may need to use flexible ureteroscopes for this procedure in small children.) If cystoscopy and video-urodynamics demonstrate an incompetent bladder neck, we discuss with the patient and his family the options of urethral reconstruction with the possible result of chronic incontinence or, alternatively, the performance of a continent abdominal stoma (appendicovesicostomy) as first-line therapy.

15. **a. apply wet-to-dry dressings and antibiotic ointment.** Penile trauma in the pediatric patient population is most commonly iatrogenic and caused by circumcision. If excess penile skin is excised during circumcision, the majority of patients can be treated by wet-to-dry dressings and antibiotic ointment. Healing by secondary intention usually results in an excellent cosmetic appearance. If the penis is totally degloved, the penile shaft skin, if salvaged, can be defatted and replaced on the penis as a full-thickness skin graft.